MW01156245

The Cowboy's Companion:

A TRAIL GUIDE FOR THE ARTHROSCOPIC SHOULDER SURGEON

The Cowboy Credo:

There's the easy way and there's the cowboy way.

The cowboy does the right thing, even if it's difficult. And arthroscopic shoulder repairs can be difficult. This book is dedicated to making them easier.

The Cowboy's Companion:

A TRAIL GUIDE FOR THE ARTHROSCOPIC SHOULDER SURGEON

STEPHEN S. BURKHART, MD
The San Antonio Orthopaedic Group
San Antonio, Texas

IAN K.Y. LO, MD, FRCSC
Department of Surgery
University of Calgary
Calgary, Alberta

PAUL C. BRADY, MD
Orthopaedic Surgeon
Tennessee Orthopaedic Clinics
Knoxville, Tennessee

PATRICK J. DENARD, MD
Southern Oregon Orthopedics
Medford, Oregon

Wolters Kluwer | Lippincott Williams & Wilkins
Health
Philadelphia • Baltimore • New York • London
Buenos Aires • Hong Kong • Sydney • Tokyo

Acquisitions Editor: Robert Hurley
Product Manager: Dave Murphy
Marketing Manager: Lisa Lawrence
Design Manager: Holly McLaughlin
Production Services: SPi Global

Two Commerce Square
2001 Market Street
Philadelphia, PA 19103

Printed in China

Library of Congress Cataloging-in-Publication Data

The cowboy's companion : a trail guide for the arthroscopic shoulder surgeon / Stephen S. Burkhart ... [et al.].

p. ; cm.

Trail guide for the arthroscopic shoulder surgeon

Companion to: Burkhart's view of the shoulder / Stephen S. Burkhart, Ian K.Y. Lo, Paul C. Brady. c2006.

Includes bibliographical references.

ISBN 978-1-60913-797-7

I. Burkhart, Stephen S., 1949- II. Burkhart, Stephen S., 1949- . Burkhart's view of the shoulder. III. Title: Trail guide for the arthroscopic shoulder surgeon.

[DNLM: 1. Shoulder—surgery. 2. Shoulder Joint—surgery. 3. Arthroscopy—methods. WE 810]

617.5'720597—dc23

2011035548

To purchase additional copies of this book, call our customer service department at (800) 638-3030 or fax orders to (301) 223-2320. International customers should call (301) 223-2300.

Visit Lippincott Williams & Wilkins on the Internet at LWW.com. Lippincott Williams & Wilkins customer service representatives are available from 8:30 am to 6 pm, EST.

10 9 8 7 6 5 4 3 2 1

RRS1111

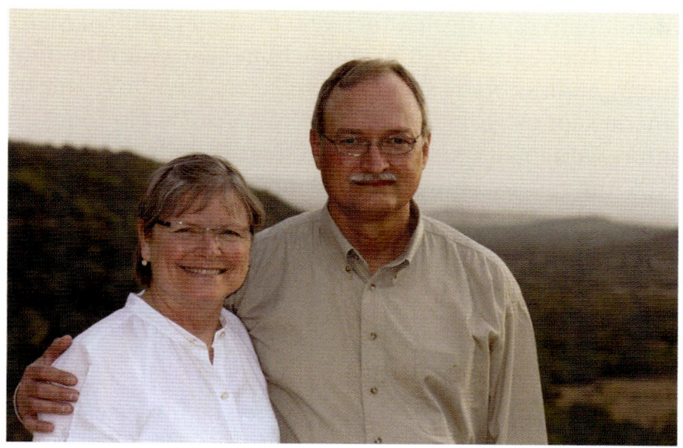

First they ignore you.
Then they laugh at you.
Then they fight you.
Then you win.
—*Mahatma Gandhi*

To Nora. Thanks for never even letting me entertain the thought of giving up, for sharing my desire to help my patients, for recognizing what has always been at stake, and for strengthening me through all the battles to victory.

To my children Zack and Sarah. Thanks for always reminding me that I need balance in life, and thanks for being that balance.

To my Fellows and to my students. You are the future of shoulder surgery. I'm glad I listened to you and took you where you wanted to go. The rest of the journey is yours.

Godspeed.

Stephen S. Burkhart, MD

To my parents, Kwan and Beatrice, whose immeasurable sacrifices I have never forgotten—I thank you. To my wife, Elaine, and my children, Katelyn, Madison, Isabella, and James, who know me best as husband and father.

Ian K.Y. Lo, MD

I am extremely thankful to my wife, Jennifer, and my four children, Meredith, Davis, Garrett, and Hayden. They encouraged me more than I can communicate in words during the seemingly endless hours spent on this book. Their love and support and their pride in me kept me going on many occasions. Thanks to my shoulder arthroscopy mentors who in addition to Dr. Burkhart include Gary Poehling, MD, and David Martin, MD, And mostly I humbly thank my savior Jesus who as the Master healer chooses to use me as a tool to help and teach others. Please keep using and sharpening me!

Paul C. Brady, MD

To Steve Burkhart for teaching me the difference between the easy way and the cowboy way.

To Marion—the real writer in the family—for her enduring love and support.

Patrick J. Denard, MD

Acknowledgments

The authors wish to thank the many individuals whose efforts made this book possible.

The artwork and the animations are simply spectacular. Our extremely talented artists for this project were Kelly Carvallis, Marco Marchionni, and Dawn Knight. The Hollywood-quality three-dimensional animations were brilliantly composed by Alvaro Villagomez. The critically important role of technical-to-artistic interfacing to ensure the accuracy of the final artwork was very capably performed by John Sodeika.

In San Antonio, we received expert technical video support from Bob Merrill, as well as tireless organizational management of all phases of the manuscript's evolution by Gina Diaz.

At Lippincott Williams & Wilkins, our sincere gratitude goes out to David Murphy for his superb work as project editor for this book; to Chris Merillo for his work as video editor; to Lisa Lawrence for her role as marketing manager; and to Bob Hurley, senior editor, for believing in the *Cowboy Way* of arthroscopic shoulder surgery when others were dubious.

For permission to use the badge photos on the menu of the DVD, we thank the professionals at http://www.thelastbestwest.com/old_west_ranger_badges.htm.

Finally, we wish to thank Reinhold Schmieding, founder and president of Arthrex, for his vision in recognizing the potential for arthroscopic shoulder surgery and for his support in our development of the techniques that are featured in this book.

Stephen S. Burkhart, MD
Ian K.Y. Lo, MD
Paul C. Brady, MD
Patrick J. Denard, MD

Contents

Preface

I never intended to write a second book on shoulder arthroscopy. Lord knows, writing the first one was painful enough to last a lifetime.

The problem is that the human memory for painful experiences is way too short. Over the past 5 years, the memory of the pain faded and was overshadowed by the success of the first book, *A Cowboy's Guide to Advanced Shoulder Arthroscopy*. The success was measured not in books sold but in its contribution to the paradigm shift that has occurred in shoulder surgery: the shift of the gold standard from open surgery to arthroscopic surgery.

In the past 5 years, the techniques of arthroscopic shoulder surgery have advanced exponentially. The basic principles remain the same, but the theories, techniques, and instrumentation have dramatically improved. So, even though we have written a new book, it is not a second edition of the first book. Instead, it is a companion book that builds on the principles of the first book and concentrates on the new theories and techniques that have developed since the first book was written. Hence the title *The Cowboy's Companion: A Trail Guide for the Arthroscopic Shoulder Surgeon*. Our reservation about writing a second edition to the first book was that second editions usually have 90% of the same material as the first edition and only 10% new material. Our goal was to produce a book that reversed those percentages, with at least 90% new material. I think we have accomplished that goal.

In producing this book, we have re-assembled most of our "Dream Team" from the first book. My original coauthors, Dr. Ian Lo and Dr. Paul Brady, have been joined by another coauthor, Dr. Patrick Denard, who was my most recent Fellow. All three of these gentlemen are extremely gifted, both as surgeons and as educators and communicators. Perhaps the greatest thrill for an educator is to be taught by his former students, and I could not be more thrilled by what I have learned from my coauthors.

I know that you as readers will appreciate the advanced interactive technology that we have been able to apply to this book. The digitally enhanced illustrations and animations, produced in association with the medical graphics team at Arthrex, are simply spectacular. Furthermore, the interactivity is maximized by means of an iPad/iPhone application, which makes this book the first of its kind among surgical textbooks.

The procedure-specific technology for shoulder arthroscopy continues to advance at a breathtaking pace. I have been privileged over the past 20 years to have worked closely with Reinhold Schmeiding, president and founder of Arthrex, and his engineering team to develop much of that technology. I remain grateful for that opportunity.

Last year, I was given one of the greatest opportunities and honors of my career when I was invited to deliver the keynote Kessel Lecture at the International Congress on Shoulder and Elbow Surgery on September 8, 2010, in Edinburgh, Scotland. In the course of my research for this address, I was struck by the potential for uniting the best ideas from disparate technologies (including biomechanics, stem cell technology, synthetic biology, RNA interference, nanotechnology, and biotechnology) to forge advances in shoulder surgery that would previously have seemed impossible. We must remember that each of these disruptive breakthrough technologies has been pioneered by persistent mavericks that continue to have the courage of their convictions. It's reassuring to know that there are still a lot of cowboys out there.

KESSEL LECTURE

Stephen S. Burkhart, MD

Presented at the 11th International Congress on Shoulder and Elbow Surgery, Edinburgh, Scotland, September 8, 2010.

Expanding the Frontiers of Shoulder Arthroscopy*

Ladies and Gentlemen,

Technology is not kind. It does not say, "Are you ready for me yet?" In particular, technology is not kind to surgeons. As much as we like to think of ourselves as the masters of technology, the truth is that rapid technologic advancement complicates our lives.

Humans find security in the routine. Patients want their surgeons to be able to say, "I've done this operation hundreds (or thousands) of times." Surgeons want to be able to reassure their patients by saying, "I've done this operation hundreds (or thousands) of times."

Change is intimidating. Adopting change can be challenging. But truly assimilating change is exhilarating.

In today's Information Age, the rapid doubling time of human knowledge makes change inevitable. In 1950, the

*This article was published in *Journal of Shoulder and Elbow Surgery* – March 2011 (Vol. 20, Issue 2, Pages 183–191, DOI: 10.1016/j.jse.2010.10.029) Copyright Elsevier (2010).

doubling time was 10 years. By 2004, the doubling time was 18 months.[9]

With knowledge increasing at rocket-like speed, we can choose either to resist the change that is the by-product of this knowledge or to ride the rocket. I would like to think our choice would be made with the same enthusiasm as Alan Shepard, the first US Mercury astronaut to be launched into space. As he sat alone in the Mercury space capsule above the gigantic Redstone rocket on the launching pad at Cape Canaveral, his last words to Mission Control before liftoff could not restrain his unbridled excitement about the threshold he was about to cross. As Mission Control counted down, Alan Shepard encapsulated the mood of the moment by shouting, "Let's light this candle!"

Disruptive technologies in shoulder surgery

Physicians and surgeons are fond of the term "paradigm shift." This is a gentle phrasing of a disruptive concept. It suggests that the familiar practices of today will gradually and peacefully transition to the kinder, gentler, more advanced practices of tomorrow. It suggests that we will barely notice the shift as we transition easily to new technologies. It may be reassuring to view paradigm shifts in terms of riding the gentle waves of change, but nothing could be further from the truth. Technological change is not gentle, it is not easy, and it is often not kind. It does not ask permission.

Clayton Christensen is an associate professor at the Harvard Business School. He coined the term "disruptive technology" and identified it as the way that rapid paradigm shifts occur. In his book *The Innovator's Dilemma*, he described the computer industry as a prime example of the contrasting means by which change can occur.[6]

In the 1970s, IBM was the undisputed world leader in computer technology. Almost every major corporation had its mainframe computers manufactured by IBM, and they used IBM's software and operating systems. IBM was incentivized to steadily upgrade and enhance its computers with incremental improvements. This is called "enhancement technology." Grateful customers would show their appreciation for these enhancements by upgrading to newer models every few years. IBM had a dominant market share with loyal customers, so there was no incentive to try to innovate a radically new computing system. Even if IBM were to develop a new transformational technology, they would simply cannibalize their own business and be no better off for their efforts. At least this was what they thought. But they were wrong.

The disruptive technology that was not recognized by IBM was spurred by the personal computer. IBM saw no need to invest research and development dollars in the low-profit realm of personal computers when they already had the majority of large corporate customers. This left the door open for small start-up companies to develop the technology required for personal computers—the technology of miniaturization and microprocessors, as well as unique operating systems and software to operate them and to allow interfacing with another new and underestimated technology, the Internet. These small companies were often started by college dropouts with very little money, who gave them goofy names like Apple, Microsoft, and Intel. They were no match for the mighty corporate culture and the unlimited resources of International Business Machines, Incorporated. Or were they?

The thing that Apple, Microsoft, Intel, and the others had, that IBM did not have, was the flexibility and the desire to target a small and barely profitable segment of the computer market. And the only way to succeed in that market was to develop a series of technologies that would ultimately become disruptive to the entire computer industry by making mainframe computers obsolete. Once IBM recognized the need to be in the minicomputer market, it was too late. By then, the upstarts were the new leaders of the industry.

You may be thinking that this example of paradigm shift by disruptive technology applies only to business and industry and not to medicine. But then you would be wrong. Medical technology is advancing at a breathtaking pace, in step with computer technology, biotechnology, and nanotechnology. There are multiple disruptive technologies that are in the process of affecting how we will practice medicine in the future. But before we speculate about the future, I think it would be instructive to examine the history of past major paradigm shifts in shoulder surgery.

The past

The further backward you look, the further forward you can see.

Winston Churchill

Early paradigm shifts were quite simple but nonetheless dramatic. The ancient Egyptians documented a modified Kocher technique for reducing an anterior shoulder dislocation over 3,000 years ago.[10] By means of this relatively simple maneuver, a human intervention could immediately relieve considerable pain and disability. This created a paradigm shift—a change in the way humans dealt with shoulder dislocations.

For chronic instability, Hippocrates initiated a paradigm shift in the fifth century BC, when he described the use of a red-hot iron in the axilla to create eschars that caused contractures that eliminated instability.[14] Although the technology was crude, Hippocrates' understanding of the anatomy allowed him to use that basic technology to create an effective treatment. His moderately invasive technique for producing thermal contractures was the precursor to modern shoulder surgery.

For hundreds of years, treatment of the shoulder did not advance. The painful shoulder was treated with poultices and herbs, heat and cold, sympathetic looks, and benign neglect. Orthopaedic interventions were limited to bone setting and amputations.

The advent of reliable anesthesia in the mid to late 1800s led to the next disruptive technology: surgical intervention in the shoulder. By the early part of the 20th century, surgeons such as Bankart, Perthes, and Nicola were performing surgery for anterior instability of the shoulder, and E. A. Codman was presenting his work on surgical repair of the torn rotator cuff.

It is tempting to assume that surgery gradually evolved through enhancement of existing medical technology. But the single disruptive event that allowed surgery to be safely done indoors was the invention of the electric light. In the most general way, Thomas Edison, the inventor of the light bulb, was the father of modern surgery!

Impossible, you must be saying to yourselves. Thomas Edison was not a surgeon. He didn't know anatomy, and he never conducted a single biological experiment. But consider this. Prior to the invention of the light bulb, much of the surgery that was done in the United States was performed outdoors on a sunny day so that the surgeon could see to operate.[7] It was necessary to operate outdoors because ether was highly flammable and the use of indoor lanterns with an open flame for lighting was extremely dangerous. Even Lipmann Kessel, for whom this lectureship is named, remarked on the alternatives to ether in his book Surgeon at Arms, in which he recounted his experiences as a surgeon during World War II.[11] "Chloroform may sound old-fashioned, but at that time, ether was the only alternative, and it was too inflammable. as I'd found out during an explosion in an operating tent in Tunisia." The invention of the electric light bulb allowed for the safe indoor use of flammable anesthetics in addition to reducing contamination and providing focused illumination into the surgical wound. Thank you, Thomas Edison, for taking surgeons out of the cow pasture and putting them into the operating room.

As the 20th century progressed, many talented shoulder surgeons contributed to the enhancement of shoulder surgery by incrementally refining operations such as rotator cuff repair. But the next orthopaedic paradigm shift, beginning in the 1960s, was the treatment of arthritis by means of arthroplasty. Dr. Charles Neer pioneered shoulder arthroplasty, and it developed into a mature technology through the efforts of many talented and creative shoulder surgeons, researchers, and engineers. A number of those innovators are in the audience today, and I salute you for your accomplishments.

As much as arthroplasty improved the treatment of arthritis of the shoulder, it was not a true global paradigm shift because it did not radically change the way that most shoulder surgery was done. Surgical procedures continued to be performed through open incisions, with knives, osteotomes, and sutures, just as they have been done for a century, with only the occasional enhancement.

The next truly global paradigm shift in shoulder surgery caught most surgeons by surprise, as all important disruptive technologies do. The arthroscope, an innocent-looking device that initially was thought to have only diagnostic capabilities (and limited ones at that), was applied to the shoulder with little fanfare and with more than a little disdain from many of the halls of orthopaedic influence. But that disdain would not last.

From disdain to disruption and transformation

First they ignore you,
then they laugh at you,
then they fight you,
then you win.

Mahatma Gandhi

How do new ideas gain widespread acceptance? How do radical new ideas create paradigm shifts? Thomas Kuhn examined this phenomenon extensively in his book *The Structure of Scientific Revolutions*.[13] Kuhn made the critical observation that, "Almost always the men who achieve these fundamental inventions of a new paradigm have been either very young or very new to the field whose paradigm they change. The resulting transition to a new paradigm is scientific revolution."

If you doubt the truth of this observation, then consider the case of a 26-year-old clerk in the Swiss patent office who published his *Theory of Special Relativity* in 1905. Albert Einstein was a young outsider to the scientific community who had the audacity to challenge the universal application of Newtonian physics. At age 26, he was undoubtedly naive, but he was persistent and relentless. He had no substantial academic credentials, and therefore he had nothing to lose by inciting the disdain and the resistance of academia.

In a similar fashion, the surgeons who pioneered shoulder arthroscopy in the 1980s and early 1990s were mostly young men in their 30s and 40s. They were in private practice with no affiliation to academic institutions, so they had little or nothing to lose by bucking the shoulder establishment. These were men like Steve Snyder, Jim Esch, and Dick Caspari, among others.

Thomas Kuhn, in describing the genesis of scientific revolutions, went on to say, "Most anomalies (i.e., potential paradigm shifts) are resolved by normal means; most proposals for new theories prove to be wrong. If, on the other hand, no one reacted to anomalies or to brand-new theories in high-risk ways, there would be few or no revolutions."

By reacting in "high-risk ways," as Kuhn put it, the early shoulder arthroscopists ensured their status as pariahs for a number of years, as they developed their techniques and their technology out of view from the shoulder establishment. By the time the establishment recognized that the new disruptive technology of shoulder arthroscopy was a threat to its dominance, it was too late. The younger generation of orthopaedic surgeons had already embraced it, and the public would soon demand it.

The shifting paradigm

Don't raise your voice; improve your argument.

Archbishop Desmond Tutu

In the early to mid 1990s, shoulder arthroscopy burst out of the blocks with rapid developments that caught mainstream shoulder surgeons by surprise. These developments were sometimes greeted with sarcastic remarks such as, "The arthroscope is the instrument of the devil." We had clearly gone past Gandhi's stage of being ignored to the stage of being laughed at, which rapidly led to the stage of conflict.

But why was conflict necessary? Thomas Kuhn said that when an existing paradigm is challenged, "resistance is inevitable and legitimate." He suggested that new paradigms undergo a process of incremental acceptance, if they are accepted at all. In *The Structure of Scientific Revolutions*, Kuhn wrote, "If a paradigm is ever to triumph it must gain some first supporters, men who will develop it to the point where hardheaded arguments can be produced and multiplied. And even these arguments, when they come, are not individually decisive. Because scientists are reasonable men, one or another argument will ultimately persuade many of them. But there is no single argument that can or should persuade them all. Rather than a single group conversion, what occurs is an increasing shift in the distribution of professional allegiances."

There were many attractive reasons to pursue shoulder arthroscopy. First, the arthroscope allowed the surgeon to view the pathology without any spatial constraints. One no longer had to view the pathoanatomy through the keyhole of an open incision, and one could visualize deeper structures without having to damage superficial structures to get there. This expanded visualization greatly enhanced diagnostic capabilities, leading to the recognition of new categories of pathology such as SLAP (superior labrum anterior-posterior) lesions. It also improved diagnostic accuracy for conditions such as subscapularis tears. In the open literature, subscapularis tears were recognized in fewer than 5% of rotator cuff tears, whereas arthroscopic studies raised that figure to the 30% to 40% range, which is more in keeping with the incidence in postmortem studies.[1,5]

Shoulder arthroscopists began to realize that their improved visualization allowed for more precise diagnostic assessment. For example, in instability cases, bone loss could be accurately measured to better assess the need for bone grafting. In rotator cuff tears, the tear pattern could be more precisely determined so that the cuff could be anatomically repaired under physiologic resting tension.

Patient outcomes were positively affected. Infection rates for arthroscopic shoulder surgery were dramatically lower than those reported for open shoulder surgery. In fact, the International Society for Arthroscopy, Knee Surgery, and Orthopaedic Sports Medicine Complications Registry in 2000 had a total of 60,000 shoulder arthroscopies registered, with only 4 infections reported, for an incidence of 1 in 15,000.[4] The rate of postoperative stiffness dropped dramatically in comparison to open techniques. Furthermore, once the techniques of arthroscopic capsular release and lysis of adhesions were developed, postoperative stiffness was no longer the looming threat that it had been in open surgery. Whereas it was difficult to improve postoperative stiffness after open surgery by either manipulation or open releases, experienced arthroscopic surgeons could always restore full motion by means of arthroscopic releases. Finally, with this minimally invasive approach, postoperative pain could easily be managed on an outpatient basis.

Patients steadily gravitated to surgeons who could do their shoulder surgery arthroscopically. They told their families, friends, and acquaintances, and over time, this created a critical mass of patients who expected and demanded that their shoulder surgery be performed arthroscopically.

So why and how did shoulder arthroscopy ultimately succeed? Like any paradigm shift, it succeeded in stages. In the earliest stages, there were a few talented surgeons who were able to do complex arthroscopic procedures with rather crude instrumentation and still obtain excellent outcomes. The fact that some surgeons were good at arthroscopy from the very beginning kept it alive. Their techniques steadily evolved as they partnered with engineers to develop new technology that made the surgery easier for the average surgeon. Suture anchors, high-strength sutures, reliable suture passers, and knot-tying techniques were developed and represented pivotal advances.

In addition to technologic advances, there were new educational initiatives, didactic courses, cadaver laboratories, and even a new journal that emphasized the technical aspects of performing arthroscopic surgery. There was a tremendous sense of mission among the pioneers in shoulder arthroscopy. That mission focused on making shoulder arthroscopy the standard of care, and it could only be accomplished by education of surgeons in the new technology. Finally, the combination of improved technology and intensive education created a new generation of surgeons who could reliably perform these techniques.

Redirecting old concepts

Make everything as simple as possible, but no simpler.

Albert Einstein

Today's technology is a constantly moving target. Just 24 hours ago, today was tomorrow. Just an instant ago, the present was the future. Change is a constant in our world. We truly live on the edge of tomorrow.

But change is not always new. It can be driven by observations of the past or by new applications of old ideas. A personal example of this type of observation occurred in 1998, when I first went to China.[3] My host in Hong Kong, Dr. James Lam, showed me some traditional bamboo scaffolding that was held together with lashings that did not contain knots. In those days, knotless bamboo scaffolding was still used to build skyscrapers, including the 100-story Bank of China building. The lives of construction workers 100 floors above the ground depended on the strength and reliability of knotless bamboo scaffolding. As I looked at the scaffolding with Dr. Lam, I realized that lashings and perhaps other mechanical constructs could be more secure than knots, and later, I learned that their strength is governed by the powerful mechanical concept of cable friction. This experience opened my eyes to the potential for secure knotless fixation, which has now been successfully applied to arthroscopic rotator cuff repair and instability repair. Obviously, one has to understand the implications and proper applications of these techniques, but they have become excellent tools for the arthroscopic shoulder surgeon.

Change is driven by technology, and technology has three components: theories, methods, and devices. In the case of shoulder arthroscopy, mechanically based theories such as margin convergence and balanced force couples led to techniques, instrumentation, and devices that permitted side-to-side tendon repair and tendon-to-bone repair.

Cynics who resist change have said that technologic change is market driven; that change is financed and marketed by companies simply to sell products. Well, by necessity, technologic change is facilitated by market forces. But think about it. If the products for the new technology are not available, then nothing will change. This criticism of market-driven change is a circular argument that, in my mind, is flawed. If a technology has no merit, the market will abandon it.

Maturing of technologies and technologic succession

The technology S-curve demonstrates how a technology matures over three stages (Fig. 1).[6] The rate of progress in performance is initially slow. As the technology improves and becomes better understood, the rate of technologic improvement accelerates. But in the mature stages, the technology approaches a natural or physical limit that it cannot exceed on its own.

Ideally, strategic technology management would identify when the present technology's inflection point has been passed and would also identify whatever successor

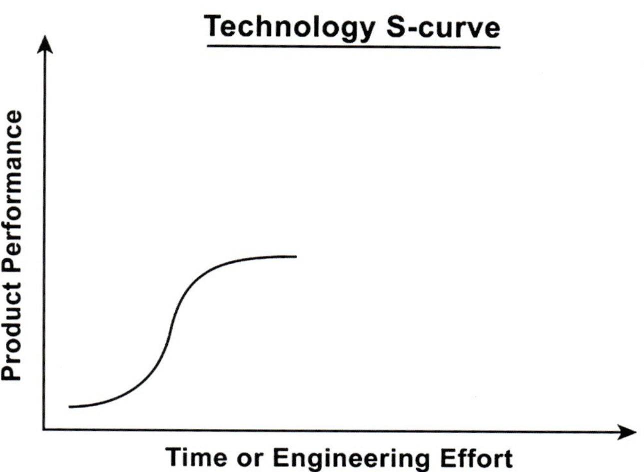

Figure 1 Technology S-curve. The rate of progress is initially slow; it then accelerates and then reaches a physical limit.

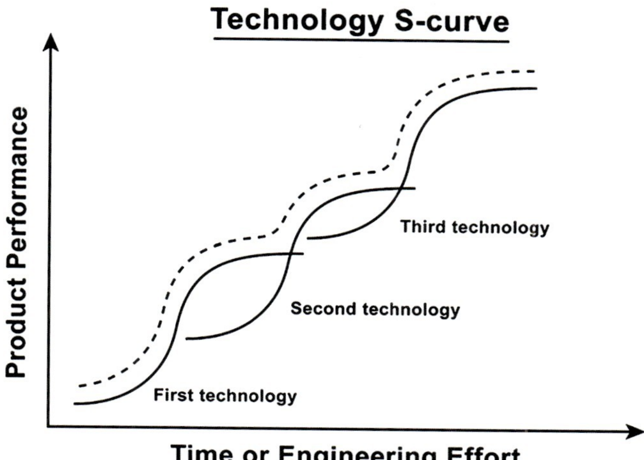

Figure 2 Enhancement technologies produce improvements by the method of stair-step intersection of S-curves.

technology rising from below will eventually supplant the current approach. The challenge is to successfully switch or merge technologies at the point where the S-curves of the old and new intersect.

Enhancement technologies, where incremental improvements are overlaid onto the basic technology within a given market, function by the method of stair-step intersection of S-curves (Fig. 2). An example would be the addition of biologic enhancement of rotator cuff healing by means of growth factors, adult stem cells, and platelet-rich plasma (technology B) layered onto the basic platform technology of optimized mechanical fixation of the torn rotator cuff (technology A).

The problem in strategic technology management comes with the difficulty—and, usually, the inability—to predict or detect potential disruptive technologies. A disruptive technology is not obvious to the market that it will eventually disrupt because it develops in an entirely different market. If and when it progresses to the point where it can satisfy the level and nature of performance demanded in another market, the disruptive technology can invade that market, knocking out the established technology and its practitioners, often with stunning speed (Fig. 3).

I keep coming back to the concept that technology is not kind. It will not ask permission. It will not say, "Are you ready for me yet?"

What's next?

It seems clear to me that the next phases of enhancement technology for shoulder arthroscopy have already begun. Biologic enhancement technology is available, in the form of platelet-rich plasma preparations and techniques of bone bed preparation (microfracture variants) and implant design (vented and cannulated suture anchors) to encourage open access of bone marrow elements to the tendon-bone interface.

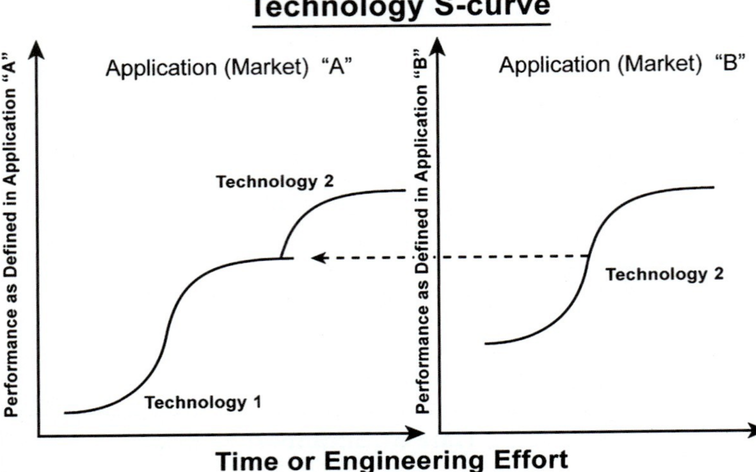

Figure 3 A disruptive technology develops in one market until it reaches the performance demands of another market. Then it invades the second market, disrupting the established technology.

Another enhancement technology has also begun, and it involves the augmentation of current fixation techniques with self-reinforcing systems. The concept of self-regulating systems has been around for a long time in the automotive industry, where there are self-balancing engine components and self-centering mechanical systems. However, biomechanical self-regulating mechanisms have only recently been identified and used. Specifically, the suture-bridge technique of rotator cuff fixation by means of linked bridging sutures between two rows of suture anchors exhibits self-reinforcement characteristics.

The term "self-reinforcement" refers to the fact that, the harder you try to make the system fail, the stronger it becomes. One example of a self-reinforcing system that most surgeons are familiar with is the Chinese finger trap. In the case of the Chinese finger trap, the harder you pull in an attempt to pull it off the finger, the tighter it grips the finger. In effect, it harnesses a potentially destructive force to make itself stronger. This is a very useful characteristic, particularly for a biologic repair construct such as a rotator cuff repair.

We first noted the self-reinforcing attributes of bridging double-row rotator cuff repair about 5 years ago while testing this fixation technique on cadavers in the biomechanics laboratory.[2] We noted that the yield load approached the ultimate load, in contradistinction to nonlinked double-row repairs. The reason this happens is that the suture-bridge fixation functions much like a Chinese finger trap.

In the unloaded situation, the suture bridge forms a rectangle of fixation around a segment of rotator cuff tendon (Fig. 4). Under load, this rectangle changes shape into a parallelogram with a decreased height of the construct and an increased normal force perpendicular to the tendon. The increased normal force translates into increased friction at the tendon-bone interface because of the relationship $f = \mu N$ (f, frictional force; μ, coefficient of friction; N, normal force). As the normal force increases, the frictional force increases. Also, because the height of the parallelogram continues to decrease under load, the tendon becomes wedged progressively more tightly under the sutures (Fig. 5). We think that the improved clinical results that are being reported with suture-bridge techniques are at least

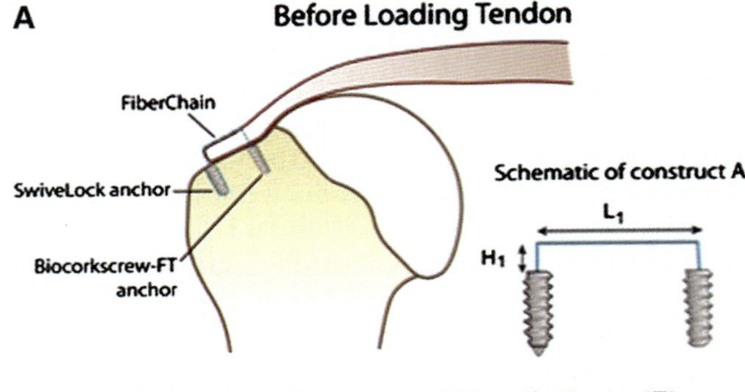

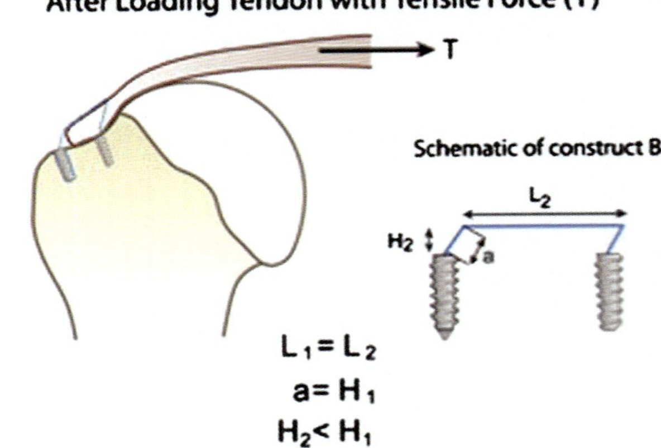

Figure 4 **A:** In the unloaded situation, the suture-bridge configuration forms a rectangle of fixation around a segment of rotator cuff tendon. (H1, thickness of rotator cuff before loading; L1, length of tendon beneath suture.) **B:** Under load, the rectangle changes shape into a parallelogram with a decreased height and an increased normal force (N) perpendicular to the tendon. (T, tensile loading force; L2, length of tendon beneath suture; a, length of suture between tendon edge and lateral anchor; H2, thickness of compressed rotator cuff under tensile load.)

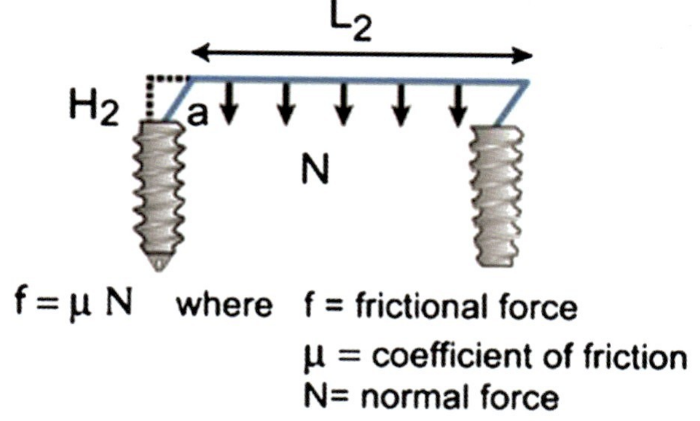

Figure 5 As the height of the parallelogram decreases under load, the frictional force increases, and the tendon becomes wedged progressively more tightly under the sutures. (f, frictional force; μ, coefficient of friction; N, normal force perpendicular to the tendon)

partly because of the enhanced fixation afforded by this self-reinforcing mechanism.

Self-reinforcement and biologic enhancement are incremental enhancing technologies that are layered onto the base technology of strong mechanical fixation. I feel certain that there are other self-reinforcing and self-regulating techniques that will be discovered to enhance fixation and thereby improve healing.

Biologic enhancement is in its infancy. Even though a variety of platelet-rich plasma preparations are available, much needs to be learned about how to optimally apply this technology. A great deal of work is currently being done to secure growth factors at the repair site. Perhaps a time-release preparation will ensure that the proper cascade of factors will occur at the proper time to enhance healing.

Further research should clarify whether patients need repeated postoperative injections to introduce specific growth factors at the correct time to optimize healing.

As the paradigm of biologic enhancement progresses, it will depend on two diametrically opposite conditions. These conditions are: order and chaos. Order must be imposed on the pathways most likely to succeed, because progress builds on its own increasing order. However, the evolution of a paradigm does not occur in a closed system, and it must draw upon the chaos in the larger system in which it takes place to enhance its options for diversity. Chaos is necessary to create options, but order must then be imposed on those options, in essence creating order from chaos.

What if?

Now for the fun part. What if we were to survey disparate technologies that are developing today, and to imagine how they might converge to affect shoulder surgery in the future? The resulting conjectures could easily be dismissed as the unfocused wanderings of a disturbed mind. And that might be very close to the truth. But it's fun to imagine, so let's take the risk.

Stem cell technologies

Despite the political rhetoric, stem cell research has moved far beyond embryonic stem cells to a process called "transdifferentiation." In this process, adult cells, usually from human skin, are transformed into a new kind of stem cell called induced pluripotent stem (iPS) cells.[8] These iPS cells are fundamentally identical to embryonic stem cells and can be programmed to grow into other cell types such as heart cells, pancreatic islet cells, or articular cartilage cells. Scientists at Rice University and at the University of California at Davis have used iPS cells from a mouse to grow its entire distal femur in the laboratory (Athanasiou KA, personal oral communication, June 2010). Imagine doing this in humans so that the patient's own skin cells are used to grow a younger version of his or her own shoulder in the laboratory, which can then be surgically implanted as a biologic autologous joint replacement. In similar fashion, focal chondral defects could be treated arthroscopically by implanting laboratory-grown autografts.

Synthetic biology

Manipulating genomes has become so commonplace today that even high schoolers do it. Craig Venter, who decoded the human genome for a fraction of the cost and in a fraction of the time that the US government had allotted, is pushing the boundaries of synthetic biology. Venter and his associates at the J. Craig Venter Institute in California have made a bacterial genome from scratch and have even turned one type of microbe into another. Venter expects to create the first artificial life form within the next year, which will essentially be a "designer bacteria."[8] His next step is to engineer a "designer algae" that will secrete high-grade hydrocarbons that can easily be refined into transportation fuels. ExxonMobil has so much faith in this concept that they have funded Venter's project with $300 million.

Other researchers have created synthetic organelles and even an entirely new organelle known as the "synthosome" to make enzymes for synthetic biology.[8] One can envision the day when synthosomes that produce enzymes and proteins that are useful in the repair process of tendons could be used to enhance rotator cuff healing or to reverse the changes of tendon degeneration.

RNA interference

Synthetic biology and stem cell strategies can be categorized under the umbrella of "regenerative medicine," which has the power to restore damaged or senescent tissues but does not attack the cause of disease. This is where RNA interference (RNAi) fits in.

RNAi is able to turn off specific genes by blocking their messenger RNA, thus preventing them from creating proteins.[8,12] RNAi provides the ability to control any of the genes in our bodies as well as the proteins they produce. This is a very powerful function. With its ability to create proteins blocked, the gene is effectively silenced. RNAi could be used to turn off the gene that allows cancers to develop capillary networks. It could turn off the protein production responsible for Alzheimer's disease. In the shoulder, RNAi could be used to turn off the genes responsible for articular cartilage degeneration or rotator cuff degeneration. This strategy could be augmented by cell therapies in which induced iPS cells are introduced into the damaged tissue to initiate healing with young healthy cells generated by the patient's own DNA.

For the first time, science is looking not just to treat symptoms, but to actually stop the gene functions that cause disease. This is truly revolutionary. The challenge right now is in the delivery of RNAi preparations to cells. These molecules are large and fragile, so they do not penetrate cell membranes easily. Right now, a number of delivery mechanisms are under investigation, and their successful development will ensure the future of RNAi.

Nanotechnology/biotechnology convergence

The role of the infinitely small is infinitely large.

Louis Pasteur

One nanometer is one one-billionth of a meter. The nanotechnology range is generally considered to be under 100 nm, which gets down to molecular and atomic levels.

Until recently, a large part of nanotechnology's resources were directed toward the creation of molecular machines. Boston College chemistry professor T. Ross Kelly reported that he had constructed a chemically powered nano-motor out of 78 atoms.[8] Another molecular-sized motor fueled by solar energy was built out of 58 atoms by Ben Feringa at the University of Groningen in the Netherlands.[8] Carbon nanotubes have been used to construct nanoscale conveyor belts.[12]

DNA is also proving to be very versatile for building molecular structures. A tiny biped robot constructed from DNA was developed at New York University. It has legs that are only 10-nm long. The robot can walk down a DNA walking track.[8] DNA was chosen as the construction material because of its ability to attach and detach itself in a controlled manner.

Nanoscale scaffolds have been used to grow biological tissues such as skin. Future therapies could use these tiny scaffolds to grow any type of tissue needed for repairs inside the body.

One fascinating application of nanotechnology is to harness nanoparticles to deliver treatments to specific sites in the body. Nanoparticles can guide drugs into cell walls and through the blood-brain barrier. Scientists at McGill University in Montreal demonstrated a "nanopill" with structures in the 25- to 45-nm range.[8] The nanopill is small enough to pass through the cell wall and deliver medication directly to targeted structures inside the cell.

Ray Kurzweil, in his book *The Singularity is Near*, envisions nanoscale robots, or nanobots, that will be able to travel through the bloodstream, going in and around our cells and performing various services, such as removing toxins, correcting DNA errors, repairing and restoring cell membranes, modifying the levels of hormones and neurotransmitters, and doing a myriad of other tasks.[12]

Enhanced arthroscopic technology

Let's come back down to earth for a moment. Let's leave nanotechnology and induced iPS cells behind and look at an example of what enhanced arthroscopic technology is capable of today. One of the new frontiers in arthroscopy of the shoulder is arthroscopic arthroplasty. In Vienna, Austria, Dr. Werner Anderl has been performing arthroscopic resurfacing of the humerus, and he is developing techniques for arthroscopic transhumeral glenoid preparation (Anderl W, personal oral communication, April 2010). Components are introduced through the rotator interval and secured by screws with a transhumeral retrograde screwdriver. The technology involved in this procedure is truly breathtaking, and I feel certain that it will ultimately lead to a new era in arthroplasty surgery.

En fuego

The future ain't what it used to be.

Yogi Berra

I hope you have found this lecture disturbing. And I hope you have found it exhilarating. At the very least, I hope it made you uncomfortable. The world of shoulder surgery is changing whether we individually change or not. It is fitting that the two essential ingredients for the evolution of a paradigm are chaos and order. Without chaos we would have no choices, without choices we would have no order, and without order we would have no progress.

Technology is not kind. It will not ask, "Are you ready yet?" But you know what? I'm ready. Let's light this candle!

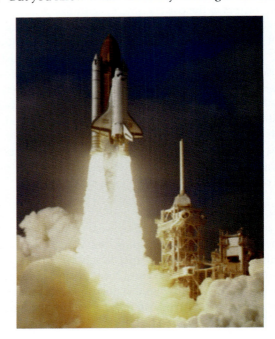

REFERENCES

1. Adams CR, Schoolfield JD, Burkhart SS. The results of arthroscopic subscapularis tendon repairs. *Arthroscopy* 2008;24:1381–1389. doi:10.1016/j.arthro.2008.08.004.
2. Burkhart SS, Adams CR, Burkhart SS, et al. Abiomechanical comparison of 2 techniques of footprint reconstruction for rotator cuff repair: the SwiveLock-FiberChain construct versus standard double-row repair. *Arthroscopy* 2009;25:274–281. doi:10.1016/j.arthro.2008.09.024.
3. Burkhart SS, Athanasiou KA. The twist-lock concept of tissue transport and suture fixation without knots: observations along the Hong Kong skyline. *Arthroscopy* 2003;19:613–625. doi:10.1016/S0749-8063(03)00396-7.
4. Burkhart SS. Report of ISAKOS Upper Extremity Committee. ISAKOS (International Society for Arthroscopy, Knee Surgery, and Orthopaedic Sports Medicine). *Newsletter* 2000;3:3–4.
5. Burkhart SS, Tehrany AM. Arthroscopic subscapularis tendon repair: Technique and preliminary results. *Arthroscopy* 2002;18:454–463. doi: 10.1053/jars.2002.30648.
6. Christensen CM. *The Innovator's Dilemma*. New York: Harper Business; 2006.
7. Cox M. Frontier medicine: Texas doctors overcome disease and despair. *Texas Med* 2003;99:19–26.
8. Cox P. The coming biotech bubble. John Mauldin's Outside the Box E-Letter 2010;6:1–15.
9. Gover M. Knowledge doubling curve and you. March 10, 2010. Available from: URL: http://ezinearticles.com/?Knowledge-Doubling-Curve-and-You&id¼3908031. Accessed on August 23, 2010.
10. Hussein MK. Kocher's method is 3,000 years old. *J Bone Joint Surg Br* 1968;50:669–671.
11. Kessel L, St John J. *Surgeon at Arms*. London, UK: Leo Cooper; 1976.
12. Kurzweil R. *The Singularity Is Near*. New York: Penguin Group; 2005.
13. Kuhn TS. The structure of scientific revolutions. Chicago: University of Chicago Press; 1962.
14. Matsen FA, Thomas SC, Rockwood CA. Anterior glenohumeral instability. In: Rockwood CA, Matsen FA, eds. *The Shoulder*. Philadelphia, PA: Saunders; 1990:526–622.

Foreword

I sincerely recommend this innovative text, photo, and video collection entitled: *The Cowboy's Companion* by Steve Burkhart, Ian Lo, Paul Brady, and Patrick Denard. Over the past 25 years, I have had the pleasure to discuss and argue the fine points of shoulder arthroscopy with Steve. I am aware of the enthusiasm, planning, and skill he brings to the operating room and to his Texas ranch. I have watched his interactions with patients, colleagues, and cowboys.

Surgeon and rancher Steve Burkhart shares the planning and skill sets necessary to be successful on the maturing ranch of shoulder arthroscopy. Dr. Burkhart's guide shows the reader the tools and moves necessary to make the complex problems of selecting the correct operation for rotator cuff repair and instability surgery. By following his recommendations, our patients will be grateful that they can return to a successful daily life. The graphic visual and video connections help visual learners like me appreciate the fine points necessary to be a successful surgeon. This *Cowboy's Companion* book enables the surgeon to be comfortable and efficient in the saddle of the operating room. I am confident your practice will improve by using this exceptional resource.

James C. Esch, MD (Urban Cowboy)
Orthopaedic Specialists of North County
Oceanside, California

Foreword

In 2006, I had the pleasure and honor to write a foreword to Dr. Stephen S. Burkhart's first comprehensive textbook, *A Cowboy's Guide to Advanced Shoulder Arthroscopy,* written with Drs. Ian Lo and Paul Brady. The book was an instant success, serving as a beacon of enlightenment to all students interested in the most up to date information in the field of shoulder arthroscopy.

In the intervening 5 years, shoulder arthroscopy has matured. There are many new procedures and products, and many older ones have been refined and improved.

Now I again have the pleasure of writing a few words as a foreword to Dr. Burkhart's second book, *The Cowboy's Companion: A Trail Guide for the Arthroscopic Shoulder Surgeon,* and again I am pleased and honored.

All who know Steve understand the meaning of his books' titles. There is a rich cultural lore in cowboy history and especially in early Texas tradition, which includes work, honesty, minimal showoff, and striving for perfection. These are all part of Steve's DNA. In preparation for writing a few words for his book, I have enjoyed reviewing some special cowboy aphorisms and have chosen a few especially meaningful examples to help me characterize my friend.

"The best sermons are lived, not preached."

Dr. Burkhart's new book is written to "update" rather than replace the initial volume. He is joined again by Drs. Lo and Brady along with the addition of Dr. Patrick Denard. These are three of Steve's former Fellows who are now proven leaders in the field, following the "Burkhart" way as well as blazing their own trails.

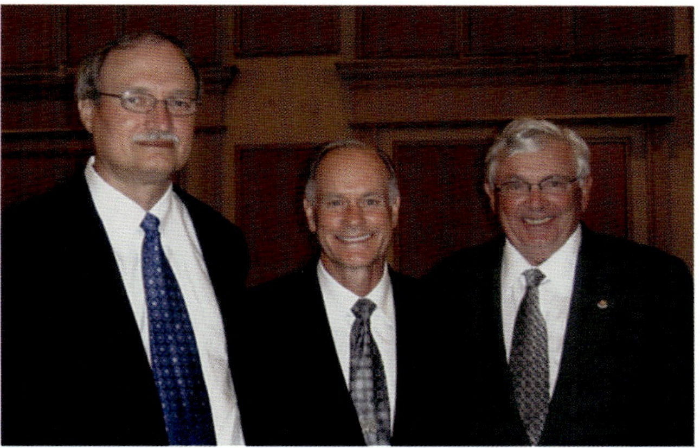

"Don't go where the path may lead. Go instead where there is no path... and you can leave a trail."

This new book takes on many of the still unresolved questions that complicate our everyday decision making in shoulder arthroscopy. Still unresolved are the most efficient and successful methods to treat massive cuff and subscapularis tears, especially those known to have retracted medially and are complicated by fatty degeneration of the muscles. Dr. Burkhart has taught us a method of performing scar and tendon release that permits repairing even apparently hopeless cases.

"Nobody ever drowned in his own sweat."

There are very few people in my circle of shoulder surgical friends and acquaintances who are as indefatigable in pursuit of excellence in our field as Steve Burkhart. His travel agenda annually takes him to all corners of the world as well as across the US. His participation in AANA, AAOS, ASES, AOSSM, ISAKOS, and TCO leaves little time for sleep and no time for golf. Hence, he excels at shoulder surgery and is mediocre at best with golf.

"Behind every successful cowboy there's a strong woman running the ranch." (slightly revised by SJS)

I place the Burkharts among a special breed of people who live life in the truest family tradition. It's a rare time indeed that Steve travels without Nora at his side. Zack, their oldest child, is a resident in opthamology and is married to Jenny. They have given Steve and Nora their first grandchild. Grandbaby number two is due later this year. Sarah is their remarkably brilliant daughter who, after completing a degree in mechanical engineering with highest honors, decided to follow her calling to join the seminary. She loves teaching and charity endeavors and shares the deep religious beliefs of her parents. Of course Mom and Dad are very proud!

"Talk slowly, think quickly."

One thing that many surgeons don't understand is that many of the tools that Dr. Burkhart uses for arthroscopic surgery and displays in this book and video were personally conceived, designed and championed by him. It may seem like a small task to some, but I can attest that it is exactly the opposite. I know that our job in the operating room would be much more difficult if it were not for Dr. Burkhart's creativity, intellect, and tenacity.

"If you're ridin' ahead of the herd, take a look back every now and then to make sure it's still there with ya."

I'm not sure this one fits, but take a look at the Three Amigos. Dr. James Esch, Dr. Steve Burkhart, and I have had a deep bond of friendship for most of our professional years. We have worked together in numerous labs, courses, seminars, meetings, and committees and always came away with our mutual respect and support strengthened. Steve is that kind of cowboy, an amigo and sidekick for life. Congratulations on this second great shoulder arthroscopy book. **Happy trails, Cowboy.**

Stephen J. Snyder, MD
Van Nuys, California

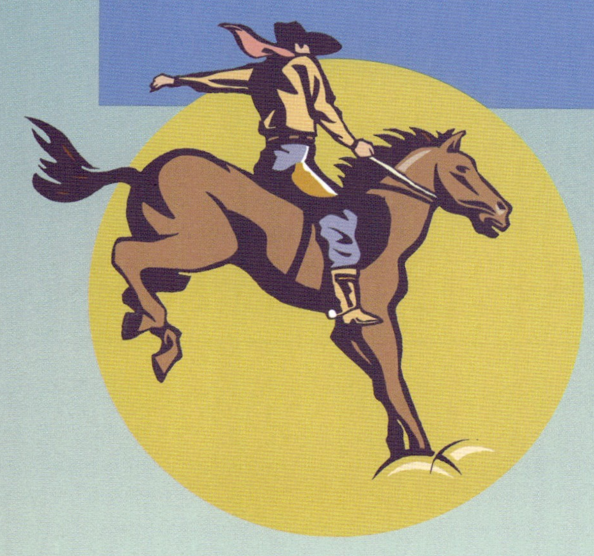

PART I

THE SHOULDER ROUND-UP

COWBOY PRINCIPLE 1

There ain't a horse that can't be rode, there ain't a man that can't be throwed.

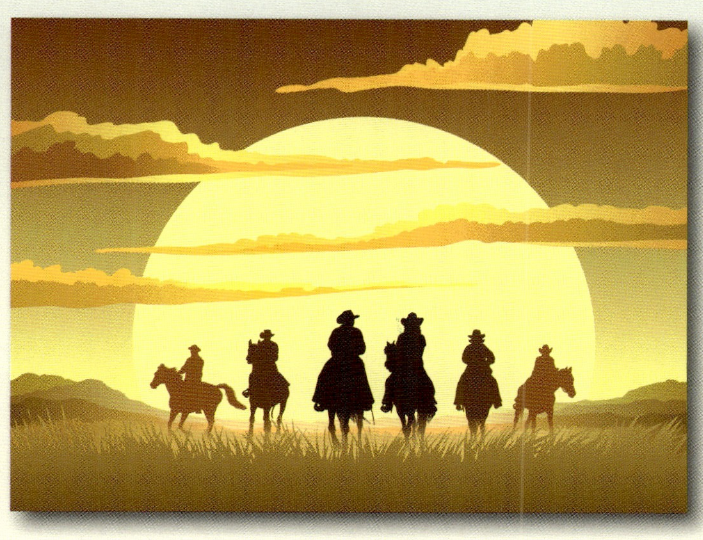

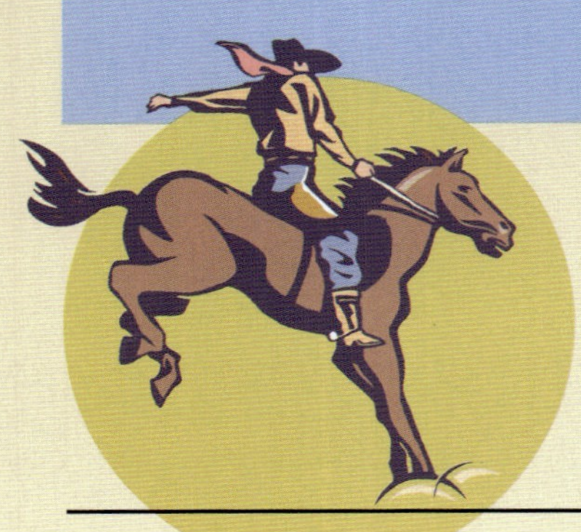

INTRODUCTION

COWBOY PRINCIPLE 2

Admire a big horse. Saddle a small one.

In the round-up, the cowboy needs to keep things simple and manageable. Riding a big horse may feed the ego, but it's sure a long way to fall.

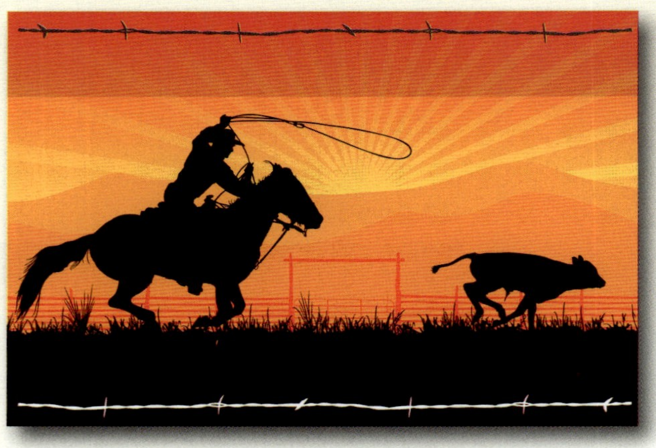

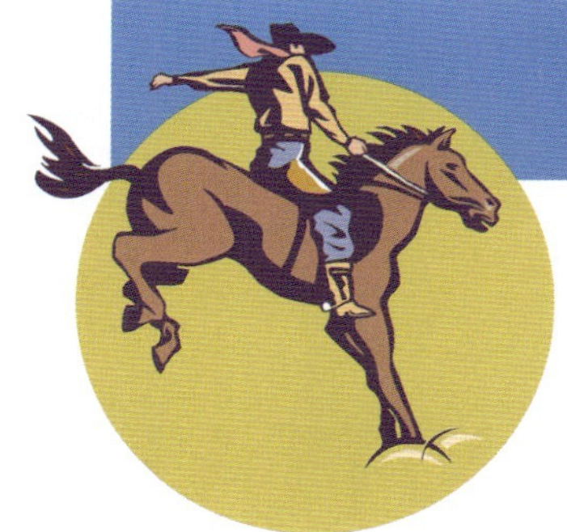

So you're back again for another roundup. A lot has happened around here since you last joined us in *"A Cowboy's Guide to Advanced Shoulder Arthroscopy"* 6 years ago. Shoulder arthroscopy has advanced faster than a Texas tornado!

Some mighty fine surgeons have signed on with our outfit and adopted the Cowboy Way. What they've discovered is that the Cowboy Way is not only the brand of surgery that we practice, but it's a whole new perspective on lookin' at life.

This book is intended as a trail guide for the arthroscopic shoulder surgeon. It's got common-sense solutions to your everyday shoulder problems and a logical approach to your once-in-a-lifetime shoulder problems. In the past 6 years, we've gotten into our fair share of surgical dilemmas, and we want to share with you the solutions and the thought processes that have helped us to manage these problems successfully. There are some powerful mechanical concepts and technological advances that have evolved over that time period, and we have tried to lay these out as clearly as possible in the text, illustrations, and videos.

In keepin' with our roots, we also wanted to share the wisdom of the Cowboy Code. So we decided to start each section of the book with a rock-solid cowboy principle to live by and to open each chapter with a pithy nugget of western wisdom. If you want to avoid lookin' like you're all hat and no cattle, you need to pay close attention to these little pearls.

So I'll be your trail boss as long as you're in this outfit. When you ride, I expect you to ride for the brand. When you're tired, just remember that no man ever drowned in his own sweat. And when you disagree with me, just be sure to saddle your horse before sassin' the boss.

—Stephen S. Burkhart, MD

SECTION I

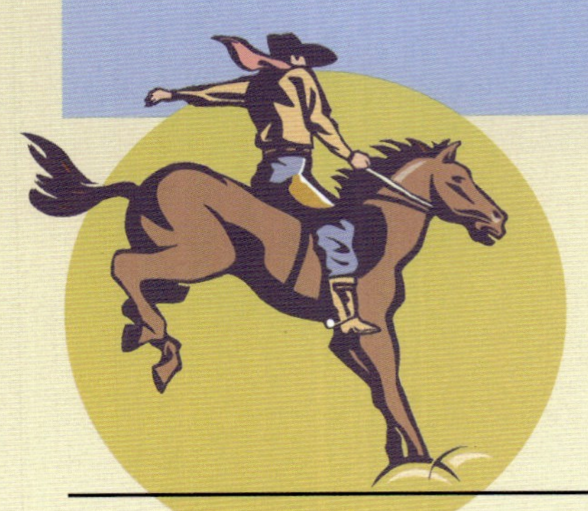

ESSENTIALS

COWBOY PRINCIPLE 3

A good horse is never a bad color.

The horse and the cowboy work in tandem as a single unit. Good cowboys teamed with good horses make the round-up go without a hitch. When the job gets done right, nobody cares about the color or the conformation of the horses that make it possible. Ugly horses don't know about mirrors.

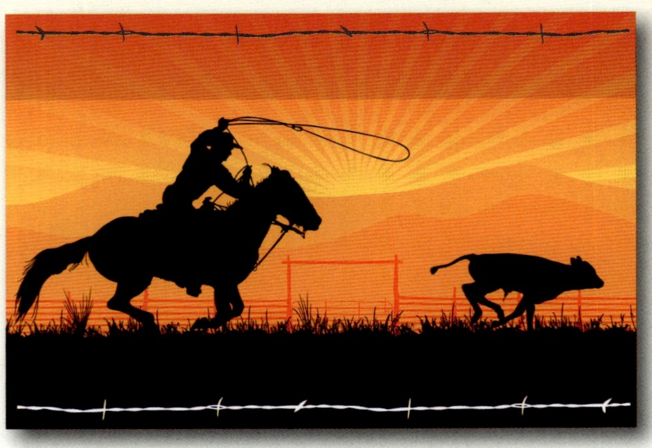

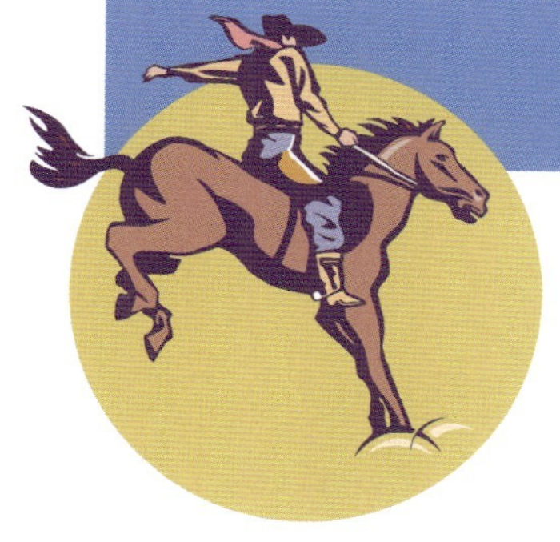

1

Advanced Shoulder Arthroscopy Essentials

WESTERN WISDOM

Advice is handy only before trouble comes.

As in all surgical procedures, the operating room setup for shoulder arthroscopy is an essential component of the procedure. Visualization is affected by patient positioning and adequate fluid management. Portal placement dictates the angle of approach and determines access to the shoulder. The details of the above have been fully outlined in *A Cowboy's Guide to Advanced Shoulder Arthroscopy*. The following is a brief review of patient positioning and setup, fluid management, and our most commonly used portals.

POSITIONING AND SETUP

We perform all shoulder arthroscopy in the lateral decubitus position. We have performed shoulder arthroscopy in both the lateral decubitus and the beach-chair positions, and there is no doubt in our minds that the lateral decubitus provides the best view of the shoulder. The beach-chair position developed at a time when surgeons were transitioning from open to arthroscopic procedures. Ironically, the inferior visualization the beach-chair position provides has slowed the transition to all-arthroscopic procedures. While this position is familiar, we recommend that for the surgeon to become an advanced shoulder arthroscopist, he or she use the lateral decubitus position exclusively. Shoulder arthroscopy relies on access to the anatomy and this should not be compromised.

To position the patient in the lateral decubitus position, an axillary roll is placed under the nonoperative arm, the legs are padded, a warming blanket is applied, and the patient is secured with a vacuum beanbag. The operative arm is placed in a Star Sleeve Balanced Suspension System (Arthrex, Inc., Naples, FL). Five to ten lbs of balanced suspension is used with the arm in 20° to 30° of abduction and 20° of forward flexion.

The surgical team consists of the surgeon, a first assistant, and two surgical technicians. The surgeon stands behind the patient's shoulder. The first assistant stands behind the patient's head. The primary surgical technician stands behind the surgeon, working from a Mayo stand and the instrument table. The second surgical technician stands in front of the patient's torso and manipulates the operative arm and manages the shaver, burr, and electrocautery that are positioned on a second Mayo stand (Fig. 1.1).

FLUID MANAGEMENT

Maintaining visualization relies upon limiting bleeding by balancing the patient's blood pressure and the arthroscopic pump pressure, as well as controlling turbulence within the shoulder. Assuming no medical contraindications, we prefer that the patient's systolic blood pressure be kept below 100 mm Hg. An arthroscopic pump infuses normal saline at 60 mm Hg. Turbulence must be minimized. Turbulence promotes bleeding according to the Bernoulli effect whereby fluid flow creates a negative pressure gradient (at right angles to the flow) that literally sucks blood from exposed vessels. This is particularly noticeable while working in the subacromial space where uncannulated

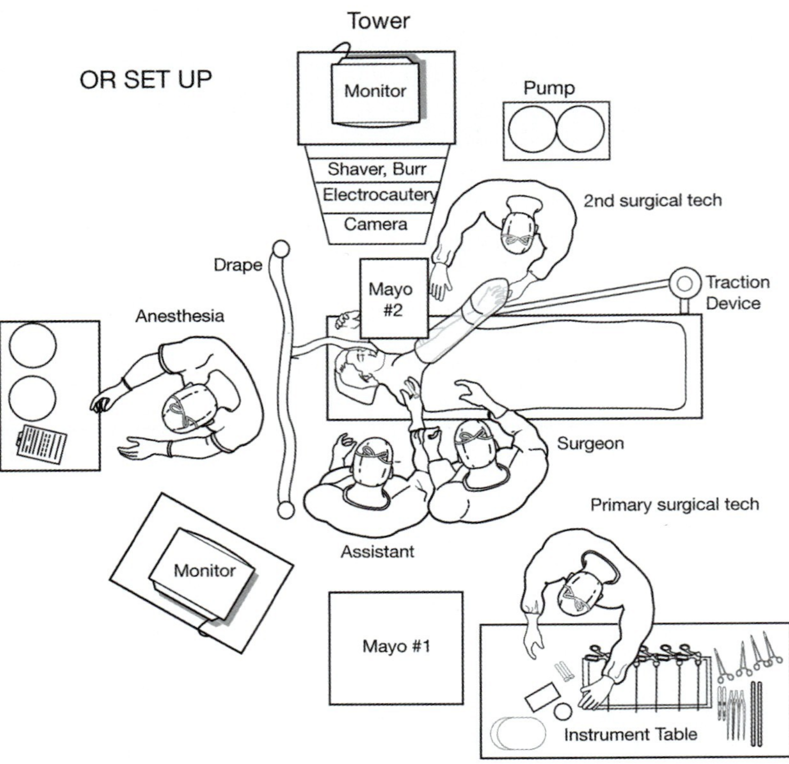

Figure 1.1 Overhead perspective of the operating room setup used by the authors for shoulder arthroscopy.

portals allow fluid to flow from a high-pressure system (inside the shoulder) to a low-pressure system (outside the shoulder), causing bleeding by virtue of the Bernoulli effect. In this scenario, it is important to resist the temptation to immediately increase the pump pressure as this will only increase the pressure gradient. Rather, the solution is to simply have an assistant plug the hole to eliminate turbulence. It is only after eliminating turbulence that we sometimes increase the arthroscopic pump pressure for a brief period of time. Using this rationale, we advise avoiding dedicated fluid outflow portals because these only exacerbate the Bernoulli effect. A final trick for maintaining fluid control for optimal visualization is to have a separate fluid inflow portal. A dedicated large-diameter inflow portal can improve fluid mechanics and is particularly useful for maintaining pressure when the arthroscope is frequently being moved between portals.

PORTAL PLACEMENT

One of the great advantages of shoulder arthroscopy over open surgery is the ability to access all areas of the shoulder from multiple angles. Accurate portal placement is vital to achieving the proper angle of approach. For this reason, with the exception of the initial posterior viewing portal, we create all portals with an outside-in approach under direct visualization. An 18-gauge spinal needle is first used to identify the location for the skin incision. Then, a switching stick or working instrument is walked down the spinal needle to enter the joint exactly as planned. In general, we use cannulas for work in the glenohumeral joint and uncannulated portals for most of our work in the subacromial space. In our experience, cannulas in the subacromial space are only necessary for performing knot tying and for antegrade suture passage. We use several portals as described below to maximize access to the shoulder but do not hesitate to make accessory portals to obtain visualization or achieve the proper angle of approach (e.g., percutaneous placement of anchors for the proper deadman angle) (Figs. 1.2 and 1.3).

Posterior Portal

The skin incision for the posterior portal is used to enter both the glenohumeral joint and the subacromial space. We have found that the often-used (by others) posterior portal 1 to 2 cm distal and 1 to 2 cm medial to the posterolateral corner of the acromion enters the shoulder too superior and too lateral. The posterior skin incision will tend to move superior as soft tissue swelling increases. A posterior portal placed only 1 to 2 cm distal to the acromion will therefore become problematic as the case progresses because the arthroscope will abut the posterior acromion and provide a poor angle of approach to the subacromial space. This is avoided by placing the skin incision more

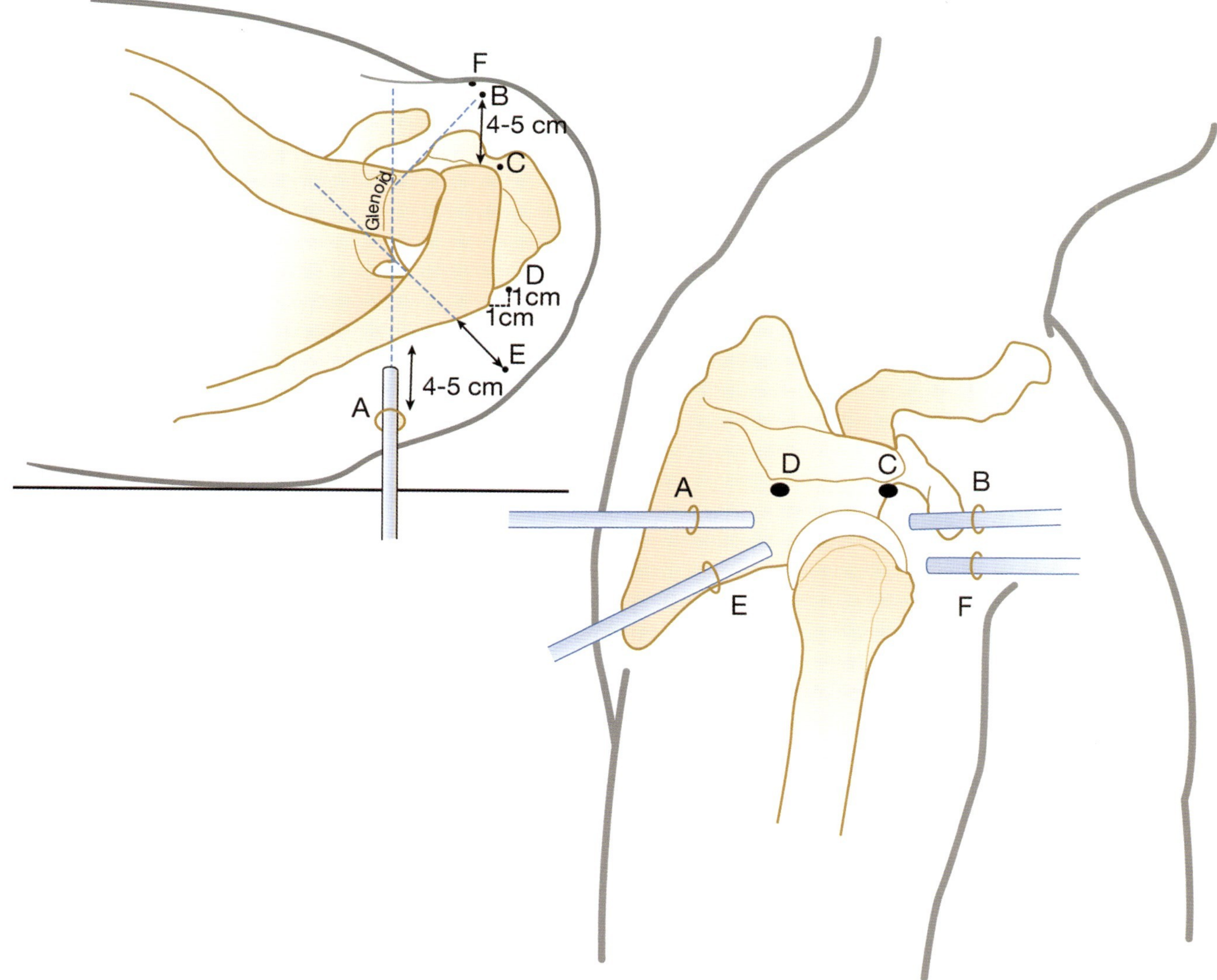

Figure 1.2 Schematic diagram demonstrating the relative positions of the most common glenohumeral portals (*A*) posterior portal; (*B*) anterior portal; (*C*) anterosuperolateral portal; (*D*) Port of Wilmington portal; (*E*) low posterolateral portal; (*F*) 5 o'clock portal.

inferior. We palpate the "soft spot" created by the glenoid medially, the humeral head laterally, and the rotator cuff superiorly and insert the arthroscope below the equator of the glenohumeral joint at about 7 o'clock. Because of this location, our skin incision is usually 4 to 5 cm distal and 3 to 4 cm medial to the posterolateral corner of the acromion (Fig. 1.4).

Anterior Portal

This portal is established just above the lateral half of the subscapularis, medial to the biceps sling. In placing the anterior portal, the trajectory of the spinal needle is typically from inferior to superior (Fig. 1.5). This orientation of the anterior portal allows access to the superior glenoid neck for superior labrum anterior and posterior (SLAP) repair, and also allows the surgeon to push down on the subscapularis tendon to obtain a 30° to 45° angle of approach for anterior glenoid anchor placement. Additionally, the location of the skin puncture for this portal is usually perfectly situated to provide a working portal for distal clavicle excision.

Anterosuperolateral

This portal is established 5 to 10 mm lateral to the anterolateral corner of the acromion and enters the glenohumeral joint through the rotator interval, just anterior to the supraspinatus, and directly above the biceps tendon. The exact position depends on the pathology, with

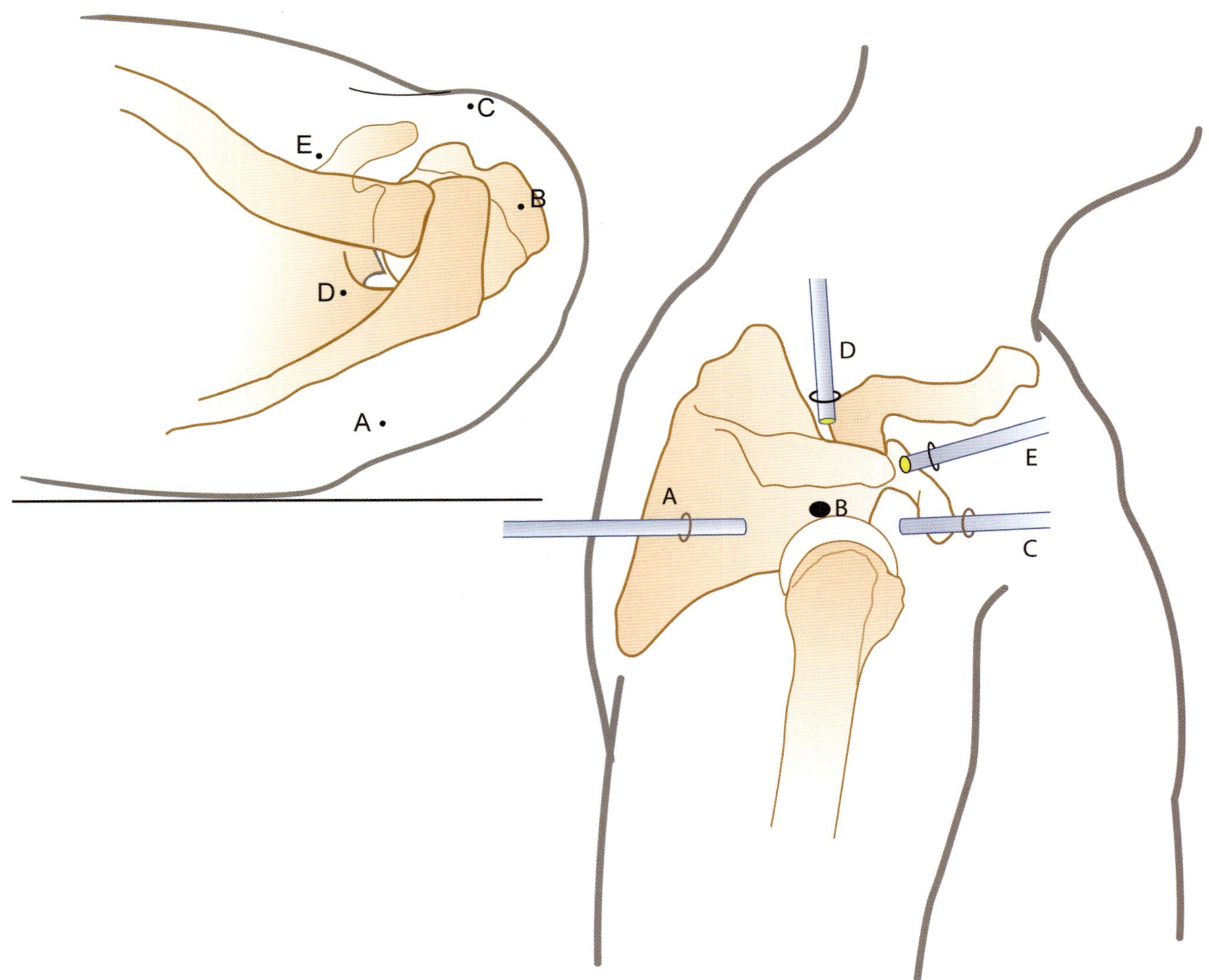

Figure 1.3 Schematic diagram demonstrating relative positions of the most common subacromial portals (*A*) posterior portal; (*B*) lateral portal; (*C*) anterior portal; (*D*) modified Neviaser portal; (*E*) subclavian portal.

a 45° angle of approach to the superior glenoid necessary for anchor placement for SLAP repair; and a 5° to 10° angle of approach to the lesser tuberosity for subscapularis repair, coracoid work, and biceps tenotomy or tenodesis. This portal becomes the primary viewing portal when addressing the anteroinferior and posteroinferior labrum and is essential to view through in ALL instability cases.

The 5 O'clock Portal

The 5 o'clock portal is created 1 cm inferior to the anterior portal through the subscapularis tendon. This portal is necessary in many Bankart repair cases to obtain an adequate angle of approach to the anteroinferior glenoid during anchor placement. This portal is used for percutaneous anchor placement only, using a Spear guide (Arthrex, Inc., Naples, FL) without establishing a standard cannula.

Port of Wilmington Portal

This portal is established 1 cm anterior and 1 cm lateral to the posterolateral acromion to provide a 45° angle of approach to the posterosuperior glenoid. This portal is used for posterior anchor placement during superior labral repairs, and similar to the 5 o'clock portal, is used without establishing a cannula. Only the Spear guide is used through this portal.

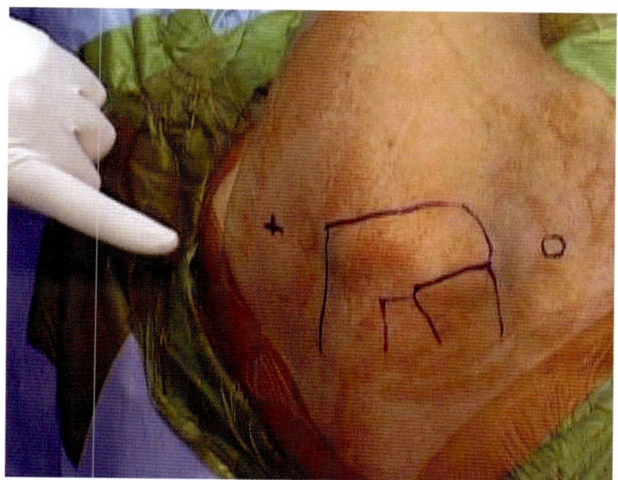

Figure 1.4 External view of a right shoulder demonstrates the location of our standard posterior portal (*X*), which is 4 to 5 cm distal to the posterolateral acromion.

Posterolateral Portal

The posterolateral portal is required when it is necessary to access the posteroinferior labrum in cases of posterior instability. It is established 4 to 5 cm distal and 4 to 6 cm lateral to the posterolateral corner of the acromion while viewing from an anterosuperolateral portal. Because of the depth of soft tissue, the portal is typically established with an 8.25 mm × 9 cm threaded clear cannula (Arthrex, Inc., Naples, FL) as opposed to the standard 8.25 × 7 cm cannula typically used for the anterior and anterosuperolateral portals.

Lateral Portal

The lateral subacromial portal is created approximately 4 cm lateral to the acromion in line with the posterior aspect of the clavicle. During rotator cuff repair, this portal can be created through a cuff defect while viewing from intra-articular and used to debride the cuff and perform bone bed preparation. In the absence of a rotator cuff tear, this portal is created while viewing subacromially and should parallel the undersurface of the acromion.

Modified Neviaser Portal

This portal is created 2 to 3 cm posteromedial to the acromioclavicular joint in the "soft spot" bordered by the posterior clavicle, medial acromion, and the scapular spine. We use this portal percutaneously to shuttle suture during superior labral repairs (MicroLasso; Arthrex, Inc., Naples, FL). We have previously used this portal for retrograde suture passage through the rotator cuff, but seldom do so anymore because the oblique angle of approach creates a tension mismatch between the superior and the

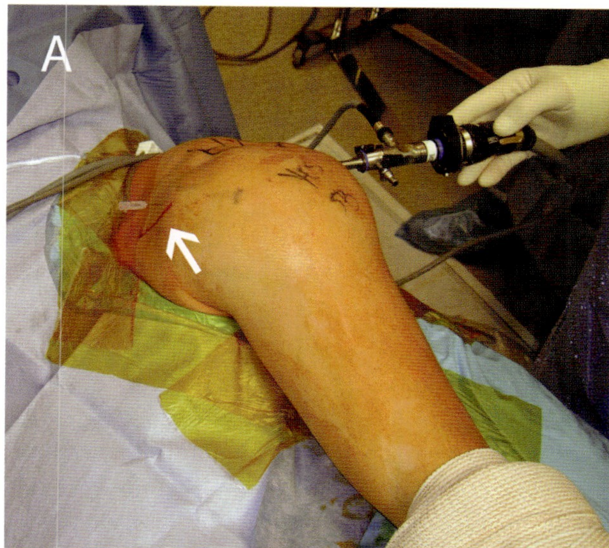

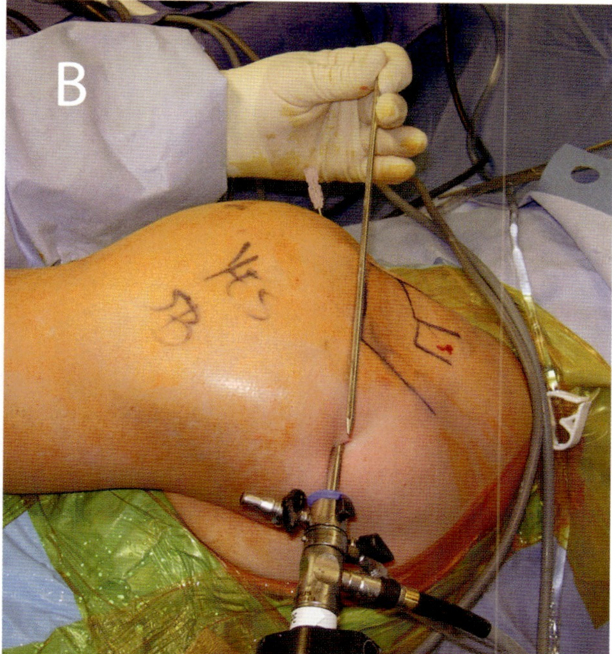

Figure 1.5 **A:** External view of a left shoulder demonstrating spinal needle localization (*white arrow*) of an anterior portal. **B:** The orientation of the spinal needle for the anterior portal is typically inferior to superior. This orientation provides an adequate angle of approach to the superior glenoid and also by beginning inferiorly, facilitates inferior displacement of the subscapularis by the Spear guide (Arthrex, Inc., Naples, FL) for placement of anterior glenoid anchors.

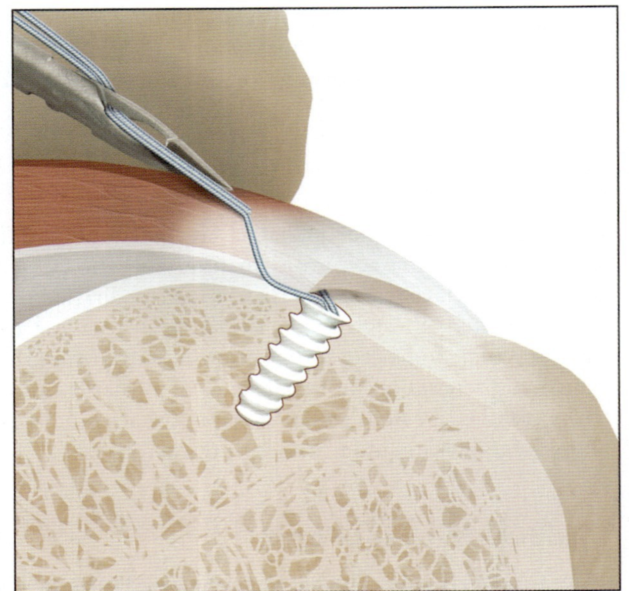

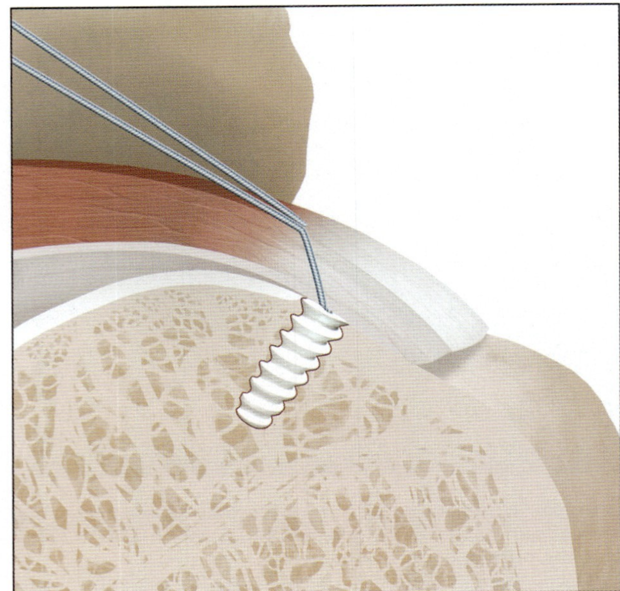

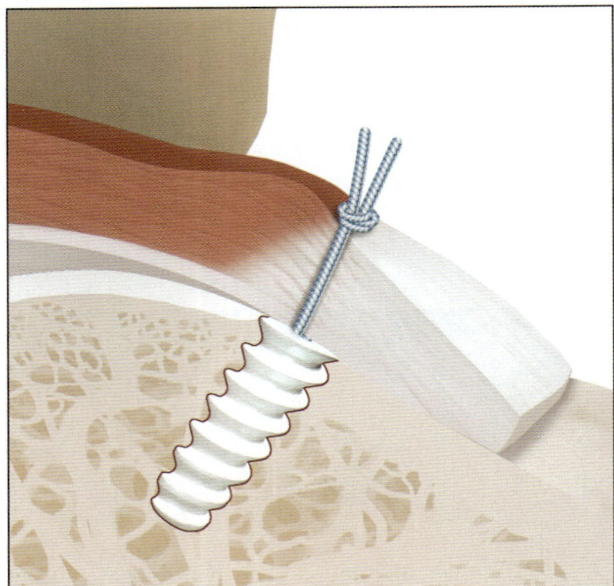

Figure 1.6 Schematic illustration of the tension mismatch created in the muscle-tendon segments of the supraspinatus if retrograde suture passage is used through a modified Neviaser portal. **A:** Retrograde suture passage is performed through a modified Neviaser portal. **B:** The suture has been passed through the rotator cuff obliquely. **C:** Tying the sutures results in a tension mismatch as the superior surface of the rotator cuff is pulled further lateral than the inferior surface.

inferior muscle-tendon segments of the supraspinatus during repair because the retrograde suture passing instrument travels from superomedial to inferolateral (Fig. 1.6). With antegrade instruments such as the Scorpion Fast-Pass (Arthrex, Inc., Naples, FL), a suture can easily be passed through the rotator cuff tendon in vertical fashion (without a tension mismatch) and retrieved in one step (Fig. 1.7).

Subclavian Portal

This portal is 1 to 2 cm medial and inferior to the acromioclavicular joint. This portal is useful for retrograde passage through the anterior supraspinatus tendon. With the improvement of antegrade suture passers, however, we rarely find it necessary to use the subclavian portal anymore.

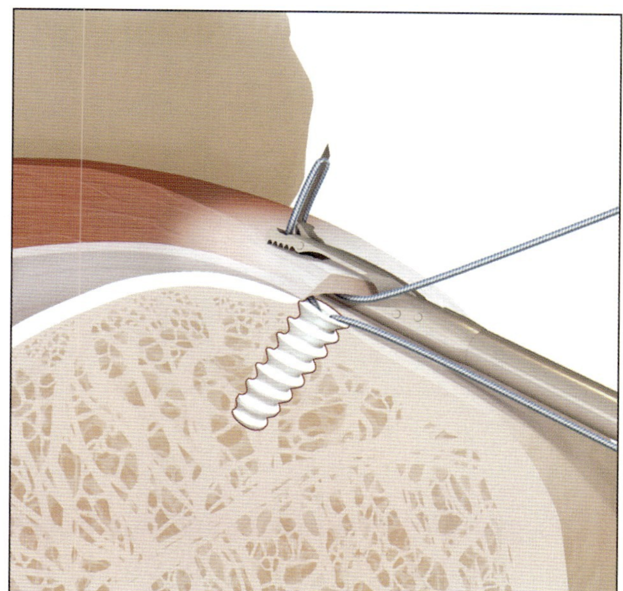

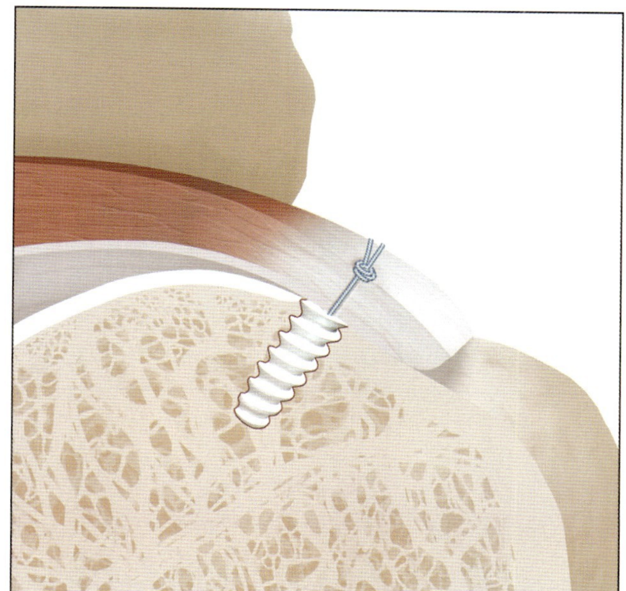

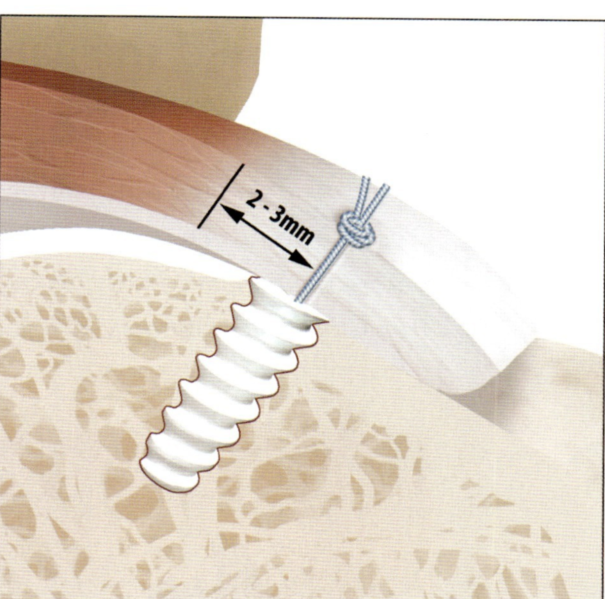

Figure 1.7 **A:** Schematic illustration of antegrade suture passage with a Scorpion suture passer (Arthrex, Inc., Naples, FL) used through a lateral working portal. Notice that the suture passes through the entire tendon at right angles to the tendon, assuring equal tension in all muscle-tendon segments from inferior to superior. **B:** Following knot tying, there is equal tension in the superior and inferior segments of the rotator cuff tendon. **C:** Up-close view demonstrates the equal tension and the placement of the sutures 2 to 3 mm lateral to the musculotendinous junction.

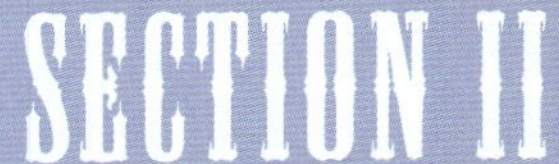

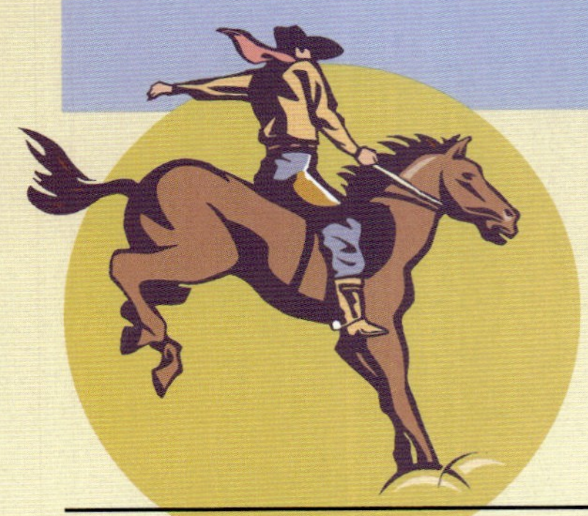

ROTATOR CUFF AND RELATED TOPICS

COWBOY PRINCIPLE 4

Don't build the gate till you've built the corral.

Construction on the ranch always proceeds in a logical and stepwise sequence. A sound basic structure must be completed before the enhancements make any sense. That's just about as true for shoulder surgery as it is for horse corrals.

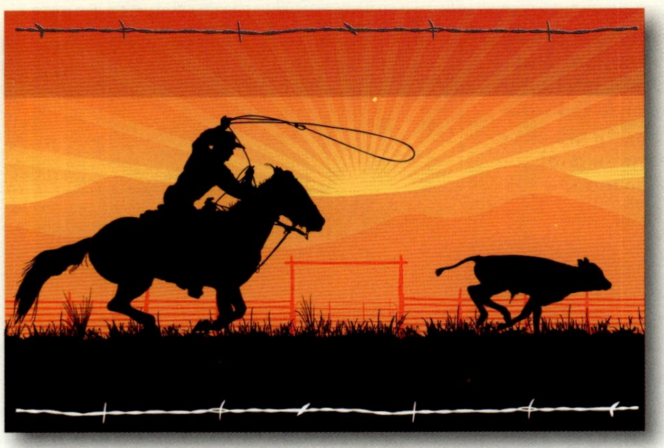

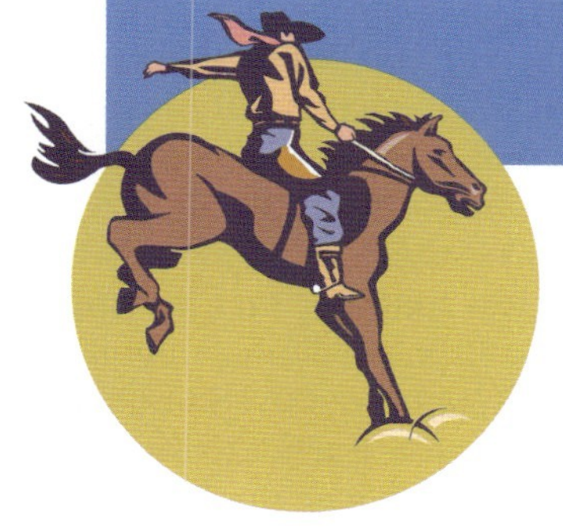

2

The Philosophy of Arthroscopic Rotator Cuff Repair

WESTERN WISDOM

When a cowboy is too old to set a bad example, he hands out good advice.

Arthroscopic rotator cuff repair has undergone dramatic advancements in the last 20 years. As with any technological paradigm shift, this rapid progress was made possible by the marriage of insight to technology. One of the great misconceptions of our time is that technology alone will advance a discipline. The reality is that technology without understanding produces mere gadgets; technology guided by insight produces tools.

To the uninitiated, arthroscopic rotator cuff repair may seem like magic. Our goal in this book is to pull back the curtain and break the magic down into tricks, teaching the reader how to systematically perform these tricks with tools rather than gadgets.

One must always bear in mind that magic is the currency of ignorance, whereas tools are the instruments of understanding. This chapter is dedicated to understanding.

BEDROCK PRINCIPLES

The overriding premise in our philosophy of arthroscopic rotator cuff repair is that almost all cuff tears are repairable, and our surgical experience confirms that assertion. In 2003, a review of one full year of the senior author's (SSB) surgical practice revealed that 97% of the rotator cuff tears that he operated on were fully repairable. The remaining 3% underwent varying degrees of partial repair. These results were achieved in a tertiary referral practice that included a large percentage of massive tears and revision repairs.

Despite our success at completely repairing the vast majority of cuff tears arthroscopically, we continue to hear presentations and read reports by other authors on their vast experience with salvage procedures (latissimus dorsi transfers, allograft patches, and even reverse total shoulder replacement) for "irreparable" cuff tears. We obviously have a difference of opinion on what is "irreparable," because our stepwise approach to restoring the anatomy is successful 97% of the time.

ANATOMY AND BIOMECHANICS

Form follows function. This basic tenet of all mechanical design is particularly true of biomechanical systems. The anatomic design produces biomechanical consequences that are specific to the anatomy, and therefore it behooves us to reconstitute the anatomy (and thereby the biomechanics) as precisely as possible.

Tear Pattern Recognition

In order to properly restore the anatomy, the surgeon must accurately recognize the cuff tear pattern. Arthroscopy offers a huge advantage over open surgery in that regard. With open surgery, there has always been a bias toward

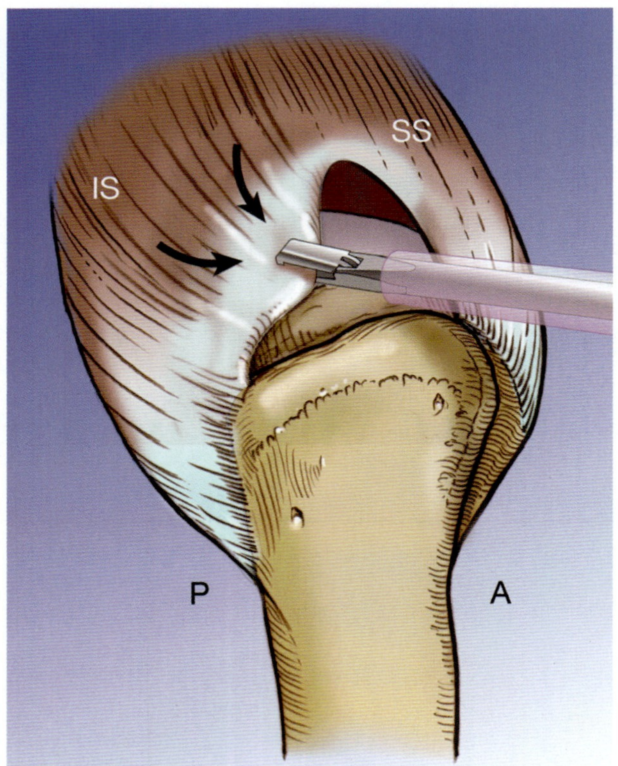

Figure 2.1 With an arthroscopic approach, rotator cuff tear pattern and mobility can be assessed from multiple angles of approach. In this schematic, a grasper introduced from an anterior portal is used to assess the anterior mobility of the posterior leaf. A, anterior; IS, infraspinatus; P, posterior; SS, supraspinatus.

medial-to-lateral mobilization of the cuff, since the open surgeon would try to bring the cuff to his window of visualization, which was an anterolateral incision. The arthroscope removes these restrictions on visualization and replaces the limited "window" of the surgical incision with an unlimited 360° field of view. This allows for a more precise determination of the tear pattern as the surgeon manipulates the cuff margins with a grasper to assess the direction of maximum cuff mobility (Fig. 2.1).

The Importance of the Subscapularis

At a recent national arthroscopy meeting in the United States, the senior author (SSB) was involved in a panel discussion that addressed the question of which subscapularis tears needed to be repaired. Some of the participants said that upper subscapularis tears would do just as well if they were debrided as if they were repaired, and they even recommended debridement. The absurdity of this recommendation is rather breathtaking, as it is so wrong on so many levels.

First of all, these panelists were inconsistent in their logic, as they were stressing the importance of completely repairing the supraspinatus and infraspinatus tendons, and at the same time they were recommending not repairing the subscapularis, as if the subscapularis were somehow less important than the other rotator cuff tendons. However, it is well documented that the subscapularis generates the largest amount of force of any rotator cuff muscle and is generally felt to be the most important single rotator cuff muscle as it is the only anterior muscle that can balance the posterior forces of the rotator cuff. Furthermore, the fact that the footprint of the upper subscapularis is much larger than that of the lower subscapularis is a clear indicator that the upper portion of that muscle-tendon unit is much more important as a force generator than the lower portion. In addition, the anterior attachment of the rotator cable extends to the upper subscapularis insertion. Therefore, repair of the upper subscapularis decreases the stress on the adjacent repair of the supraspinatus, thereby protecting the supraspinatus repair. For these reasons, debridement of this very important upper subscapularis tendon should be contraindicated in all cases.

The corollary to the principle of repairing all subscapularis tears is that the surgeon must adequately address the biceps pathology that accompanies subscapularis tears. Our experience has been that almost all tears of the upper subscapularis have a concomitant medial subluxation of the long head of the biceps. This subluxation is sometimes subtle, but is usually present on critical examination, and it must be dealt with by tenodesis or tenotomy of the long head of the biceps. If it is not dealt with at the time of subscapularis repair, the biceps will continue to sublux medially onto the edge of the repaired subscapularis and will eventually cause failure of that repair.

We believe that a large number of subscapularis tears are not recognized arthroscopically, even by experienced surgeons, because the footprint is not fully visualized. We have found that, using a posterior viewing portal, the subscapularis footprint can only be fully visualized by using a 70° arthroscope combined with a posterior lever push (see Chapter 6, "Subscapularis Tendon Tears") (Fig. 2.2). Furthermore, the 70° scope allows the surgeon to see the upper 2.5 cm of the bicipital groove, so that he can assess for irregularities or osteophytes within the groove as well as for occult tears of the lower subscapularis. In addition, abrasive changes on the medial aspect of the biceps tendon at the level of the medial sling are a clear indication of biceps subluxation (Fig. 2.3).

The Importance of Differentiating Tendon from Bursal Leaders

Many large rotator cuff tears will scar down rather extensively to the acromion, the scapular spine, and the deltoid. Dense "bursal leaders" will often extend from the tendon margins to the deltoid fascia (Fig. 2.4). These bursal leaders can be quite thick and robust, and can be confused with tendon. The surgeon may be reluctant to debride these bursal leaders for fear of debriding tendon, but this must be done because a repair of bursa to tendon or bursa to bone will fail 100% of the time. The key to finding the true edge of the tendon is to first identify the bursal leader by following the tissue laterally. If the tissue inserts into the

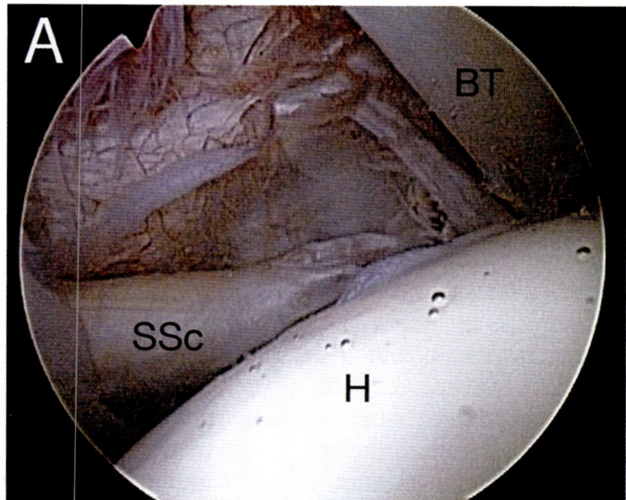

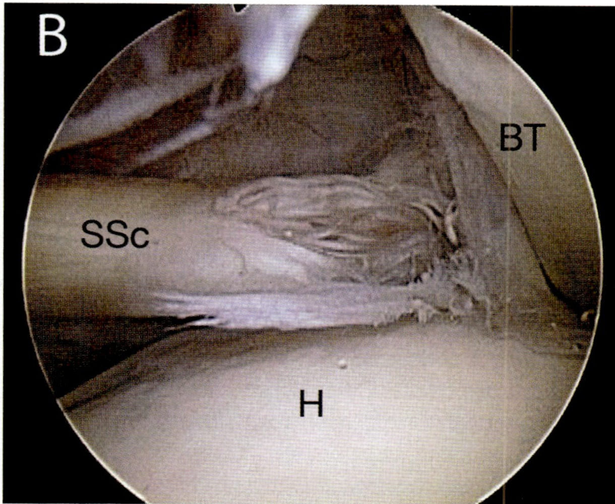

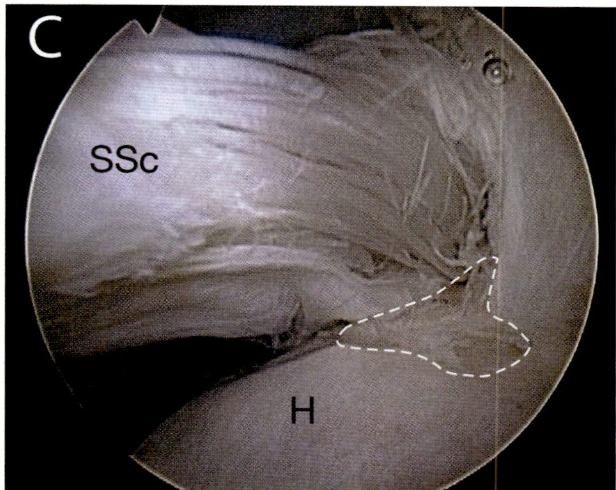

Figure 2.2 Right shoulder, posterior viewing portal comparing views obtained of the subscapularis tendon with **(A)** a 30° arthroscope and **(B)** a 70° arthroscope. With the 30° arthroscope, it is difficult to ascertain if there is a subscapularis tendon tear. The 70° arthroscope provides an "aerial view" of the footprint, and it becomes obvious that there is a tear of the upper subscapularis. **C:** Same shoulder viewed with 70° arthroscope and a posterior lever push. This maneuver dramatically increases the exposure of the subscapularis footprint, providing much more room for visualization, instrumentation, and bone bed preparation. In this case, an exposed subscapularis footprint (*white hashed area*) is quite evident at the 4 o'clock position of this picture. BT, biceps tendon; H, humeral head; SSc, subscapularis tendon.

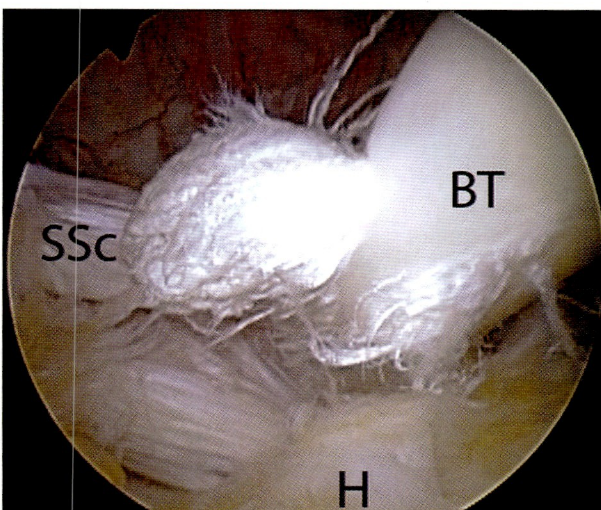

Figure 2.3 Right shoulder, viewed from a posterior portal with a 70° arthroscope, demonstrates abrasion of the medial biceps tendon. Abrasive changes of the medial biceps tendon are indicative of a subscapularis tendon tear. BT, biceps tendon; H, humerus; SSc, subscapularis tendon.

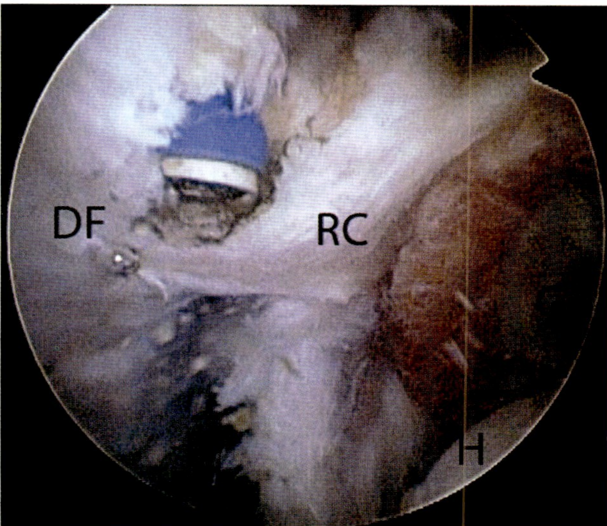

Figure 2.4 Right shoulder, viewed from a lateral subacromial portal demonstrating a bursal leader that is being separated from the deltoid fascia (DF). The bursal leader must be debrided in order to identify the intact rotator cuff (RC) margin. G, glenoid; H, humeral head.

bone of the greater tuberosity, it is tendon and should not be debrided. If the tissue extends past the greater tuberosity to insert into the deltoid fascia, it is bursal leader and must be debrided. The bursal leaders are debrided back to good tendon, which will be recognizable as dense parallel collagen fibers inserting into the greater tuberosity.

In a broader sense, we believe in doing a complete subacromial bursectomy in all cases of arthroscopic rotator cuff repair in order to fully visualize the tear margins. Even if there are not dense bursal leaders, the subacromial bursa can obscure the cuff margins. We have heard some surgeons recommend that the bursa be preserved in order to enhance the blood supply to the cuff repair site. We disagree with this approach for three reasons. First of all, the surgeon must be sure he is repairing tendon and not just bursa, but he cannot fully visualize the tendon without first removing the overlying bursa. Secondly, the blood supply for healing that is potentially provided by the bursa is inconsequential in comparison to the blood supply from the bone bed (1). The bone bed provides growth factors and marrow elements for healing that are not available from the bursa. Thirdly, the advantage of blood supply from an intact bursa is offset by the distinct disadvantage of retaining the various degradative enzymes that are present in the bursa and which may actually retard or prevent healing if the bursa is not thoroughly debrided and excised.

Critical Biomechanical Requirements: Balancing the Force Couples and Repairing the Rotator Cable Attachments

The cornerstone of our philosophy of arthroscopic rotator cuff repair is that force couples must be restored and balanced in the coronal and axial planes (Fig. 2.5). By recognizing the tear pattern and achieving an anatomic repair, the surgeon will automatically balance the force couples unless the muscle quality is so poor that it cannot generate sufficient force to produce balanced force couples.

In general, our experience has been that if a given muscle has up to 75% fatty infiltration (as judged on the T-1 parasagittal MRI images), it will have enough elasticity to be fully repairable to its anatomic insertion (2). If there is not enough elasticity in the muscle-tendon unit for repair, and if interval slide releases fail to provide enough additional lateral excursion for repair, we simply repair as much as possible in order to achieve the best partial repair that we can. We do not believe in trying to "cover the hole" with latissimus dorsi transfers or allograft patches.

There is another critical biomechanical aspect to rotator cuff repair that is too often overlooked, and that is the importance of a secure repair of both ends of the rotator cable. In 1993, the senior author (SSB) described the cable–crescent complex of the rotator cuff (Fig. 2.6) (3). The majority of rotator cuff tears begin within the rotator crescent. As long as the rotator cable attachments are intact, the cuff muscles can produce a distributed load along the cable that gets transferred to bone at the cable attachments. In this way, a torn rotator cuff can still function by load transmission through a construct that is analogous to a suspension bridge (Fig. 2.7) (4). We have recently completed a clinical study (unpublished data) that shows that all patients who have pseudoparalysis (inability to actively elevate the shoulder above 90°) have disruption of one or both ends of the rotator cable.

The rotator cable attachments are so important to overhead function that we believe it is important to reinforce their repair during arthroscopic rotator cuff repair.

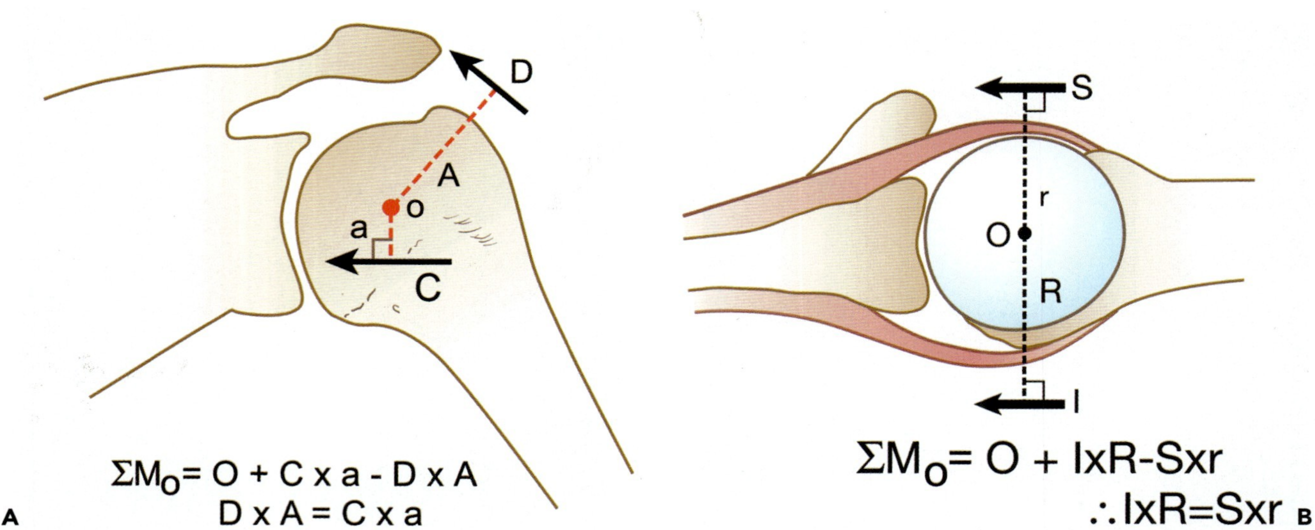

Figure 2.5 **A:** Balanced force couples are required to maintain the normal glenohumeral relationship. *A:* In the coronal plane, the combined inferior rotator cuff force (*C*) is balanced against the deltoid (*D*). **B:** In the axial plane, the subscapularis (*S*) is balanced against the infraspinatus and teres minor (*I*). *O*, center of rotation; *A*, moment arm of the deltoid; *a*, moment arm of the inferior rotator cuff; *r*, moment arm of the subscapularis; *R*, moment arm of the infraspinatus and teres minor.

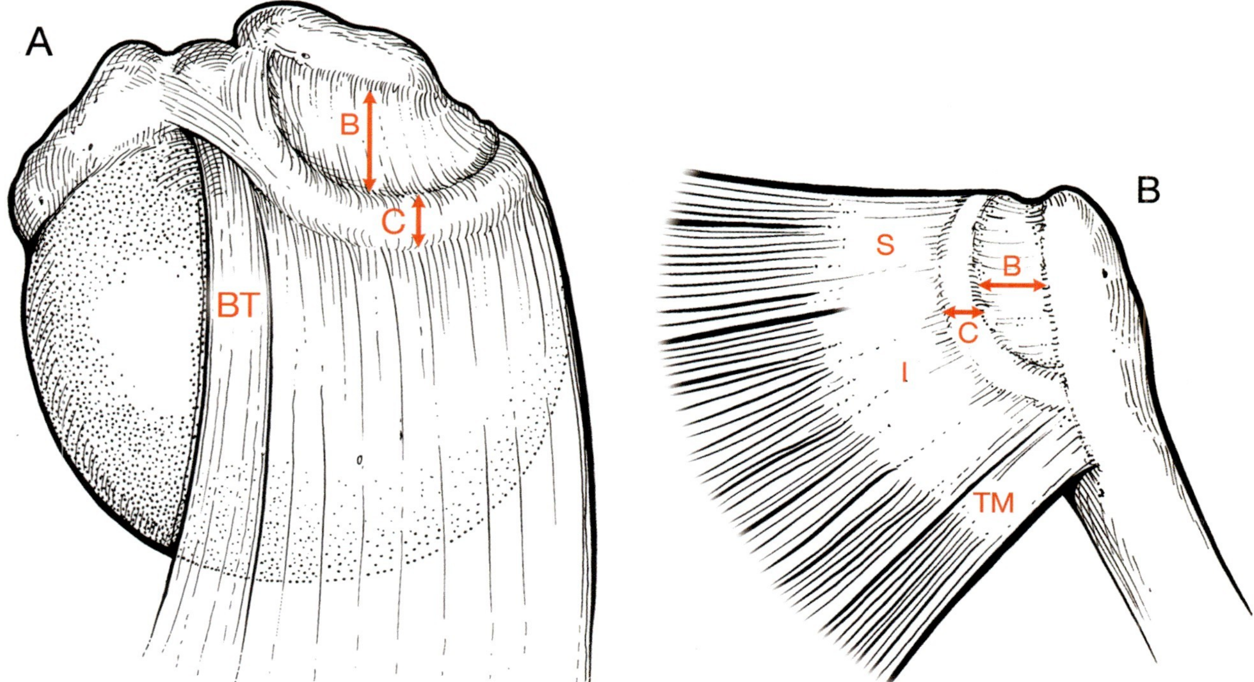

Figure 2.6 Superior (**A**) and posterior (**B**) projections of the rotator cable and crescent. The rotator cable extends from the biceps to the inferior margin of infraspinatus, spanning the supraspinatus and infraspinatus insertions. C, width of rotator cable; B, mediolateral dimension of rotator crescent; S, supraspinatus; I, infraspinatus; TM, teres minor; BT, biceps tendon.

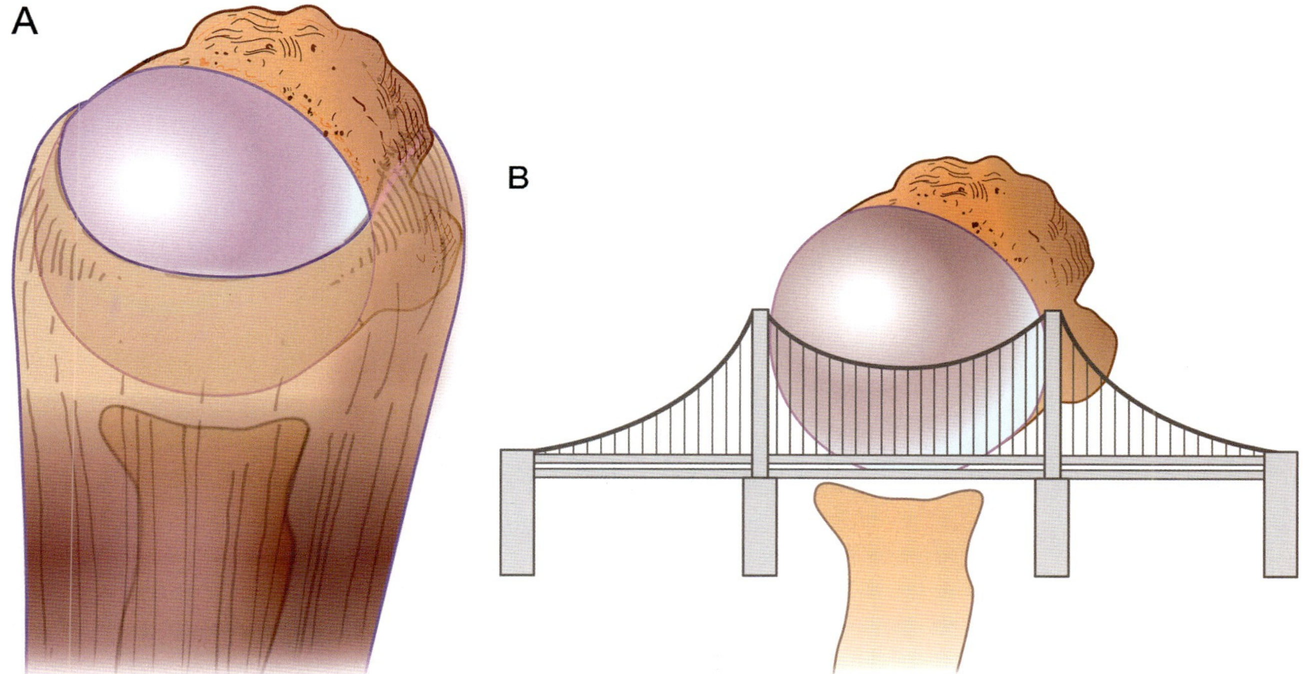

Figure 2.7 A rotator cuff tear (**A**) can be modeled after a suspension bridge. **B:** The free margin corresponds to the cable, and the anterior and posterior attachments of the tear correspond to the supports at each end of the cable's span. A preserved rotator cable can exert a compressive force sufficient to stabilize the humeral head in the setting of a large rotator cuff tear.

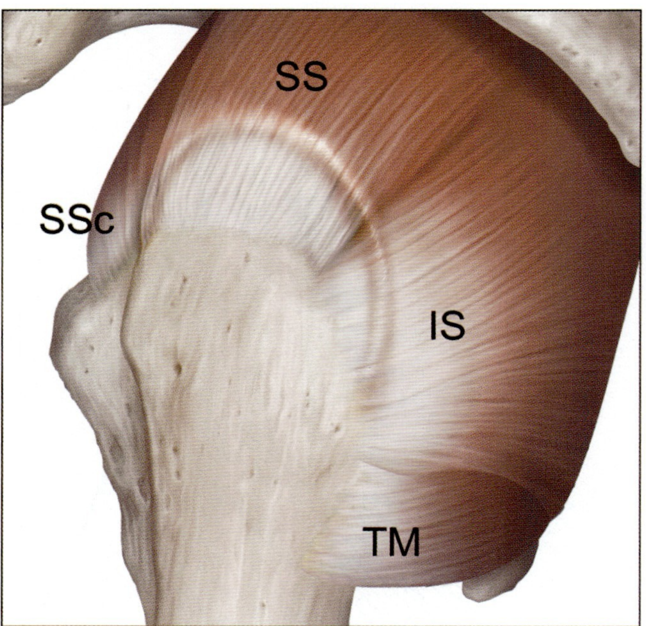

Figure 2.8 Schematic of the rotator cable in a left shoulder. The rotator cable has three attachment points that consist of the upper subcapularis and anterior supraspinatus anteriorly and the lower infraspinatus posteriorly. IS, infraspinatus; SS, supraspinatus; SSc, subscapularis; TM, teres minor.

The posterior cable attachment corresponds to the attachment of the lower infraspinatus. The anterior cable attachment bifurcates around the top of the bicipital groove, with part of the anterior cable attachment corresponding to the anterior attachment of the supraspinatus and the other part corresponding to the upper attachment of the subscapularis. We believe that healing of these three attachment points of the rotator cable (lower infraspinatus, anterior supraspinatus, and upper subscapularis) are crucial to optimal function of the shoulder (Fig. 2.8). Because of this crucial role, we reinforce these three points with cinch-loop sutures (infraspinatus and supraspinatus) and rip-stop sutures (subscapularis). Interestingly, a standard SutureBridge repair (two medial anchors and two lateral anchors) of a tear involving the supraspinatus and infraspinatus will frequently leave "dog ears" at the anterior and posterior margins of the repair. Placing cinch-loop sutures at the anterior and posterior margins to reinforce the repair at the anterior and posterior cable attachments will also eliminate the dog-ears (Figs. 2.9 and 2.10).

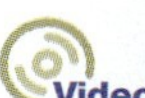

Footprint Reconstruction

We strongly believe in bridging double-row footprint repair for rotator cuff tears. This belief is an extension of our philosophy of always restoring the anatomy and always restoring the biomechanics.

The rationale is easy to understand. The normal insertions of the rotator cuff tendons comprise wide footprints on the bone bed, and we believe that an important part of an anatomic repair is to restore the footprint anatomy of the insertion. However, there are some cases where the tendon tears and leaves a stump

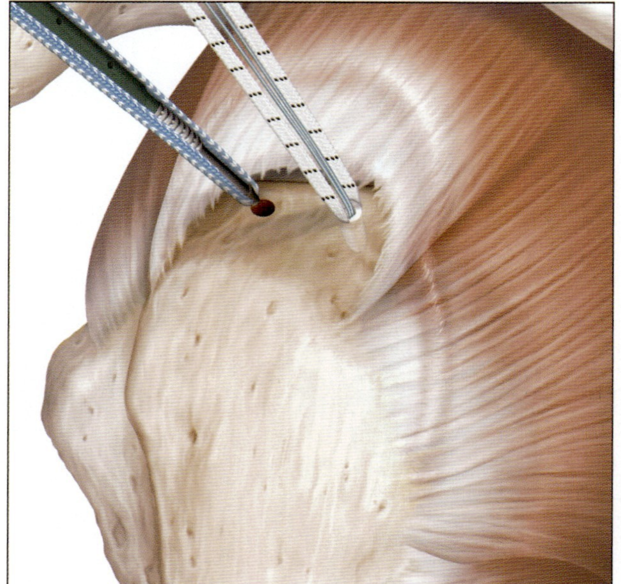

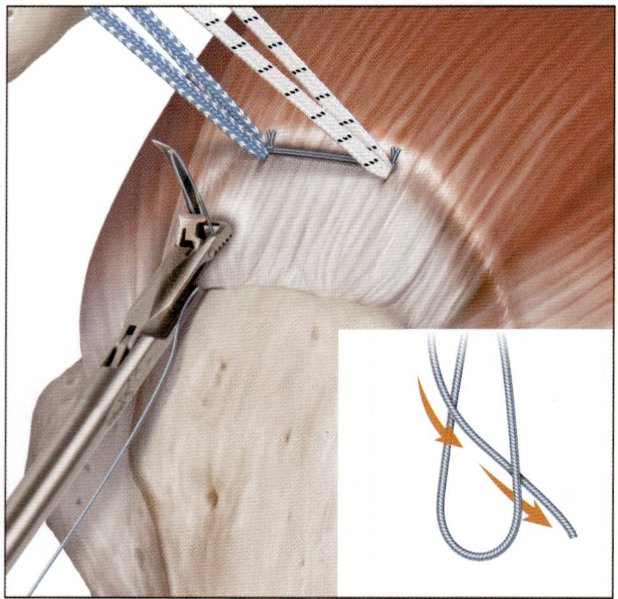

Figure 2.9 Schematic of a SpeedBridge (Arthrex, Inc., Naples, FL) rotator cuff repair with FiberLink (Arthrex, Inc., Naples, FL) dog-ear reduction. **A:** Two medial anchors are placed for a SpeedBridge repair. **B:** After the medial sutures are passed, the closed end of a FiberLink is passed through the rotator cuff at the margin of the tear. The closed end will be retrieved out the same portal as used for insertion. Inset: Extracorporeally, the closed end of the FiberLink is passed through the looped end to create a cinch loop.

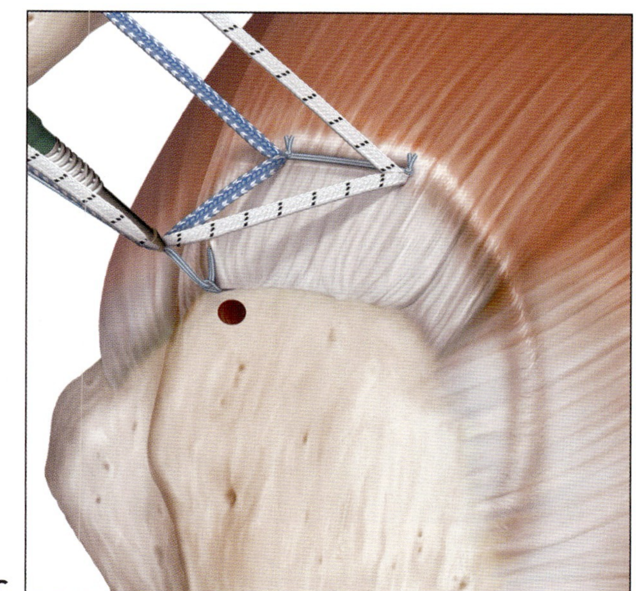

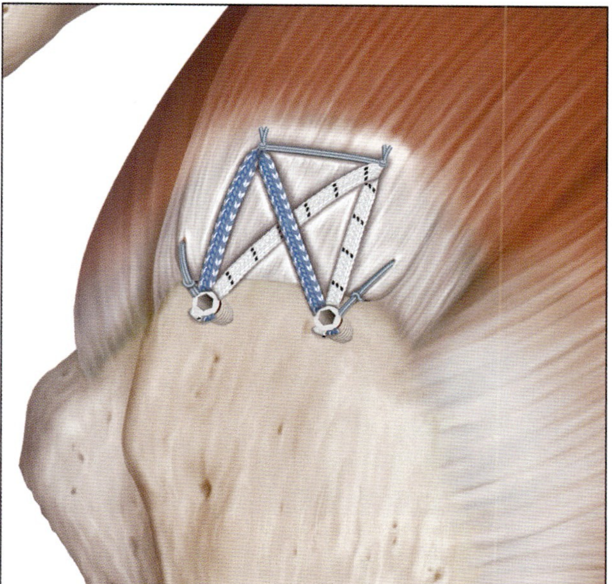

Figure 2.9 *(Continued)* **C:** The cinch loop, a suture from the anteromedial anchor, and a suture from the posteromedial anchor are secured laterally with a BioComposite SwiveLock C anchor. **D:** Final appearance after placement of a posterior FiberLink and a posterolateral anchor.

on the greater tuberosity. In such a case, pulling the tendon to the lateral part of the tuberosity would not be an anatomic repair and it would also tend to overtension the repair. So, if there is tendon loss we do not do a footprint reconstruction. However, we are careful to put the medial tendon margin back to its anatomic insertion on the medial part of the footprint in order to preserve the normal length–tendon relationship of the muscle-tendon unit.

We have a simple way of restoring the normal length–tendon relationship, even in the case of tendon loss, in order to achieve an anatomic repair with normal biomechanical characteristics. Our method is based on the fact that an anatomic and properly tensioned double-row footprint

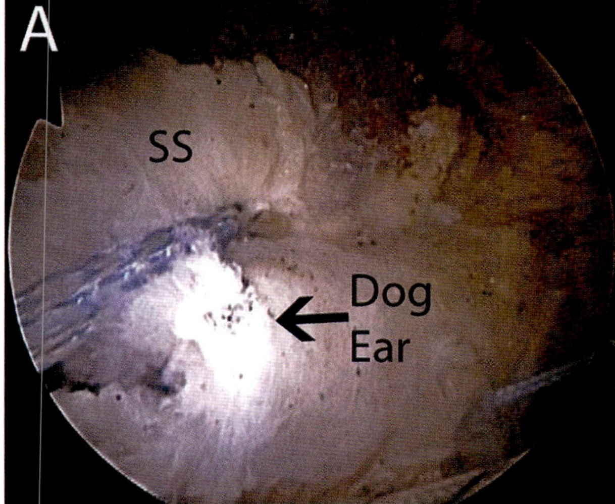

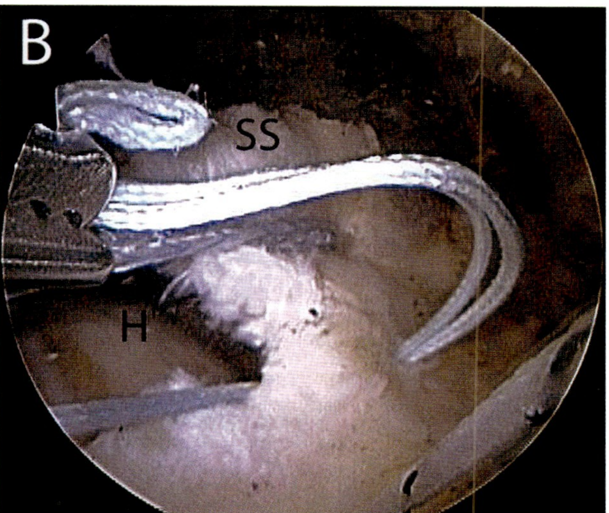

Figure 2.10 Left shoulder, posterior viewing portal demonstrating use of a cinch loop for "dog-ear" reduction. **A:** After placement of a posterior stitch for repair of a supraspinatus (SS) tear, lateral traction demonstrates that fixation would result in a dog ear (*black arrow*). **B:** A FiberLink (Arthrex, Inc., Naples, FL) is placed at the apex of the dog ear. FiberLink has a looped end and a straight end. The straight end is passed through the rotator cuff.

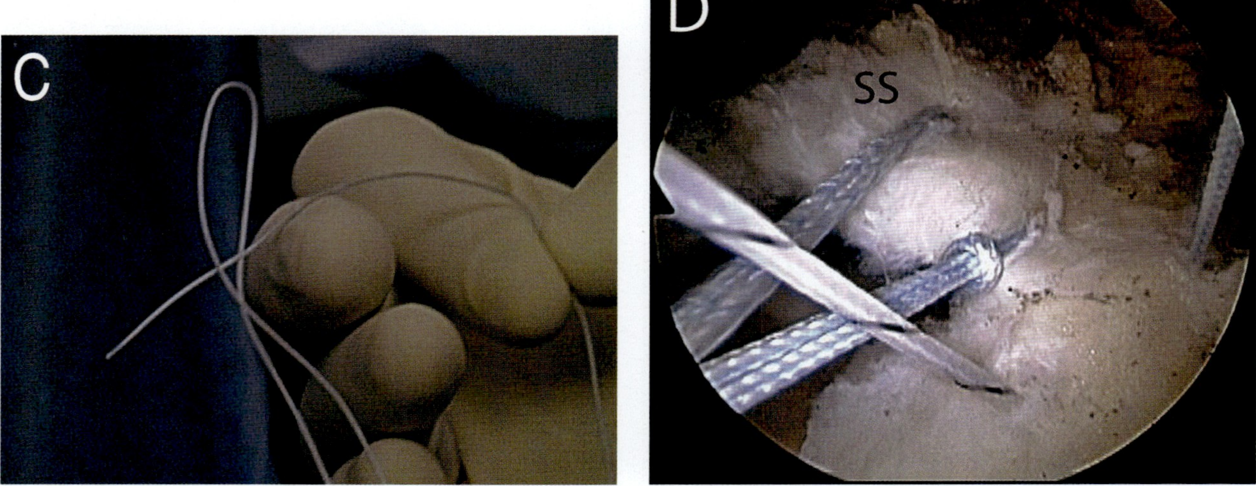

Figure 2.10 *(Continued)* **C:** Extracorporeally, the retrieved straight end of the FiberLink is passed through the loop to create a cinch loop. **D:** The cinch loop is brought down to the rotator cuff by tensioning the straight end. Lateral tension now demonstrates that the dog ear will be effectively reduced with the cinch loop. H, humeral head.

reconstruction (in a case without tendon loss) can virtually always be obtained if the surgeon passes his medial row sutures 2 to 3 mm lateral to the musculotendinous junction. This always restores the proper length–tendon relationship. In the case of tendon loss in which only a single-row repair is possible, anchors are placed about 4 mm lateral to the articular margin. Therefore, the sutures are placed through the tendon approximately 6 to 7 mm lateral to the musculotendinous junction so that when the sutures are tied, the musculotendinous junction will lie approximately 2 mm medial to the articular margin of the humerus (Figs. 2.11 and 2.12).

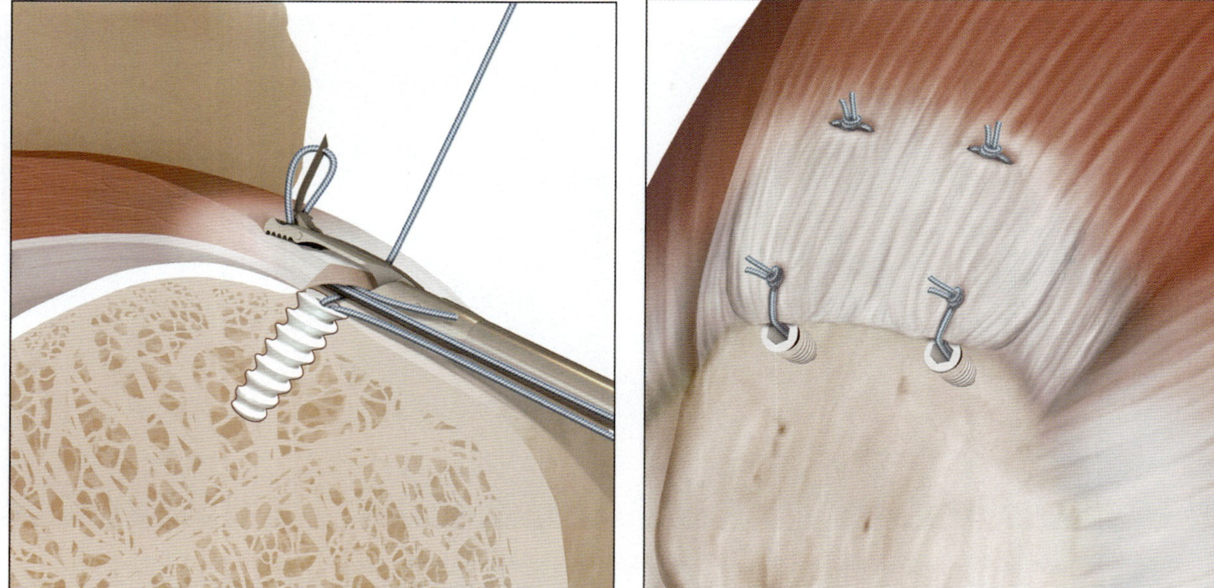

Figure 2.11 Schematic of correct placement of medial sutures. **A:** Medial sutures have been properly placed 2 to 3 mm lateral to the musculotendinous junction. **B:** View following knot tying.

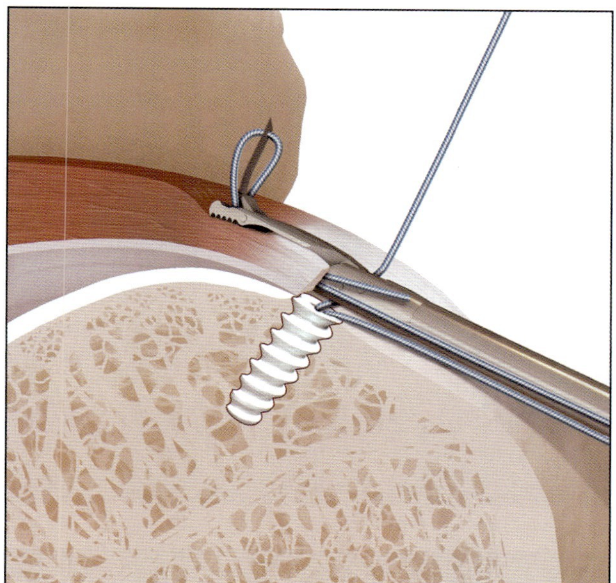

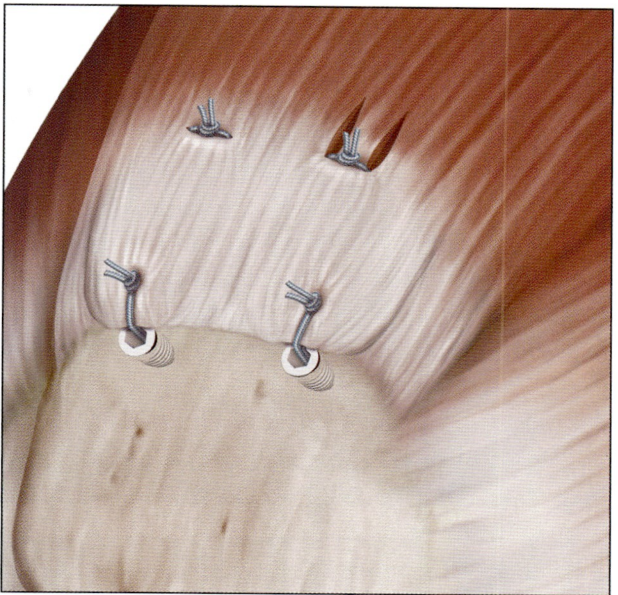

Figure 2.12 Schematic of improper placement for medial sutures. **A:** Medial sutures have been passed medial to the musculotendinous junction. **B:** When sutures are placed too far medial into the rotator cuff muscle, under tension they will pull through laterally until they reach an equilibrium of muscle–tendon tension by cutting through to a point lateral to the musculotendinous junction.

PHILOSOPHY OF SURGICAL TECHNIQUE

Our philosophy of surgical technique is centered on the belief that details are important. In fact, surgery is all about the details, each of which is important in creating the optimal repair construct.

Angles

The two important categories of arthroscopic angles are *angle of visualization* and *angle of approach*.

The angle of visualization is influenced by the position of the portal through which the surgeon is viewing as well as the angle of the arthroscope (30° vs. 70°). In performing arthroscopic rotator cuff repair, we frequently switch the scope through various viewing portals, and we also frequently alternate between 30° and 70° arthroscopes. The 70° scope is much like a periscope in that it allows the surgeon to look around corners. This is helpful in many situations, but it is essential in adequately visualizing the subscapularis.

The *angle of approach* refers to the angle at which the arthroscopic instruments approach the tissue that is being worked on. This is influenced by the position of the working portal, and to a lesser extent by any angles or curves in the shaft or tip of the instrument. Furthermore, the internal deltoid fascia can restrict the surgeon's ability to move the working instrument to various locations within the subacromial space of the shoulder. For that reason, we routinely release the internal deltoid fascia in order to achieve greater freedom of motion for our instruments (Fig. 2.13). Similarly, a rigid cannula will restrict the freedom of angular motion of the instruments, so we frequently do much of our subacromial work without a cannula in the working portal. However, when we pass sutures or tie knots, we typically use a cannula to avoid entrapping deltoid muscle between the suture pairs. Video

A major tenet to successful arthroscopic rotator cuff repair is that if you can see it (*angle of visualization*) and reach it with your instruments (*angle of approach*), you can repair it.

Adequate Preparation of Soft Tissue and Bone Bed

Soft tissue preparation involves, first of all, a complete bursectomy. This allows the surgeon to see the entire margin of the cuff tear. This is essential, because you can't repair it if you can't see it. Secondly, it removes the potentially harmful degradative enzymes that reside in the subacromial bursa. In addition to the bursectomy, the surgeon must debride any bursal leaders that attach to the internal deltoid fascia, and he must debride friable tendon edges while retaining robust tendon even if it appears poorly vascularized. Revascularization will occur from the "bone side" of the repair.

As for bone bed preparation, we prefer a uniformly bleeding bone bed. It is useful to remove soft tissues from the greater tuberosity with electrocautery (which creates a charcoal-like film on the bone surface) and then use a high-speed burr to "burr off the charcoal"

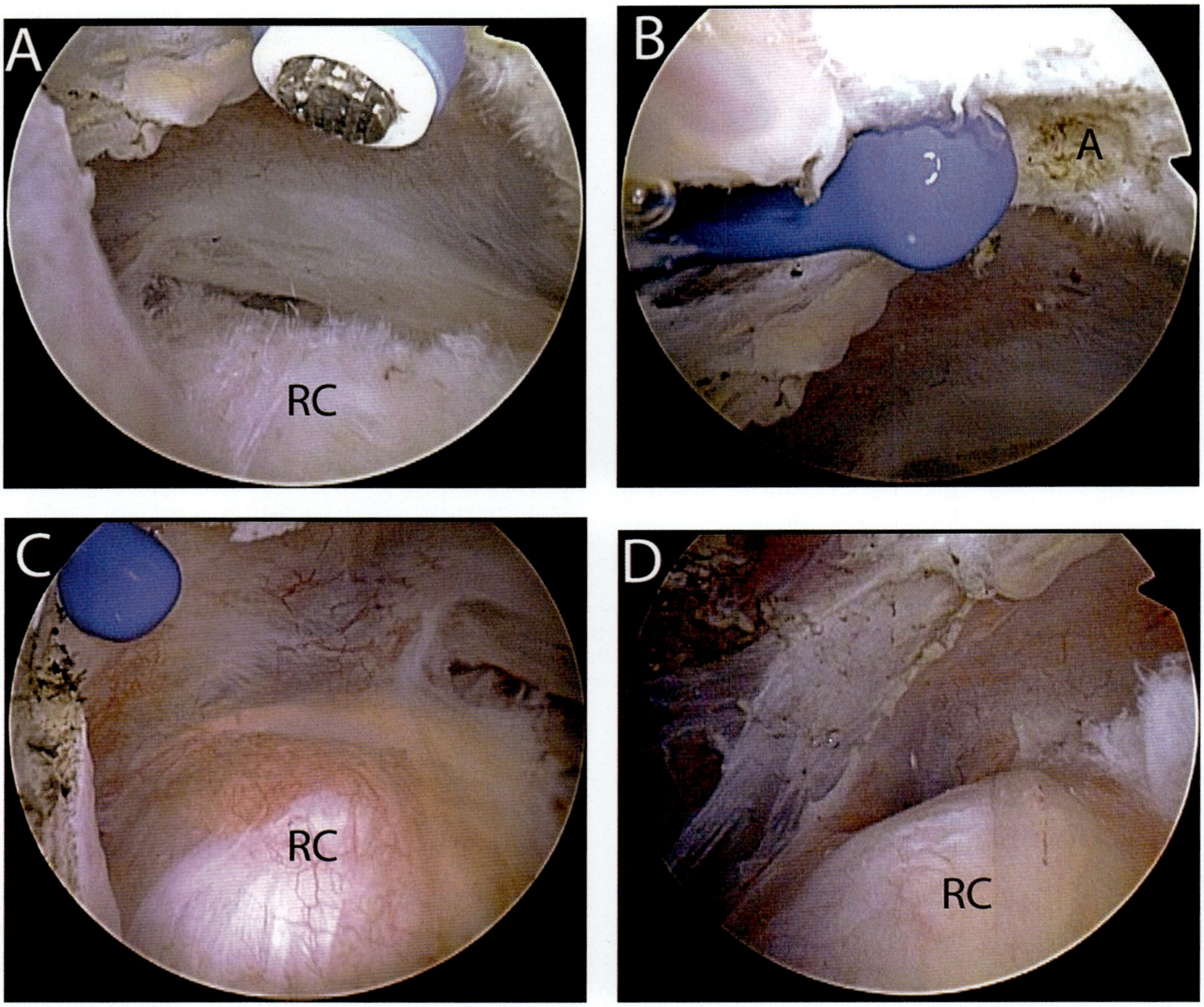

Figure 2.13 Splitting the deltoid fascia allows greater freedom of motion for instruments and also provides access to the lateral rotator cuff for double-row repair. **A:** Prior to splitting the deltoid fascia, there is limited instrument mobility and visualization of the lateral rotator cuff (RC). **B:** The internal deltoid fascia is split superiorly to the edge of the acromion (A). **C:** The fascial split is carried inferiorly to the reflection of the bursa. **D:** After the complete split of the internal deltoid fascia, the lateral rotator cuff is clearly seen.

(Fig. 2.14). Ample evidence now exists that the blood supply for rotator cuff healing comes from the bone. In order to enhance the amount of blood and bone marrow products that reach the tendon–bone interface, we prefer to use vented suture anchors that have side vents in addition to the longitudinal cannulation whereby blood products from the bone marrow can reach the repair interface at the bone surface (BioComposite Vented Corkscrew FT and BioComposite Vented SwiveLock suture anchors; Arthrex, Inc., Naples, FL). These vents also allow bone formation within the anchor channels (Fig. 2.15). In addition, we frequently perform two or three microfracture perforations on the greater tuberosity with a chondropick or drill (PowerPick; Arthrex, Inc., Naples, FL) (Fig. 2.16).

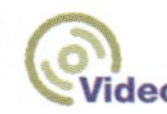

Utilize Mechanical Principles to Optimize the Repair Construct

From the very beginning, we have emphasized sound mechanical principles to create strong repair constructs, and we have spent a great deal of effort in the lab to identify the optimal components of fixation for our repairs. For example, we showed that the best combination of knot security and loop security is achieved by tying a six-throw surgeon's knot in which the fourth and the sixth throws are flipped (optimizing knot security), and by tying the knot with a Surgeon's Sixth Finger Knot Pusher (Arthrex, Inc., Naples, FL) to optimize loop security (5,6). We frequently use FiberTape (a 2-mm. high-strength suture

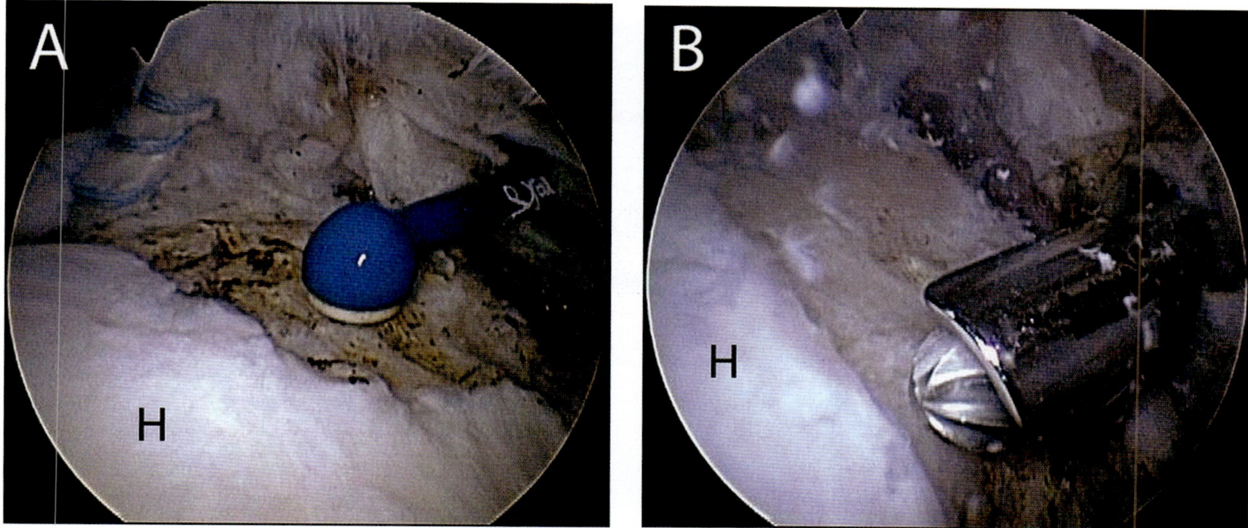

Figure 2.14 Right shoulder, posterior viewing portal demonstrates preparation of the greater tuberosity bone bed for rotator cuff repair. **A:** Soft tissue is cleared off the greater tuberosity with an electrocautery. **B:** A burr is then used to "clear the charcoal" and create a viable bone bed for rotator cuff repair. H, humeral articular surface.

tape) (Arthrex, Inc., Naples, FL) instead of suture, since FiberTape has a 20% greater load to failure in tendon than #2 FiberWire.

In U-shaped and L-shaped cuff tears, we utilize *margin convergence* (7) to enhance the strength of our construct by means of strain reduction at the "converged" cuff margin (Figs. 2.17 and 2.18). This is a very powerful mechanical property for protecting the integrity of these types of tears.

Harnessing the *self-reinforcing* characteristics of the SutureBridge (Arthrex, Inc., Naples, FL), footprint repair construct has been a huge breakthrough in arthroscopic rotator cuff repair. These constructs function much like the Chinese finger trap mechanism, whereby a potential disruptive force is transformed into a mechanism that reinforces the strength of the repair.

Reestablishing the normal length–tension relationship of the rotator cuff muscle-tendon units is critically important. In all our cuff repairs, both double-row and single-row, we strive to have the tendon contact the medial articular margin of the bone bed at a distance of 2 to 3 mm. lateral to the musculotendinous junction. In some cases of retracted tendons, interval slide procedures can give additional lateral excursion to the tendons for repairs that restore the normal length–tension relationships.

Tissue quality influences the types of repair that we perform. If the tissue quality is poor, we try to incorporate more suture passes through the tendon and more knots to strengthen the construct. For good tissue with a small cuff tear, we usually use a knotless SpeedBridge technique with FiberTape and two rows of BioComposite SwiveLock C suture anchors (Arthrex, Inc., Naples, FL) (Fig. 2.19). For fair tissue, we utilize a SpeedBridge repair augmented with a medial double mattress suture (double-pulley technique) (Fig. 2.20). For poor tissue and large

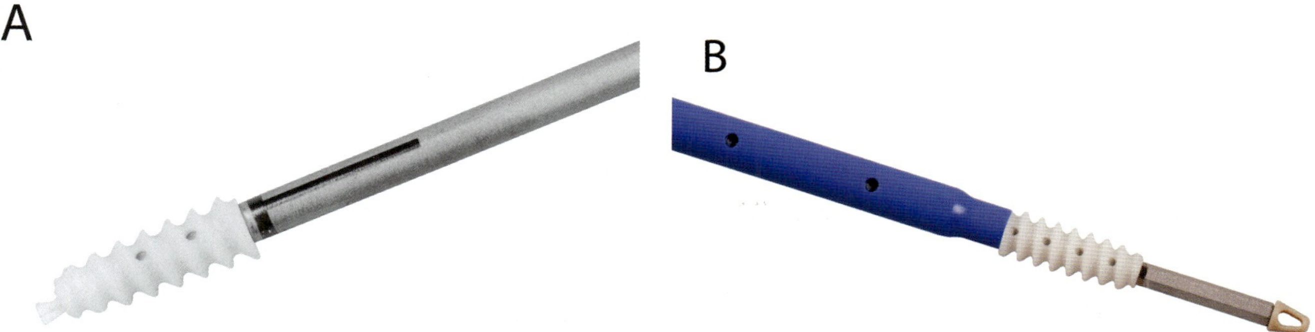

Figure 2.15 The BioComposite Corkscrew FT **(A)** and the BioComposite SwiveLock C **(B)** anchors (Arthrex, Inc., Naples, FL) contain side vents in addition to the longitudinal cannulation that allow blood products from the bone to reach the rotator cuff repair interface at the bone surface and that also allow bone formation within the vents.

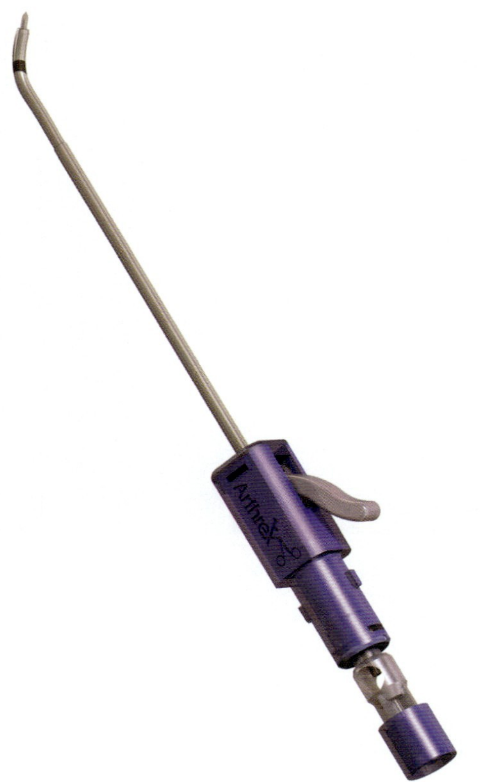

Figure 2.16 The PowerPick device (Arthrex, Inc., Naples, FL) can be used during rotator cuff repair to create vents in the greater tuberosity to provide access of the marrow elements and blood to the bone–tendon repair interface to encourage tendon to bone healing.

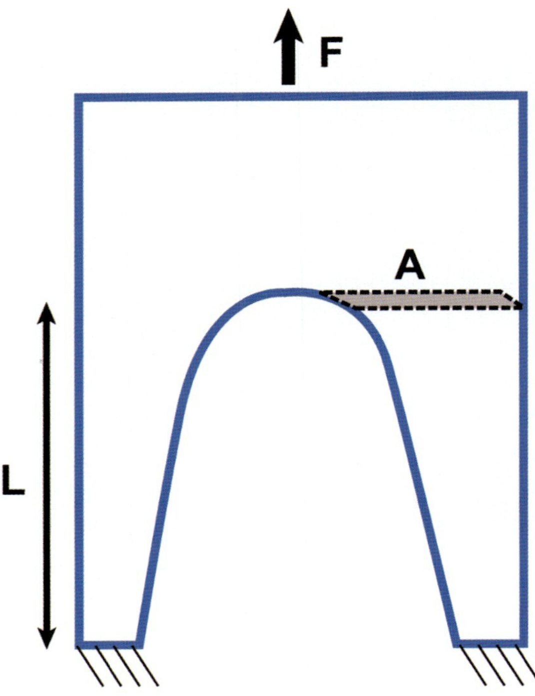

Figure 2.17 Diagrammatic representation of linear strain and elongation. A force (F) applied to a rotator cuff tear of length (L) will cause an elongation of the tear (ΔL). Elongation is related to strain according to the formula:

$$\varepsilon\,(\text{strain}) = \frac{\Delta L}{L} = \frac{F}{AE}$$

A, cross-sectional area of intact cuff at the level of strain measurement; E, modulus of elasticity (Young's modulus). ε, strain.

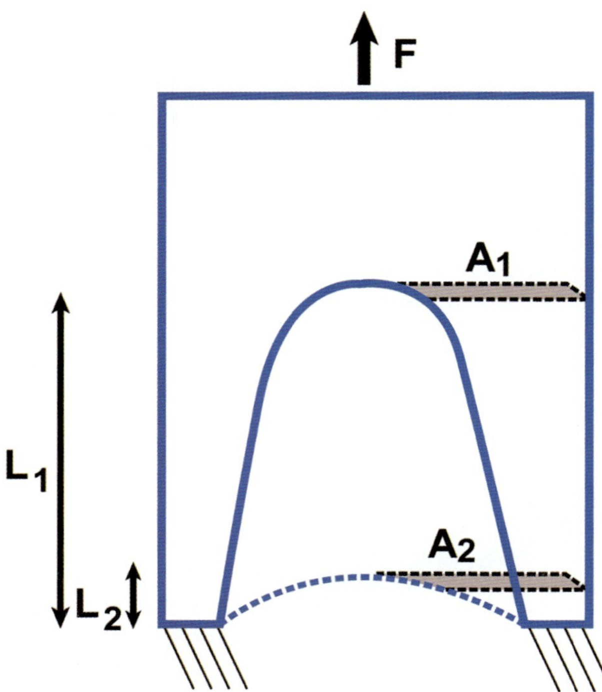

Figure 2.18 Free body diagram showing the mechanical conditions before and after partial side-to-side repair. The length of the tear has been reduced from L_1 to L_2, and the cross-sectional area of the cuff tissue at the apex of the margin of the tear has been increased from A_1 to A_2. These changes decrease the elongation of the tear and decrease the strain at the tear margin.

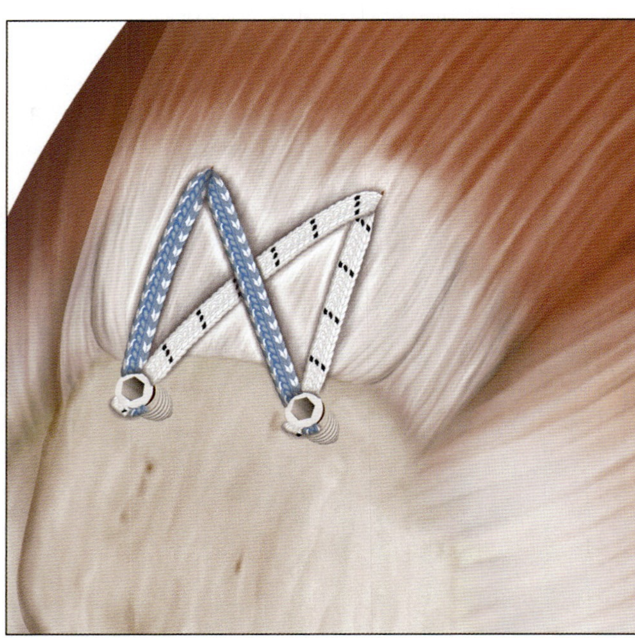

Figure 2.19 Schematic of a SpeedBridge (Arthrex, Inc., Naples, FL) rotator cuff repair. Two BioComposite SwiveLock C anchors are placed medially and the FiberTape sutures are passed through the rotator cuff. Then, FiberTape sutures from the medial anchors are crisscrossed and secured laterally with two BioComposite SwiveLock C suture anchors.

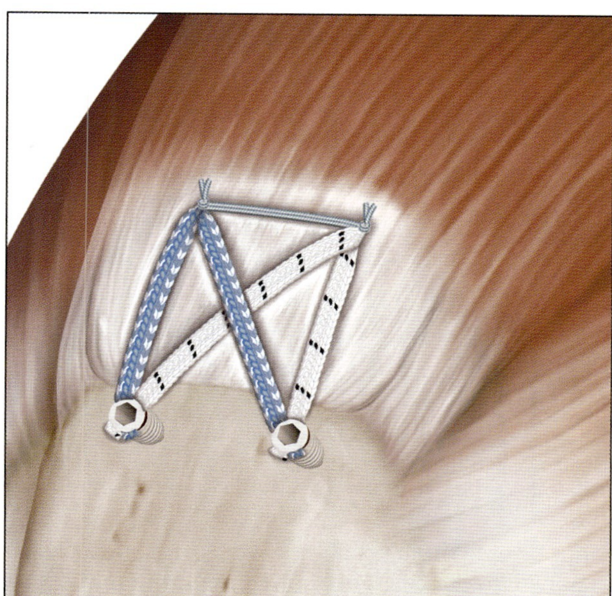

Figure 2.20 Schematic of a SpeedBridge (Arthrex, Inc., Naples, FL) rotator cuff repair with a medial double mattress. Two BioComposite SwiveLock C anchors are placed medially and the FiberTape sutures are passed through the rotator cuff. Then, the #2 FiberWire eyelet safety sutures are tied as a medial double mattress using a double-pulley technique. These sutures are cut. The FiberTape sutures from the medial anchors are then crisscrossed and secured laterally with two BioComposite SwiveLock C suture anchors.

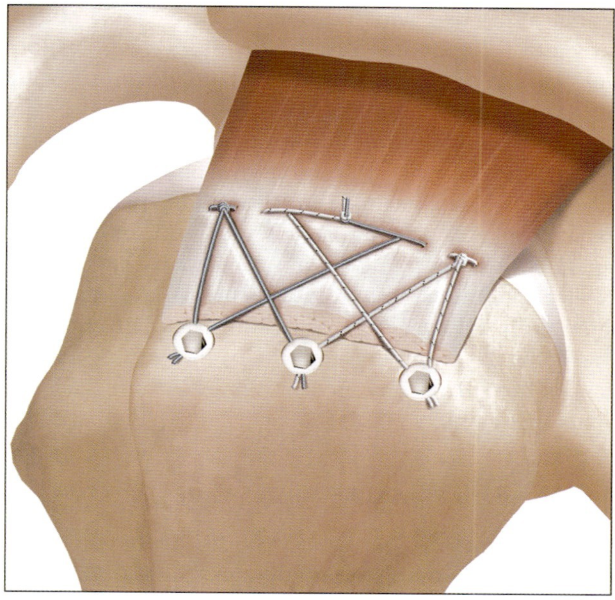

Figure 2.21 Schematic of the Diamondback repair. Two double-loaded anchors medially are linked to three anchors laterally. This repair configuration provides twice as many linked diagonal compressive sutures as are possible with a standard transosseous equivalent technique. Thus, this technique provides greater footprint compression and is useful for large rotator cuff tears or those with poor tissue quality.

tears, we use an extended SutureBridge or diamondback repair configuration (Fig. 2.21). This technique utilizes medial anchors with double-pulley augmentation, or multiple mattress sutures medially to increase the number of fixation points in the tendon.

Biologic Considerations

In general, the biologic environment for healing is enhanced by strong biomechanical fixation. A large footprint with strong fixation will maximize the area of bleeding bone that is in contact with the repaired tendon. Vented anchors (BioComposite Corkscrew FT and BioComposite SwiveLock C anchors; Arthrex, Inc., Naples, FL) and bone vents placed in the greater tuberosity facilitate delivery of blood and marrow products (e.g., adult stem cells) to the tendon–bone interface. We prefer biocomposite anchors composed of PLA polymers and β-TCP (tricalcium phosphate). This composition has a more physiologic pH upon degradation than standard PLA anchors.

We see a definite role for platelet-rich plasma (PRP) in some cases of cuff repair as discussed below.

We do not believe that routine suprascapular nerve releases are helpful to the final function of the muscle, as anatomic repair of the tendon restores the anatomic course of the suprascapular nerve. Even if only a partial cuff repair is possible (e.g., repair of the infraspinatus can be done, but not the supraspinatus), release of the suprascapular nerve at the notch will not relieve any tethering of the nerve that occurs at the base of the scapular spine.

PLATELET-RICH PLASMA

We use PRP (Arthrex ACP; Naples, FL) at the time of repair of massive cuff tears as well as all revision repairs. The application of exogenous growth factors to enhance the healing potential of soft tissue injuries and disorders has long been proposed. Platelet-rich preparations comprise one such autologous category and are characterized by their increased concentration of platelets compared to whole blood. Platelet-rich preparations have been highly valued due to their ability to retain their alpha and dense granules and to deliver a balanced preparation of healing factors. When activated in vivo or in vitro, various growth factors or cytokines are released including platelet-derived growth factors, transforming growth factor beta (TGFβ), insulin-like growth factor, basic fibroblast growth factor, and vascular endothelial growth factor. By concentrating platelets, the concentration of these growth factors increases linearly. Each of these growth factors is then free to bind to various receptors in local or circulating cells and initiate intracellular signaling. From there, a cascade of events may result in cellular chemotaxis, differentiation, and proliferation. Other nongrowth factors are present in dense granules including calcium, adenosine, dopamine, histamine, and serotonin. These noncytokine molecules play fundamental roles during the biological phases of healing including the inflammation, proliferation, and remodeling phases.

One distinct advantage of platelet-rich preparations over delivery of a single exogenous recombinant cytokine (e.g., bone morphogenic protein) is that a whole host of biologically active cytokines may be delivered simultaneously and at their native proportions seen in whole blood. While some cytokines may be potentially more beneficial than others, one must recognize that wound healing is a very complex process, and no single "magical" factor likely exists. The exact concentration required for enhancement of soft tissue healing is unclear. While likely different preparations, concentrations, volumes, and timing will be dependent on the particular application, it appears that a platelet concentration two to four times baseline is associated with enhancement of healing (8,9). It should be considered, however, that the role of PRP in the enhancement of healing of acute injuries versus chronic tendinosis is likely different.

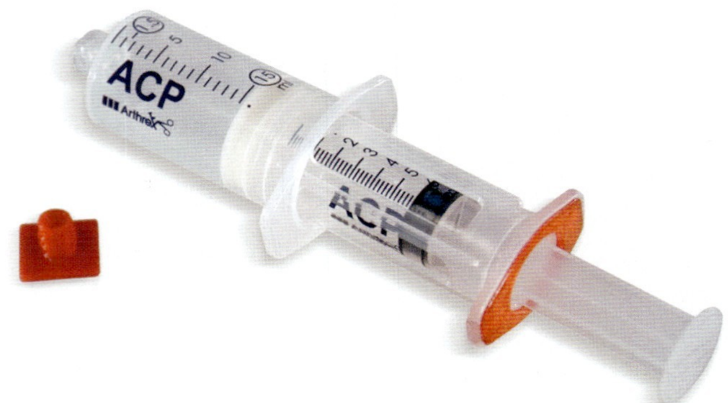

Figure 2.22 The double-syringe system for ACP (Arthrex, Inc, Naples, FL) facilitates extraction of ACP for patient use. Patient blood is withdrawn into an outer large syringe and, after centrifugation, ACP supernatant can be extracted into the small inner syringe for patient use.

Platelet-Rich Plasma Preparation

Although a number of methods of PRP preparation exist, our preference is to use the autologous conditioned plasma (ACP) system (Arthrex, Inc., Naples, FL). In addition to its efficacy, it has many other advantages including its ease of use, short preparation time, cost-effectiveness, and the ability to use the technique both in the clinic setting and operating room setting under sterile conditions.

Approximately 10 ml of venous blood is drawn from the nonaffected arm and placed in a uniquely designed double syringe (Fig. 2.22). If the ACP is not going to be used within 30 minutes, 1 ml of anticoagulant citrate dextrose solution A is first drawn into the larger outer syringe to bind free calcium and prevent the clotting of blood. Clotted whole blood cannot be used during platelet-rich preparation since platelets adhere to the clot. Furthermore serum cannot be used due to the low native concentration of platelets in serum. However, in most cases, we use ACP within 30 minutes of blood extraction and therefore do not add the anticoagulant.

Following extraction of blood, a centrifugation step is performed separating red blood cells and white blood cells from the plasma and platelets. The syringe is sealed with a cap and centrifuged for 5 minutes at 1,500 rpm, separating the red and white blood cells from the platelet-rich supernatant (Fig. 2.23A). The supernatant is withdrawn from the outer syringe and into the inner syringe by pulling up the plunger on the inner syringe (Fig. 2.23B). The inner syringe

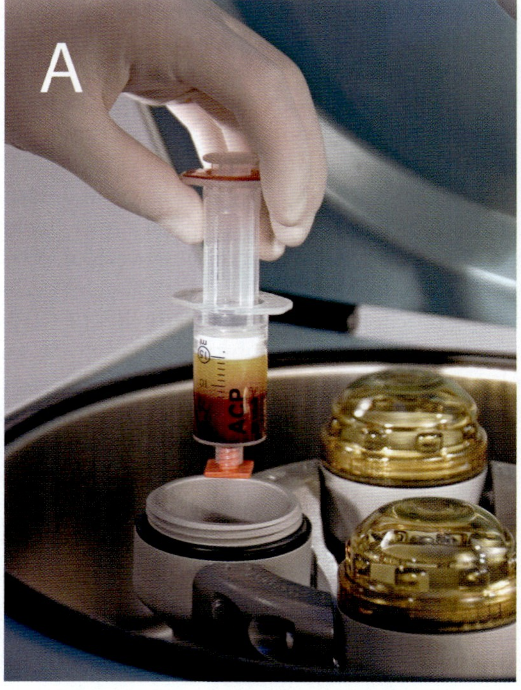

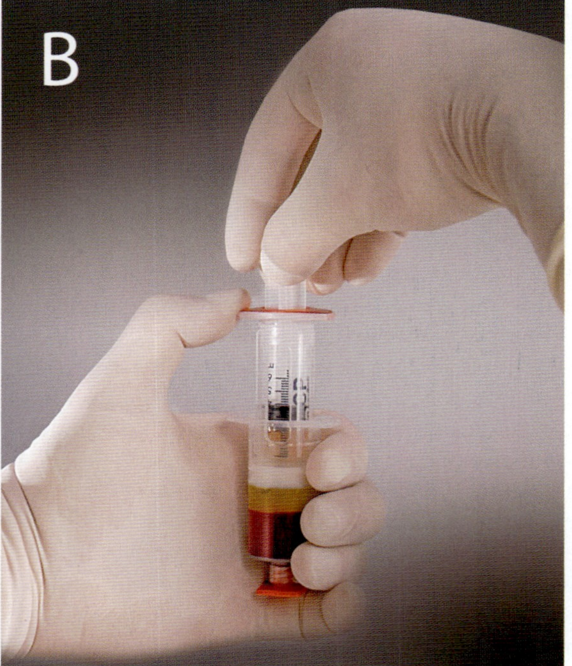

Figure 2.23 **A:** Blood from the patient is run in a centrifuge to separate supernatant (*yellow*) from whole blood (*red*). **B:** The supernatant is transferred for patient use by pulling up on the plunger of the small inner syringe.

is then unscrewed from the outer syringe and may now be delivered using a needle.

Approximately 3 to 5 ml of concentrated platelets is obtained from 10 ml of venous blood. Even when using a small volume of venous blood, growth factor concentrations of epidermal growth factor, vascular endothelial growth factor, TGFβ-1, TGFβ-2, platelet-derived growth factor-AB, and platelet-derived growth factor-BB have been demonstrated to be 5 to 25 times greater when compared to whole blood. Importantly, using the double-syringe method, white blood cells are eliminated from the preparation. White blood cells are known to harbor various proteases and hydrolases that can degrade PRP preparations. In addition, while other preparations may produce higher concentrations of growth factors, many of these preparations require more initial blood volume, and various studies have demonstrated that higher concentrations do not necessarily produce a superior end effect (e.g., cellular proliferation). These studies suggest that there may be a therapeutic window whereby higher concentrations may have no more effect or may be potentially detrimental.

PRP may then be delivered to the repair site by direct injection at the tendon–bone interface or simply into the subacromial space (Fig. 2.24). There is no firm evidence that injection into the tendon–bone interface is any more effective than simple injection into the subacromial space. Injection is performed as the final procedure during arthroscopic rotator cuff repair of large and massive tears, as well as in revision cases, under dry conditions.

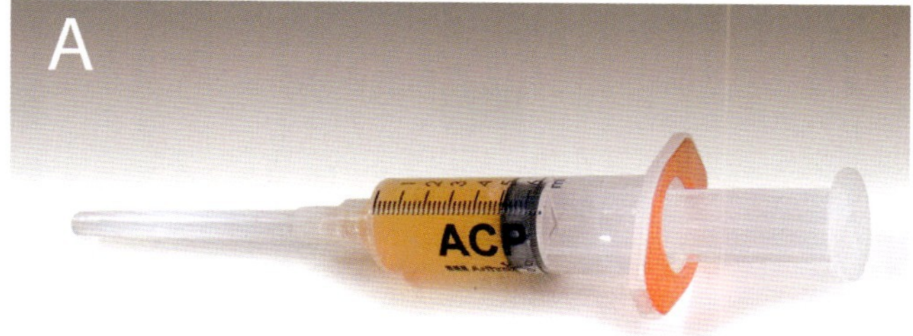

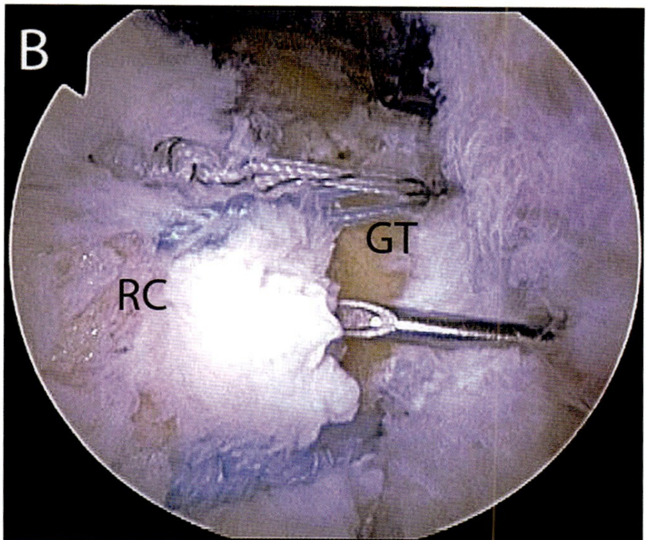

Figure 2.24 **A:** Photo of ACP supernatant (Arthrex, Inc., Naples, FL) that has been separated from whole blood for patient use. **B:** Arthroscopic view of a right shoulder from a posterior viewing portal demonstrates injection of ACP at the site of a rotator cuff repair. GT, greater tuberosity; RC, rotator cuff.

PHILOSOPHY OF REHABILITATION

Arthroscopic rotator cuff repair has brought about a paradigm shift in the postoperative rehabilitation of rotator cuff repairs. Research has shown that *passive* elevation can cause strains great enough to cause failure of rotator cuff repairs. We have no doubt that many failures of cuff repair are brought about by too-aggressive stretching and strengthening exercises in the early postoperative period. One could argue that, with open cuff repair, early motion is necessary to prevent postoperative stiffness. But with arthroscopic cuff repair, where postoperative stiffness is rare, we have the luxury of enforcing early immobilization (6 weeks in a sling) without undue risk of stiffness. If a shoulder does develop postoperative stiffness, we can always restore motion almost immediately with an arthroscopic capsular release and lysis of adhesions. Therefore, the threat of stiffness is not as intimidating as it was in the era of open cuff repair.

We have identified categories of patients who are at risk for developing postoperative stiffness (patients with single-tendon tears; combined labral and cuff repair; calcific tendinitis) (10). In these patients, we initiate table slides the day after surgery as a closed-chain stretch to prevent stiffness (Fig. 2.25).

The other component to rehabilitation is strengthening. We have noted that many surgeons begin strengthening exercises at 6 to 8 weeks after rotator cuff repair. However, Sonnabend et al. (11) showed, in an excellent primate study, that it takes 3 months for the repaired tendon to form Sharpey fibers to bone. Therefore, we wait until 3 months postoperative to begin strengthening exercises. In the case of massive tears and revision repairs, we do not begin strengthening until 4 months postoperative.

REFLECTIONS

What about the surgeon and his skill level? How does that relate to results? Nobody has adequately defined what makes a great technical surgeon. It probably comes down to a mix of focus, knowledge base, judgment, speed, efficiency of motion, and seamless transition from one segment of an operation into the next. We may not

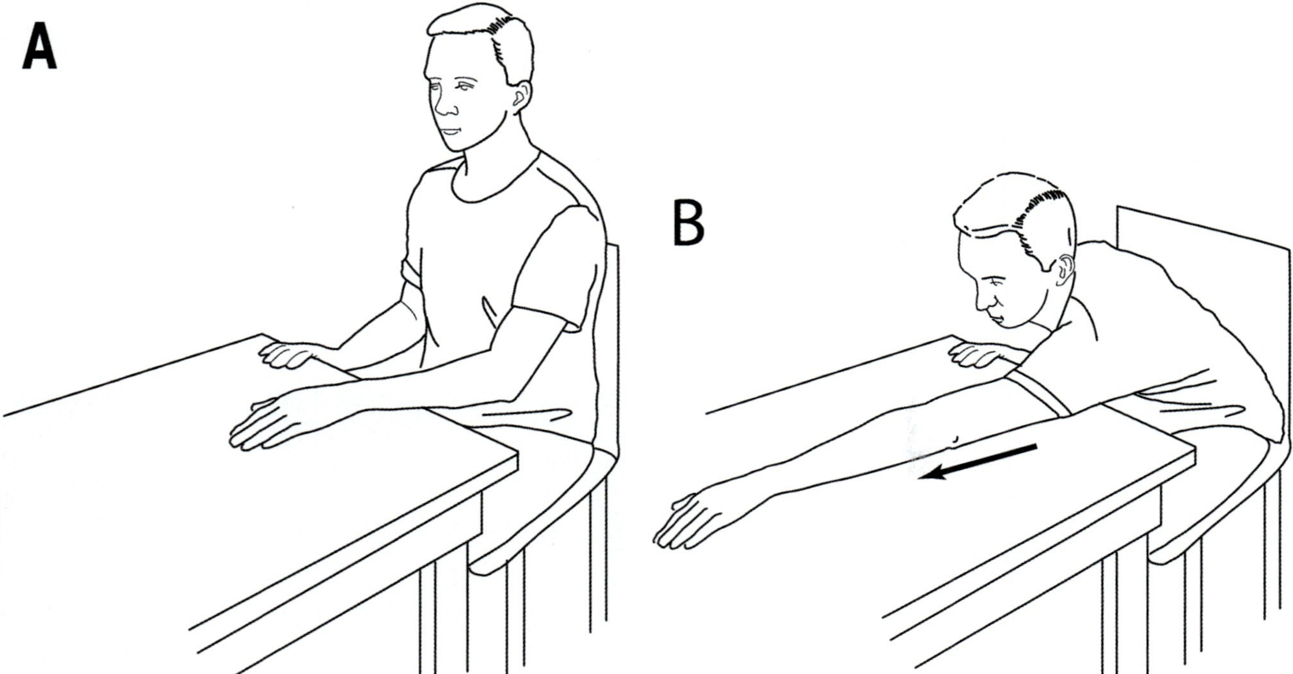

Figure 2.25 Table slide. **A:** Starting position. While seated at a table, the patient places the hand of the affected shoulder on a sliding surface (e.g., a magazine that slides over a smooth table surface). **B:** Ending position. The patient slides the hand forward, maintaining contact with the table, while the head and chest advance toward the table.

be born with an abundance of all of these skills, but we can always strive to cultivate and improve our own God-given abilities, so that we apply sound principles to our surgical techniques.

We have long drawn the analogy between cowboys and arthroscopic shoulder surgeons, and we believe now more than ever that this is true. For the credo of the cowboy and the credo of the surgeon have always been the same: Always strive to do what's right.

REFERENCES

1. Gamradt SC, Gallo RA, Adler RS, et al. Vascularity of the supraspinatus tendon three months after repair: characterization using contrast-enhanced ultrasound. *J Shoulder Elbow Surg*. 2010;19:73–80.
2. Burkhart SS, Barth JR, Richards DP, et al. Arthroscopic repair of massive rotator cuff tears with stage 3 and 4 fatty degeneration. *Arthroscopy*. 2007;23:347–354.
3. Burkhart SS, Esch JC, Jolson RS. The rotator crescent and rotator cable: an anatomic description of the shoulder's "suspension bridge". *Arthroscopy*. 1993;9:611–616.
4. Burkhart SS. Fluoroscopic comparison of kinematic patterns in massive rotator cuff tears. A suspension bridge model. *Clin Orthop Relat Res*. 1992:144–152.
5. Burkhart SS, Wirth MA, Simonick M, et al. Loop security as a determinant of tissue fixation security. *Arthroscopy*. 1998;14:773–776.
6. Lo IK, Burkhart SS, Chan KC, et al. Arthroscopic knots: determining the optimal balance of loop security and knot security. *Arthroscopy*. 2004;20:489–502.
7. Burkhart SS, Athanasiou KA, Wirth MA. Margin convergence: a method of reducing strain in massive rotator cuff tears. *Arthroscopy*. 1996;12:335–338.
8. Anitua E, Sanchez M, Zalduendo MM, et al. Fibroblastic response to treatment with different preparations rich in growth factors. *Cell Prolif*. 2009;42:162–170.
9. Graziani F, Ivanovski S, Cei S, et al. The in vitro effect of different PRP concentrations on osteoblasts and fibroblasts. *Clin Oral Implants Res*. 2006;17:212–219.
10. Huberty DP, Schoolfield JD, Brady PC, et al. Incidence and treatment of postoperative stiffness following arthroscopic rotator cuff repair. *Arthroscopy*. 2009;25:880–890.
11. Sonnabend DH, Howlett CR, Young AA. Histological evaluation of repair of the rotator cuff in a primate model. *J Bone Joint Surg Br*. 2010;92:586–594.

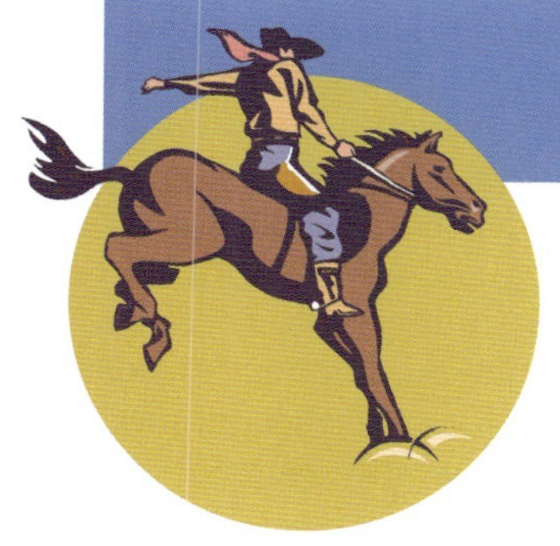

3

Double-row versus Single-row Cuff Repair*

WESTERN WISDOM

Stay away from a man who's all gurgle and no guts.

This book is intentionally oriented toward surgical techniques, emphasizing tips and tricks. In general, we believe it is more important to discuss techniques than controversies. However, a controversy has recently developed in the realm of arthroscopic rotator cuff repair to which we believe we should devote a chapter. That controversy revolves around single-row versus double-row arthroscopic rotator cuff repair. Two recently published clinical studies, one by Franceschi et al. (1) and one by Burks et al. (2) concluded that single-row techniques offered the same clinical and anatomic outcomes as double-row techniques. We believe these conclusions are erroneous.

First of all, one must recognize that contemporary state-of-the-art double-row repair differs from earlier-generation double-row techniques. The current suture-bridge technique (or transosseous-equivalent technique) (3,4) has bridging self-reinforcing sutures between the medial and the lateral rows. The first-generation double-row repair construct consisted of medial mattress sutures and lateral simple sutures without linkage between the two rows (5). The first-generation double-row constructs had superior biomechanical parameters compared to single-row constructs (6,7). However, they did not adequately resist rotational effects nor did they distribute forces across the entire rotator cuff insertional footprint.

Biomechanical testing has consistently demonstrated the superiority of a linked double-row construct (such as SutureBridge) to both unlinked double-row and single-row constructs. Currently, testing techniques that emphasize cyclic loading as well as resistance to shear, show that linked double-row constructs are the strongest.

We recently did a biomechanical study (8) on a linked double-row construct that showed that it possesses self-reinforcing properties similar to the Chinese finger trap. The self-reinforcing features of the linked suture bridge indicate that in vivo destructive forces can be neutralized and even harnessed to make the construct stronger under load.

It is ironic that we find ourselves in the awkward position of having to rationalize the use of a repair construct that is biomechanically superior to other constructs and that has been shown in several studies to improve tendon-to-bone healing (9–11). However, the aforementioned level I studies by Franceschi et al. (1) and by Burks et al. (2) have cast some doubt on the clinical superiority of linked double-row self-reinforcing constructs. Therefore, it is essential that we critically analyze these two studies to see if that doubt can be justified.

The study by Franceschi et al. (1) utilized a double-row repair technique with medial mattress sutures and lateral simple sutures, a construct devoid of suture linkage or bridging between the two rows. This first-generation double-row suture anchor repair technique, as previously discussed, embodies an inferior mechanical profile compared to the contemporary double-row linked bridging technique. The authors reported the use of an average of 1.9 suture anchors for single-row repairs and 2.3 suture

*Note: much of this chapter is adapted from an article by Stephen Burkhart, MD, and Brian Cole, MD (Burkhart SS, Cole BJ. Bridging self-reinforcing double-row rotator cuff repair: we really are doing better. *Arthroscopy.* 2010;26:677–680. Adapted with permission.)

anchors for double-row repairs. In general, one would expect that the double-row repairs would have had twice the number of suture anchors as the single-row repairs. However, in this study, the average number of suture anchors were nearly identical and it becomes difficult to differentiate these as truly differing repair techniques. As this is a level I study, the authors should be commended for conducting it in a randomized and controlled fashion. However, it suffers from a fatal flaw and essentially prevents one from deriving a valid conclusion based upon the results. Although the authors concede that a limitation to their study is that no formal power analysis was performed, reporting on 26 patients in each group provides a study that is clearly grossly underpowered when healing is the primary outcome variable (12). Thus, it becomes, even in the best of procedure comparisons (i.e., a true first-generation double-row compared to a single-row repair technique), impossible to conclude that differences do not exist between these two populations of patients. The study offers little to our knowledge or ability to compare a single-row to a double-row technique and does not speak in any way to the merit of the self-reinforcing linked bridging suture technique.

As for the study by Burks et al. (2), the repair technique was not a bridging double-row construct nor a true double-row technique as it was initially described, but rather, a "triangle" repair with one medial anchor and two lateral anchors. Mazzocca et al. (14) have previously tested this "triangle" configuration and found its strength to be equivalent to single-row repairs. So, it is no surprise that this older generation nonbridging double-row repair construct was not superior to the single-row technique. Once again, these authors should be commended for conducting a level I randomized controlled trial. But, similar to the study by Francheschi et al. (1), the authors presented a grossly underpowered study (12) whereby valid comparisons of these techniques cannot be made. In essence, the authors predicted a 20% retear rate, yet only demonstrated a 10% retear rate in both groups and thus committed a type II error whereby 20 patients analyzed in each group cannot render a valid comparison of two surgical techniques. To summarize, while both of these studies are often quoted as substantive evidence that there are "no differences between single-row and double-row techniques," they both suffer from an inability to make valid comparisons because they are grossly underpowered in addition to utilizing older-generation nonbridging repair constructs for their double-row repairs. Making the argument that differences do not exist between these repair techniques is no different than the historical argument that arthroscopic suture anchor repairs for instability should not be done because the earlier arthroscopic transglenoid instability repairs had very high failure rates.

Furthermore, multiple studies have shown that tendon-to-bone healing occurs in significantly greater numbers of patients who have had double-row cuff repairs than in those with single-row repairs (9–11). In the systematic review of the existing literature performed by Duquin et al. (11) that included more than 1,100 rotator cuff repairs, the authors demonstrated a statistically significant reduction in anatomic retear rates for true double-row repairs compared to single-row repairs for all tears >1 cm in length. While this study supports what some might believe to be a self-evident finding considering the biomechanical comparisons of these techniques, this review does not separate or discuss the results of the self-reinforcing bridging suture technique.

Recently, at the Closed Shoulder and Elbow Meeting (New York, NY, November, 2009), Gartsman et al. (14) presented a Level I prospective randomized comparison using ultrasound evaluation of single-row repairs of isolated supraspinatus tendon tears compared to the suture-bridge transosseous repair technique, a self-reinforcing bridging suture technique. The authors performed a power analysis and determined that for an 80% power, assuming a 12% difference between groups with $p = 0.05$, that 50 patients in each group would suffice. The authors used two anchors medially and two anchors laterally, with bridging sutures linking the two rows of anchors, and demonstrated that the single-row retear rate was 20% versus the transosseous equivalent suture-bridge technique that was 6%, a highly significant difference between the two groups. The limitations of this study include that it is not yet formally published and no functional outcomes were reported.

A consistent problem with existing literature is that aggregate scores (University of California at Los Angeles [UCLA], American Shoulder and Elbow Surgeons [ASES], Constant) and outcomes do not separate out strength as a primary outcome variable. Arguably, comparisons in strength following different repair techniques might yield additional findings not yet considered by current literature. We believe that the magnitude of improvement in external rotation strength and forward elevation strength after self-reinforcing suture-bridging double-row repair has been greater than that seen previously with single-row techniques. Most recently, Cole and associate authors have demonstrated a statistically significant improvement in forward elevation strength as used to, in part, calculate the Constant score when comparisons were made between double-row and single-row repair techniques (personal communication, November 2009).

Let's take this line of reasoning a bit further. We have long known that arthroscopic debridement and decompression for the treatment of rotator cuff tears lead to significant pain relief and improvement in postoperative UCLA scores even in the face of little or no gain in strength. But is that level of functional improvement the benchmark that we want for evaluating our rotator cuff tears? Surely not!

In our opinion, the great advantage of cuff repair over cuff debridement is the ability to improve strength, yet

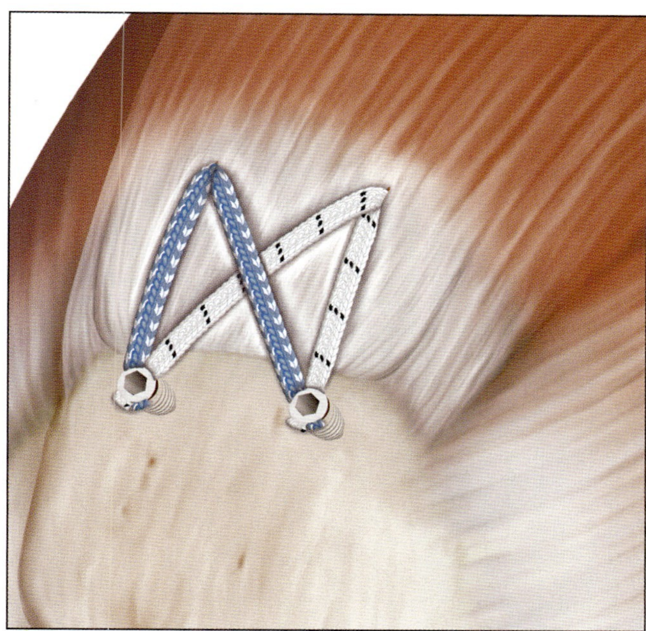

Figure 3.1 Schematic of a SpeedBridge (Arthrex, Inc., Naples, FL) rotator cuff repair. Two BioComposite SwiveLock C anchors preloaded with FiberTape are placed medially. The FiberTape sutures are passed through the rotator cuff 2 to 3 mm lateral to the musculotendinous junction. The FiberTape sutures from the medial anchors are crisscrossed and secured laterally with two BioComposite SwiveLock C suture anchors.

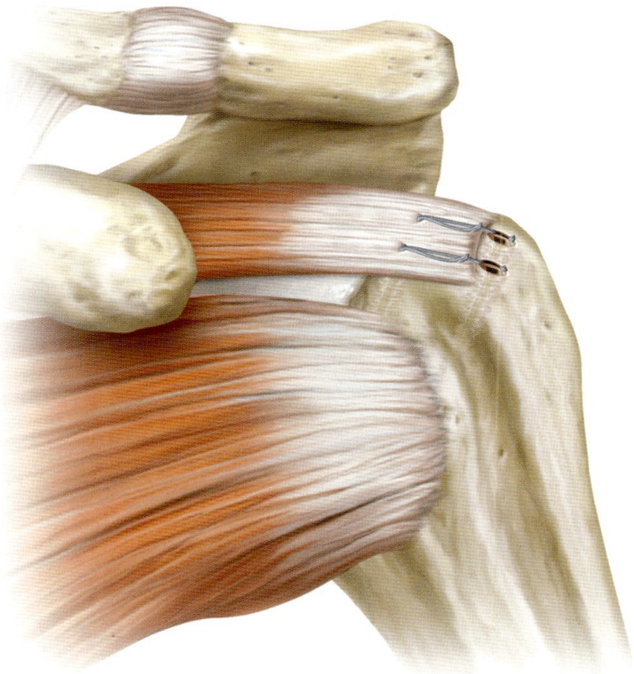

Figure 3.2 Schematic of a SwiveLock-FiberChain (Arthrex, Inc., Naples, FL) double-row rotator cuff repair. Two Bio-Corkscrew FT anchors preloaded with FiberChain are placed medially. The FiberChain sutures are passed through the rotator cuff 2 to 3 mm lateral to the musculotendinous junction. The FiberChain sutures from the medial anchors are then secured laterally with two Bio-SwiveLock suture anchors.

strength is not properly (or at all) weighted in our current scoring systems. In light of this, we are currently evaluating the relative importance of strength return to patients in the outcome following rotator cuff repair and are developing a new outcome tool that adequately addresses strength by quantifying postoperative gains in strength. This is the only way that we can assess the clinical improvement that is directly attributable to tendon healing with improved transmission of muscle forces to the joint.

So what is the self-reinforcing bridging rotator cuff repair technique? Arguably, it can be achieved in multiple ways. The authors use variations of bridging constructs tailored to the patient's tear pattern and tissue quality. Two totally knotless techniques are frequently used, one that utilizes a suture tape (SpeedBridge with FiberTape; Arthrex, Inc., Naples, FL) with four screw-in anchors (SwiveLock; Arthrex, Inc.; Naples, FL) (Fig. 3.1) and the other that utilizes a chain-link suture and screw-in anchors (FiberChain-SwiveLock system; Arthrex, Inc.; Naples, FL) (Fig. 3.2). Similarly, by tying knots medially and effectively neutralizing the forces that are transmitted laterally, a knotless device (i.e., PushLock Anchor or SwiveLock Anchor; Arthrex, Inc.) can effectively create the self-reinforcing suture-bridge technique with total rotator cuff tendon apposition (Fig. 3.3). Furthermore, a "double-pulley" double mattress suture tied with suture limbs from the two medial anchors can seal the medial footprint from the potentially deleterious effects of joint fluid (15,16). In the SpeedBridge technique, the two medial anchors (SwiveLock C; Arthrex, Inc.; Naples, FL) have each been preloaded with FiberTape. After tying the double-pulley sutures medially, the FiberTape limbs are then crisscrossed in a standard SpeedBridge configuration and linked to two lateral SwiveLock-C anchors. This creates a compressive footprint that is sealed off medially from synovial fluid (Fig. 3.4).

Unfortunately, the recent studies by Franceschi et al. (1) and Burks et al (2) are being used by some to justify the use of less expensive procedures that are inferior to self-reinforcing bridging suture double-row techniques. But the path of least resistance in orthopedics is not always the best way. Or, as we have said so many times, the easy way is not usually the cowboy way. We should not apologize for using a superior construct while others try to minimize its importance. On the contrary, we should celebrate its superiority and recognize its importance as a significant advancement in the treatment of rotator cuff tears.

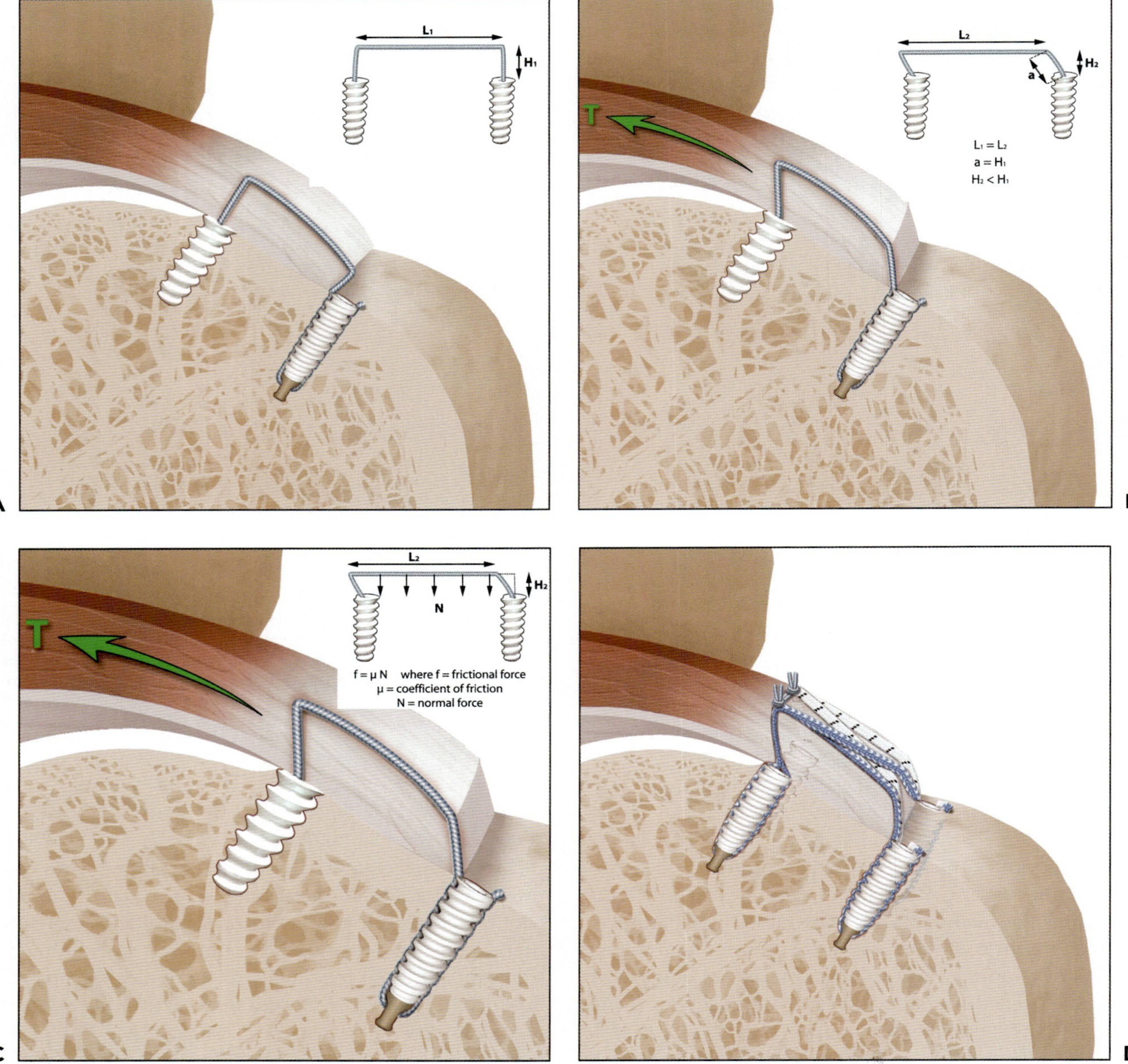

Figure 3.3 Schematic of self-reinforcing suture-bridge technique. **A:** Linked double-row construct before loading. **Inset:** Free-body diagram of the construct. H_1, thickness of rotator cuff before loading; L_1, length of tendon beneath suture. **B:** Loading of the linked double-row construct results in compression of the rotator cuff footprint. **Inset:** Free-body diagram of the construct. T, tensile loading force; L_2, length of tendon beneath suture; a, length of suture between tendon edge and lateral anchor; H_2, thickness of compressed rotator cuff under tensile load. **C:** Up-close view of the linked double-row construct after loading. **Inset:** Free-body diagram showing distributed normal force (N) resulting from elastic deformation of tendon beneath the suture. The frictional force (f) increases as the normal force (N) increases under load. **D:** Linked double-row construct with two medial anchors linked to two lateral anchors provides maximal footprint compression under loading. Additionally, a medial double-mattress stitch in this case provides a seal to joint fluid.

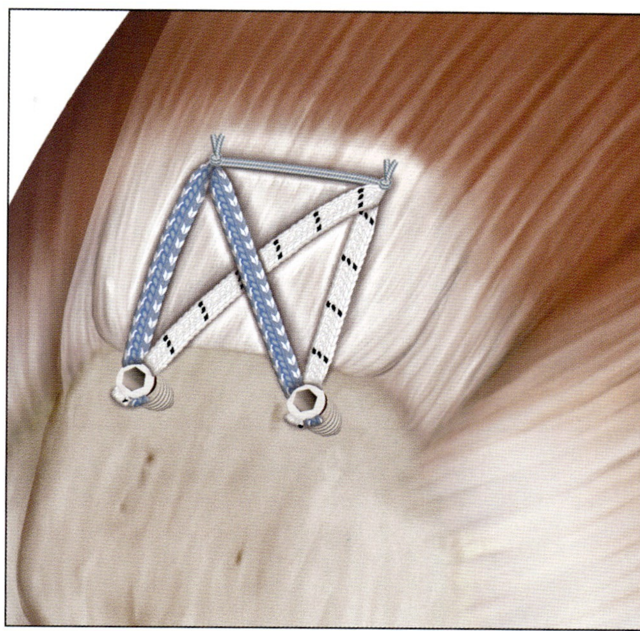

Figure 3.4 Schematic of a SpeedBridge (Arthrex, Inc., Naples, FL) rotator cuff repair with a medial double mattress. Two BioComposite SwiveLock C anchors are placed medially and the FiberTape sutures are passed through the rotator cuff. Then, the #2 FiberWire eyelet safety sutures are tied as a medial double mattress using a double-pulley technique. These sutures are cut. The FiberTape sutures from the medial anchors are then crisscrossed and secured laterally with two BioComposite SwiveLock C suture anchors.

REFERENCES

1. Franceschi F, Ruzzini L, Longo U, et al. Equivalent clinical results of arthroscopic single-row and double-row suture anchor repair for rotator cuff tears: a randomized controlled trial. *Am J Sports Med.* 2007;35:1254–1260.
2. Burks RT, Crim J, Brown N, et al. A prospective randomized clinical trial comparing arthroscopic single-and double-row rotator cuff repair. *Am J Sports Med.* 2009;37:674–682.
3. Park MC, ElAttrache NS, Tibone JE, et al. Part I: footprint characteristics for a transosseous-equivalent rotator cuff repair technique compared with a double-row repair technique. *J Shoulder Elbow Surg.* 2007;16:461–468.
4. Park MC, Tibone JE, ElAttrache NS, et al. Part II: biomechanical assessment for a footprint-restoring transosseous-equivalent rotator cuff repair technique compared with a double-row repair technique. *J Shoulder Elbow Surg.* 2007;16:469–476.
5. Lo IKY, Burkhart SS. Double-row arthroscopic rotator cuff repair: re-establishing the footprint of the rotator cuff. *Arthroscopy.* 2003;19: 1035–1042.
6. Kim DH, ElAttrache NS, Tibone JE, et al. Biomechanical comparison of a single-row versus double-row suture anchor technique for rotator cuff repair. *Am J Sports Med.* 2006;34:407–414.
7. Meier SW, Meier JD. The effect of double-row fixation on initial repair strength in rotator cuff repair: a biomechanical study. *Arthroscopy.* 2006;22:1168–1173.
8. Burkhart SS, Adams C, Burkhart SS. A biomechanical comparison of 2 techniques of footprint reconstruction for rotator cuff repair: The SwiveLock-FiberChain construct versus standard double-row repair. *Arthroscopy.* 2009;25:274–281.
9. Sugaya H, Maeda K, Matsuki K, et al. Functional and structural outcome after arthroscopic full-thickness rotator cuff repair: single-row versus dual-row fixation. *Arthroscopy.* 2005;21:1307–1316.
10. Frank JB, ElAttrache NS, Dines JS, et al. Repair site integrity after arthroscopic transosseous-equivalent suture-bridge rotator cuff repair. *Am J Sports Med.* 2008;36:1496–1503.
11. Duquin TR, Buyea C, Bisson LJ. Which method of rotator cuff repair leads to the highest rate of structural healing? *Am J Sports Med.* 2010; 38: 835–841
12. Wall LB, Keener JD, Brophy RH. Systematic review: clinical outcomes of double-row versus single-row rotator cuff repairs. *Arthroscopy.* 2009;25: 1312–1318.
13. Mazzocca AD, Millett PJ, Guanche CA, et al. Arthroscopic single-row versus double-row suture anchor rotator cuff repair. *Am J Sports Med.* 2005;33:1861–1868.
14. Gartsman GM, Drake G, Edwards TB, et al. Ultrasound evaluation of arthroscopic full-thickness supraspinatus rotator cuff repair: single-row versus double-row suture bridge (transosseous equivalent) fixation—results of a randomized, prospective study. Presented at the 2009 Closed Meeting of the American Shoulder and Elbow Surgeons; October 25, 2009, New York, NY.
15. Lo IK, Burkhart SS. Transtendon arthroscopic repair of partial-thickness, articular surface tears of the rotator cuff. *Arthroscopy.* 2004;20: 214–220.
16. Arrigoni P, Brady PC, Burkhart SS. The double-pulley technique for double-row rotator cuff repair. *Arthroscopy.* 2007;23:675.e1–675.e4.

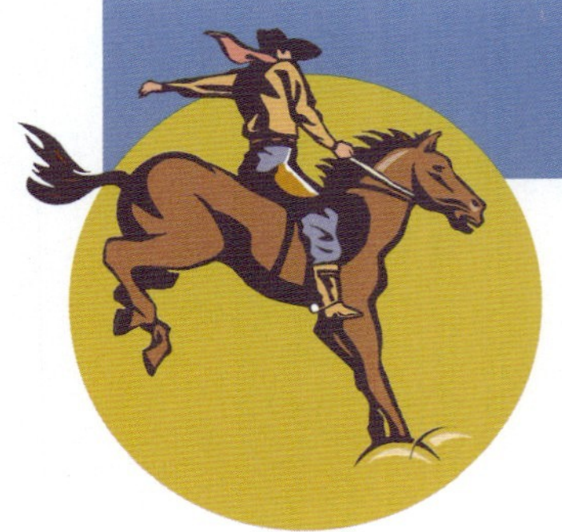

4

Complete Rotator Cuff Tears

WESTERN WISDOM

You can cut your throat with a sharp tongue!

Rotator cuff tears are one of the most common disorders in shoulder practice. Despite a long history of surgical treatment, the optimal rotator cuff repair continues to evolve. Our approach to rotator cuff repair was fully described in Chapter 2, "Philosophy of Rotator Cuff Repair." This chapter describes our preferred repair techniques for complete rotator cuff tears.

CRESCENT TEARS

Single-row Rotator Cuff Repair (SpeedFix Repair)

Although we prefer double-row repair over single-row repair, in some cases a single-row repair when performed correctly will still yield excellent clinical results with anatomic healing. In general, we reserve single-row repair for cases where there is insufficient mobility to perform a double-row repair (i.e., massive contracted rotator cuff tears). In addition, in patients with partial-thickness bursal surface rotator cuff tears where only a small bursal leaf must be repaired to the bone bed, a single-row repair may also be performed (see Chapter 5, "Partial-thickness Rotator Cuff Tears").

Similar to double-row repair, many different suture configurations are possible for a single-row repair. We prefer in many cases to perform a SpeedFix repair, which utilizes inverted mattress FiberTape stitches (Arthrex, Inc., Naples, FL) coupled to a 4.75-mm BioComposite SwiveLock C anchor (Arthrex, Inc., Naples, FL) (Figs. 4.1 and 4.2). An inverted mattress configuration is utilized since it provides superior fixation in the cuff when compared to a simple stitch and provides compression of the rotator cuff tendon against the footprint.

Following diagnostic arthroscopy, the subacromial space is evaluated and a subacromial decompression is performed as indicated. The rotator cuff margins are evaluated and the mobility is assessed. Tears amenable to this type of repair demonstrate good mobility from a medial-to-lateral direction indicating a crescent-shaped tear and are small, with a footprint that measures only 10 to 12 mm from medial to lateral. For full-thickness tears, our primary indication for a single-row SpeedFix repair is when medial bone quality is insufficient to place a medial anchor. In this setting, fixation can always be achieved in the lateral cortex using a SwiveLock anchor (Fig. 4.3).

While viewing through a posterior portal, a shaver or burr is introduced through the lateral portal, and the footprint of the rotator cuff is debrided to a bleeding bone surface. Since an anchor will only be placed along the lateral aspect of the footprint, a number of bone vents can be created with a punch or PowerPick (Arthrex, Inc., Naples, FL) along the medial aspect of the footprint to encourage infiltration of marrow elements containing cells beneficial for rotator cuff healing.

An inverted mattress stitch is placed in the rotator cuff using either a FastPass or MultiFire Scorpion device (Arthrex, Inc., Naples, FL). The #2 FiberWire leader (Arthrex, Inc., Naples, FL) of a FiberTape suture is loaded

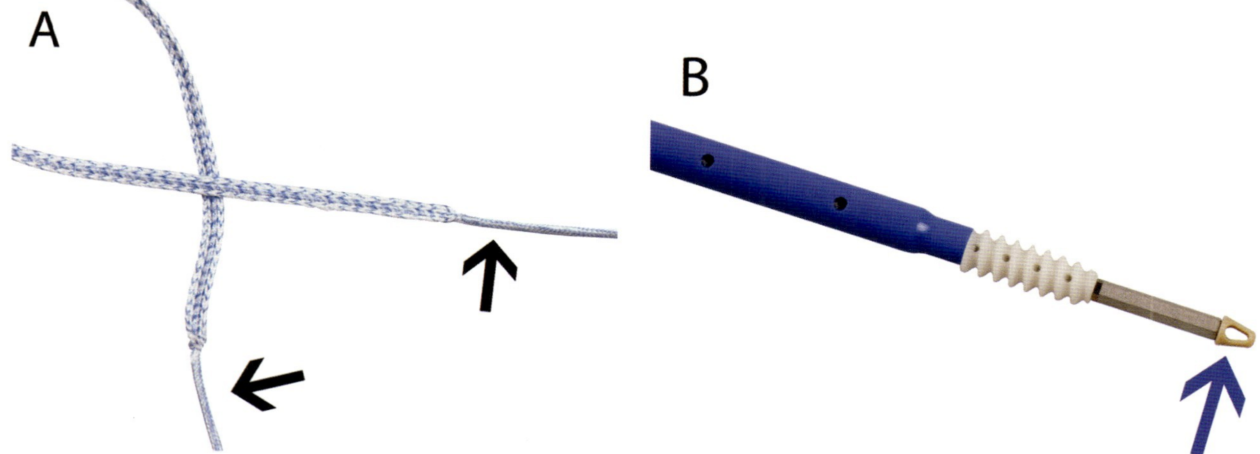

Figure 4.1 The SpeedFix (Arthrex, Inc., Naples, FL) utilizes **(A)** a FiberTape suture coupled to a **(B)** SwiveLock anchor. The FiberTape suture has #2 FiberWire leaders (*black arrows*) that facilitate passing through the rotator cuff. The FiberTape is threaded through the eyelet (*blue arrow*) of a SwiveLock anchor to secure the suture to bone.

onto the Scorpion. While viewing through the posterior portal, the Scorpion is introduced through the lateral portal. A #2 FiberWire leader is passed antegrade through the anterior aspect of the tear (Fig. 4.4A), and then the opposite FiberWire leader is passed antegrade through the posterior aspect. The FiberWire leaders are then retrieved and the FiberTape is pulled through the tendon creating an inverted mattress stitch (Fig. 4.4B).

The suture limbs are tensioned and the cannula is used as a guide to determine the position for the lateral anchor. The punch for a 4.75-mm BioComposite SwiveLock C is then used to create a bone socket in the lateral aspect of the greater tuberosity approximately perpendicular to the bone (Fig. 4.5). Extracorporeally, the FiberTape sutures are fed through the distal eyelet of the BioComposite SwiveLock C anchor. The anchor is then inserted and the sutures are appropriately tensioned to remove slack from the construct and reduce the tendon to the bone socket. It is helpful to maintain the location and orientation of the bone socket by keeping the punch in place until just prior to insertion of the loaded anchor. The eyelet of the anchor is seated into the bone socket and advanced until the leading threads of the anchor just contact the bone socket. While holding the thumb pad on the SwiveLock driver, the anchor is inserted

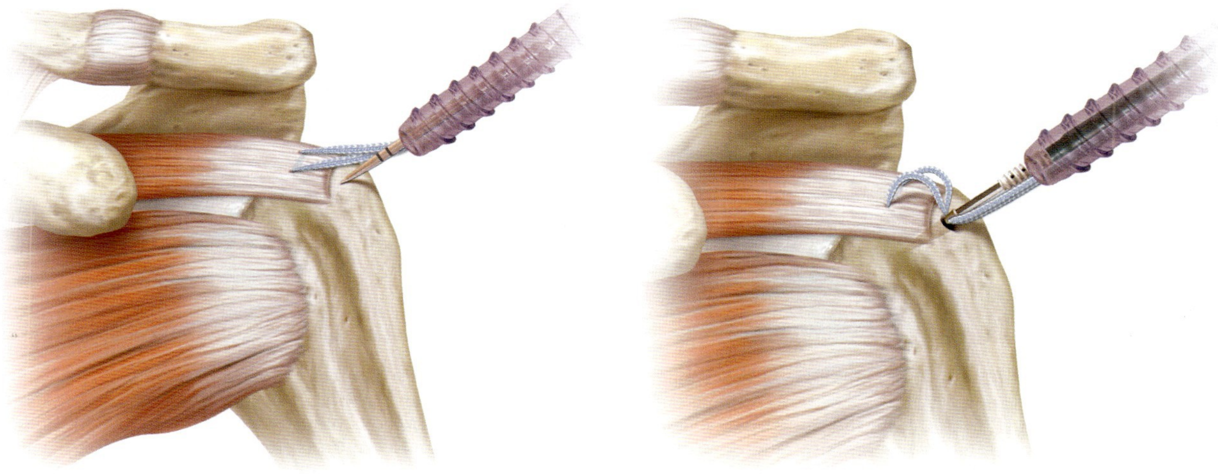

Figure 4.2 Schematic of the SpeedFix (Arthrex, Inc., Naples, FL) rotator cuff repair. **A:** A FiberTape suture is placed as an inverted mattress stitch in the rotator cuff and the suture limbs are retrieved out a lateral portal. Then, a punch is used to create a bone socket in the lateral cortex. **B:** Extracorporeally, the suture limbs are threaded through the eyelet of a BioComposite SwiveLock C anchor. Then, the eyelet of the anchor is seated into the prepared bone socket.

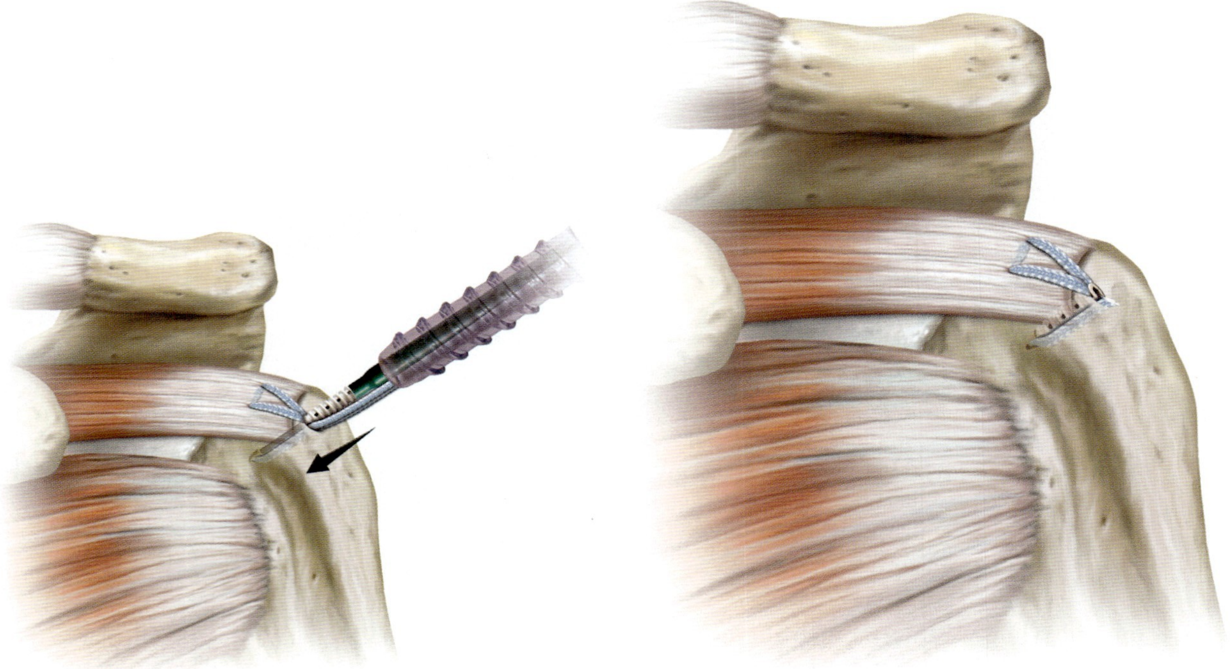

Figure 4.2 (*Continued*) **C:** The suture limbs are tensioned and the eyelet is seated until the anchor is just in contact with the bone. Manual tension on the suture limbs is released and the anchor is advanced until it is fully seated. **D:** Final repair. The suture limbs have been cut flush with the anchor.

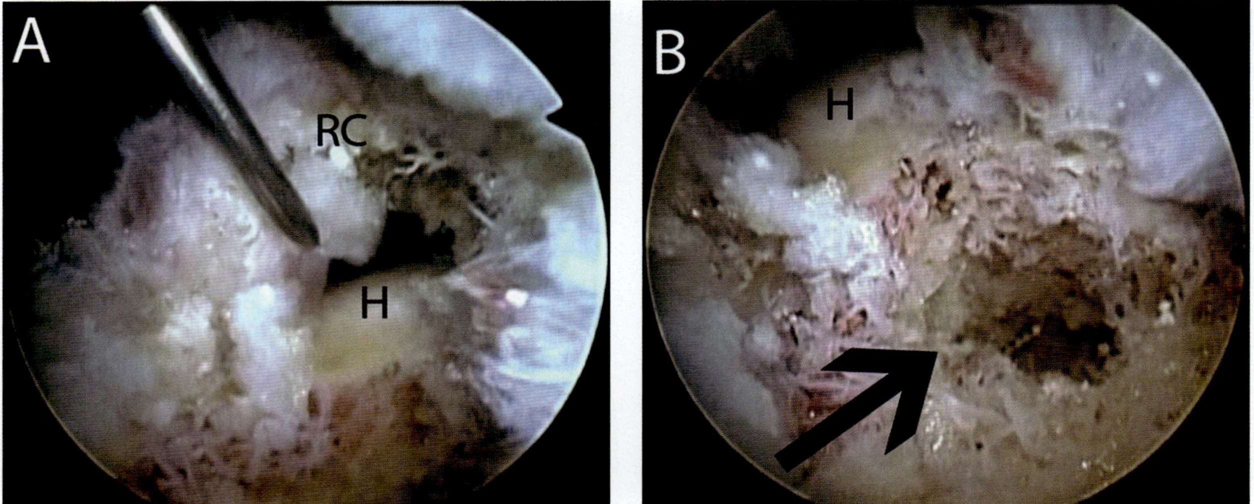

Figure 4.3 **A:** Right shoulder, lateral subacromial viewing portal, demonstrates a crescent-shaped rotator cuff tear. **B:** View of the proximal humerus bone bed in the same shoulder demonstrates a large cyst. In this case, the bone quality was very poor. Despite multiple techniques including bone graft, a buddy anchor, and use of a tenodesis screw, medial fixation could not be achieved. A Speed-Fix repair (Arthrex, Inc., Naples, FL) is indicated that achieves lateral cortical fixation. H, humerus; RC, rotator cuff.

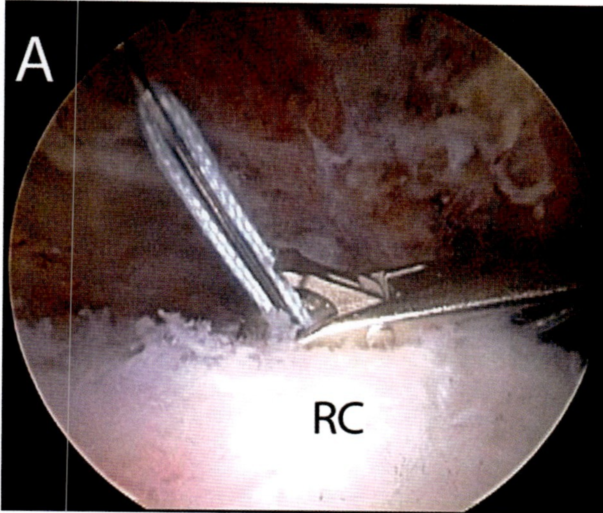

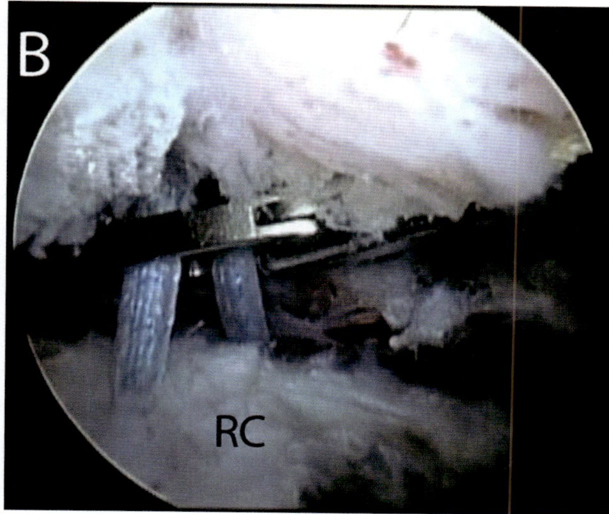

Figure 4.4 **A:** Right shoulder, posterior subacromial viewing portal demonstrates use of a Scorpion FastPass suture passer (Arthrex, Inc., Naples, FL) to pass a #2 FiberWire leader of a FiberTape (Arthrex, Inc., Naples, FL) through the rotator cuff. To place an inverted mattress stitch, the opposite limb of the FiberTape will similarly be passed through the rotator cuff **B:** A FiberTape suture has been placed as an inverted mattress stitch. The two limbs are seen exiting the rotator cuff and are retrieved out a lateral working cannula for lateral cortical fixation. RC, rotator cuff.

into the bone. With self-punching versions, the anchor itself (4.75-mm BioComposite SwiveLock SP; Arthrex, Inc., Naples, FL) may be used in a similar fashion without preparing a bone socket (Fig. 4.6). The final repair demonstrates secure tendon fixation to bone and adequate coverage of the medial aspect of the footprint (Fig. 4.7).

SutureBridge Double-row Repair

Double-row rotator cuff repair may be performed in many different configurations with the advantages of each configuration described previously (see Chapter 2, "Philosophy of Arthroscopic Rotator Cuff Repair"). When originally

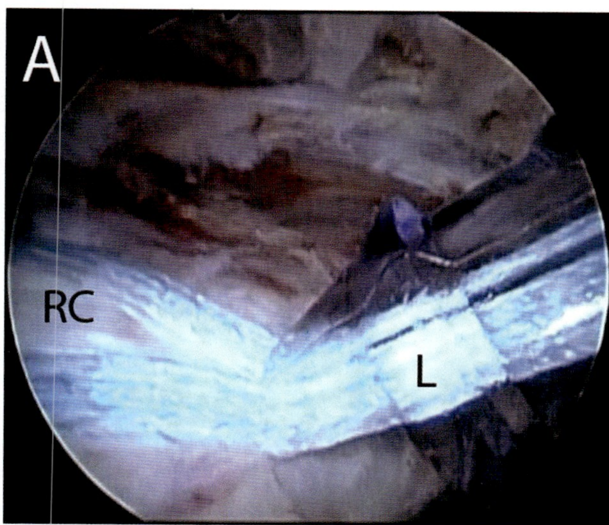

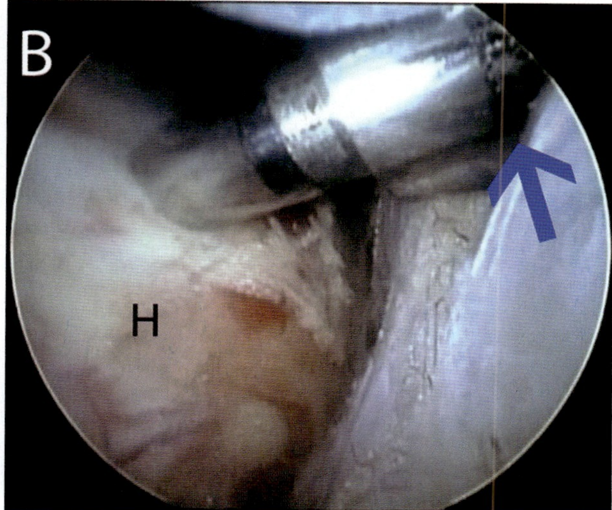

Figure 4.5 Right shoulder, posterior subacromial viewing portal, demonstrates creation of a lateral bone socket for a SwiveLock C anchor (Arthrex, Inc., Naples, FL). **A:** After sutures are retrieved, the cannula is used as a guide to determine the position for a lateral anchor bone socket. By tensioning the sutures and placing the cannula adjacent to the humerus, the proper position for the bone socket is determined. **B:** A punch has been introduced and will be impacted to the second line (*blue arrow*) to create a bone socket for the SwiveLock C anchor. H, humerus; L, lateral portal cannula; RC, rotator cuff.

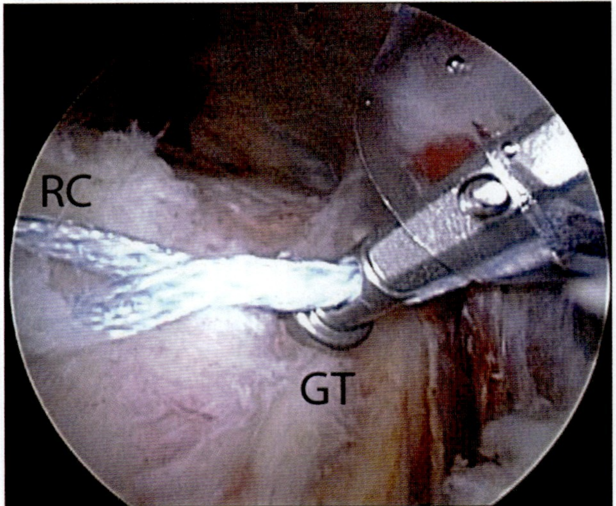

Figure 4.6 Right shoulder, posterior subacromial viewing portal. As an alternative to using a cannula to determine the location for lateral anchor placement, in one step a self-punching anchor (SwiveLock SP; Arthrex, Inc., Naples, FL) can be used to tension the sutures and determine the location. GT, greater tuberosity; RC, rotator cuff.

described, arthroscopic double-row rotator cuff repair was performed using two rows of unlinked anchors, with sutures passed in a mattress configuration for the medial row and simple stitches for the lateral row (Fig. 4.8). Linking the medial and lateral rows when performing a double-row rotator cuff repair has improved our biomechanical constructs and has demonstrated lower retear rates following rotator cuff repair. In this methodology, two rows of anchors are utilized. However, in this technique after the

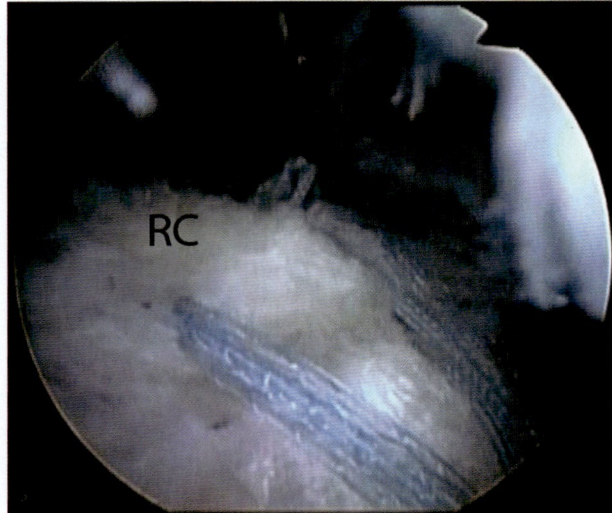

Figure 4.7 Right shoulder, posterior subacromial viewing portal, demonstrates a SpeedFix repair (Arthrex, Inc., Naples, FL) of a full-thickness crescent-shaped rotator cuff tear in which medial fixation could not be achieved. (Compare to Fig. 4.3. RC, rotator cuff.)

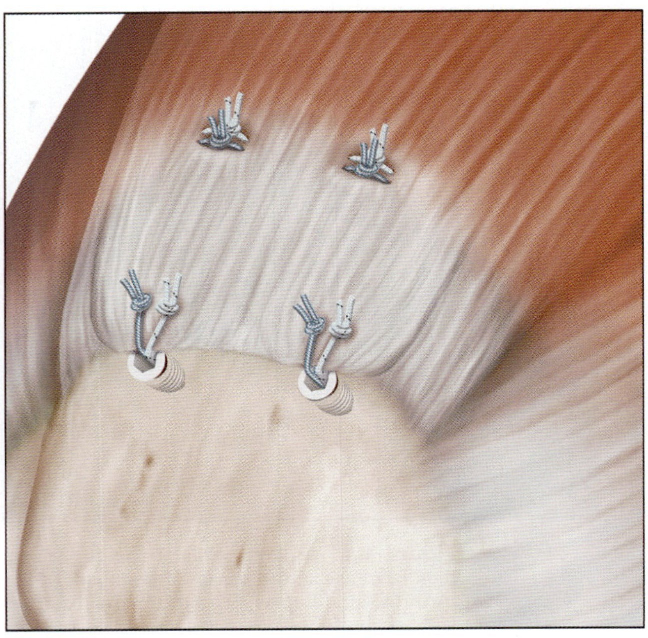

Figure 4.8 With the original double-row rotator cuff repair, two medial anchors were placed, sutures were individually passed and tied as mattress stitches, and then the suture limbs were cut. Two lateral anchors were also placed, sutures were passed and tied as simple stitches, and the suture limbs were cut.

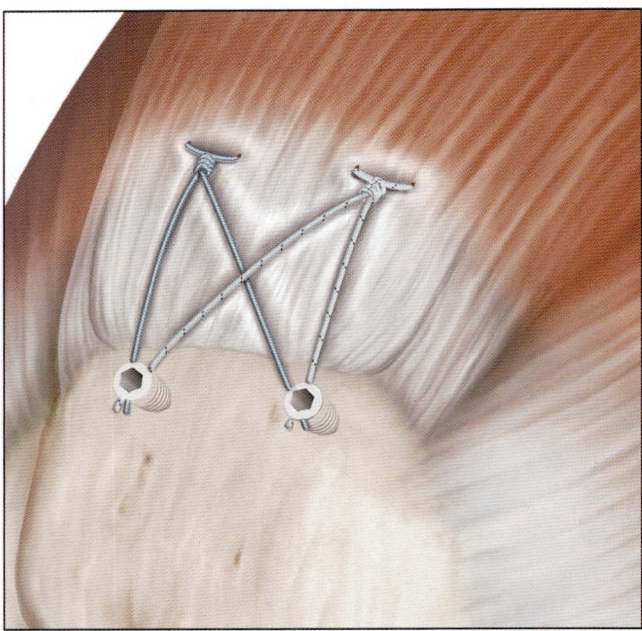

Figure 4.9 The SutureBridge (Arthrex, Inc., Naples, FL) rotator cuff repair represents an advancement over the traditional double-row repair, whereby the medial and lateral rows are linked. Two medial suture anchors are placed and sutures from these anchors are individually passed and tied as mattress stitches. Rather than cutting the suture limbs, however, the sutures are crisscrossed and secured laterally to two knotless anchors. This repair mechanically links the two rows and provides enhanced footprint compression to encourage rotator cuff healing.

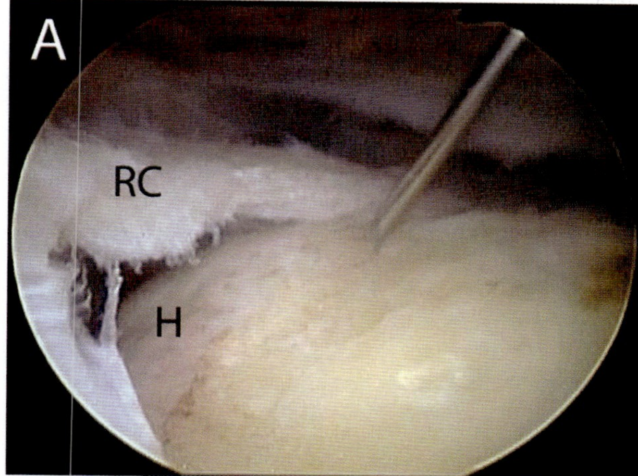

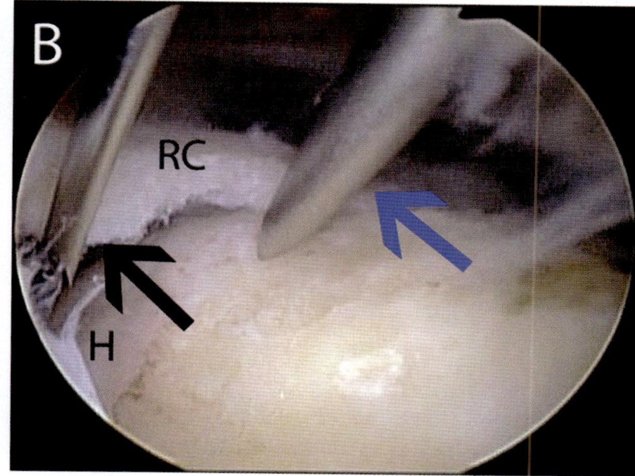

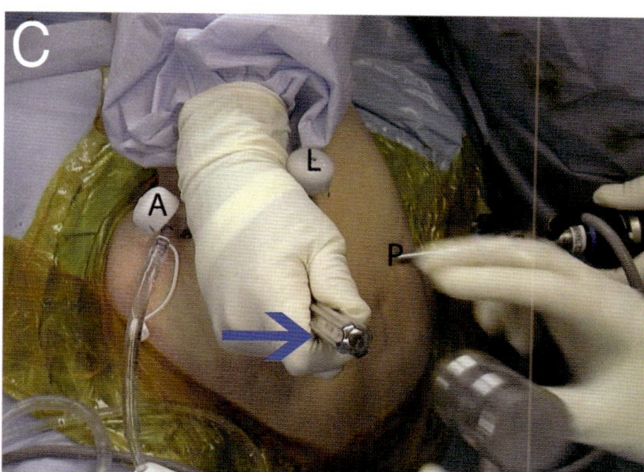

Figure 4.10 **A:** Right shoulder, posterior subacromial viewing portal, demonstrates use of a spinal needle as a guide to determine an adequate angle of approach for placement of **(B)** a punch that is placed through the same incision. The punch is used to create a bone socket for an anteromedial anchor. **C:** Outside view of a right shoulder demonstrates the percutaneous position of the punch (*blue arrow*) that is placed just lateral to the acromion. A, anterior portal; H, humerus; L, lateral portal; P, posterior portal; RC, rotator cuff.

#2 FiberWire sutures from the medial-row anchors have been passed through the medial rotator cuff and tied, the tails from the knotted medial anchors are individually crisscrossed, then placed through the distal eyelet of the lateral-row anchors, and secured into the lateral tuberosity (Fig. 4.9).

Threaded, double-loaded anchors (5.5-mm BioComposite Corkscrew FT, Arthrex, Inc., Naples, FL) are placed medially. Using a spinal needle as a guide, a punch is inserted into the anteromedial aspect of the footprint just lateral to the articular margin through a separate percutaneous incision (Fig. 4.10). The anchor is similarly inserted through the same incision, reproducing the same angle of insertion. A second medial anchor is then placed in the posteromedial aspect of the footprint. To improve visualization of the posteromedial aspect of the footprint, a 70° arthroscope may be utilized while viewing from a posterior subacromial portal. Alternatively, a posterolateral or lateral viewing portal may improve visualization (Fig 4.11). Finally, it is also sometimes necessary to place the posteromedial anchor while viewing intra-articularly (Fig. 4.12). For suture management, sutures are temporarily retrieved through the corresponding percutaneous puncture that the anchors were inserted through (Fig. 4.13).

Following placement of both anchors, mattress sutures are passed through the rotator cuff. It is important again to place sutures 2 to 3 mm lateral to the musculotendinous junction and to pass wide mattress sutures to avoid suture cut through. In addition, when performing any suture bridge technique, the location of the medial sutures and anchors will dictate the tendon reduction. Inaccurate anchor or suture placement will cause malreduction of the tendon and poor footprint reconstruction. For example, sutures passed more medially than described above will result in excessive tension and risk for failure. Once again, we emphasize that the sutures should be passed 2 to 3 mm lateral to the musculotendinous junction. Sutures are passed individually using a SureFire Scorpion needle in a FastPass Scorpion suture passer (that has a spring-loaded trapdoor in the upper jaw that captures the suture) (Arthrex, Inc., Naples, FL)

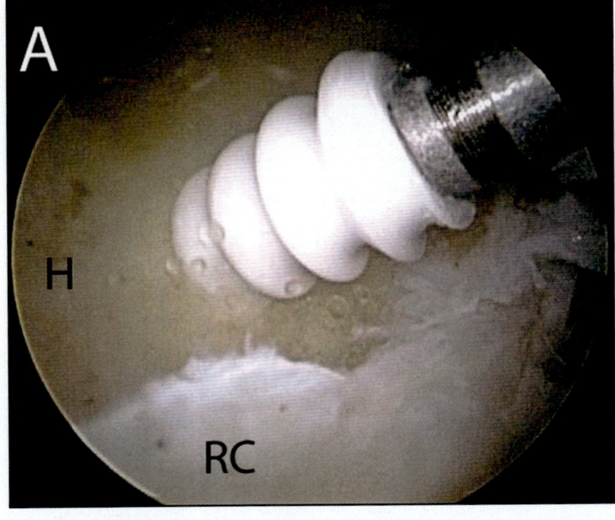

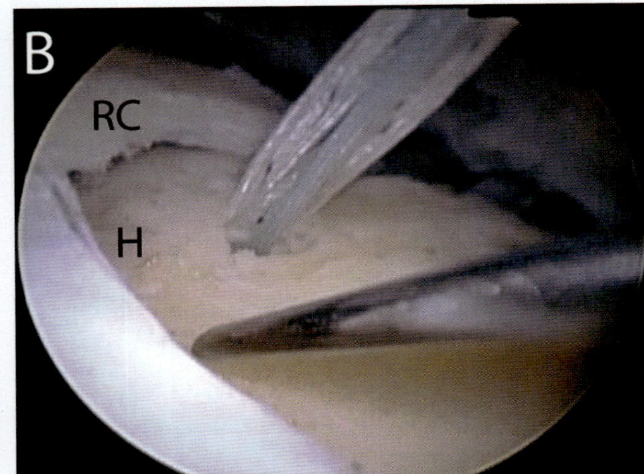

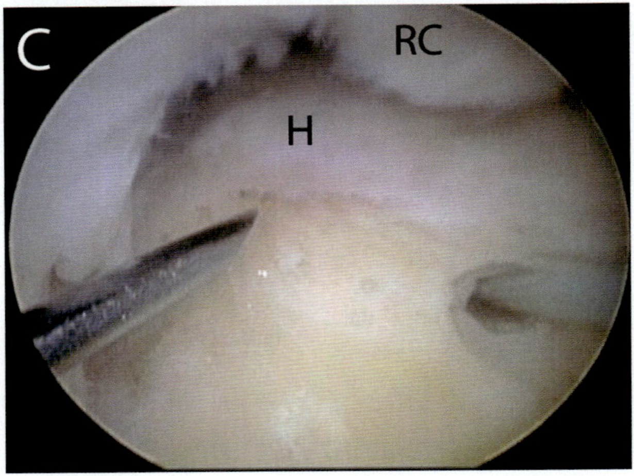

Figure 4.11 Right shoulders viewed with a 70° arthroscope demonstrate visualization for posteromedial anchor placement. **A:** A posteromedial anchor can be placed while viewing from a posterior subacromial portal with a 70° arthroscope. **B:** For many crescent-shaped tears, however, it difficult to visualize the posteromedial articular margin while viewing from a posterior subacromial portal. In this case, an anteromedial anchor has been placed and a spinal needle is used as a guide for a posteromedial anchor. But visualization is obstructed by the posterior margin of the crescent tear. **C:** Same shoulder as in previous image demonstrates how moving the arthroscope to the lateral subacromial portal may provide improved visualization of the posteromedial articular margin for placement of a posteromedial anchor. H, humerus; RC, rotator cuff.

(Figs. 4.14 and 4.15). As the suture passage moves more posteriorly, retrograde suture passage through the posterior portal using a Penetrator suture passer (Arthrex, Inc., Naples, FL) can provide the correct angle of approach (Fig. 4.16). Final medial suture passage should demonstrate equal spacing and complete coverage of the medial tendon (Fig. 4.17). Although the classic SutureBridge technique utilizes only one suture pair from each medial anchor, the second suture in each anchor may be preserved and utilized for additional security, particularly if the tendon is of poor quality.

The medial mattress sutures are then tied compressing the medial cuff against the footprint (Fig. 4.18). Sutures are tied with a static six-throw Surgeon's knot using a Surgeon's Sixth Finger Knot Pusher (Arthrex, Inc., Naples, FL). Suture tails are not cut but are left long for subsequent incorporation into the lateral-row anchors. Although skipping tying the medial sutures is an option, tying the medial mattress sutures has shown improved biomechanical characteristics when using #2 FiberWire suture.

Once the medial sutures have been tied, the potential for any dog-ear during lateral fixation can be judged. We commonly prevent dog-ears by placing a cinch-loop stitch at both the anterior and posterior margins of the tear using a FiberLink suture (Arthrex, Inc., Naples, FL) (see Chapter 2, "Philosophy of Rotator Cuff Repair"). FiberLink is a #2 FiberWire suture that has a closed loop on one end. To place a cinch loop, the free end of the suture is loaded onto a Scorpion and passed through the rotator cuff. Then, the free end is retrieved and threaded through the looped end of the suture. Tensioning the free end delivers the loop down to the rotator cuff, creating a cinch-loop stitch (Fig. 4.18C).

To secure the tendon laterally, the medial suture limbs are retrieved and secured with two 4.75-mm BioComposite SwiveLock C anchors. In most cases, one suture limb is retrieved from each anchor in a crisscross fashion through the lateral cannula. However, the number of sutures incorporated into each anchor and the number of lateral anchors should be dictated by the tear configuration and provide complete lateral fixation and

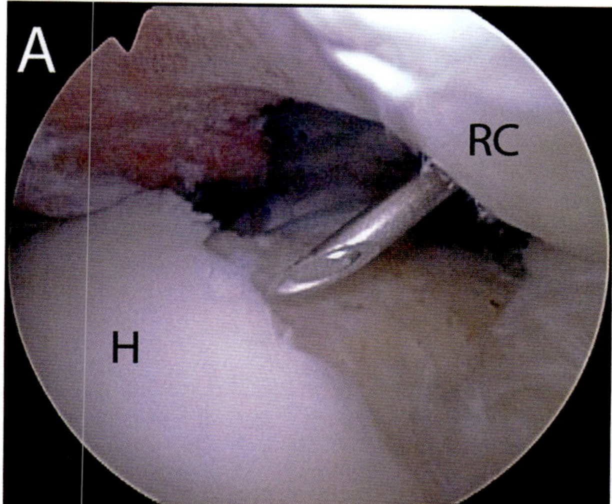

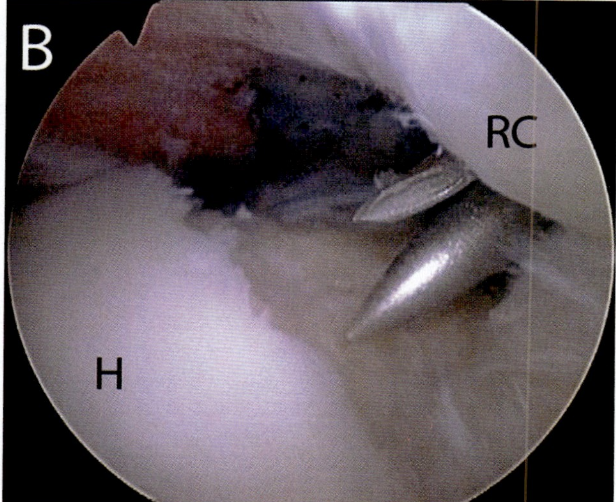

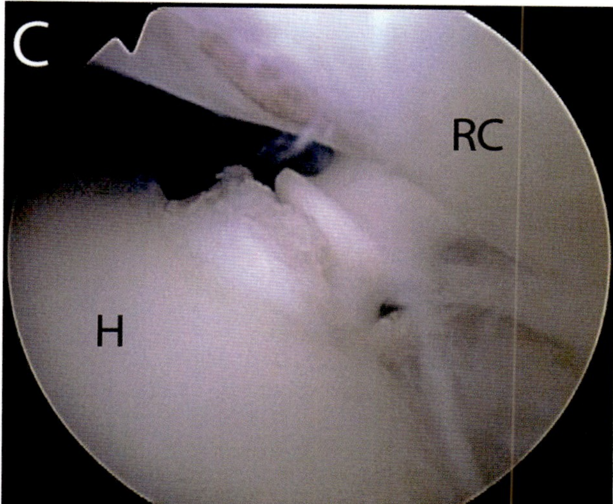

Figure 4.12 Right shoulder, posterior glenohumeral intra-articular viewing portal with a 70° arthroscope, demonstrates placement of a posteromedial anchor for a SutureBridge (Arthrex, Inc., Naples, FL) rotator cuff repair. This posterior glenohumeral view is useful if the posteromedial articular margin cannot adequately be seen with either posterior or lateral subacromial viewing portals. **A:** A spinal needle is used as a guide to determine an adequate angle of approach to the posteromedial bone bed. **B:** After an incision is made adjacent to the spinal needle, a punch is walked down the spinal needle to create a bone socket. **C:** A BioComposite Corkscrew FT anchor is inserted into the bone socket. H, humerus; RC rotator cuff.

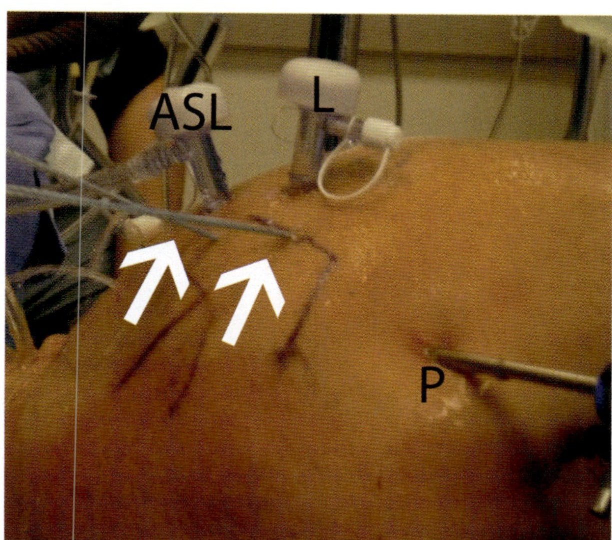

Figure 4.13 External view of a right shoulder in the lateral decubitus position. After placement of anchors via stab incisions, suture management is facilitated by keeping the sutures (*white arrows*) in the percutaneous incisions until suture passing is performed. ASL, anterosuperolateral portal; L, lateral subacromial portal; P, posterior portal.

footprint compression. If cinch loops have been placed, the posterior cinch loop is typically secured with the posterolateral anchor and the anterior cinch loop is secured with the anterolateral anchor. Prior to anchor insertion, tensioning the sutures through the cannula is useful to evaluate the proposed anchor location (Fig. 4.19). The lateral anchors are placed just lateral to the "corner" of the greater tuberosity, in the metaphyseal cortex: one anterior and one posterior.

A bone socket is then punched into the humerus (Fig. 4.20A). The suture limbs are threaded through the eyelet of a BioComposite SwiveLock C anchor (Fig. 4.20B) and the eyelet of the anchor is placed into the bone socket (Fig. 4.20C). Prior to completely seating than eyelet, the sutures are tensioned to remove slack from the construct (Fig. 4.20D). If the eyelet does not fully seat manually by pushing on the inserter, the inserter handle is gently impacted until the anchor just reaches the top of the bone socket (Fig. 4.20E). While holding the thumb pad, the inserter handle is then turned to advance the SwiveLock anchor (Fig. 4.20F). Sutures are then cut flush with the

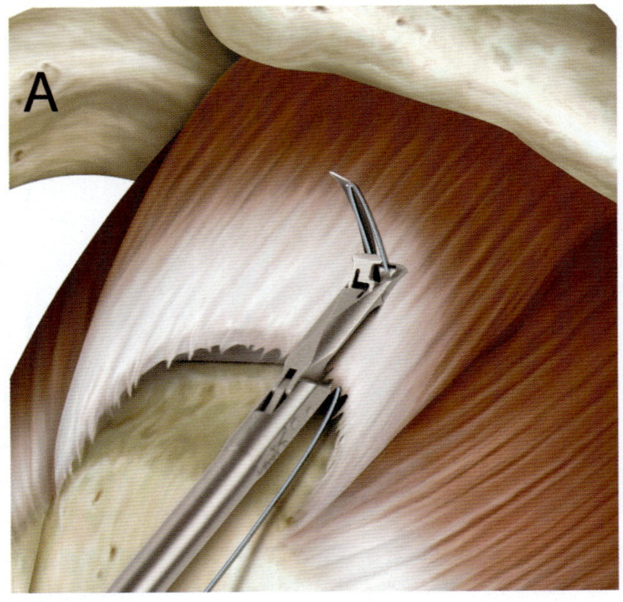

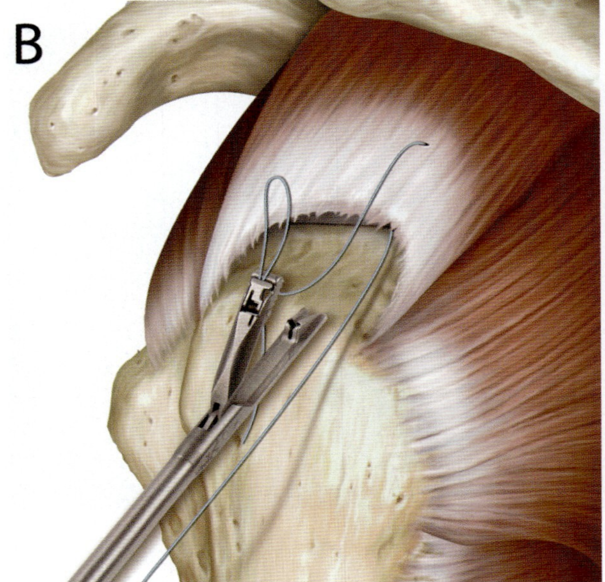

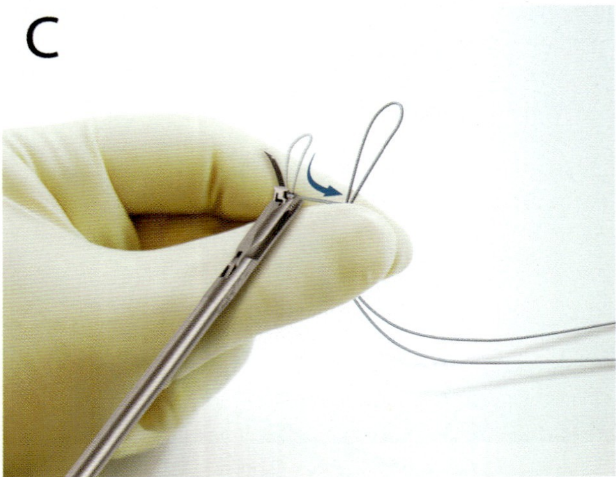

Figure 4.14 Schematic illustration of the Scorpion FastPass (Arthrex, Inc., Naples, FL). **A:** A suture is passed through the rotator cuff. **B:** A trapdoor on the instrument captures the suture, allowing suture passage and retrieval in one step. **C:** Extracorporeally, the suture is unloaded by firing the needle again, which raises the trap door so that the suture may be removed.

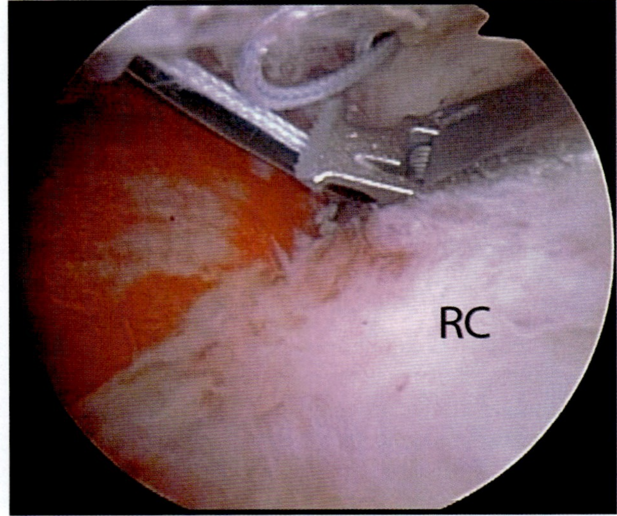

Figure 4.15 Arthroscopic photo of a right shoulder viewing from a posterior subacromial portal demonstrates suture passage with a Scorpion FastPass (Arthrex, Inc., Naples, FL).

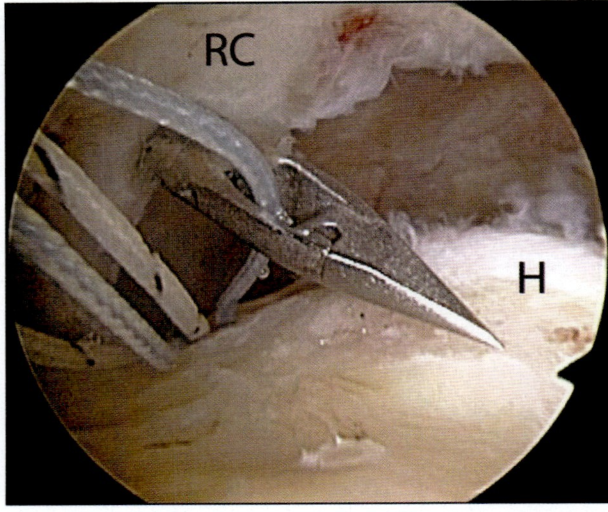

Figure 4.16 Right shoulder, lateral subacromial viewing portal, demonstrates use of a Penetrator (Arthrex, Inc., Naples, FL) to pass sutures from a posteromedial anchor. H, humerus; RC, rotator cuff.

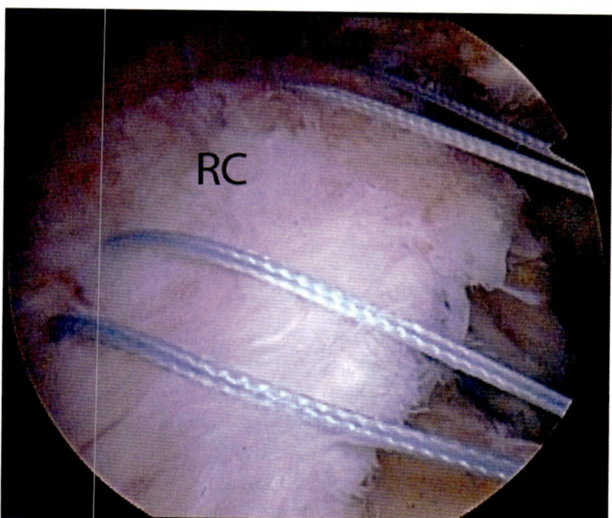

Figure 4.17 Right shoulder, posterior viewing portal, demonstrates placement of equally spaced mattress stitches that were placed from medial anchors for a SutureBridge (Arthrex, Inc., Naples, FL) rotator cuff repair.

anchor using an open-ended knot cutter or a closed FiberTape cutter (Arthrex, Inc., Naples, FL). The steps are then repeated for the second lateral anchor. Any unused sutures are then cut.

The final construct is evaluated for fixation and footprint reconstruction (Fig. 4.21).

SutureBridge with Medial Double Pulley

In most cases, we prefer to perform a variation of the standard SutureBridge technique in which medial mattress sutures are tied between the two medial anchors to create a seal from the joint (Fig. 4.22). In this variation, medial suture passage and knot tying are carried out quickly with a double-pulley technique. The double-pulley technique creates a double mattress stitch between the anteromedial and posteromedial anchors. The steps for medial anchor placement are performed exactly as previously described. However,

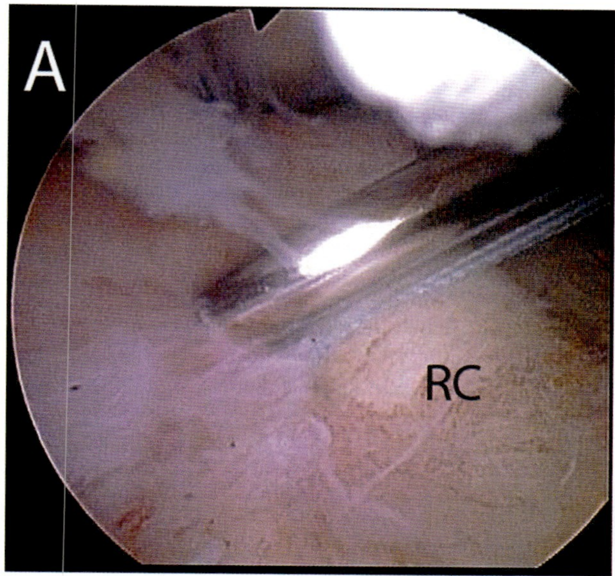

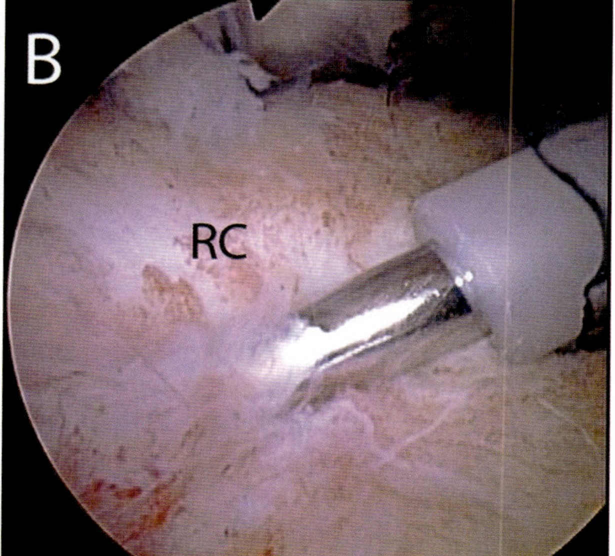

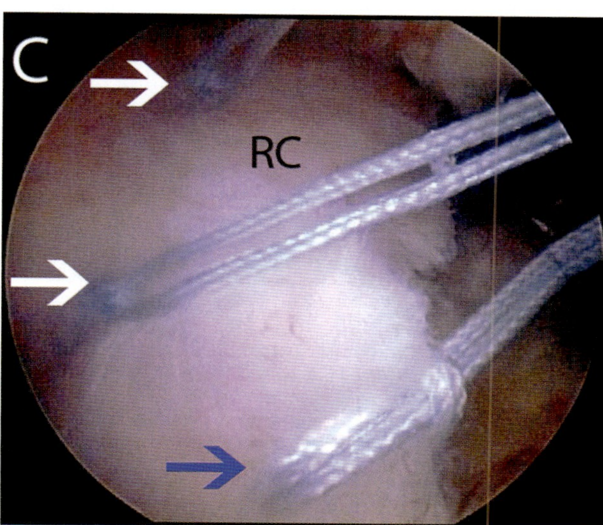

Figure 4.18 Right shoulder, posterior viewing portal. **A, B:** In the standard SutureBridge (Arthrex, Inc., Naples, FL) technique, medial mattress knots are tied after sutures are passed from two medial anchors. **C:** Appearance after medial mattress stitches (*white arrow*) have been tied. In this case, a FiberLink (Arthrex, Inc., Naples, FL) was also placed posteriorly (*blue arrow*) for dog-ear reduction during lateral-row fixation. RC, rotator cuff.

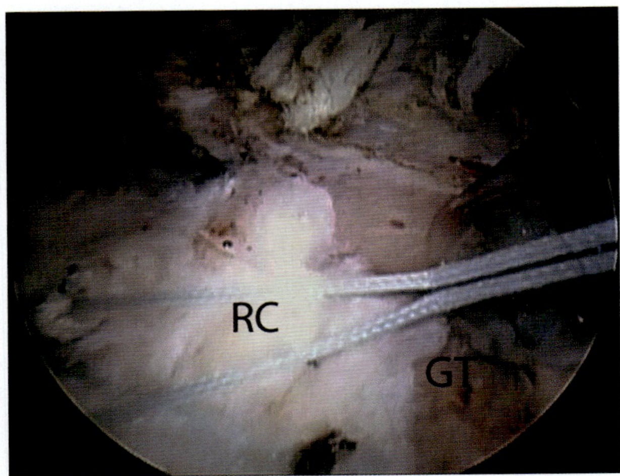

Figure 4.19 Right shoulder, posterior subacromial viewing portal, demonstrates use of a cannula as a guide, with tensioning of the sutures within the cannula, to determine the position of a lateral anchor. GT, greater tuberosity; RC, rotator cuff.

rather than passing each suture limb individually, all four sutures from a single anchor are shuttled through the rotator cuff in one pass with a FiberLink suture loop. The free end of the FiberLink suture is loaded onto a Scorpion (Fig. 4.23A), inserted through a lateral working portal, and passed through the rotator cuff (Fig. 4.23B). This free end is retrieved out an anterior portal while the looped end is held outside the lateral portal (Fig. 4.23C). The sutures from the anteromedial anchor are retrieved out the lateral portal and threaded through the looped end of the FiberLink (Fig. 4.23D). Then, by pulling the free end the FiberLink (Fig. 4.23E), these sutures are shuttled through the rotator cuff (Fig. 4.23F). This step is repeated for the sutures from the posteromedial anchor. To shuttle the suture from the posteromedial anchor, we often retrieve the closed end of the FiberLink out the same percutaneous portal used for anchor placement so that there will be a less acute angle of pull and less chance of the sutures cutting the tendon (by means of a cheese-cutter effect) as they are shuttled through.

A double-pulley technique is then used to tie double medial mattress stitches between the two medial anchors. A suture limb of the same color is retrieved from both the anteromedial anchor and posteromedial anchor (Fig. 4.24A,B). Extracorporeally, a Surgeon's knot is tied over an instrument (Fig. 4.24C). The knot security is checked by pulling on the sutures beneath the knot to ensure that the knot does not slide (Fig. 4.24D). The suture limbs are then cut above the knot. The knot is delivered into the subacromial space and seated onto the rotator cuff by pulling on the opposite ends of the sutures that exit through percutaneous portals used for anchor placement (Fig. 4.24E). Then, the opposite ends of the suture limbs are retrieved and the double mattress stitch is completed by tying a static knot in the subacromial space with a Surgeon's Sixth Finger Knot Pusher (Fig. 4.24F). The suture limbs from this knot are cut. The steps are repeated with the opposite colored suture limbs. With the knots from this second double-pulley construct, however, the suture limbs are

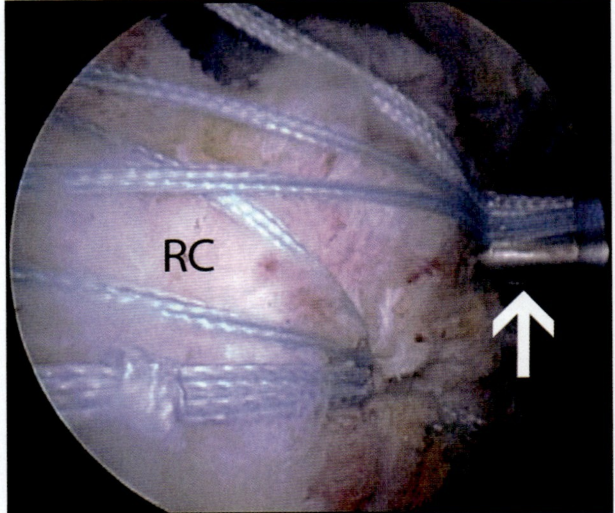

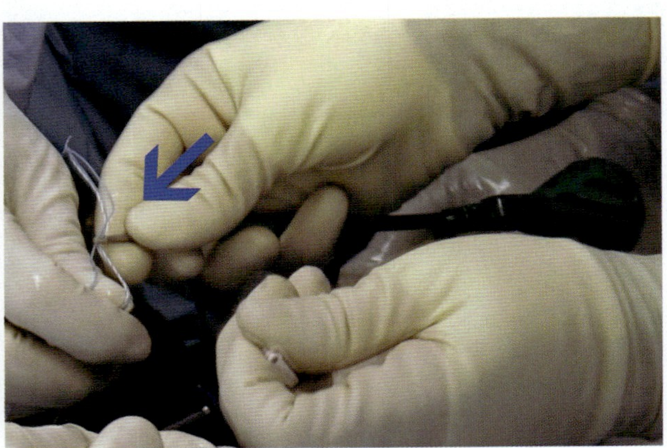

Figure 4.20 Right shoulder, posterior subacromial viewing portal, demonstrates lateral anchor placement for a SutureBridge (Arthrex, Inc., Naples, FL) rotator cuff repair. **A:** A posterolateral anchor has previously been placed. The remaining suture limbs from the anteromedial and posteromedial anchors, as well as an anterior FiberLink (Arthrex, Inc., Naples, FL) placed for dog-ear reduction, have been retrieved out a lateral subacromial portal. A punch (*white arrow*) is inserted through this portal and used to create a bone socket for an anterolateral anchor. **B:** The suture limbs are threaded through the eyelet (*blue arrow*) of a BioComposite SwiveLock anchor.

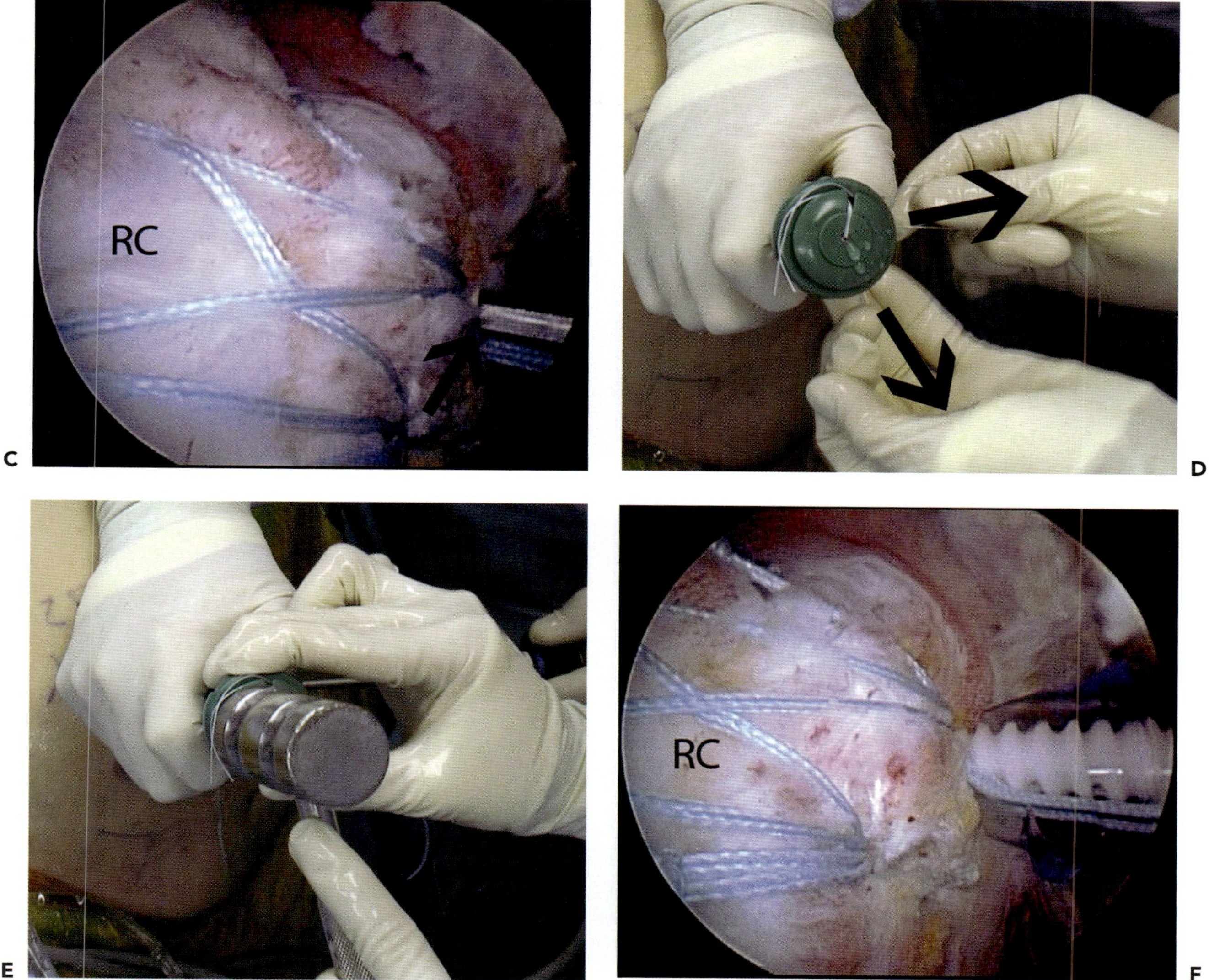

Figure 4.20 (*Continued*) **C:** The eyelet of the anchor is seated into the prepared bone socket. **D:** Prior to advancing the eyelet, an assistant individually tensions the suture limbs (*black arrows*). **E:** The eyelet is advanced manually, or by gently impacting the inserter handle as in this case, until **(F)** the anchor just contacts the bone. Then, the anchor is screwed into the desired depth. RC, rotator cuff.

preserved so that they can be incorporated into a lateral-row repair.

Lateral anchor placement then proceeds exactly as described for the standard SutureBridge repair. The final repair is not only a transosseous equivalent repair, but also provides a medial seal from the joint via the medial double mattress stitch (Fig. 4.25).

Diamondback SutureBridge Transosseous Equivalent

Although most suture bridge transosseous equivalent repairs utilize only one pair of sutures from each anchor medially and two lateral-row knotless anchors, the technique may be altered to improve biomechanical fixation.

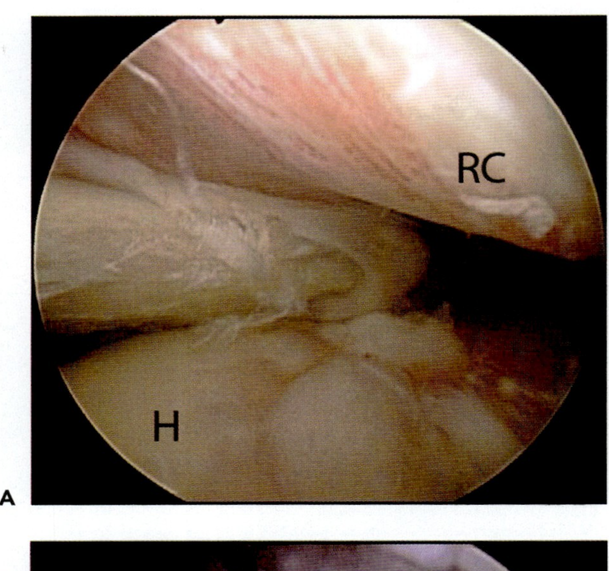

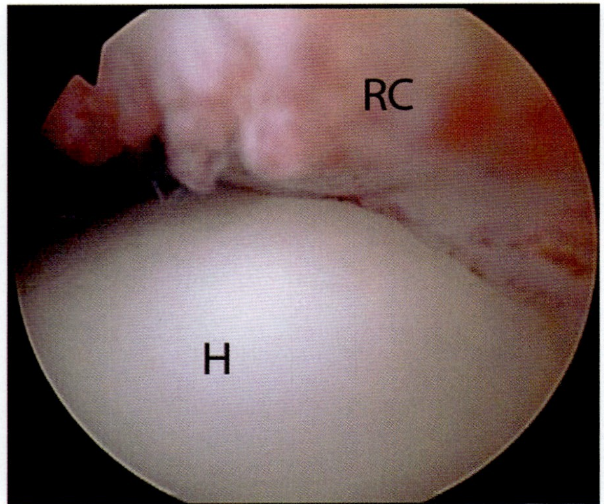

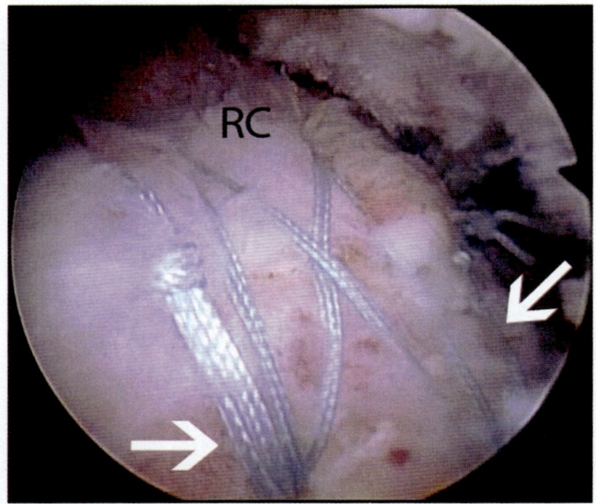

Figure 4.21 Completed SutureBridge (Arthrex, Inc., Naples, FL) rotator cuff repair in a right shoulder. **A:** Posterior glenohumeral viewing portal of the rotator cuff tear prior to repair. **B:** Same shoulder and view postrepair demonstrates medial footprint restoration. **C:** Lateral subacromial viewing portal demonstrates the SutureBridge repair. Suture limbs from anteromedial and posteromedial anchors have been crisscrossed and secured laterally with two anchors. In addition, FiberLink cinch-loop stitches (*white arrows*) have been used posteriorly and anteriorly to prevent dog-ears. H, humerus; RC, rotator cuff.

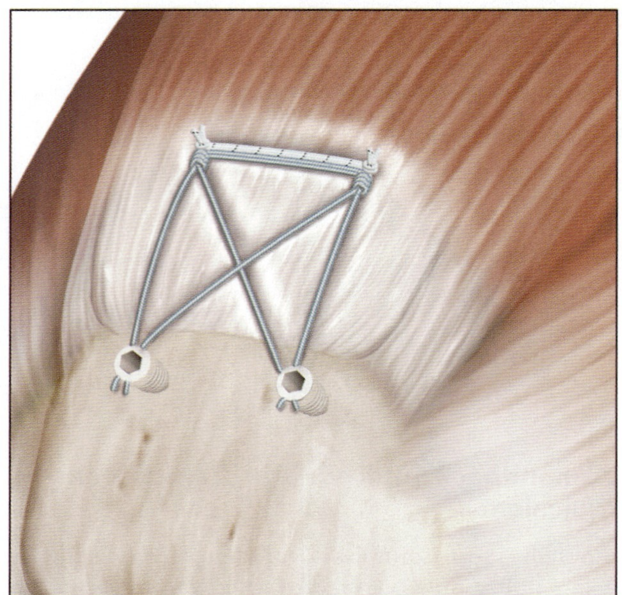

Figure 4.22 Schematic of a SutureBridge (Arthrex, Inc., Naples, FL) rotator cuff repair with medial mattress stitches that have been tied using a double-pulley technique. This variation on the standard SutureBridge repair creates a medial seal from the degradative enzymes in the glenohumeral joint.

In essence, this technique may be modified to utilize multiple anchors and sutures medially and multiple anchors and sutures laterally according to the tear size and tear configuration at hand. Furthermore, the number of sutures incorporated into each anchor laterally may be varied (one to four sutures) to provide complete lateral fixation and footprint compression.

In a large crescent-shaped tear, two medial anchors are utilized and sutures are passed in a mattress fashion 2 to 3 mm lateral to the musculotendinous junction (Figs. 4.26 and 4.27). However, due to the larger size of this tear, three anchors will be utilized laterally using varying number of sutures. Starting anterolaterally, three sutures are retrieved to secure the anterolateral cuff (Fig. 4.28A), two sutures are retrieved to secure the midlateral cuff (Fig. 4.28B) and three sutures are retrieved to secure the posterolateral cuff (Fig. 4.28C).

Final evaluation of the construct demonstrates secure tendon fixation, footprint reconstruction and a diamond-back appearance of the spanning sutures (Fig. 4.29).

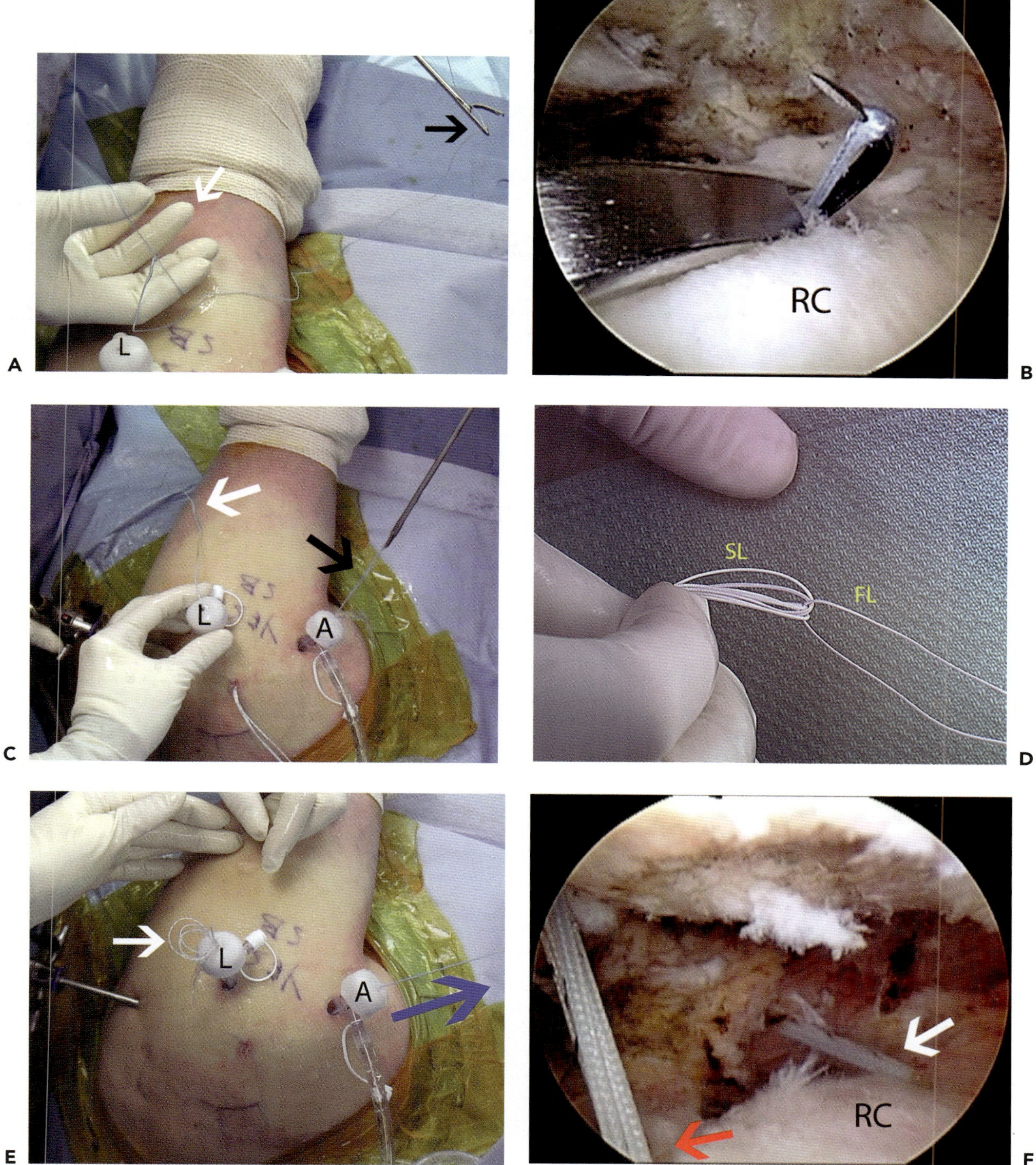

Figure 4.23 Left shoulder demonstrating use a FiberLink (Arthrex, Inc., Naples, FL) to shuttle sutures through the rotator cuff. **A:** FiberLink has a looped end (*white arrow*) and a closed end. The closed end of a FiberLink suture is loaded onto a Scorpion (*black arrow*). **B:** Posterior subacromial viewing portal, demonstrates passage of the free end of a FiberLink through the rotator cuff. **C:** The closed end of a FiberLink (*black arrow*) has been passed through the rotator cuff and is retrieved out an anterior portal. The closed end is kept in a different portal from the one used for passing (*white arrow*). **D:** The suture limbs from a previously placed medial anchor are retrieved out the same portal used for passing the FiberLink. Then, extracorporeally the suture limbs (SL) are threaded through the looped end of the FiberLink (FL). **E:** Pulling on the closed end of the FiberLink (*blue arrow*) shuttles the suture limbs (*white arrow*) through the rotator cuff. **F:** Posterior viewing portal demonstrates sutures from an anteromedial anchor (*white arrow*) that have been shuttled through the rotator cuff using the Fiberlink loop. Sutures from a posteromedial anchor (*red arrow*) are also visible and will be shuttled with the same technique through a different spot in the rotator cuff. A, anterior portal; L, lateral portal; RC, rotator cuff.

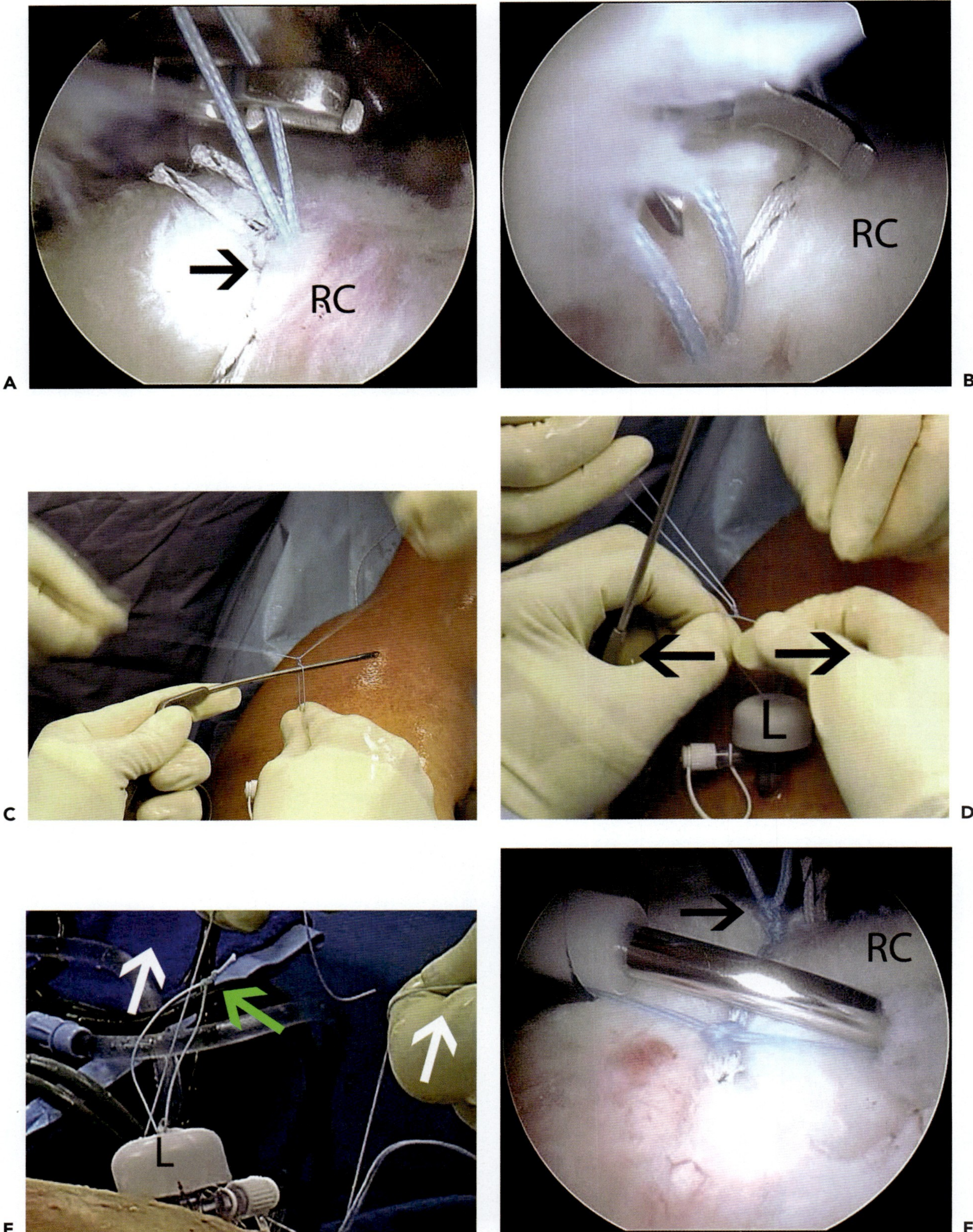

Figure 4.24 Left shoulder demonstrates the double-pulley technique for medial knot tying. **A:** While viewing from a posterior subacromial portal, a suture limb is retrieved from the anteromedial anchor. The *black arrow* points to a TigerWire (Arthrex, Inc., Naples, FL) mattress stitch previously tied with a double-pulley technique. **B:** A suture of the same color is retrieved from the posteromedial anchor. **C:** Extracorporeally, a static knot is tied over an instrument. **D:** The security of the knot is checked by pulling the loop (*black arrows*). **E:** The externally tied knot (*green arrow*) is delivered into the subacromial space by pulling on the opposite suture limbs (*white arrows*). Pulling the opposite suture limbs uses the eyelets of the two medial anchors as pulleys, thus the phrase double pulley. **F:** The mattress knot is completed by tying a static knot between the opposite suture limbs using a Surgeon's Sixth Finger Knot Pusher (Arthrex, Inc., Naples, FL). Note: Because the externally tied suture was brought down anteriorly (*black arrow*) over the rotator cuff, the second knot is tied to lie down posteriorly. L, lateral portal; RC, rotator cuff.

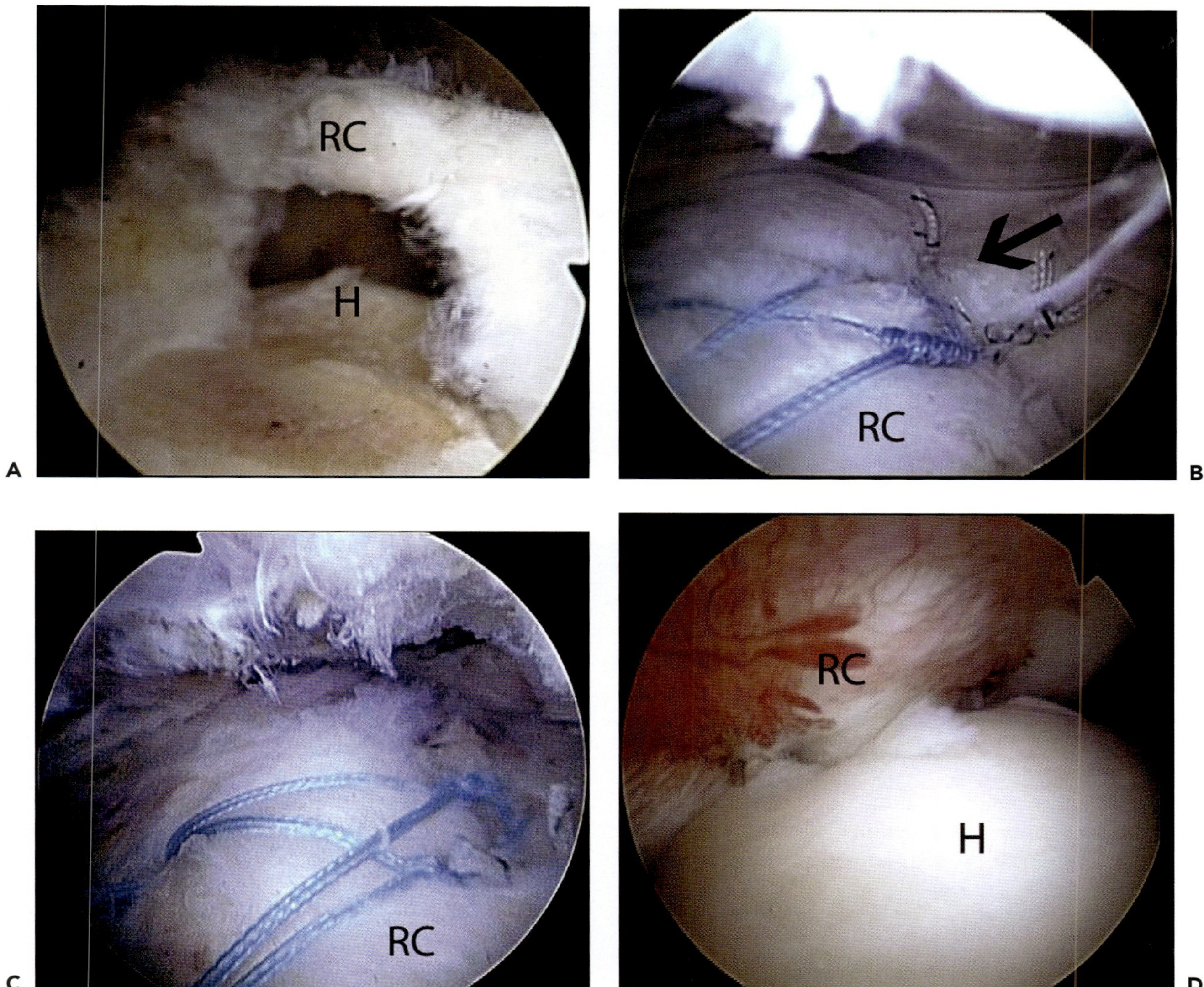

Figure 4.25 Left shoulder demonstrates repair of a crescent-shaped rotator cuff tear with a SutureBridge (Arthrex, Inc., Naples, FL) and medial double-pulley technique. **A:** Prerepair view from a lateral subacromial portal. **B:** Postrepair view from a posterior subacromial portal demonstrates the SutureBridge repair and an up-close view of the medial mattress stitches (*black arrow*). **C:** Profile view from a posterior subacromial viewing portal demonstrates crisscrossed sutures that have been secured laterally with knotless anchors. **D:** Intra-articular view of the repair from a posterior glenohumeral portal demonstrates restoration of the medial rotator cuff footprint. H, humerus; RC, rotator cuff.

SpeedBridge Transosseous Equivalent Double-row Rotator Cuff Repair

The SpeedBridge technique is a double-row variant of the SpeedFix FiberTape repair. This is a knotless repair that utilizes two BioComposite SwiveLock C anchors medially and two BioComposite SwiveLock C anchors laterally with FiberTape linking the two rows of anchors (Fig. 4.30). Similar to the SutureBridge technique, a double-pulley technique can also be added medially using the safety stitches from the SwiveLock C anchors (Fig. 4.31). Following bone bed preparation, an anteromedial bone socket is prepared adjacent to the articular margin for a SwiveLock C anchor (Fig. 4.32A). A SwiveLock C anchor is preloaded with FiberTape suture (Fig. 4.32B) and is placed through the same percutaneous portal used for punch insertion (Fig. 4.32C). The eyelet is seated until the anchor just contacts the bone. While holding the thumb pad of the inserter, the screwdriver handle is turned to advance the screw into the bone socket (Fig. 4.32D). Because the inserter sheath is flush with the anchor, the sheath must be backed off to confirm the depth of insertion. This is accomplished by holding the screwdriver handle and turning the thumb pad clockwise (Figs. 4.32E,F).

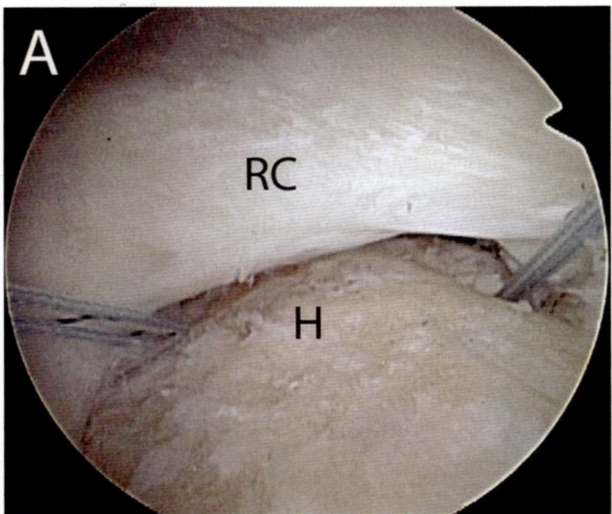

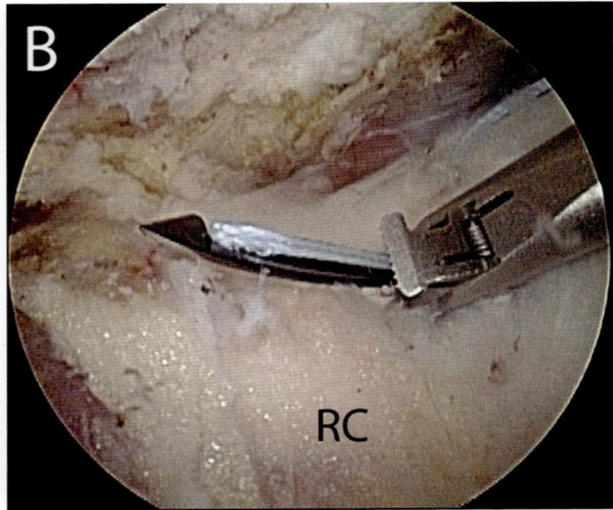

Figure 4.26 **A:** Right shoulder, lateral subacromial viewing portal, demonstrates a large crescent-shaped rotator cuff tear. Two medial anchors have been placed in preparation for a diamondback repair. **B:** Each suture limb from the medial anchors is individually passed through the rotator cuff 2 to 3 mm lateral to the musculotendinous junction. H, humerus; RC, rotator cuff.

A posteromedial anchor is then inserted in the same fashion (Fig. 4.33). A free FiberLink suture is used to shuttle the FiberTape and the FiberWire safety sutures through the rotator cuff. While viewing from a posterior portal, a Scorpion is used to pass the closed end of a FiberLink through the anteromedial rotator cuff, 2 to 3 mm lateral to the musculotendinous junction. The free end of the FiberLink is retrieved through an accessory portal while the looped end is kept out the lateral portal. Then, the FiberTape and FiberWire safety sutures from the anteromedial anchor are retrieved out the lateral portal and passed through the looped end of the FiberLink. The FiberTape is then shuttled through the rotator cuff by pulling the closed end of the FiberLink. This sequence is then repeated for the posteromedial anchor sutures (Fig. 4.34).

In most cases, prior to obtaining lateral fixation, we prefer to tie medial mattress stitches with a double-pulley technique using the #2 FiberWire safety eyelet sutures from the SwiveLock anchors (Fig. 4.35). This medial mattress stitch provides a medial seal between the glenohumeral joint and the rotator cuff.

Once the medial sutures have been placed, the anterior and posterior margins of the tear are assessed for the potential for dog ears following lateral-row fixation. If this is anticipated, FiberLink sutures can be used to create cinch loops at the apex of each dog ear as previously described (Chapter 2, "Philosophy of Rotator Cuff Repair") (Fig. 4.36).

To complete the repair, the FiberTape limbs are crisscrossed and secured laterally with two additional SwiveLock anchors (Fig. 4.37). A suture limb from the anteromedial anchor and a suture limb from the posteromedial anchor are retrieved out a lateral portal. While maintaining tension on the suture limbs, the lateral cannula is used to determine the appropriate position for an anterolateral anchor. A punch is inserted to create a bone socket, the FiberTape is threaded through the eyelet of a BioComposite SwiveLock C anchor, the anchor is inserted, and the sutures are cut flush with the anchor. The remaining FiberTape suture limbs are retrieved and the steps are repeated with a posterolateral anchor. The final repair is observed subacromially and intra-articularly (Fig. 4.38).

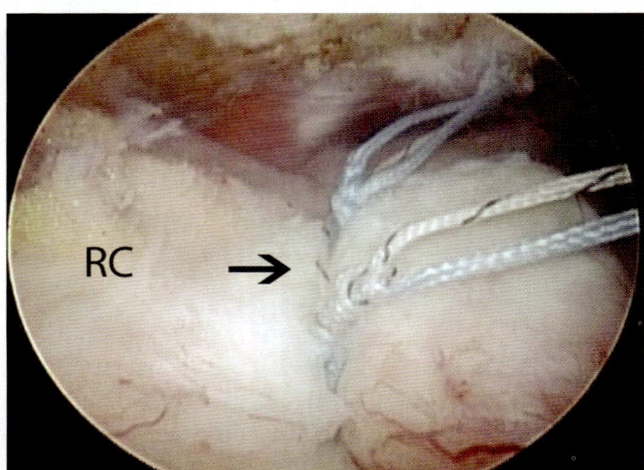

Figure 4.27 Right shoulder, posterior subacromial viewing portal, demonstrates appearance after all medial knots have been tied for a diamondback repair. Note: A static bridging mattress knot (*black arrow*) has been tied between the anteromedial and posteromedial anchors. All eight sutures will be incorporated into a lateral repair using three anchors (Fig. 4.28). RC, rotator cuff.

(Text continued on page 59)

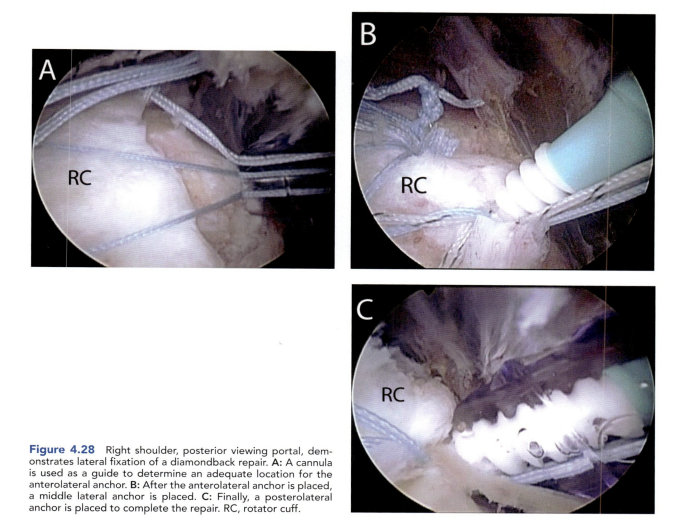

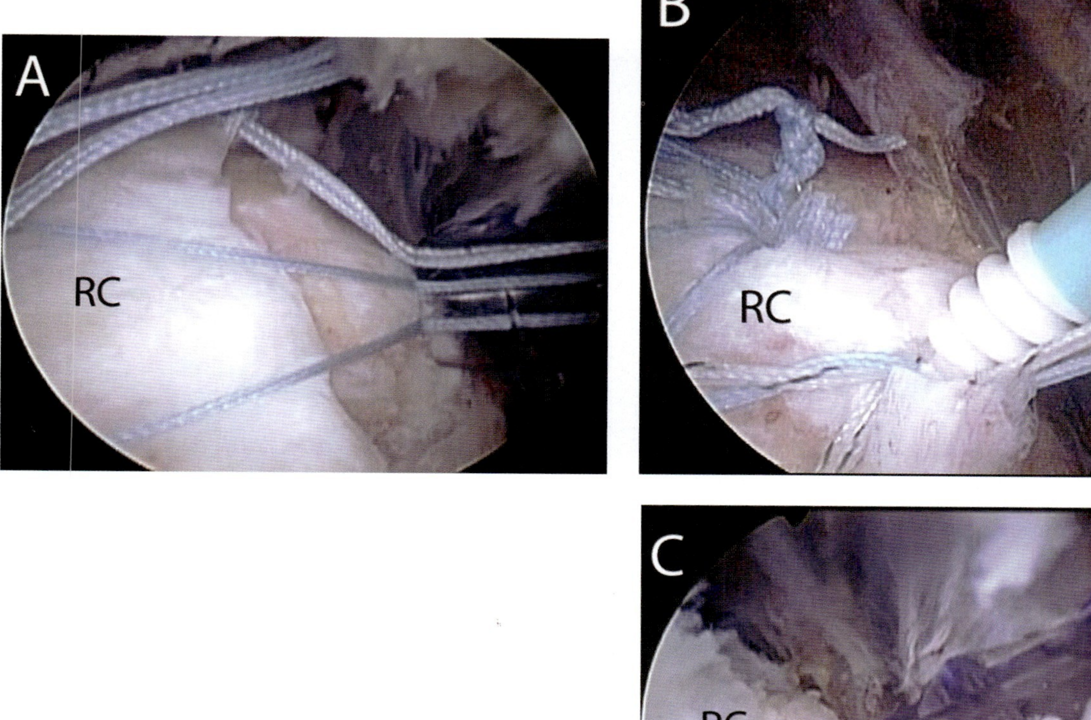

Figure 4.28 Right shoulder, posterior viewing portal, demonstrates lateral fixation of a diamondback repair. **A:** A cannula is used as a guide to determine an adequate location for the anterolateral anchor. **B:** After the anterolateral anchor is placed, a middle lateral anchor is placed. **C:** Finally, a posterolateral anchor is placed to complete the repair. RC, rotator cuff.

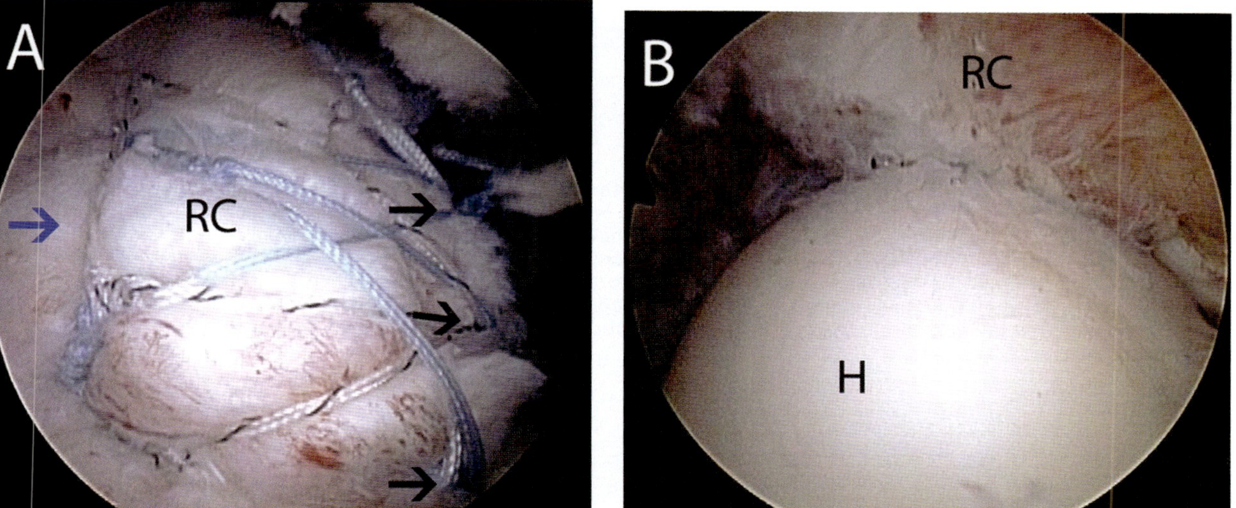

Figure 4.29 **A:** Right shoulder, posterior subacromial viewing portal demonstrates final appearance after a diamondback repair. Medially, multiple knots have been tied, including a static bridging mattress knot between the two medial anchors (*blue arrow*). Laterally, the suture limbs have been secured with three anchors (*black arrows*) to provide maximal footprint compression. B: Final repair viewed from a posterior glenohumeral portal. H, humerus; RC, rotator cuff.

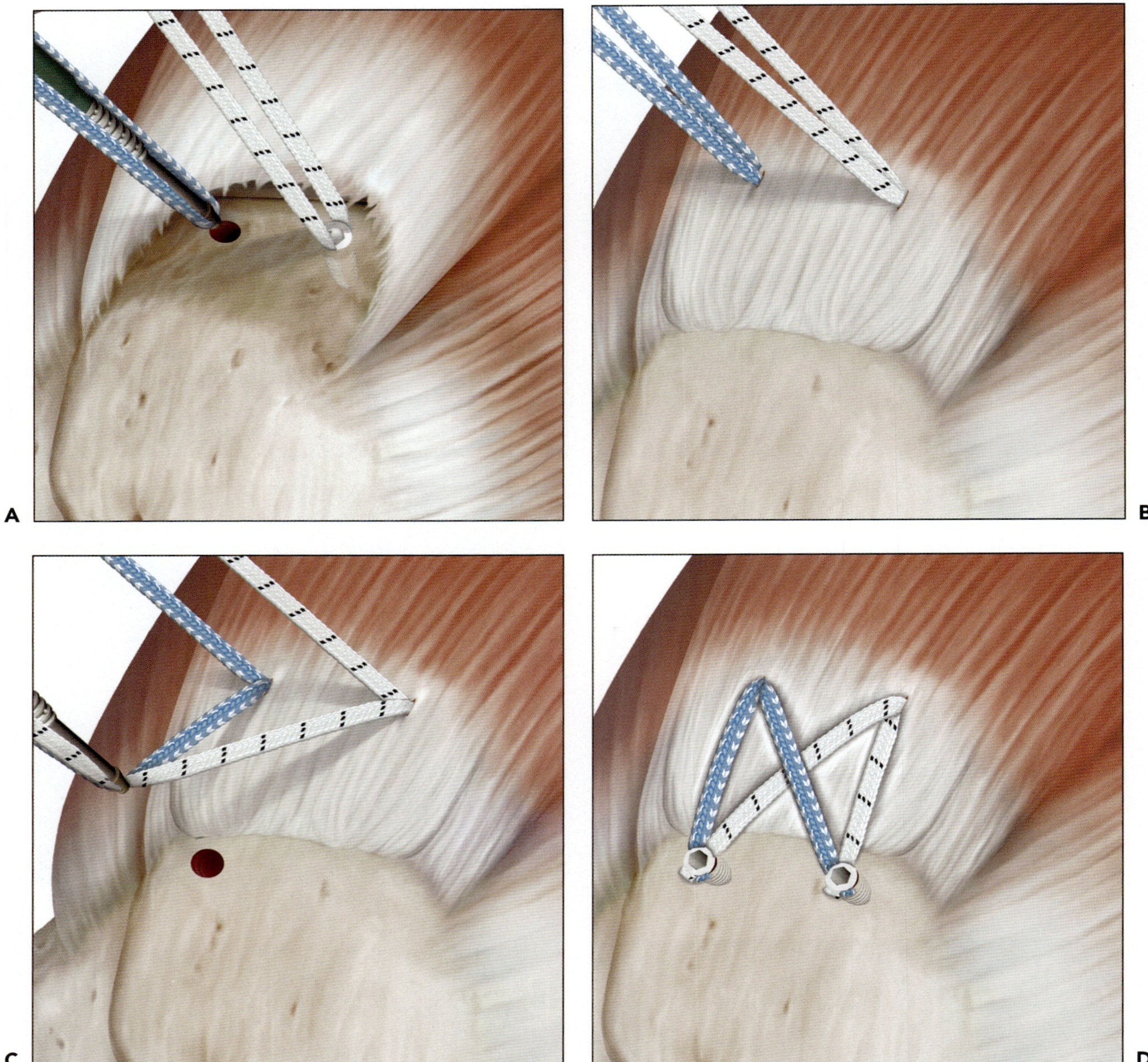

Figure 4.30 Schematic of a SpeedBridge (Arthrex, Inc., Naples, FL) rotator cuff repair. **A:** Two BioComposite SwiveLock C anchors preloaded with FiberTape are placed medially adjacent to the articular margin. **B:** The FiberTape sutures have been shuttled through the rotator cuff with a FiberLink. Alternatively, the preloaded FiberTape with a merged FiberWire leader between the two ends of the tape can be passed with a Scorpion suture passer, achieving passage of both tails of the FiberTape simultaneously. **C:** The medial FiberTape suture limbs are crisscrossed and secured laterally with two BioComposite SwiveLock C anchors. **D:** Final construct of this knotless rotator cuff repair.

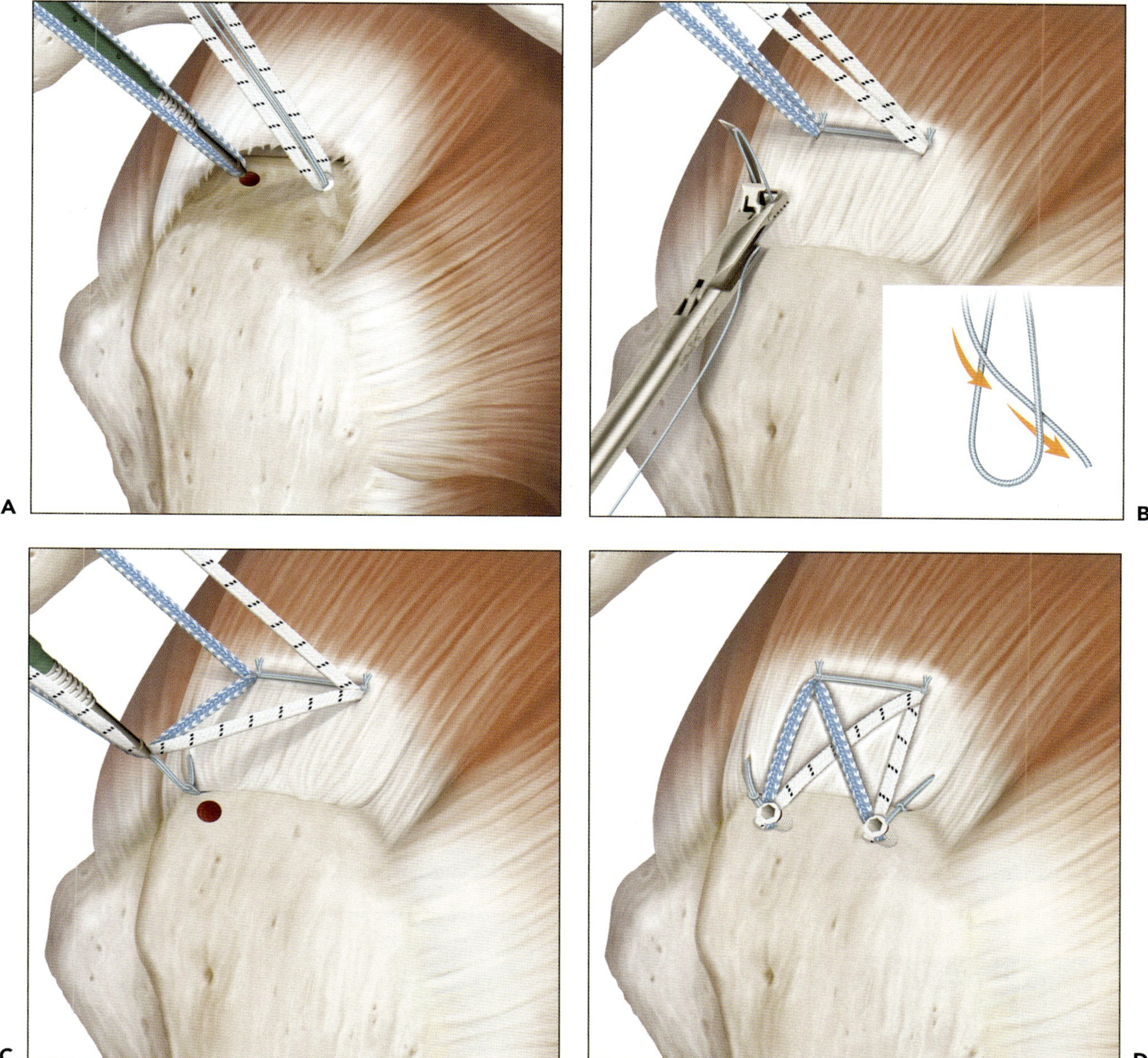

Figure 4.31 Schematic of a SpeedBridge (Arthrex, Inc., Naples, FL) rotator cuff repair with medial double-pulley and dog-ear reduction. **A:** Two medial anchors are placed for a SpeedBridge repair. **B:** Medial sutures are passed through the rotator cuff in a single pass using a FiberLink (Arthrex, Inc., Naples, FL). Then, a mattress stitch is tied between the two anchors using the #2 FiberWire eyelet safety stitches with a double-pulley technique. The FiberLink can then be used for dog-ear reduction. The closed end of the FiberLink is passed through the rotator cuff at the margin of the tear and is retrieved out the same portal as used for insertion. Inset: Extracorporeally, the closed end of the FiberLink is passed through the looped end to create a cinch loop. **C:** The cinch loop, a suture from the anteromedial anchor, and a suture from the posteromedial anchor are secured laterally with a BioComposite SwiveLock C anchor. **D:** Final appearance after placement of a posterior FiberLink and a posterolateral anchor.

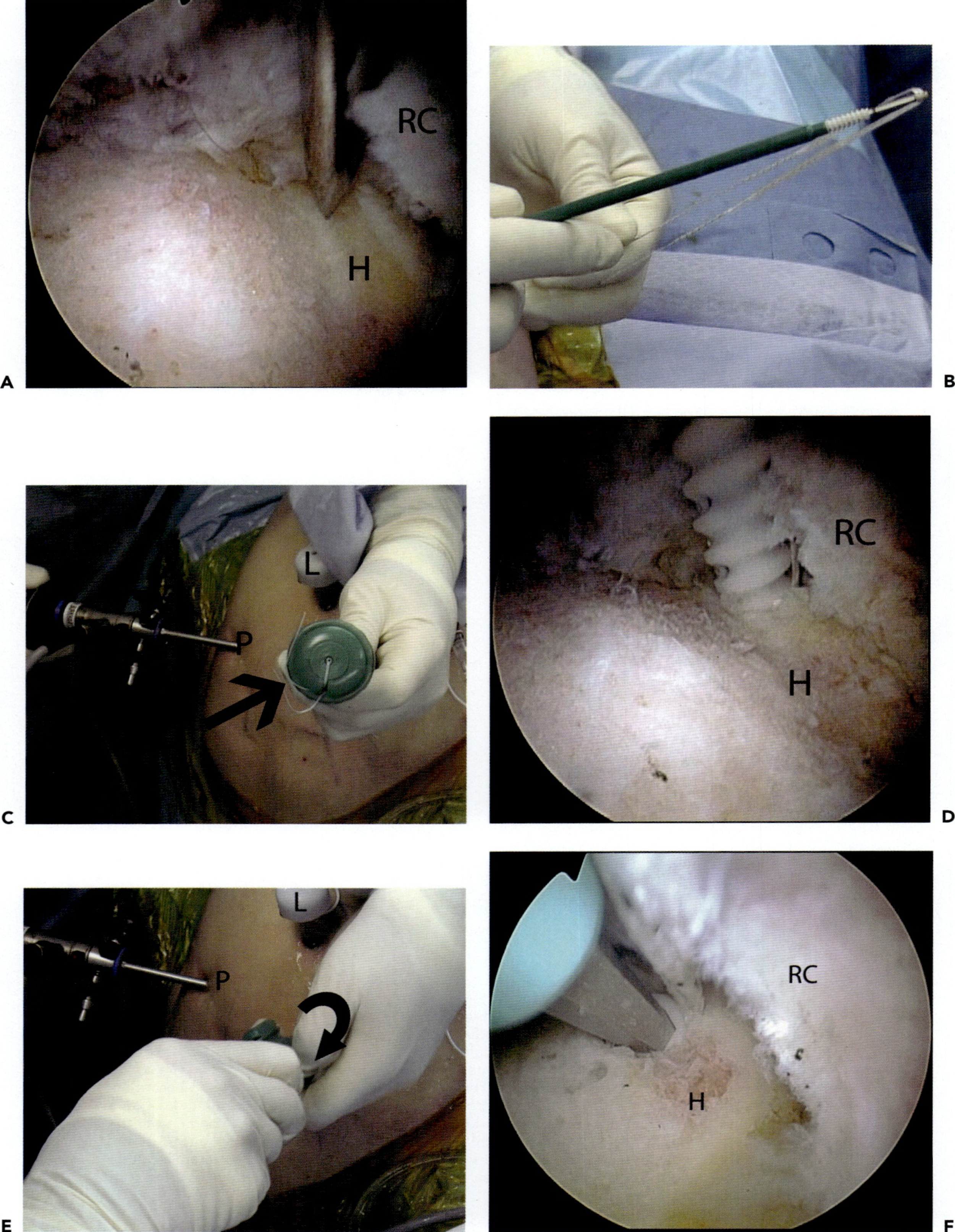

Figure 4.32 Left shoulder, demonstrates placement of an anteromedial anchor for a SpeedBridge (Arthrex, Inc., Naples, FL) rotator cuff repair. **A:** Viewing from a posterior subacromial portal, a punch is used to create a bone socket for an anteromedial anchor. **B:** A BioComposite SwiveLock C anchor is preloaded with FiberTape suture. **C:** The anchor is inserted (*black arrow*) into the subacromial space using the same percutaneous portal used to create the bone socket. **D:** After the eyelet is completely seated, the anchor is screwed into place. **E:** After the anchor is screwed into place, the depth of insertion is checked by backing off the inserter. This is accomplished by holding the driver handle, while the thumb pad is turned clockwise (*curved black arrow*). **F:** Arthroscopic view demonstrates checking anchor insertion depth by backing of the inserter. H, humerus; L, lateral portal; P, posterior portal; RC, rotator cuff.

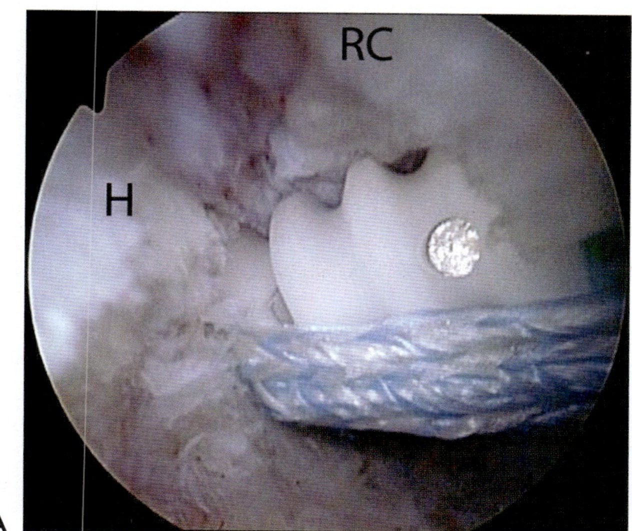

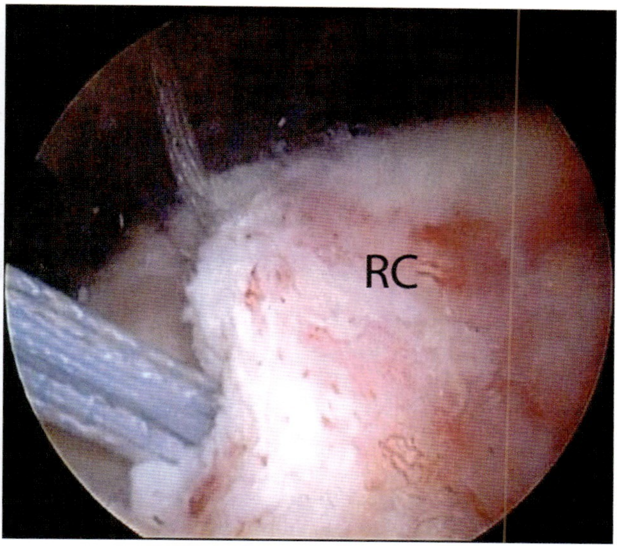

Figure 4.33 **A:** Left shoulder, lateral subacromial viewing portal, demonstrates placement of a posteromedial anchor for a SpeedBridge (Arthrex, Inc., Naples, FL) rotator cuff repair. **B:** Posterior subacromial viewing portal in the same shoulder demonstrates appearance after placement of both an anteromedial and a posteromedial anchor. H, humerus; RC, rotator cuff.

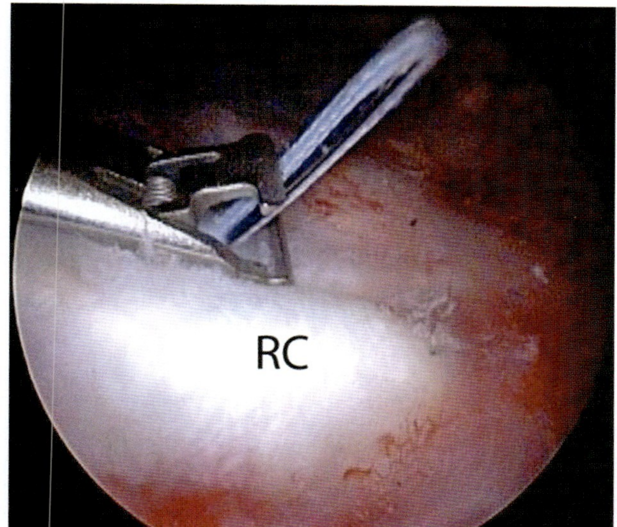

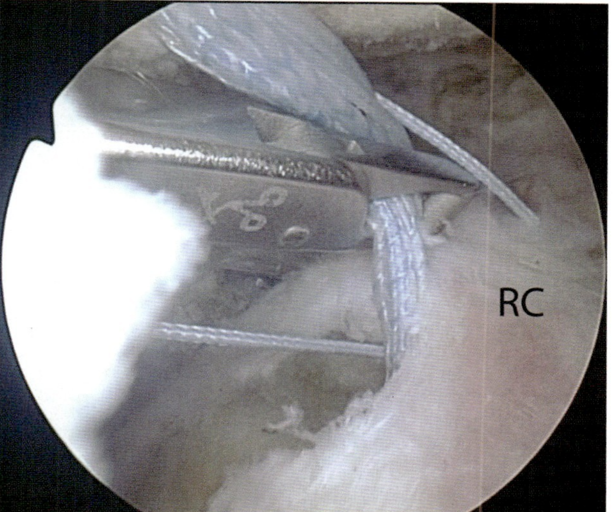

Figure 4.34 Left shoulder, posterior subacromial viewing portal, demonstrates medial suture passage for a SpeedBridge (Arthrex, Inc., Naples, FL) rotator cuff repair. **A:** The free end of a FiberLink suture is passed through the rotator cuff, 2 to 3 mm lateral to the musculotendinous junction. **B:** The free end of the suture is retrieved out an anterior portal, while the looped end is maintained in a lateral portal. FiberTape sutures and FiberWire safety sutures from the anteromedial anchor are then retrieved out the lateral portal with a FiberTape suture retriever (Arthrex, Inc., Naples, FL).

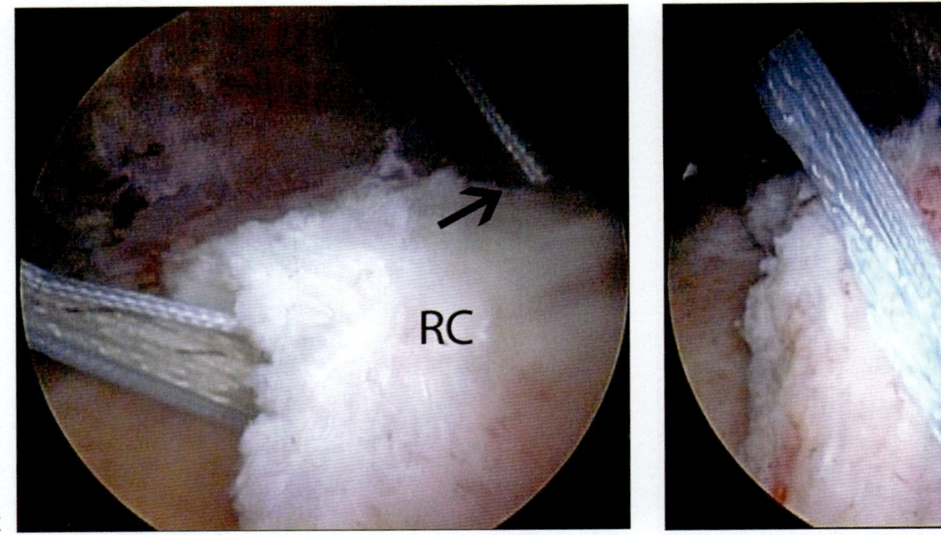

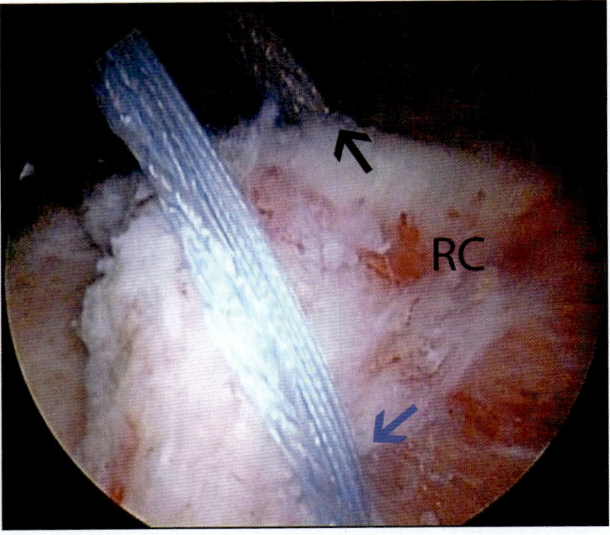

Figure 4.34 (*Continued*) **C:** Appearance prior to shuttling demonstrates the free end of the FiberLink that has been retrieved out an anterior portal (*black arrow*). Extracorporeally, the FiberTape and FiberWire sutures will be threaded through the looped end of the FiberLink suture in order to shuttle them through the rotator cuff. **D:** Appearance after the anteromedial sutures (*black arrow*) and posteromedial sutures (*blue arrow*) have been shuttled through the rotator cuff. RC, rotator cuff.

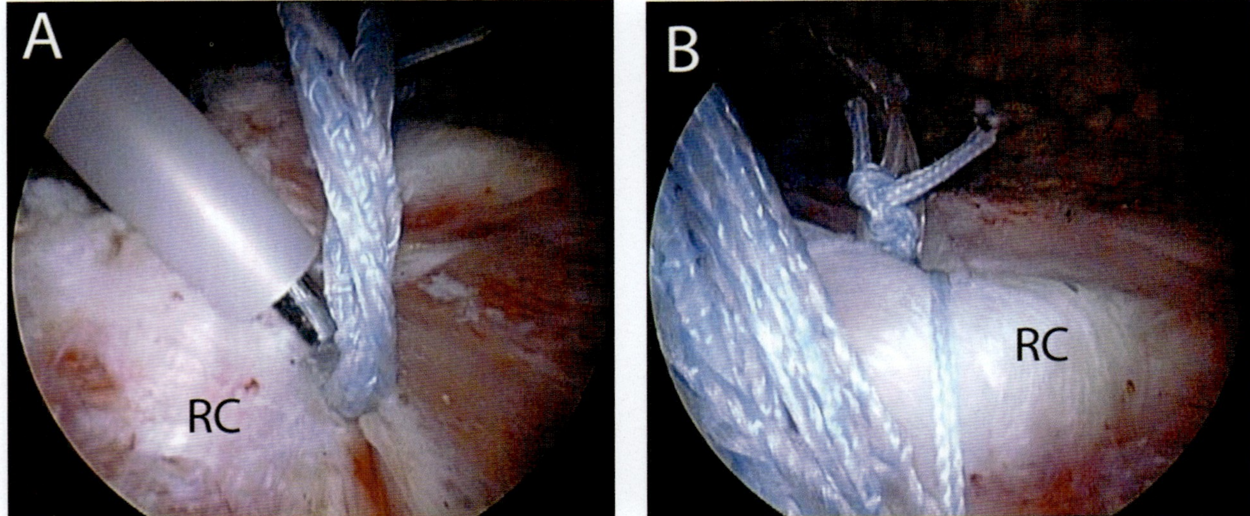

Figure 4.35 Left shoulder, posterior subacromial viewing portal, demonstrates **(A)** knot tying for a medial mattress suture using the #2 FiberWire (Arthrex, Inc., Naples, FL) eyelet safety stitches from a SwiveLock C anchor (Arthrex, Inc.). **B:** Appearance after the medial mattress stitch has been tied. RC, rotator cuff.

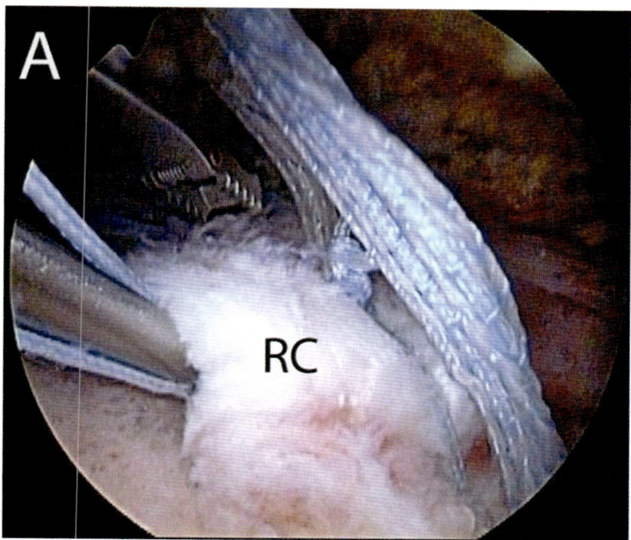

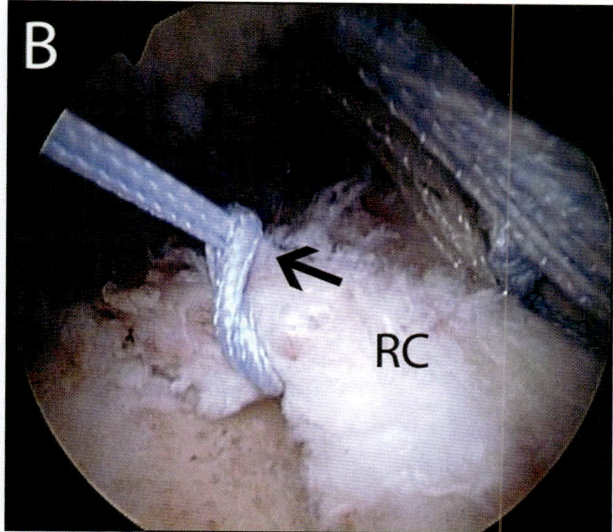

Figure 4.36 Left shoulder, posterior subacromial viewing portal, demonstrates a technique for dog-ear reduction using a FiberLink suture (Arthrex, Inc., Naples, FL). **A:** Prior to securing the lateral row, the free end of the FiberLink is passed through the rotator cuff, anterior to the previously placed sutures. This free end is retrieved out the same portal using for passing, and is threaded through the looped end of the FiberLink to create a cinch loop. **B:** Final view of the cinch loop (*black arrow*) that will prevent dog-ears during lateral-row fixation. RC, rotator cuff.

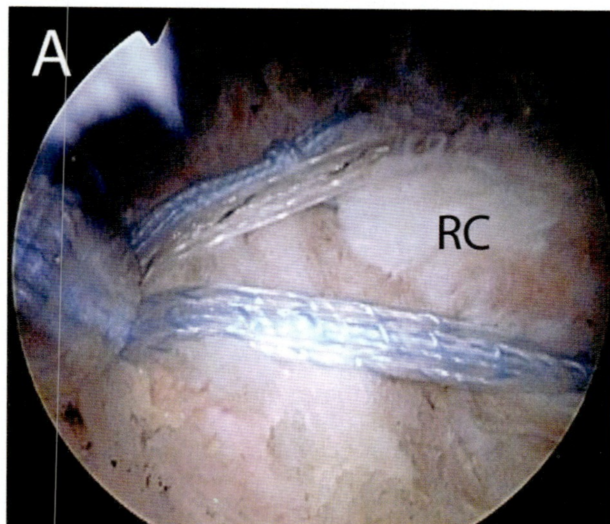

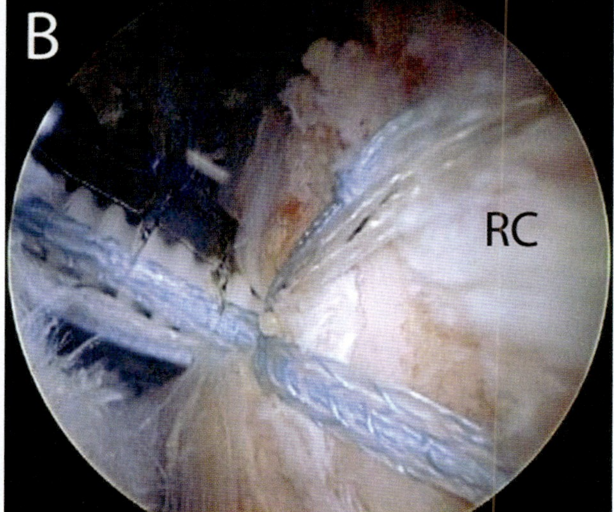

Figure 4.37 Left shoulder, posterior subacromial viewing portal, demonstrates lateral-row fixation for a SpeedBridge (Arthrex, Inc., Naples, FL) rotator cuff repair. **A:** A cannula is used as a guide to determine the proper position for an anterolateral anchor. **B:** Insertion of an anterolateral BioComposite SwiveLock C anchor.

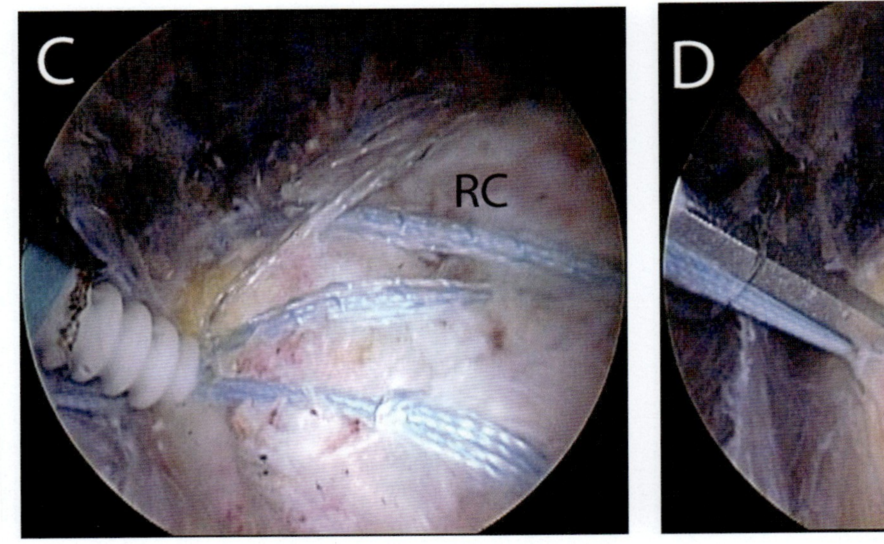

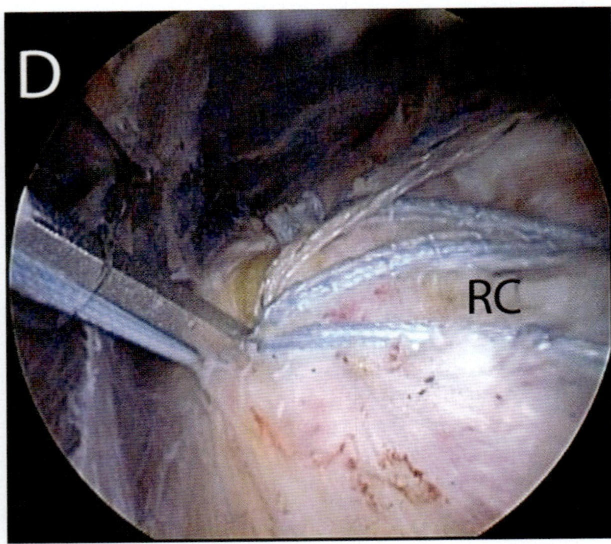

Figure 4.37 (*Continued*) **C:** Insertion of a posterolateral anchor. **D:** The thumb pad on the SwiveLock driver can be unscrewed to confirm that the anchor is fully seated prior to removing the handle. RC, rotator cuff.

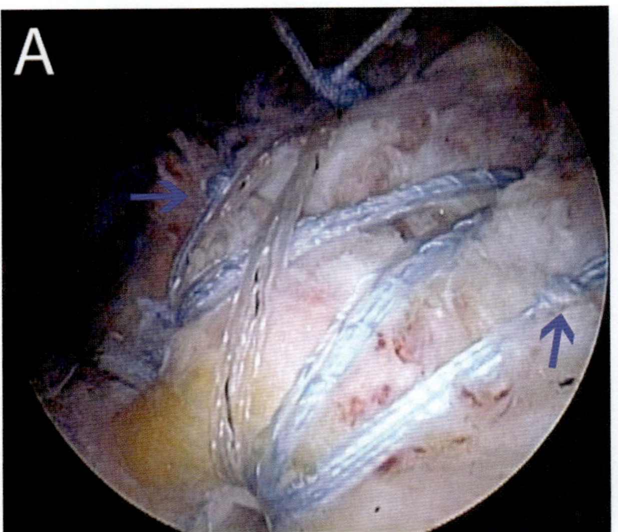

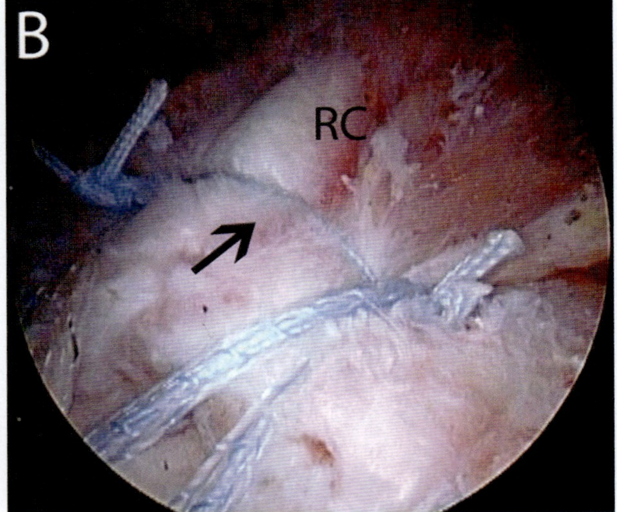

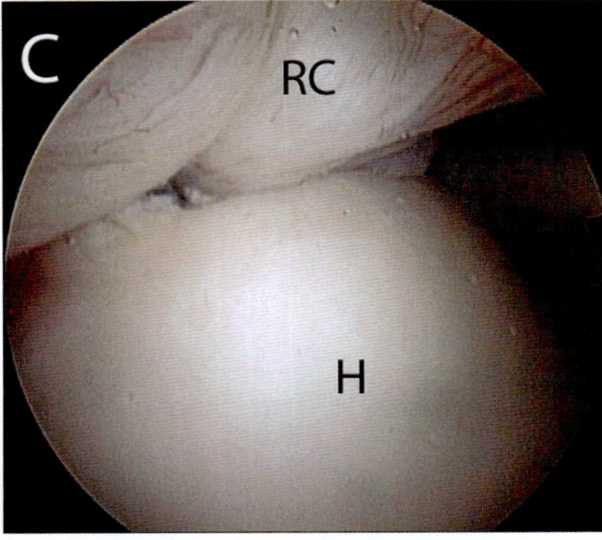

Figure 4.38 Left shoulder demonstrating final appearance of a rotator cuff repair using a SpeedBridge (Arthrex, Inc., Naples, FL) technique. **A:** Posterior subacromial viewing portal demonstrates the double-row repair with FiberTape sutures that crisscross the rotator cuff to provide footprint compression. Cinch-loop sutures (*blue arrows*) are also seen that have been used anteriorly and posteriorly to prevent dog ears. **B:** A close-up demonstrates a medial mattress stitch (*black arrow*) that was tied using a double-pulley technique in order to seal the medial repair. **C:** Intra-articular view from a posterior portal demonstrates restoration of the medial rotator cuff footprint. H, humerus; RC, rotator cuff.

FiberChain Transosseous Equivalent Double-row Rotator Cuff Repair

The double-row SwiveLock-FiberChain system was devised by the senior author (SSB) (Fig. 4.39). This type of repair is indicated in crescent tears and can provide a quick double-row repair. This is particularly useful in patients with multiple comorbidities where anesthesia time and fluid inflow must be minimized; that is, patients in which speed is of the essence. The medial-row anchors are BioComposite Corkscrew FT suture anchors that are preloaded with FiberChain (Arthrex, Inc., Naples, FL). FiberChain is a flexible

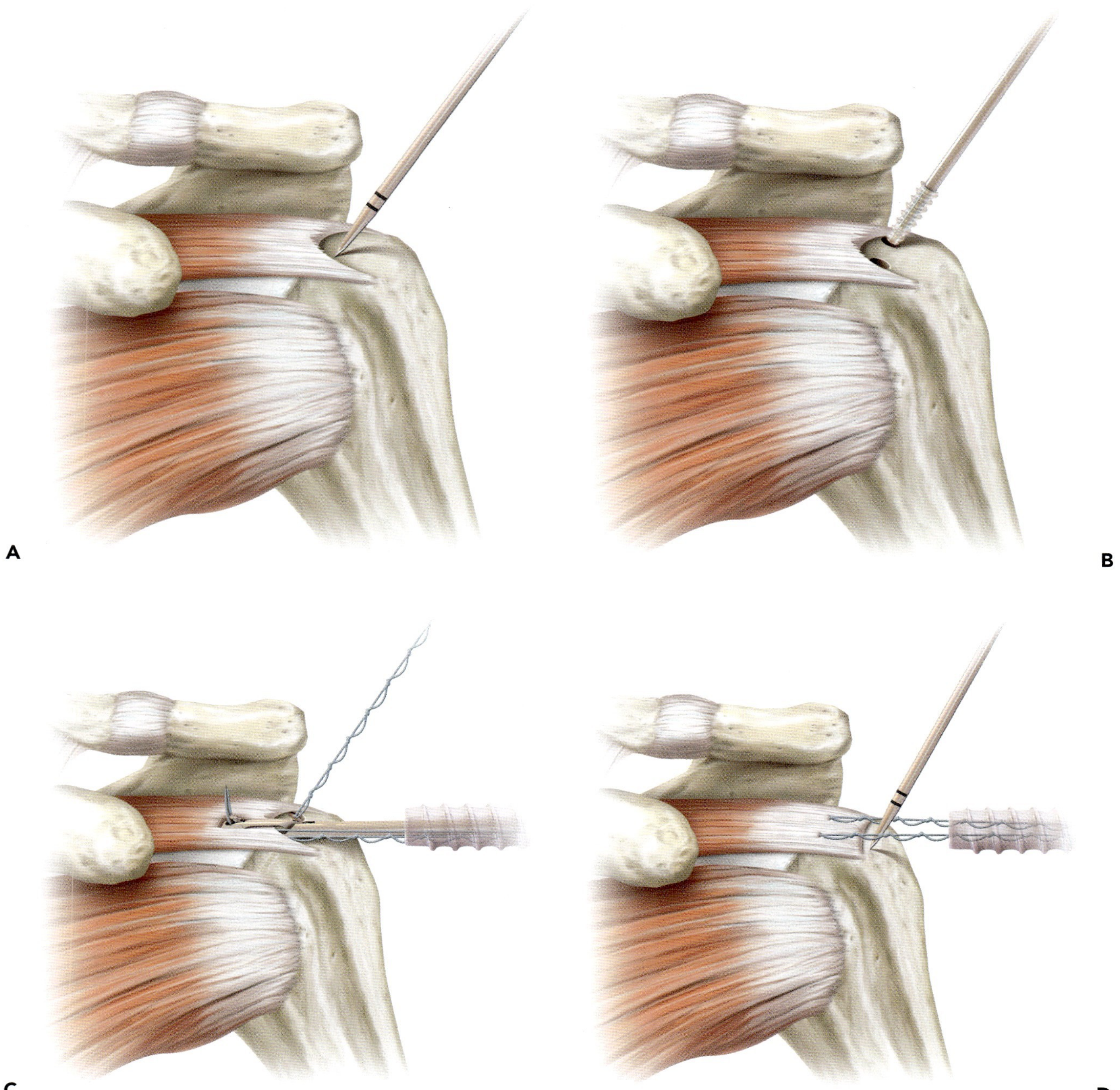

Figure 4.39 Schematic demonstrating SwiveLock-FiberChain (Arthrex, Inc., Naples, FL) repair technique. **A:** A punch is used to create a bone socket for a medial anchor. **B:** A Bio-Corkscrew FT anchor preloaded with FiberChain is inserted into the bone socket. **C:** Two medial anchors have been placed. The FiberChain is passed through the rotator cuff tendon. **D:** The FiberChain is retrieved out a lateral portal and a punch is used to create a bone socket for a lateral anchor.

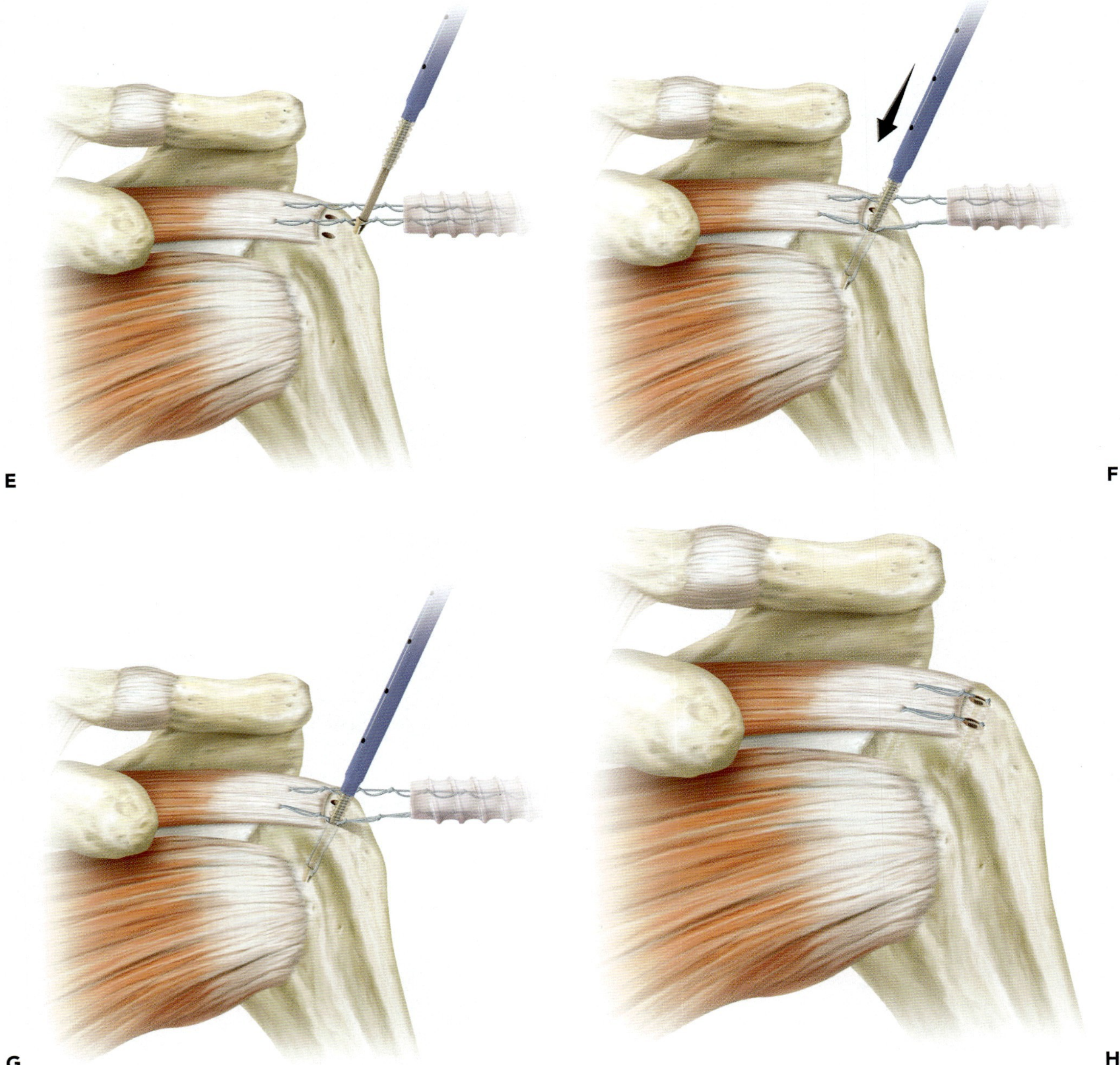

Figure 4.39 (*Continued*) **E:** The forked eyelet tip of a Bio-SwiveLock C anchor captures the second link from the lateral edge of the torn rotator cuff. **F:** The eyelet of the anchor is seated until the anchor is just in contact with the bone. **G:** The SwiveLock anchor is advanced by screwing it into the bone socket. **H:** Final repair of this knotless linked double-row repair.

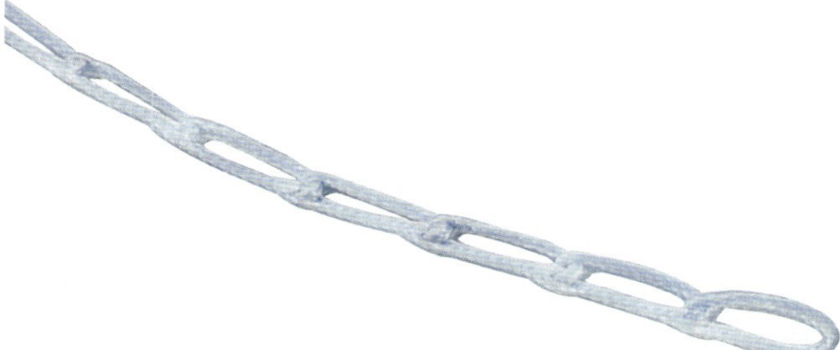

Figure 4.40 FiberChain (Arthrex, Inc., Naples, FL) is a flexible chain of woven FiberWire suture links, in which each link is 6 mm in length.

chain of woven FiberWire suture links, in which each link is 6 mm in length (Fig. 4.40). The linked end of the FiberChain is preassembled into a Bio-Corkscrew anchor eyelet in a nonsliding manner, and the free end has a FiberWire leader that can be loaded onto standard suture-passing instruments for ease of passage through the tendon.

Two suture anchors are placed at the articular margin, anteromedially and posteromedially (Fig. 4.41). Then, the FiberWire leader of the preloaded FiberChain is passed through the rotator cuff tendon 2 to 3 mm lateral to the musculotendinous junction (Fig. 4.42A). To achieve lateral fixation, the suture link must be captured with a lateral anchor that enters the subacromial space above the FiberChain. Therefore, the FiberChain is first retrieved through a lateral portal (Fig. 4.42B). A small stab incision is made and a punch is percutaneously inserted to create a bone socket just lateral to the free edge of the rotator cuff. With the FiberChain suture remaining in the lateral portal, a Bio-SwiveLock anchor with a forked eyelet tip is inserted through the stab incision. The forked eyelet tip of the anchor then captures the second link from the lateral edge of the tendon and fixates it at the bottom of the bone socket beneath the screw-in portion of the anchor (Fig. 4.43). This system provides fixation with a "hard stop" as a result of captured chain links on each end of the FiberChain's span. The final repair is a knotless, low-profile, double-row repair (Fig. 4.44).

L-SHAPED TEARS

General Principles

When repairing L-shaped or U-shaped tears, a number of general principles should be considered. These tear patterns are more complex than standard crescent-shaped tears and complete understanding of the tear mobility must be appreciated for tension-free repair to bone. In either case, careful traction on the tear margins (usually in an oblique fashion) is required to determine the appropriate reduction maneuver. Furthermore, planning anchor placement and suture passage early in the procedure is critical to avoid malpositioning or mismanaging fixation options.

When a standard L-shaped (or U-shaped tear) is encountered, it is important to identify the apex of the tear and the corner of the L to ensure proper closure of the rotator cuff defect (Fig. 4.45). While we have concentrated on closing this defect by advancing the posteromedial apex to the anterolateral corner (in a standard L-shaped tear) (Fig. 4.46), it is also important to ensure the posterolateral rotator cuff/

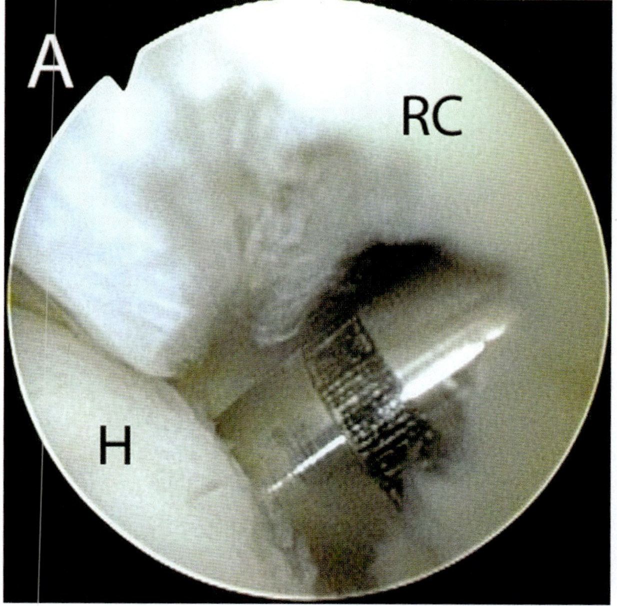

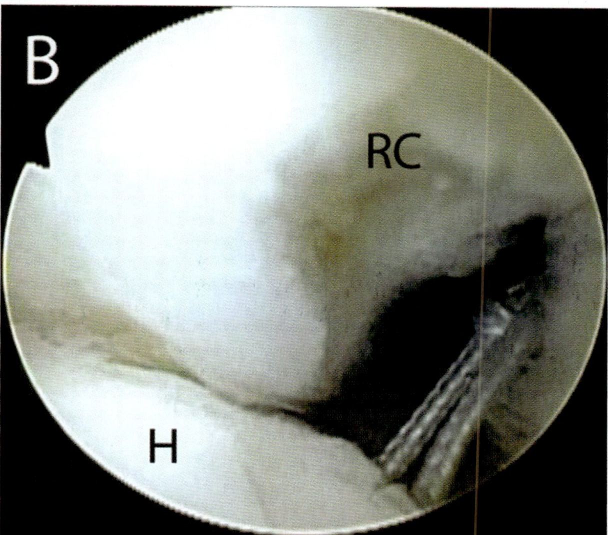

Figure 4.41 Right shoulder, posterior glenohumeral viewing portal, demonstrates **(A)** creation of a bone socket for an anteromedial anchor and **(B)** an anteromedial anchor in place preloaded with FiberChain (Arthrex, Inc., Naples, FL) suture. H, humerus; RC, rotator cuff.

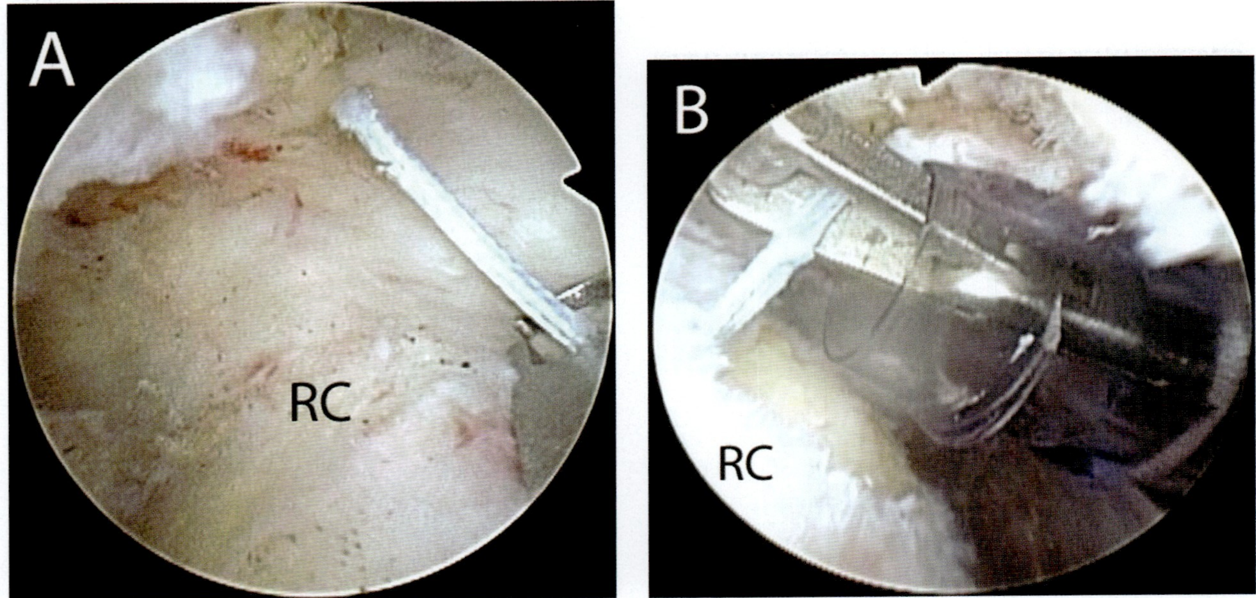

Figure 4.42 Right shoulder, posterior subacromial viewing portal, demonstrates **(A)** antegrade passage of a #2 FiberWire leader of a FiberChain suture (Arthrex, Inc., Naples, FL), and **(B)** retrieval of the suture out a lateral working portal. RC, rotator cuff.

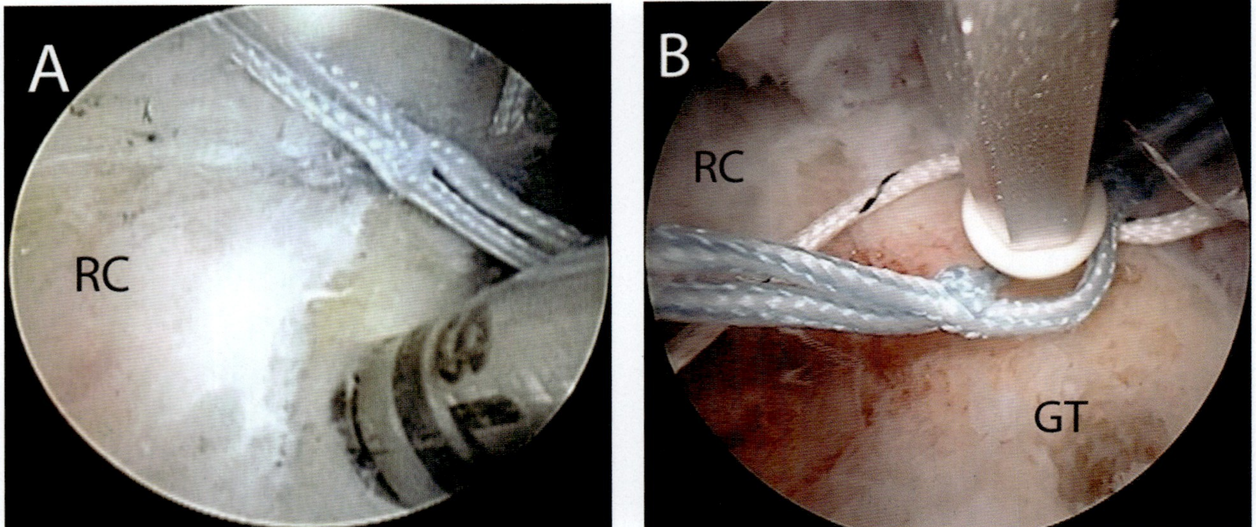

Figure 4.43 Right shoulder, posterior subacromial viewing portal, demonstrates **(A)** creation of a lateral bone socket via a percutaneous portal, and **(B)** insertion of an anchor with a forked eyelet that captures a link of a FiberChain suture (Arthrex, Inc., Naples, FL). GT, greater tuberosity; RC, rotator cuff.

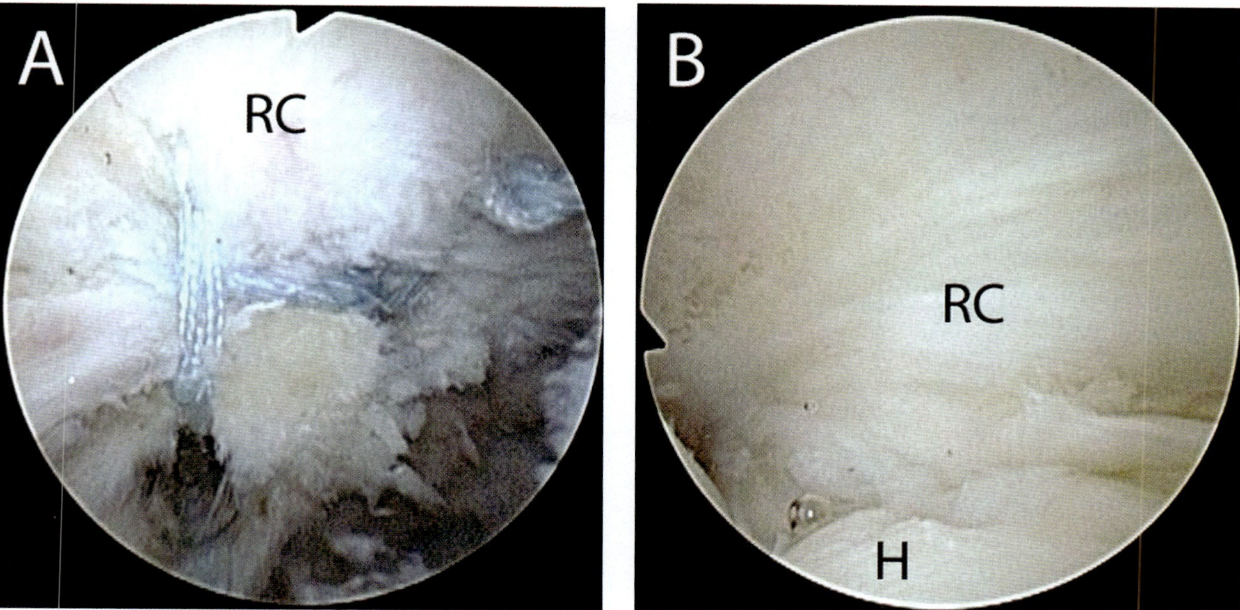

Figure 4.44 **A:** Right shoulder, lateral subacromial viewing portal, demonstrates completed rotator cuff repair using FiberChain (Arthrex, Inc., Naples, FL). **B:** Intra-articular view from a posterior glenohumeral portal in the same shoulder. H, humerus; RC, rotator cuff.

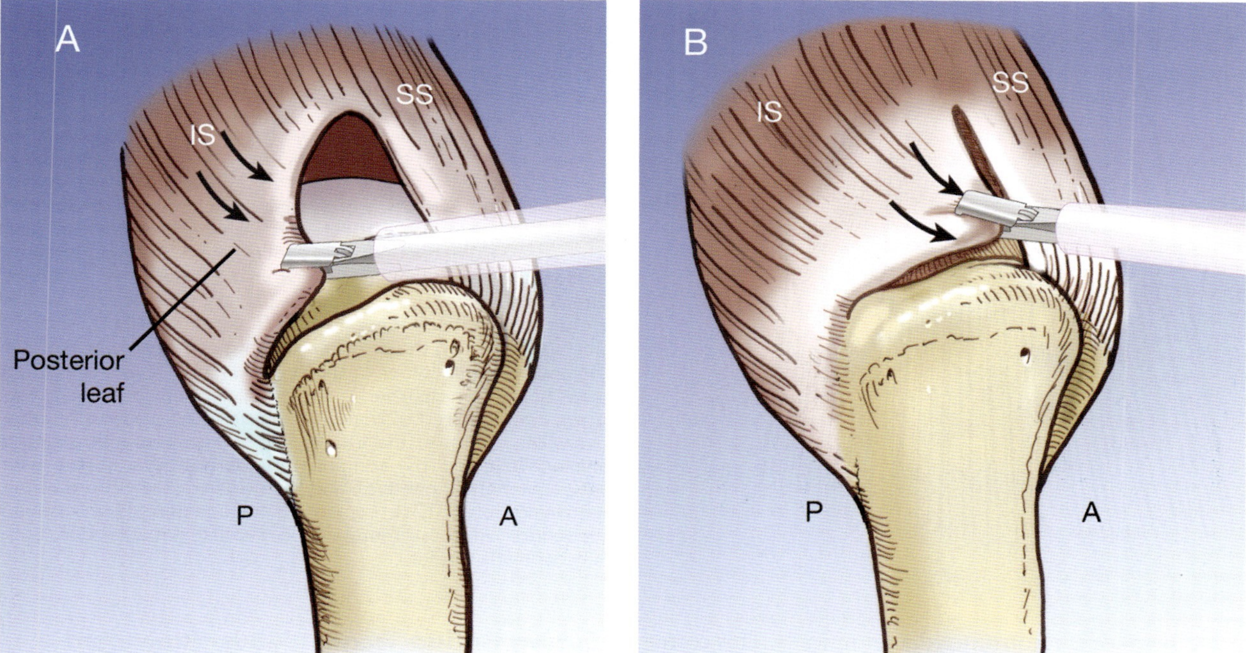

Figure 4.45 Schematic of an L-shaped rotator cuff tendon tear. **A:** A tendon grasper introduced through an anterior arthroscopic portal is used to grasp a point on the posterior leaf of a rotator cuff tendon tear. **B:** The tendon margin is pulled anteriorly and laterally toward the bone bed, demonstrating an L-shaped tear. A, anterior; P, posterior; IS, infraspinatus tendon; SS, supraspinatus tendon.

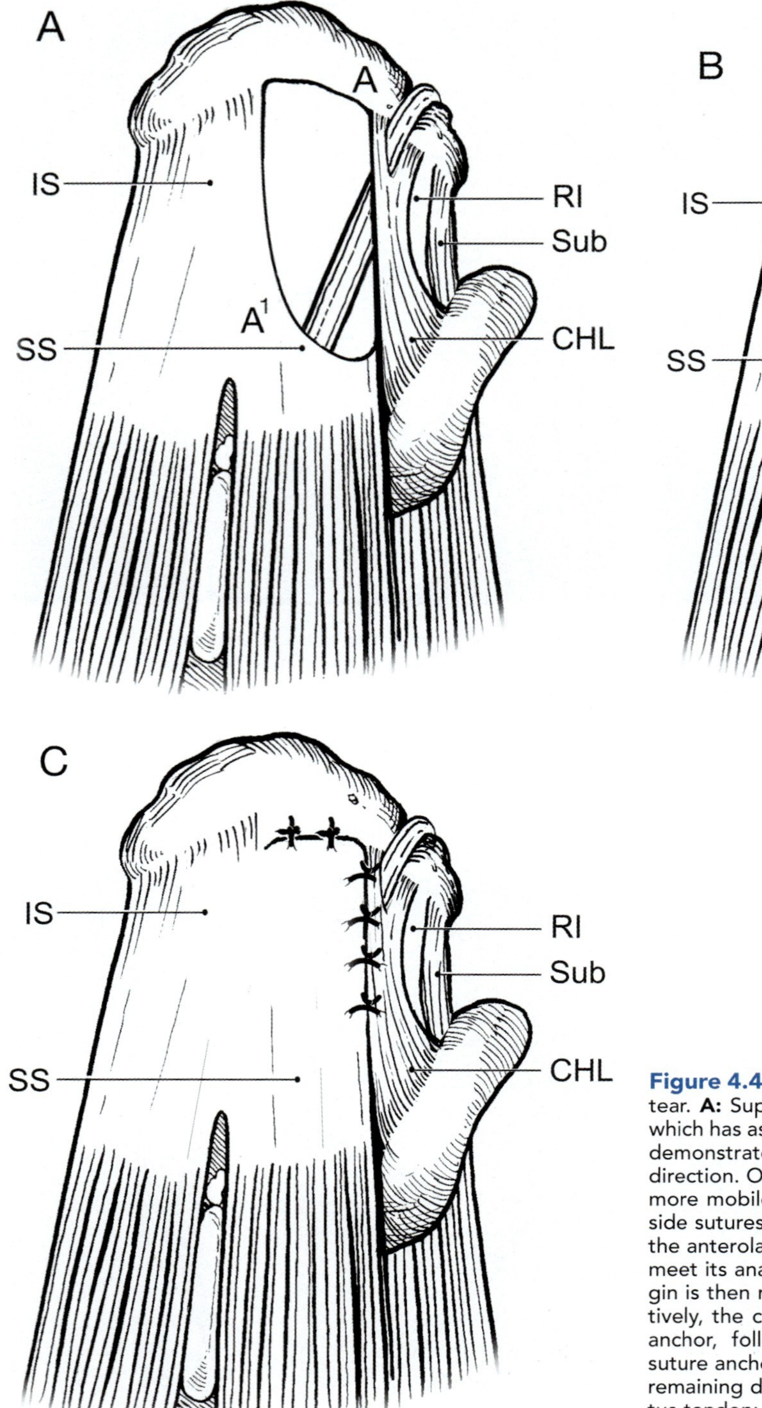

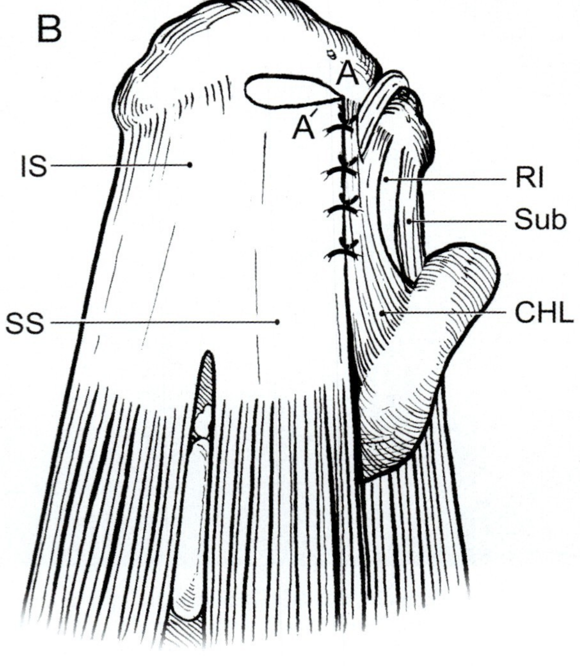

Figure 4.46 Schematic of a repair of an L-shaped rotator cuff tear. **A:** Superior view of a chronic L-shaped rotator cuff tear, which has assumed a U-shaped configuration. **B:** L-shaped tears demonstrate excellent mobility from an anterior to posterior direction. One of the tear margins (usually the posterior leaf) is more mobile. These tears may be repaired initially by side-to-side sutures using the principle of margin convergence so that the anterolateral corner of the supraspinatus (A,) converges to meet its anatomical insertion point (A). **C:** The converged margin is then repaired to bone in a tension-free manner. Alternatively, the corner of the L may first be repaired with a suture anchor, followed by additional tendon-to-bone repair with suture anchors (if needed), and then side-to-side closure of the remaining defect. CHL, coracohumeral ligament; IS, infraspinatus tendon; RI, rotator interval; SS, supraspinatus tendon; Sub, subscapularis tendon.

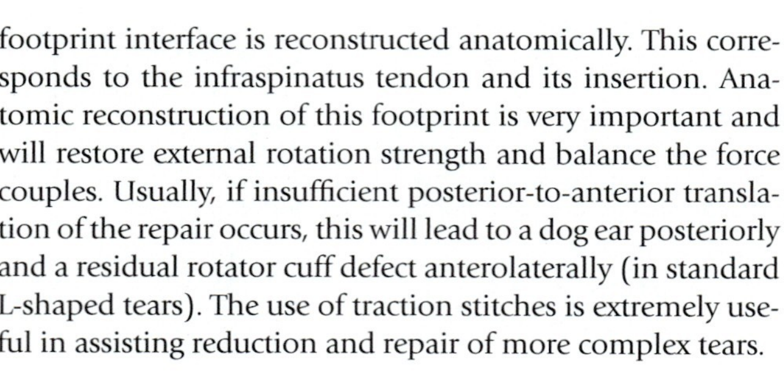

footprint interface is reconstructed anatomically. This corresponds to the infraspinatus tendon and its insertion. Anatomic reconstruction of this footprint is very important and will restore external rotation strength and balance the force couples. Usually, if insufficient posterior-to-anterior translation of the repair occurs, this will lead to a dog ear posteriorly and a residual rotator cuff defect anterolaterally (in standard L-shaped tears). The use of traction stitches is extremely useful in assisting reduction and repair of more complex tears.

Suture Bridge Transosseous Equivalent

Following initial debridement and bursectomy, the medial-to-lateral and anterior-to-posterior mobility of the tear margins is evaluated. In an L-shaped tear, the posteromedial apex of the tear can be advanced to the bone anterolaterally. In a reverse L-shaped tear, the anteromedial apex of the tear can be advanced to the bone posterolaterally (Fig. 4.47). Sometimes, it is useful to place a traction stitch in the apex of the tear, which corresponds to the corner of the L. The traction stitch is then retrieved through a separate stab incision or portal (i.e., anterolateral stab incision for an L-shaped tear) (Fig. 4.48). Keeping the stab incision low against the tuberosity will help to draw the rotator cuff against the footprint, assisting in tendon reduction. The traction stitch and its reduction are then evaluated through the posterior and lateral portals to ensure anatomic reduction may be achieved (Fig. 4.49). The exact position of the corner of the L can be adjusted as necessary.

Medial anchors are placed next, beginning at the apex of the tear (i.e., posteromedial anchor for an L-shaped tear). The first anchor is placed at the apex of the tear because visualization of this will be obscured as fixation progresses. If a traction stitch is used, it is allowed to retract so that the bone bed will be exposed. A 5.5-mm BioComposite Corkscrew FT is placed adjacent to the articular margin. Then, tension can be reapplied to the traction stitch for suture passage. Sutures are passed in a mattress fashion using a Scorpion suture passer through a lateral portal. If the tear has a large anterior-posterior dimension, two anchors are placed and sutures are passed with a FiberLink in preparation for a double-pulley technique as previously discussed (Fig. 4.50). Care is taken to ensure the sutures are 2 to 3 mm lateral to the musculotendinous junction and that the mattress sutures will restore the medial footprint of the infraspinatus insertion. When using the suture bridge technique, it should be remembered that the reduction of the lateral margin of the rotator cuff is dependent on the position of both the margin convergence sutures and the medial mattress sutures. Spanning sutures that cross to the lateral-row anchors provide no medial-to-lateral reduction and generally provide only compression of the rotator cuff against the footprint. These medial sutures are tied by a double-pulley technique with a Surgeon's Sixth Finger Knot Pusher. The suture limbs are preserved for lateral incorporation into a lateral-row repair. To assist in suture management, sutures are retrieved through the percutaneous stab incision that was used for the corresponding anchor insertion.

A BioComposite Corkscrew FT suture anchor is placed in the medial aspect of the footprint near the longitudinal split (i.e., anteromedial anchor for an L-shaped tear). Sutures from this anchor are passed in a side-to-side fashion to close the longitudinal split. Generally, the sutures are first passed through the anterior leaf using a Scorpion through the lateral portal for antegrade passage and subsequently through the posterior leaf using a Penetrator suture passer for retrograde passage. Since the sutures from the anchor are being passed to achieve side-to-side closure in addition to bone fixation, we call this the "margin convergence to bone" technique (Fig. 4.51). If a traction stitch was previously placed, it may be removed at this point. Alternatively, if the traction stitch is felt to be in a good location for a suture from this anchor, it can be used to shuttle the suture through the rotator cuff by a "suture-through-a-suture" technique. The humeral-sided (inferior) suture limb from the traction stitch and a suture from the anchor are retrieved out a lateral portal. The anchor suture is passed through the traction stitch limb using a Graft Preparation Needle (Arthrex, Inc., Naples, FL), which is a straight needle with a Nitinol wire loop on the end. Then, the opposite end of the traction stitch is pulled to shuttle the suture through the rotator cuff.

The next step of the repair is to perform margin convergence of the remaining portion of the longitudinal split. Although we have previously described performing margin convergence as the first step in the repair, we now often delay this step of the procedure until after the sutures from medial anchors have been passed. Performing margin convergence first can be difficult because of the floppiness of the margins. Additionally, we have found that anatomic reduction of the rotator cuff is more reliably obtained by placing the medial anchors first. If margin convergence sutures have been placed prior to anchors, these sutures should not be tied until after

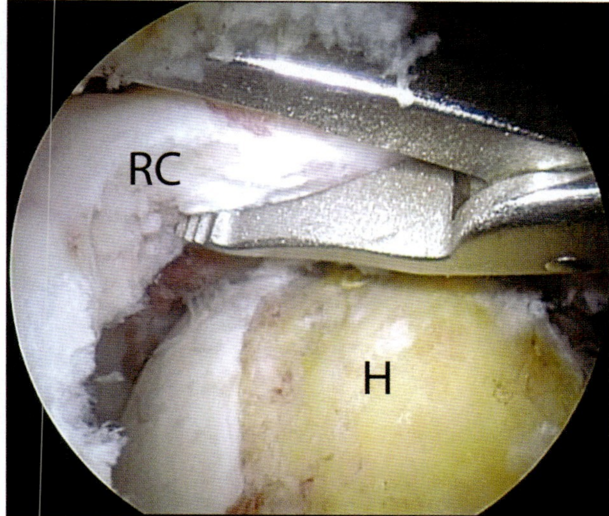

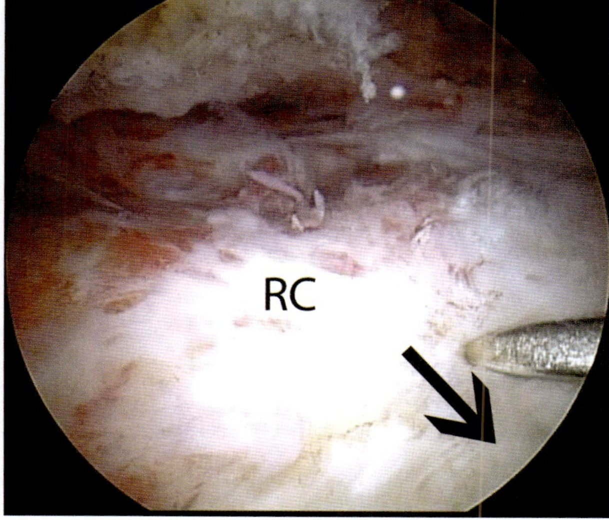

Figure 4.47 **A:** Right shoulder, posterior subacromial viewing portal. A grasper is introduced from a lateral working portal to assess the mobility of a rotator cuff tear. **B:** The tear reduces to bone with a posterolateral pull (*black arrow*), indicating a reverse L-shaped tear. H, humerus; RC, rotator cuff.

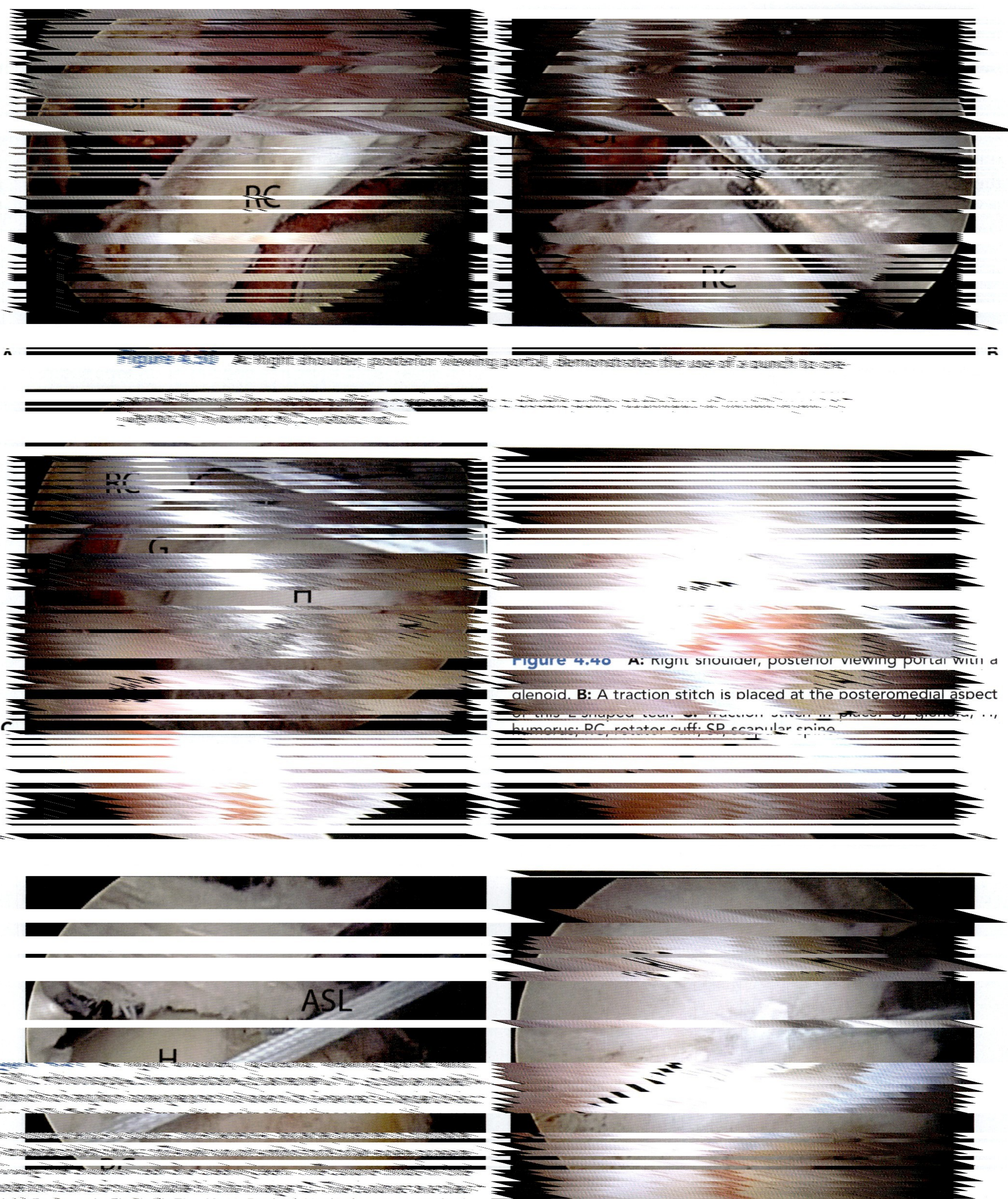

Figure 4.48 **A:** Right shoulder, posterior viewing portal with a [illegible] glenoid. **B:** A traction stitch is placed at the posteromedial aspect of this L-shaped tear. **C:** Traction stitch in place. G, glenoid; H, humerus; RC, rotator cuff; SP, scapular spine.

Figure 4.49 **A:** Right shoulder, posterior viewing portal [illegible] traction stitch that has been placed (Fig. 4.48) in the posteromedial apex of an L-shaped tear and retrieved out an antero[illegible] the L-shaped pattern of the tear. ASL, anterosuperolateral portal; H, humerus; RC, rotator cuff.

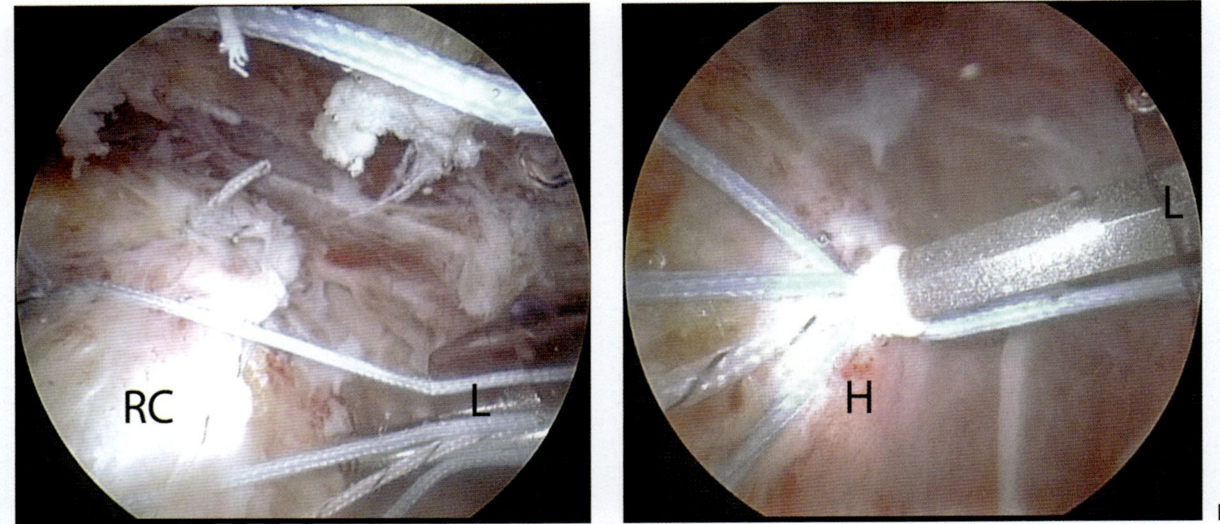

Figure 4.52 **A:** Right shoulder, posterior viewing portal. Sutures have been crisscrossed and retrieved through a lateral portal. A punch is used to create a bone socket for an anterolateral anchor. **B:** The sutures have been threaded through the eyelet of a BioComposite SwiveLock C anchor (Arthrex, Inc., Naples, FL) and the eyelet is seated into the previously created bone socket. H, humerus; RC, rotator cuff; L, lateral subacromial portal.

the sutures from the anchors are passed. We generally pass side-to-side sutures while viewing through a lateral portal. Through a posterior working portal, a #2 FiberWire suture is passed antegrade through the anterior leaf of the rotator cuff tendon using a Scorpion suture passer. A Penetrator suture passer is then passed retrograde through the posterior leaf to retrieve the suture, completing the margin convergence stitch. Depending on the size of the longitudinal split, one to three side-to-side sutures may be required. After all side-to-side sutures have been placed, they are sequentially tied from medial to lateral using a Surgeon's Sixth Finger Knot Pusher.

Following medial suture passage and margin convergence, fixation of the lateral rotator cuff proceeds as described above for crescent tears. Dog-ear reduction sutures (FiberLink cinch loops) can be placed if needed. Lateral fixation is accomplished with two BioComposite SwiveLock C anchors with sutures retrieved from each anchor in a crisscross fashion through the lateral cannula (Fig. 4.52). Final evaluation demonstrates secure tendon fixation to bone and reconstruction of the rotator cuff footprint (Fig. 4.53).

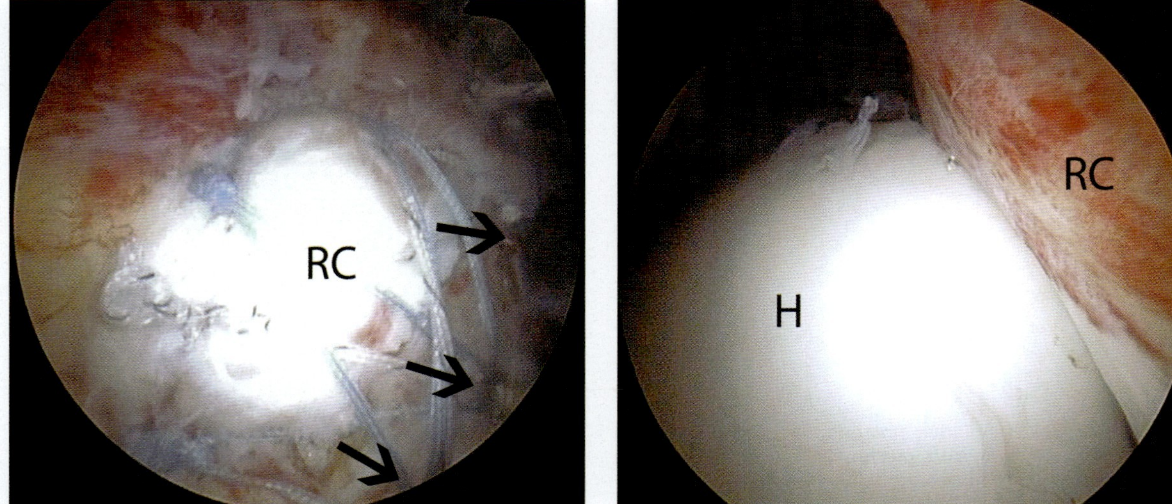

Figure 4.53 **A:** Right shoulder, posterior subacromial viewing portal, demonstrates final repair of a reverse L-shaped tear (compare to Fig. 4.47). In this case, because of the large anterior–posterior dimension of the tear, three lateral anchors (*black arrows*) were used in a diamondback configuration. **B:** Same shoulder, posterior glenohumeral viewing portal, demonstrates restoration of the medial footprint. H, humerus; RC, rotator cuff

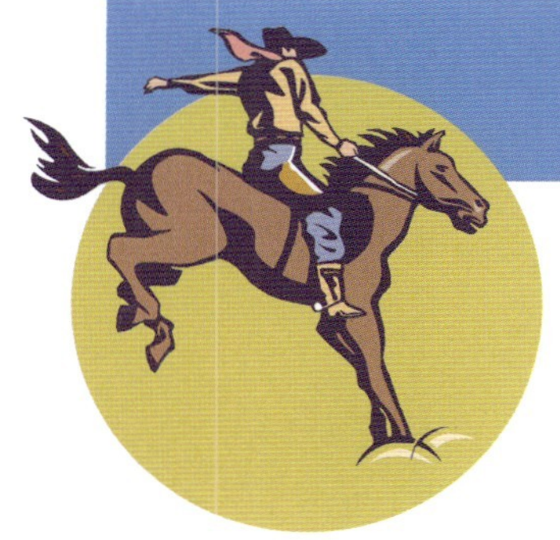

5

Partial-thickness Rotator Cuff Tears

WESTERN WISDOM

Suspicion ain't proof.

Partial-thickness rotator cuff tears are a common cause of pain and disability in the adult shoulder. Despite this, the indications for various types of nonoperative and operative treatment of partial-thickness tears (e.g., debridement vs. repair) remain controversial. Partial-thickness tears are approximately twice as common as full-thickness tears of the rotator cuff, and they may be associated with significant concomitant pathology including superior labral lesions, biceps pathology, chondromalacia/osteoarthritis, acromioclavicular joint derangement, and adhesive capsulitis. Furthermore, many partial tears may present as incidental magnetic resonance imaging (MRI) findings and therefore should be correlated to the patient's history and physical findings.

Partial tears are generally classified by tendon location (e.g., supraspinatus, infraspinatus), anatomic location (e.g., bursal surface, articular surface, interstitial), and the percentage of tendon thickness torn. While no clear consensus exists, the indications for surgical repair of the tendon (following failure of nonoperative treatment) are generally based on the percentage of tendon thickness torn. In patients with a tear involving 50% or more of the tendon thickness, surgical reattachment of the tendon is usually indicated. However, other factors should also be strongly considered and may be more influential than the percentage of thickness torn. These factors include age, activity level, vocation, sports participation, chronicity of symptoms, and associated pathology.

Once surgical repair has been selected, several different surgical repair techniques and configurations may be chosen. The specific technique is largely based upon the pathology at hand.

COMPLETION OF THE TEAR

In a patient with a significant articular-sided partial-thickness rotator cuff tear, converting the partial-thickness into a full-thickness rotator cuff tear is an option. After that, standard arthroscopic rotator cuff repair techniques may be utilized for tendon fixation to bone. We use this technique only when >80% to 90% of the tendon thickness is torn and/or the residual intact rotator cuff tendon tissue is of poor quality with minimal structural integrity. However, in patients with good-quality residual tendon remaining, conversion to a full-thickness rotator cuff tear should be avoided. As will be discussed in the following sections, our strong preference is to preserve as much residual cuff as possible and perform transtendon anchor placement if tissue quality allows.

When performing the repair after completion of the tear, a double-row rotator cuff repair should be performed to restore full footprint coverage (1). Since single-row rotator cuff repair results in poor footprint coverage (particularly medially), single-row repair may merely recreate the preoperative partial-thickness tear anatomy (Fig. 5.1). For this reason, a double-row rotator cuff repair should be performed to restore the normal anatomy (Fig. 5.2).

Once the rotator cuff tear has been debrided, its location is marked using a suture. The arthroscope is redirected

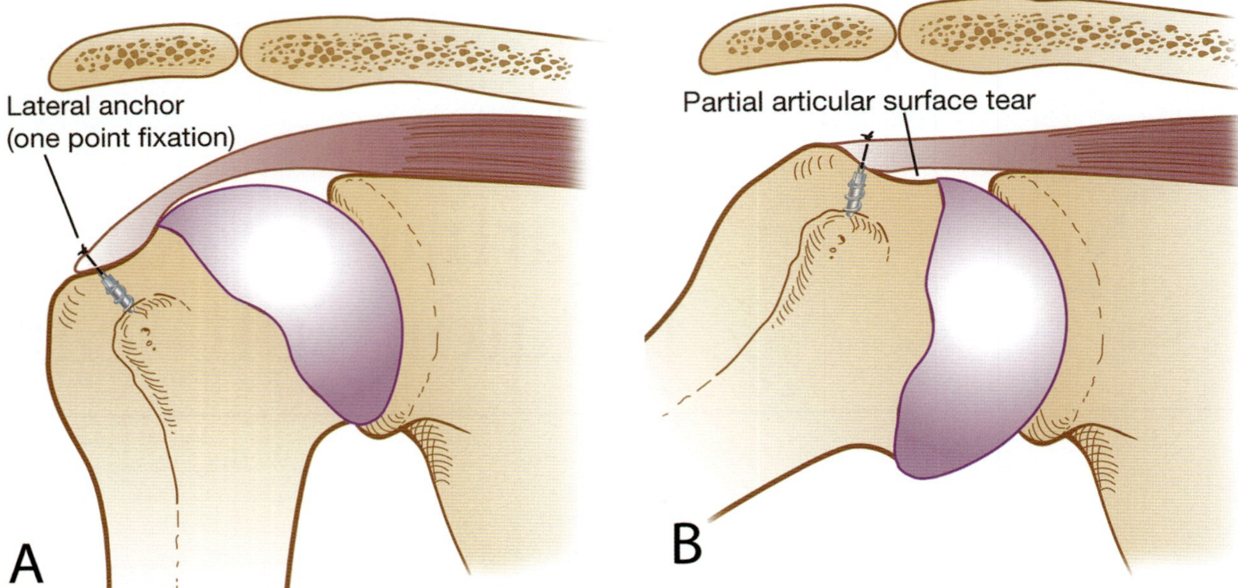

Figure 5.1 Schematic drawing of a single-row suture anchor repair for a partial-thickness articular surface rotator cuff tear (PASTA). **A:** Point fixation is achieved with only a lateral row repair. **B:** When the shoulder is abducted, a similar PASTA lesion, with lifting of the medial footprint, is created, despite lateral repair.

into the subacromial space and a lateral portal is created. A subacromial bursectomy and decompression are performed and the marking suture is identified in the subacromial space. The integrity of the residual rotator cuff is evaluated, and if it is estimated that >80% to 90% of the tendon thickness is torn, the tear may be completed.

A shaver, scissor, or #11 scalpel blade inserted tangential to the footprint may be used to accurately release the residual lateral tendon and potentially preserve as much tendon length as possible. A shaver is subsequently used to debride degenerative tissue that has little residual biomechanical integrity.

A full-thickness tear has now been created and standard rotator cuff repair techniques may be utilized. Bone bed preparation is followed by assessment of the tear mobility and pattern. In most cases, the tear pattern will be crescent and repair will proceed with direct suture anchor repair to bone.

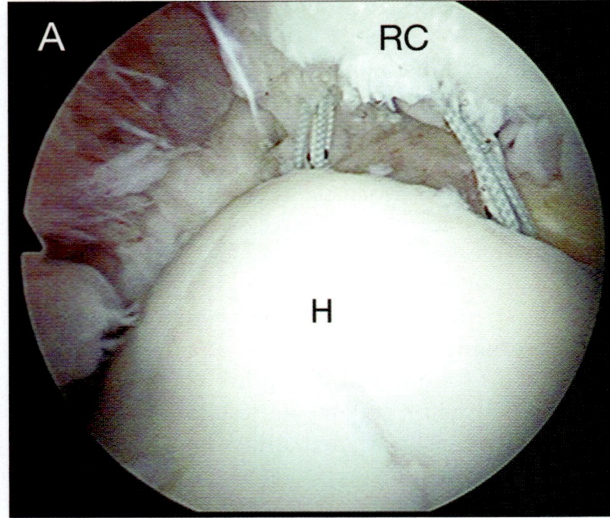

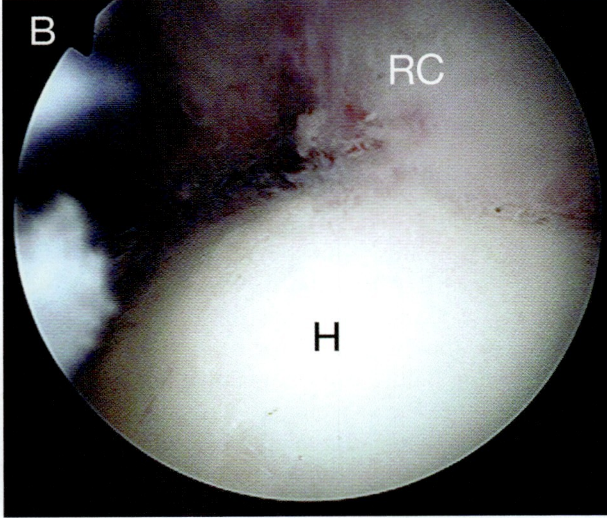

Figure 5.2 Arthroscopic views through a posterior glenohumeral viewing portal of a right shoulder demonstrating a double-row rotator cuff repair, following tying of the lateral row of sutures **(A)** and following tying of the lateral and medial row of sutures **(B)**. Note: Tying only the lateral row of sutures leaves the rotator cuff elevated off the medial footprint. With tying of the medial sutures, the rotator cuff is compressed against the medial footprint. H, humeral head; RC, rotator cuff.

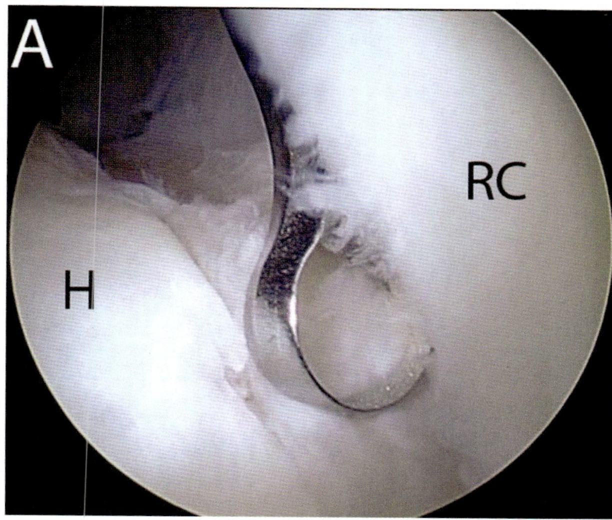

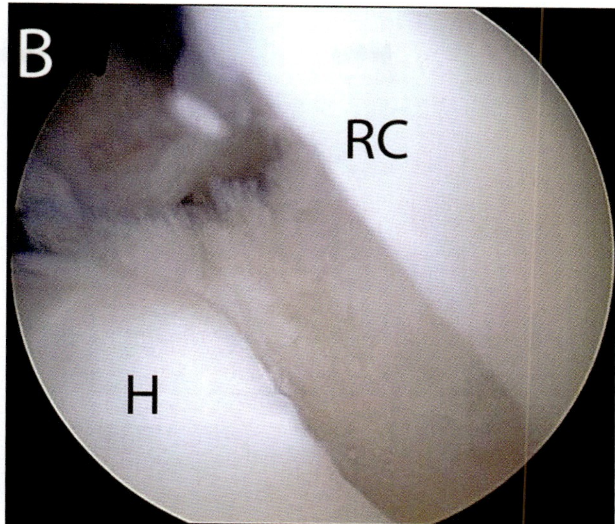

Figure 5.3 **A:** Right shoulder, posterior glenohumeral viewing portal, demonstrates use of a curette introduced from an anterior portal to prepare the bone bed for repair. **B:** Soft tissue has been removed and the bone bed is exposed to a bleeding base to encourage healing following repair. For anterior lesions such as this case, complete preparation can typically be achieved through an anterior portal H, humerus; RC, rotator cuff.

TRANSTENDON ROTATOR CUFF REPAIR OF PASTA LESIONS

In cases where a partial articular surface tendon avulsion (PASTA) lesion has been determined and where significant tendon substance remains, preservation of the intact rotator cuff has several theoretical advantages, including maintenance of the normal length–tendon relationship of the rotator cuff, preservation of the integrity of the glenohumeral joint, provision of an intrinsic source of native tendon cells, and improved biomechanics. In a cadaveric study of similar partial-thickness rotator cuff tears, transtendon rotator cuff repair with preservation of the intact lateral cuff was biomechanically superior to completion of the tear with double-row rotator cuff repair (2).

One challenge in transtendon repair is achieving adequate tendon debridement and bone bed preparation in the face of an intact lateral cuff. We typically begin debridement and bone bed preparation with the use of an instrument introduced through an anterior portal (Fig. 5.3). Variations in abduction/adduction and internal/external rotation help deliver the bone bed to the instrument. Posterior access, however, is often limited from an anterior portal because of the convexity of the humeral head. In the setting of a PASTA lesion involving the posterior rotator cuff (i.e., infraspinatus), we commonly work through the rotator cuff lesion. A spinal needle is used as a guide to pass through the lesion with an adequate angle of approach to reach the bone bed. Then, a shaver is walked down the spinal needle and pushed through the rotator cuff (Fig. 5.4). In this way, only a small 4 to 5 mm defect is created in the rotator cuff, allowing debridement and bone bed preparation without completing the rotator cuff tear.

Transtendon repair can be performed with anywhere from 1 to 4 anchors, depending upon the anterior-to-posterior and medical-to-lateral dimensions of the tear. Maybe not essential, but might help orient the ready to these two variables that we highlight later as when to increase the number of anchors.

Single-anchor Mattress

Once a partial-thickness articular surface tear has been debrided, the bone bed is debrided to a bleeding bone surface. The arthroscope is redirected into the subacromial space using the same posterior skin incision and a lateral subacromial portal is established. The subacromial space is then cleared of fibrofatty tissue and bursa and a subacromial decompression with acromioplasty may be performed if indicated. It is critical to completely clear the subacromial space prior to insertion of anchors to facilitate subsequent retrieval and tying of sutures in the subacromial space. Additionally, failure to clear the space first may lead to inadvertent damage to the sutures when a shaver is used to subsequently clear the subacromial space. Following subacromial bursectomy, the rotator cuff is evaluated on its bursal surface.

If significant tendon tissue and quality is present to warrant preservation, a transtendon approach may be utilized. A transtendon repair is generally indicated when 10% to 90% of the tendon thickness remains. In partial articular surface tears with only a small portion of the tendon involved from an anterior-to-posterior direction(i.e., <1.5 cm), a single-anchor mattress technique may be utilized (Fig. 5.5).

The arthroscope is reintroduced into the posterior glenohumeral portal and the anterior portal is reestablished if necessary. An anchor is then inserted transtendon while viewing through the posterior glenohumeral portal. In some cases, if an anterosuperolateral portal has been

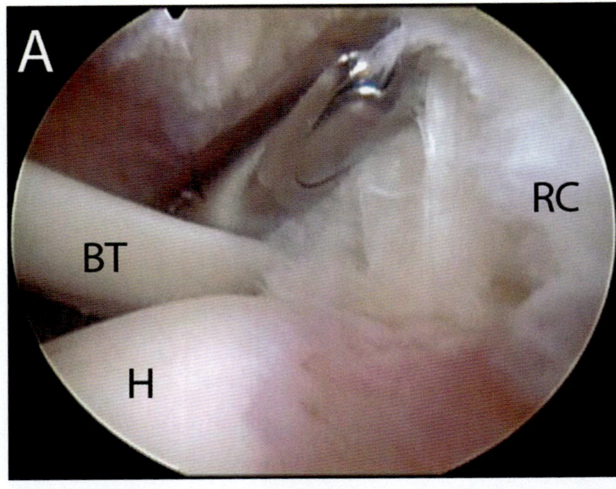

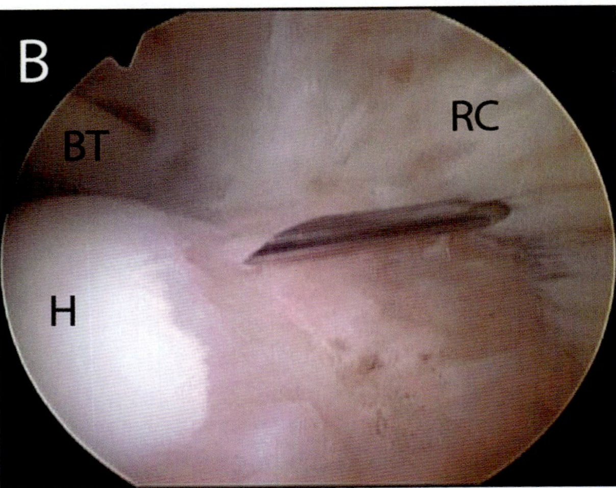

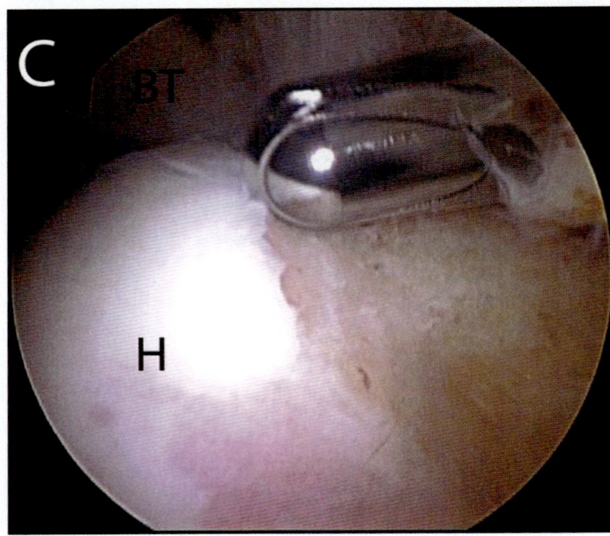

Figure 5.4 Right shoulder, posterior viewing portal demonstrates bone bed preparation of a PASTA lesion with posterior involvement. **A:** With an anterior working portal, the angle of approach prevents access to the posterior bone bed for preparation. Transtendon preparation is required. **B:** A spinal needle is used to penetrate the center of the lesion with an angle of approach that allows access to the entire bone bed. **C:** A shaver is walked down the spinal needle and is used to perform bone bed preparation. BT, biceps tendon; H, humerus; RC, rotator cuff.

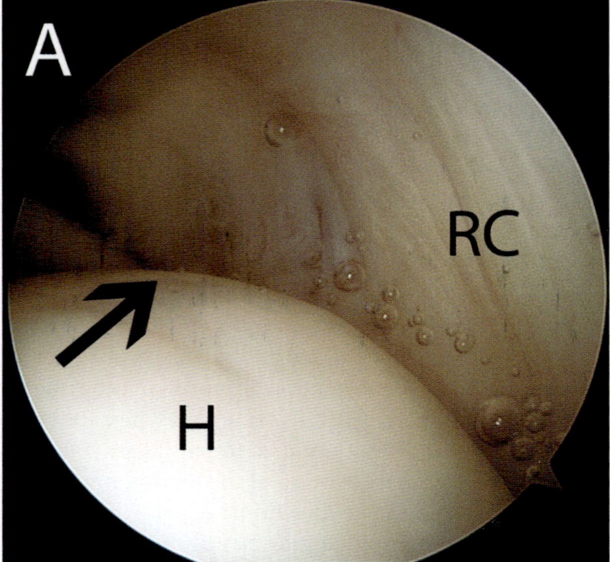

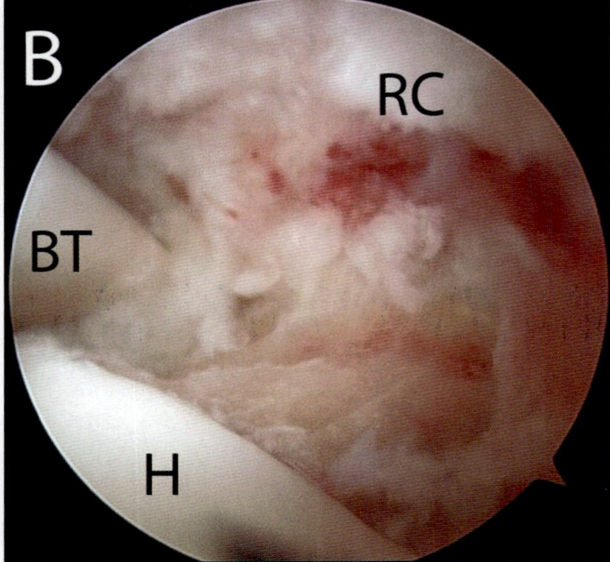

Figure 5.5 **A:** Right shoulder, posterior glenohumeral viewing portal, demonstrates a small PASTA (*black arrow*). Note: In this case, the tear is amenable to a single-anchor repair because it only involves a small portion of the footprint in the anterior-to-posterior dimension and the posterior supraspinatus is intact (**right**). **B:** Same shoulder demonstrating a prepared bone bed. BT, biceps tendon; H, humerus; RC, rotator cuff.

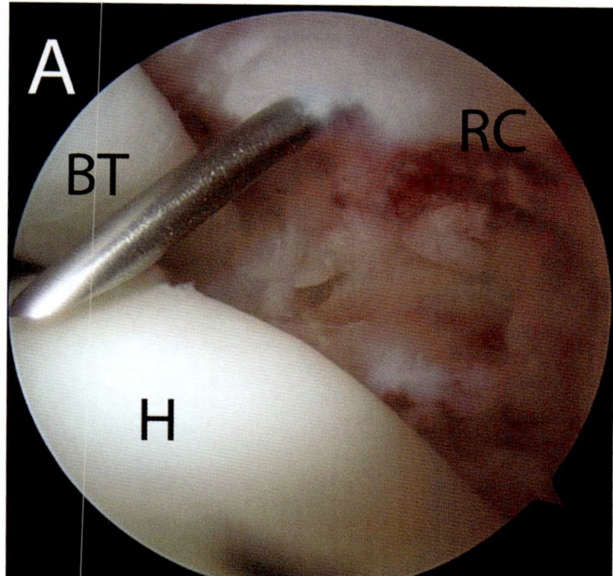

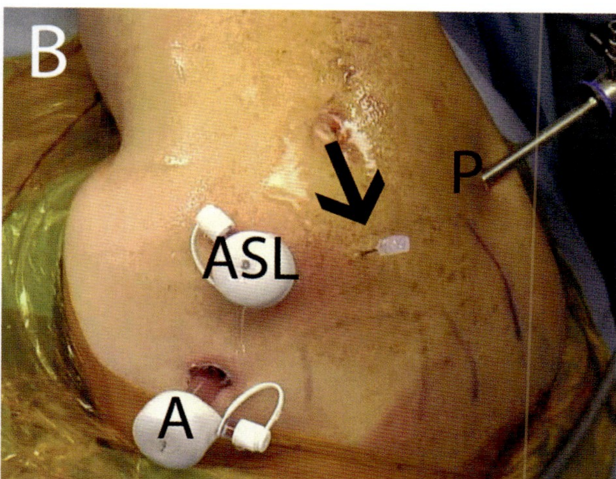

Figure 5.6 **A:** Right shoulder, posterior glenohumeral viewing portal, demonstrates use of a spinal needle to determine an adequate angle of approach for transtendon anchor placement for repair of a partial-thickness rotator cuff tear. **B:** External view shows the spinal needle location. A, anterior portal; ASL, anterosuperolateral portal; BT, biceps tendon; H, humerus; P, posterior portal; RC, rotator cuff.

created superior and lateral in the rotator interval, the anchor may be placed through the anterosuperolateral portal. However, in many cases, this will not provide the correct angle of approach to the medial aspect of the footprint. To assist in anchor insertion, a spinal needle is used to determine the correct angle of approach (Fig. 5.6). It is important to maintain the position of the needle during the entire anchor insertion step to provide a guide for the correct angle of approach. A skin puncture is then made and a punch is inserted parallel to the spinal needle in a transtendon approach (Fig. 5.7A). To assist in visualization of the punch during impaction, passing the entire punch through the tendon beyond the laser marking prior to bone insertion will dilate the transtendon hole and prevent "sticking" of the rotator cuff against the punch (Fig. 5.7B). The punch is then tapped to its laser marking at the medial margin of the footprint (Fig. 5.7C)

A 4.5-mm BioComposite Corkscrew FT anchor (Arthrex, Inc., Naples, FL) is then passed transtendon through the same hole and inserted into the bone socket (tapping of the bone

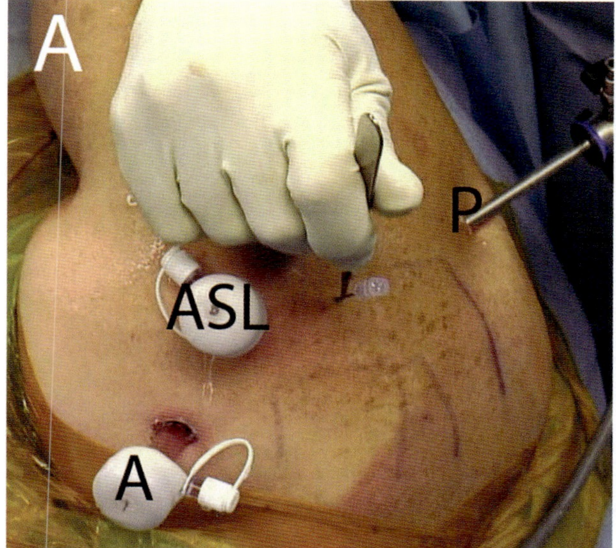

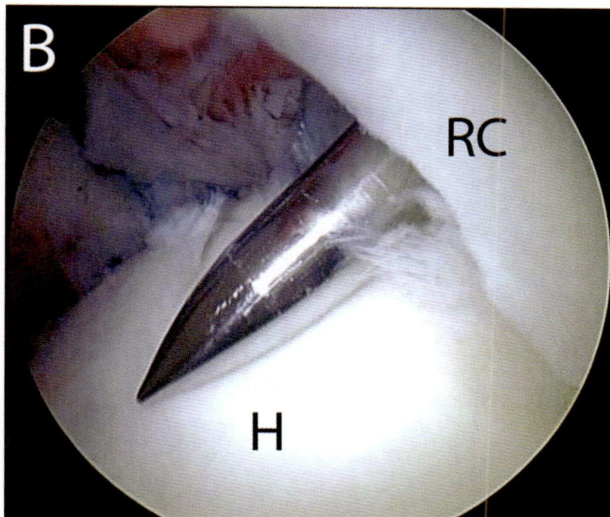

Figure 5.7 Punch insertion for transtendon anchor placement in a right shoulder. **A:** A stab incision is made adjacent to a previously placed spinal needle. **B:** Posterior glenohumeral viewing portal demonstrates insertion of a punch for bone socket preparation. The punch is inserted beyond the bone bed to dilate the hole in the tendon and prevent the rotator cuff from "sticking" to the punch.

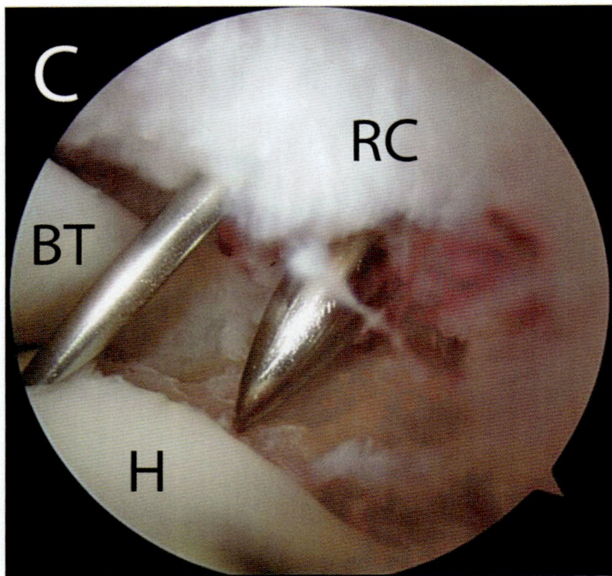

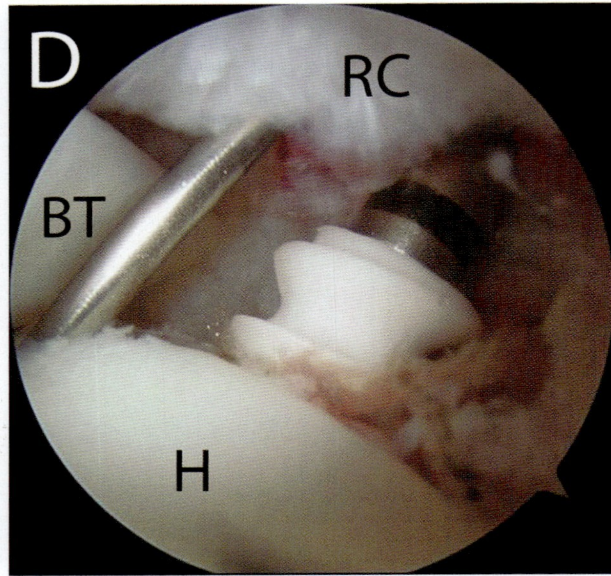

Figure 5.7 *(Continued)* **C:** The punch is withdrawn slightly and positioned for creation of a bone socket. **D:** An anchor is then placed using the same path as the punch. Note: The spinal needle has been left in place to serve as a guide for insertion of the anchor. A, anterior portal; ASL, anterosuperolateral portal; BT, biceps tendon; H, humerus; P, posterior portal; RC, rotator cuff.

bed is rarely required) (Fig. 5.7D). A 5.0-mm transtendon metal cannula (Arthrex, Inc., Naples, FL) can simplify anchor insertion by preserving the same channel for insertion of the punch and the anchor (Fig. 5.8). In some cases, it may also be simpler to directly insert a metallic anchor (4.5-mm Corkscrew FT; Arthrex, Inc., Naples, FL) through the rotator cuff and bone since no punch is required. Once anchor insertion and stability have been confirmed, suture passage proceeds.

Sutures are passed through the rotator cuff in a mattress fashion. Suture passage may be accomplished in a retrograde manner with a Penetrator (Arthrex, Inc., Naples, FL) (Fig. 5.9), or using a shuttling technique (Micro SutureLasso; Arthrex, Inc., Naples, FL) (Fig. 5.10). Shuttling is simple, accurate, and minimally traumatizes the rotator cuff. The rotator cuff is penetrated percutaneously through a lateral approach. The shuttle is then advanced through the Micro SutureLasso and one suture limb and the shuttle are retrieved through the anterior portal. The suture is then shuttled through the rotator cuff and out through the skin. The steps are repeated for the other suture limbs creating a spread of mattress sutures.

In either technique, it is important to penetrate the rotator cuff through robust tissue. However, penetrating the rotator

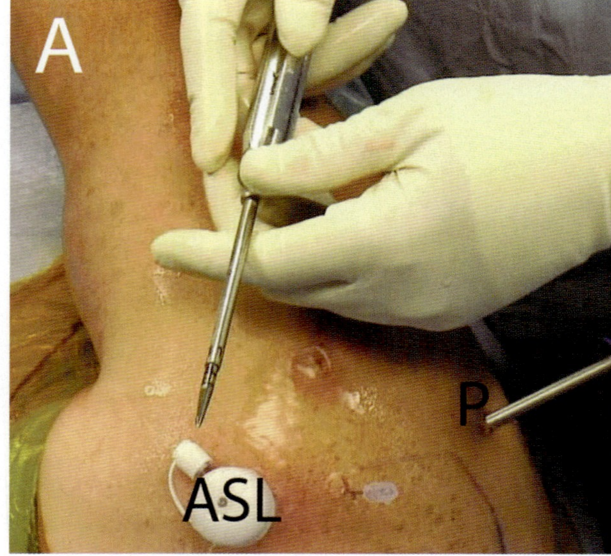

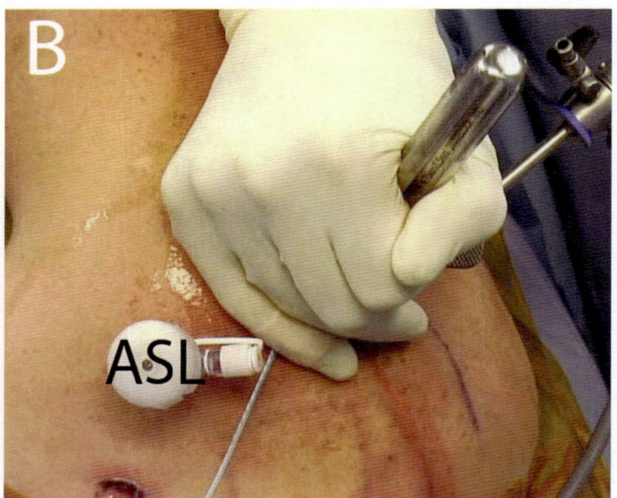

Figure 5.8 Using a metal cannula for transtendon anchor placement in a right shoulder. **A:** External view demonstrates a 5.0-mm metal cannula (Arthrex, Inc., Naples, FL). **B:** The cannula is inserted transtendon adjacent to a previously placed spinal needle.

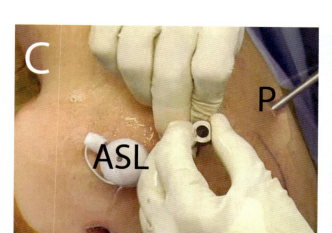

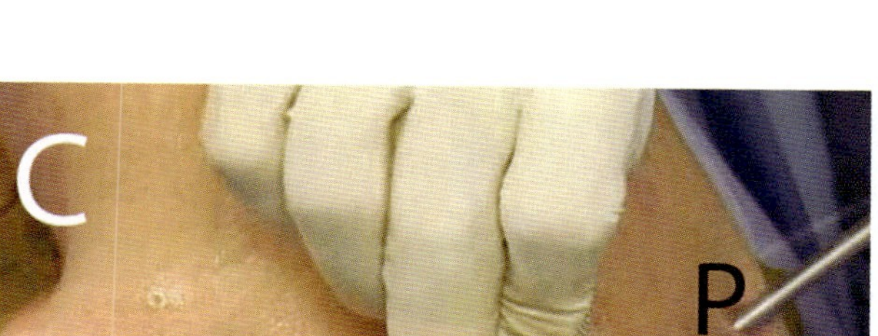

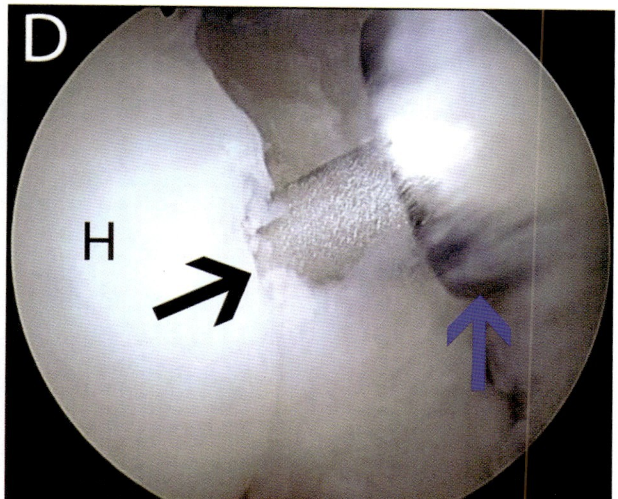

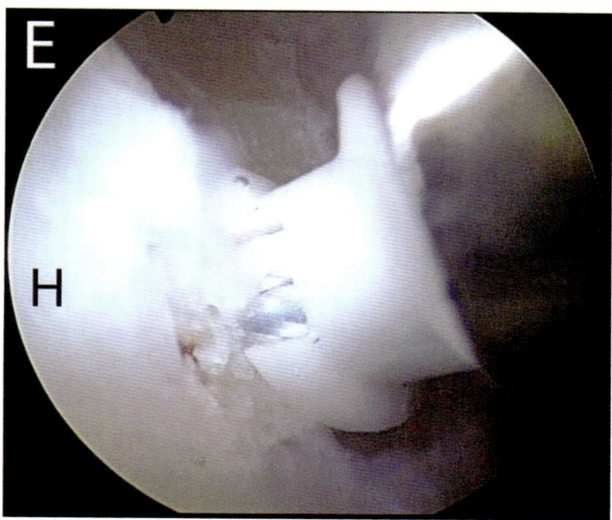

Figure 5.8 *(Continued)* **C:** The inner trochar is removed for punch placement. **D:** Arthroscopic view from a posterior glenohumeral portal demonstrates punch placement (*black arrow*) for creation of a bone socket. Note: The metal cannula (*blue arrow*) preserves the channel, simplifying bone socket creation and anchor placement. **E:** A 4.5-mm BioComposite Corkscrew FT anchor (Arthrex, Inc., Naples, FL) is inserted. ASL, anterosuperolateral portal; H, humerus; P, posterior portal.

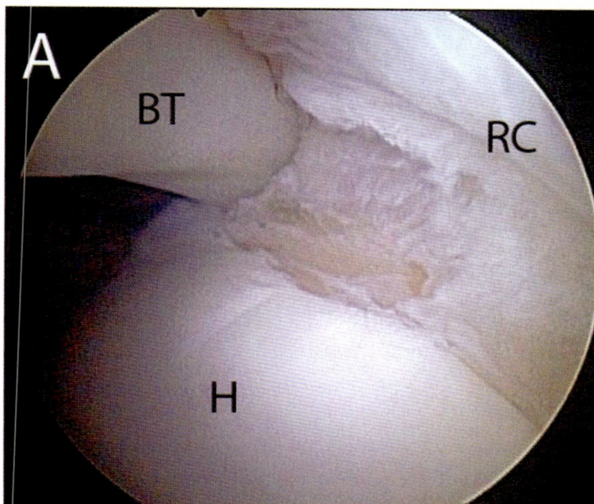

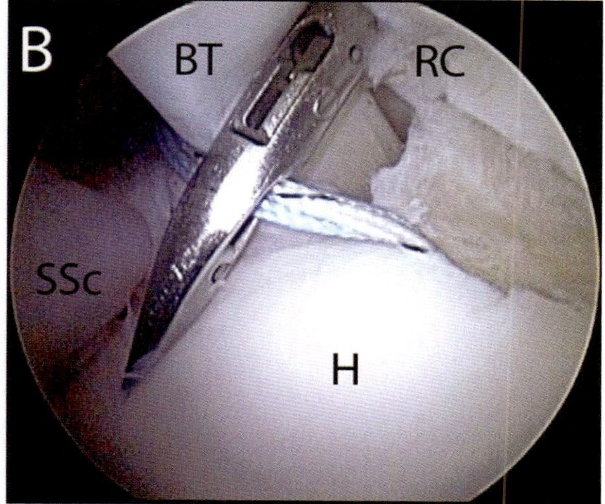

Figure 5.9 **A:** Right shoulder, posterior viewing portal, demonstrates a small articular-sided rotator cuff tear amenable to a single-anchor repair. **B:** After placement of a transtendon anchor, sutures can be passed retrograde with a Penetrator (Arthrex, Inc., Naples, FL).

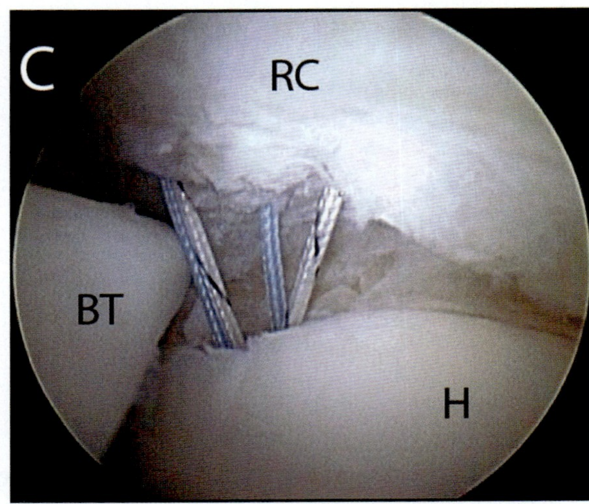

Figure 5.9 *(Continued)* **C:** The sutures are passed to create a spread that will maximize footprint coverage. BT, biceps tendon; H, humerus; RC, rotator cuff; SSc, subscapularis tendon.

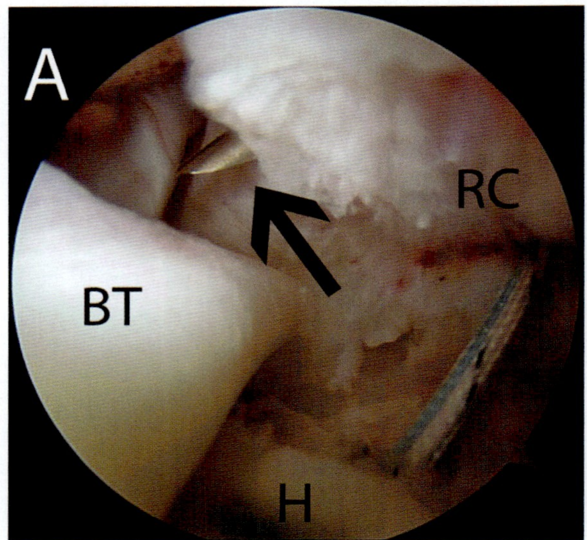

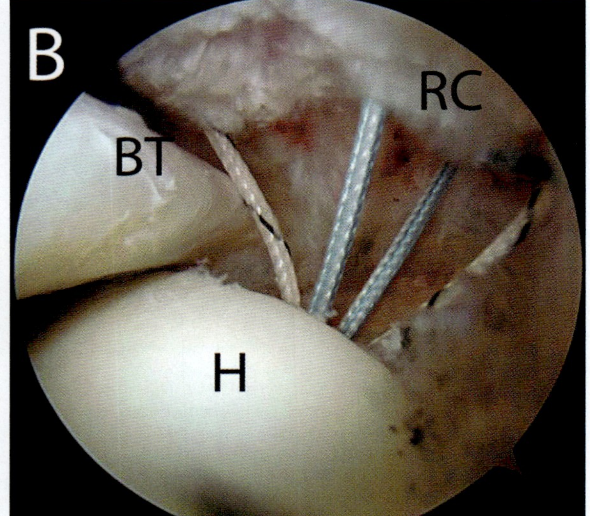

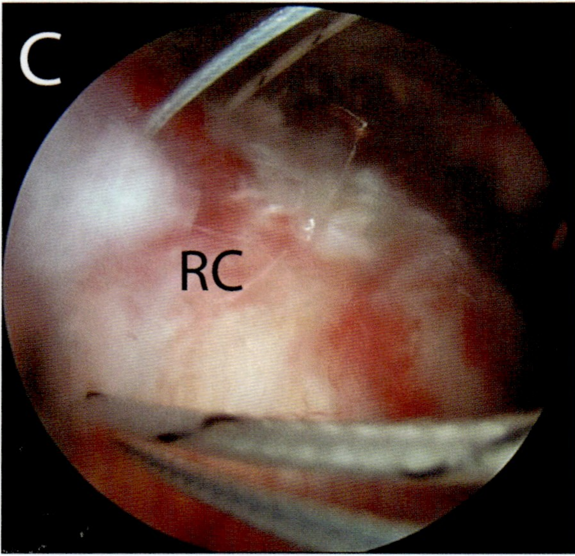

Figure 5.10 **A:** Right shoulder view from a posterior portal demonstrates a MicroLasso (*black arrow*), which has been passed through the anterior rotator cuff to shuttle sutures for a PASTA. **B:** Sutures that have been individually passed to create a spread of sutures for a single-anchor repair of a PASTA. **C:** Subacromial view from a posterior portal in the same shoulder. BT, biceps tendon; H, humerus; RC, rotator cuff.

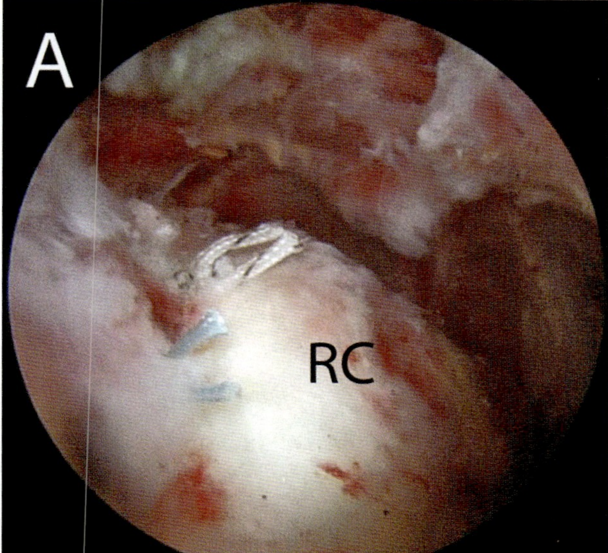

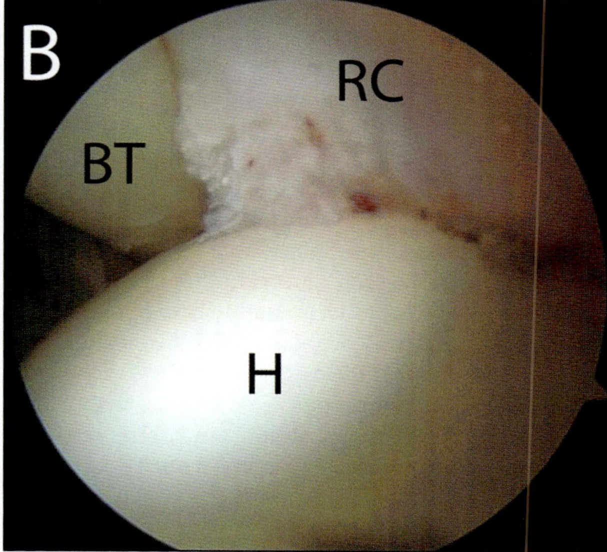

Figure 5.11 **A:** Right shoulder, posterior subacromial viewing portal, demonstrates final single-anchor repair of a PASTA. Note: The knots have been purposely tied to maximize the spread between contact points and thus maximize fixation. **B:** Intra-articular view from a posterior portal in the same shoulder demonstrates restoration of the medial footprint (Compare to Fig. 5.5B). BT, biceps tendon; H, humerus; RC, rotator cuff.

cuff too far medially can lead to an oblique passage through the rotator cuff and potentially a bursal-articular surface tension mismatch. Perpendicular passage through the rotator cuff is preferable and may be accomplished by adducting the arm.

After passing sutures, the arthroscope is reintroduced into the subacromial space. The sutures are identified in the subacromial space and tied. To prevent "buckling" the tendon, the arm is brought into adduction and the sutures tied. The final construct should be viewed both on the bursal side and from the articular side to ensure tendon reduction to bone (Fig. 5.11).

Video

Two Anchor Double-pulley Technique

In patients with more extensive partial articular surface rotator cuff tears, two or more anchors may be required. Usually two anchors are required if >1.5 cm of the anterior-to-posterior footprint is involved. A subacromial bursectomy or decompression is performed prior to anchor insertion. In patients with extensive partial-thickness articular surface tears, two anchors are placed (e.g., BioComposite Corkscrew FT) transtendon as described previously, one anterior and one posterior in the medial aspect of the footprint (Fig. 5.12).

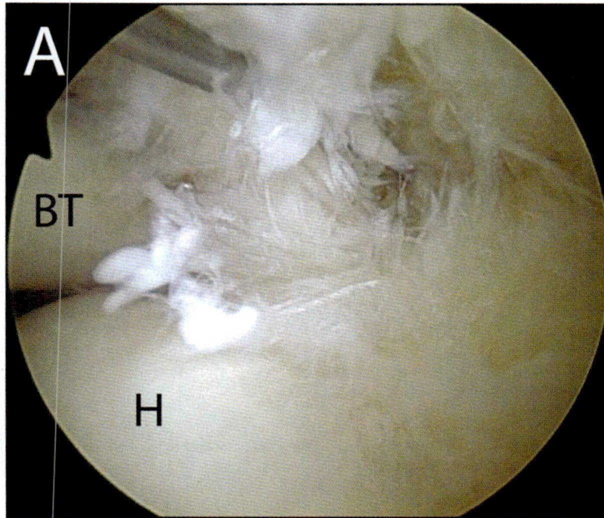

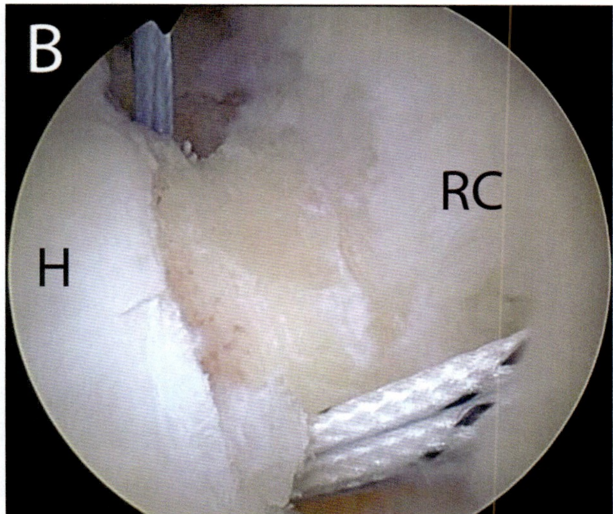

Figure 5.12 Right shoulder, posterior viewing portal. **A:** A partial-thickness rotator cuff tear is visualized. **B:** Anteromedial and posteromedial anchors have been placed in a transtendon fashion. BT, biceps tendon; H, humerus; RC, rotator cuff.

When using two or more anchors, the arthroscopist may choose to individually pass mattresses sutures as described previously. However, when two anchors are used, a "double-pulley" technique is possible. A suture from the anterior anchor may be tied to a suture from the posterior anchor to create a large mattress stitch between the anchors. One or both sutures pairs from each anchor may be used to create a mattress suture between the anchors.

Following transtendon placement of two medial anchors, the arthroscope is reintroduced into the subacromial space and a cannula is established in the lateral portal. The suture limbs are then identified exiting the rotator cuff. To perform the double-pulley technique, one limb from each suture pair (i.e., one from the anterior anchor, one from the posterior anchor) is retrieved through the lateral cannula. A Surgeon's knot is then tied extracorporeally and the tails cut. Using the anchor eyelets as pulleys, traction is applied to the opposite ends of the sutures, pulling the knot through the cannula, into the subacromial space and against the rotator cuff. The sutures are pulled until the knot lies taut against the rotator cuff. The opposite ends of the suture are then retrieved through the lateral portal and a static knot is tied using the Surgeon's Sixth Finger (Arthrex, Inc., Naples, FL), closing the suture loop (Fig. 5.13). Because these latter sutures can no longer move between the anchor eyelets, a sliding knot is not possible and a static knot must be tied. This creates a double-mattress knot between anchors, the largest mattress loop possible, and compresses the rotator cuff along its entire anterior-to-posterior footprint. It also seals the medial margin of the footprint against synovial fluid (Fig. 5.14).

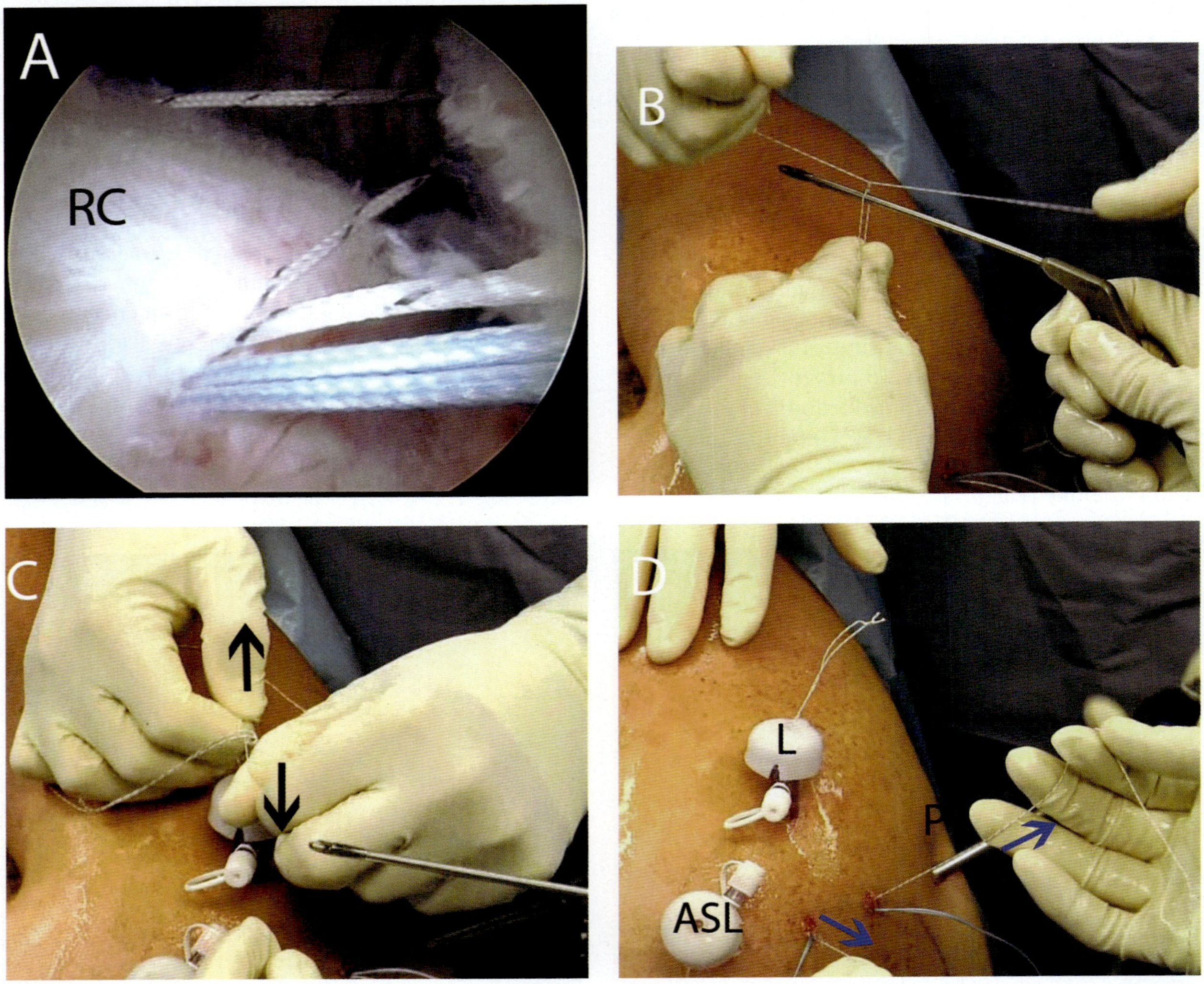

Figure 5.13 Double-pulley technique in a right shoulder. **A:** While viewing from a posterior subacromial portal, a suture from an anterior anchor and a suture from a posterior anchor are retrieved out a lateral portal. **B:** Extracorporeally, a surgeon's knot is tied over an instrument. **C:** After the knot is tied, the surgeon pulls on the loop (*black arrows*) to ensure that the knot does not slide. **D:** The suture tails at the knot are cut. Then, an assistant pulls on the opposite suture limbs (*blue arrows*) to deliver the knot into the subacromial space.

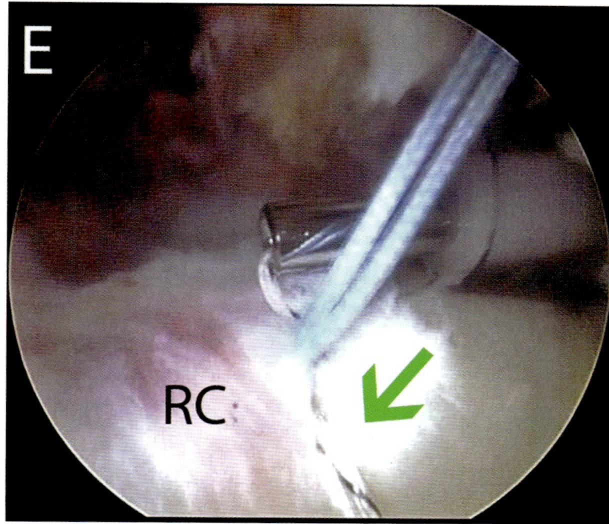

Figure 5.13 *(Continued)* **E:** The double-mattress knot is completed by tying the opposite suture limbs as a static knot with a Surgeon's Sixth Finger Knot Pusher (Arthrex, Inc., Naples, FL). The first mattress knot is also seen (*green arrow*). ASL, anterosuperolateral portal; L, lateral subacromial portal; P, posterior portal; RC, rotator cuff.

Double-pulley PASTA-bridge Technique

Repair of PASTA lesions is very adequately treated by the transtendon double pulley technique in many cases, particularly if the medial-to-lateral dimension of the tear is ≤50% of the width of the entire footprint. However, when the medial-to-lateral tear dimension exceeds 50%, the standard double-pulley technique may not provide compression to the lateral part of the PASTA lesion.

We believe that compression over the entire tendon–bone interface of the cuff repair construct is important in promoting tendon healing. Therefore, in most PASTA repairs, we currently use a double-row bridging technique called

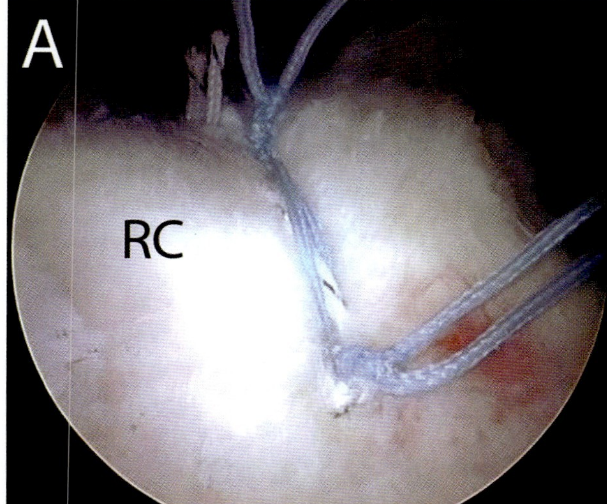

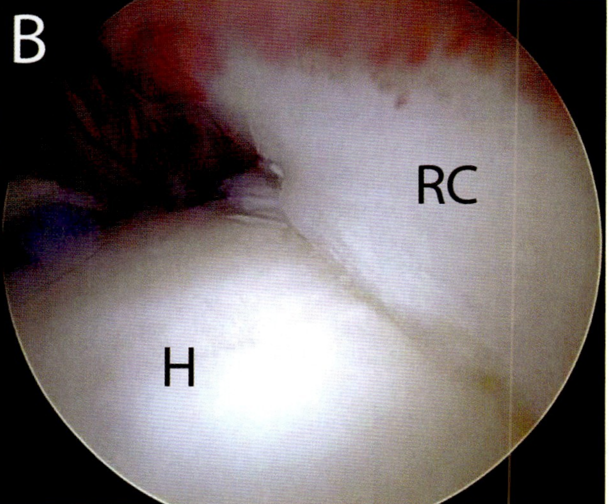

Figure 5.14 **A:** Right shoulder, posterior subacromial portal, demonstrating completed double-pulley mattress stitch for repair of a PASTA rotator cuff tear. **B:** Intra-articular view from a posterior portal demonstrates restoration of the medial rotator cuff footprint (compare to Fig. 5.12). H, humerus; RC, rotator cuff.

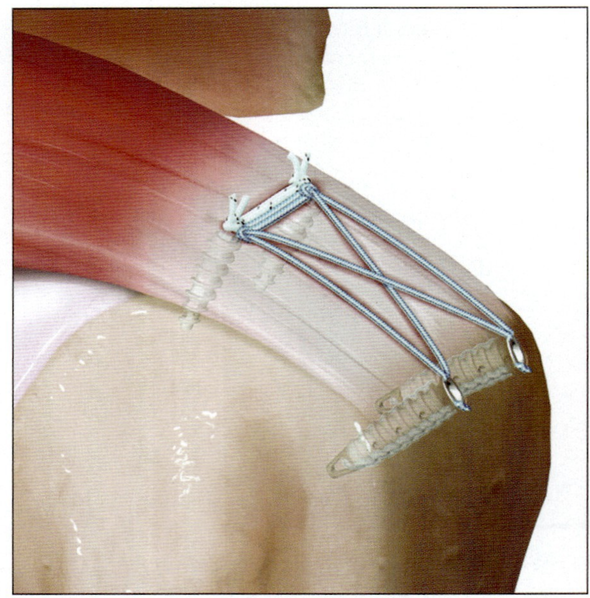

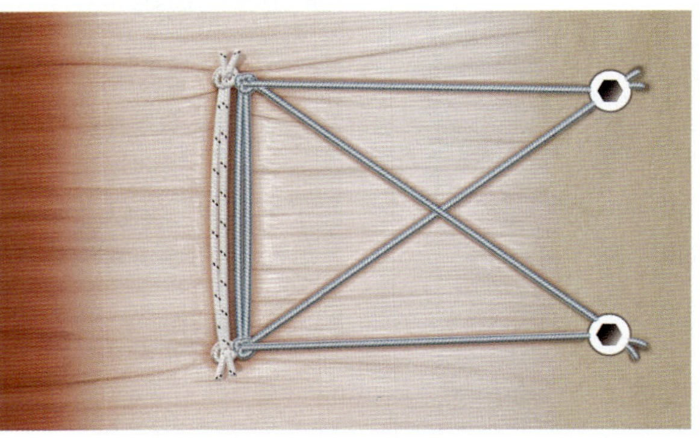

Figure 5.15 **A:** Schematic of a completed PASTA-bridge repair. Mattress knots tied between two medial anchors (BioComposite Corkscrew FT; Arthrex, Inc., Naples, FL) seal off the rotator cuff footprint from synovial fluid. Blue suture limbs have been crisscrossed and secured laterally to two lateral BioComposite SwiveLock C anchors (Arthrex, Inc., Naples, FL). **B:** Aerial view demonstrates the double-medial mattress, as well as the crisscross pattern.

the *PASTA bridge*. In this technique, we use two transtendon medial anchors, and tie two sets of double-mattress sutures between the two anchors, using the *double-pulley* technique to recreate the medial border of contact between tendon and bone. These medial mattress sutures effectively seal the footprint from synovial fluid and its potential deleterious effects on healing. After tying the medial knots, one set of sutures, with tails left long, is used to create a *suture bridge in situ* (PASTA bridge) configuration that bridges across to a lateral row of two anchors, creating a linked compressive construct over the PASTA lesion(Fig. 5.15).

After the PASTA lesion has been identified, the bone bed is prepared with a combination of power shaver, power burr, and ring curettes so that there is a bleeding base of bone. In many cases, the anterior working portal is sufficient to access the entire footprint. However, in some of the large PASTA lesions, a lateral transtendon mini-puncture may be necessary to reach all parts of the footprint. One should not complete the entire cuff tear from anterior to posterior, but only make a small 4-mm puncture that barely admits the instrumentation. In this way, almost all of the lateral tendon attachments are preserved and standard PASTA repair techniques can be used without disrupting these important intact lateral tendon attachments.

After the bone bed has been prepared, the arthroscope is transferred from the intra-articular space to the subacromial space, and a thorough subacromial bursectomy is performed. It is important to do the bursectomy prior to placing the transtendon suture anchors so that the sutures can be easily visualized in the subacromial space and retrieved later during the repair. If the bursectomy is done after anchor placement, the sutures can be inadvertently damaged or destroyed by the shaver blade. In doing the bursectomy, the posterior gutter should be cleared of fibrofatty tissue, since anchor placement is often in a relatively posterior position. In addition, the lateral gutter is cleared to approximately 12 to 15 mm below the corner of the greater tuberosity in order to provide adequate visualization for placement of the lateral anchors.

A spinal needle is used to determine the correct transtendon placement of the anteromedial suture anchor while viewing intra-articularly. This anchor should be placed just posterior to the top of the bicipital groove. A transtendon 5-mm cannula with a silicon-dam diaphragm is placed alongside the spinal needle. Through this cannula, a punch is introduced to create the bone socket for the anchor. Then, a 4.5-mm BioComposite Corkscrew FT suture anchor is placed (Fig. 5.16).

Next, the spinal needle is used to determine optimal placement of the posteromedial anchor. In general, a 70° arthroscope affords a better view for performing this part of the procedure. The 5-mm cannula is again passed transtendon alongside the spinal needle, the bone socket is made, a second 4.5-mm BioComposite Corkscrew FT is placed, and the cannula is removed. At this point, there are two medial anchors, and the suture strands from each individual anchor are passing through one of two

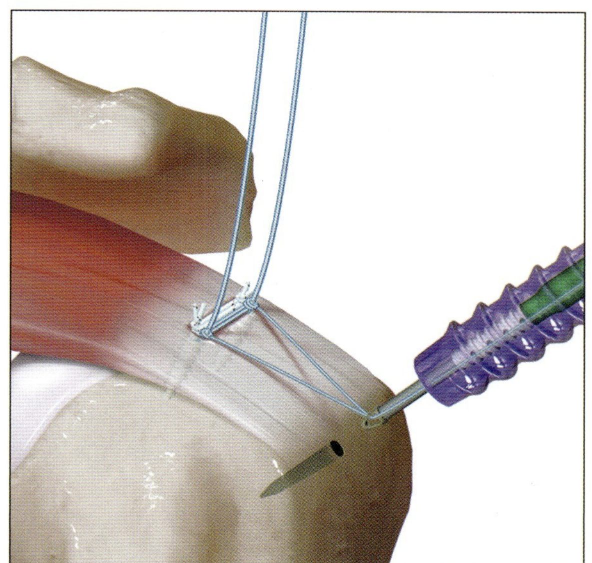

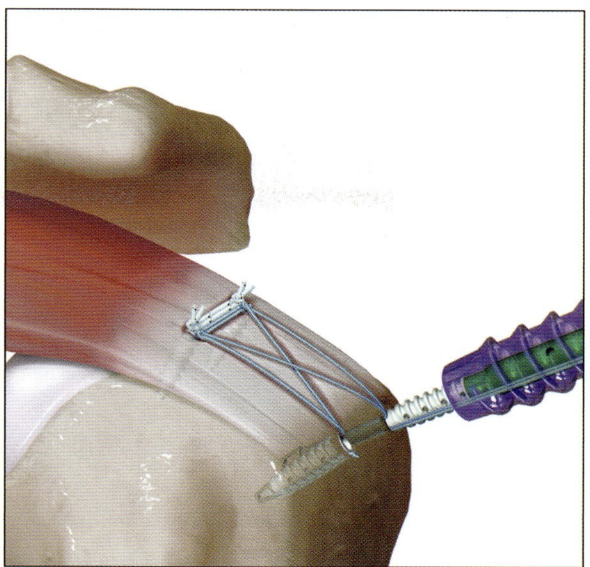

Figure 5.19 Schematic of lateral row fixation during a PASTA-bridge repair. **A:** Medial mattress knots have been tied using a double-pulley technique. Suture limbs from the second medial mattress knot have been preserved. One limb from the anteromedial anchor and one limb from the posteromedial anchor are retrieved and secured with a posterolateral BioComposite SwiveLock C anchor (Arthrex, Inc., Naples, FL). **B:** The steps are repeated with an anterolateral anchor.

(Fig. 5.21). Then the two suture tails are threaded through the eyelet of a 4.75-mm BioComposite SwiveLock C anchor (Arthrex, Inc., Naples, FL) (Fig. 5.22A). The anchor eyelet is slid along the sutures and positioned at the bottom of the bone socket, then the suture tails are tensioned and the screw is inserted by turning the inserter handle while holding the thumb pad to prevent its rotation (Fig. 5.22B). This causes the reverse-threaded sleeve on the inserter to advance the screw to the bottom of the bone socket while the eyelet and suture tails are held stationary during screw insertion (Fig. 5.22C). The safety suture for the eyelet is then unwrapped from the base of the driver handle and the inserter is removed. The safety suture is a #2 FiberWire that may be used to reduce dog-ears, if necessary, by

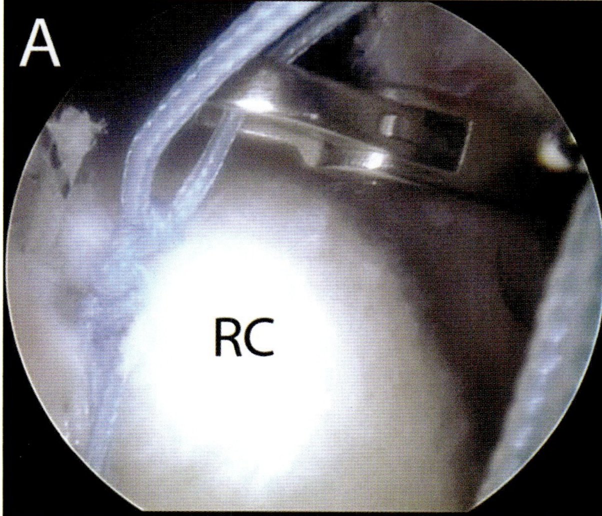

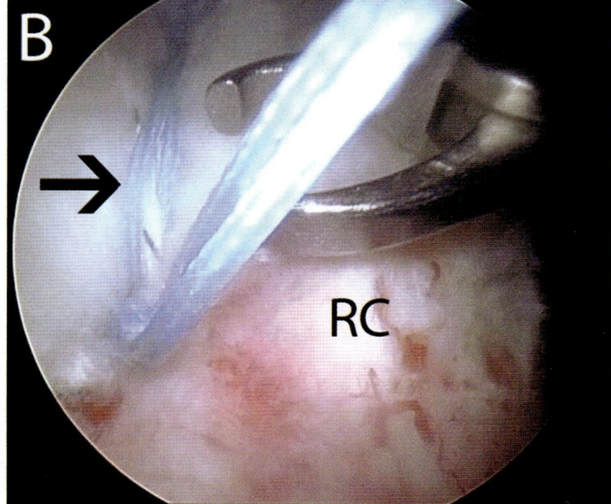

Figure 5.20 Right shoulder, posterior subacromial viewing portal, demonstrates **(A)** retrieval of a suture limb from an anterior anchor, and **(B)** retrieval of a suture limb from a posterior anchor in preparation for a lateral bridge for repair of a PASTA. A double-mattress stitch (*black arrow*) is also seen that was tied using a double-pulley technique. RC, rotator cuff.

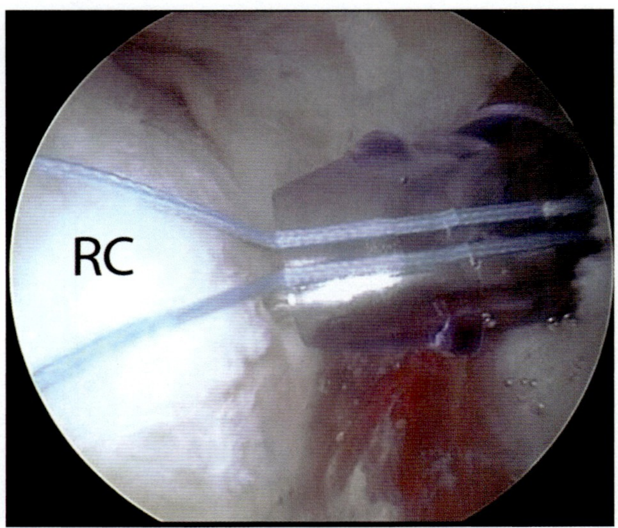

Figure 5.21 Right shoulder, posterior subacromial viewing portal, demonstrates use of a punch to create a bone socket for an anterolateral anchor. Note: By tensioning the suture limbs, the cannula can be used as a guide to determine the adequate position prior to placement of the punch. RC, rotator cuff.

passing one limb through the redundant tendon tissue and securing the tendon with a six-throw Surgeon's knot. The two suture tails that have been wedged between the anchor and the bone as a knotless lateral fixation are cut flush with the bone.

The remaining two FiberWire suture limbs are retrieved through the lateral portal, and they are tensioned against the mouth of the lateral cannula to determine optimal placement of the posterolateral anchor. Another BioComposite SwiveLock C anchor is placed posterolaterally in the same manner as the anterolateral anchor (Fig. 5.23). This four-anchor construct creates a *suture bridge in situ*, or a *PASTA bridge* (Fig. 5.24A). The arthroscope is once again placed inside the joint to confirm that the footprint contact has been anatomically restored (Fig. 5.24B).

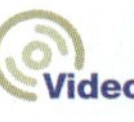

It should be noted that, for lateral fixation, we sometimes prefer the self-punching SwiveLock anchors (BioComposite SwiveLock SP; Arthrex, Inc., Naples, FL). This anchor has a pointed metal eyelet that allows the driver itself to be used as a punch, eliminating punching as a separate step.

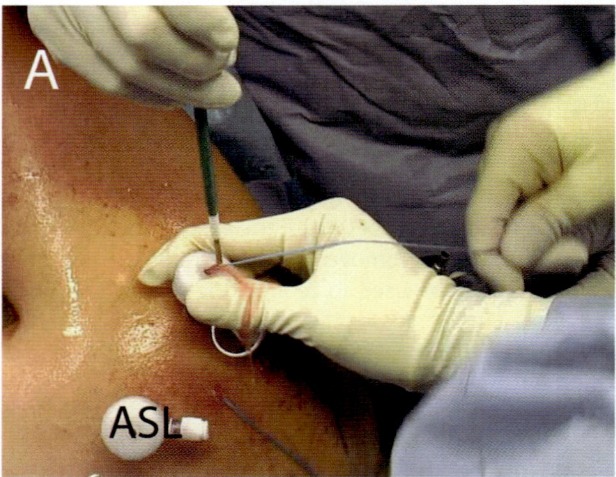

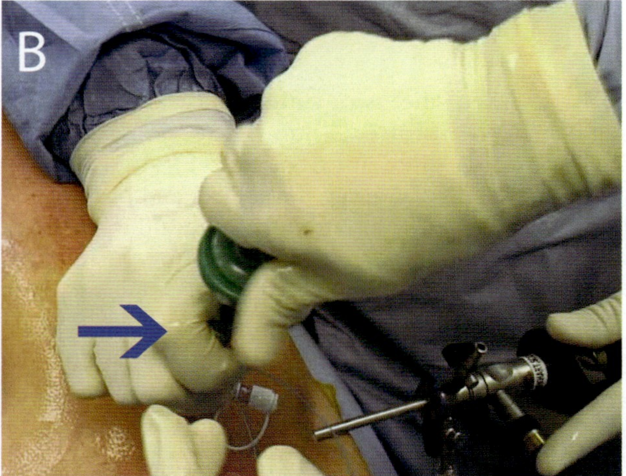

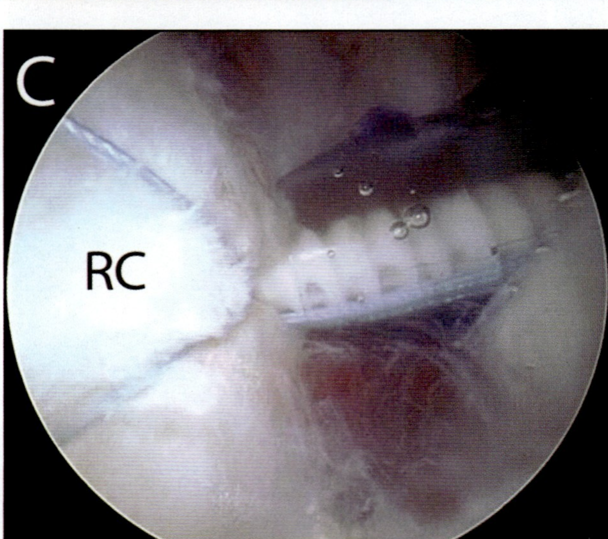

Figure 5.22 Lateral anchor placement for a PASTA-bridge repair in a right shoulder. **A:** Following creation of a bone socket, sutures limbs are extracorporeally threaded through the eyelet of a BioComposite SwiveLock C anchor (Arthrex, Inc., Naples, FL). **B:** After seating the eyelet, the surgeon holds the thumb pad of the driver stationary (*blue arrow*), while an assistant turns the handle to advance the anchor. **C:** Arthroscopic view from a posterior subacromial portal demonstrates insertion of the anchor. ASL, anterosuperolateral portal; RC, rotator cuff.

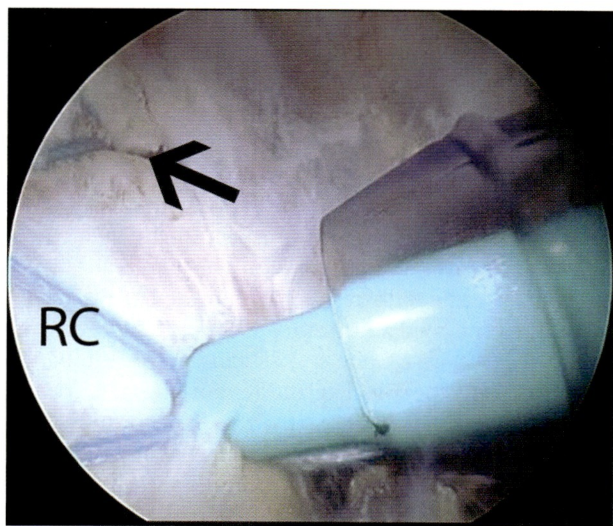

Figure 5.23 Right shoulder, posterior subacromial viewing portal, demonstrates placement of posterolateral anchor for a PASTA-bridge rotator cuff repair. The suture limbs from an anterolateral anchor can be seen as well (*black arrow*). RC, rotator cuff.

Combined PASTA Bridge and Biceps Tenodesis

If the biceps is determined to require tenodesis due to partial tearing or to subluxation, the sutures from the tenodesis construct can be incorporated into the PASTA bridge as a minor modification. This requires that the biceps tenodesis be performed prior to rotator cuff repair, using a BioComposite Tenodesis screw (Arthrex, Inc., Naples, FL) at the anterior aspect of the greater tuberosity. This creates a construct in which the BioComposite Tenodesis screw essentially performs the same function as an anteromedial anchor. The only difference is that the four suture limbs from this construct are fixed within the tenodesis construct and will not slide.

The fact that the anteromedial sutures will not slide necessitates a small modification in the double-pulley technique. First of all, the four suture limbs must be passed through the anterior portion of the supraspinatus tendon, since the BioComposite Tenodesis screw would have been placed through the upper part of the rotator interval tissue. Secondly, the sutures cannot be tied outside the body as in

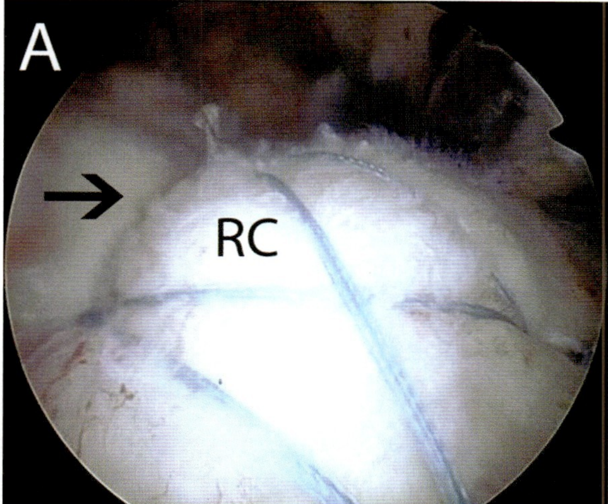

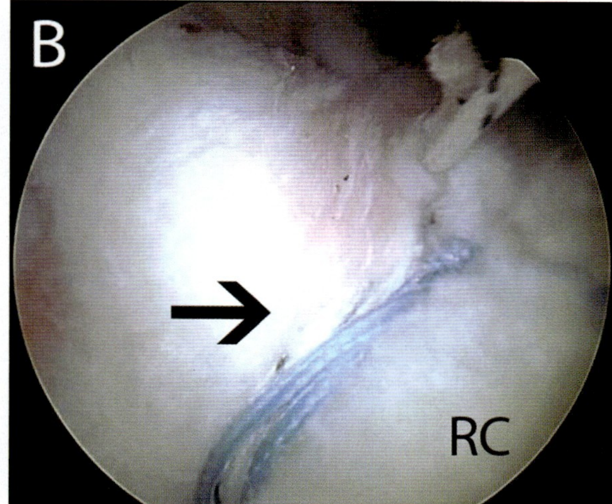

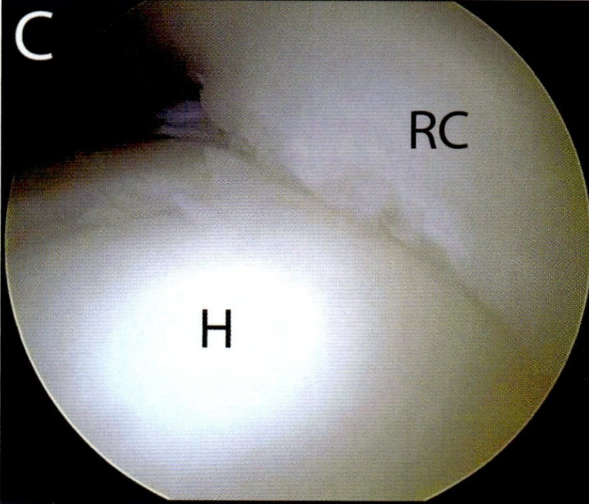

Figure 5.24 **A:** Right shoulder, posterior subacromial viewing portal, demonstrates final PASTA-bridge repair with a medial double-mattress stitch (*black arrow*) and criss-crossed sutures from medial anchors that have been secured laterally with knotless anchors. **B:** Up-close view of the medial double-mattress portion of the repair (*black arrow*). **C:** Intra-articular view from a posterior viewing portal demonstrates restoration of the medial rotator cuff footprint. H, humerus; RC, rotator cuff.

the standard double-pulley technique because the sutures cannot slide and therefore an exteriorized knot cannot be delivered back into the subacromial space. Static knots are tied between sutures from the BioComposite Tenodesis construct and the posteromedial anchor, and then the tails are used to connect to lateral bridging BioComposite SwiveLock C anchors in the same way as in the double-pulley technique.

INTRA-ARTICULAR REPAIR OF PASTA LESIONS

In patients with PASTA lesions, an intra-articular repair provides a low-profile repair, which reduces the articular flap to the footprint without theoretically altering the tension of the bursal surface of the rotator cuff. In this technique, knots and sutures are avoided in the subacromial space with repair performed using a knotless anchor (PushLock; Arthrex, Inc., Naples, FL). The ideal candidate is a young patient with an acute partial articular surface tear, whereby the articular surface flap is still intact, with good-quality tissue that is purely avulsed from the bone bed (Fig. 5.25).

The bone bed is similarly debrided to a bleeding bone surface. Attention is briefly turned to the subacromial space and a thorough bursectomy is performed. Then, the arthroscope is returned to the intra-articular space and one or two sutures are placed through the edge of the articular surface flap in either a simple or mattress fashion. Depending on the angle of approach, a Scorpion (Arthrex, Inc., Naples, FL) or SutureLasso (Arthrex, Inc., Naples, FL) may be used to pass a #2 FiberWire suture. Care is taken to ensure an adequate bite of tissue is obtained without inadvertently entrapping the bursal aspect of the rotator cuff. Usually one or two sutures are required (Fig. 5.26).

A spinal needle is then used to find the correct angle of approach to the medial aspect of the footprint. A punch is then used to create a bone socket transtendon through the rotator cuff using the spinal needle as a guide (Fig. 5.27). If the angle of approach allows, the punch and anchor may also be inserted through the rotator interval to avoid any violation of the rotator cuff. After creation of the bone socket, the sutures are then retrieved through the same percutaneous incision, via the same transtendon or transrotator interval hole (Fig. 5.28).

The sutures are fed through the PushLock anchor eyelet and the anchor is slid down the sutures to the proximal portion of the bone socket (Fig. 5.29). At this time, the anchor eyelet is inserted into the bone socket with the sutures untensioned. This is to ensure that the anchor eyelet will easily "bottom out" in the bone socket with minimal tension and therefore there will be no prominence of the anchor when subsequently inserted. If another anchor is required, the bone socket is punched and the anchor eyelet

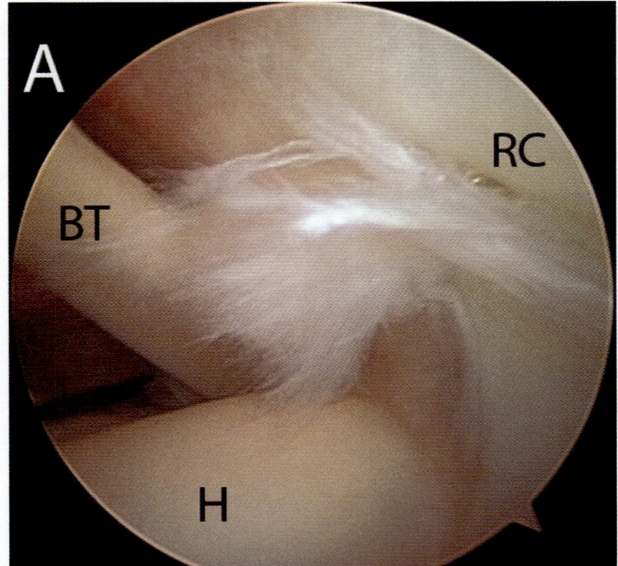

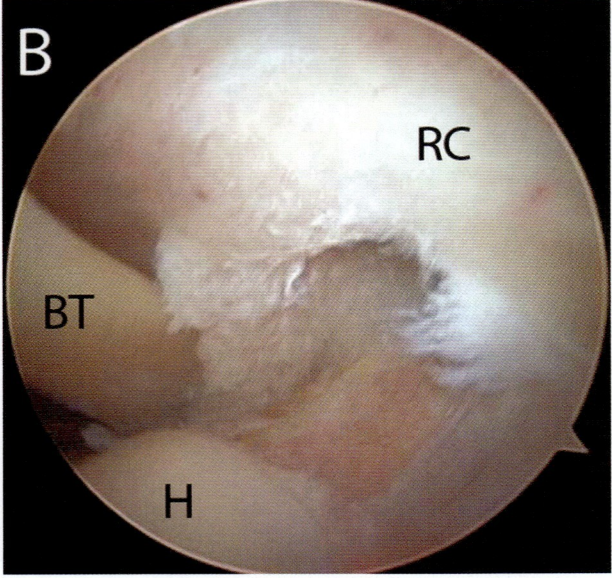

Figure 5.25 **A:** Right shoulder, posterior viewing portal, demonstrates a small partial-thickness articular surface tendon avulsion. In this young patient with good-quality tissue, the tear is amenable to an intra-articular repair technique. **B:** Same shoulder after the rotator cuff margins have been debrided. BT, biceps tendon; H, humerus; RC, rotator cuff.

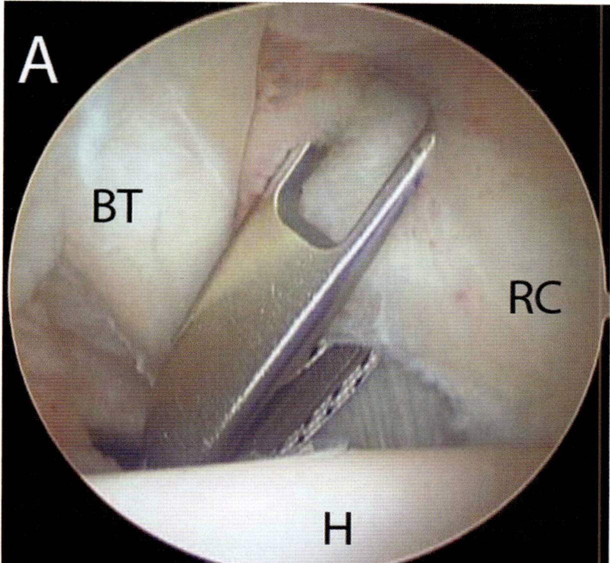

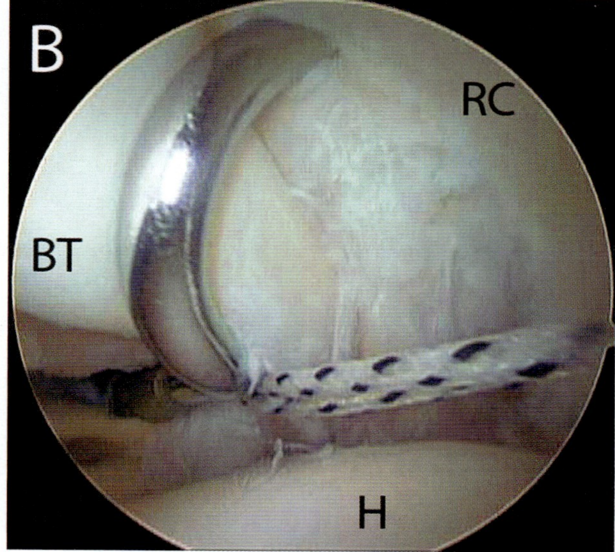

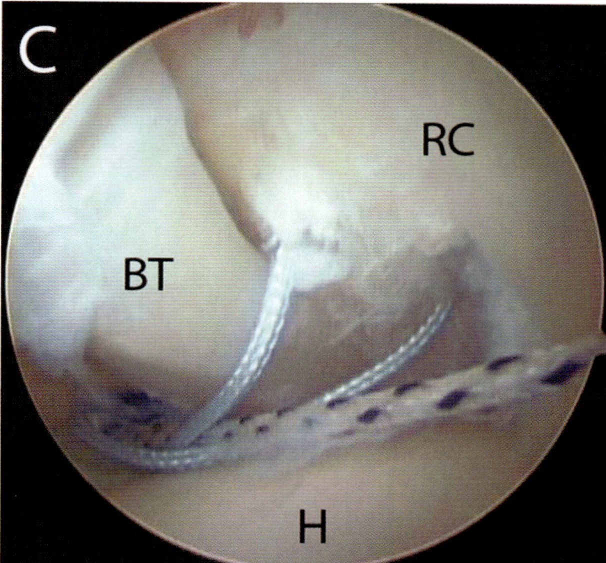

Figure 5.26 **A:** Right shoulder, posterior viewing portal. A Scorpion (Arthrex, Inc., Naples, FL) has been introduced through an anterior working portal to pass a simple stitch through the posterior margin of a partial-thickness articular-sided rotator cuff tear. **B:** A SutureLasso (Arthrex, Inc., Naples, FL) is used to pass a simple stitch through the anterior margin of the rotator cuff tear. **C:** Appearance after both sutures have been placed. BT, biceps tendon; H, humerus; RC, rotator cuff.

provisionally inserted. This is performed since reduction of the tendon (with the first anchor) will obscure visualization for placement of the second anchor and subsequent anchors.

The PushLock anchor is then impacted into place, securing the sutures and tendon to bone. The sutures are then retrieved and cut in the subacromial space as short as possible against the rotator cuff. The final construct should demonstrate articular flap reduction to bone with no sutures visible in the subacromial space (Fig. 5.30).

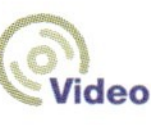

BURSAL TEARS

Bursal surface tears of the rotator cuff are less common than their PASTA counterpart but nonetheless demand special considerations. Because of their association with extrinsic impingement, an acromioplasty should be performed in nearly all cases of a bursal surface rotator cuff tear. Arthroscopic repair may be accomplished with completion of the tear and double-row repair for high-grade lesions (as described previously), or with repair in situ. This section describes in situ repair.

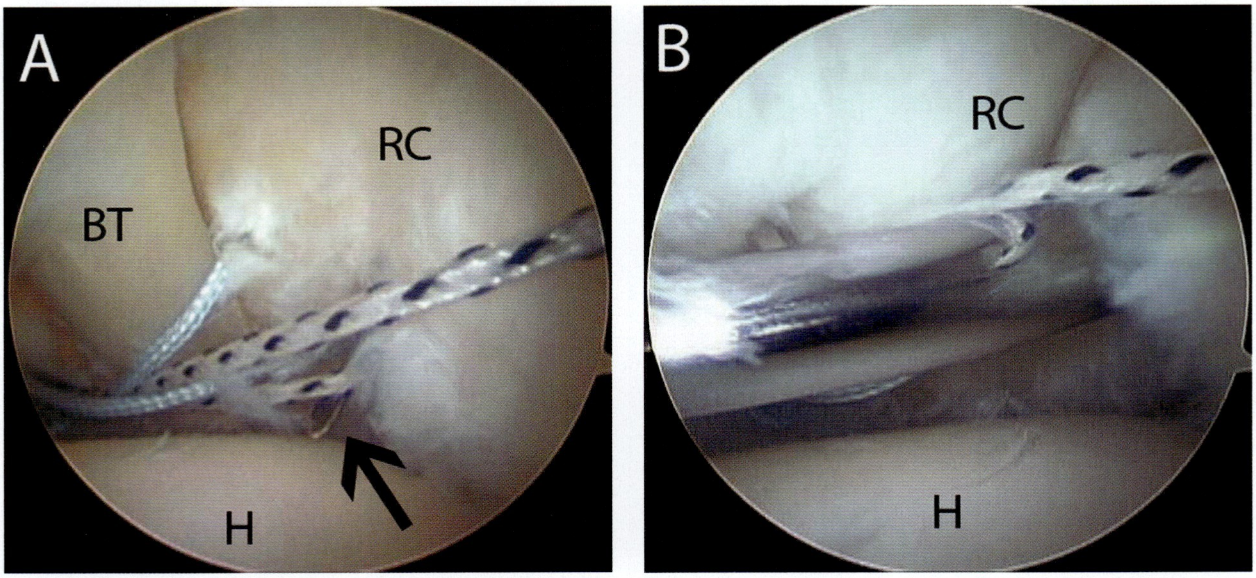

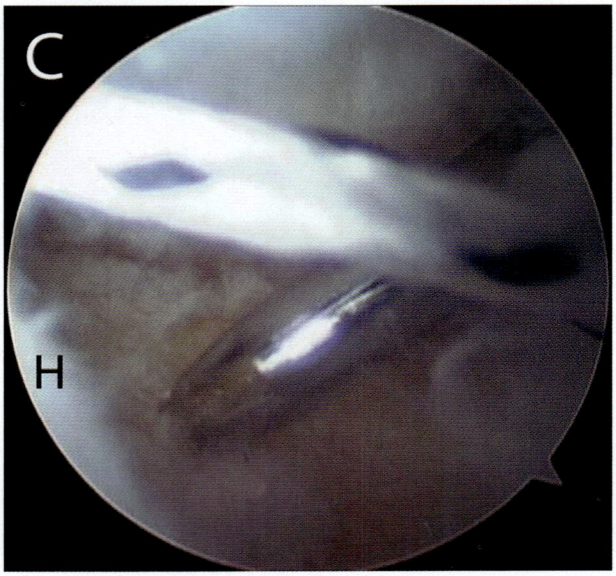

Figure 5.27 **A:** Right shoulder, posterior viewing portal, demonstrates use of a spinal needle (*black arrow*) as a guide to determine an angle of approach to create a bone socket for an intra-articular rotator cuff repair. **B:** A punch has been inserted adjacent to the spinal needle. Note: The punch is pushed past the articular margin to ensure that the rotator cuff margins are free from the tip. **C:** Then, the punch is seated on the bone bed to create a bone socket for a PushLock anchor (Arthrex, Inc., Naples, FL). BT, biceps tendon; H, humerus; RC, rotator cuff.

Small bursal surface rotator cuff tears with good-quality tissue are amenable to a SpeedFix repair (see Chapter 4, "Complete Rotator Cuff Tears"). The tear is identified and a probe is used to confirm that the medial wall of the rotator cuff is intact (Fig. 5.31). The rotator cuff margins are debrided to healthy tissue. The lateral greater tuberosity bone bed is prepared to a bleeding surface with a combination of ring curette, electrocautery, and a motorized burr. A mattress stitch of FiberTape is then placed with a Scorpion suture passer (Arthrex, Inc., Naples, FL) by passing the two FiberWire leaders from inferior to superior through the rotator cuff (Fig. 5.32). This stitch is then secured in the greater tuberosity with a BioComposite SwiveLock C anchor (Arthrex, Inc., Naples, FL) (Fig. 5.33).

For large bursal surface tears with poor tissue quality, we prefer to perform a variant of the SutureBridge double-row repair with multiple knots tied medially (Fig. 5.34). Tying multiple knots improves the construct strength by increasing the resistance to pull out in poor-quality rotator cuff tissue. Following debridement of the tear margins, the bone bed is prepared (Fig. 5.35). Two double-loaded BioComposite Corkscrew FT anchors (Arthrex, Inc., Naples, FL) are placed (Fig. 5.36A). If the footprint is narrow, 4.5-mm suture anchors may be required as opposed to the standard 5.5-mm anchors. Each suture end is passed

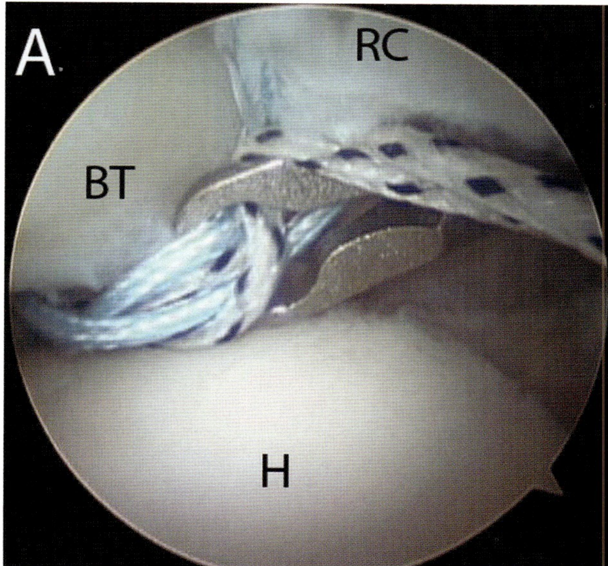

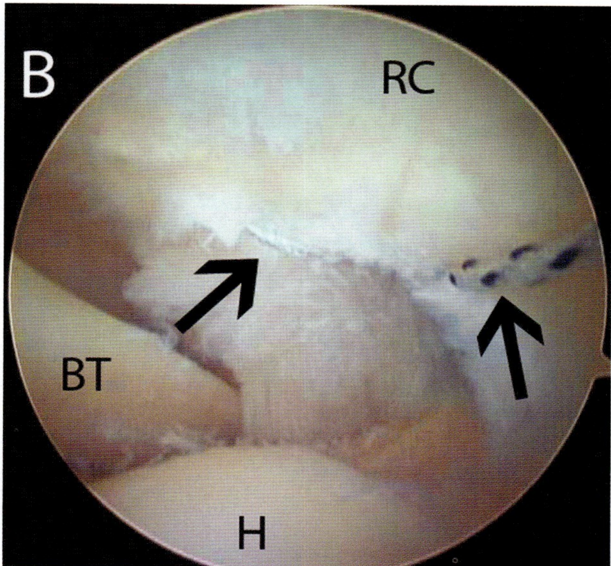

Figure 5.28 **A:** Right shoulder, posterior viewing portal. After creating a bone socket, sutures are retrieved through the rotator cuff. **B:** Sutures (*black arrows*) have been retrieved through the rotator cuff tear. BT, biceps tendon; H, humerus; RC, rotator cuff.

through the tear edge with a Scorpion suture passer, for a total of eight passes through the rotator cuff. The sutures are tied as mattress stitches, resulting in four mattress stitches through the medial rotator cuff (Fig. 5.36B). The suture tails are preserved. The free suture ends are then crisscrossed and secured laterally with two knotless Bio-Composite SwiveLock C anchors. The lateral row not only increases the footprint, but also lays the medial knots down on the rotator cuff surface to create a low-profile repair (Fig. 5.37).

Figure 5.29 Right shoulder, posterior viewing portal. A Push-Lock anchor (Arthrex, Inc., Naples, FL) is seated into a previously placed bone socket for an intra-articular repair. H, humerus; RC, rotator cuff.

PARTIAL-THICKNESS INTERSTITIAL ROTATOR CUFF TEARS

While the recognition and treatment of partial-thickness bursal-sided or articular-sided rotator cuff tears has been thoroughly discussed in the literature, a lesser recognized pattern of rotator cuff pathology is the partial-thickness interstitial rotator cuff tear pattern. The rotator cuff tendon complex is composed of parallel layers of collagen fibrils that attach to the greater tuberosity (Fig. 5.38A). While the majority of rotator cuff tears occur at the tendinous attachment to the bone, occasionally a shear force between the layers of the tendon can cause a tear between these layers. In this situation, there can be a tear between the layers of tendon as well as partial detachment of tendon from the bone. This detachment can be hidden between the articular and bursal layers of intact cuff thus making it impossible to visualize. (Fig. 5.38B, C)

This interstitial tear pattern has been termed the *PITA tear*. This term was conceived by Burkhart fellow #4, Dr. Peter Parten, and stands for Partial Interstitial Tendon Avulsion (PITA). This term is also appropriate as the tear ends up looking like pita bread. Both outer rotator cuff surfaces (bread layers) are intact but there is a hollow space between the layers (pita pocket) (Fig. 5.39).

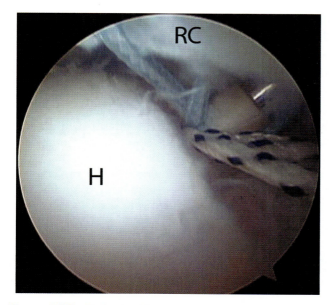

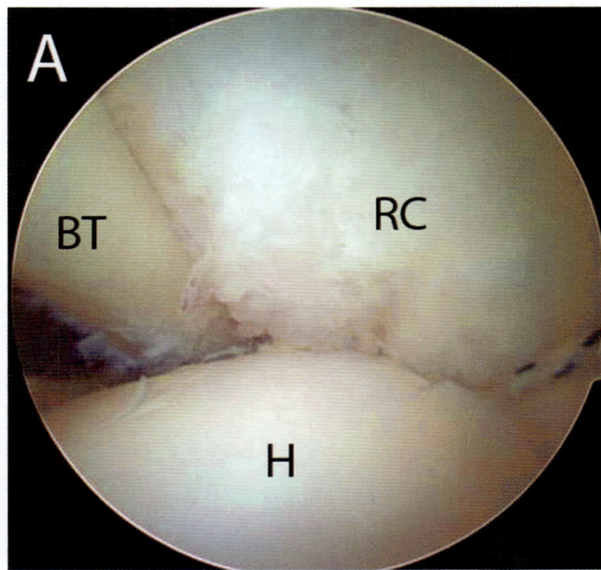

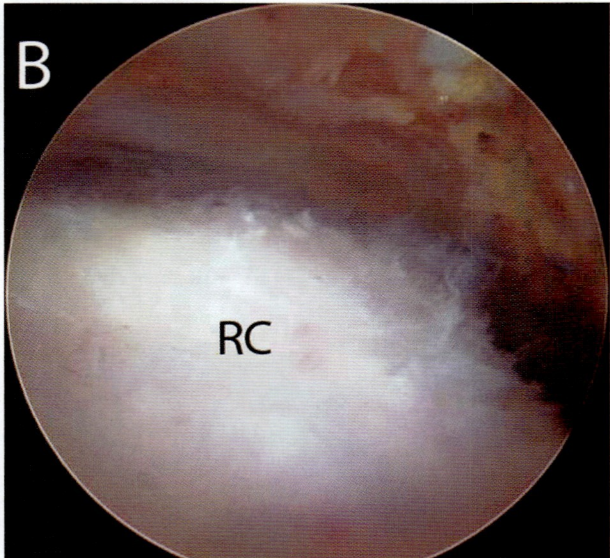

Figure 5.30 **A:** Right shoulder, posterior glenohumeral viewing portal, demonstrates final intra-articular repair of a partial-thickness articular-sided rotator cuff tear (Compare to Fig. 5.25). **B:** Posterior subacromial viewing portal in the same shoulder demonstrates a knotless repair. BT, biceps tendon; H, humerus; RC, rotator cuff.

This entity can mimic the symptoms and clinical exam of a complete-thickness rotator cuff tear. While it may be visualized on MRI (Fig. 5.40), it can be frequently missed because of the patient position in the MRI scanner. With the arm adducted by the side, the collagen layers that make up the rotator cuff tendon are all tensioned such that they are compressed against one another and thus may not be visualized as a tear on MRI. Also since the tear is within the layers, there may be little or no joint fluid extravasation into the defect. When the arm is in a more functional position however, these layers can separate causing abnormal force distribution and propagation of the tear—even within the bone bed in the middle of the cuff tendon insertion site.

Figure 5.31 Left shoulder, posterior subacromial viewing portal demonstrating a bursal surface rotator cuff tear. A probe is introduced from a lateral portal to confirm that the medial wall is intact. GT, greater tuberosity; RC, rotator cuff.

Interstitial tears can be quite difficult to diagnose with standard arthroscopy. As visualized from both the articular and bursal vantage points, the tendinous attachments appear intact. Even with palpation with a probe, these peripheral layers of cuff tendon feel attached. Some tricks we have developed to assist in the discovery of such tears are the dimple sign, sliding-layers sign, bubble sign, probe push, and the slit test

Dimple Sign

The dimple sign is an intra-articular arthroscopic finding that can clue the surgeon into a potential PITA tear. When visualizing the supraspinatus insertion at the articular margin of the humerus, pay close attention to the area between the rotator cable and the articular margin. If there is a dimpling of the tendon in this area, this is considered a positive Dimple sign (Fig. 5.41). It is not diagnostic for a PITA tear but it should heighten your suspicion for such a possibility.

Sliding-layers Sign

We recommend that you palpate EVERY rotator cuff from the bursal surface with a probe. Only by palpating completely normal rotator cuff tendons will you develop the kinesthetic feel to know when something does not "feel right." Remember that surgery (like cowboyin') is still

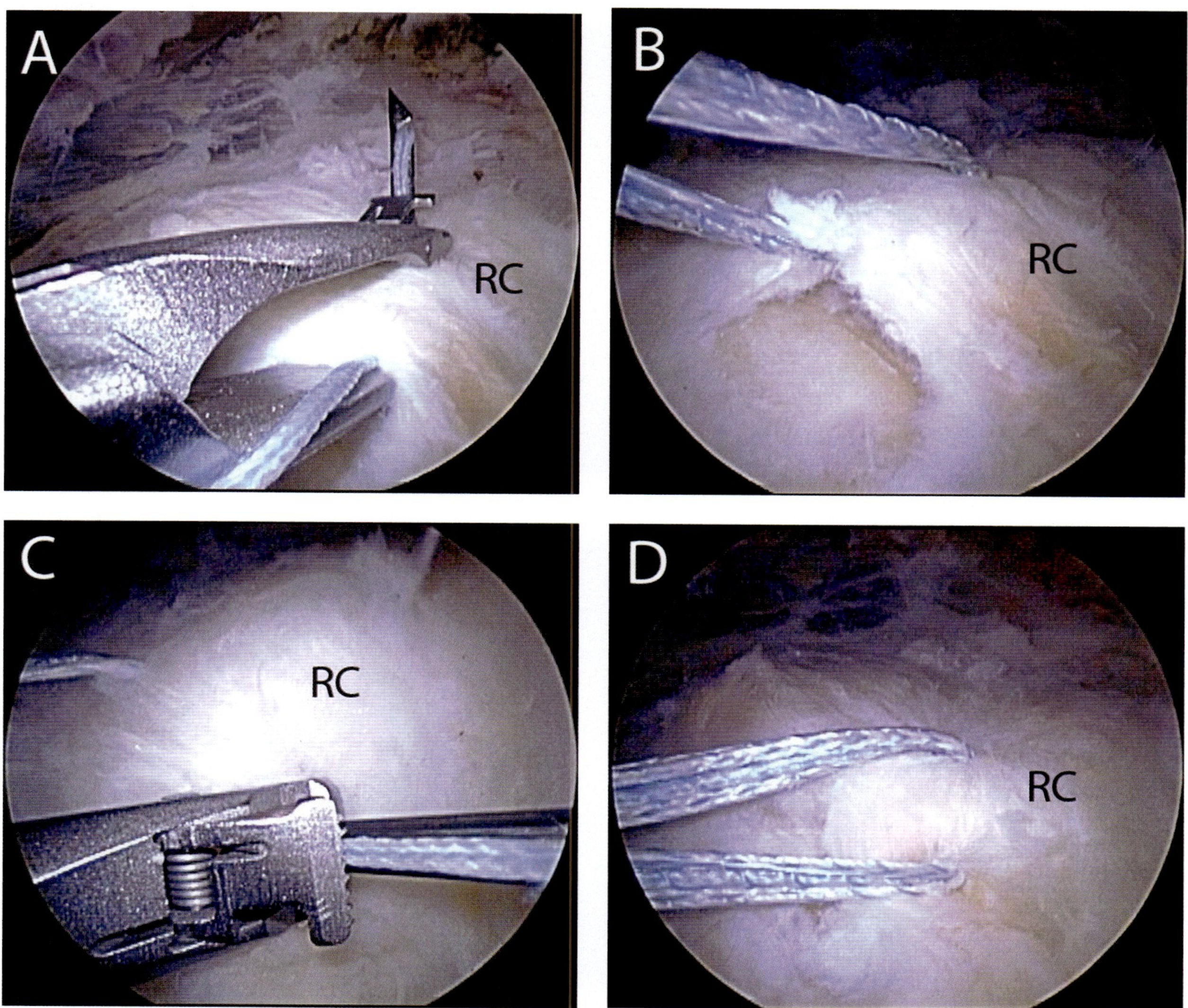

Figure 5.32 Mattress stitch placement for SpeedFix (Arthrex, Inc., Naples, FL) repair of a bursal surface rotator cuff tear in a left shoulder viewed from a posterior subsacromial portal. **A:** A #2 FiberWire leader of a FiberTape suture is passed with a Scorpion FastPass through the anterior aspect of the tear and **(B)** retrieved out the lateral portal. **C:** The FiberWire leader of the suture that exits the rotator cuff inferiorly is loaded onto the Scorpion and passed through the posterior aspect of the tear. **D:** View after placement of an inverted mattress stitch. RC, rotator cuff.

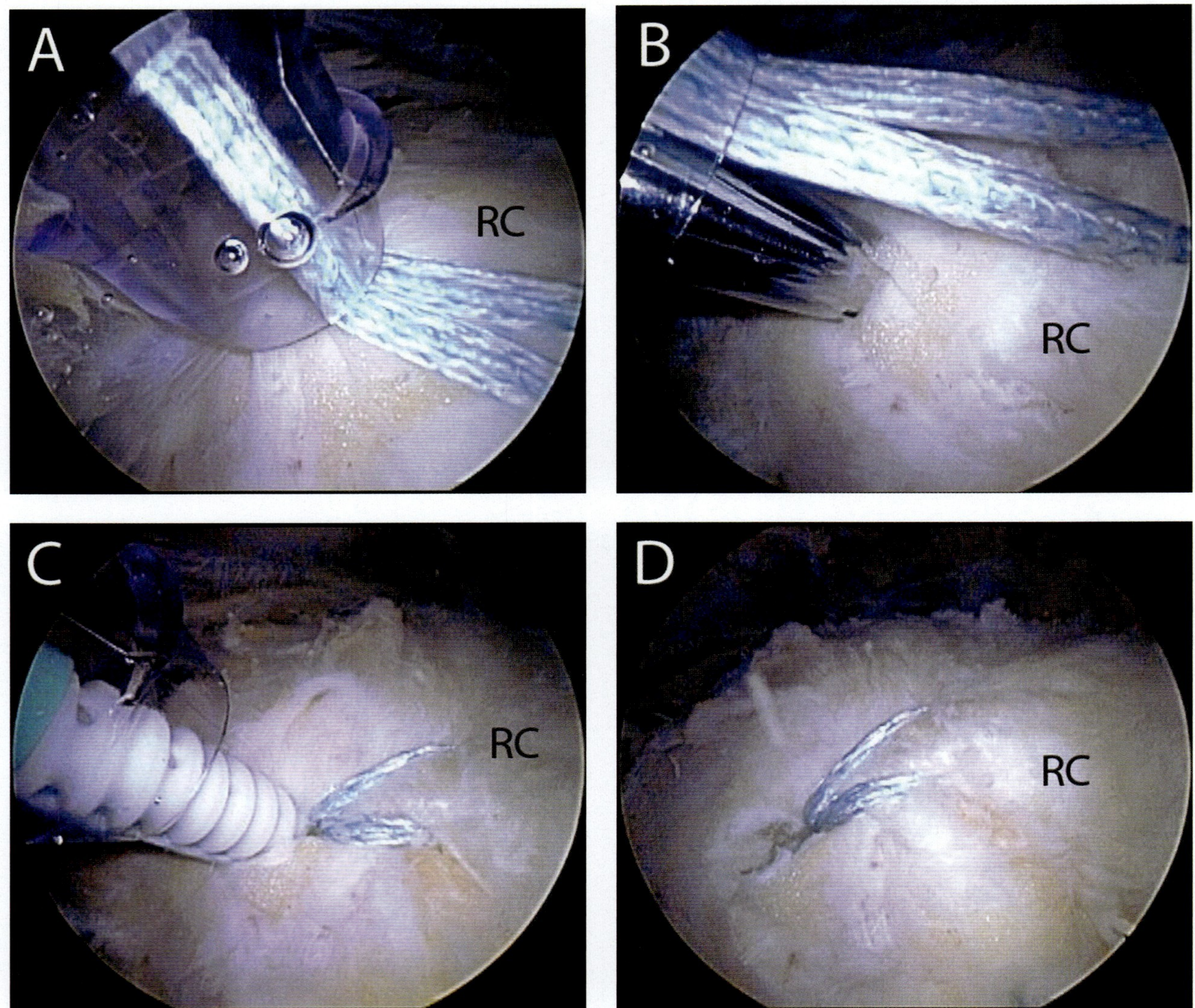

Figure 5.33 Completion of SpeedFix (Arthrex, Inc., Naples, FL) repair of a bursal surface rotator cuff tear in a left shoulder viewed from a posterior subacromial portal. **A:** Using a cannula as a guide, the rotator cuff is tensioned with the FiberTape to determine the appropriate anchor position. **B:** A punch is inserted to create a bone socket. **C:** After threading the FiberTape sutures through the eyelet of a Bio-Composite SwiveLock C anchor, the anchor is inserted into the prepared bone socket. **D:** Completed repair demonstrates restoration of the rotator cuff footprint (compare to Fig. 5.31). RC, rotator cuff.

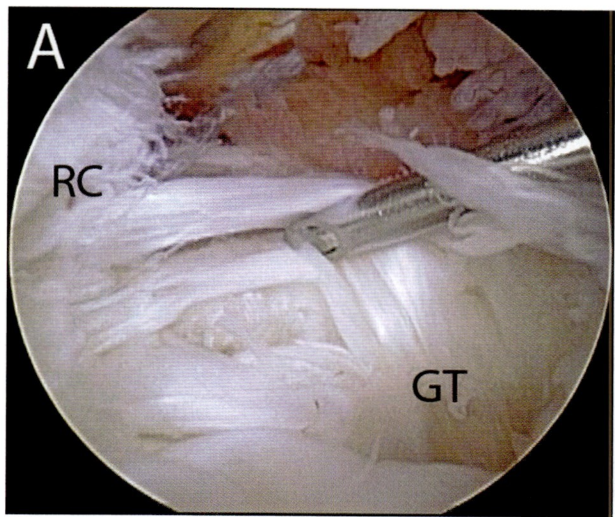

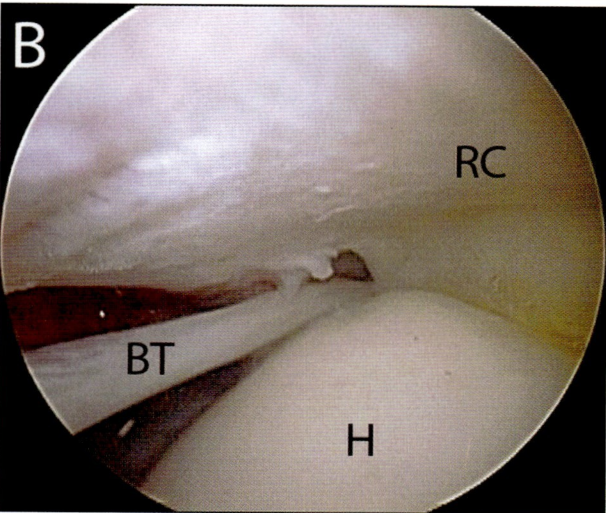

Figure 5.34 **A:** Right shoulder, posterior subacromial viewing portal demonstrates a large bursal surface rotator cuff tear with poor-quality remaining rotator cuff tissue. **B:** Intra-articular view from a posterior view in the same shoulder demonstrates an intact medial footprint. BT, biceps tendon; GT, greater tuberosity; H, humerus; RC, rotator cuff.

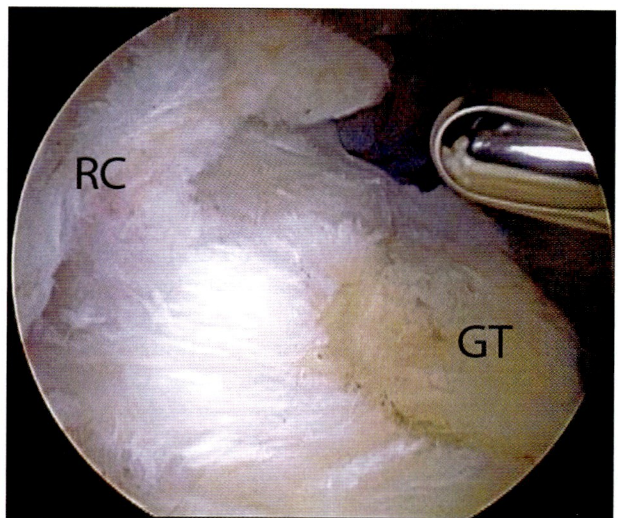

Figure 5.35 Right shoulder, posterior subacromial viewing portal demonstrates a large bursal surface rotator cuff tear after debridement and preparation of the bone bed for repair (compare to Fig. 5.34A). GT, greater tuberosity. RC, rotator cuff.

an art—always work on your skills. During palpation of a cuff with an interstitial tear, the PITA tear can often be appreciated in that it feels like there is a gap inside the layers of tendon. It feels as if you are sliding one layer of tendon over the top of another layer (sliding-layers sign) (Fig. 5.42)

Bubble Sign

If the dimple sign or the sliding-layers sign produces suspicion that interstitial pathology may exist, the next step is to perform the bubble test. In this test, an 18-gauge spinal needle is inserted into the area of suspicion through the intact bursal cuff fibers. Then, a syringe full of arthroscopy fluid is attached to the spinal needle and the plunger gently compressed. A positive bubble sign occurs when a localized area of tendon "bubbles up" (Fig. 5.43). If performed correctly, only a few ccs of fluid can be injected into the PITA lesion before feedback resistance is met, preventing the injection of more fluid. Then, when the plunger is pulled back, one should be able to pull the

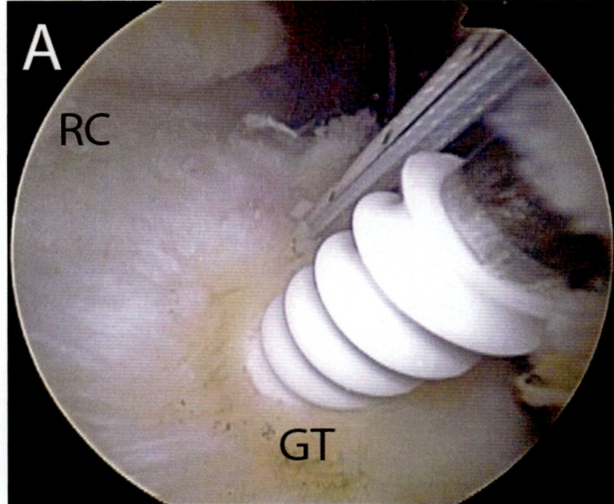

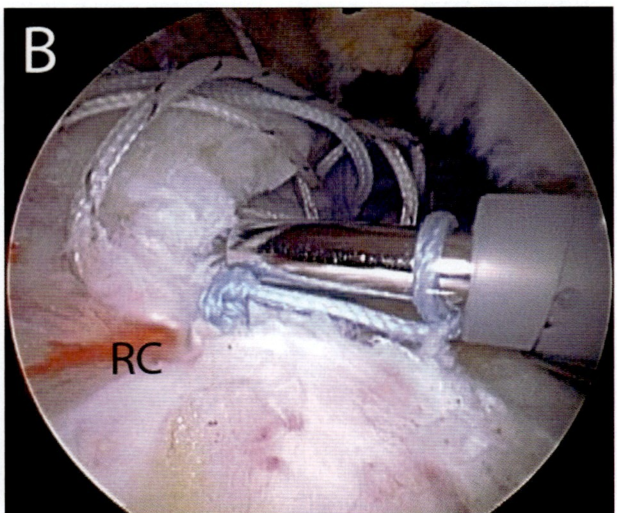

Figure 5.36 Right shoulder, posterior subacromial viewing portal demonstrates repair of a large bursal surface rotator cuff tear. **A:** Following bone bed preparation, two anchors are placed. **B:** After individual passage of all suture limbs through the rotator cuff, knots are tied with a Surgeon's Sixth Finger Knot Pusher (Arthrex, Inc., Naples, FL) to complete each mattress stitch. GT, greater tuberosity; RC, rotator cuff.

fluid back out of the defect and the bubble should deflate. If the syringe plunger is gently pressed and fluid does not flow easily, then either a PITA tear does not exist or the needle is not in the interstitial defect. Reposition the spinal needle and try again. If, after several tries, the bubble sign is negative, then a PITA tear is likely not present. If the syringe plunger is gently pressed and more than just a few ccs of fluid are injected, then the needle is likely all the way through the cuff and positioned intra-articularly or else there is communication with the joint through a small PASTA lesion. In this situation, one may see the entire cuff elevate momentarily, then go back down spontaneously without pulling back on the syringe plunger. This is NOT a positive bubble sign. Reposition the spinal needle and try again.

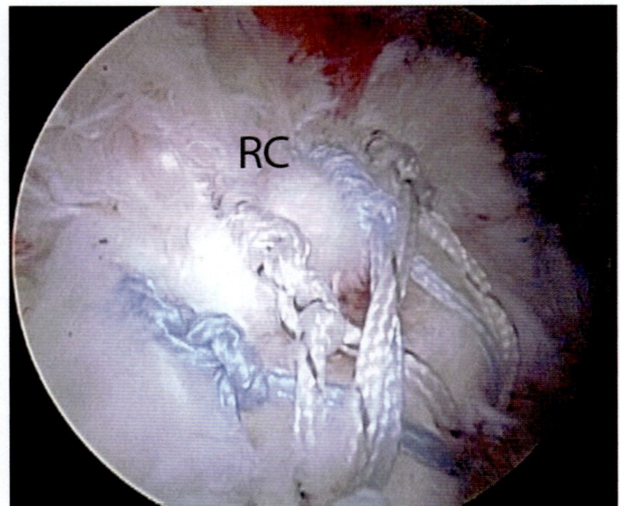

Figure 5.37 Right shoulder, posterior subacromial viewing portal demonstrates repair of a large bursal surface rotator cuff tear with compression to bone. Medial mattress stitches based off two medial anchors have been placed and then compressed to the bone in a crisscross pattern using two lateral anchors (compare to Fig. 5.33A). RC, rotator cuff.

The Probe Push

If, after some or all of the aforementioned tests, there is still suspicion of a PITA tear, the probe push test may be useful. With this test, the surgeon puts a probe on the suspicious part of the tendon and pushes firmly on the bursal layer of the cuff with the probe tip, trying to penetrate the bursal layers of the cuff. If the probe "falls" into a defect, it will be obvious (Fig. 5.44). Then, the surgeon can palpate with the tip of the probe and get a good sense of whether some cuff detachment from the bone bed exists.

The Slit Test

A final test to determine if a PITA tear exists is the slit test. We utilize this test for three specific situations:

1. At least two of the above tests are positive.
2. MRI demonstrates a likely PITA lesion and one of the above tests are positive.
3. Clinical symptoms are striking for a rotator cuff tear, other pathologies for weakness (such as a spinoglenoid cyst or suprascapular neuropathy) are ruled out, and one of the above tests is positive.

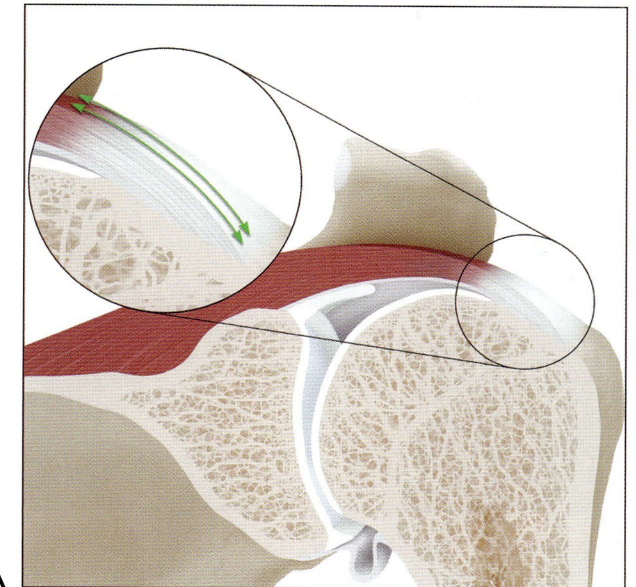

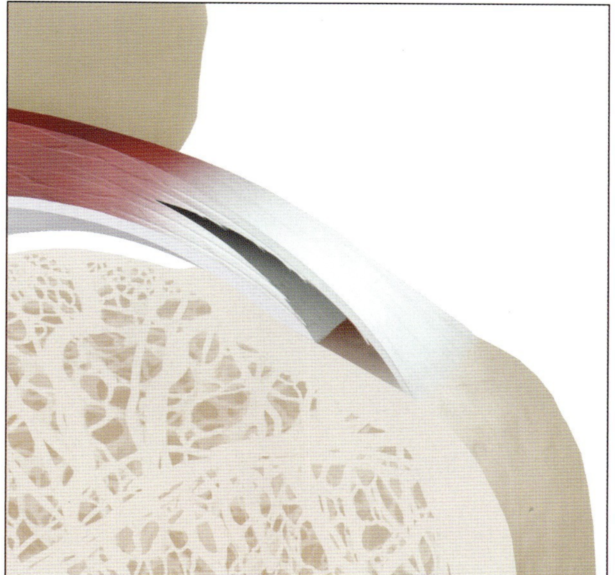

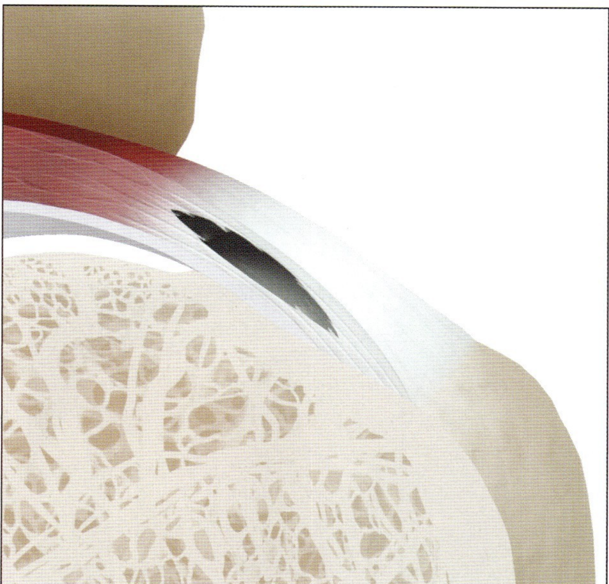

Figure 5.38 Schematic of the supraspinatus attachment. **A:** The supraspinatus tendon fibers are parallel when they insert onto the greater tuberosity. Interstitial tears can occur as a split between the parallel fibers **(B)** with or **(C)** without avulsion of the tendon from the bone. In either case, the tear will be hidden from view from both the articular and bursal surfaces.

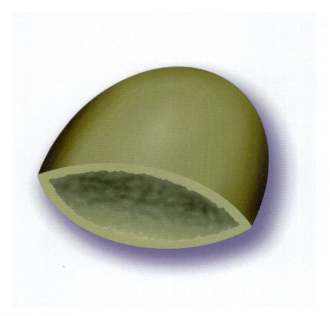

Figure 5.39 An interstitial rotator cuff tear can be likened to pita bread in which there is a separation between two intact layers (bursal side and articular side).

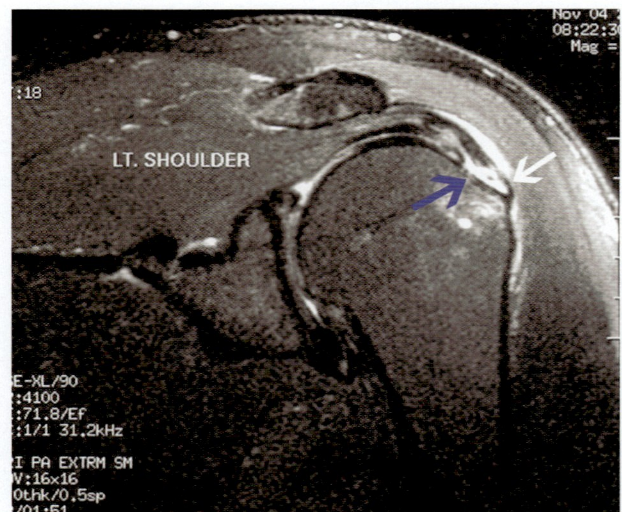

Figure 5.40 T2 coronal MRI of a left shoulder demonstrates an interstitial rotator cuff tear. Note: The medial rotator cuff attachment (*blue arrow*) and lateral rotator cuff attachment (*white arrow*) are intact, which will conceal this interstitial rotator cuff tear to a casual arthroscopic view.

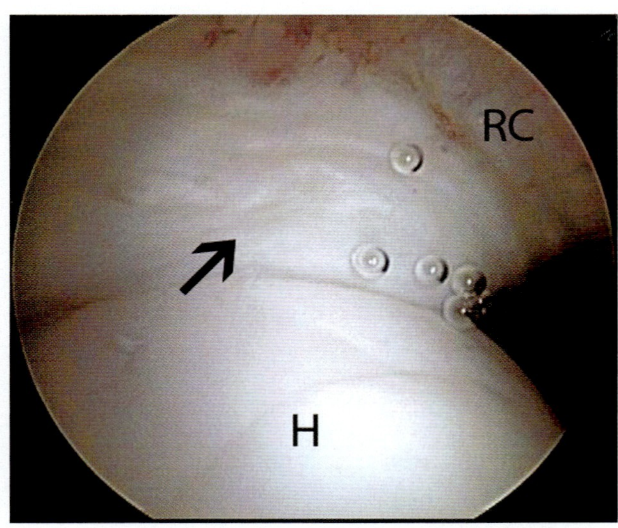

Figure 5.41 The dimple sign. Left shoulder, posterior glenohumeral viewing portal demonstrates a medial bulge (*black arrow*) of the rotator cuff that is indicative of an interstitial rotator cuff tear. H, humerus; RC, rotator cuff.

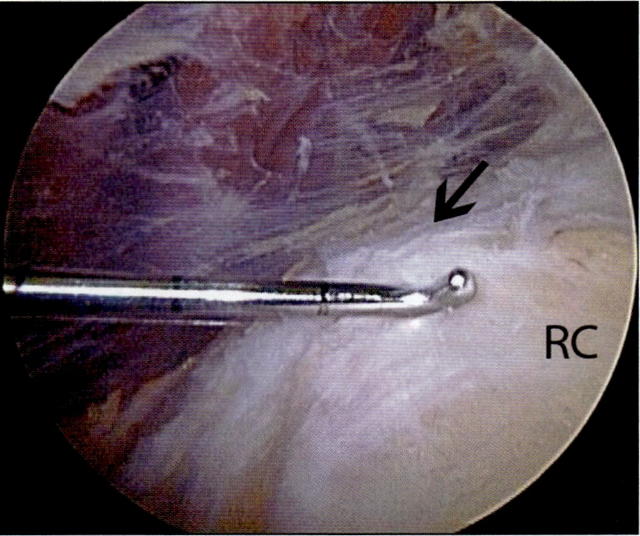

Figure 5.42 Sliding-layers sign. Left shoulder, posterior subacromial viewing portal demonstrates use of a probe to palpate the rotator cuff for the presence of an interstitial rotator cuff tear. Note: As the probe is slid over, the rotator cuff the tendon bulges on itself (*black arrow*), indicating an interstitial rotator cuff tear at this location. RC, rotator cuff.

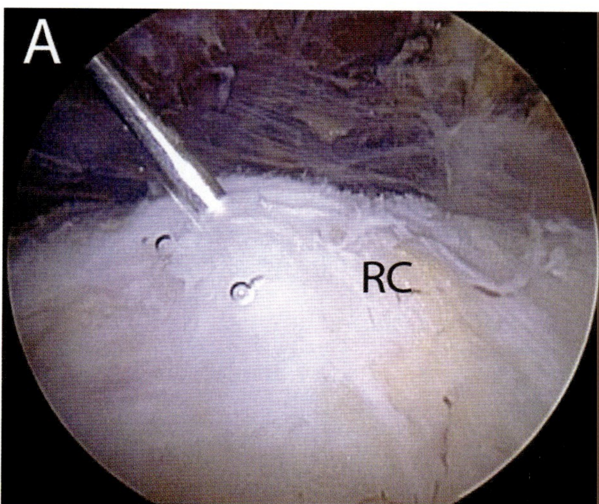

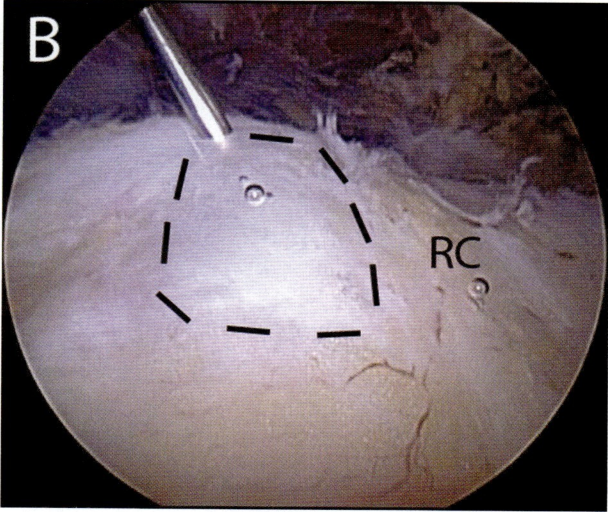

Figure 5.43 Bubble sign in left shoulder, viewed from a posterior subacromial portal. **A:** A spinal needle is inserted into the rotator cuff at the site of a suspected interstitial rotator cuff tear. **B:** As normal saline is injected, the interstitial defect fills and creates a visible bubble (*dashed black lines*), confirming an interstitial rotator cuff tear. RC, rotator cuff.

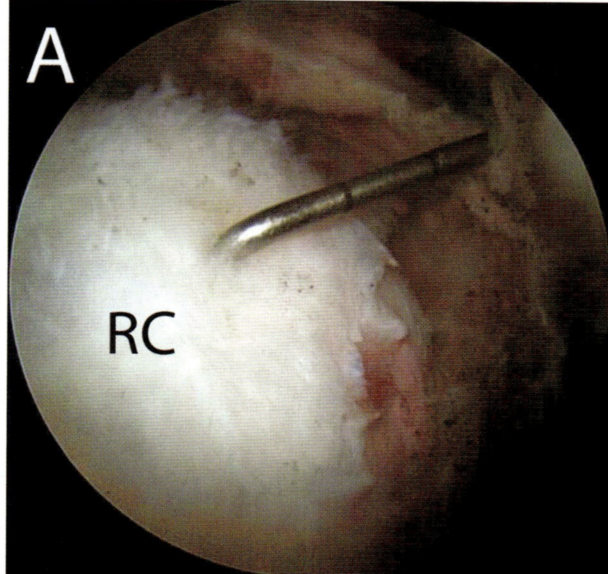

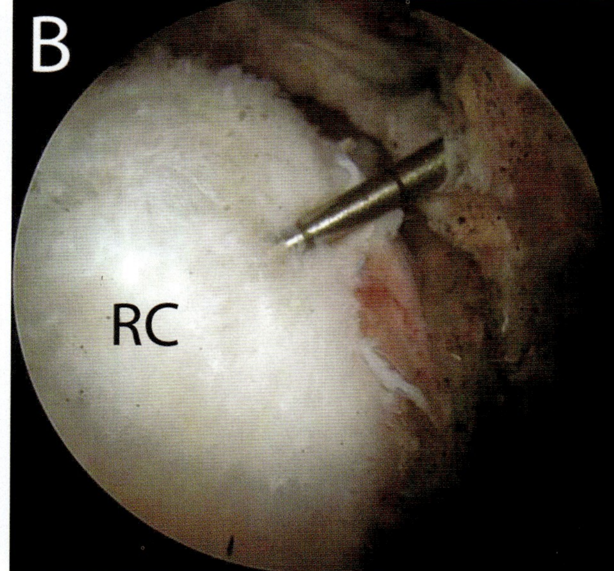

Figure 5.44 Probe push test. **A:** Right shoulder, posterior subacromial viewing portal demonstrates use of a probe to palpate a suspected interstitial rotator cuff tear. **B:** With manual pressure, the probe easily falls into a defect, indicating an interstitial rotator cuff tear. RC, rotator cuff.

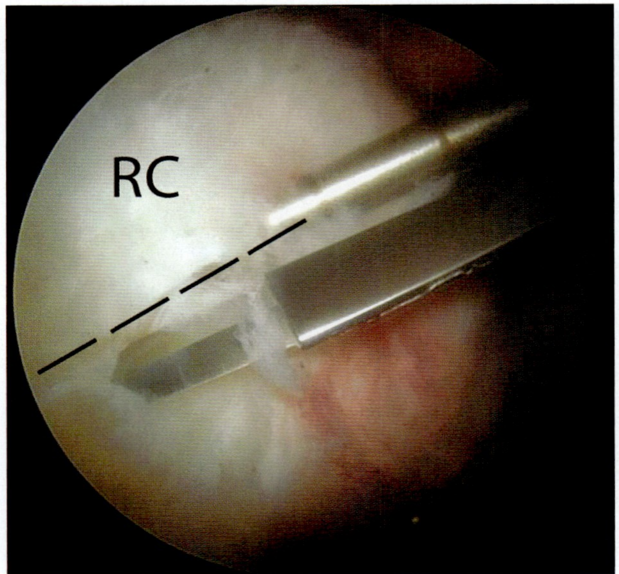

Figure 5.45 Right shoulder, posterior subacromial viewing portal, demonstrates the slit test. A knife blade is inserted near a probe that previously confirmed an interstitial tear. The knife blade is used to create a slit in the rotator cuff along the *dashed lines*. RC, rotator cuff.

Using a knife blade or arthroscopic scissors, a small slit in the bursal fibers of the cuff is created. This slit should be in line with the rotator cuff tendon fibers (Fig. 5.45). An arthroscopic grasper is inserted into the slit and opened allowing for better visualization within the defect (Fig. 5.46). Then a probe is used to palpate the interstitial layers of the cuff and the greater tuberosity attachment to search for a potential PITA tear. If the slit test is negative, then place a single suture in a side-to-side manner through the small slit to close the created slit.

PITA Repair

If a PITA tear is discovered, the defect is opened from the bursal side. The site of detachment on the greater tuberosity bone bed should be prepared with electrocautery and a burr to create a bleeding bone bed. If the bursal layer is extremely thin, it may be beneficial to proceed with detaching the bursal layer and preparing the bone bed all the way laterally to the tuberosity "drop off." If the bursal layer is healthy however, then just a slit in the cuff will allow preparation of the tuberosity bone bed. The resultant tear is then repaired in an appropriate manner as indicated by the pattern of the tear. Often this includes one or more anchors in the base of the PITA bone bed (Fig. 5.47). After these sutures are passed and

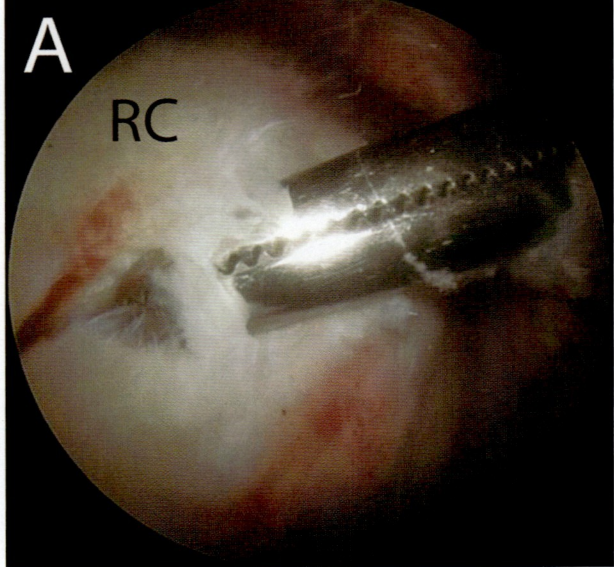

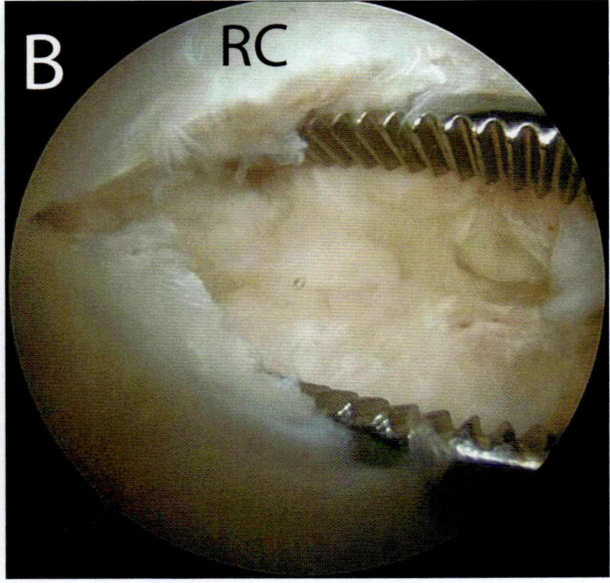

Figure 5.46 **A:** Right shoulder, posterior subacromial viewing portal. After a slit is created in the lateral rotator cuff, a grasper is introduced in the slit and (**B**) the jaws are opened, exposing an interstitial rotator cuff tear. RC, rotator cuff.

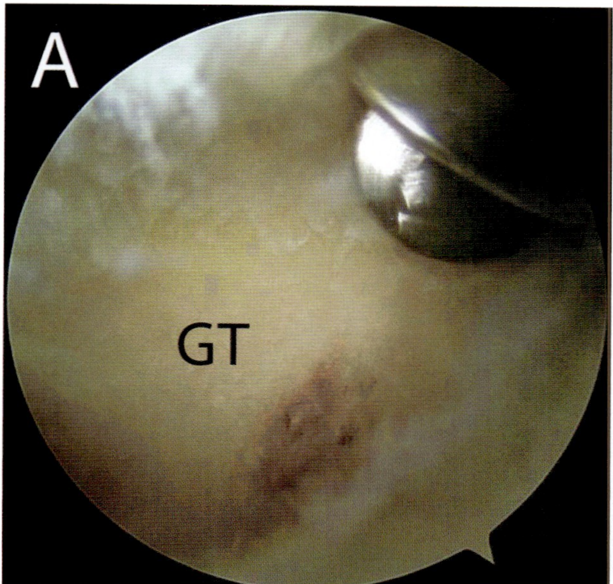

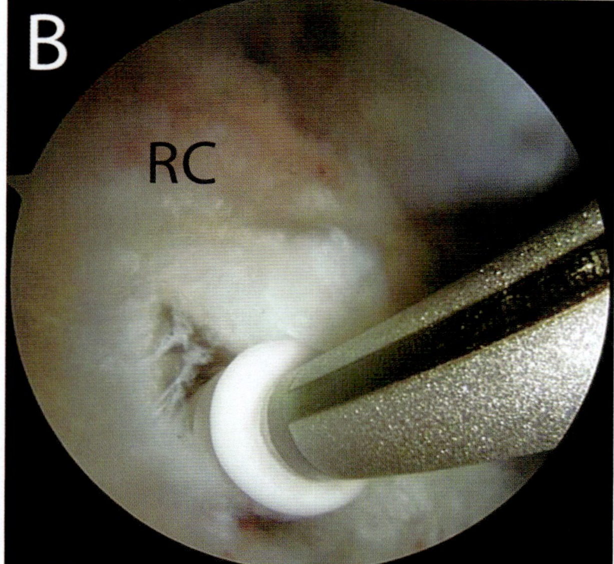

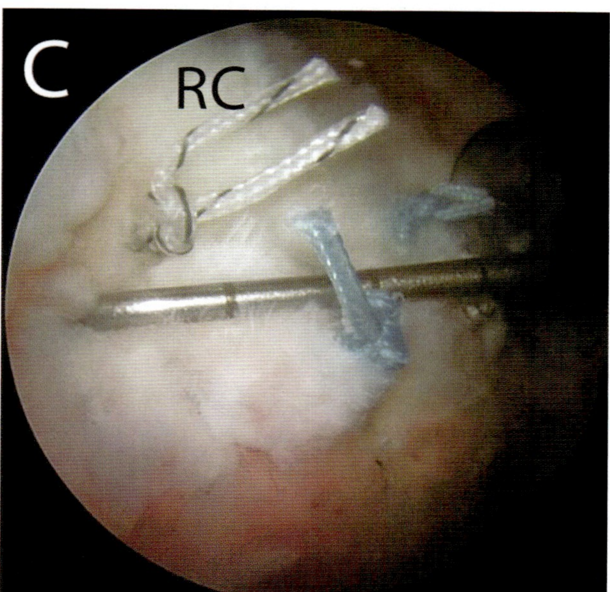

Figure 5.47 Right shoulder, posterior subacromial viewing portal, demonstrates **(A)** bone bed preparation, **(B)** insertion of a BioComposite Corkscrew FT anchor (Arthrex, Inc., Naples, FL), and **(C)** final repair of an interstitial rotator cuff tear. GT, greater tuberosity; RC, rotator cuff.

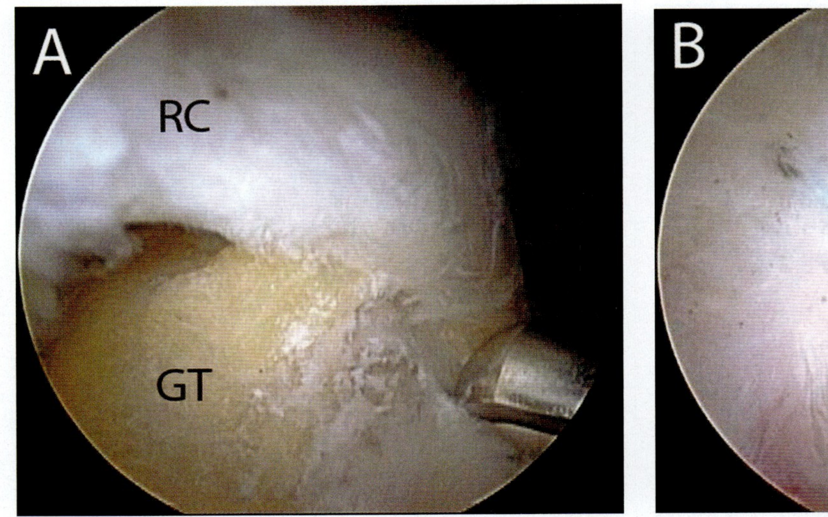

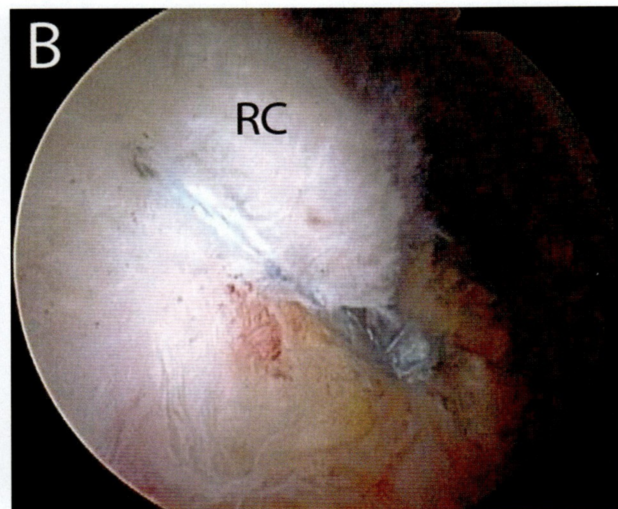

Figure 5.48 Right shoulder, posterior subacromial viewing portal demonstrates repair of an interstitial rotator cuff tear with a SpeedFix technique (Arthrex, Inc., Naples, FL). **A:** The interstitial defect has been exposed and a bone bed has been prepared for repair. **B:** Completed repair with an inverted mattress stitch secured to a lateral BioComposite SwiveLock C anchor. GT, greater tuberosity; RC, rotator cuff.

tied (but before they are cut), it is frequently helpful to bring the tails of these sutures laterally and compress them into the bone over the lateral drop-off of the greater tuberosity (via a BioComposite SwiveLock C) to accomplish a double-row repair and allow for cross row compression of the cuff against the bone bed. Alternatively, small tears can be repaired with a SpeedFix technique as previously described (Fig. 5.48)

Summary

Interstitial tears comprise an important entity that must be recognized. Because of the nature of these tears, their recognition can be extremely difficult. We believe that a significant number of failed arthroscopic procedures can be attributed to the failure to recognize interstitial rotator cuff tears. Utilizing the above techniques, the arthroscopic shoulder surgeon will significantly diminish the incidence of failure to recognize an interstitial rotator cuff tear. Once recognized, the tear can be appropriately addressed and fixed via standard arthroscopic means.

REFERENCES

1. Brady PC, Arrigoni P, Burkhart SS. Evaluation of residual rotator cuff defects after in vivo single- versus double-row rotator cuff repairs. ***Arthroscopy***. 2006;22:1070–1075.
2. Gonzalez-Lomas G, Kippe MA, Brown GD, et al. In situ transtendon repair outperforms tear completion and repair for partial articular-sided supraspinatus tendon tears. *J Shoulder Elbow Surg*. 2008;17:722–728.

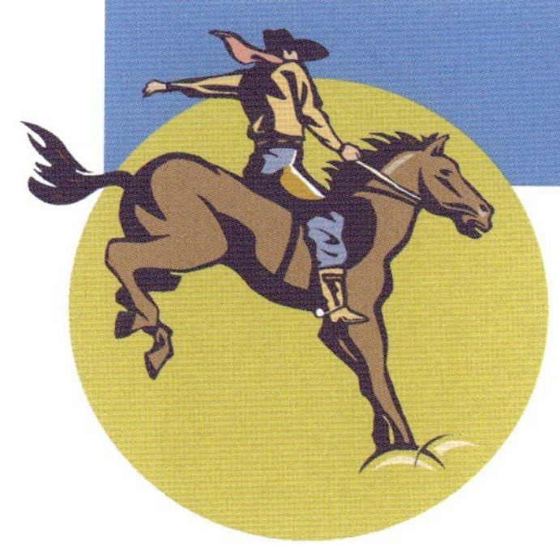

6

Subscapularis Tendon Tears

WESTERN WISDOM

You need spurs on a borrowed horse.

The torn subscapularis tendon has several unique aspects that make it difficult to repair. First of all, the "comma sign" and its relation to the intact anatomic structures must be understood in order to achieve an anatomic repair. Secondly, complete tears of the subscapularis tend to retract more than other cuff tears, necessitating significant dissections and releases in order to mobilize the tendon and get it back out to length. Third, the retracted subscapularis tends to scar against the coracoid in close proximity to important neurovascular structures, so mobilization can be daunting. Finally, the dissection and repair must be performed in the tightly packed subcoracoid space, necessitating specific techniques, positioning maneuvers, and instrumentation. Because this space can become compromised rapidly by soft tissue swelling from extravasation of arthroscopic irrigant fluid, it is essential to address the subscapularis prior to repairing the rest of the cuff.

ANATOMY OF THE SUBSCAPULARIS TEAR AND THE COMMA SIGN

In order to understand the anatomy of the torn retracted subscapularis, the surgeon must first understand the complex interrelated anatomy of the subscapularis, the medial sling of the biceps, and the biceps tendon. He must also understand how best to visualize this rather inaccessible area.

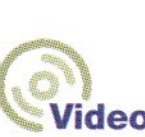

We perform all of our arthroscopic subscapularis repairs in the lateral decubitus position. In order to "open up" the subcoracoid space, we typically have an assistant provide a "posterior lever push" in which he pushes posteriorly on the proximal humerus while pulling the distal humerus anteriorly (Fig. 6.1). This maneuver also draws the tightly draped subscapularis tendon away from its bone bed on the lesser tuberosity, showing partial articular surface tears or nonretracted tears that otherwise might have been missed (Fig. 6.2). Viewing with a 70° arthroscope will give a more complete view of the inferior footprint of the subscapularis (Fig. 6.3). Forward flexion and internal rotation of the shoulder can also provide a more complete view; however, this maneuver is more useful with the patient in the beach-chair position.

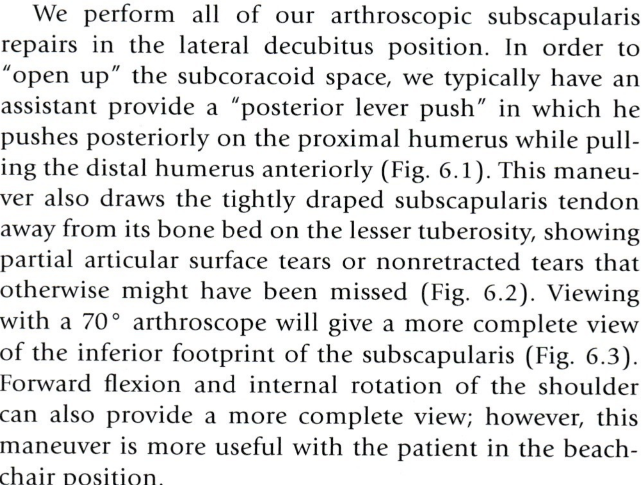

It is critical to understand the normal anatomy at the confluence of the superolateral subscapularis, the medial sling of the biceps, and biceps tendon (Fig. 6.4).The medial sling, composed of a robust deep layer (medial head of the coracohumeral ligament) and a thin superficial layer (superior glenohumeral ligament), has an insertional footprint at the top of the lesser tuberosity that is directly adjacent to the footprint of the superolateral subscapularis on the lesser tuberosity. As such, when the upper subscapularis tears away from its bone attachment, the medial sling (which is directly adjacent to it) also tears away from the bone. The torn medial sling forms a distinctive comma-shaped arc of soft tissue (*comma sign*) at the superolateral corner of the subscapularis (Fig. 6.5).

The *comma sign* is an extremely useful anatomic landmark during dissections and releases for retracted

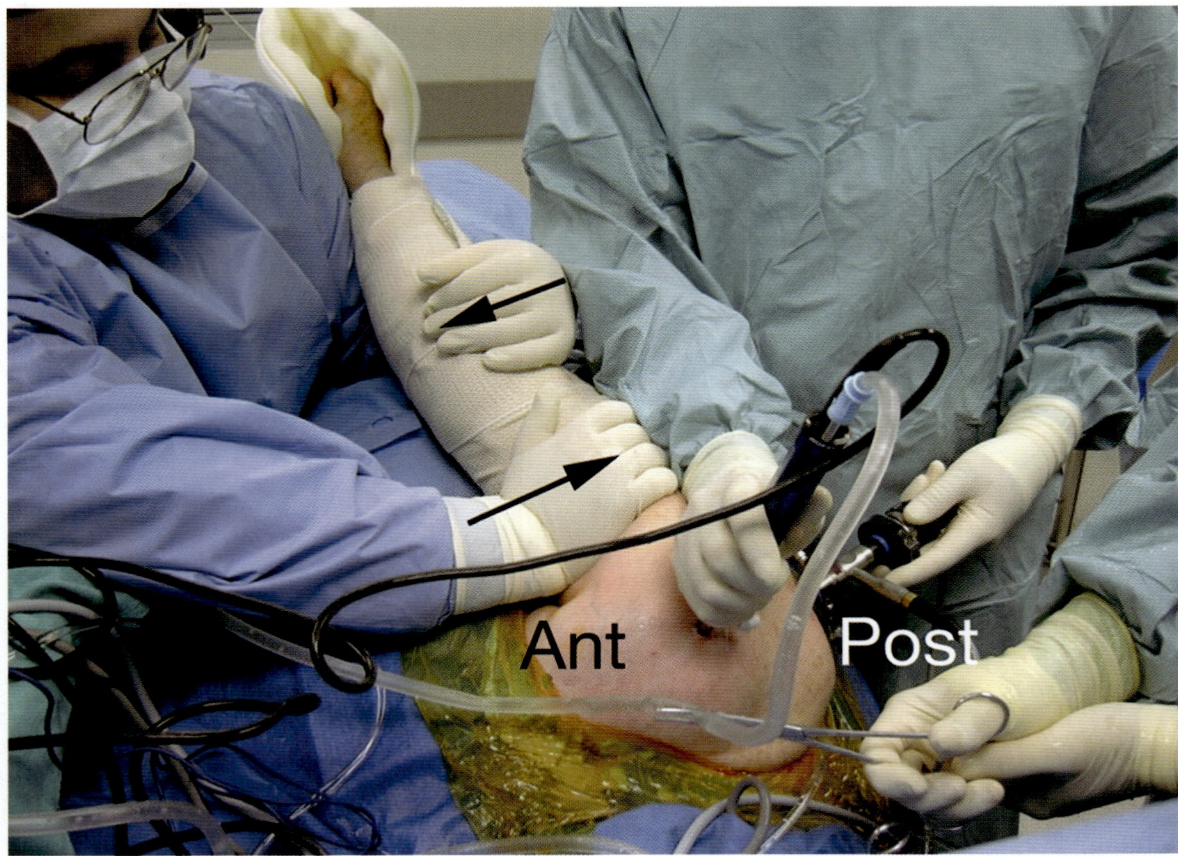

Figure 6.1 Posterior lever push. The second assistant simultaneously pushes the proximal humerus posteriorly and pulls the distal humerus anteriorly (*black arrows*). This maneuver effectively increases the working space in the anterior shoulder as the humeral head is subluxed posteriorly.

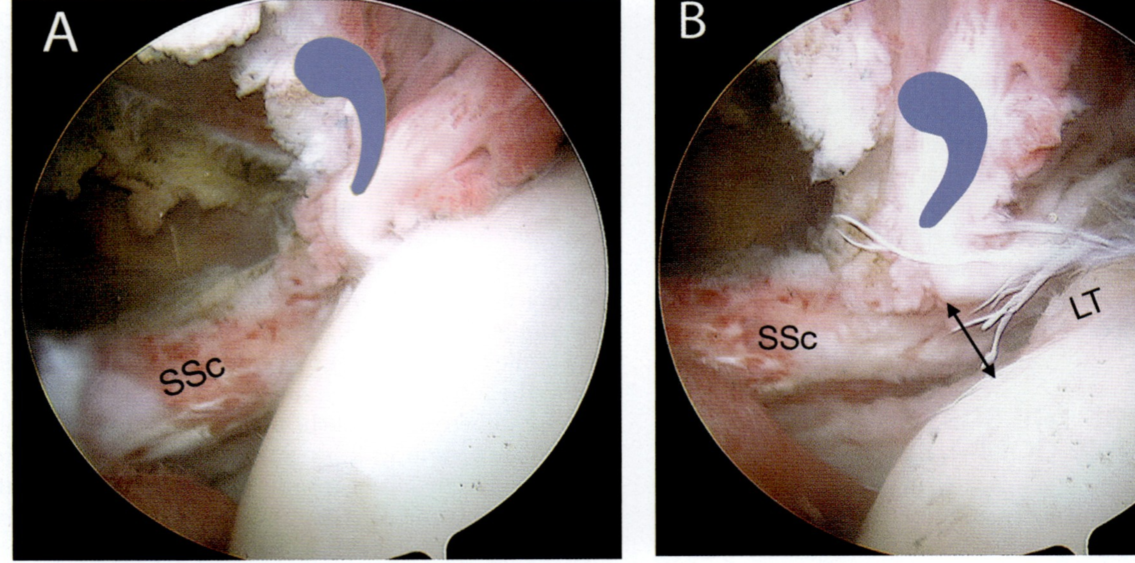

Figure 6.2 Right shoulder. Posterior viewing portal with 70° arthroscope. **A:** Exposure of the subscapularis is limited prior to a posterior lever push. **B:** Same shoulder with a posterior lever push. This maneuver dramatically increases the exposure of the subscapularis (SSc) footprint, providing much more room for visualization, instrumentation, and bone bed preparation. LT, lesser tuberosity; blue comma symbol, "comma sign".

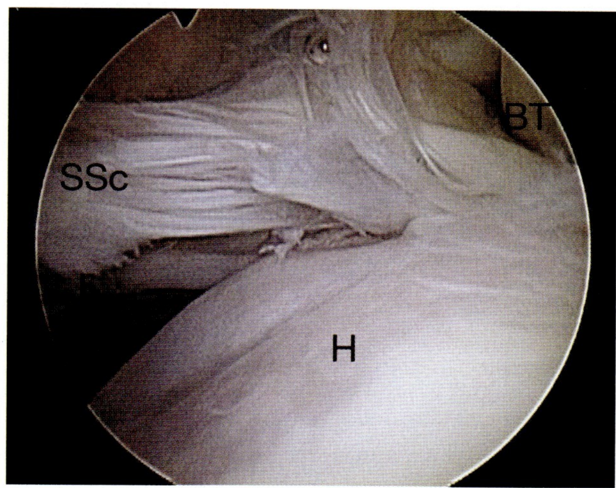

Figure 6.3 Right shoulder, posterior viewing portal demonstrates view of the subscapularis with a 70° arthroscope and a posterior lever push. The 70° arthroscope provides an "aerial view" of the subscapularis and gives a more complete view of the subscapularis footprint than that possible with a 30° arthroscope, particularly of the middle to inferior aspect. BT, biceps tendon; H, humeral head; SSc, subscapularis tendon.

subscapularis tendons. Even if the *comma sign* is extremely retracted, all the way to the rim of the glenoid or beyond, it can always be located and can be followed to its confluence with the superolateral subscapularis. The constancy of this relationship will leave no doubt as to the location of the lateral border of the subscapularis, even in cases of extreme scarring and retraction (Fig. 6.6).

After the subscapularis has been repaired, the *comma sign* is very useful for locating the anterolateral corner of the supraspinatus tendon, to which it remains attached (Fig. 6.7). Once again, this relationship is particularly useful in cases where the supraspinatus is retracted and scarred to the acromion.

NONRETRACTED SUBSCAPULARIS TEARS

Recognition of nonretracted subscapularis tears is critically important. Since a torn but nonretracted tendon can lie tightly draped across the lesser tuberosity, it may not be

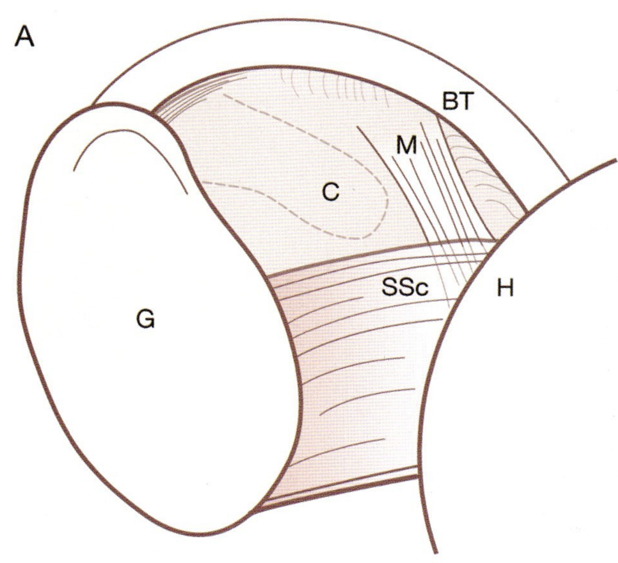

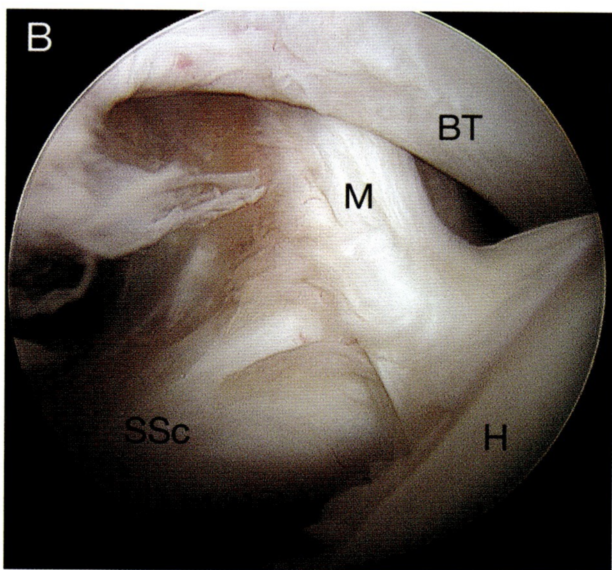

C

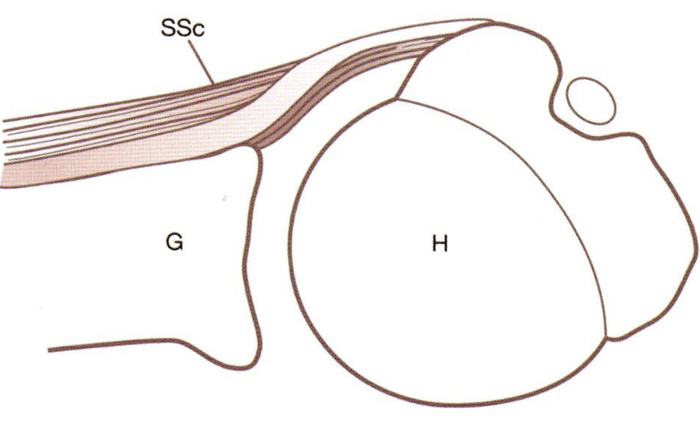

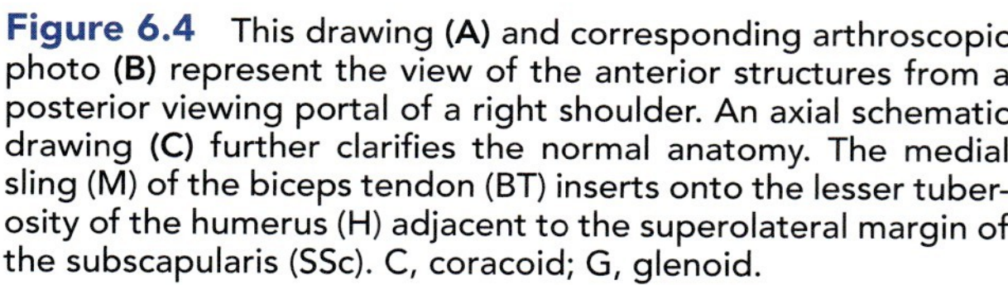

Figure 6.4 This drawing **(A)** and corresponding arthroscopic photo **(B)** represent the view of the anterior structures from a posterior viewing portal of a right shoulder. An axial schematic drawing **(C)** further clarifies the normal anatomy. The medial sling (M) of the biceps tendon (BT) inserts onto the lesser tuberosity of the humerus (H) adjacent to the superolateral margin of the subscapularis (SSc). C, coracoid; G, glenoid.

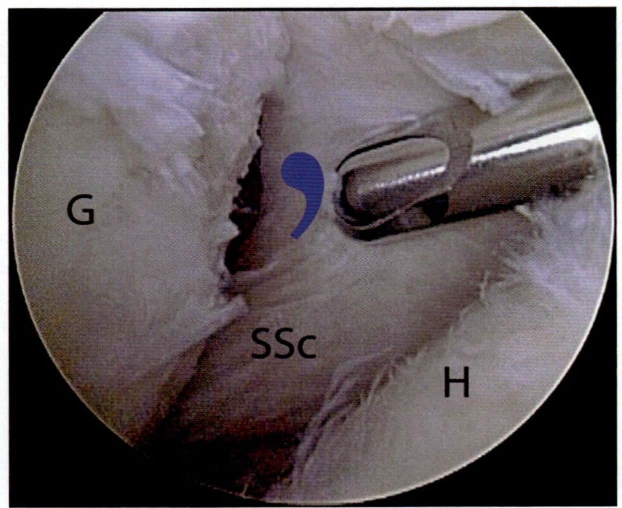

Figure 6.5 Right shoulder, posterior viewing portal. In the setting of a retracted subscapularis tear, the medial sling tears away from the bone with the subscapularis tendon. The medial sling forms a distinctive *comma-shaped arc* of soft tissue (*blue comma shape*) at the superolateral corner of the subscapularis. As demonstrated in this photo, the *comma sign* serves as a landmark for locating a retracted subscapularis tendon. G, glenoid; H, humeral head, SSc, subscapularis tendon.

detectable on casual inspection with a 30° arthroscope (Fig. 6.8A). Viewing such a tear with a 70° arthroscope while a posterior lever push is applied will usually demonstrate the tear (Fig. 6.8B, C). Nonretracted tears may be either full-thickness tears or partial articular surface tendon avulsion (PASTA) lesions.

WORKING PORTALS

During subscapularis tendon repair, we view exclusively through a posterior portal, switching between 30° and 70° arthroscopes as necessary. We use two working portals, an anterior portal (for suture anchor placement) and an anterosuperolateral portal (for everything else) (Fig. 6.9). While viewing from an anterosuperolateral portal is an option in cases of complete subscapularis tears, this portal does not provide adequate visualization of partial thickness articular-sided tears. Furthermore, using this portal for visualization can create crowding with the anterior working portals used in repair. For these reasons, we prefer to view exclusively through the posterior portal when repairing the subscapularis.

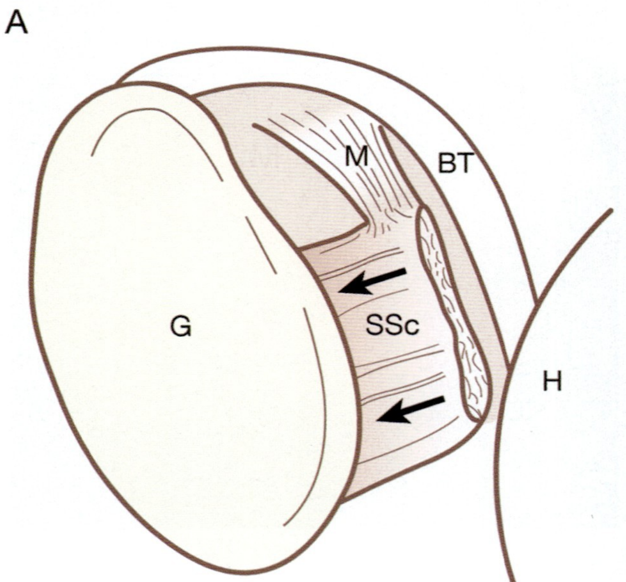

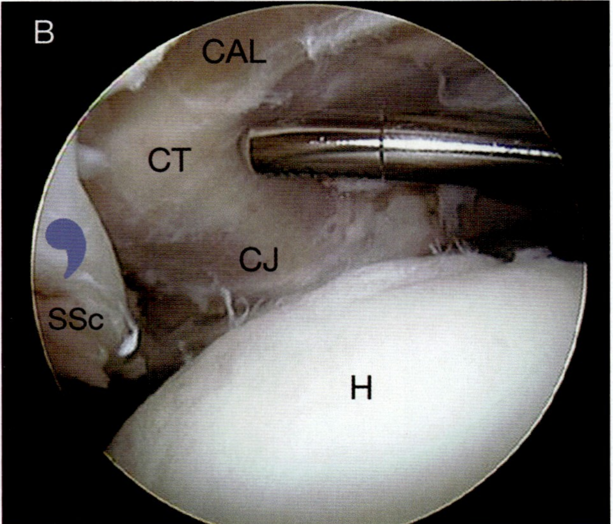

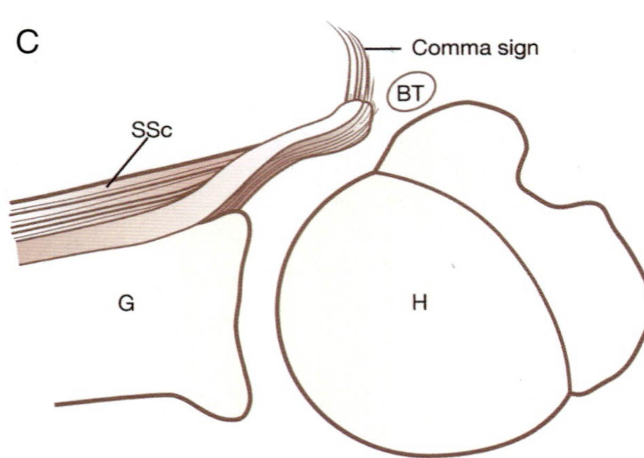

Figure 6.6 This drawing **(A)** and corresponding arthroscopic photo **(B)** represent a complete subscapularis tendon (SSc) tear with medial retraction (*black arrows*) almost to the level of the glenoid (G) in association with a medially dislocated biceps tendon (BT). An axial projection is also shown in **(C)**. In this situation, the comma sign (*blue comma symbol*) leads to the superolateral border of the subscapularis tendon. CAL, coracoacromial ligament; CT, conjoined tendon; CT, coracoid tip; H, humerus; M, medial sling.

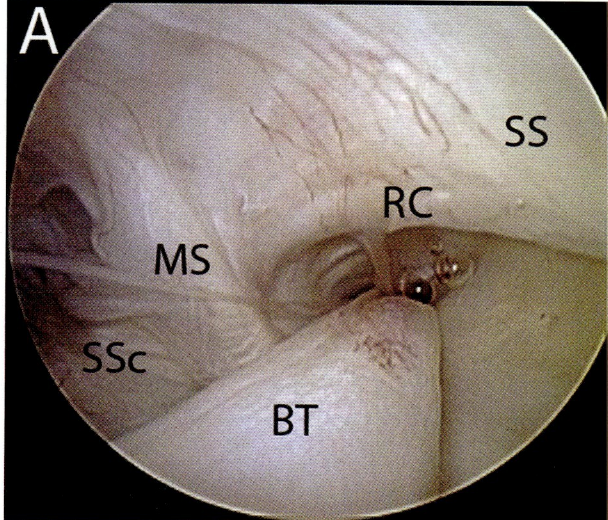

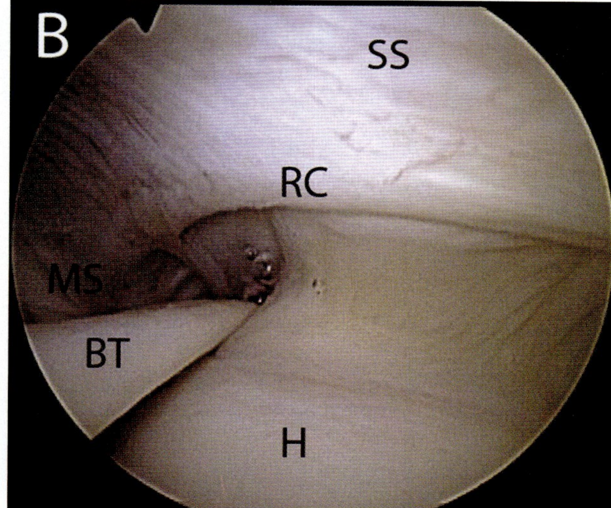

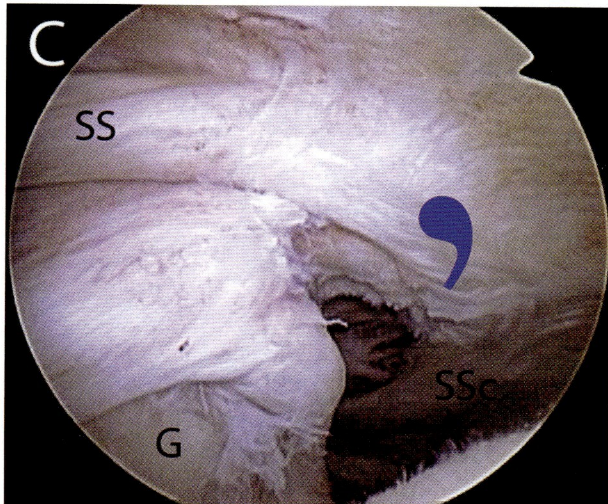

Figure 6.7 Right shoulder, posterior viewing portal, demonstrating the connection between the subscapularis (SSc) and the supraspinatus (SS) via the medial sling (MS). **A:** The rotator cable (RC) of the rotator cuff merges with the medial sling anteriorly. As such, when the medial sling detaches during a subscapularis tear, the comma sign may be followed to locate the anterolateral corner of the supraspinatus tendon. **B:** A profile view of the rotator cable further shows this constant relationship. **C:** In the case of a massive contracted rotator cuff tear, the relationship between the subscapularis and the supraspinatus is maintained and the comma sign (*blue comma symbol*) can be used to identify the anterolateral supraspinatus tendon. BT, biceps tendon; G, glenoid; H, humerus.

The anterosuperolateral portal is truly the "workhorse" portal for subscapularis repair. To create this portal, start by placing an 18-gauge spinal needle adjacent to the anterolateral corner of the acromion and direct it toward the lesser tuberosity. Ideal placement will direct the needle at a 5° to 10° angle of approach toward the lesser tuberosity (Fig. 6.10). This angle of approach is perfect for preparing the lesser tuberosity, performing a coracoplasty, dissecting a retracted subscapularis, and placing antegrade sutures into the subscapularis.

The anterior portal is usually a percutaneous stab that is used only for insertion of suture anchors and for retrograde suture passage after anchor insertion. A spinal needle is used to determine the proper "deadman angle" of approach while viewing through a posterior portal. This portal is typically somewhat medial to a standard anterior portal because of the retroversion of the humeral neck as a factor in the angle of approach for suture anchor placement (Fig. 6.11).

WHAT TO DO WITH THE BICEPS

In almost all cases of a subscapularis repair, we do a biceps tenodesis. Since most tears of the upper subscapularis also involve a tear of the medial sling of the biceps, there is biceps instability that we feel cannot be adequately addressed by simply repairing the sling. Therefore, we typically perform a biceps tenodesis with an interference screw technique (BioComposite Tenodesis Screw; Arthrex, Inc., Naples, FL) at the top of the bicipital groove. For elderly low-demand patients, we sometimes do a biceps tenotomy rather than a tenodesis. For all other patients, we begin the tenodesis procedure by placing two half-racking sutures

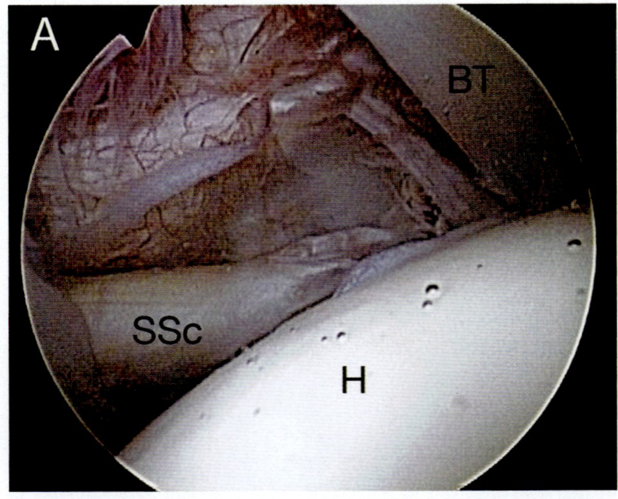

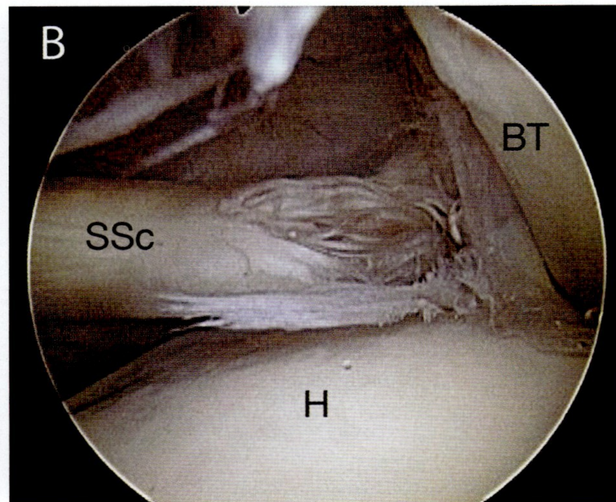

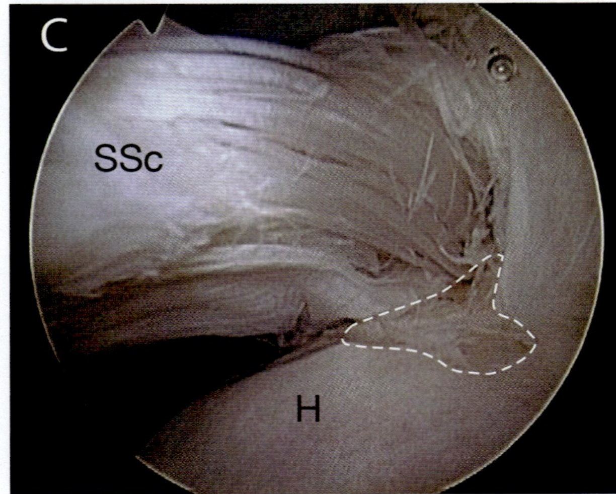

Figure 6.8 **A:** Right shoulder, posterior viewing portal with 30° arthroscope. The footprint of the subscapularis (SSc) is poorly visualized. **B:** Same shoulder. The use of a 70° arthroscope improves visualization, but in the standard lateral decubitus position, the subscapularis tendon is draped over the lesser tuberosity, obstructing the view of the lesser tuberosity footprint. **C:** Same shoulder viewed with 70° arthroscope and a posterior lever push. This maneuver dramatically increases the exposure of the subscapularis footprint, providing much more room for visualization, instrumentation, and bone bed preparation. In this case, an exposed subscapularis footprint (*white hashed area*) is quite evident at the 4 o'clock position of this picture. BT, biceps tendon; H, humeral head.

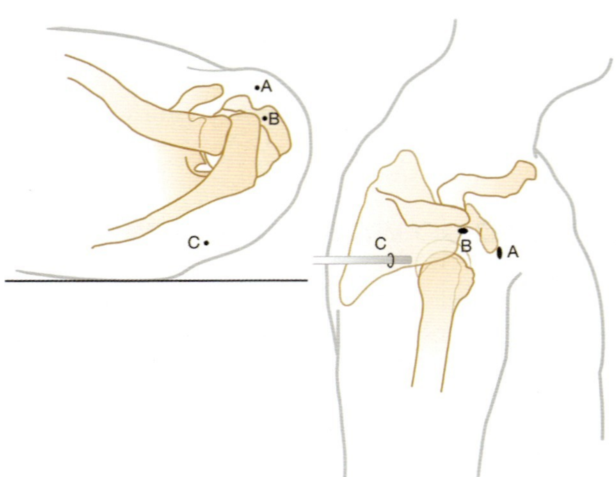

Figure 6.9 Portals for arthroscopic subscapularis tendon repair. The anterior portal (*A*) is used for anchor placement and retrograde suture passage. The anterosuperolateral portal (*B*) is used for subscapularis tendon mobilization, preparation of the bone bed, antegrade suture passage, and coracoplasty. The posterior portal (*C*) is used as an arthroscopic viewing portal.

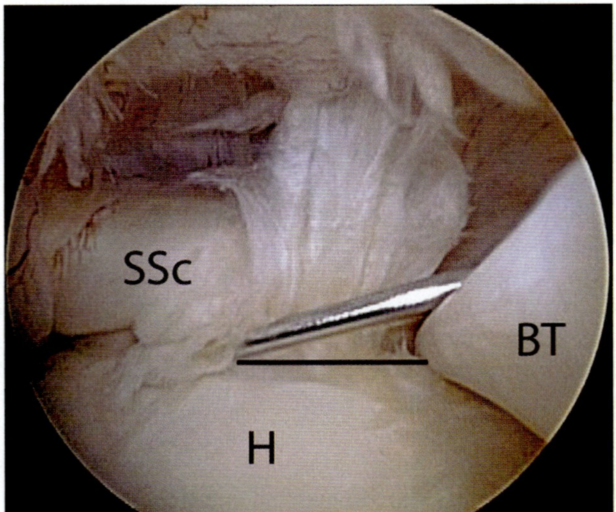

Figure 6.10 Right shoulder, posterior viewing portal with a 70° arthroscope, demonstrates spinal needle localization of an anterosuperolateral portal. Note: For subscapularis tendon repair, this portal should provide a 5° to 10° angle of approach to the lesser tuberosity (*black line*). BT, biceps tendon; H, humerus; SSc, subscapularis tendon.

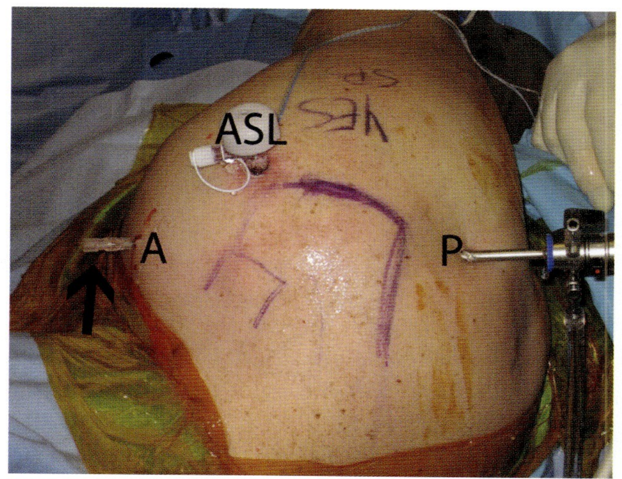

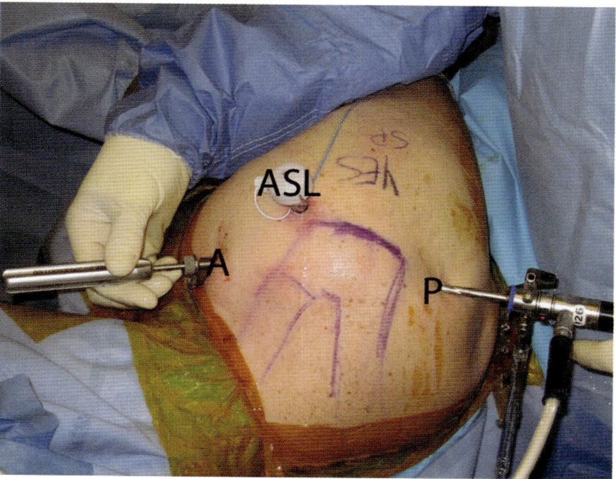

Figure 6.11 **A:** External view of a right shoulder demonstrates spinal needle placement (*black arrow*) for an anterior portal. **B:** During subscapularis tendon repair, this portal is used for anchor placement (as shown in the figure) as well as retrograde suture passage (not shown). A, anterior portal; ASL, anterosuperolateral portal; P, posterior portal.

through the intra-articular portion of the biceps to securely hold it while we tenotomize the tendon at its root, adjacent to the anterosuperior labrum. Then, we exteriorize the biceps through the anterosuperolateral portal and place a whipstitch (Fig. 6.12). By flexing the elbow and the shoulder, one can exteriorize a greater length of biceps tendon, making it easier to place the whipstitch. The tendon is then allowed to retract back into the shoulder, and the biceps tenodesis is performed after doing the subscapularis repair. Visualization of the subscapularis is greatly improved after the biceps tenotomy (in preparation for tenodesis). We believe that biceps tenodesis or tenotomy in the face of subscapularis repair is very important because the force from a persistently subluxed biceps tendon will cause the subscapularis repair to ultimately fail.

ORDER OF STEPS

In general, when the subscapularis is torn, the order of steps is as follows:

1. Do arthroscopic evaluation.
2. Place biceps whipstitch and do biceps tenotomy in preparation for tenodesis.
3. Make window in rotator interval.
4. If subscapularis tendon is adhesed, then skeletonize posterolateral coracoid, mobilize tendon, and do a three-sided release.
5. Do coracoplasty if indicated (i.e., if subcoracoid coracohumeral distance is <7 mm).
6. Prepare bone bed on lesser tuberosity.
7. Repair subscapularis.
8. Do biceps tenodesis.
9. Repair the rest of the rotator cuff.

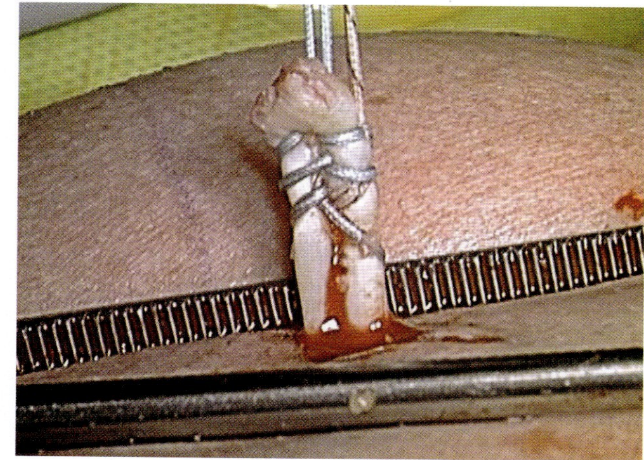

Figure 6.12 The cut end of the biceps tendon is pulled externally out of the joint through the anterosuperolateral portal by means of two half-racking sutures. Then, a whipstitch is placed and the tip of the biceps is contoured to prepare it for tenodesis.

RELEASES FOR THE RETRACTED ADHESED SUBSCAPULARIS

Using a 30° arthroscope through a posterior viewing portal, the *comma sign* is visualized and followed inferiorly to locate and identify the superolateral corner of the subscapularis. A traction suture is placed with an antegrade suture passer (FastPass Scorpion; Arthrex, Inc., Naples, FL) through the superolateral rolled edge of the subscapularis. While pulling laterally on the traction suture, a shaver or cautery electrode is introduced through the anterosuperolateral portal and is used to make a window in the rotator interval, just medial to the *comma sign*. The coracoid is identified through the window.

Then the arthroscope is pushed through the window in the rotator interval in order to view the coracoid, and the shaver and cautery are alternately passed anterior to the comma to skeletonize the coracoid tip and coracoid neck, continuing around to the coracoid base (anterior release) (Fig. 6.13). Then a 30° arthroscopic elevator is used to lyse the adhesions between the coracoid neck and the subscapularis tendon (superior release) (Fig. 6.14). The elevator is inserted only to the base of its blade, which is enough to release the adhesions to the coracoid. Contrary to some other arthroscopic surgeons, we have not found it necessary to dissect any farther medially than that, and we certainly do not feel that it is necessary to dissect and visualize any of the neurovascular structures during the releases.

The third part of the release is the posterior release of the subscapularis tendon. A 15° elevator is introduced into the plane between the posterior subscapularis tendon and the anterior glenoid neck, freeing the adhesions between tendon and bone (Fig. 6.15). This is a safe, relatively avascular plane in which the elevator can safely be manipulated blindly to do the posterior release. This completes the three-sided release (anterior, superior, posterior) (see "Bonus Videos," Disc 2). Video

We have not found it necessary to do an inferior release. By doing a three-sided release, we have found that we can always mobilize the subscapularis to the lesser tuberosity, or at the very worst to within 5 mm of the lesser tuberosity. In cases where mobilization does not create enough lateral excursion for an arthroscopic repair of the subscapularis, we medialize the footprint 5 to 7 mm (Fig. 6.16). We have noted excellent subscapularis function at follow-up of over 6 years following repair in this somewhat medialized position (Unpublished data).

CORACOPLASTY

After the three-sided release, the subcoracoid space is evaluated to see if it is stenotic enough to warrant a coracoplasty. If the coracohumeral distance is <7 mm

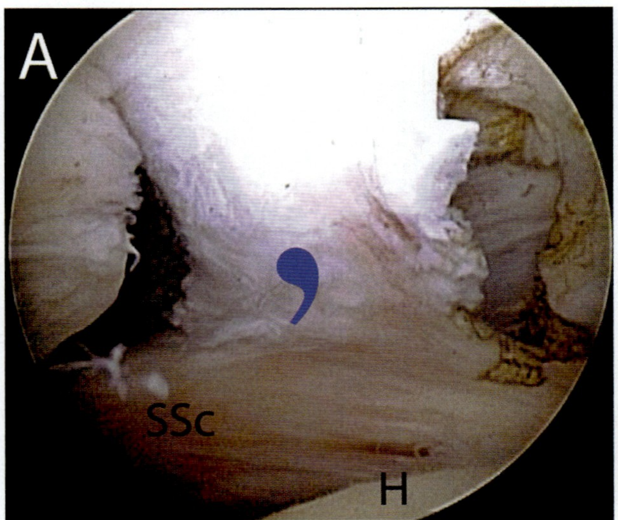

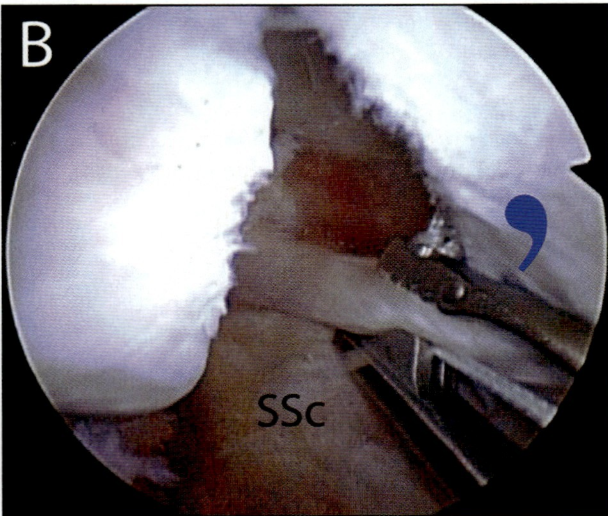

Figure 6.13 Anterior release of a retracted adhesed subscapularis tendon tear in a right shoulder, viewed from a posterior glenohumeral portal. **A:** While viewing with a 30° arthroscope, the comma sign is identified. **B:** A traction stitch is placed in the upper subscapularis tendon.

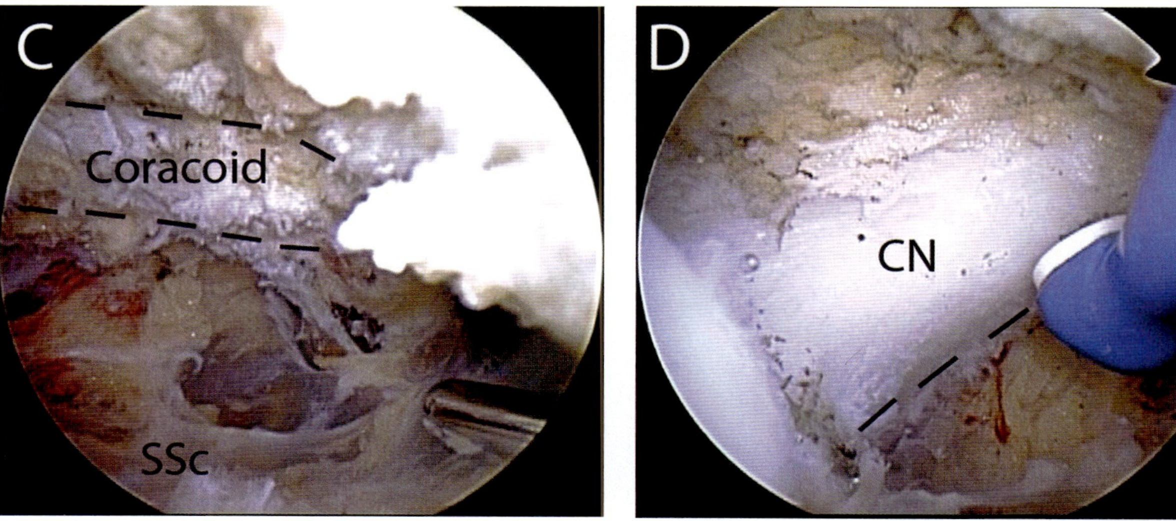

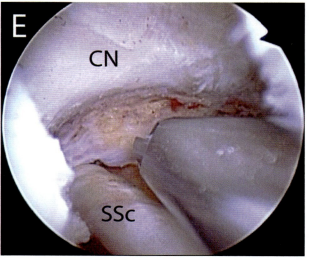

Figure 6.13 *(Continued)* **C:** The arthroscope is placed through a window in the rotator interval to identify the coracoid (*dashed black lines*). **D:** While viewing with a 70° arthroscope, the posterolateral coracoid is skeletonized to the level of the coracoid neck (*dashed black lines*) and coracoid base using an electrocautery. **E:** After the anterior release is completed, the coracoid neck and underlying subscapularis tendon are clearly visualized. CN, coracoid neck; H, humerus; SSc, subscapularis tendon; blue comma symbol, comma sign.

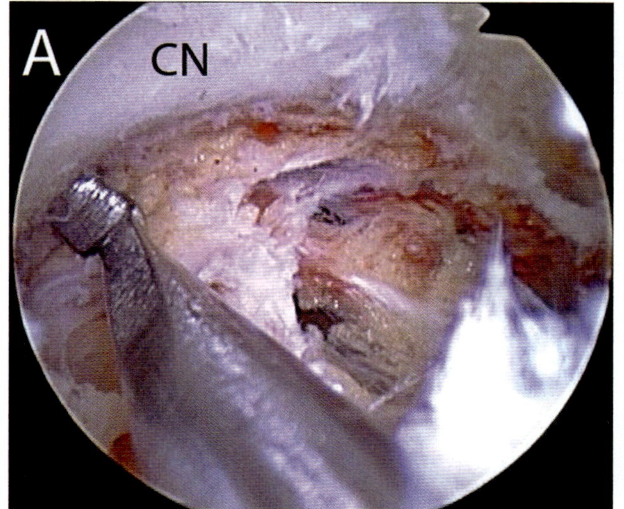

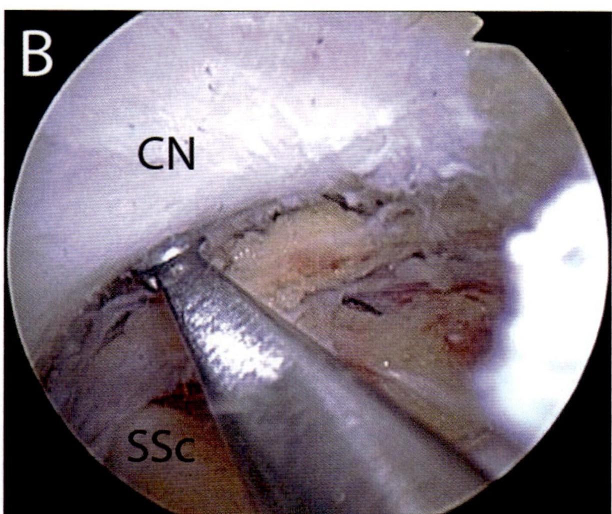

Figure 6.14 Superior release of a retracted adhesed subscapularis tendon tear in a right shoulder viewed from a posterior portal with a 70° arthroscope. **A:** A 30° elevator is introduced from an anterosuperolateral working portal. **B:** Adhesions between the superior subscapularis and the coracoid neck are released. The elevator is inserted only to the base of its blade, which is enough to release the adhesions to the coracoid. CN, coracoid neck; SSc, subscapularis tendon.

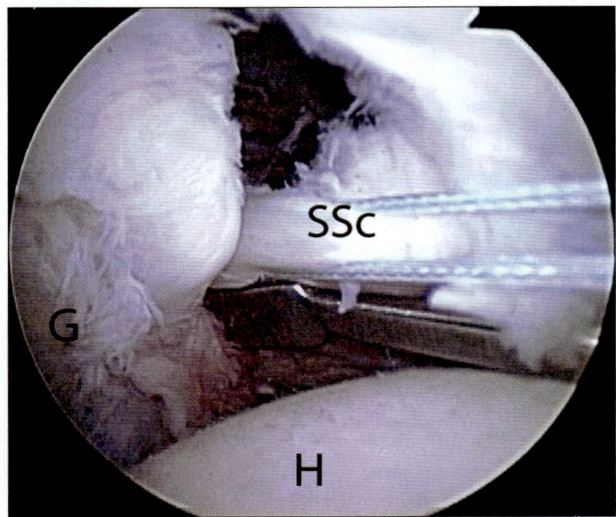

Figure 6.15 Posterior release of a retracted adhesed subscapularis tendon tear in a right shoulder viewed from a posterior portal. A 15° elevator, introduced from an anterosuperolateral portal, frees the subscapularis from adhesions between its posterior border and the glenoid. G, glenoid, H, humerus, SSc, subscapularis tendon.

(approximately 1½ diameters of the barrel-shaped burr), then a coracoplasty should be performed through the anterosuperolateral portal to create a subcoracoid space that is at least 7 mm deep (Fig. 6.17).

SUBSCAPULARIS REPAIR

Next, the bone bed on the lesser tuberosity is prepared to a bleeding base using a high-speed burr or ring curettes. For retracted tears, footprint restoration of the subscapularis tendon depends upon defining the medial and lateral margins of the lesser tuberosity. The normal medial subscapularis insertion begins 2 to 3 mm lateral to the articular margin, which is usually easy to locate. Defining the lateral margin of the lesser tuberosity can be more difficult. The key to delineating the lateral margin is to identify the bicipital groove that marks the lateral border of the lesser tuberosity, and thus the normal lateral insertion of the subscapularis tendon (Fig. 6.18). Even though there is usually a 2- to 3-mm gap between the articular cartilage

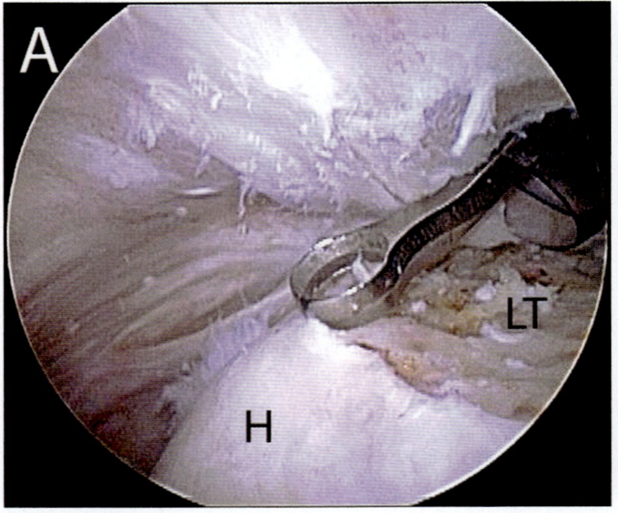

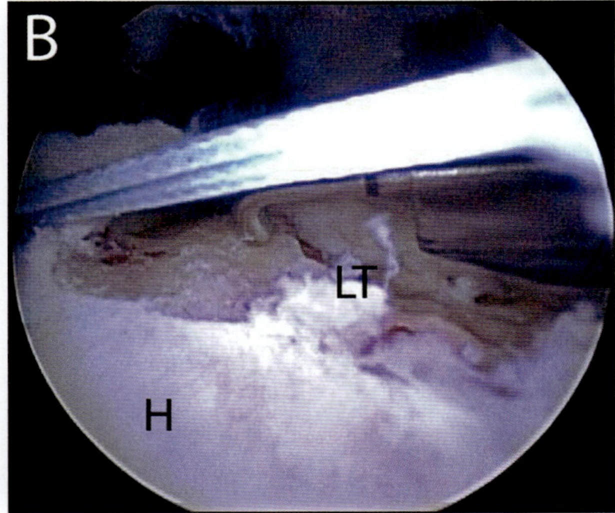

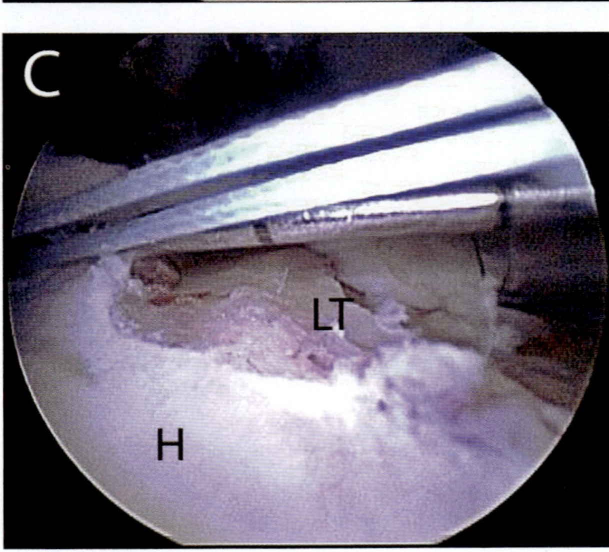

Figure 6.16 Right shoulder, posterior glenohumeral viewing portal with a 70° arthroscope demonstrates medialization of the subscapularis footprint for repair of a subscapularis tendon tear with decreased lateral excursion after a three-sided release. **A:** The medial margin of the subscapularis footprint is further medialized by using a ring curette. **B:** The tip of a probe introduced from an anterosuperolateral portal demonstrates the native medial margin of the footprint. **C:** A probe demonstrates that the footprint has been medialized approximately 5 mm to accomplish this repair. H, humerus; LT, lesser tuberosity.

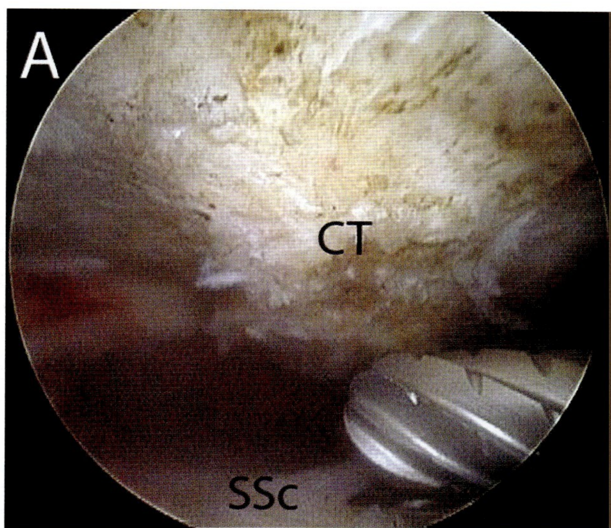

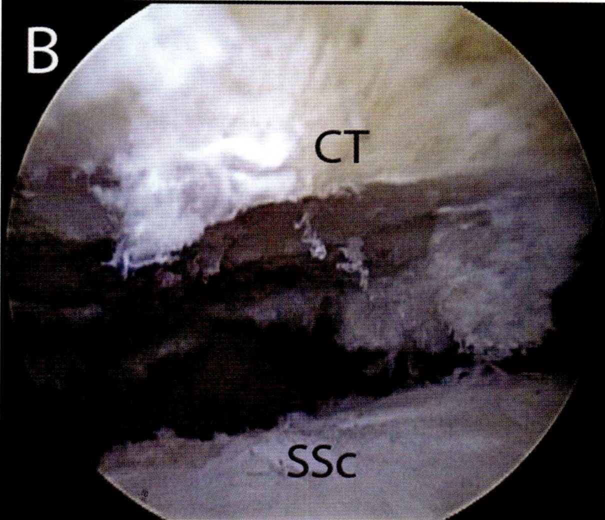

Figure 6.17 Coracoplasty in a right shoulder, viewed from a posterior glenohumeral portal through a window in the rotator interval. **A:** The coracohumeral interval is assessed by comparing to the known width of an instrument introduced from an anterosuperolateral working portal. In this case, the interval is approximately the width of a 5-mm burr. **B:** A coracoplasty has been performed to create a coracohumeral interval that is at least 7 mm deep. CT, coracoid tip; SSc, subscapularis tendon.

and the anatomic footprint of the subscapularis, we prepare the lesser tuberosity footprint for repair by creating a bleeding bone bed all the way to the articular margin. If the subscapularis tendon cannot be lateralized adequately, then the bone bed for the repair footprint is medialized up to 7 mm.

In >90% of chronic subscapularis tears, footprint coverage will only be adequate enough for single-row suture anchor repair. Naturally, if double-row repair is possible, we will do it, but if it is not possible we accept single-row repair. With single-row repair, one must place one anchor for each centimeter of tear in the superior-to-inferior dimension. Since the average subscapularis footprint is 25 mm from top to bottom (Fig. 6.19), this means that even 100% tears of the subscapularis can usually be repaired with two to three suture anchors. We prefer double-loaded fully threaded biocomposite suture anchors (BioComposite Corkscrew FT; Arthrex, Inc., Naples, FL). Sutures from the lower anchor are passed antegrade or retrograde approximately 10 to 15 mm medial to the lateral border of the subscapularis. For nonretracted tears, retrograde suture passage for mattress-configuration repair of the lower anchor sutures is often done. The sutures from the superior anchor are placed antegrade at the junction of the comma sign with the superolateral subscapularis. By placing the sutures there, the tendon edge inverts against the bone bed and the comma tissue acts as a rip-stop to suture cut-out through soft tissue (since the fibers of the comma tissue are oriented at right angles to the fibers of the subscapularis tendon) (Fig. 6.20).

Although sutures may be passed retrograde through the tendon with BirdBeak or Penetrator suture passers (Arthrex, Inc., Naples, FL), the lateral overhang of the coracoid is an obstacle to retrograde passage. For that reason, we most often perform antegrade suture passage with Viper or Scorpion suture passers (Arthrex, Inc., Naples, FL). The FastPass Scorpion is particularly useful for antegrade suture passage in the subscapularis. Its spring-loaded trapdoor in the upper jaw allows for "blind" capture of the suture, even with limited visualization in the subcoracoid space.

After the subscapularis has been repaired, the biceps tenodesis is performed at the top of the bicipital groove with a BioComposite Tenodesis screw. Then, the comma sign can be followed to the anterolateral border of the supraspinatus tendon, which can then be mobilized and repaired.

FATTY DEGENERATION OF THE SUBSCAPULARIS

Although our experience has been that most rotator cuff tears with <75% fatty infiltration will improve significantly after repair (1), we have specifically found that subscapularis tears with up to 100% fatty infiltration can heal and provide significant clinical improvement

(Text continued on page 114)

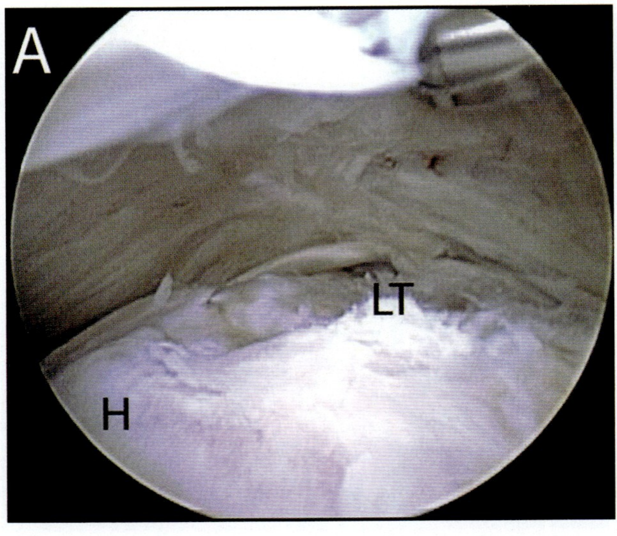

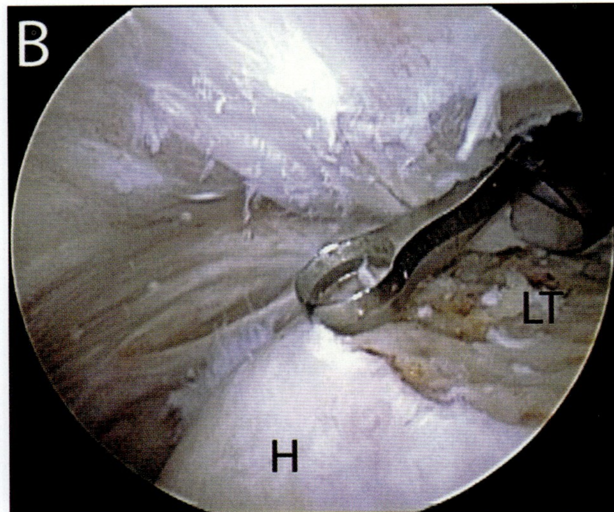

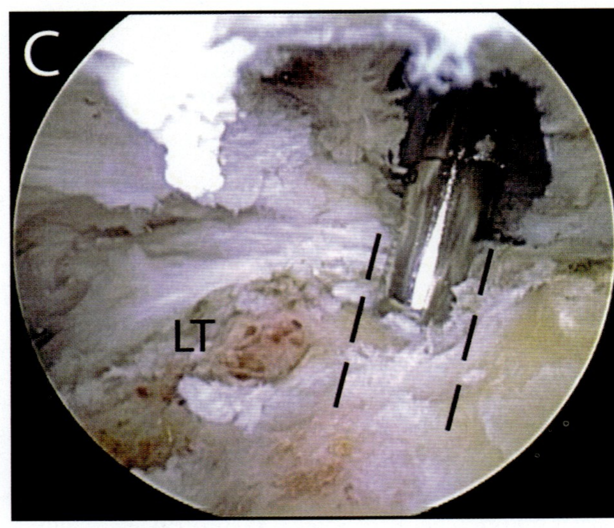

Figure 6.18 **A:** Right shoulder, posterior viewing portal with a 70° arthroscope, demonstrates a bare lesser tuberosity in an individual with a retracted subscapularis tendon tear and a chronically retracted long head of the biceps, with an "empty" bicipital groove. Restoration of the footprint depends upon defining the margins of the lesser tuberosity. **B:** The medial margin of the lesser tuberosity is easily defined adjacent to the articular margin. **C:** Defining the lateral margin of the lesser tuberosity requires identification of the bicipital groove (outlined by *dashed black lines*). H, humerus; LT, lesser tuberosity.

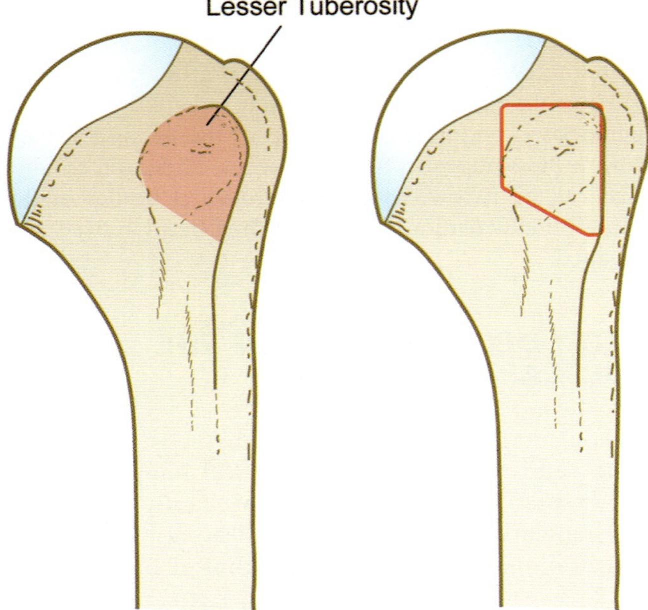

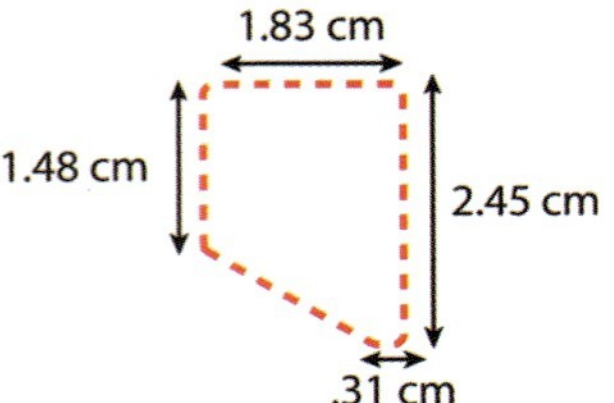

Figure 6.19 Schematic of the normal subscapularis tendon footprint. Since the average subscapularis footprint is approximately 2.5 cm from top to bottom, two to three anchors are needed to repair a completely retracted subscapularis tendon tear. Note that the footprint is wider proximally than distally, indicating a relatively more important force-generating function for the upper subscapularis than for the lower.

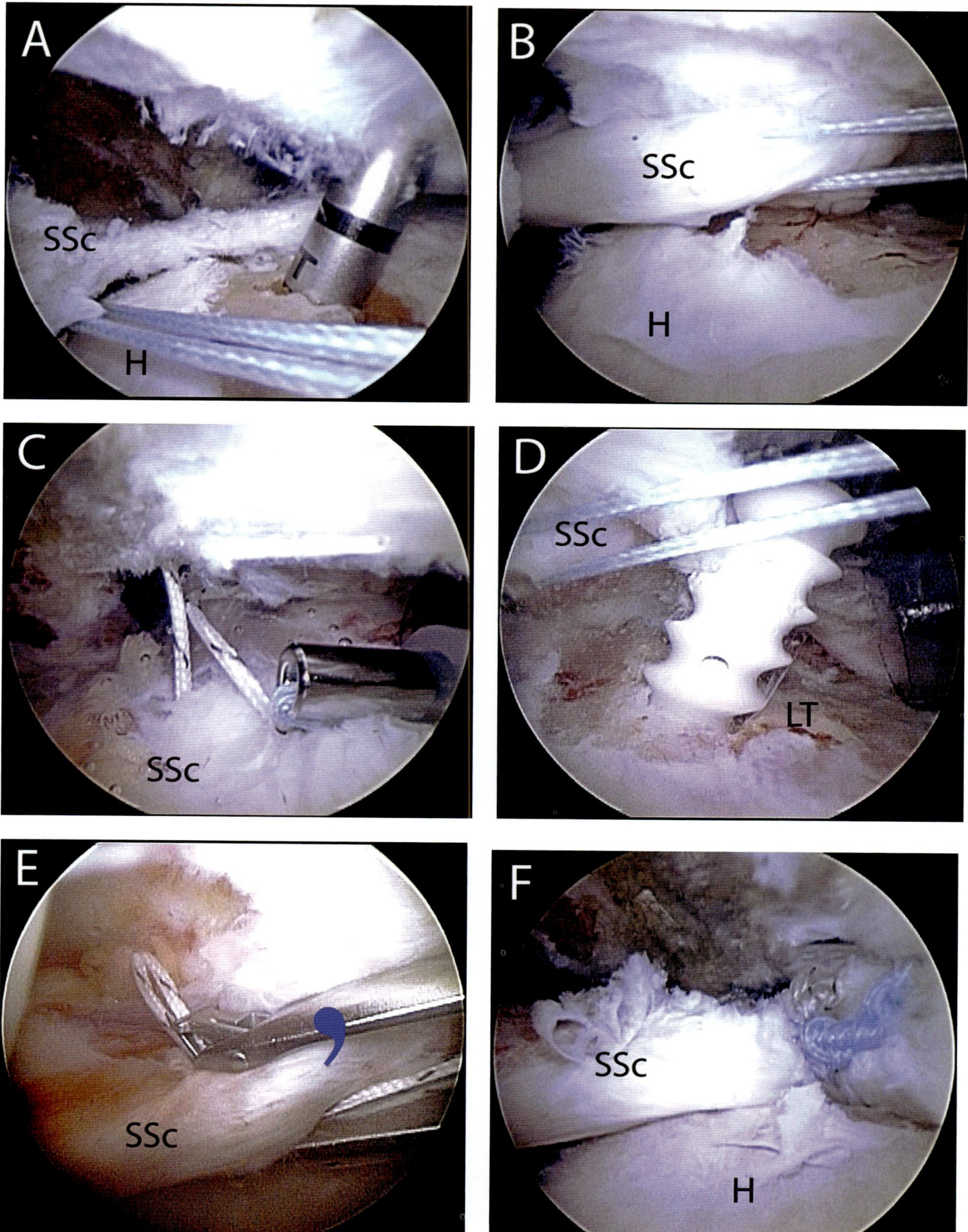

Figure 6.20 Two-anchor repair of a retracted full-thickness subscapularis tendon tear in a right shoulder viewed from a posterior glenohumeral portal. **A:** A bone socket is created in the inferior lesser tuberosity for placement of a BioComposite Corkscrew FT suture anchor (Arthrex, Inc., Naples, FL). **B:** After suture passage, a provisional reduction is obtained with a traction stitch in the upper subscapularis tendon. **C:** The arthroscope is placed through a window in the rotator interval and the sutures from the inferior anchor are tied while tension is maintained on the traction stitch. **D:** A second anchor is then placed in the superior lesser tuberosity. **E:** Sutures from the superior anchor are passed antegrade, medial to the comma tissue. **F:** Completed repair, demonstrating restoration of the subscapularis footprint (compare to Fig. 6.11A). H, humerus; LT, lesser tuberosity; SSc, subscapularis tendon; blue comma symbol, comma sign.

(Fig. 6.21). The subscapularis appears to be unique among the rotator cuff tendons in that a significant part of its function is a tenodesis effect, and it is needed as an anterior restraint whether the muscle is functional or not. Therefore, it can provide a stable fulcrum of motion even if it functions only as a tenodesis without contractile activity. Because of this, we believe that all subscapularis tears should be repaired regardless of chronicity and the degree of fatty degeneration. Based on this repair philosophy, we have noted dramatic improvements in overhead function after repair of subscapularis tears that had virtually complete fatty degeneration of the subscapularis.

SPECIFIC REPAIR TECHNIQUES

Repair of PASTA Lesions of the Subscapularis

The normal subscapularis footprint is bordered medially by a 2- to 3-mm strip of bare bone (*bare strip*) (Fig. 6.22A). A partial-thickness articular surface tendon avulsion (PASTA lesion) of the subscapularis involves actual tendon disruption from the lesser tuberosity, lateral to the *bare strip* (Fig. 6.22B). Some of these PASTA lesions are accompanied by a partial avulsion of the medial sling.

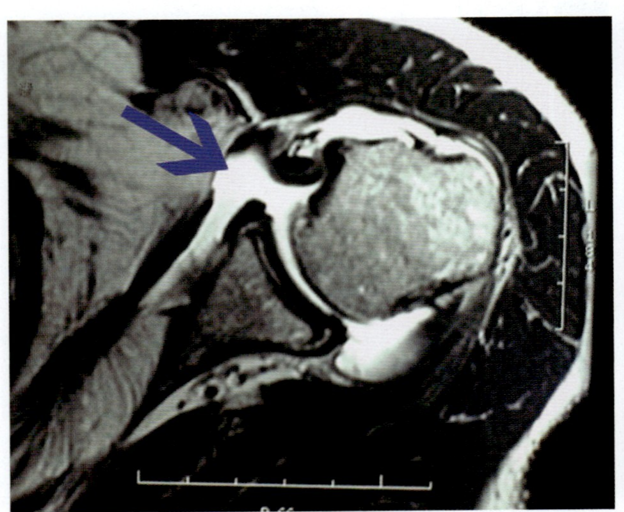

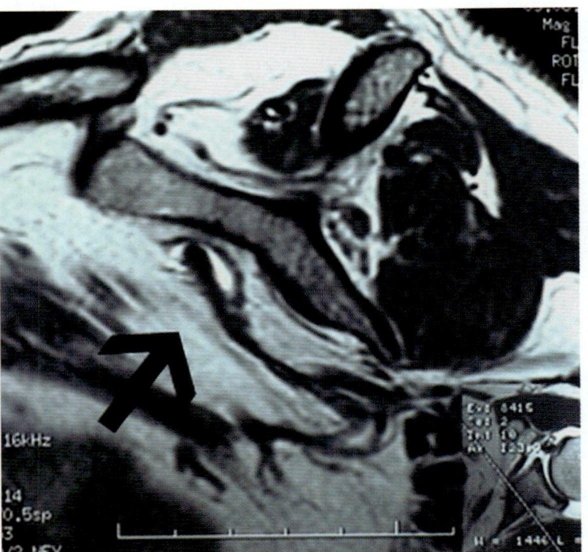

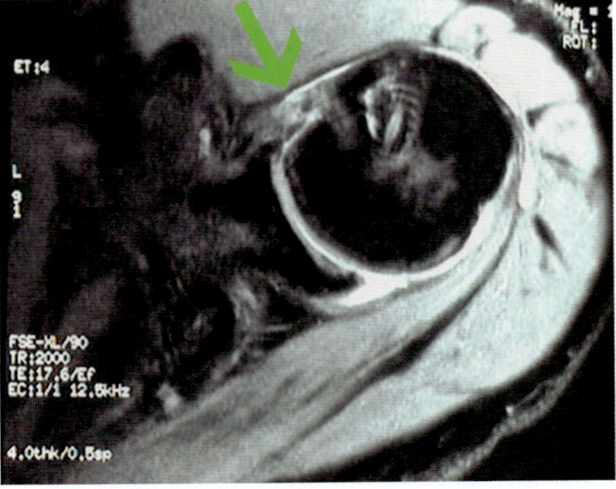

Figure 6.21 MRI of a left shoulder demonstrates **(A)** a complete retracted subscapularis tendon tear (*blue arrow*) with **(B)** nearly 100% fatty infiltration (*black arrow*). **C:** A postoperative MRI demonstrates healing of the tendon (*green arrow*). The subscapularis serves an important tenodesis function and should be repaired regardless of fatty infiltration.

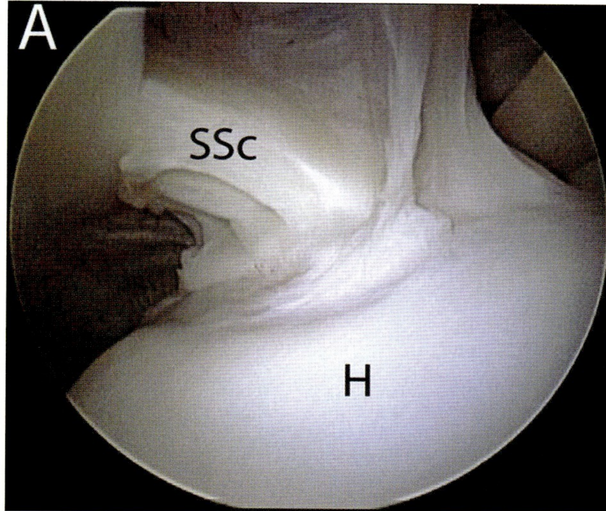

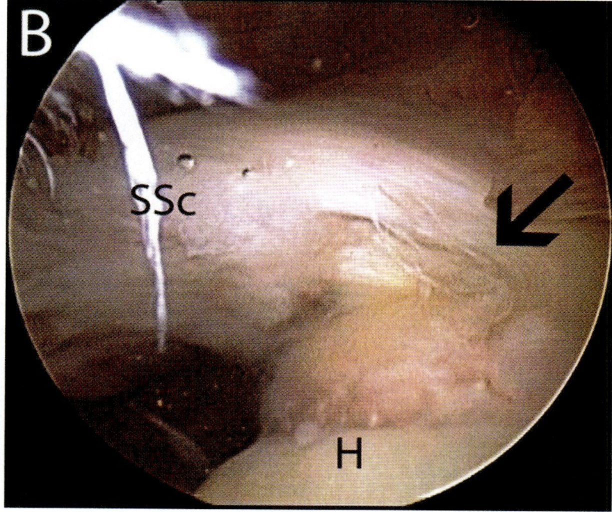

Figure 6.22 **A:** Right shoulder, posterior viewing portal. The normal subscapularis footprint **(A)** is bordered medially by a 2- to 3-mm strip of bare bone (*bare strip*). **B:** Right shoulder, posterior viewing portal, demonstrates a partial-thickness articular surface tendon avulsion of the subscapularis involving actual tendon disruption (*black arrow*) from the lesser tuberosity, lateral to the *bare strip*. H, humeral head; SSc, subscapularis tendon.

These tears can be repaired with a fully threaded double-loaded suture anchor (BioComposite Corkscrew FT) placed at the superomedial aspect of the prepared lesser tuberosity. Sutures are passed antegrade or retrograde at or near the junction of the subscapularis with the medial sling (Fig. 6.23).

Alternatively, a knotless technique (SpeedFix; Arthrex, Inc., Naples, FL) can be used to avoid the need for knot tying. In this technique, a FiberTape (Arthrex, Inc., Naples, FL) is passed through the superolateral subscapularis via an anterosuperolateral portal (Fig. 6.24A). This suture is then retrieved through the anterior portal. Through the anterior portal, a bone socket is made in the superomedial portion of the lesser tuberosity. The two limbs of the FiberTape are passed through the eyelet of the SwiveLock C anchor, which is then inserted into the bone socket after tensioning the two FiberTape limbs (Figs. 6.24B, C). This method is so reliable that it has become our current technique of choice for PASTA lesions of the subscapularis.

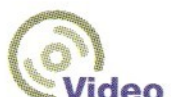

Repair of Full-thickness Tears of the Subscapularis

Most full-thickness tears of the subscapularis involve a full-thickness disruption of the medial sling, resulting

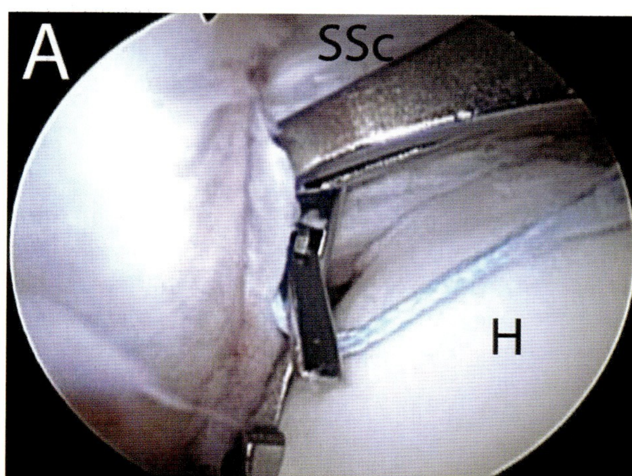

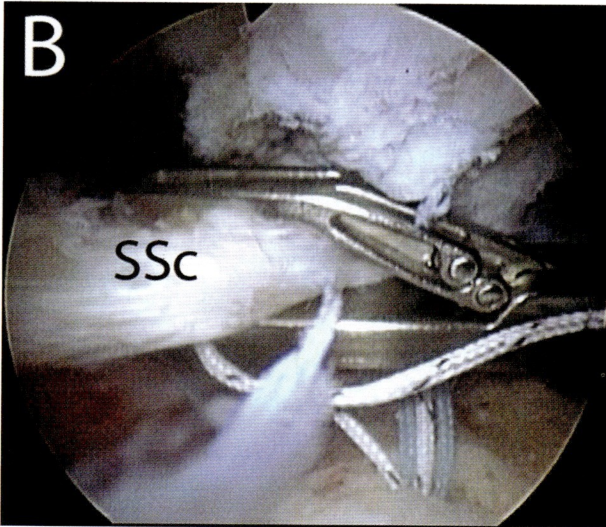

Figure 6.23 Right shoulder, posterior viewing portal. After placement of a double-loaded anchor, suture passage for repair of an upper subscapularis tear can be performed with a retrograde technique **(A)** or with an antegrade instrument **(B)**. In the case of retrograde suture passage, an additional instrument can be used to hand-off suture from the anchor. H, humerus; SSc, subscapularis tendon.

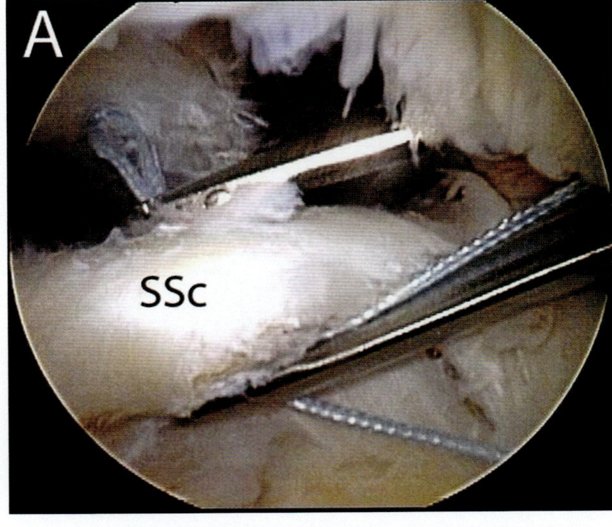

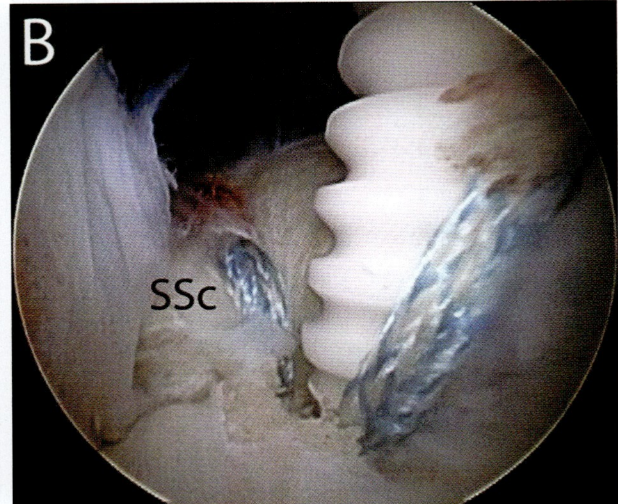

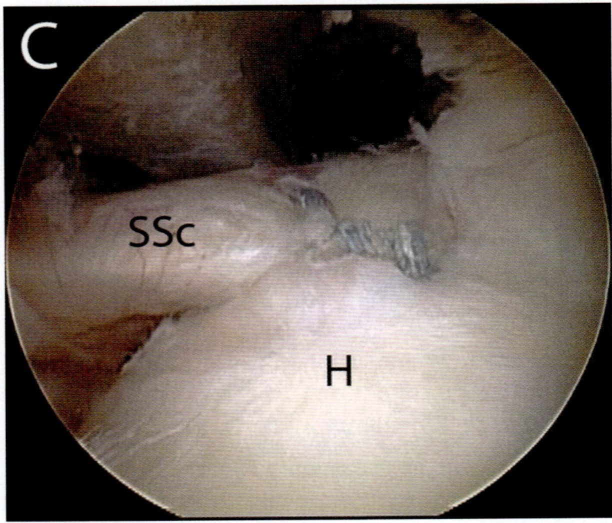

Figure 6.24 Right shoulder, posterior viewing portal demonstrating knotless repair of an upper subscapularis tendon tear. **A:** A FiberTape suture (Arthrex, Inc., Naples, FL) is passed antegrade through the upper subscapularis tendon. **B:** The tape is secured to the prepared bone bed with a BioComposite SwiveLock C anchor (Arthrex, Inc.). **C:** Final view demonstrates restoration of the footprint with a low-profile knotless repair. H, humerus; SSc, subscapularis tendon.

in an unstable biceps tendon. In such cases, the biceps is addressed by tenotomy or tenodesis as previously described in this chapter. These cases always demonstrate a *comma sign* that will lead the surgeon to the superolateral subscapularis.

If the subscapularis is minimally retracted or not retracted, double-row repair is sometimes possible, though we have found this to be possible in <25% of cases.

If the full-thickness tear involves more than the upper 1.5 cm of the subscapularis, the double-row repair will need two medial anchors (BioComposite Corkscrew FT or BioComposite SwiveLock C) and two lateral anchors (BioComposite SwiveLock C), with an intervening suture-bridge technique. For medial row fixation with a BioComposite Corkscrew anchor, usually the suture limbs from the inferomedial anchor are separately passed retrograde and tied in mattress fashion. The limbs are left long so that they can be incorporated into the lateral row. The sutures from the superomedial anchor are passed antegrade or retrograde at the junction of the subscapularis tendon with the comma sign. They are then tied as simple sutures, and then passed laterally to be incorporated into the SutureBridge (Arthrex, Inc., Naples, FL) (Fig. 6.25). Alternatively, a FiberLink (Arthrex, Inc., Naples, FL) can be used to pass the sutures from the medial anchors and a double-pulley technique can be used to tie a double mattress stitch between the two medial anchors as previously described (see Chapter 4, "Complete Rotator Cuff Tears").

In a variant of the SpeedBridge technique, SwiveLock anchors preloaded with a FiberTape can also be used for the medial row repair. In this scenario, the inferomedial anchor is placed transtendon (Fig. 6.26). The superomedial anchor is then placed and the sutures are passed retrograde with a FiberTape Penetrator (Arthrex, Inc., Naples, FL), which has a radiused lower jaw that allows for low-friction retrieval of FiberTape (Fig. 6.27). The FiberWire safety sutures from the SwiveLock anchors are then tied in a mattress fashion with a double-pulley technique between

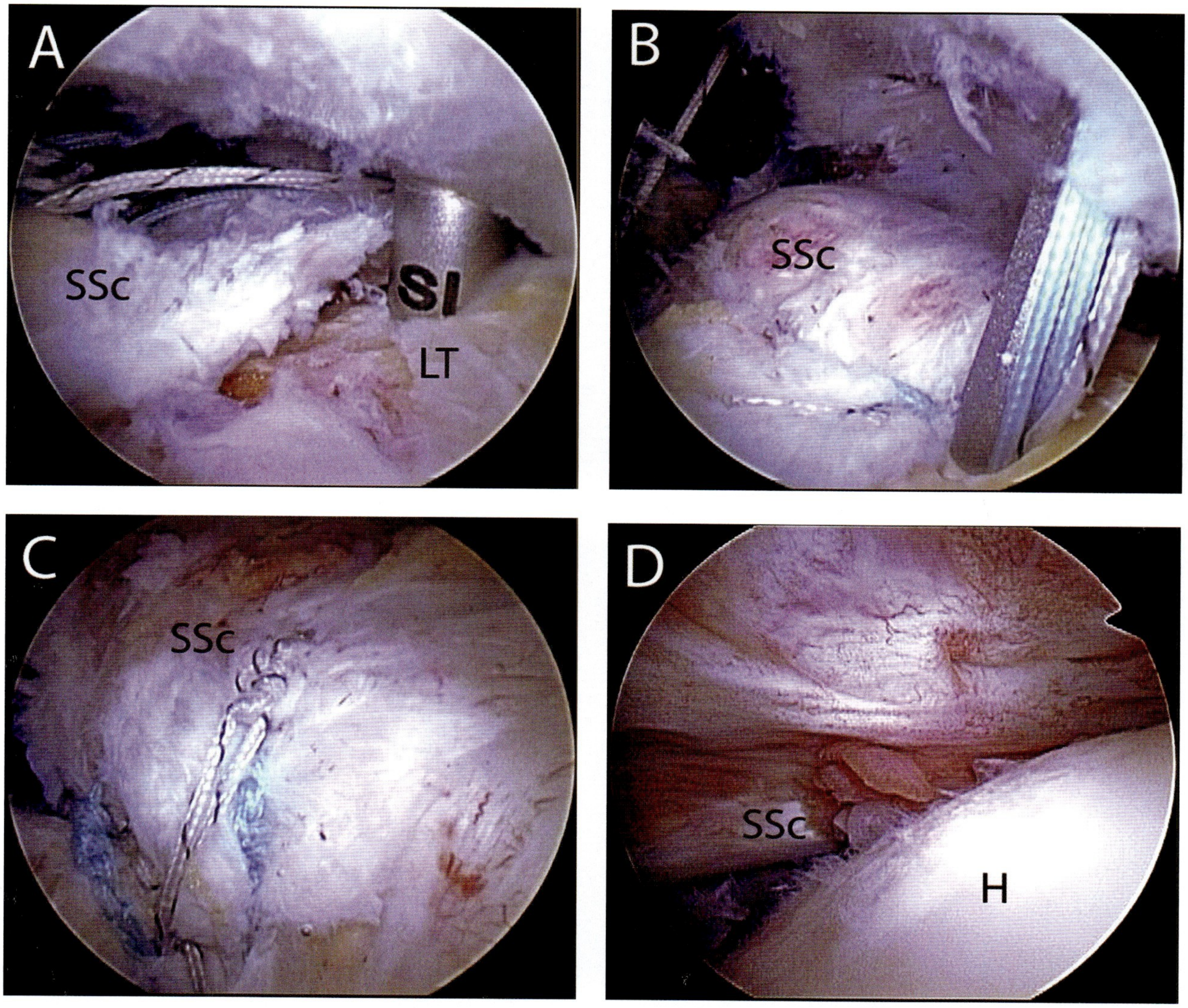

Figure 6.25 Double-row repair of a subscapularis tendon tear in a right shoulder using a SutureBridge technique (Arthrex, Inc., Naples, FL). **A:** After completing the medial row repair, suture limbs are retained and a bone socket for a SwiveLock anchor is prepared in the lateral lesser tuberosity. **B:** Suture limbs from the medial row are threaded through the eyelet of a SwiveLock anchor and secured laterally in a crisscross pattern. **C:** Completed SutureBridge repair viewed from an anterosuperolateral portal demonstrates a low-profile repair with compression of the subscapularis footprint. **D:** Completed repair viewed from a posterior glenohumeral viewing portal. H, humerus; LT, lesser tuberosity; SSc, subscapularis tendon.

the two medial anchors. This portion of the repair creates a medial seal that restricts synovial fluid penetration into the tendon–bone interface. These FiberWire suture limbs are then cut after knot tying. The FiberTape suture limbs are then incorporated into a lateral row repair with two additional SwiveLock anchors (Fig. 6.28).

For short full-thickness tears of the upper subscapularis, one can employ a knotless double-row technique using FiberTape with two BioComposite SwiveLock C anchors. A FiberTape is placed through the superolateral aspect of the subscapularis and secured with a SwiveLock C anchor as described above. However, instead of cutting the residual limbs of the FiberTape, these limbs are then passed anterior to the comma sign tissue and fixed superolaterally with another SwiveLock C anchor into a bone socket after appropriate tensioning (Fig. 6.29). This is a variant of the SpeedBridge technique.

Double-row Repair Incorporated into Biceps Tenodesis

Lateral row fixation of a subscapularis repair can be accomplished by incorporating the medial sutures into a biceps tenodesis construct. This technique is particularly useful

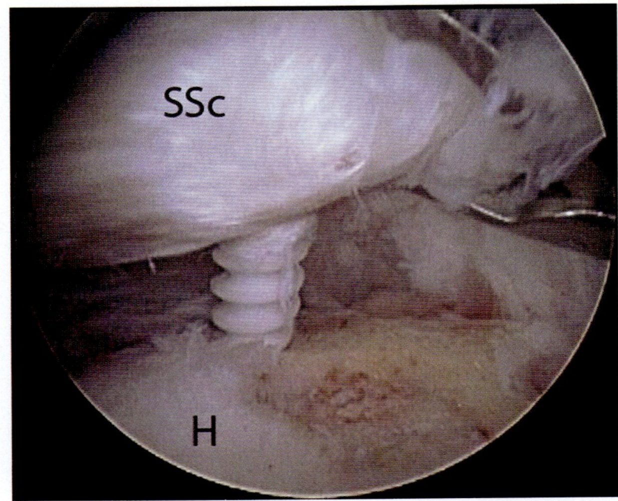

Figure 6.26 Right shoulder, posterior viewing portal demonstrates transtendon placement of an inferomedial BioComposite SwiveLock C anchor (Arthrex, Inc., Naples, FL) that has been preloaded with FiberTape (Arthrex, Inc., Naples, FL) for a double-row repair of a full-thickness subscapularis tendon (SSc) tear. H, humeral head.

for full-thickness subscapularis tendon tears when there is limited space for a lateral anchor (in addition to the biceps tenodesis). The medial repair is performed as previously described, usually with a FiberTape and SwiveLock technique, and the sutures limbs from the medial repair are preserved (Fig. 6.30).

A guide pin is placed through the anterosuperolateral portal to determine the appropriate position for tenodesis (Fig. 6.31A). A cannulated drill equal in diameter to the biceps tendon (usually 7 or 8 mm) is reamed to a depth of 25 mm to prepare a bone socket for the BioComposite Tenodesis screw (Arthrex, Inc., Naples, FL) that is 23 mm in length (Fig. 6.31B). The bone socket is cleared of debris to ensure an unobstructed path for the biceps tendon (Fig. 6.31C).The tails of the FiberTape from the medial row, which had been preserved, are now retrieved out the anterosuperolateral portal anterior to the subscapularis. Recall that in preparation for biceps tenodesis a FiberWire whipstitch has previously been placed in the biceps tendon. Extracorporeally, the tails of the FiberTape are passed between the two FiberWire suture ends exiting the biceps tendon (Fig. 6.32). Next, the FiberWire tails from the biceps whipstitch are passed through the Tenodesis screwdriver. This sequence not only delivers the biceps tendon to the tip of the screwdriver, but also creates an "eyelet" that captures the tails of the FiberTape from the medial row. The biceps tendon and screw are guided into the bone socket with the end of the screwdriver (Fig. 6.33). After the screwdriver tip is "bottomed out," any slack in the FiberTape suture is removed by tensioning the FiberTape ends. The BioComposite Tenodesis screw is then advanced down the shaft of the screwdriver. It is important to maintain tension on both the FiberWire sutures from the biceps tendon and the FiberTape sutures from the medial row repair. An interference fit secures both the biceps tendon and the FiberTape in the bone socket, completing the

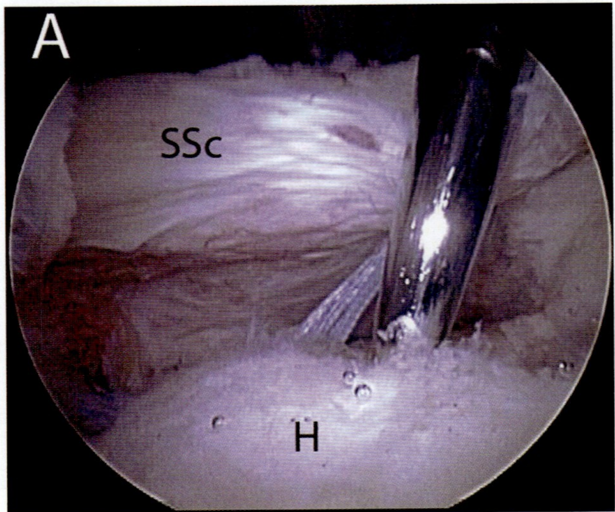

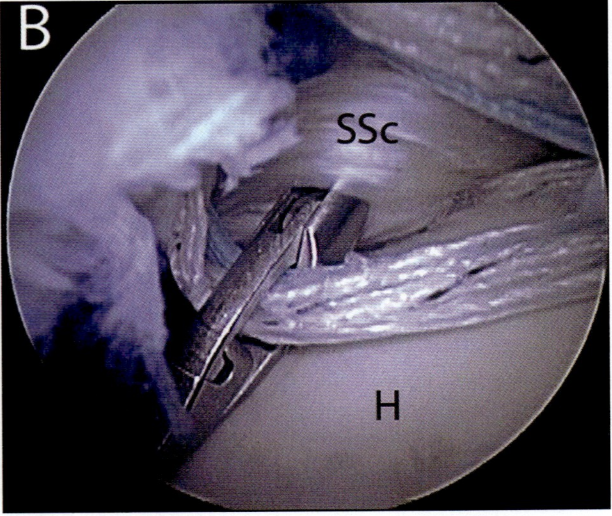

Figure 6.27 Right shoulder, posterior viewing portal. **A:** A bone socket is prepared for placement of a superomedial SwiveLock anchor (Arthrex, Inc., Naples, FL). Note the inferior sutures from the previously placed inferomedial anchor. **B:** After anchor placement, the superomedial anchor sutures are passed retrograde through the upper subscapularis using a radiused FiberTape Penetrator (Arthrex, Inc., Naples, FL). H, humeral head. SSc, subscapularis tendon.

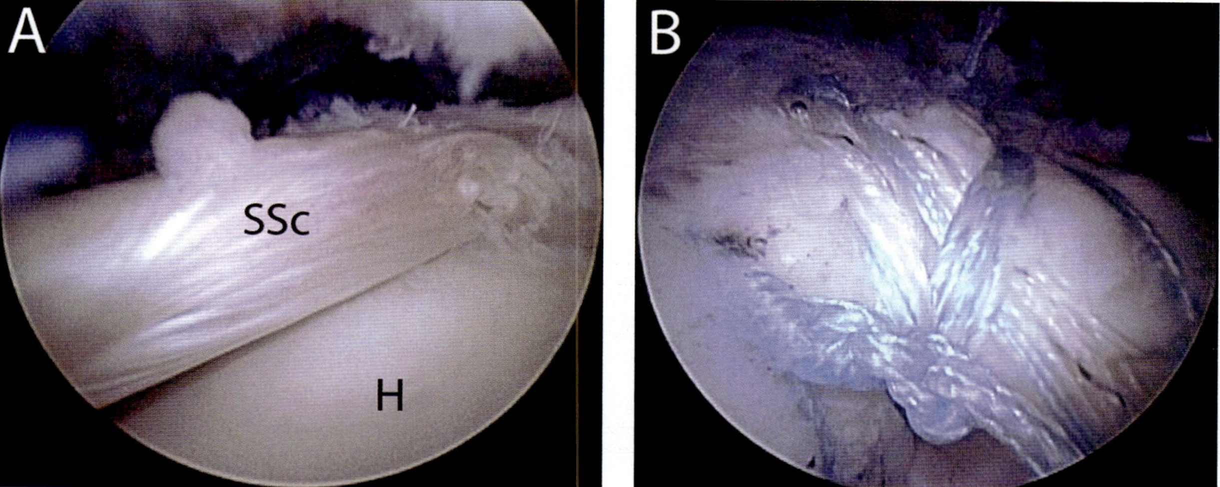

Figure 6.28 Double-row SpeedBridge (Arthrex, Inc., Naples, FL) repair of a full-thickness subscapularis tendon (SSc) tear in a right shoulder. **A:** Posterior viewing portal demonstrates low-profile restoration of the medial footprint. **B:** Lateral subacromial viewing portal demonstrates compression of the lateral footprint and an overview of the SpeedBridge repair.

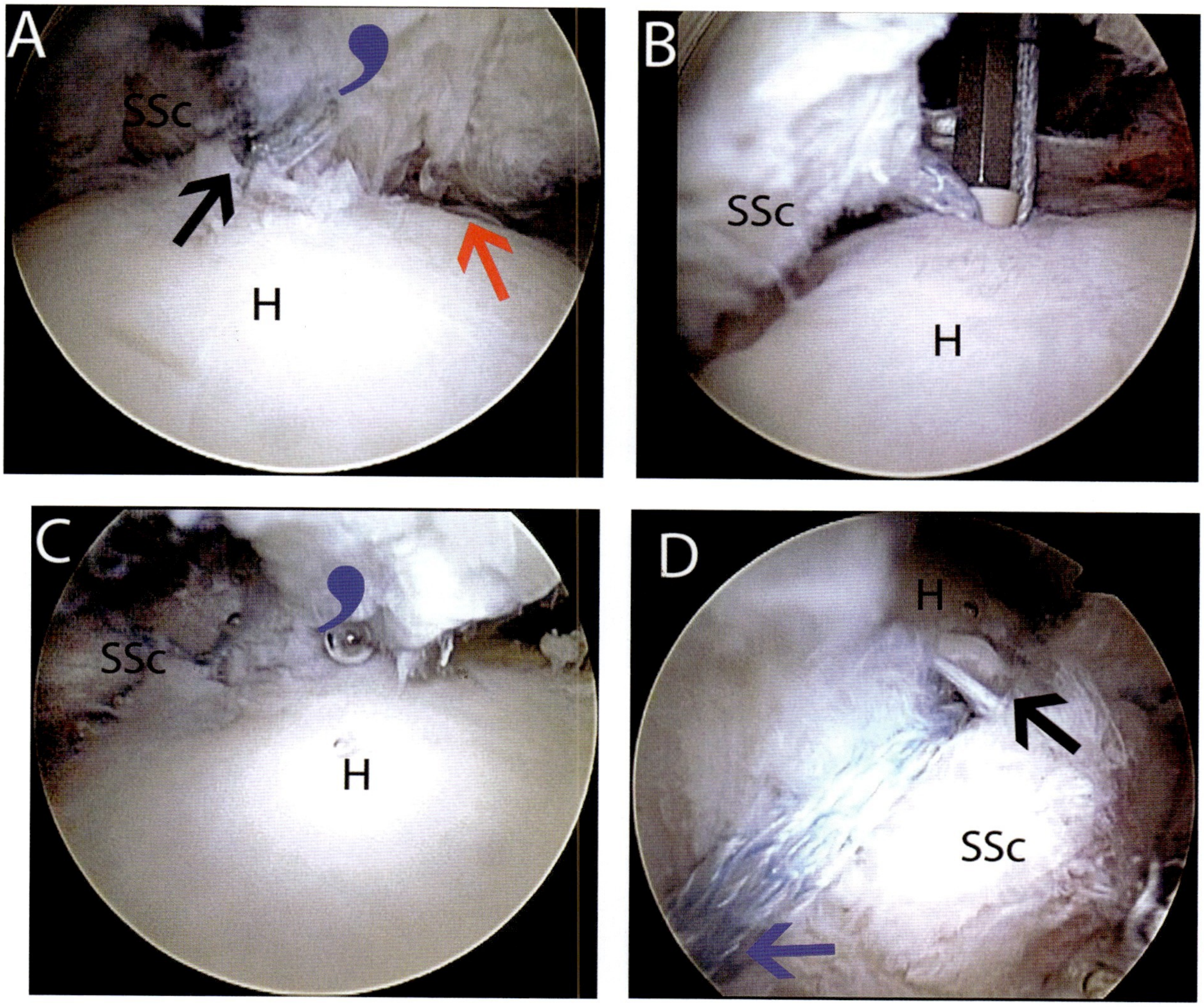

Figure 6.29 Double-row repair of an upper full-thickness subscapularis tendon tear using a SpeedBridge (Arthrex, Inc., Naples, FL) technique in a right shoulder viewed with a 70° arthroscope. **A:** Posterior viewing portal. The medial footprint (*black arrow*) of a subscapularis tendon tear has been repaired with a FiberTape and SwiveLock C anchor. However, the lateral footprint (*red arrow*) is not yet restored. The FiberTape limbs from the medial row are preserved for a double-row repair. **B:** The FiberTape limbs are passed anterior to the comma tissue and secured with a lateral SwiveLock C anchor. **C:** Following placement of the lateral anchor, both the medial and lateral footprints have been restored. **D:** Anterosuperolateral viewing portal provides an aerial view of the double-row repair, consisting of a FiberTape secured with a medial anchor (*black arrow*) and a lateral anchor (*blue arrow*). H, humerus; SSc, subscapularis tendon; blue comma symbol, comma sign.

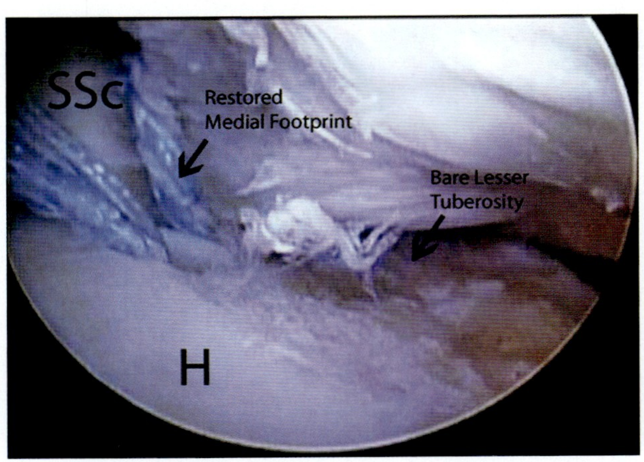

Figure 6.30 Right shoulder, posterior glenohumeral viewing portal with a 70° arthroscope. The medial subscapularis tendon has been repaired with a FiberTape and SwiveLock C anchor (Arthrex, Inc., Naples, FL). While the medial footprint has been restored, the lateral footprint remains uncovered. Lateral row fixation is therefore required. H, humerus; SSc, subscapularis tendon.

biceps tenodesis and simultaneously achieving lateral row fixation of the double-row subscapularis tendon repair (Fig. 6.34).

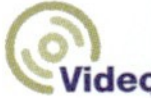

OCCULT TEARS OF THE SUBSCAPULARIS

Most tears of the subscapularis can be easily identified by viewing with both the 30° and 70° arthroscopes while an assistant applies a posterior lever push. However, there are two occult tear patterns that we have observed that can easily be missed if the surgeon does not specifically look for them. Both of these occult tear patterns require the use of a 70° arthroscope for visualization.

The first of these occult tear patterns is a distal bursal-surface tear that can only be seen while looking directly down the bicipital groove with a 70° arthroscope. This should be a routine part of every diagnostic arthroscopy, as it is an excellent way to visualize additional pathology

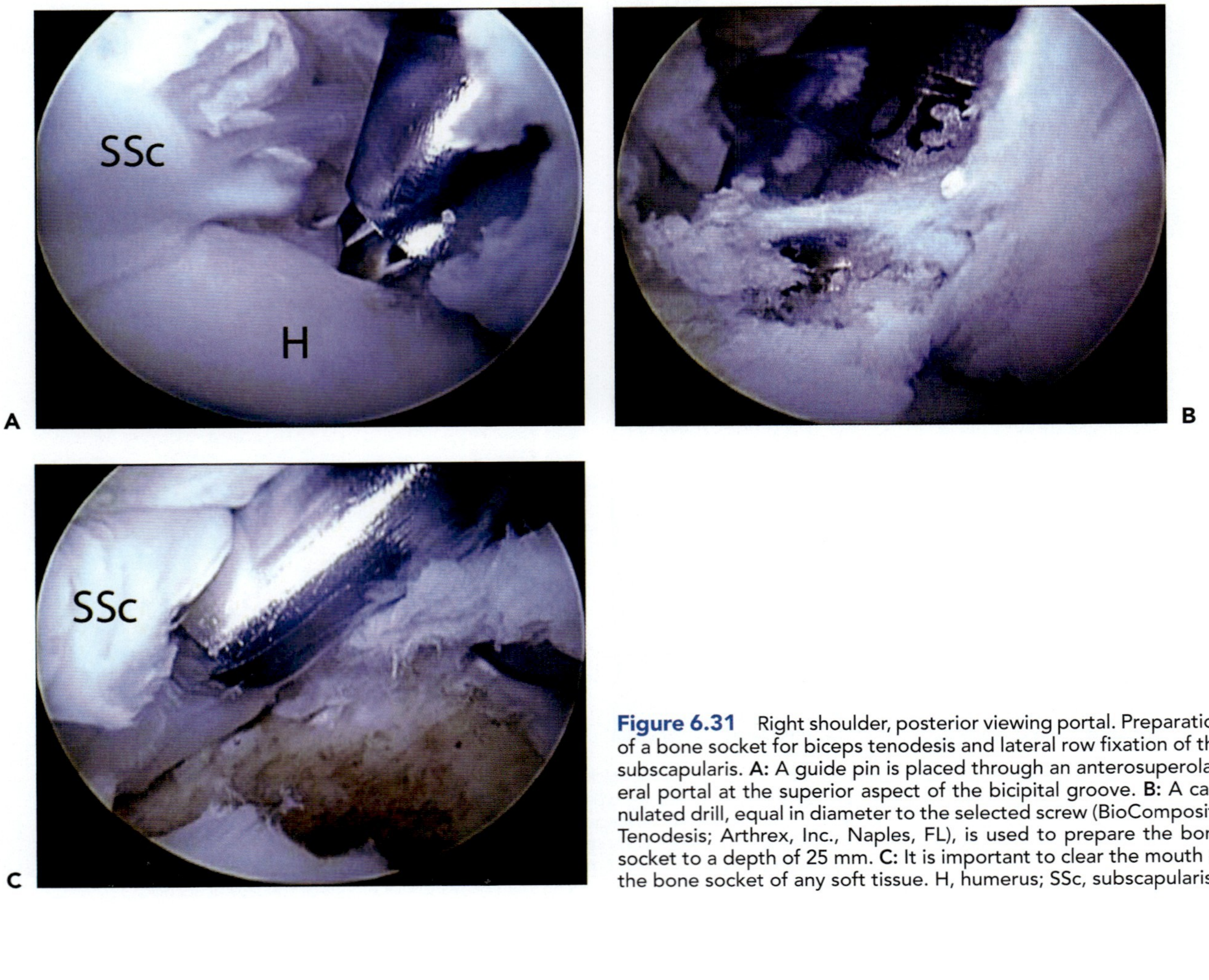

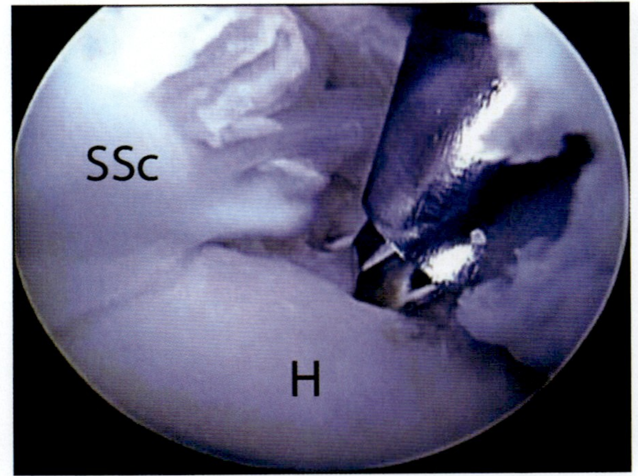

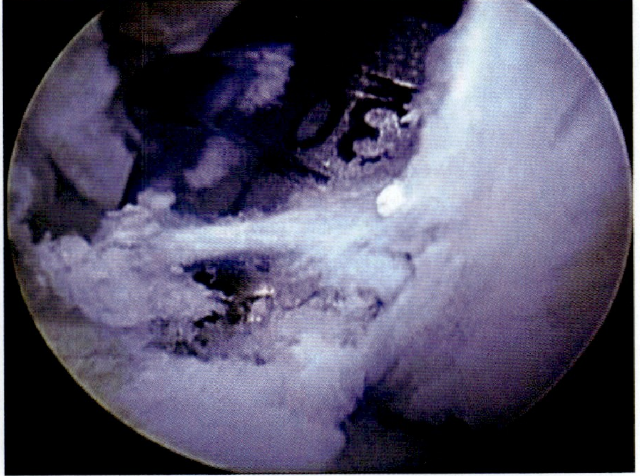

SSc

C

Figure 6.31 Right shoulder, posterior viewing portal. Preparation of a bone socket for biceps tenodesis and lateral row fixation of the subscapularis. **A:** A guide pin is placed through an anterosuperolateral portal at the superior aspect of the bicipital groove. **B:** A cannulated drill, equal in diameter to the selected screw (BioComposite Tenodesis; Arthrex, Inc., Naples, FL), is used to prepare the bone socket to a depth of 25 mm. **C:** It is important to clear the mouth of the bone socket of any soft tissue. H, humerus; SSc, subscapularis.

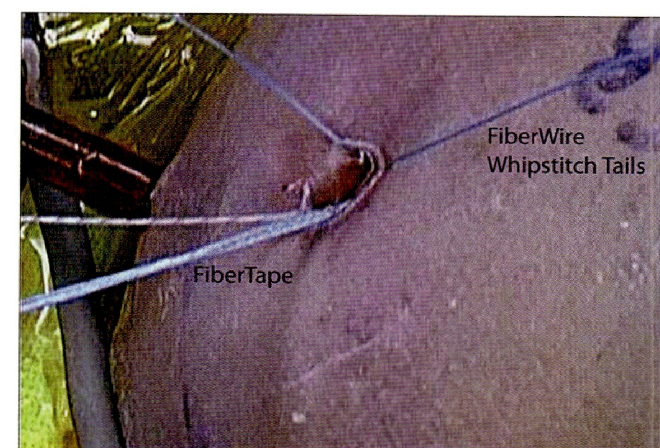

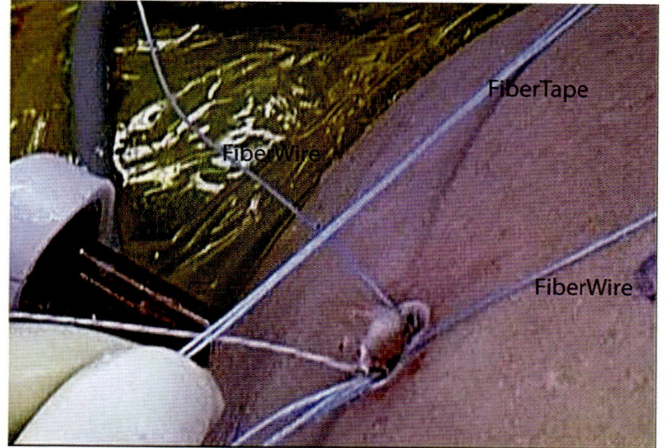

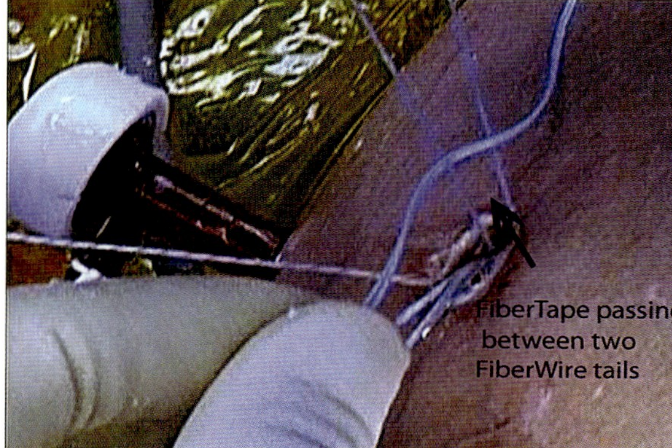

Figure 6.32 External view of a right shoulder demonstrating incorporation of medial row sutures into biceps tenodesis. **A:** Sutures are seen exiting from an anterosuperolateral portal. To the right are the two tails of FiberWire (Arthrex, Inc., Naples, FL) suture that have been previously placed as a whipstitch in the biceps tendon. To the left are retained tails of a FiberTape suture (Arthrex, Inc., Naples, FL) following medial row fixation of an upper subscapularis tear. **B:** The FiberTape is passed between the two FiberWire sutures. **C:** The FiberTape is seen passing between the FiberWire sutures. Subsequently, the FiberWire ends are passed through the cannulation of the Tenodesis screwdriver. This delivers the biceps tendon to the tip of the screwdriver and also secures the FiberTape.

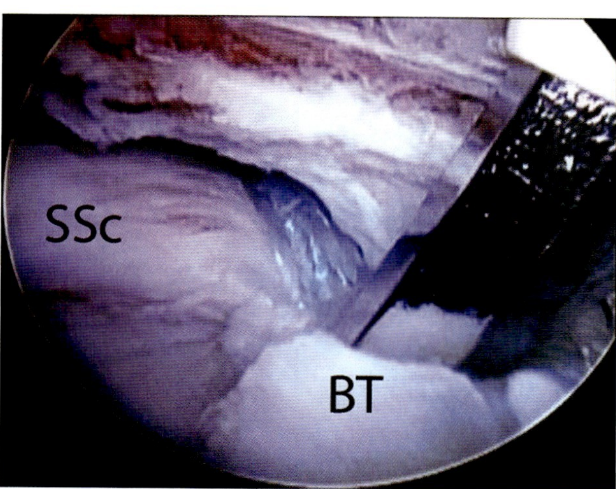

Figure 6.33 Right shoulder, posterior viewing portal demonstrating technique for incorporating medial row subscapularis sutures into a biceps tenodesis. The biceps (BT) seen at the tip of the screwdriver is delivered into a previously prepared bone socket. To the left of the screwdriver, FiberTape (Arthrex, Inc., Naples, FL) sutures are seen that pass over the superolateral edge of the subscapularis (SSc). These sutures have been threaded between the biceps tenodesis sutures so that the biceps tenodesis construct also obtains lateral row fixation of the subscapularis tendon.

within the bicipital groove (e.g., partial tears of the biceps; osteophytes within the bicipital groove; entrapped loose bodies). On a few occasions, we have noted substantial tears or "cracks" in the medial sidewall of the bicipital groove that, on probing with a hooked probe, revealed a portion of bare footprint on the lesser tuberosity at varying distances from the top of the footprint (Figs. 6.35 and 6.36). We have seen such lesions in the proximal, middle, and distal thirds of the footprint. When such tears are identified, they should be repaired like any other bursal-surface or interstitial tear, by preparing the bone bed and placing suture anchors in the lateral portion of the lesser tuberosity for repair of the tear (Fig. 6.37).

Another type of occult subscapularis tear is a variant of a short PASTA lesion at the upper subscapularis combined with an intact medial sling. In most instances of articular-sided tears of the upper subscapularis, the medial sling tears as well. This creates the easily identifiable comma sign that directs the surgeon's attention to the tear of the upper subscapularis. However, if the medial sling is completely intact, it can effectively block the visualization of an upper subscapularis tear. In such cases, the 70° arthroscope must be used to "look around the corner" of

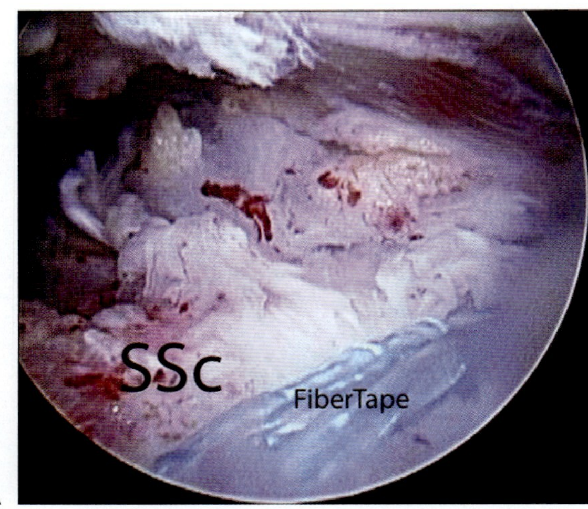

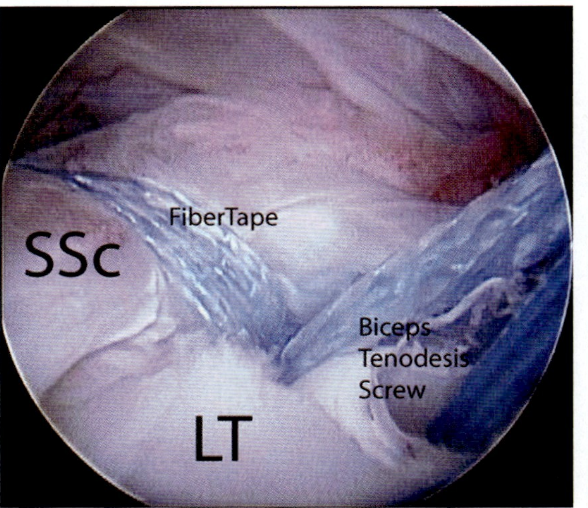

Figure 6.34 Right shoulder, posterior viewing portal. Completed double-row repair of a subscapularis tear with a single-suture anchor plus a BioComposite Tenodesis screw (Arthrex, Inc., Naples, FL). **A:** With the arthroscope placed through a window in the rotator interval, a FiberTape (Arthrex, Inc., Naples, FL) is seen securing an upper subscapularis tear in a transosseous equivalent fashion. (To the left is medial) **B:** Lateral row fixation of the subscapularis tear anatomically reestablishes the footprint. Note that lateral fixation is achieved with interference between the FiberTape, bone socket, and biceps tenodesis screw. LT, lesser tuberosity; SSc, subscapularis.

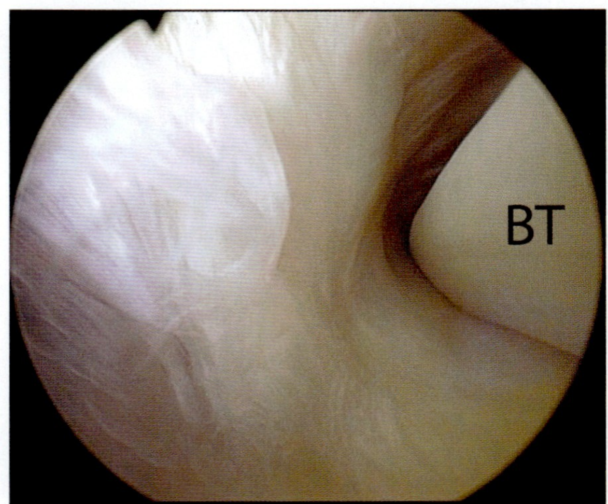

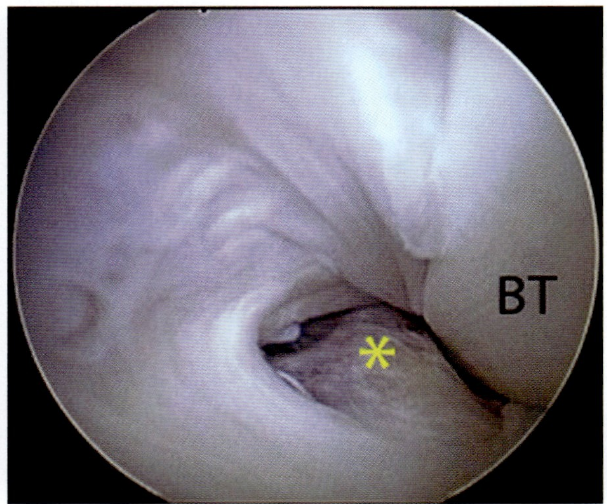

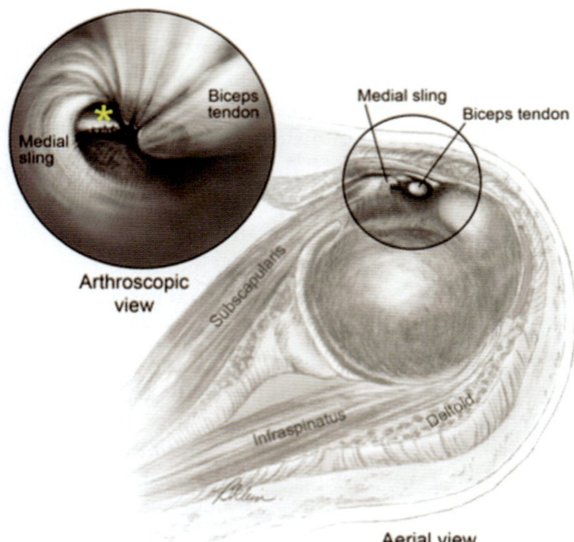

Figure 6.35 **A:** Right shoulder, posterior viewing portal with a 70° arthroscope, shows approximately 2.5 cm of the floor and sidewalls of the bicipital groove in this normal right shoulder. **B:** In a different right shoulder, there is disruption in the medial sidewall with a bare lesser tuberosity footprint distally. **C:** Depiction of the same view as Fig 6.28B, showing a disrupted medial sidewall, indicating a mid to distal tendon tear of the subscapularis. asterisk, disrupted medial sidewall; BT, biceps tendon.

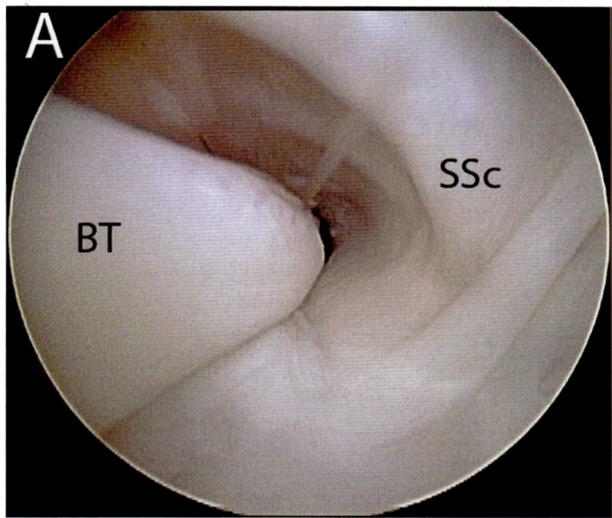

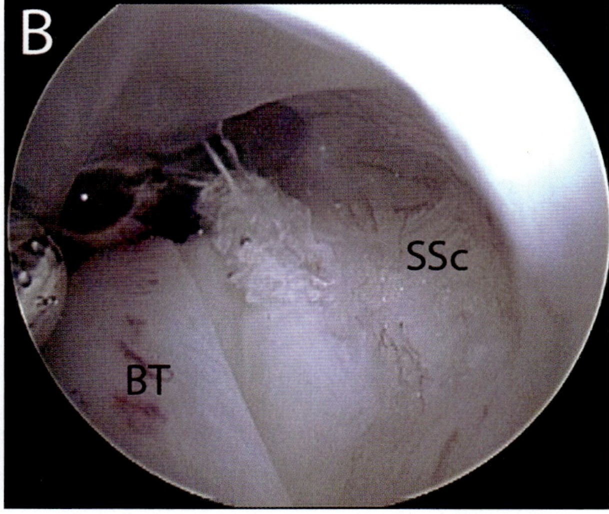

Figure 6.36 Left shoulders, posterior viewing portal with a 70° arthroscope demonstrates **(A)** normal medial sidewall of the bicipital groove, and **(B)** a different shoulder with cracks in the medial sidewall with disruption indicative of an occult subscapularis tendon tear. BT, biceps tendon; SSc, subscapularis tendon.

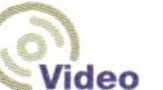

the intact medial sling in order to observe the bare footprint under the torn subscapularis (Fig. 6.38).

UNUSUAL CAUSES OF SUBSCAPULARIS TENDON DEFECTS REQUIRING REPAIR

Most cases of calcific tendinitis that involve the subscapularis tendon will reveal an inflammatory calcific deposit located posterior to the coracoid tip (Fig. 6.39). This causes a very painful subcoracoid impingement as the calcific deposit repetitively strikes the coracoid tip during internal and external rotation, particularly when combined with some degree of forward flexion. After arthroscopic evacuation and debridement of these calcific deposits, there is typically a significant bursal-surface subscapularis defect that is best treated by suture anchor repair.

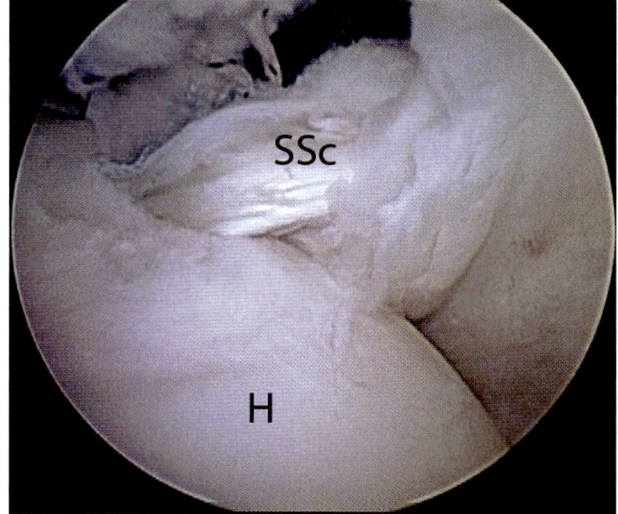

Figure 6.37 Left shoulder, posterior viewing portal demonstrating repair of the occult subscapularis tendon (SSc) tear seen in Fig. 6.36B. H, humeral head.

Another interesting subscapularis problem can occur as a result of an injury or repetitive overhead trauma (e.g., competitive swimming), in which an ossicle forms within the subscapularis tendon (Fig. 6.40). Such an ossicle can be very disabling, particularly to a swimmer who will experience painful subcoracoid impingement of the ossicle against the coracoid tip with every stroke. Such ossicles can be arthroscopically dissected and extracted from the subscapularis tendon, followed by suture anchor repair of the tendon defect (see "Arthroscopic Rodeo").

SUBCORACOID IMPINGEMENT

Anterior shoulder pathology encompasses multiple etiologies. Not uncommonly, evaluation of this area can reveal significant abnormalities of the upper subscapularis and/or the rotator interval. The pathoanatomy can include a partial upper subscapularis tear as well as significant synovitis of the rotator interval tissue. We believe that one of the major causes of these abnormalities is subcoracoid impingement.

Abnormal stresses on the articular side of the subscapularis can be caused by subcoracoid impingement and the resultant *roller-wringer* effect on the subscapularis (Fig. 6.41) (2). If the tip of the coracoid impinges on the

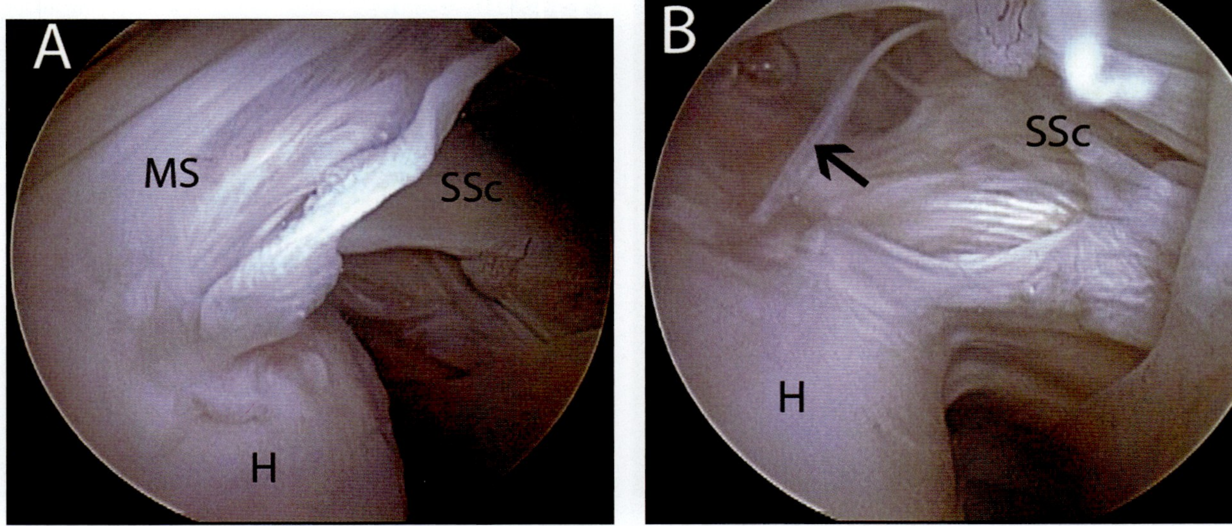

Figure 6.38 Left shoulder, posterior viewing portal demonstrates an occult tear of the subscapularis tendon. **A:** On initial inspection, the medial sling obscures the view and the subscapularis tendon appears intact. **B:** With use of a 70° to "look around the corner," disruption of the subscapularis insertion is seen with a bare footprint (*black arrow*). H, humerus; MS, medial sling; SSc, subscapularis tendon.

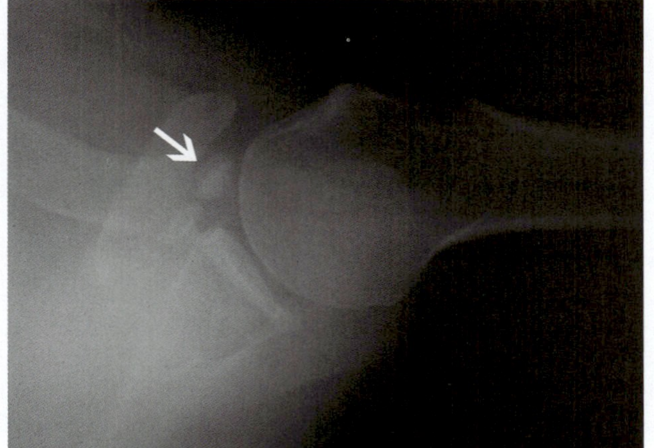

Figure 6.39 Axillary lateral radiograph in a right shoulder demonstrates calcific tendonitis (*white arrow*) posterior to the coracoid.

anterior subscapularis/rotator interval tissue, this can cause both inflammation of this area and undersurface tearing of the upper subscapularis tendon. With rotation of the arm as well as cross body adduction, the impingement can be exacerbated. No specific clinical exam tests are reliable for isolating the diagnosis of subcoracoid impingement. Hence, we heavily rely on an arthroscopic assessment of the coracohumeral interval to diagnose subcoracoid impingement.

We have observed that the most reliable arthroscopic sign of significant subcoracoid impingement, in patients without frank tearing of the subscapularis from its footprint, is the presence of linear longitudinal tearing of the upper subscapularis near its insertion. These occur as the result of a repetitive "battering-ram" effect from the coracoid tip. Repetitive compression of the tendon fibers in the anterior-to-posterior direction by the coracoid tip causes spreading of the fibers in the superior-to-inferior direction, with resultant longitudinal splits between fiber bundles (Fig. 6.42).

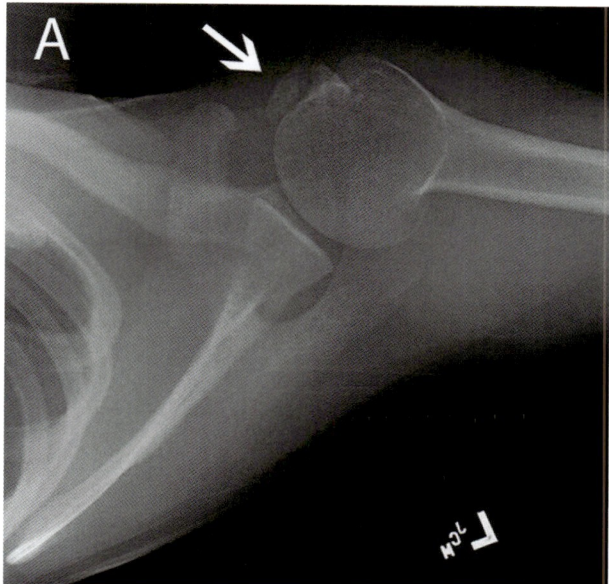

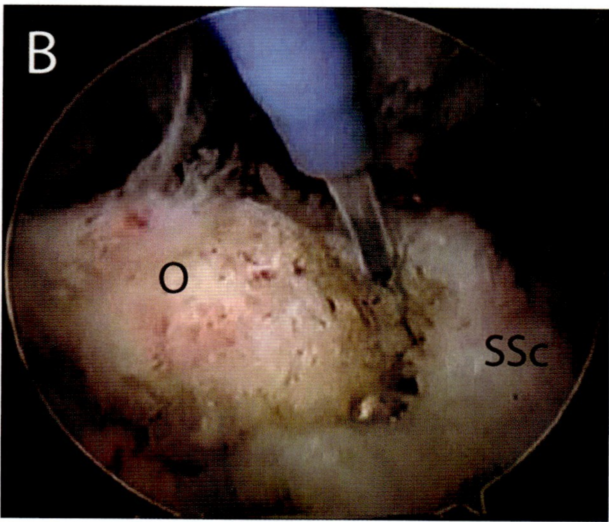

Figure 6.40 Left shoulder demonstrating an ossicle within the subscapularis tendon. **A:** On an axillary radiograph, the ossicle (*white arrow*) can seen within the subscapularis tendon adjacent to the lesser tuberosity. There is also an osteophyte on the lesser tuberosity. **B:** Arthroscopic appearance from a posterior subacromial viewing portal with a 70° arthroscope. The ossicle (O) is shelled out of the subscapularis tendon (SSc) and the tendon is then repaired with sutures anchors.

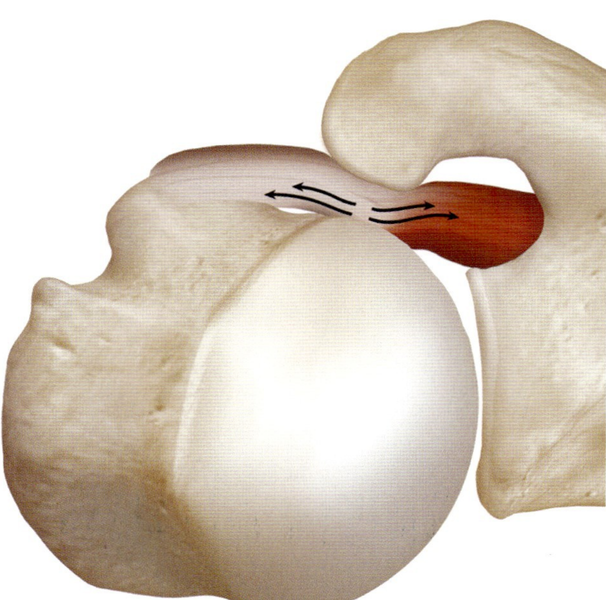

Figure 6.41 Schematic drawing of the roller-wringer effect. In patients with subcoracoid impingement, the prominent coracoid tip indents the superficial surface of the subscapularis tendon. This creates tensile forces on the convex, articular surface of the subscapularis tendon and can lead to failure of the subscapularis fibers (i.e., tensile undersurface fiber failure (TUFF) lesion.)

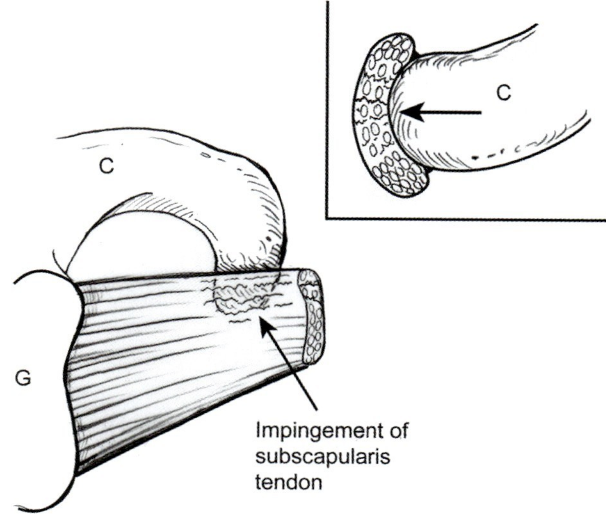

Figure 6.42 Schematic of subcoracoid impingement. Repetitive compression of the subscapularis tendon fibers in the anterior-to-posterior direction by the coracoid tip causes spreading of the fibers in the superior-to-inferior direction, with resultant longitudinal splits between subscapularis tendon fiber bundles. C, coracoid; G, glenoid.

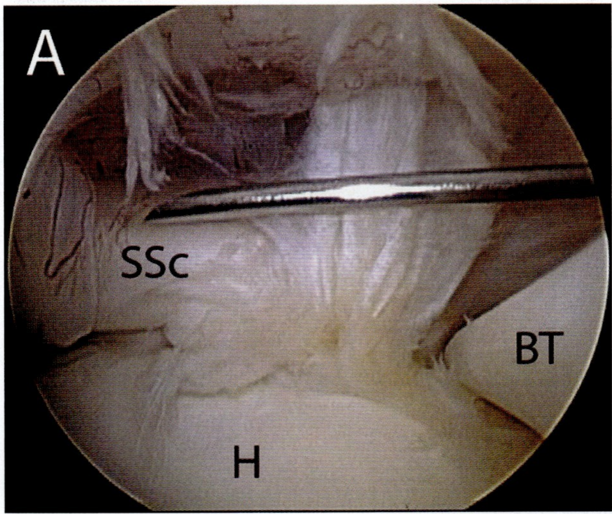

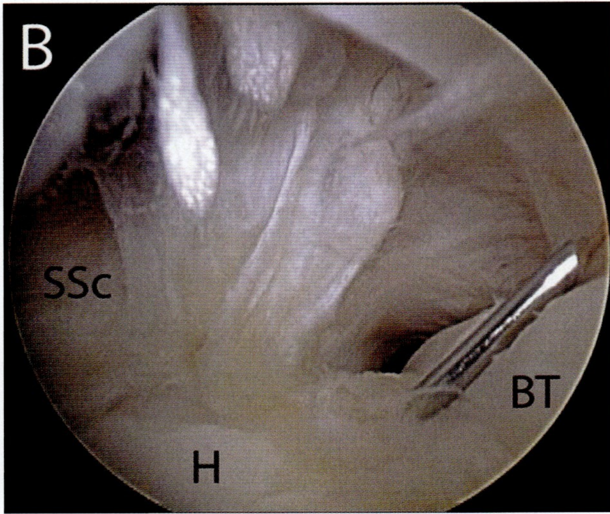

Figure 6.43 Right shoulder, posterior viewing portal demonstrates use of a spinal needle to place an anterosuperolateral portal that allows both **(A)** a proper angle of approach to address the subcoracoid space, as well **(B)** easy access to the bicipital groove in the event that treatment of the biceps tendon is also required. BT, biceps tendon; H, humerus; SSc, subscapularis tendon.

Whenever we observe any pathology of the subscapularis or rotator interval tissue, we feel that an evaluation of the subcoracoid space is essential. This must also include the biceps tendon and medial sling. An anterosuperolateral portal is created appropriately such that it allows a good approach to the upper portion of the lesser tuberosity and the subcoracoid space (Fig. 6.43). While viewing with a 30° arthroscope, a window is created in the rotator interval and the bony prominence of the coracoid tip is located by palpation with an instrument (Figs. 6.44 and 6.45). Once the coracoid tip is located, a 70° arthroscope provides an enhanced view of the coracoid, which is skeletonized with an electrocautery device (Fig. 6.46). The coracohumeral interval is assessed by comparing to the known width of an arthroscopic instrument (Fig. 6.47A)

Internal and external rotation of the arm can also be helpful as sometimes the impingement worsens with these maneuvers. If subcoracoid impingement is encountered, a burr is used to remove the tip of the coracoid until there is a 7-mm space between the subscapularis and the coracoid (Fig. 6.47B). After the coracoplasty is completed, cautery is used to diminish bone bleeding from the cut coracoid.

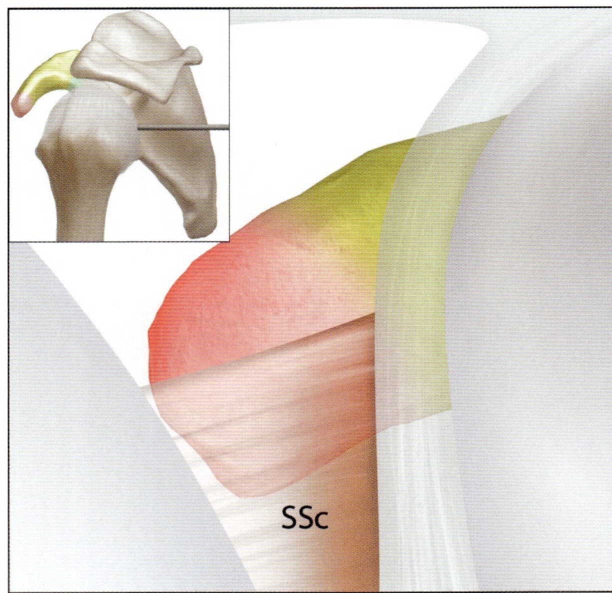

Figure 6.44 When viewing from a posterior glenohumeral portal, the coracoid tip (colored in *red*) can be identified anterior to the upper subscapularis tendon. The inset demonstrates the view from the posterior glenohumeral viewing portal. SSc, subscapularis tendon.

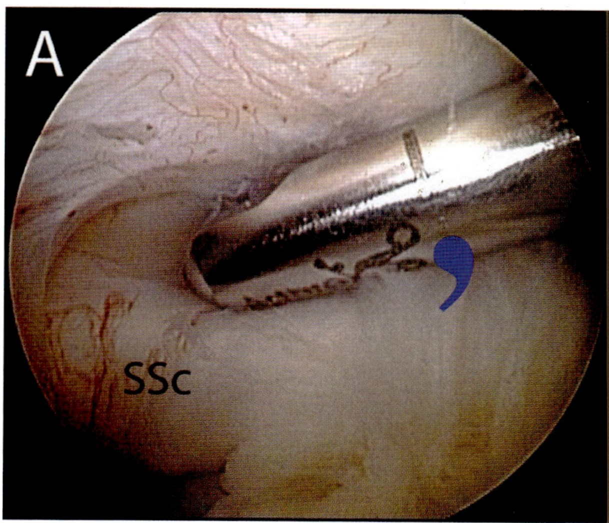

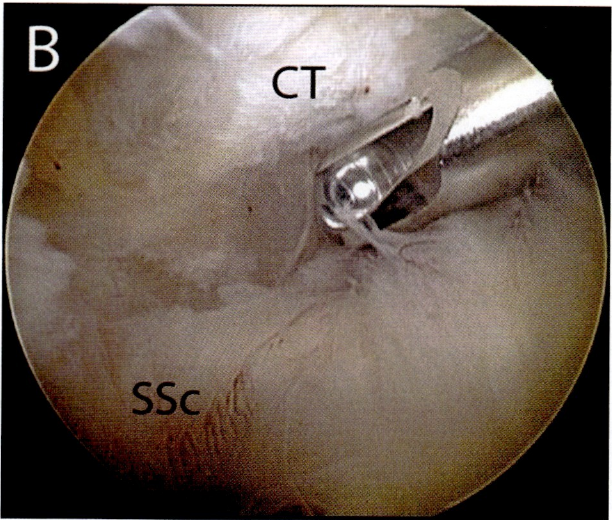

Figure 6.45 Right shoulder, posterior viewing portal. **A:** A shaver is used to make a window in the rotator interval medial to the comma tissue. **B:** The coracoid tip is located by palpation with the shaver. CT, coracoid tip; SSc, subscapularis tendon; blue comma symbol, comma sign.

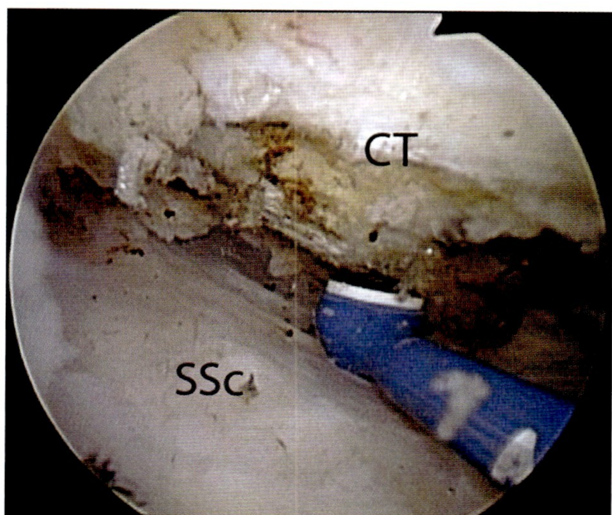

Figure 6.46 Right shoulder, posterior viewing portal with a 70° arthroscope demonstrates skeletonization of the coracoid tip with an electrocautery device. CT, coracoid tip; SSc, subscapularis tendon.

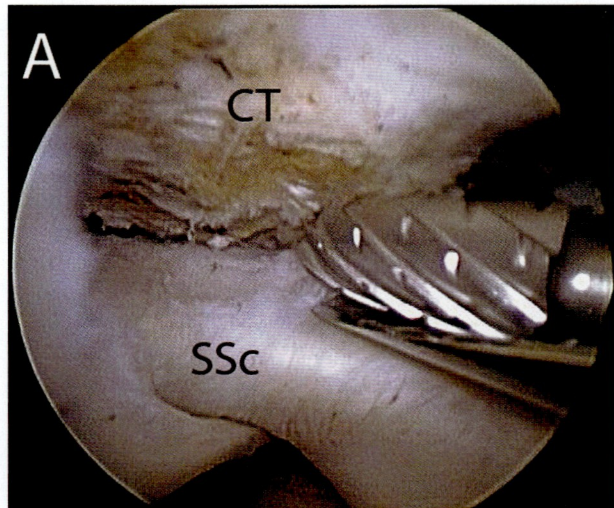

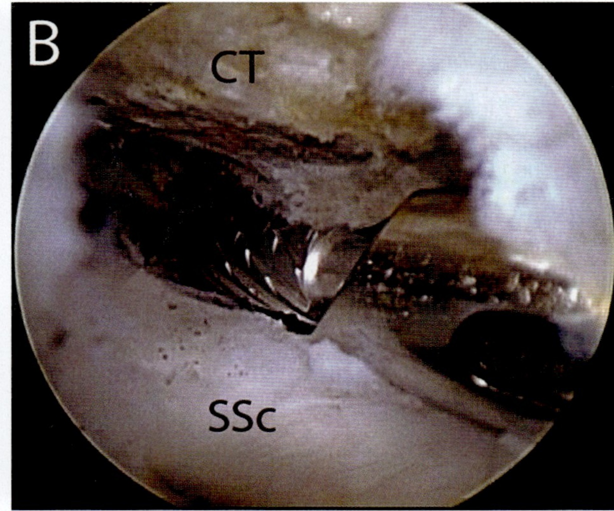

Figure 6.47 Evaluation of the coracohumeral interval in a right shoulder, viewed from a posterior glenohumeral portal with a 70° arthroscope. **A:** The native coracohumeral interval is estimated by comparison to the known width of an instrument. In this case, the width of the interval is less than that of a 5-mm burr. **B:** A coracoplasty has been performed to create a coracohumeral interval of at least 7 mm. CT, coracoid tip; SSc, subscapularis tendon.

Typically subcoracoid stenosis is found in patients with anterior shoulder pathology such as an upper subscapularis tear. However, occasionally in a patient with anterior shoulder pain, no obvious initial pathology is encountered during diagnostic arthroscopy. In this situation, it is particularly important to evaluate for subcoracoid stenosis. Failure to evaluate the coracohumeral interval for possible subcoracoid stenosis in this situation is to overlook a readily treatable pathology.

REFERENCES

1. Burkhart SS, Barth JR, Richards DP, et al. Arthroscopic repair of massive rotator cuff tears with stage 3 and 4 fatty degeneration. *Arthroscopy*. 2007;23:347–354.
2. Lo IK, Burkhart SS. The etiology and assessment of subscapularis tendon tears: a case for subcoracoid impingement, the roller-wringer effect, and TUFF lesions of the subscapularis. *Arthroscopy*. 2003;19:1142–1150.

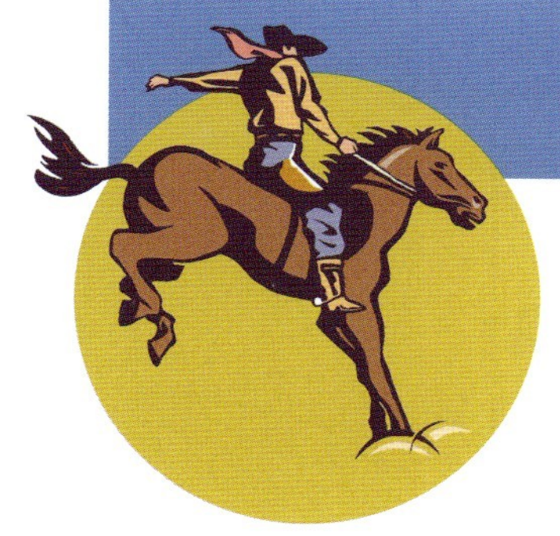

7

Large and Massive Rotator Cuff Tears

WESTERN WISDOM

A man don't get thirsty till he can't get water.

BIOMECHANICS OF LARGE AND MASSIVE ROTATOR CUFF TEARS

The goal of arthroscopic rotator cuff repair is to anatomically repair the rotator cuff with a biomechanically sound construct while respecting the biology of the tissues. While historically these principles have largely been adhered to, in some instances heroic measures have been undertaken to "close the defect." These have included large tendon transfers (e.g., subscapularis tendon transfer, latissimus dorsi transfer), allograft or autograft transplantations (e.g., fascia lata), and aggressive slides and elevations (e.g., supraspinatus slide). Although in rare cases these procedures may provide some benefit, in many instances a biomechanically sound repair without complete closure of the defect may suffice, that is, a partial rotator cuff repair.

The major function of the rotator cuff is to compress and depress the humeral head into the glenoid to provide a stable fulcrum of glenohumeral motion. For this to occur, the rotator cuff must be balanced in the transverse (axial) and sagittal planes (Fig. 7.1). With a stable fulcrum of glenohumeral motion, the major muscle movers of the shoulder (i.e., deltoid, pectoralis major, latissimus dorsi) can exert their moments about the shoulder, providing global functional motion.

With a significant rotator cuff tear, the transverse and/or sagittal plane force couples are no longer balanced, resulting in an unstable fulcrum of motion and painful dysfunction of the shoulder (Fig. 7.2). However, not all rotator cuff tears will result in an unstable fulcrum of motion with pain and disability. In fact, many tears, particularly those in the avascular crescent region of the rotator cuff (i.e., supraspinatus tendon and anterior half of the infraspinatus tendon), may be minimally symptomatic with relatively preserved strength. This is due to the ability of the torn rotator cuff to transmit a distributed load to the humeral head by utilizing the cable region of the rotator cuff, an anatomic thickening of the rotator cuff.

The rotator cable is an anatomic thickening of collagen fibers within the rotator cuff, seen best arthroscopically (Fig. 7.3) and is formed anatomically by an extension of the coracohumeral ligament. This cable extends from a bifurcated insertion on both sides of the long head of the biceps tendon and continues posteriorly to the inferior margin of the infraspinatus (Fig. 7.4). Enclosed within the arc of the rotator cable is the classical crescent region of the rotator cuff, the area where the majority of rotator cuff tears begin. When a rotator cuff tear occurs in this region, the muscle may still exert its force on the humeral head through the rotator cable in much the same way that a suspension bridge exerts its force through a distributed load from its cable to its columns (Fig. 7.5). Because of this preserved function, most tears that are contained within the rotator cable region will still have a stable fulcrum of motion, preserved clinical motion, and minimal strength deficit on manual muscle testing.

In contrast, tears that extend through the rotator cable attachments usually will result in an unstable fulcrum, loss

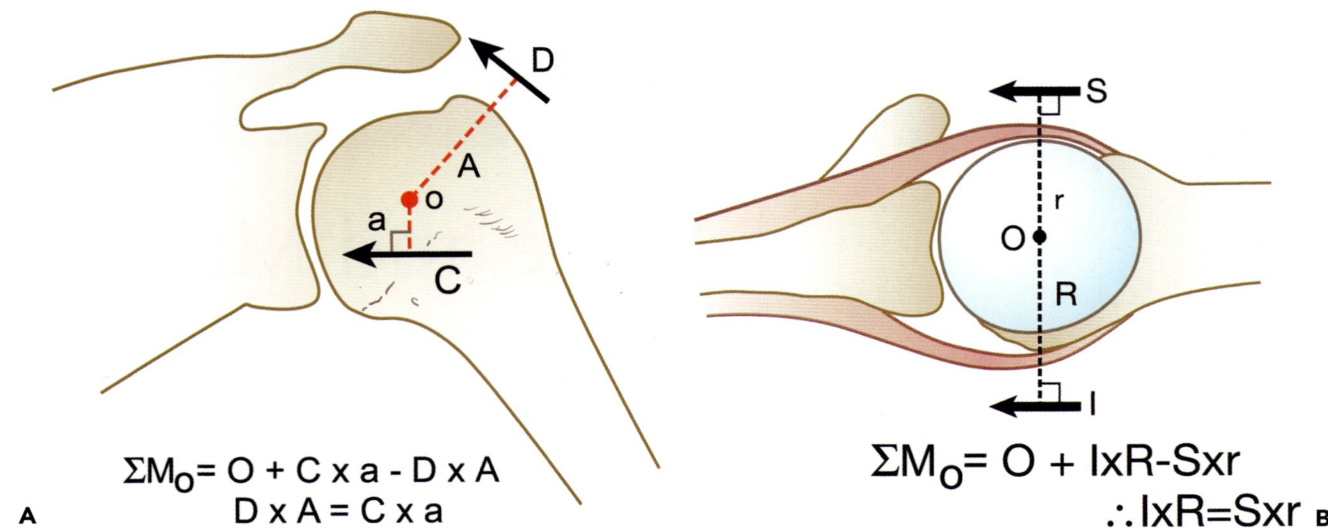

Figure 7.1 Balanced force couples are required to maintain the normal glenohumeral relationship. **A:** In the coronal plane, the combined inferior rotator cuff force (*C*) is balanced against the deltoid (*D*). **B:** In the transverse plane, the subscapularis (*S*) is balanced against the infraspinatus and teres minor (*I*). O, center of rotation; A, moment arm of the deltoid; a, moment arm of the inferior rotator cuff; r, moment arm of the subscapularis; R, moment arm of the infraspinatus and teres minor.

of motion, and significant strength deficit. This clinical picture generally conforms anatomically to tears extending anteriorly into the upper half of the subscapularis tendon or posterior tears that extend through the inferior half of the infraspinatus tendon. This has led to the conventional wisdom that, although single-tendon tears may have preserved function or even be asymptomatic, tears extending into a second tendon are usually poorly tolerated.

The consequence of the cable-crescent architecture in patients with massive rotator cuff tears is that, if a complete repair is not possible, a partial repair focusing on reattachment of the subscapularis and infraspinatus tendons can provide significant clinical improvement due to restoration of the cable attachment, preservation of rotator cuff function, restoration of balanced force couples, and reestablishment of a stable fulcrum of motion. This principle respects the natural anatomy and biomechanical function of the rotator cuff and precludes the natural tendency to simply "close the defect" using the heroic measures as described above.

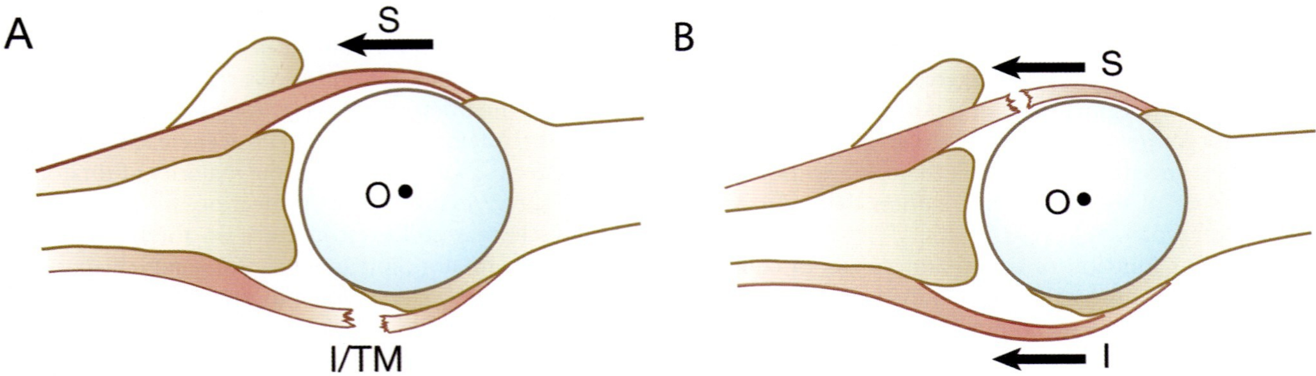

Figure 7.2 **A:** The transverse plane force couple is disrupted because of a massive rotator cuff tear involving the posterior rotator cuff (infraspinatus and teres minor). **B:** An alternative pattern of disruption of the transverse plane force couple. The transverse plane force couple is disrupted by a massive tear involving the anterior rotator cuff (i.e., subscapularis). I, infraspinatus; TM, teres minor; O, center of rotation; S, subscapularis.

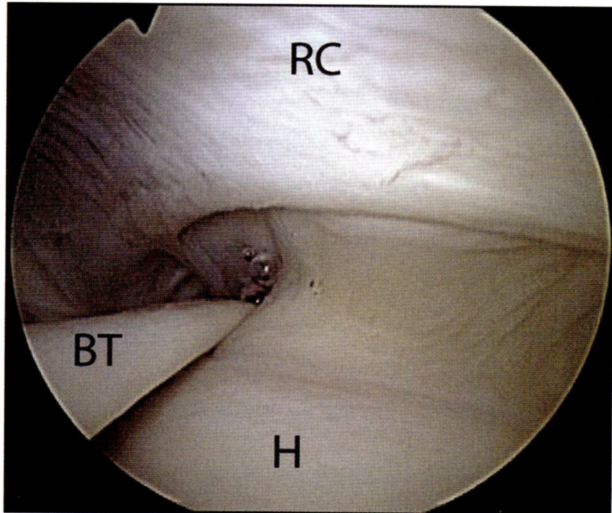

Figure 7.3 Arthroscopic view of a right shoulder demonstrating a cablelike thickening of the capsule surrounding a thinner crescent of tissue that inserts into the greater tuberosity of the humerus. BT, biceps tendon; H, humerus; RC, rotator cuff.

TEAR PATTERNS

Clearly, if a complete rotator cuff repair is possible, this is more desirable than a partial rotator cuff repair. Furthermore, a complete rotator cuff repair that respects the natural mobility of the tear will inherently result in a low-tension, anatomic repair. For this reason, it is critical to exhaustively evaluate the medial-to-lateral and anterior-to-posterior mobility of the tear margins. That is to say, if a tear may be repaired from a medial-to-lateral direction (i.e., crescent-shaped tear) or by an anterior-to-posterior margin convergence technique (i.e., U-shaped, or reverse-L-shaped tears), then it should be performed. A complete anatomic rotator cuff repair will result in restoration of the cable region with resultant improvement in function.

In severe chronic cases, particularly cases in which the margins of the rotator cuff are scarred to the internal deltoid fascia (e.g., massive adhesed immobile rotator cuff tears), there may be no mobility from a medial-to-lateral and an anterior-to-posterior direction. This precludes repair by direct tendon to bone repair or by margin convergence. These cases represent approximately 10% of massive rotator cuff tears and repair in such cases may be attempted using interval slide techniques.

ADVANCED RELEASES FOR THE ROTATOR CUFF

In clinical practice, rotator cuff tears may present with a wide spectrum of size and mobility. Although a tear may be massive in size, the necessity for complex releases is purely dependent on its inherent mobility. Many massive rotator cuff tears may be reparable without releases after proper evaluation of their natural mobility. This natural mobility defines its tear pattern and therefore its repair pattern.

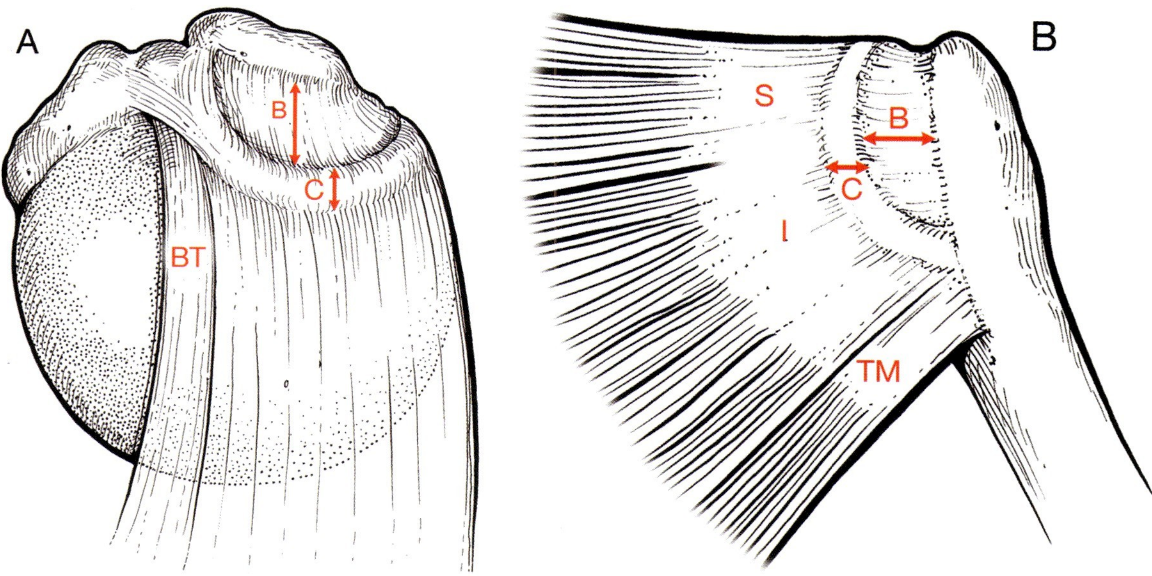

Figure 7.4 Superior (A) and posterior (B) projections of the rotator cable and crescent. The rotator cable extends from the biceps to the inferior margin of infraspinatus, spanning a crescent-shaped area of tendon composed of the supraspinatus and half of the infraspinatus insertions. The cable inserts into the humerus posteriorly at the lower margin of the infraspinatus. C, width of rotator cable; B, mediolateral dimension of rotator crescent; S, supraspinatus; I, infraspinatus; TM, teres minor; BT, biceps tendon.

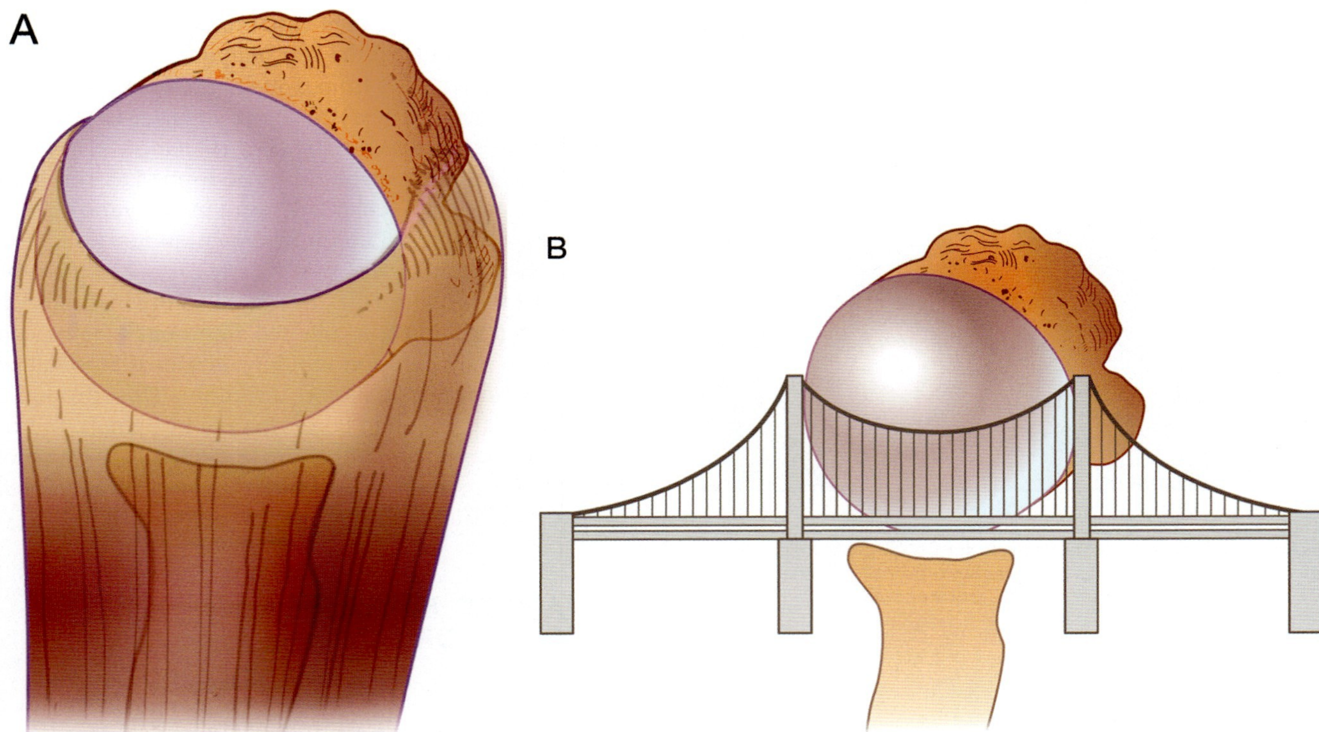

Figure 7.5 A rotator cuff tear (**A**) can be modeled after a suspension bridge. **B:** The free margin corresponds to the cable, and the anterior and posterior attachments of the tear correspond to the supports at each end of the cable's span. A preserved rotator cable can exert a compressive force sufficient to stabilize the humeral head in the setting of a large rotator cuff tear.

In contrast, some small rotator cuff tears may require releases particularly in the presence of concurrent disorders (e.g., adhesive capsulitis or revision surgery). When a tear can be anatomically reduced to the footprint, advanced releases are not required and can unnecessarily increase the complexity of the procedure.

Rotator cuff releases may be divided into bursal-sided releases, articular-sided releases (i.e., capsular releases), and interval slides (see "Bonus Videos," Disc 2). Releases associated with the subscapularis tendon are covered in Chapter 6.

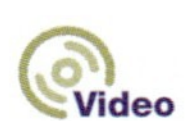

ARTICULAR-SIDED RELEASES—THE CAPSULAR RELEASE

When a rotator cuff tear will not quite reach the bone bed, or is reducible to the bone bed only with significant tension, a capsular release may provide sufficient mobility for tension-free repair to bone. In most scenarios, capsular release is most beneficial in crescent-type tears where the direction of repair is generally from a medial-to-lateral direction. Capsular release generally provides 1 to 1.5 cm of additional mobility.

When performing a capsular release for increasing mobility of the tear margins, one must be cognizant of the proximity of the suprascapular nerve. The suprascapular nerve lies approximately 1.5 to 2.0 cm medial to the glenoid rim and therefore any releases should not be performed more than 1 to 1.5 cm medial to the glenoid rim. By applying traction to the margins of the rotator cuff tear, the rotator cuff and capsule can be lateralized and therefore increase the margin of safety when performing a capsular release.

When performing a capsular release, it is easiest to view through a lateral portal. One or two traction sutures are placed along the margin of the rotator cuff tear using a Scorpion (Arthrex, Inc., Naples, FL) suture passer. The traction stitches are retrieved through lateral stab incisions that are created close to the edge of the acromion. In this fashion when traction is applied, it draws the tendon laterally and superiorly to improve access to the medial capsule. In some cases, a switching stick or grasper may be used to "lift" the rotator cuff away from the glenoid labrum to further maximize visualization.

Using a combination of an elevator and pencil-tip electrocautery, the medial capsule underneath the margin of the rotator cuff and just above the glenoid labrum is carefully incised. It is important to incise the capsule completely until the muscular fibers of the rotator cuff are exposed to ensure maximum tendon excursion. The rotator cuff margin can then be reassessed for mobility. If sufficient mobility is obtained for tendon repair to bone, rotator cuff repair may proceed. However, if inadequate mobility is obtained, then one may proceed with interval slides.

INTERVAL SLIDES

The need for interval slides is based upon the mobility of the rotator cuff tendon margins. Many U-shaped and L-shaped tears, despite their size, have adequate mobility and may be repaired using the principles of margin convergence. Understanding and elucidating tear patterns is one of the most important principles of successful performance of routine arthroscopic rotator cuff repair.

When a tear has been determined to be irreparable despite standard capsular release, proceeding with interval slides to improve mobility should be considered. The decision is based upon patient age, patient symptoms (i.e., pain vs. weakness), tissue quality, and initial tear mobility. Young patients, with a primary complaint of weakness, who have adequate tissue quality and moderate tear mobility, should be strongly considered for interval slides. In contrast, older patients (e.g., age >70), with a primary complaint of pain, who have poor tissue quality, and minimal to no medial-to-lateral mobility may be candidates for a partial repair or for debridement alone. This is particularly relevant when a prolonged rehabilitation program may be poorly tolerated or in patients with >75% fatty atrophy on MRI.

Two slides are relevant to repairs of the posterosuperior rotator cuff: the anterior interval slide and the posterior interval slide. The anterior interval slide is a release of the anterior leading edge of the supraspinatus from the rotator interval and can improve mobility of the rotator cuff by approximately 2 cm. This same release can be accomplished without dividing the tissue adjacent to the anterior leading edge of the subscapularis. This is done by using an elevator to lyse the underlying soft tissue attachments to the coracoid base. This is called an anterior interval slide in-continuity, and we prefer this method when an anterior interval slide is indicated. In contrast, the posterior interval slide is a release of the posterior edge of the supraspinatus from the infraspinatus and can also increase mobility by a further 2 to 4 cm.

When only one release is performed, this is commonly referred to as a single-interval slide, whereas when both releases are performed, this is referred to as a double-interval slide. Although classically the anterior interval slide is performed prior to the posterior interval slide, choosing which slide to perform first and whether a single or a double-interval slide is necessary is based upon the tear mobility. In general, the releases are performed first in the location with the most severe restriction of mobility. If sufficient mobility may be obtained with a single release, this may be advantageous since the residual flaps of rotator cuff are larger and more robust than if a second release is performed. A second release is performed only if insufficient mobility is obtained with the initial release.

If the tendon mobility is equally restricted anteriorly and posteriorly, then the arthroscopist may perform either release first. However, in general, the authors have noted that the posterior interval slide provides more mobility than the anterior interval slide, and importantly improves mobility of both the supraspinatus and infraspinatus. Many times, only a posterior interval slide is required and will provide sufficient mobility for repair of both the supraspinatus and infraspinatus. Furthermore, maintaining the continuity of the leading edge of the supraspinatus to the rotator interval facilitates repair of the anterior rotator cuff.

The keys to expedient and effective use of interval slides are exposing the critical landmarks, utilizing the correct angle of approach, and employing traction stitches appropriately. Standard anterior, posterior, and lateral subacromial portals will have already been established. A posterolateral viewing portal is also created. A complete subacromial bursectomy should be performed. Formal subacromial decompression with release or excision of the coracoacromial ligament is not performed to avoid the risk of iatrogenic anterosuperior escape.

THE BONY LANDMARKS

In doing interval slides, the two key bony landmarks are the scapular spine and the base of the coracoid. The scapular spine is easiest to identify while viewing through the lateral portal. Using a combination of a shaver and cautery through the posterior portal, the undersurface of the acromion is debrided. As the exposure is continued posteriorly and medially, the scapular spine may be identified as a keel-shaped structure, posterior to the acromioclavicular joint (Fig. 7.6). In cases of massive rotator cuff tears, the scapular spine is actually easier to identify than in cases with an intact cuff where the bulk of the rotator cuff

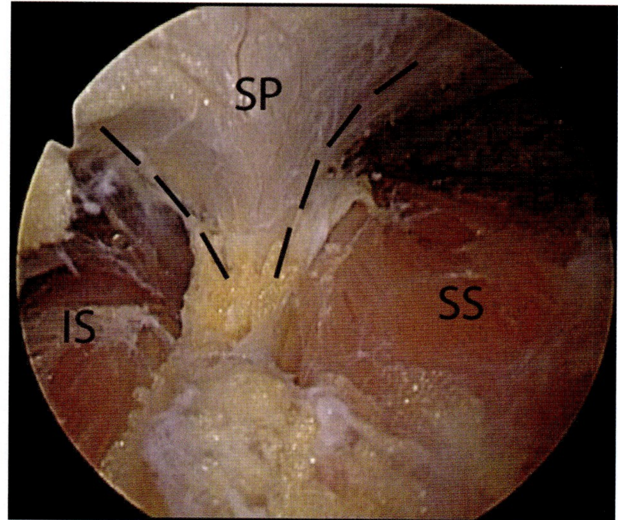

Figure 7.6 Arthroscopic view of the scapular spine in a right shoulder viewed from a lateral portal. The scapular spine (outlined by *dashed black lines*) defines the margin between the supraspinatus (**right**) and the infraspinatus (**left**). IS, infraspinatus; SP, scapular spine; SS, supraspinatus.

muscle may obscure medial visualization. Exposure of the scapular spine should proceed inferiorly toward the glenoid. Exposure should be carefully performed due to risk of injury to the suprascapular nerve, and should stop upon reaching the tendinous bridge of tissue connecting the infraspinatus and supraspinatus. Exposure of the scapular spine is vital to performing posterior interval slides since this keel-shaped structure delineates the interval between the supraspinatus and infraspinatus tendons.

The second key bony landmark is the coracoid base. It is easiest to identify this landmark while viewing through the lateral portal. Using an accessory lateral portal, a switching stick or similar instrument is used to palpate the coracoid base. The coracoid base can be palpated as a bony prominence just anteromedial to the biceps root. Although one may choose to formally expose the coracoid base, this is usually not required and only its location needs to be identified. The coracoid base is critical to discern the location and direction of the anterior interval slide.

TRACTION STITCHES

Once the bony landmarks have been identified, tractions stitches are placed through the supraspinatus and infraspinatus tendons. Generally speaking, one stitch is placed at the anterior leading edge of the infraspinatus tendon and another stitch is placed in the midpoint to posterior leading edge of the supraspinatus tendon. Traction stitches are critical and should be used routinely. Differential tensioning of the traction stitches can help align the interval to the arthroscopic scissor during release and can spread apart the interval during release to maximize visualization.

While viewing through a posterolateral portal, an antegrade suture-passing instrument is introduced through the lateral portal (e.g., Scorpion) and a #2 FiberWire (Arthrex, Inc., Naples, FL) stitch is placed through the supraspinatus tendon. The supraspinatus traction stitch is then retrieved through an anterior portal. A second traction stitch is similarly placed through the infraspinatus tendon (Fig. 7.7). As an alternative to an antegrade pass, a retrograde suture-passing instrument (e.g., Penetrator; Arthrex, Naples, FL) can be used. The Penetrator is preloaded with a traction stitch (usually of a different color (e.g., #2 TigerWire; Arthrex, Inc., Naples, FL). The Penetrator is first used to pass a suture loop through the infraspinatus tendon. The Penetrator is then carefully retracted back out of the infraspinatus tendon leaving the suture loop in situ. The suture loop can then be retrieved by the Penetrator, completing passage and retrieval of the traction stitch.

POSTERIOR INTERVAL SLIDE

It is easiest to perform the posterior interval slide while viewing through a lateral or posterolateral subacromial portal. The traction stitches are retrieved through corresponding portals to spread the posterior interval apart—the supraspinatus traction stitch through an anterior or anterolateral portal and the infraspinatus traction stitch through a posterior or posterolateral portal (Fig. 7.8).

A spinal needle is used to identify the correct angle of approach in line with the posterior interval and toward the spine of the scapula. An arthroscopic scissor is then introduced through the accessory portal and begins the

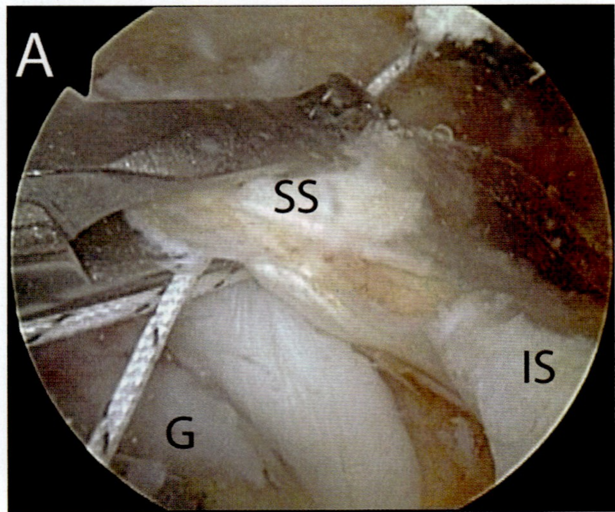

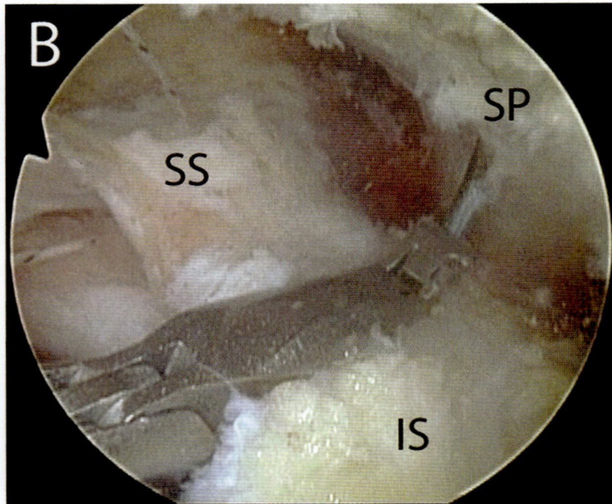

Figure 7.7 Arthroscopic view of a left shoulder viewed from a lateral portal demonstrating **(A)** placement of a traction stitch in the supraspinatus, and **(B)** placement of a traction stitch in the infraspinatus. G, glenoid; IS, infraspinatus tendon; SP, scapular spine; SS, supraspinatus tendon.

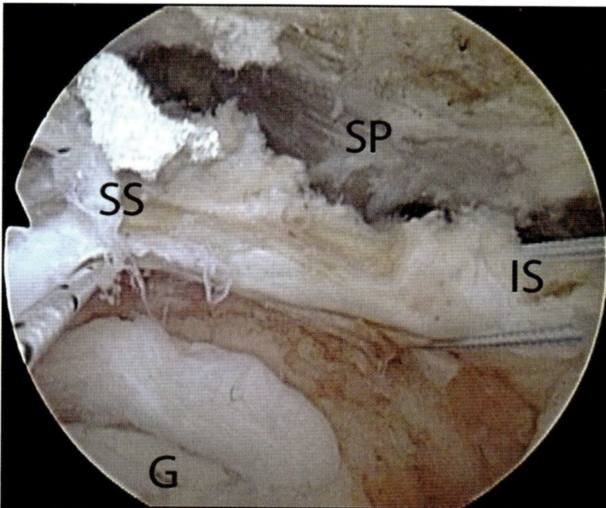

Figure 7.8 Arthroscopic view of a left shoulder viewed from a lateral portal showing traction sutures placed in preparation for a posterior interval slide. G, glenoid; IS, infraspinatus tendon; SP, scapular spine; SS, supraspinatus tendon.

posterior interval slide along the lateral margin of the rotator cuff tendon directing the incision toward the base of the scapular spine. By using a combination of straight or curved arthroscopic scissors, the release is continued toward the base of the scapular spine (Fig. 7.9A). Instead of an accessory working portal, one may view through a posterolateral portal and use the scissors through a lateral portal, or vice versa. When performing the slide, it is critical to place traction on both the anterior supraspinatus tendon stitch and the posterior infraspinatus tendon stitch to spread the tissues apart as the release progresses, facilitating release and maximizing visualization of the apex of the release. Furthermore, differential tensioning of the traction stitches can help position the interval in line with the arthroscopic scissors.

When performing the release, it is important to incise the tissue full thickness as it can sometimes appear as though there are two separate layers. Failure to do so will result in an incomplete release and insufficient mobility. The release is continued toward the scapular spine until the fat pad lateral to the bony spine is encountered. This fat pad heralds the proximity of the suprascapular nerve (Fig. 7.9B). Once the posterior interval release is completed, care is taken to ensure that the capsular release underlying the infraspinatus and supraspinatus is also complete and connected to the posterior interval release.

The supraspinatus and infraspinatus tendons are then assessed for mobility (Fig. 7.10A–C). Usually with an isolated posterior interval slide, mobility of the infraspinatus tendon is sufficient for tendon repair to bone. If there is also sufficient mobility for supraspinatus tendon repair to bone, then an anterior interval slide is avoided to maintain the anterosuperior rotator cuff as a single sleeve facilitating repair (Fig. 7.10D). In more severe cases, however, where mobility is insufficient, an anterior interval slide may be required for mobilization of the supraspinatus tendon as well. After repair of the tendon to bone, the separation between the supraspinatus and infraspinatus is closed with margin convergence sutures (Fig. 7.10E).

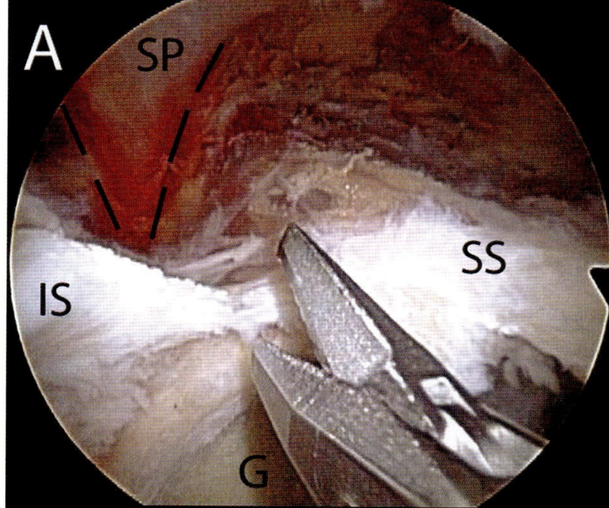

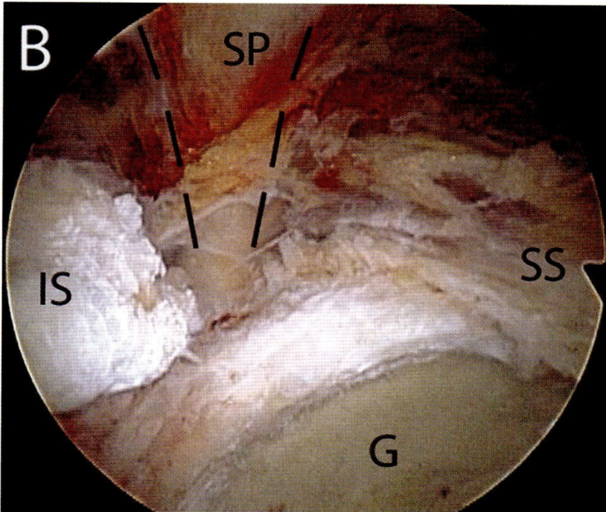

Figure 7.9 **A:** Arthroscopic view of a right shoulder viewed from a posterolateral portal demonstrating a posterior interval slide performed with arthroscopic scissors. **B:** The interval slide is completed when the supraspinatus and infraspinatus are completely separated and the perineural fatty tissue at the base of the scapular spine (outlined by *dashed black lines*) is visualized. G, glenoid; IS, infraspinatus tendon; SP, scapular spine; SS, supraspinatus tendon.

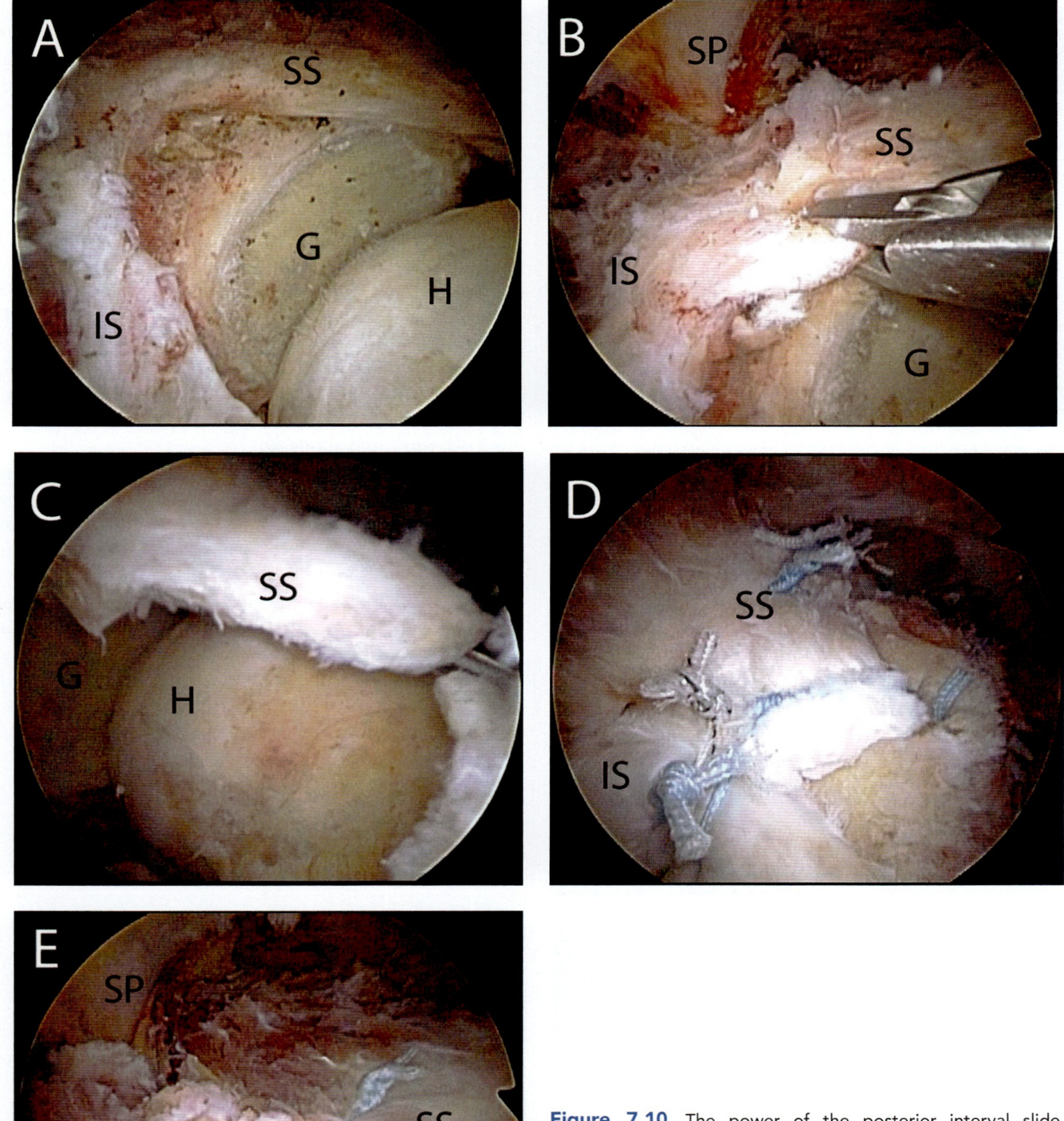

Figure 7.10 The power of the posterior interval slide. **A:** Right shoulder viewed with a 70° arthroscope from a posterior portal demonstrates a massive rotator cuff tear retracted medially beyond the glenoid rim. **B:** Initial assessment shows limited mobility. **C:** Following a posterior interval slide (Fig. 7.9), the mobility of the supraspinatus is dramatically increased and can now reach the greater tuberosity bone bed. **D:** Final repair shows the rotator cuff secured to the greater tuberosity. **E:** The separation created by the posterior interval slide has been closed with margin convergence sutures. G, glenoid; H, humerus; IS, infraspinatus tendon; SP, scapular spine; SS, supraspinatus tendon.

ANTERIOR INTERVAL SLIDE

When performing the anterior interval slide, it is easiest to perform the release while viewing through a lateral or posterolateral subacromial portal. The anterior supraspinatus traction stitch is retrieved through the posterior portal to again assist in visualizing the tear apex and positioning the anterior interval. A traction stitch through the rotator interval or subscapularis tendon is not required since these tissues are either intact or have been previously repaired.

The release is performed along the leading edge of the supraspinatus tendon toward the coracoid base, separating the tendon from the rotator interval and subscapularis (Fig. 7.11). The location of the coracoid is again confirmed by palpation using a switching stitch and a spinal needle is used to locate the correct angle of approach in line with the anterior interval. In many instances, the same two lateral

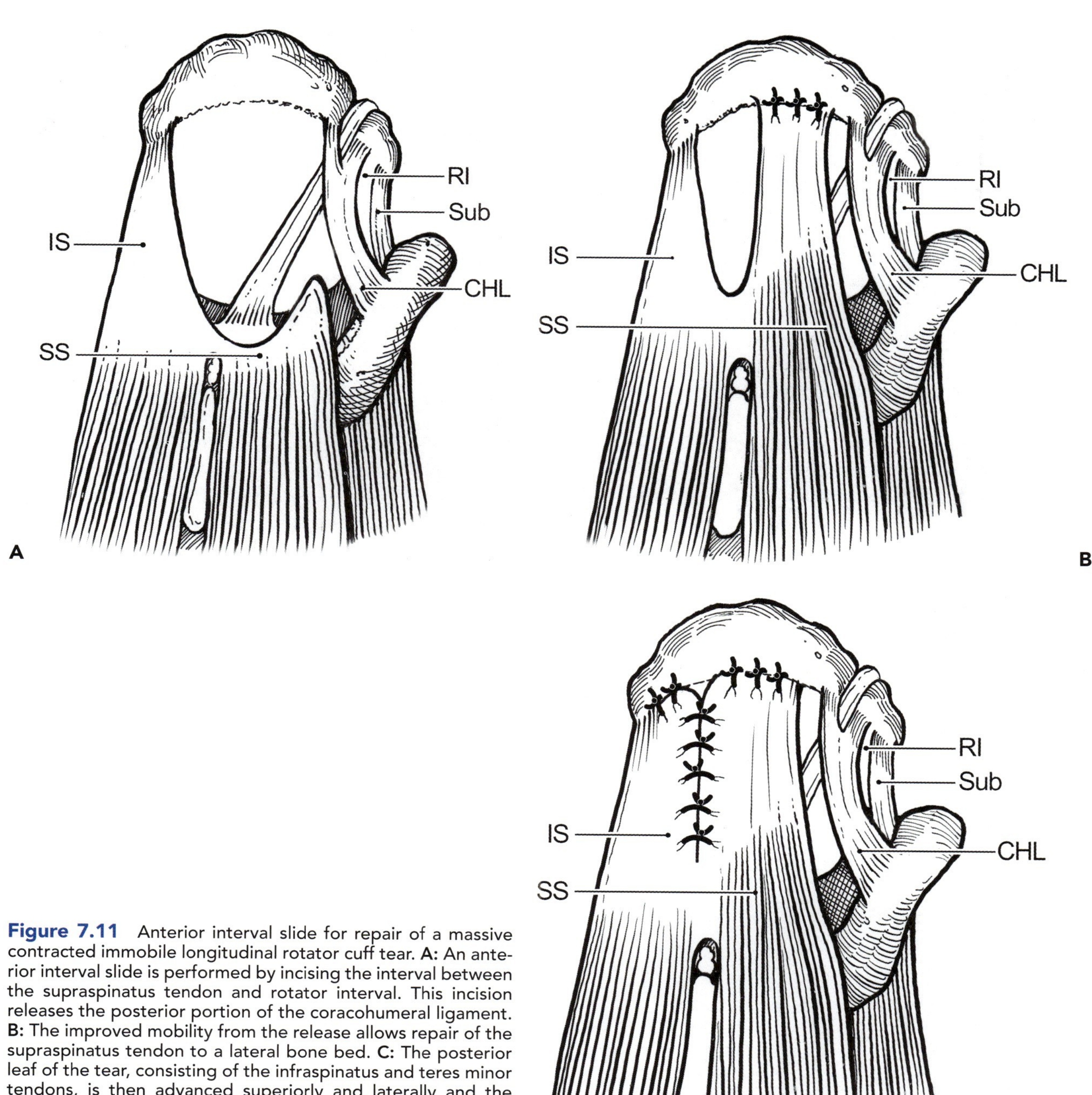

Figure 7.11 Anterior interval slide for repair of a massive contracted immobile longitudinal rotator cuff tear. **A:** An anterior interval slide is performed by incising the interval between the supraspinatus tendon and rotator interval. This incision releases the posterior portion of the coracohumeral ligament. **B:** The improved mobility from the release allows repair of the supraspinatus tendon to a lateral bone bed. **C:** The posterior leaf of the tear, consisting of the infraspinatus and teres minor tendons, is then advanced superiorly and laterally and the residual longitudinal defect is closed by side-to-side sutures. CHL, coracohumeral ligament; IS, infraspinatus; RI, rotator interval; SS, supraipnatus; Sub, subscapularis.

portals may be utilized (that were used during the posterior interval slide) and the arthroscope is simply switched to the more posterior lateral portal and the arthroscopic scissors are used through the more anterior lateral portal. However, we do not hesitate to establish another portal if required.

Similar to the posterior interval slide, the anterior interval slide is begun at the margin of the rotator cuff tendon and proceeds toward the bony landmark—in this case, the base of the coracoid. The traction stitch is used posteriorly to distract and improve visualization of the apex and position the anterior interval in line with the arthroscopic scissors. The release is completed when the fat pad medial to the coracoid base is encountered and the coracoid is palpated. Care is taken to ensure that the slide is performed lateral to the coracoid base to avoid injury to the suprascapular nerve.

This anterior interval slide can also be performed without incising the interval tissue (see next section on Anterior Interval Slide in Continuity). This is currently our preferred technique, as it avoids the floppiness of a supraspinatus tendon that has been released on both sides. The one situation in which we will perform a traditional anterior interval slide is when, after a posterior interval slide and an anterior interval slide in continuity, the anterolateral margin of the supraspinatus tendon does not quite reach the bone bed and it is felt that with additional mobility a complete repair will be possible. Once the slide is complete, the capsule underlying the supraspinatus tendon is reevaluated to ensure a complete release has been performed. The supraspinatus tendon is then evaluated for its mobility and reparability.

THE ANTERIOR INTERVAL SLIDE IN CONTINUITY

In patients with combined tears of the subscapularis tendon and supraspinatus tendon (+/− infraspinatus tendon), an interval slide in continuity is preferable to the complete anterior interval slide. By releasing the soft tissues at the base of the coracoid, the coracohumeral ligament is released. It is this ligament that restricts the excursion of a medially retracted supraspinatus tendon. In contrast to a standard anterior interval slide, the interval slide in continuity maintains the connection laterally between the subscapularis and supraspinatus tendon, which simplifies repair of the anterosuperior rotator cuff (Fig. 7.12)

In patients with combined tears of the subscapularis tendon and the supraspinatus tendon, it is important to first address the anterior structures (i.e., subscapularis, biceps, coracoid) prior to proceeding with supraspinatus tendon repair (see Chapter 6, "Subscapularis Tendon Tears" for a complete discussion). It may be necessary to tag and release the long head of the biceps tendon prior to performing the interval slide in continuity.

To perform the interval slide in continuity, it is easiest to view through a posterior glenohumeral portal. An anterosuperolateral portal is established, the comma sign is identified, and a traction stitch is placed in the superolateral corner of the subscapularis tendon if the subscapularis is torn and retracted; if the subscapularis is not torn the following steps are still performed with the only differences being that a traction stitch is not necessary and a posterior release of the subscapularis is not required (Fig. 7.13). The subscapularis tendon is then placed under traction,

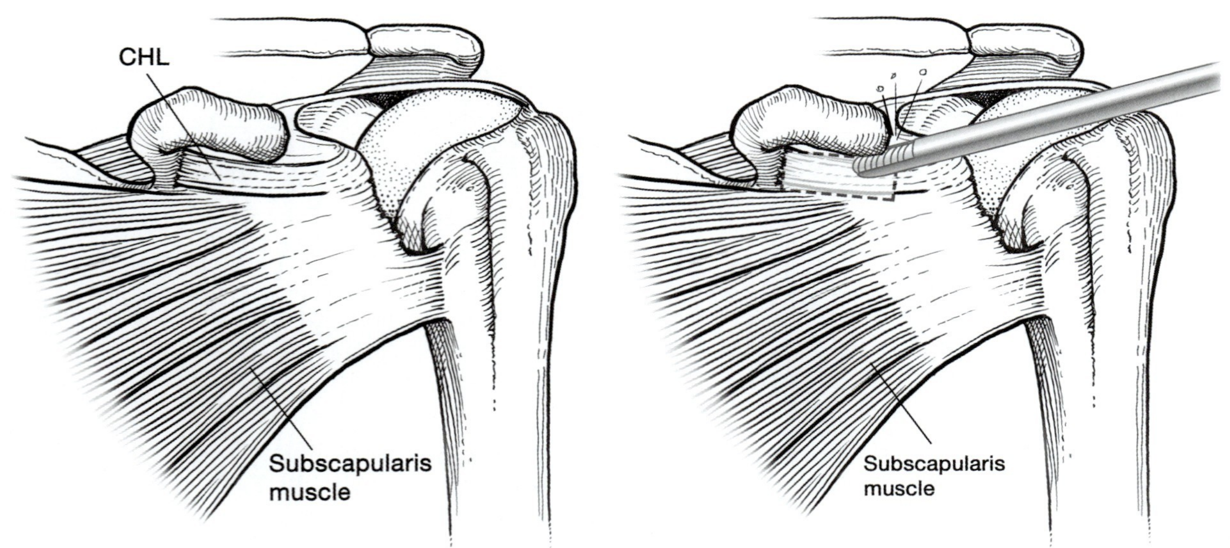

Figure 7.12 Anterior interval slide in continuity. **A:** An anterosuperior rotator cuff tear involving 50% of the subscapularis tendon and a massive tear of the supraspinatus and infraspinatus tendons. **B:** A coracoplasty is performed. The *dotted box* outlines the proposed area for resection of a portion of the rotator interval for the interval slide in continuity.

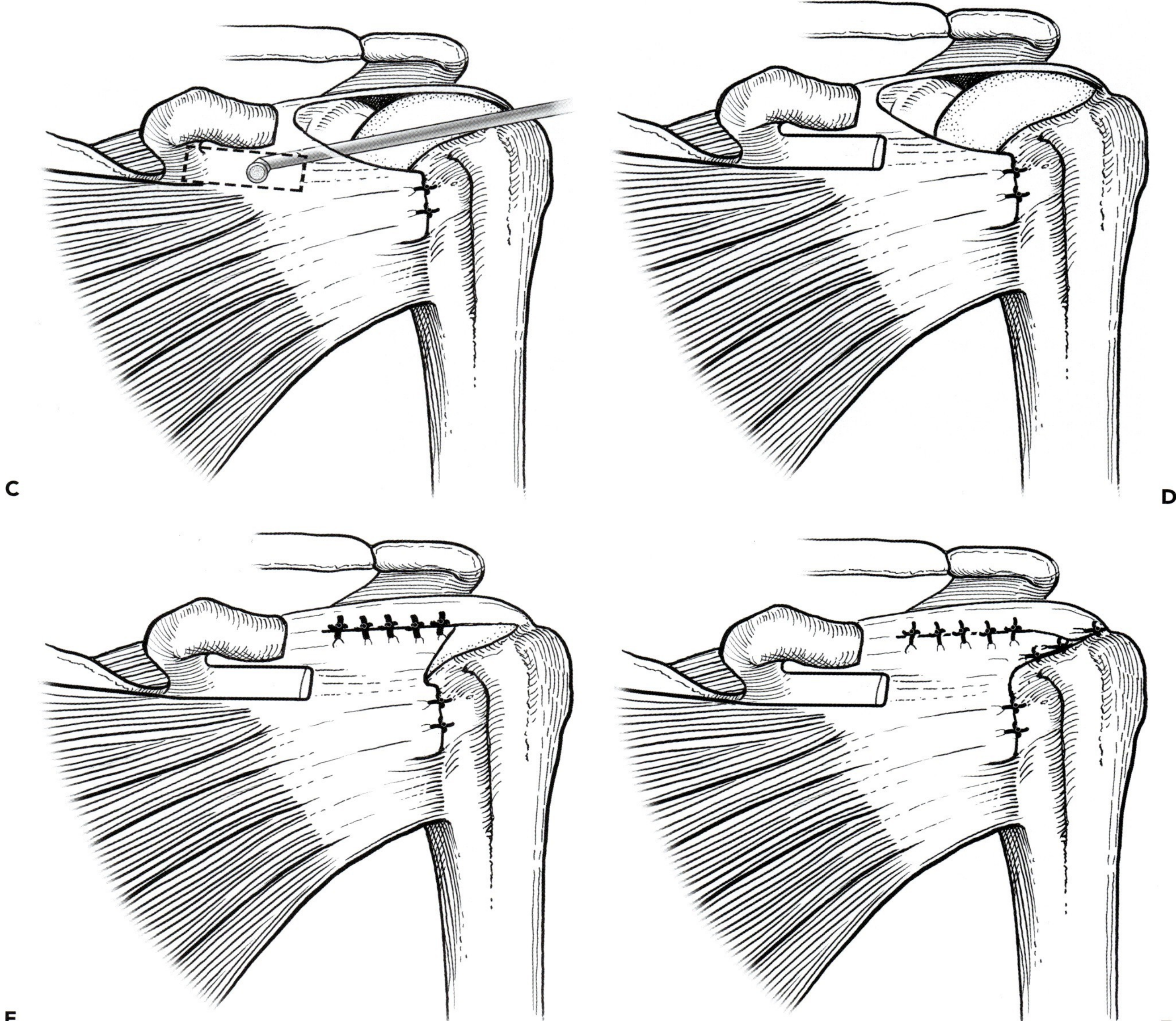

Figure 7.12 *(Continued)* **C:** An interval slide in continuity is performed by first exposing the posterolateral aspect of the coracoid all the way to the coracoid neck, releasing any adhesions between the subscapularis tendon and the inferolateral coracoid. Then, the medial rotator interval tissue is excised, creating a "window" through the rotator interval, partially releasing and excising the coracohumeral ligament. Care is taken to ensure that the lateral margin of the rotator interval remains intact, maintaining the continuity between the subscapularis and the supraspinatus tendons. Then, soft tissues are debrided and released from the posterolateral base of the coracoid while viewing through the "window" with a 70° arthroscope. This completes the release of the coracohumeral ligament without creating separate tissue flaps. **D:** Following an interval slide in-continuity, mobility of the subscapularis tendon is improved. The subscapularis tear can now be repaired to bone, leaving a U-shaped posterosuperior rotator cuff tear to be repaired. **E:** The residual U-shaped posterosuperior rotator cuff tear is repaired with side-to-side sutures using the principle of margin convergence. **F:** The converged margin is then repaired to bone in a tension-free manner. *CHL*, coracohumeral ligament.

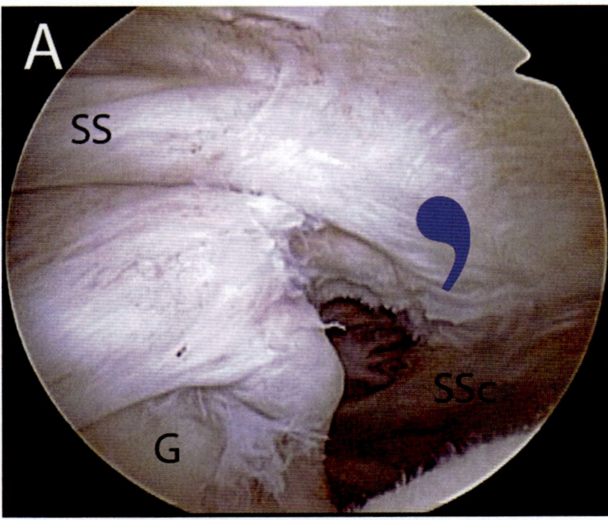

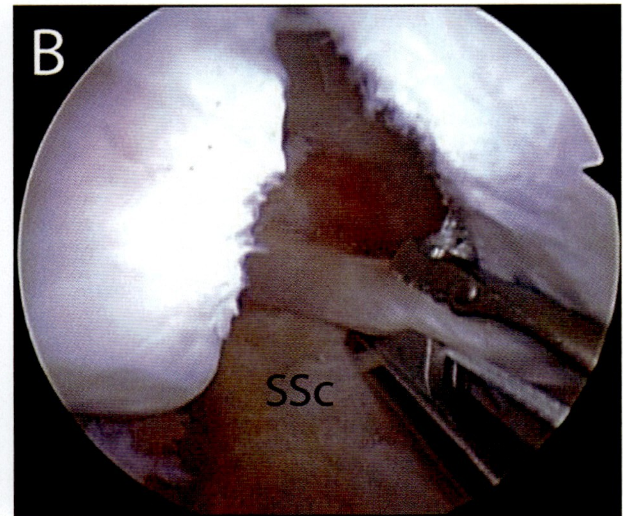

Figure 7.13 Right shoulder, posterior viewing portal demonstrates a massive contracted rotator cuff tear. **A:** The comma sign, which leads to the superolateral border of the subscapularis tendon, is identified. **B:** A traction stitch is placed in the upper subscapularis tendon. G, glenoid; SS, supraspinatus tendon; SSc, subscapularis tendon; blue comma symbol, comma sign.

drawing the subscapularis tendon and rotator interval out from behind the glenoid neck. Starting just above the upper subscapularis tendon border, the rotator interval is then excised using a combination of a shaver and electrocautery (Fig. 7.14A, B). As the dissection proceeds, the hard bony prominence of the coracoid tip can be felt through the rotator interval.

When performing this release, it is important to maintain the integrity of the lateral rotator interval (i.e., the comma sign) that maintains the connection laterally between the subscapularis tendon and supraspinatus tendon. The excision of the rotator interval continues until the coracoid tip and base are exposed (Fig. 7.14C). The posterolateral aspect of the coracoid is then skeletonized using a combination of electrocautery and an elevator to maximize excursion by releasing the coracohumeral ligament. With the interval slide in continuity completed, excursion of both the subscapularis tendon and supraspinatus tendon should be improved.

Next, the arthroscopist should proceed with further release of the subscapularis tendon posteriorly (between the glenoid neck and subscapularis tendon) to maximize subscapularis tendon excursion. The repair of the subscapularis tendon proceeds prior to repair of the supraspinatus tendon.

Once the subscapularis tendon is repaired, supraspinatus tendon mobility is reassessed. If insufficient mobility is obtained, the arthroscopist may proceed with capsular release or a posterior interval slide. In rare cases, if insufficient mobility of the supraspinatus tendon is obtained despite capsular release and posterior interval slide, the anterior interval slide may be completed (i.e., incision of the comma sign) and may provide modest mobility improvement.

BURSAL-SIDED RELEASES: EXCAVATION OF THE ROTATOR CUFF

In some patients, the rotator cuff may become adhesed and scarred to the undersurface of the acromion and internal deltoid fascia. This is particularly relevant in massive recurrent tears of the rotator cuff and some massive tears in association with adhesive capsulitis. In these patients, the margins of the rotator cuff become obscured and scarred to the undersurface of the acromion and internal deltoid fascia, and on initial diagnostic arthroscopy it may first appear as though there is no rotator cuff to repair (Fig. 7.15).

In this scenario, it is important to initially enter the subacromial space through a lateral portal. While viewing through a posterior glenohumeral portal, a standard lateral subacromial portal is created. The arthroscope is then introduced through the lateral subacromial portal and a diagnostic arthroscopy is again performed. Usually again, the margins of the rotator cuff are obscured and scarred to the undersurface of the acromion. To begin delineating the margins of the rotator cuff, a shaver or an electrocautery device is introduced through the posterior portal in the interval between the rotator cuff and undersurface of the acromion. To perform this, the instrument is passed through the skin and deltoid, and the posterior acromion is palpated with the tip of the instrument. The instrument is then "blindly" passed just deep to the undersurface of

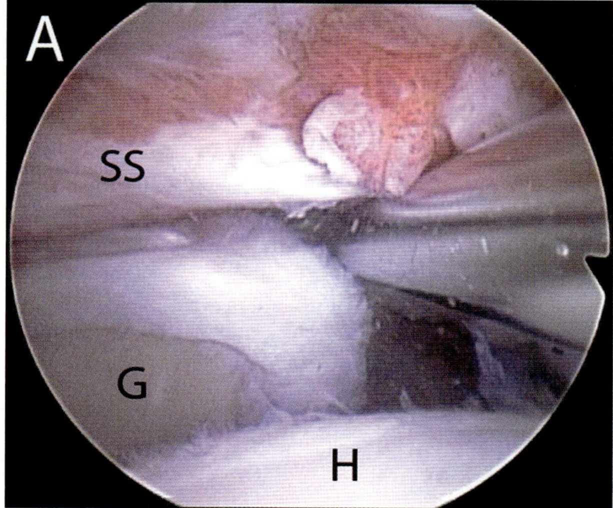

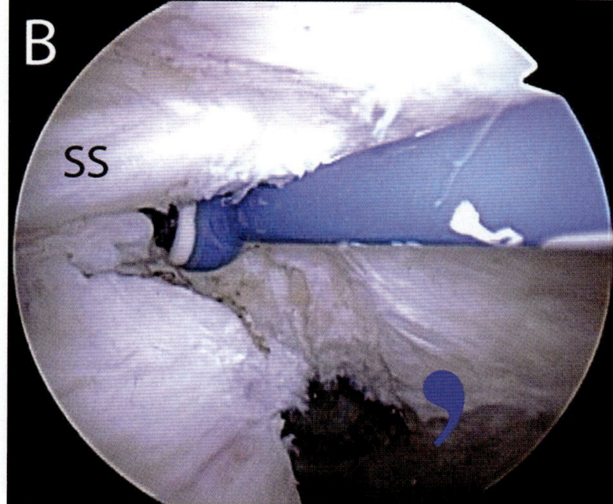

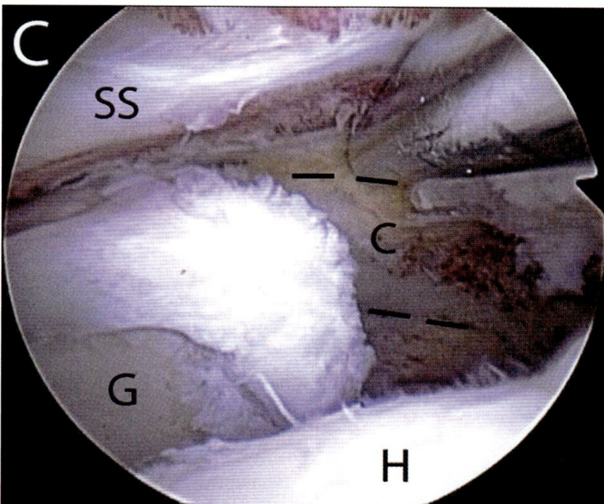

Figure 7.14 Right shoulder, posterior viewing portal demonstrating an anterior interval slide in continuity. **A:** After identifying the comma sign and placing a traction stitch (Fig. 7.13), a window is created in the rotator interval with a shaver. **B:** The rotator interval tissue is excised and dissection is carried medially, excising the coracohumeral ligament, until **(C)** the base of the coracoid (out lined by *dashed black lines*) is palpated or seen. C, coracoid; G, glenoid; H, humerus; SS, supraspinatus tendon; SSc, subscapularis tendon; blue comma symbol, comma sign.

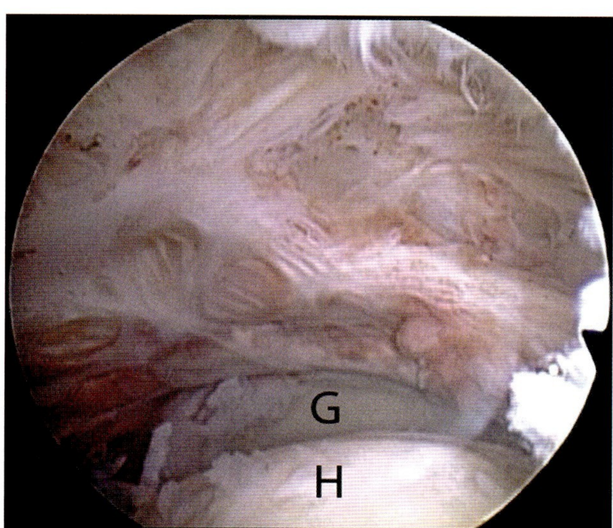

Figure 7.15 Right shoulder, lateral subacromial viewing portal demonstrating a massive contracted rotator cuff tear that is adhesed to the undersurface of the acromion. G, glenoid; H, humerus.

the acromion and medial enough to "bounce off" the scapular spine and remain just lateral to the scapular spine. It is then pushed anterolaterally so that it can be seen as a bulge under the overlying soft tissue of the acromion. Using the electrocautery device or shaver, the soft tissue is then carefully dissected off the undersurface of the acromion starting medially just posterior to the acromioclavicular joint and working laterally and posteriorly toward the arthroscope (Fig. 7.16).

As the dissection proceeds laterally, the rotator cuff (with an extended bursal leader) is lifted away from the undersurface of the deltoid and inner deltoid fascia. Eventually, as the lateral dissection continues, the instrument will exit through the bursal leader and the lateral border of the "rotator cuff" is established. The instrument can now be visualized and the dissection is completed. With the rotator cuff now dissected off the undersurface of the acromion, the margins now must be delineated. Usually, the rotator cuff margins are still obscured due to a large bursal leader.

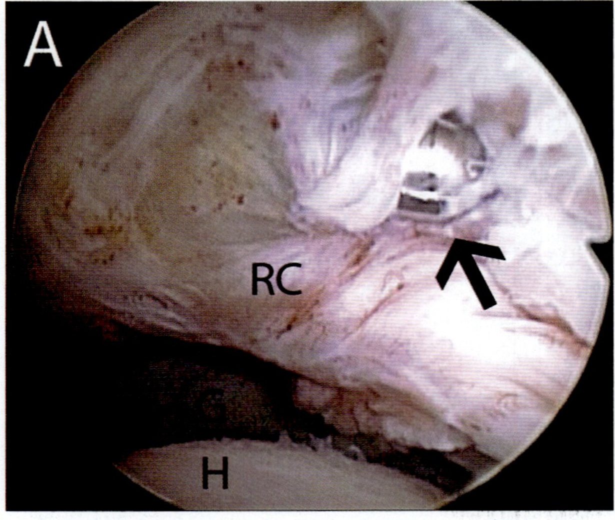

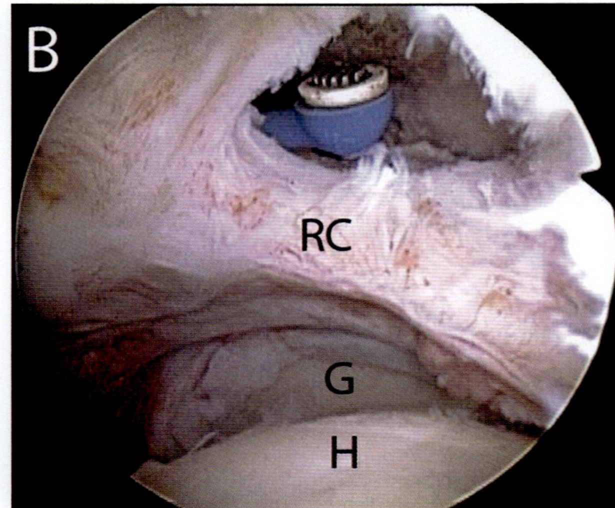

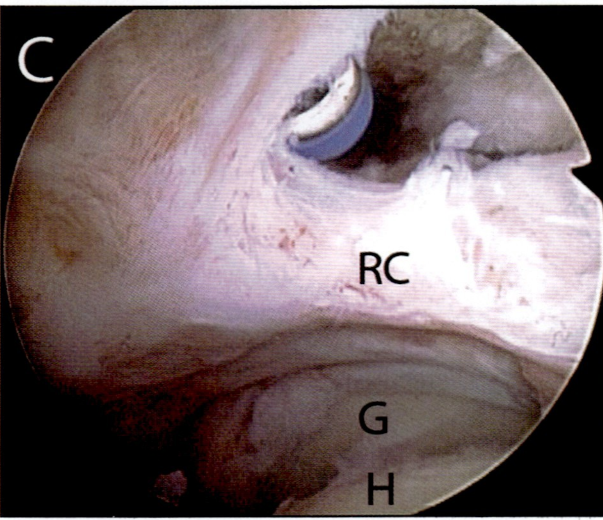

Figure 7.16 Right shoulder, lateral subacromial viewing portal demonstrating excavation of massive contracted rotator cuff tear that is adhesed to the undersurface of the acromion (Fig. 7.15). **A:** A shaver (*black arrow*) is inserted through a posterior portal and used to "bounce off" the scapular spine, just lateral to the bone. **B:** A window has been created above the rotator cuff. **C:** Dissection carries laterally to excavate the rotator cuff from acromial adhesions. G, glenoid; H, humerus; RC, rotator cuff.

To delineate the true cuff margins, it is easiest to first define the posterior margin. While viewing through the lateral portal, the footprint of the rotator cuff is viewed until the most posterior and inferior insertion of the rotator cuff is identified. This intact cuff insertion is seen more easily if the arm is internally rotated. The loose fibrous sheet superior to this is the bursal leader. Using the electrocautery probe or shaver, the bursal leader is debrided until the true posterior margin of the rotator cuff is revealed as parallel collagen fibers. The posterior bursal leader is then debrided beginning laterally and working medially toward the medial margin of the tear (Fig. 7.17).

In some cases, the medial margin of the rotator cuff may still be adhered to the medial acromion and acromioclavicular joint. The rotator cuff is then dissected off until the rotator cuff tendon and muscle belly are exposed. The dissection is continued anteriorly until the anterior margins are exposed. During the anterior dissection, it is important not to inadvertently release the coracoacromial ligament.

Once the posterior, medial, and anterior margins have been delineated, the mobility of the tendon is assessed and further releases are performed if necessary.

PARTIAL ROTATOR CUFF REPAIR

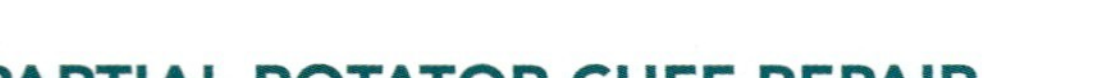

Following single- or double-interval slides, approximately 70% of massive immobile tears may be completely repaired. However, in approximately 30% of cases, despite releases, a complete rotator cuff repair is not possible and a partial balanced rotator cuff repair is the goal. In this scenario, it is important to restore the anterior and posterior rotator cable attachments, that is, the upper subscapularis tendon and the infraspinatus tendon.

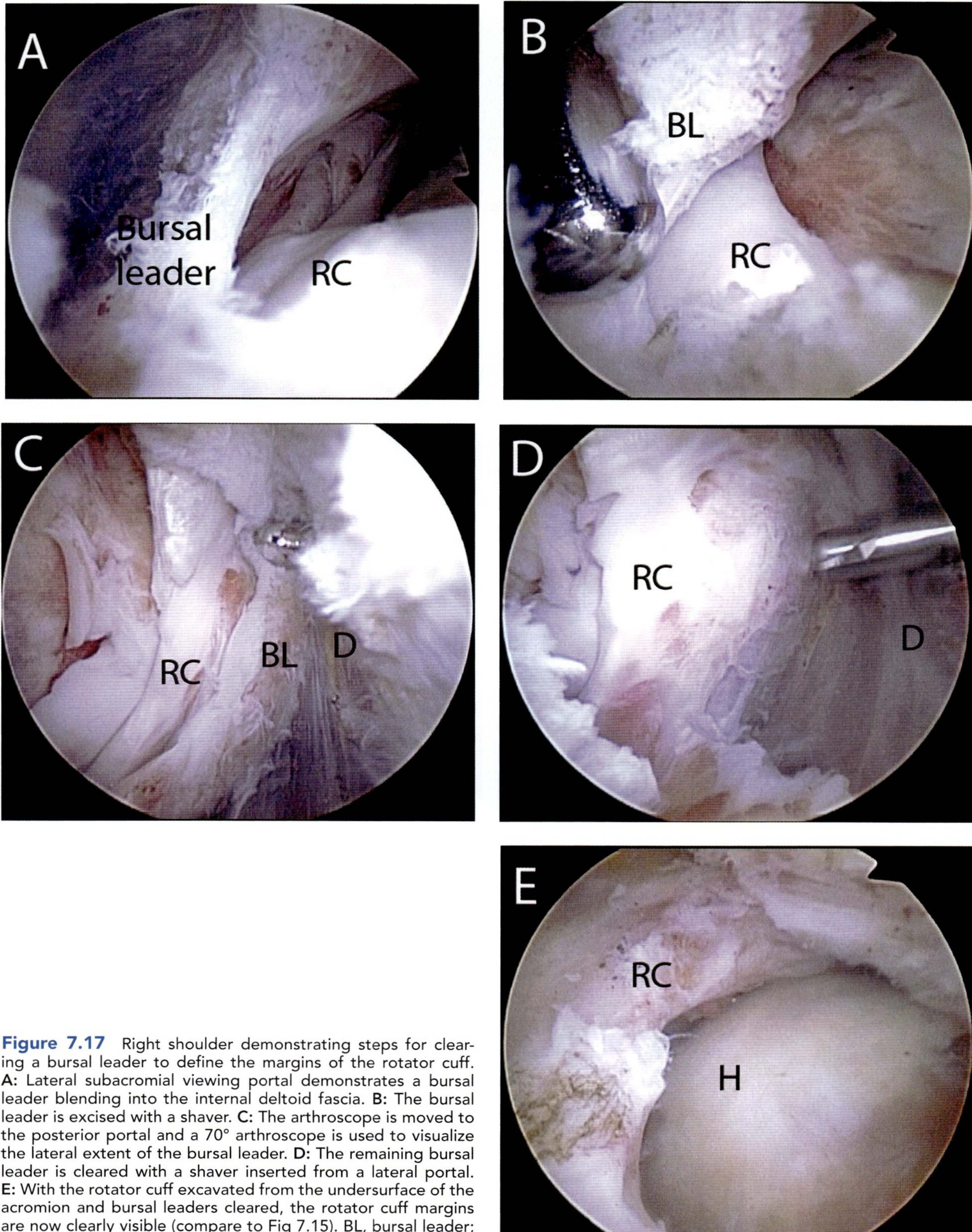

Figure 7.17 Right shoulder demonstrating steps for clearing a bursal leader to define the margins of the rotator cuff. **A:** Lateral subacromial viewing portal demonstrates a bursal leader blending into the internal deltoid fascia. **B:** The bursal leader is excised with a shaver. **C:** The arthroscope is moved to the posterior portal and a 70° arthroscope is used to visualize the lateral extent of the bursal leader. **D:** The remaining bursal leader is cleared with a shaver inserted from a lateral portal. **E:** With the rotator cuff excavated from the undersurface of the acromion and bursal leaders cleared, the rotator cuff margins are now clearly visible (compare to Fig 7.15). BL, bursal leader; D, internal deltoid fascia; H, humerus; RC, rotator cuff.

The technique of partial rotator cuff repair applies the principles of subscapularis tendon mobilization with a posterior interval slide, and results from the inability to obtain adequate mobilization for a complete repair. The most common scenario is in patients with combined subscapularis, supraspinatus, and infraspinatus tendon tears. Patients with triple-tendon tears generally present with pain, poor active range of motion, and weakness. Although proximal humeral migration is not a contraindication to rotator cuff repair, chronic radiographic changes of cuff tear arthropathy including acetabularization of the acromion, thinning or fragmentation of the acromion, and femoralization of the humeral head are poor prognostic signs for function improvement even when partial repair is possible.

MRI will usually demonstrate massive tears of the supraspinatus, infraspinatus, and subscapularis tendons with retraction to the level of the glenoid (Fig. 7.18). Combined tear length >2 cm on coronal images and width >2 cm on the sagittal images suggest that interval slides or partial repair will be necessary in over 75% of cases. Combined length and width >3 cm predicts the need for interval slides or partial repair in all cases (1,2). Advanced degrees of atrophy and fatty infiltration may be present on non-fat-suppressed T1 parasagittal images medial to the glenoid. In general, MRI scans in which the infraspinatus muscle

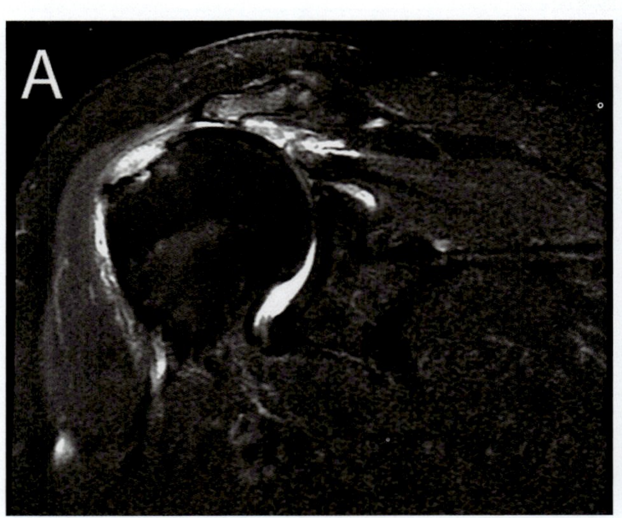

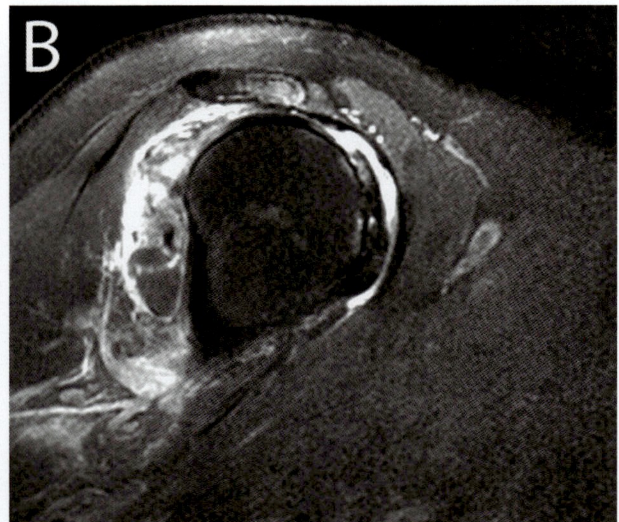

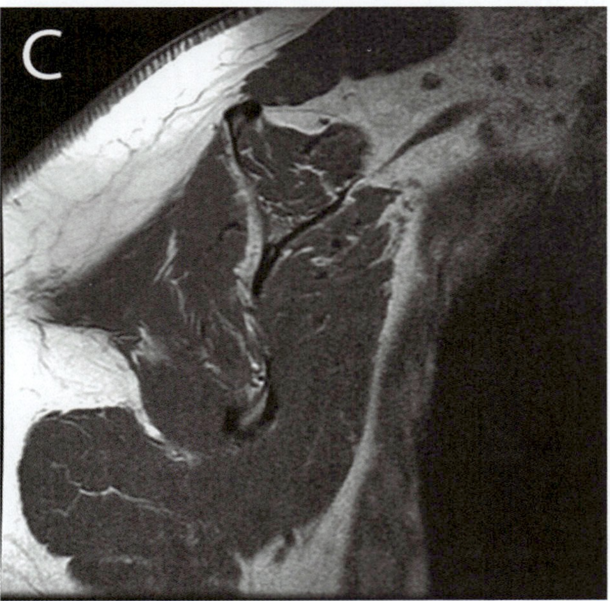

Figure 7.18 MRI of a right shoulder demonstrating a massive rotator cuff tear. **A:** T2 Coronal image shows retraction of the rotator cuff to the level of the glenoid. **B:** T2 Sagittal shows that the tear extends posteriorly to include all of the infraspinatus tendon. The large dimensions of the tear predict the need for an interval slide in this case. **C:** T1 parasagittal image demonstrates only mild fatty infiltration, suggesting a reasonable expectation for functional improvement with arthroscopic repair.

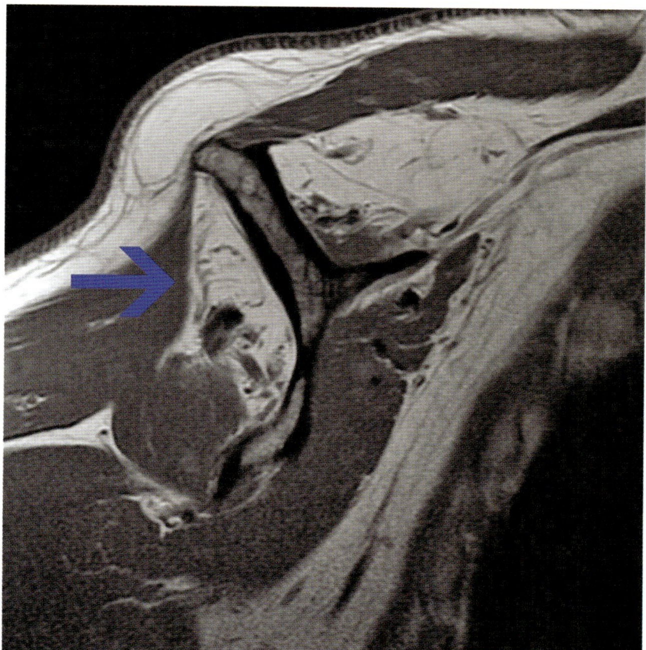

Figure 7.19 T1 parasagittal magnetic resonance image demonstrates >75% fatty infiltration of the infraspinatus (*blue arrow*). Individuals with this degree of fatty infiltration have a poor prognosis following rotator cuff repair.

has >75% fatty infiltration are a poor prognostic sign for significant functional improvement following repair (Fig. 7.19). In patients with less fatty infiltration than this, an arthroscopic repair may be attempted with reasonable expectations of improvement in pain and function (3).

Diagnostic arthroscopy will demonstrate massive tearing of the rotator cuff with retraction of the tendon margins medial to the glenoid (Fig. 7.20). Close evaluation of secondary changes of the glenohumeral joint (e.g., chondromalacia), and subacromial space (e.g., eburnation of the undersurface of the acromion) is performed. As in all combined tears of the rotator cuff, attention is initially focused anteriorly to the biceps tendon and subscapularis tendon.

An anterosuperolateral portal is created and the biceps tendon is tagged with two half-racking stitches and released from its insertion on the superior labrum. Extracorporeally, a whip stitch is placed. Throughout the rest of the procedure (prior to tenodesis), gentle traction is applied to the biceps tendon through the anterosuperolateral portal (outside the cannula) to pull the tendon out of the anterior working space improving visualization. For a complete discussion of biceps tenodesis, see Chapter 10, "The Biceps Tendon."

RESTORATION OF THE ANTERIOR MOMENT

After initial treatment of the biceps tendon, the subscapularis tendon is approached. The comma sign is identified, leading to the superolateral corner of the subscapularis tendon, and a traction stitch is placed (Fig. 7.21). Initial mobility of the subscapularis tendon is assessed and a three-sided release of the subscapularis tendon is performed, progressing superiorly, anteriorly, and posteriorly. It is critical in three-tendon tear cases to obtain as much mobility of the subscapularis tendon as possible since repair of the subscapularis restores the anterior moment of the transverse force plane couple and facilitates repair of the anterior supraspinatus tendon. Failure to repair the

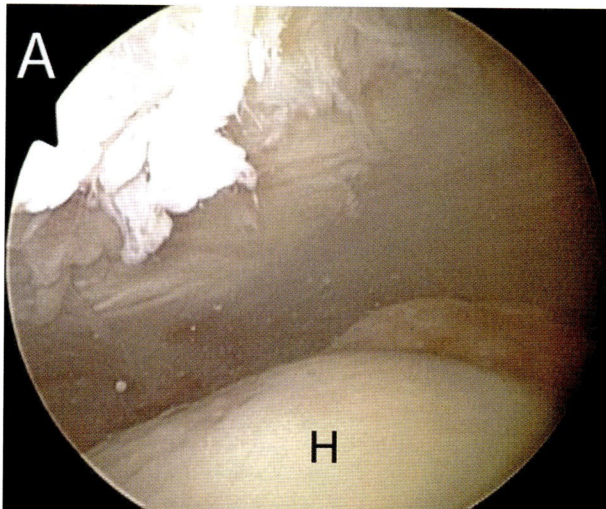

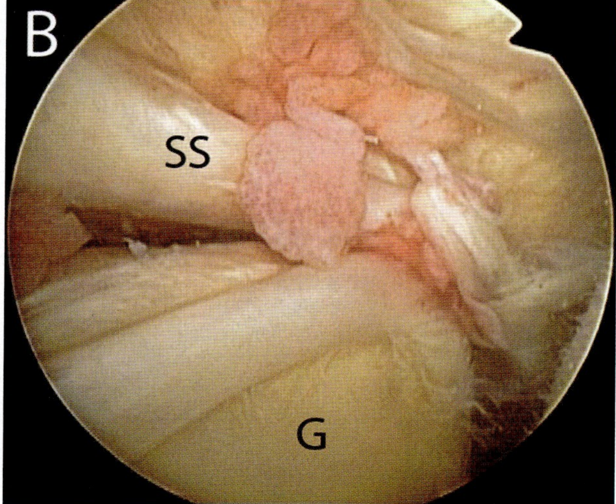

Figure 7.20 Right shoulder, posterior viewing portal demonstrating a massive rotator cuff tear. **A:** The greater tuberosity footprint is bare. **B:** There is retraction of the rotator cuff medial to the glenoid. G, glenoid; H, humerus; SS, supraspinatus tendon.

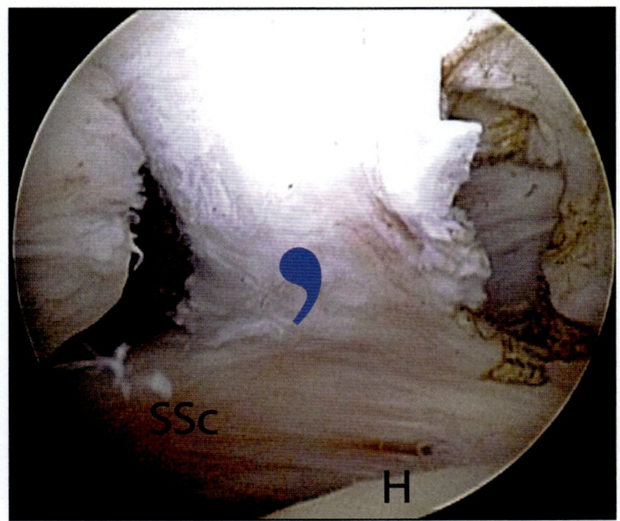

Figure 7.21 Right shoulder, posterior viewing portal demonstrating a retracted subscapularis tendon tear in the same shoulder as Fig. 7.20. Repair begins with identification of the comma sign (*blue comma symbol*). H, humerus; SSc, subscapularis tendon.

subscapularis will place the anterior supraspinatus tendon under tension leading to repair failure (Fig. 7.22)

When sufficient mobility is obtained, the subscapularis tendon is repaired anatomically to the lesser tuberosity. It is important to repair the subscapularis tendon with reference to the local anatomy including the lesser tuberosity, greater tuberosity and bicipital groove. The subscapularis tendon is then repaired to the lesser tuberosity starting from inferior to superior. Standard suture anchor (5.5-mm Bio-Composite Corkscrew FT; Arthrex, Inc., Naples, FL)–based techniques are utilized, passing sutures using an antegrade technique (Scorpion). The superior border is restored to its anatomic position, repairing the comma sign (i.e., medial biceps sling) adjacent to the bicipital groove (Fig. 7.23). Definitive treatment of the biceps tendon with tenodesis in the bicipital groove is then performed.

If sufficient mobility is obtained, a double-row subscapularis repair may be performed. In many chronic cases, a double-row repair is not possible and excursion is at a premium. In these cases, medialization of the bone bed by 5 to 7 mm may be performed to improve tendon to bone contact. For a complete discussion of subscapularis repair, see Chapter 6, "Subscapularis Tendon Tears."

RESTORATION OF THE POSTERIOR MOMENT

Once the subscapularis tendon has been repaired, with restoration of the anterior moment, the posterosuperior (i.e., supraspinatus, infraspinatus) rotator cuff is then approached. It is critical during repair of the subscapularis tendon to maintain the integrity of the lateral rotator interval (i.e., the comma sign), which may facilitate repair of the posterosuperior rotator cuff.

The margins of the rotator cuff are assessed for mobility (Fig. 7.24). If the posterosuperior rotator cuff has excellent medial-to-lateral mobility, then it may be repaired in a crescent-shaped fashion. If there is excellent anterior-to-posterior mobility, the posterosuperior rotator cuff may be repaired in a side-to-side fashion initially, using the principles of margin convergence. Then, the converged margin is repaired to bone (Fig. 7.25). When evaluating the anterior-to-posterior mobility of the tear margins, it is important to remember that the anterior leaf (i.e., residual comma sign) will have inherently excessive mobility due to the previous dissection and rotator interval resection. Therefore, tear mobility and tear classification must be largely based on the mobility of the medial and the posterior margins.

In cases with poor anterior-to-posterior, and medial-to-lateral mobility, we routinely progress to capsular release with interval slides. In patients with concomitant retracted subscapularis tears, an interval slide in continuity (i.e., resection of the rotator interval) has already been performed along with subscapularis tendon mobilization and takes the place of the anterior interval slide. Thus, only a posterior interval slide is required and may be performed in isolation. Otherwise, a double-interval slide may be considered.

In chronic adhesed cases, the margins of the posterosuperior rotator cuff are obscured by scar tissue and the rotator cuff must be dissected from the undersurface of the acromion and internal deltoid fascia. Usually when this aggressive mobilization is required, the rotator cuff cannot be repaired by direct tendon repair to bone or by margin convergence, and interval slides will be required.

Once capsular releases and interval slides have been performed, the rotator cuff tendon mobilization has been maximized. There are essentially no other major releases that can be performed to improve mobilization. A final assessment of the mobility of the infraspinatus and supraspinatus tendons is performed. In most cases, both the supraspinatus and infraspinatus tendon may now be repaired (Fig. 7.26). However, in severe cases, repair of only a portion of the posterosuperior rotator cuff may be achievable. In the vast majority of these cases, repair of the infraspinatus tendon is possible but the supraspinatus tendon is of either poor quality, has poor mobility or both (Fig. 7.27).

When this occurs, attention is focused completely on the infraspinatus tendon. The bone bed for the infraspinatus tendon is prepared. It is not uncommon to incorporate the bare area of the humeral head as part of the bone bed during bone preparation to augment tendon to bone contact.

The traction stitch is usually retrieved through an anterolateral percutaneous portal along the bone bed to advance the infraspinatus tendon anteriorly and superiorly. Repair in this position restores the infraspinatus

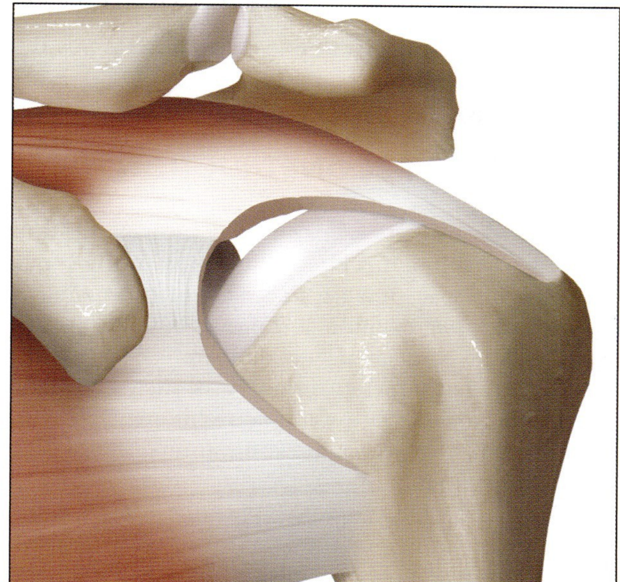

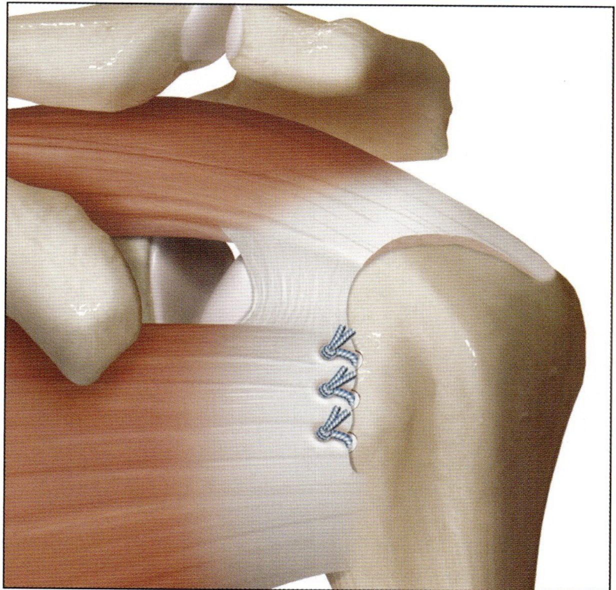

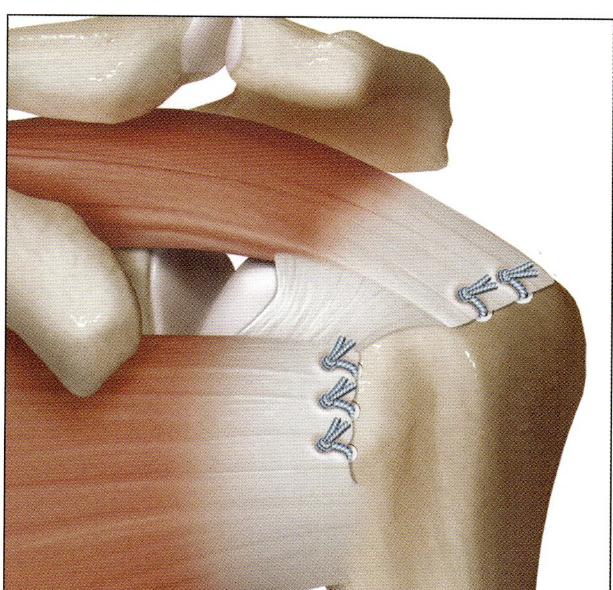

Figure 7.22 Schematic of the relationship between subscapularis repair and the supraspinatus. **A:** Massive retracted and contracted tear of the subscapularis and supraspinatus tendons. **B:** Repair of the subscapularis partially reduces the supraspinatus retraction. **C:** Repair of the supraspinatus can then be accomplished with minimal tension.

tendon to its anatomic position and restores its lever arm and mechanical advantage. For repair of the infraspinatus tendon, two anchors are usually required (5.5-mm Bio-Composite Corkscrew FT) and are positioned to repair the lateral margin of the infraspinatus tendon (Fig. 7.28A). Sutures are passed in an antegrade fashion (Scorpion) while viewing through a posterior portal (Fig. 7.28B) or retrograde fashion while viewing through a lateral portal (Fig. 7.28C). Placing traction on the traction stitch while passing sutures can help position the sutures to recreate the anterolateral infraspinatus advancement.

Sutures are then tied from posterior to anterior using a Surgeon's Sixth Finger Knot Pusher (Arthrex, Inc., Naples, FL) and static knot tying (Surgeon's knot) (Fig. 7.29). In rare cases, a double-row infraspinatus tendon repair may be performed, utilizing medial anchors with medial mattress stitches or a suture bridge transosseous equivalent technique (Fig. 7.30). Once the infraspinatus tendon has been repaired, the posterior moment has been restored and the force couples are balanced in the transverse and sagittal planes (Fig. 7.31).

The supraspinatus tendon is again assessed for repairability. If, despite interval slides, the supraspinatus does not have sufficient mobility to reach the greater tuberosity, then the supraspinatus is sutured side to side to the infraspinatus after the infraspinatus has been advanced

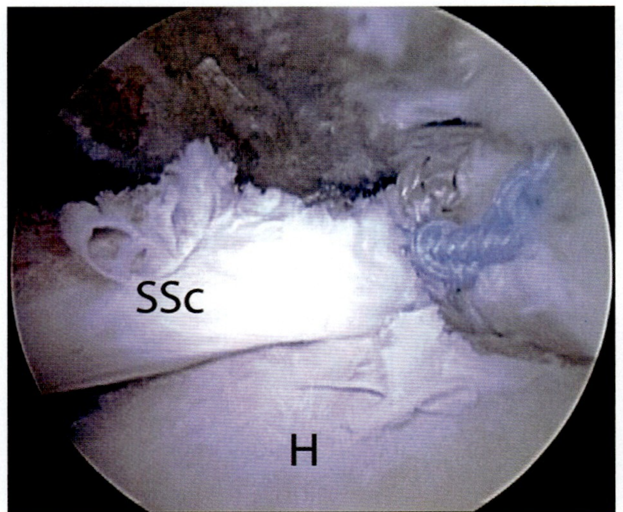

Figure 7.23 Right shoulder, posterior viewing portal. Repair of the subscapularis tendon restores the anterior moment (compare to Fig. 7.21). H, humerus; SSc, subscapularis tendon.

and repaired to bone (Fig. 7.32). These efforts are made to reestablish the rotator cable and do as much as possible to rebalance force couples.

ALLOGRAFT RECONSTRUCTION

Allograft reconstruction for massive tears of the rotator cuff has had a long history of utilization in the shoulder. Recently, however, the development of processing technologies and sterilization techniques has decreased the complications associated with allograft reconstruction and enhanced the postoperative viability of such. Furthermore, the advancement of arthroscopic techniques has allowed the use of such technologies with minimal morbidity and superior outcomes.

In patients with massive tears of the rotator cuff, our primary goal is to repair the rotator cuff with the patient's own tissue using the principles of tendon mobilization,

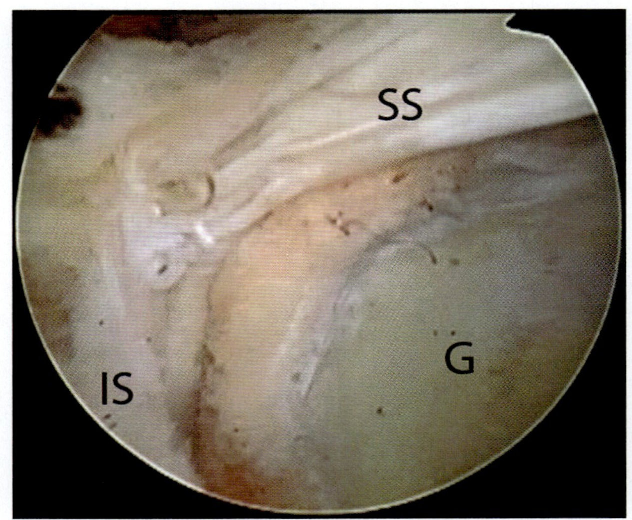

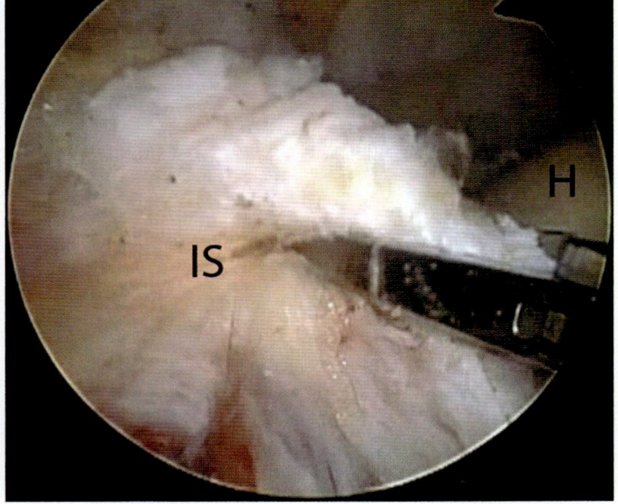

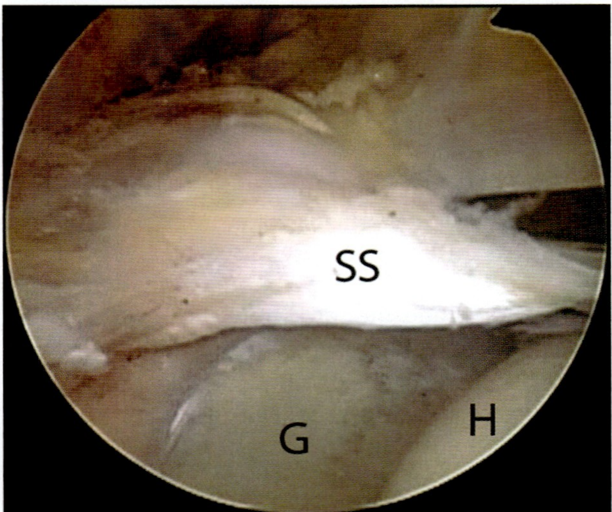

Figure 7.24 Right shoulder, posterior viewing portal with a 70° arthroscope demonstrates **(A)** a massive rotator cuff tear with medial retraction to the glenoid. **B:** The mobility of the posterior and **(C)** anterior tear margins is assessed with a grasper introduced from a lateral subacromial portal. In this case, there is good anterior-to-posterior mobility of the tear margins, indicating a U-shaped tear that should be repaired with margin convergence. G, glenoid; H, humerus; IS, infraspinatus tendon; SS, supraspinatus tendon.

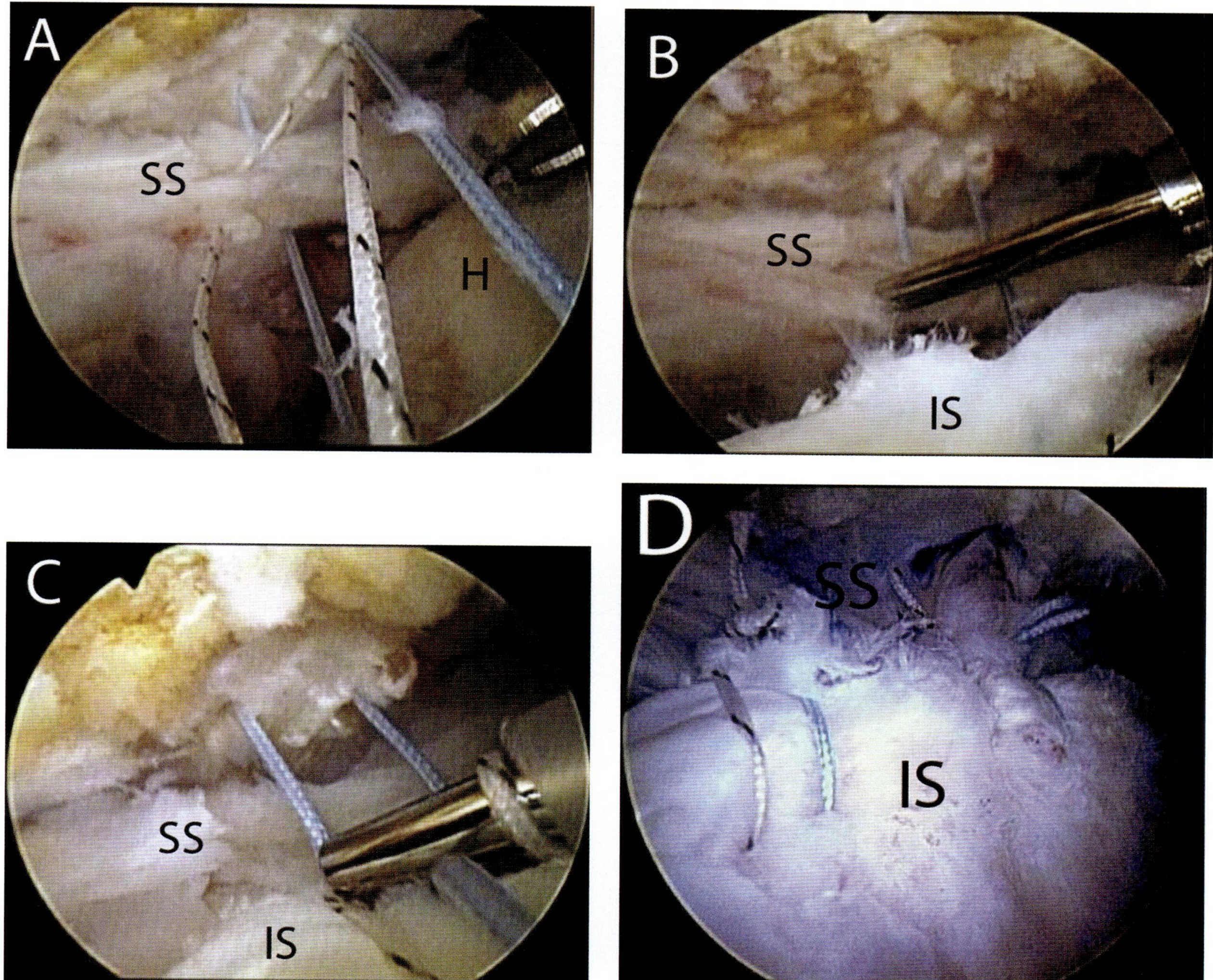

Figure 7.25 Margin convergence in a right shoulder viewed from a posterior subacromial portal. **A:** Margin convergence sutures in place. **B:** The double-diameter knot pusher (Surgeon's Sixth Finger, Arthrex Inc., Naples, FL) is introduced. **C:** With the Surgeon's Sixth Finger, reduction of the two leaves of the tear is obtained and can be maintained while subsequent throws are completed. **D:** Appearance of the same tear following placement of side-to-side sutures and margin convergence to bone (Compare to Fig. 7.24). H, humerus; IS, infraspinatus tendon; SS, supraspinatus tendon.

tear pattern recognition, and obtaining a secure and stable construct. The vast majority of patients, particularly in primary cases, may be repaired using standard and advanced (e.g., interval slide) techniques as described elsewhere in this book. In this scenario, we rarely augment a primary repair with allograft. Furthermore the results of partial rotator cuff repair have demonstrated excellent results particularly when the subscapularis and infraspinatus tendon are repaired to balance the force couples about the glenohumeral joint and provide a stable fulcrum of motion. Although the "cowboy philosophy" has not embraced allografts for rotator cuff repair, one of us (IKYL) has some experience in their use, and his allograft experience constitutes the basis for this section.

The major indications for allograft reconstruction are for augmentation of arthroscopic rotator cuff repair where there is a concern for postoperative rotator cuff integrity and in patients with irreparable tears of the rotator cuff where the allograft is used to span a defect. The preferred allograft is an acellular dermal allograft (ArthroFlex; Arthrex, Inc., Naples, FL). It should be noted that in general, most commercially available allografts are only Food and Drug Administration (FDA) approved for augmentation of rotator cuff repair and to span defects of <1 cm. However, their

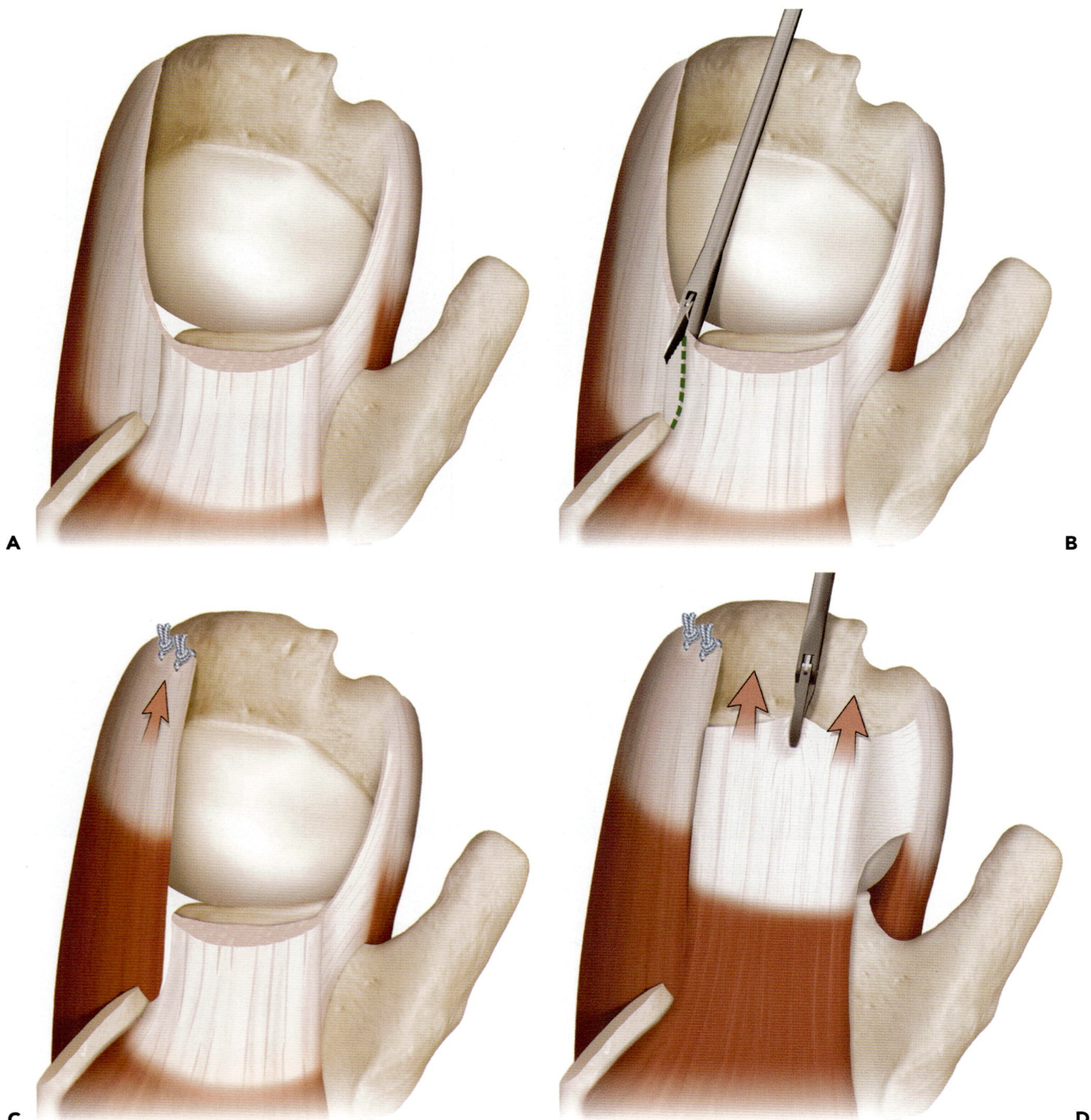

Figure 7.26 Schematic of a massive contracted tear amenable to repair to bone after interval slides. **A:** Superior view. **B:** A posterior interval slide is performed. Additionally, an anterior slide in continuity is performed (not visualized). **C:** The infraspinatus is advanced and repaired to bone. **D:** Reassessment of mobility demonstrates that the supraspinatus has sufficient mobility to reach the greater tuberosity following the modified double-interval slide.

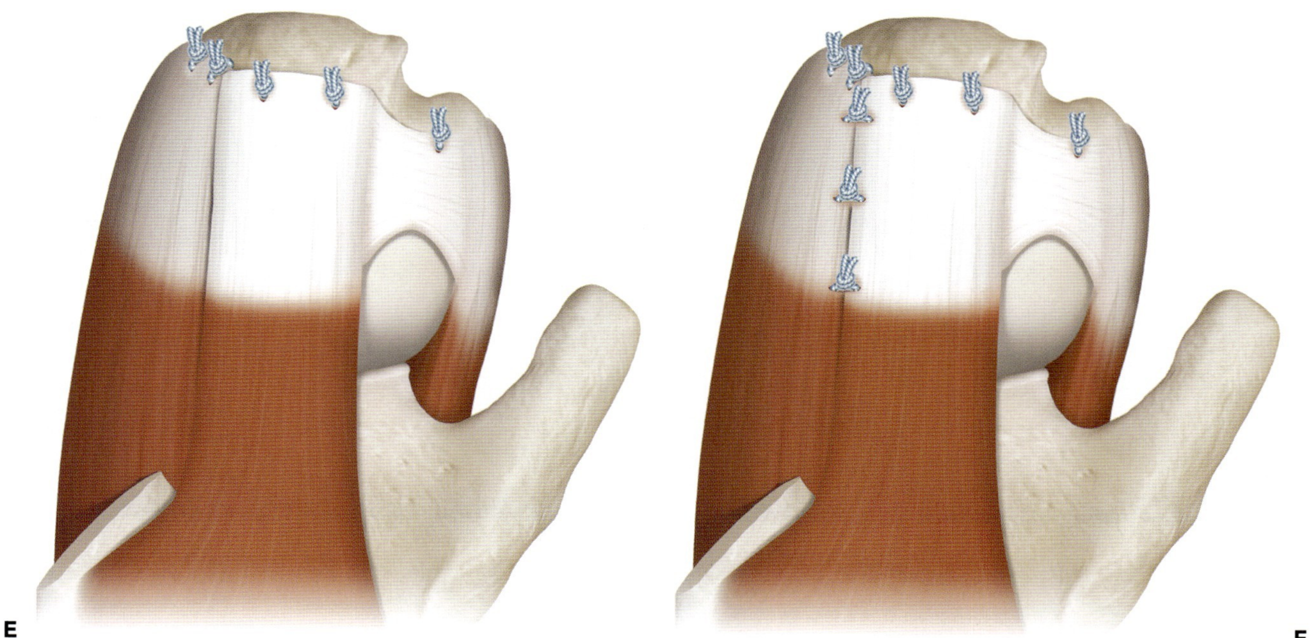

Figure 7.26 *(Continued)* **E:** The supraspinatus tendon is repaired to bone. **F:** Margin convergence sutures are then placed following repair of the supraspinatus and the infraspinatus tendons.

clinical use by some surgeons has expanded beyond these indications.

ALLOGRAFT REPLACEMENT

In general, one may consider patients with massive, irreparable rotator cuff tears who have failed to obtain pain relief after a previous partial repair as candidates for allograft replacement. Most candidates for this treatment have previously failed a rotator cuff repair and have evidence of retraction, muscle atrophy, and fatty infiltration on MRI. However, advanced cuff tear arthropathy (e.g., proximal humeral migration with obliteration of the acromiohumeral interval, acetabularization of the acromion, femoralization of the humeral head), or significant arthritic changes are considered contraindications for allograft replacement. Furthermore, in patients with extreme external rotation weakness and loss of overhead elevation, postoperative improvement in active range of motion and strength over and above pain relief is unlikely (unless a significant partial repair is obtained). For these reasons, patients must be educated preoperatively on reasonable postoperative outcomes (i.e., pain relief).

Following standard diagnostic glenohumeral arthroscopy, the subacromial space is entered. Standard posterior and lateral portals are established. A thorough subacromial bursectomy is performed. The margins of the rotator cuff are delineated and any previous fixation is removed. A limited smoothing of the undersurface of the acromion is performed but care is taken to preserve the coracoacromial arch to avoid iatrogenic anterosuperior escape.

Defining the Margins

In many cases, particularly revision cases, the margins of the rotator cuff are obscured and scarred to the internal deltoid fascia and undersurface of the acromion. In these patients, the rotator cuff must be dissected and excavated from the overlying scar tissue as discussed earlier in this chapter.

The rotator cuff tendon tear must be assessed for tissue quality and mobility. If a partial rotator cuff repair is possible, then it should be performed. Restoration of the anterior moment (i.e., subscapularis tendon) and posterior moment (i.e., infraspinatus and teres minor tendons) is essential for restoring force couples and will make the eventual allograft size smaller. It should be noted, however, that excessive tension should not be applied to any portion of the partial rotator cuff repair. Tension overload will result in failure of the partial rotator cuff repair and therefore failure of the allograft reconstruction.

When performing allograft reconstruction of the rotator cuff, the preparation of the margins of the rotator cuff tendon tear is critical. This includes the anterior, lateral, and posterior margins. Anteriorly (similar to the prerequisites for a latissimus dorsi transfer), the best-case scenario is an intact subscapularis tendon and a complete, intact

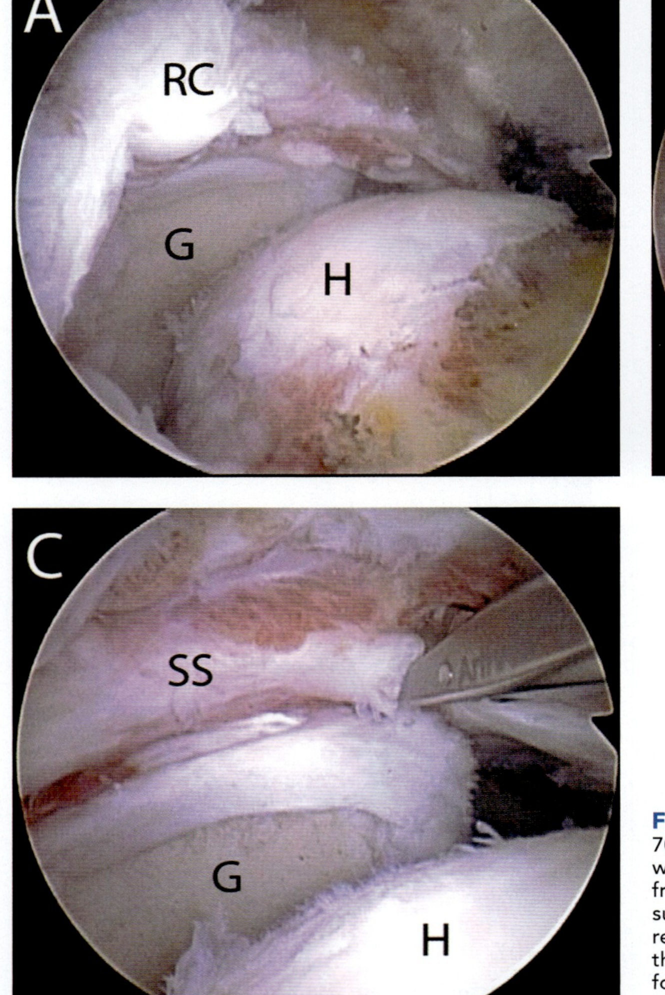

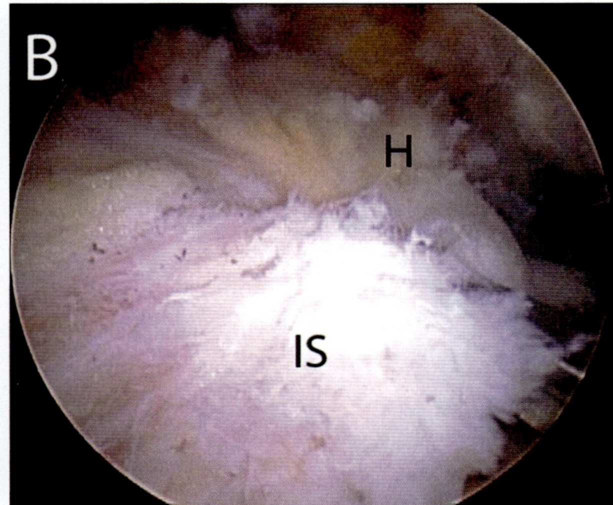

Figure 7.27 Right shoulder, posterior viewing portal with a 70° arthroscope demonstrates **(A)** a massive rotator cuff tear with medial retraction to the glenoid. **B:** A grasper introduced from a lateral subacromial portal demonstrates that there is sufficient mobility of the infraspinatus tendon to perform a repair to bone. **C:** There is very limited mobility, however, of the supraspinatus tendon. Thus, only a partial repair will be performed. G, glenoid; H, humerus; IS, infraspinatus tendon; RC, rotator cuff; SS, supraspinatus tendon.

rotator interval. This maintains the anterior moment of the transverse plane force couple and the lateral rotator interval (comma tissue) will serve as the attachment point for the allograft anteriorly.

In the case of a subscapularis tendon tear, the subscapularis should be repaired first to restore the anterior moment. When dissecting the anterior margins, particularly in revision cases, it is important to ensure that the coracoacromial ligament is not violated and that the subscapularis tendon is identified using the principles as described in Chapter 6. During repair, maintenance of the lateral rotator interval (or comma tissue) is critical as this will serve as the anterior attachment of the allograft. In addition, a secure repair of the superior margin of the subscapularis tendon to maximize healing of the superolateral border will help to assure that retearing of the subscapularis and thus avulsion of the leading edge of the allograft does not occur.

For the uppermost subscapularis anchor, we place a triple-loaded 5.5-mm BioComposite Corkscrew FT (Arthrex, Inc., Naples, FL) in the superior footprint of the lesser tuberosity. Two sutures are used to secure the upper border of the subscapularis tendon. The third set of sutures is used to secure the subsequent allograft as a side-to-side stitch through the subscapularis upper border and the anterolateral edge of the allograft. If no repair of the subscapularis is required, then anchors may be inserted later during fixation of the allograft.

In the rare case where the subscapularis is not repairable, multiple options exist. One may choose to leave the leading edge of the allograft free. However, due to the theoretical risk of abrasion of the free leading edge, it is our preference to secure the allograft anteriorly in some fashion. If the long head of the biceps is present, the anterior margin of the allograft may be secured to the intra-articular biceps tendon. If this is performed, we generally also secure

(Text continued in page 156)

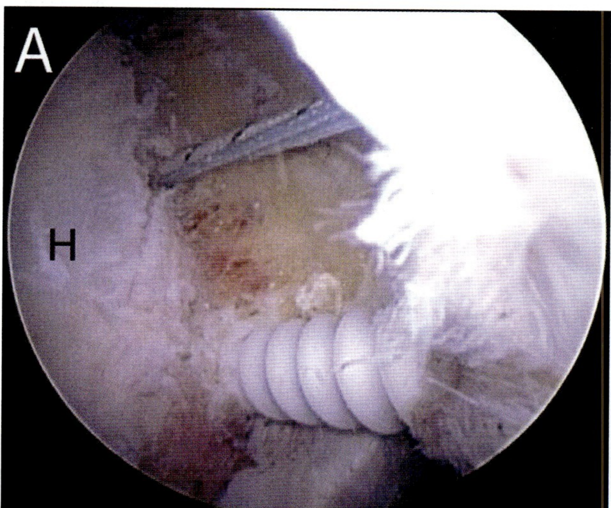

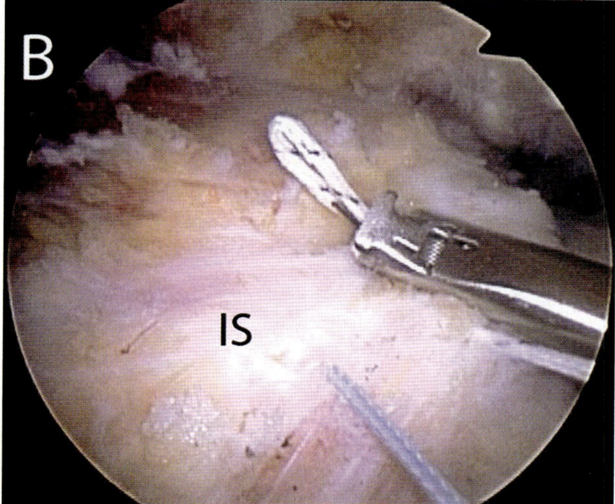

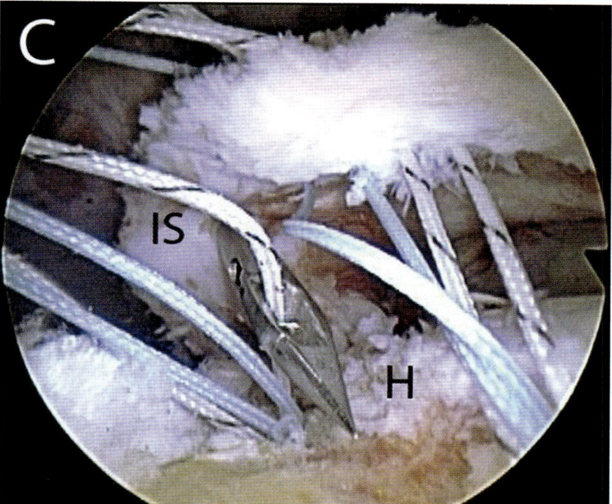

Figure 7.28 **A:** Right shoulder, posterior viewing portal demonstrates placement of two anchors for repair of the infraspinatus. **B:** Sutures from the anterior anchor are passed with an antegrade suture passer while continuing to view from the posterior portal. **C:** Sutures from the posterior anchor are passed retrograde while viewing from a lateral subacromial portal. In this case, sutures have been passed as mattress stitches for subsequent incorporation into a lateral row repair. H, humerus; IS, infraspinatus tendon.

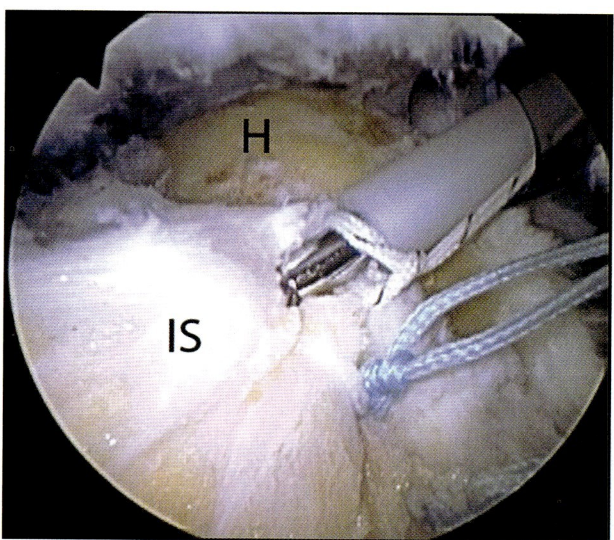

Figure 7.29 Right shoulder, posterior viewing portal demonstrating knot tying for infraspinatus tendon repair using a Surgeon's Sixth Finger Knot Pusher (Arthrex, Inc., Naples, FL). H, humerus; IS, infraspinatus tendon.

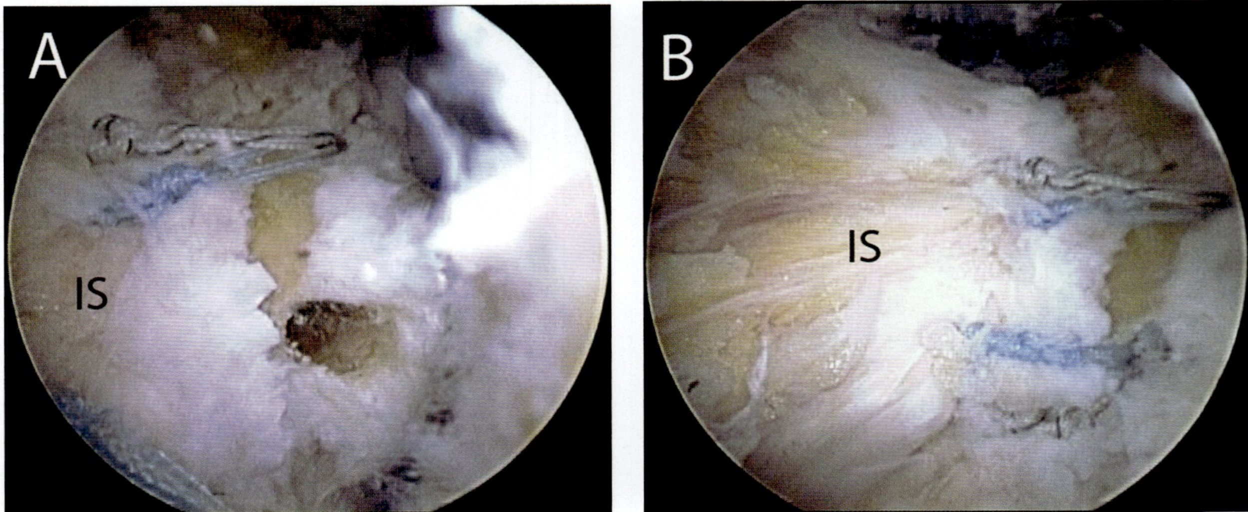

Figure 7.30 Right shoulder, posterior viewing portal. **A:** After knot tying (Fig. 7.29), the suture limbs are secured laterally with knotless anchors (BioComposite SwiveLock C; Arthrex, Inc., Naples, FL) to reinforce the repair. **B:** Final view of the double-row infraspinatus tendon repair. IS, infraspinatus tendon.

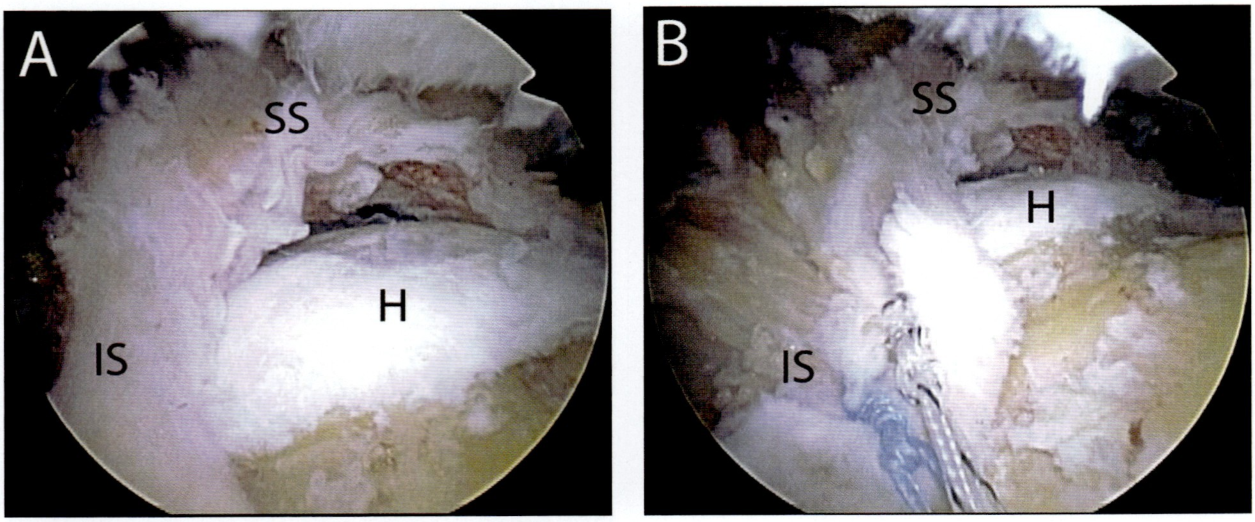

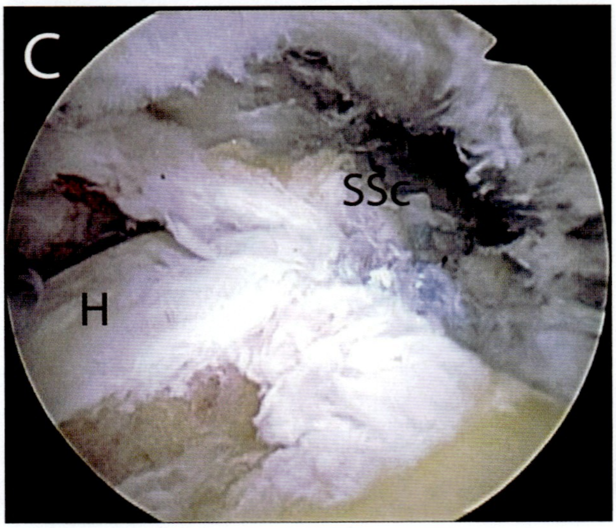

Figure 7.31 Right shoulder, posterior subacromial viewing portal demonstrating **(A)** a partial rotator cuff repair with restoration of the **(B)** posterior (infraspinatus repair) and **(C)** anterior moments (subscapularis repair) (compare to Fig. 7.20). H, humerus; IS, infraspinatus tendon; SS, supraspinatus tendon; SSc, subscapularis tendon.

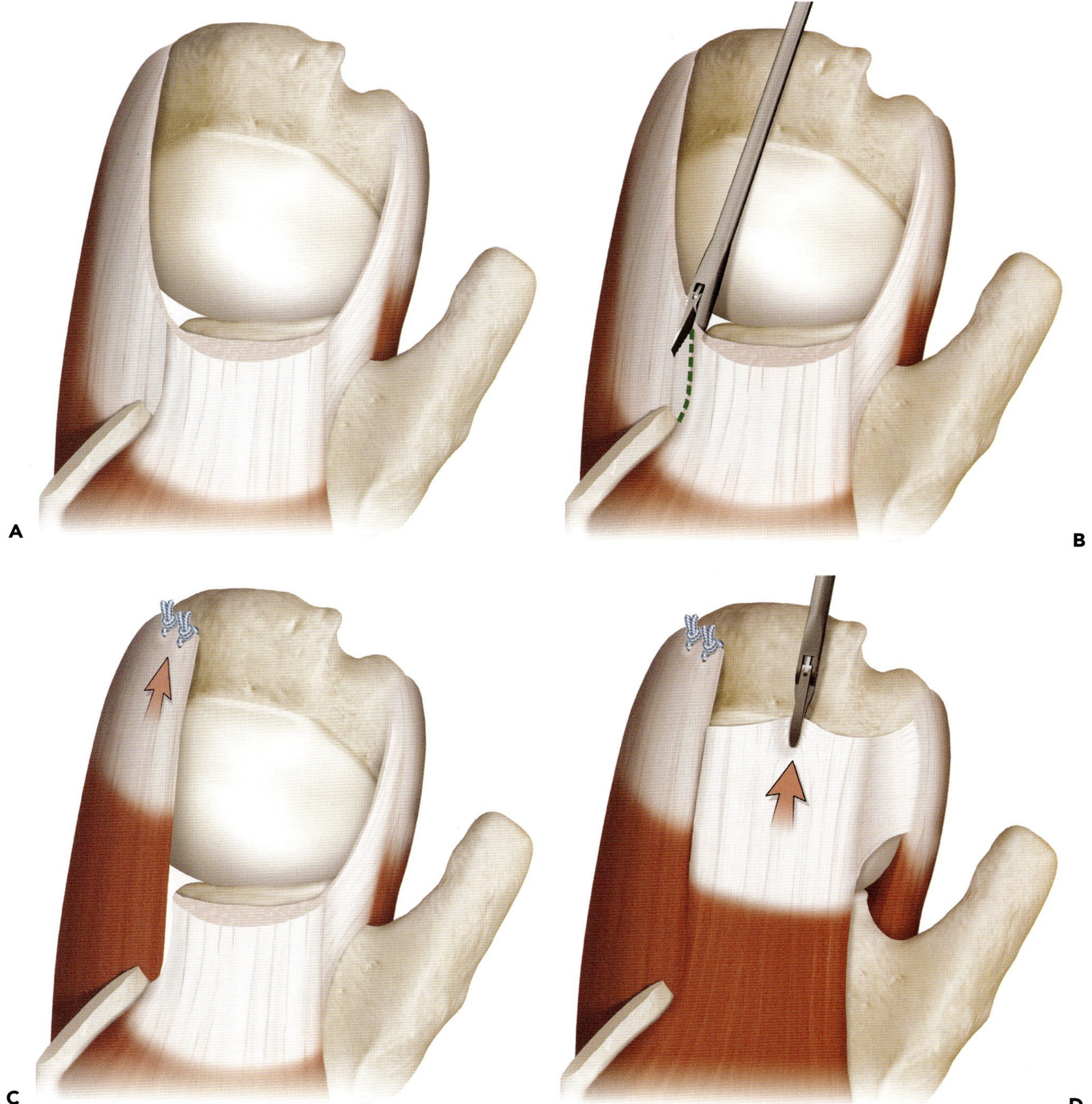

Figure 7.32 Schematic of a massive contracted tear amenable to partial repair only. **A:** Superior view with rotator cuff retracted to the level of the glenoid. **B:** An anterior interval slide in continuity (not visualized) is performed followed by a posterior interval slide (as seen in the figure). **C:** The infraspinatus is then repaired to bone. **D:** Despite double–interval slides, the supraspinatus does not have sufficient mobility to obtain a repair to bone.

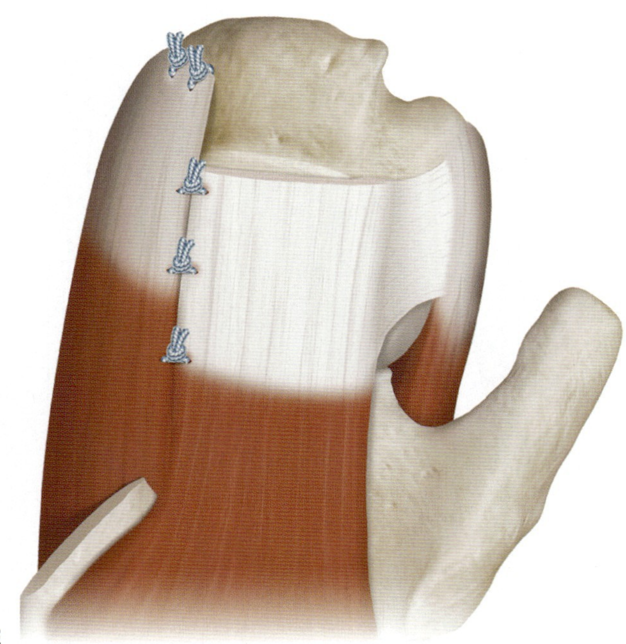

Figure 7.32 *(Continued)* **E:** The supraspinatus is advanced as much as possible and sutured side to side into the infraspinatus to reestablish the rotator cable.

the biceps tendon laterally to the greater tuberosity so that there will be no tension on the graft during early rehabilitation with elbow motion.

Alternatively, the allograft may be extended over the humeral head anteriorly and secured to the stump of the subscapularis tendon anteromedially. We use this approach when the biceps tendon is absent or has been released during subscapularis tend mobilization. Usually, there is a small portion of the subscapularis tendon attached inferiorly (e.g., lower 20%) where the anterior inferior margin of the allograft may be secured. When the graft is extended anteriorly, this increases the complexity of the procedure, and the size of the graft should be measured carefully since graft size will commonly exceed 5 cm (from an anterior to posterior direction).

Posteriorly, it is important to locate and define the "keel" of the scapular spine. This will determine the position of the supraspinatus and infraspinatus tendons and therefore the amount of tearing and residual tendon attachment. Usually, tears will involve the supraspinatus and at least a portion of the infraspinatus tendon attachment. It is again important to remove any bursal leaders posteriorly to define the true tendon margins.

Similar to the subscapularis tendon, if there is any posterior attachment to be repaired it is performed first. A triple-loaded 5.5-mm BioComposite Corkscrew is used if repair is required. If no repair is required, then separate anchors may be inserted later when securing the allograft to bone. Delamination of the posterior rotator cuff is easiest to identify and address prior to allograft insertion.

The lateral margin of the rotator cuff tear is commonly scarred and obscured to the undersurface of the medial aspect of acromion. This margin should be dissected off the medial aspect of the acromion until the tendon substance is identified and the rotator cuff muscle is free of overlying fibrofatty tissue. In many instances, the lateral margin of the rotator cuff tendon is medial to the superior glenoid. In this situation, a capsular release is commonly required along the superior aspect of the glenoid. This not only improves mobilization, but also ensures that an adequate amount of tissue is available for securing the allograft medially.

Measuring the Defect

Once the margins of the rotator cuff tear have been identified and any partial repairs have been performed, the size of the defect may be measured. A suture is used rather than a straight arthroscopic probe to measure length since its malleable shape allows the dimensions to be measured across curved objects (e.g., humeral head).

The anterior, posterior, medial, and lateral dimensions are measured using a #1 PDS suture (Ethicon, Somerville, NJ) knotted on one side. For example, to measure the length of the medial dimension, the rotator cuff defect is viewed through the lateral portal. A grasper is used to introduce the PDS suture through the posterior portal and the knot is placed in the posteromedial corner of the defect accounting for overlap of the graft onto the rotator cuff. A second grasper is then introduced through the anterior portal, grasping the PDS suture in the anteromedial corner of the defect. The posterior grasper is released from the suture and the suture is retrieved through the anterior portal while maintaining the position of the anterior grasper

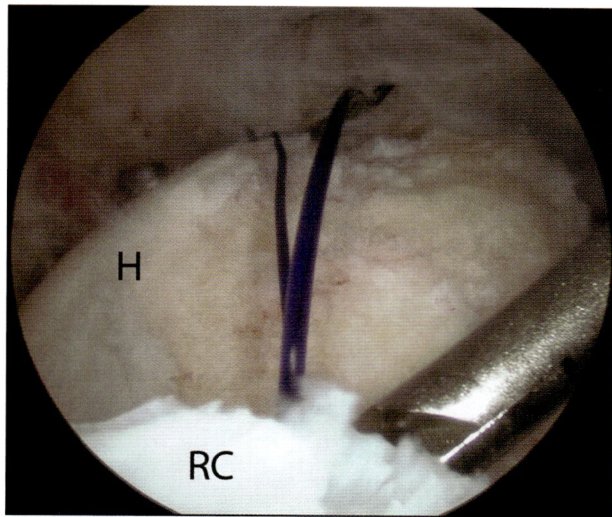

Figure 7.33 Right shoulder, posterior subacromial viewing portal, demonstrates use of a suture to measure the anterior-to-posterior dimension of a rotator cuff defect in preparation for a dermal allograft replacement. H, humerus; RC, rotator cuff.

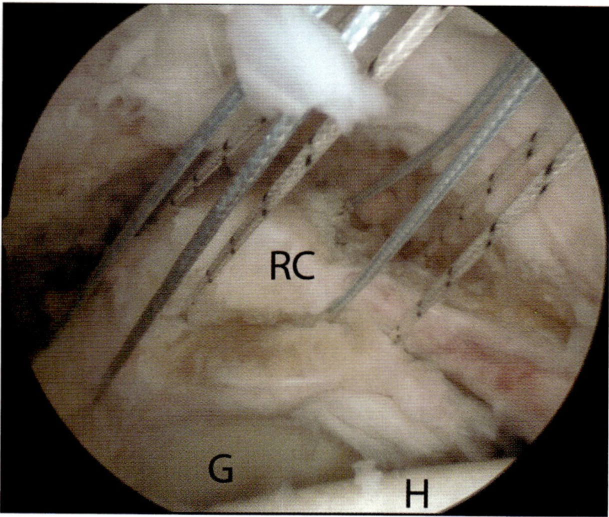

Figure 7.34 Right shoulder, lateral subacromial viewing portal, demonstrates sutures that have placed in the medial margin of a massive retracted rotator cuff tear in preparation for shuttling a dermal allograft. G, glenoid; H, humerus; RC, rotator cuff.

on the suture. The length of suture is then measured extracorporeally using a ruler. The dimensions anteriorly, posteriorly, and laterally are similarly measured (Fig. 7.33).

Graft Preparation

Prior to graft insertion, some acellular dermal grafts require rehydration with normal saline. During preparation, the graft is kept moist. Specific graft requirements should be followed according to the manufacturer's instructions. The graft should be handled carefully and gently as inadvertent pulling or overzealous grasping of the allograft can lead to tearing and indentation of the graft.

The dimensions of the graft are then marked out over the allograft and the allograft is trimmed to the appropriate size and shape. The direction of insertion (i.e., medial/lateral, anterior/posterior, bursal/articular) is also marked.

It is important to preplan the number of sutures that will be placed along each side to ensure there will be secure and balanced fixation. It is particularly important to assess laterally, where any previously placed suture anchors used to repair the anterior or posterior rotator cuff should be accounted for, as well as whether any double- or triple-loaded sutures anchors will be used for lateral fixation. We generally use double-loaded anchors to secure the lateral margin to bone as triple-loaded anchors can cause wrinkling of the graft by drawing to a single point.

Preparation of Shuttling Sutures

A number of methods may be used to insert the graft into the subacromial space. One should generally place four to five medial sutures into the residual cuff arthroscopically. The sutures are then retrieved through the lateral portal and then passed extracorporeally through the allograft. These sutures are used to shuttle the graft into the joint. Although one may chose to place all the sutures through the cuff tissue and graft simultaneously (including those through the anterior, posterior, and lateral margins), too many sutures can make suture management difficult and lead to tangling of the graft and sutures. For this reason, we generally place four to five sutures maximum.

While viewing through the posterior portal, sutures are placed through the lateral margin of the native rotator cuff tendon, starting anteriorly and working posteriorly. A Scorpion suture passer is inserted through a lateral portal and penetrates the lateral margin of the rotator cuff. Sutures are retrieved through an accessory anterior portal and subsequent sutures are sequentially passed. Sutures are evenly spaced along the lateral margin (Fig. 7.34). The number of sutures passed should match the number of holes planned in the medial margin of the allograft. Depending on the size, this is usually four or five sutures.

Starting from the most anterior suture, the undersurface limb of each suture is retrieved through a lateral cannula (Fig. 7.35). It is extremely important to keep the sutures organized with no overlapping or twists. When performing this retrieval, we insert the suture retriever along the posterior aspect of the cannula and retrieve the suture (without crisscrossing adjacent sutures) along the anterior aspect of the suture. This maneuver helps keep the sutures organized without any twists.

As each suture is retrieved, it is passed extracorporeally through the allograft using a straight needle or Scorpion suture passer. A mulberry knot is tied at the end of each suture to prevent the suture from pulling through the allograft (Fig. 7.36). Each suture is carefully handled to ensure there is no tangling or crisscrossing of sutures. Once

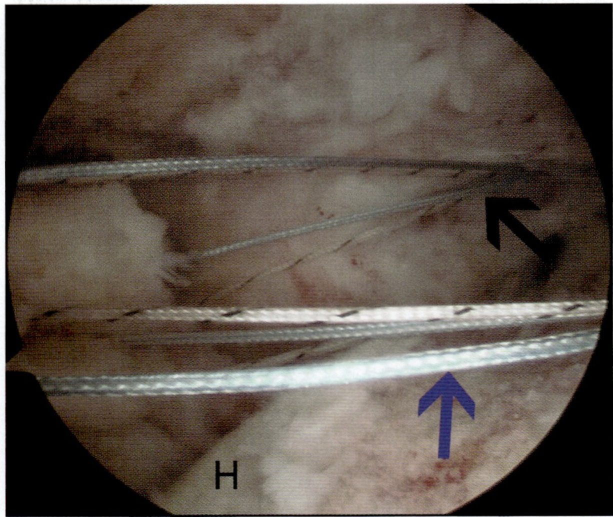

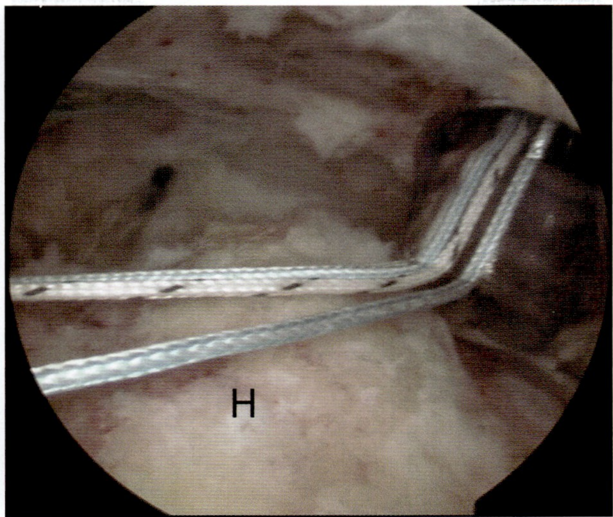

Figure 7.35 **A:** Right shoulder, posterior subacromial viewing portal. The undersurface limbs of sutures previously placed in the lateral rotator cuff margin have been retrieved out a lateral portal (*blue arrow*). The opposing suture limbs have been retrieved out an anterior portal (*black arrow*) to facilitate graft shuttling. **B:** View of the lateral portal demonstrates the sutures that have retrieved without tangling. H, humerus.

the suture passage has been completed, the corresponding sutures limbs (exiting the anterior portal) are organized. Sutures are then passed through each of the corners of the lateral aspect of the allograft. These sutures will assist in spreading out the allograft and keeping the allograft under tension during insertion and fixation.

During preparation of the shuttling sutures, we use an 8.25-mm clear cannula to retrieve sutures. This assists in ensuring there is no tangling of sutures. However, when the allograft size is large (e.g., >5 cm × 5 cm), the allograft may be too large to shuttle through the cannula. For this reason, when the allograft size is large, all the sutures are retrieved and organized in a similar fashion through a cannula without passing the sutures through the allograft. The cannula is then slowly removed from the subacromial space keeping the sutures organized and each suture is individually pulled out of the cannula, keeping the sutures organized without tangles.

Shuttling the Allograft into the Subacromial Space

Once the sutures have all been organized, the graft is shuttled into the subacromial space. The allograft is rolled into the shape of a tube, gently grasped with a grasper, and pushed through the cannula into the subacromial space (Fig. 7.37). The rubber dam of the cannula may be removed to facilitate graft passage. The graft is then

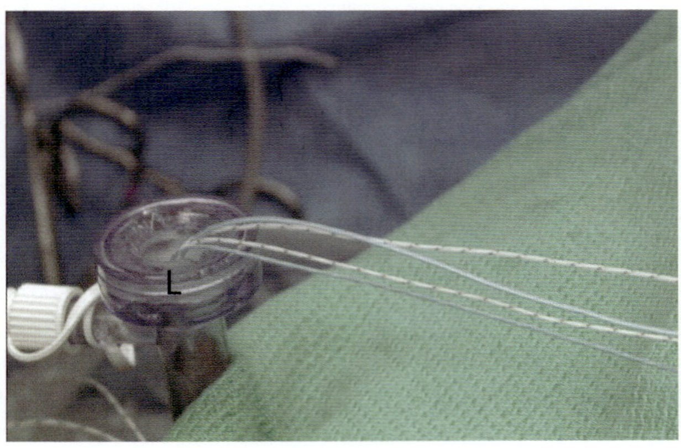

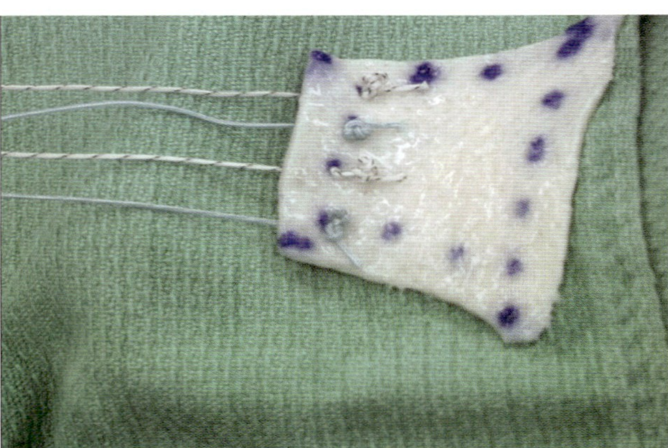

Figure 7.36 **A:** External photo demonstrates suture limbs that have been retrieved out a lateral portal (L). **B:** The suture limbs have been passed through a dermal allograft and mulberry knots have been tied to assist in graft shuttling.

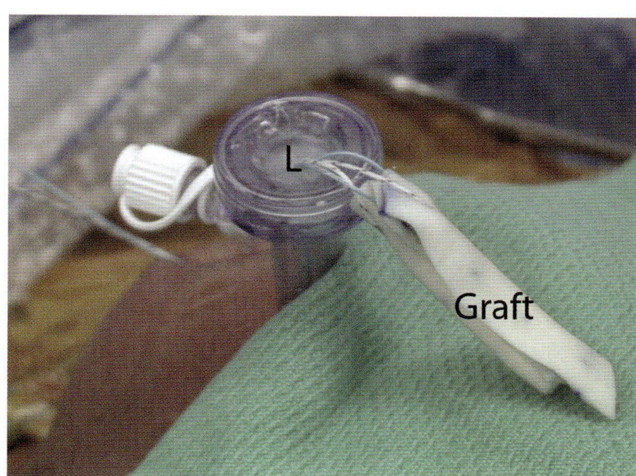

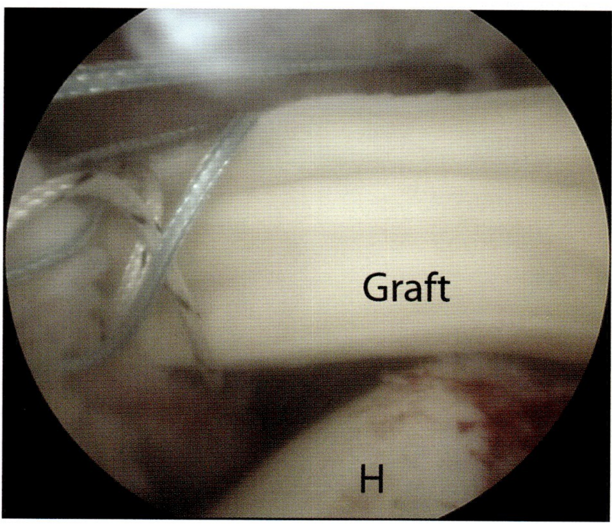

Figure 7.37 **A:** External view demonstrates a dermal allograft that has been rolled on itself and is about to be shuttled into the subacromial space via a lateral portal. **B:** Arthroscopic view of a right shoulder viewed from a posterior subacromial portal demonstrates the graft that has been shuttled into the subacromial space. H, humerus; L, lateral portal.

unrolled in the subacromial space, and with gentle traction on the shuttling sutures, the graft is pulled against the lateral margin of the rotator cuff (Fig. 7.38). Care is taken to pay meticulous attention to graft orientation and suture organization since any twisting of the graft or sutures will lead to significant tangling and surgical delay.

Trailing sutures in the lateral margin of the graft may be retrieved through separate percutaneous subacromial portals to tension the graft and reduce the graft laterally against the greater tuberosity.

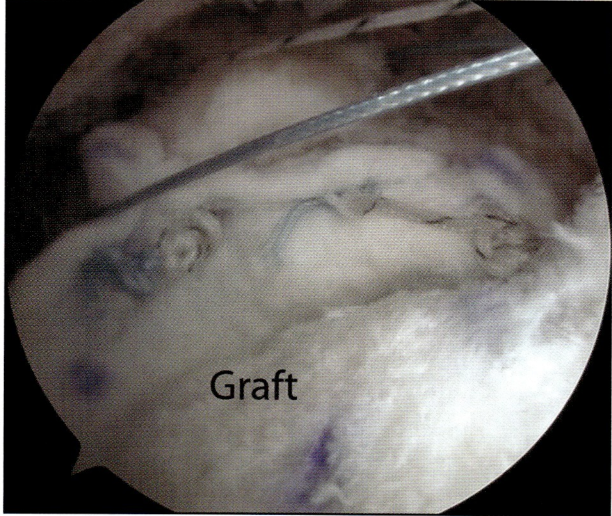

Figure 7.38 Right shoulder, lateral subacromial viewing portal, demonstrates a dermal allograft that has been shuttled into the subacromial space and unfolded. Mulberry knots (seen medially) have been used to bring the graft to the lateral rotator cuff margin by pulling on opposing suture limbs that exit an anterior portal.

Securing the Graft

Once the graft has been seated medially, the graft is secured medially, anteriorly, and posteriorly to the rotator cuff tear margins. The subacromial space is viewed from a lateral portal and the shuttling sutures are sequentially retrieved through a posterior cannula. We generally secure the graft starting posteromedially and advancing anteriorly. A corresponding suture pair is retrieved and the mulberry knot on the graft side is cut. A Surgeon's Sixth Finger Knot Pusher is used to roll the graft up onto the rotator cuff margin, maximizing graft-tendon contact, and static knots are then tied. Static knots are used in order to minimize sliding of the suture against the graft, which can cause graft abrasion and "guillotine" the suture through the graft. The remaining sutures are subsequently tied until the medial margin is secure.

The anterior and posterior margins of the graft are then secured. We generally start posteriorly although either is reasonable. The number and placement of the sutures will vary. Usually three or four sutures are required. Using a combination of antegrade (Scorpion), retrograde (Penetrator), and shuttling techniques (SutureLasso; Arthrex, Inc., Naples, FL), side-to-side sutures are passed through the rotator cuff margin and graft.

We generally use only the Scorpion for suture passage through the graft itself. The graft's elasticity combined with its tight, tough collagen structure makes it very difficult to pass sutures retrograde through the graft. When using the Scorpion, only a single pass is used to pass the suture with no "ratcheting" to avoid multiple punctures through the graft, which may damage its integrity. Sutures are sequentially tied. The anterior and posterior margins of the graft are subsequently secured. As the suturing

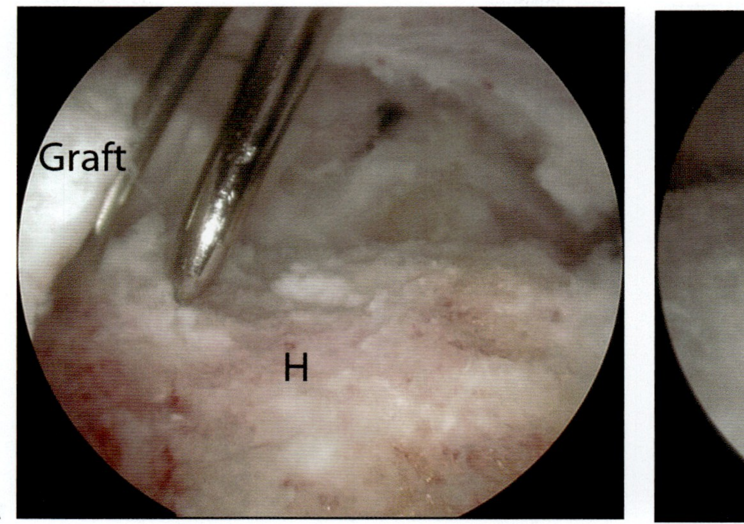

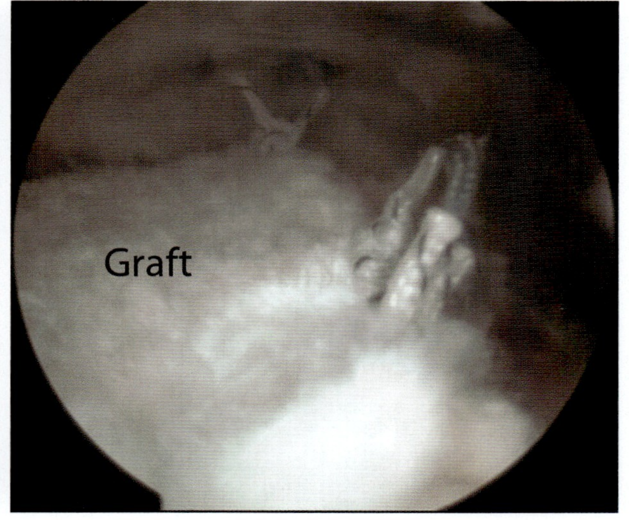

Figure 7.39 **A:** Right shoulder, posterior subacromial viewing portal. Using a spinal needle as a guide, a punch creates a bone socket for anchors in the proximal humerus that will be used to secure the lateral margin of a dermal allograft. **B:** Same shoulder. Sutures have been passed and tied to secure the lateral graft margin to the proximal humerus. H, humerus.

proceeds laterally, it is important to account for any previously placed suture anchors with remaining sutures that may be used for side-to-side stitches or for direct graft attachment to bone.

The final step is to secure the graft to bone. Depending on the size of the graft, the size of the greater tuberosity, and the number of previously placed anchors, the number of anchors may vary, but two or three anchors are usually used to secure the graft. In the central portion of the graft, we generally only use double-loaded anchors (5.5-mm Bio-Composite Corkscrew FT) since triple-loaded anchors tend to draw too much graft toward a single point, wrinkling the graft. Suture anchor positioning is carefully planned in the greater tuberosity. Depending on the resting length of the graft, anchor positioning is usually into the midpoint of the medial-to-lateral dimension of the greater tuberosity.

Anchors are then inserted into the greater tuberosity in the same manner as for a standard rotator cuff repair (Fig. 7.39). Sutures are subsequently passed using the Scorpion. Prior to tying the sutures, multiple puncture holes are placed in the greater tuberosity both medially and laterally using an anchor punch or a motorize PowerPick (Arthrex, Inc., Naples, FL) to maximize marrow infiltration of the dermal allograft. Care is taken to ensure that anchor fixation is not compromised. The final repair is evaluated for coverage, fixation, and tension (Fig. 7.40).

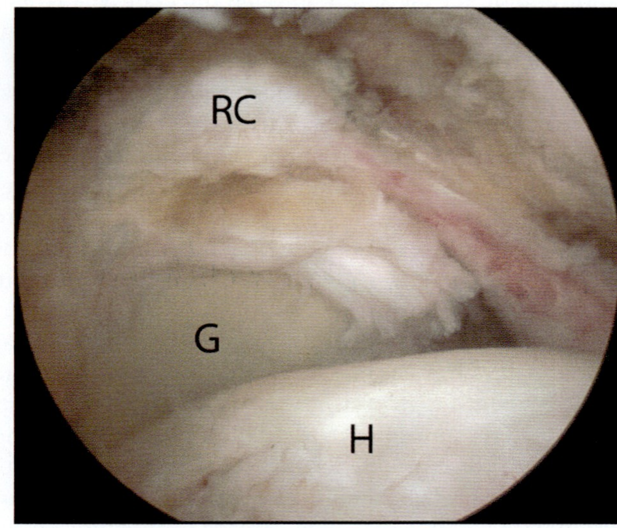

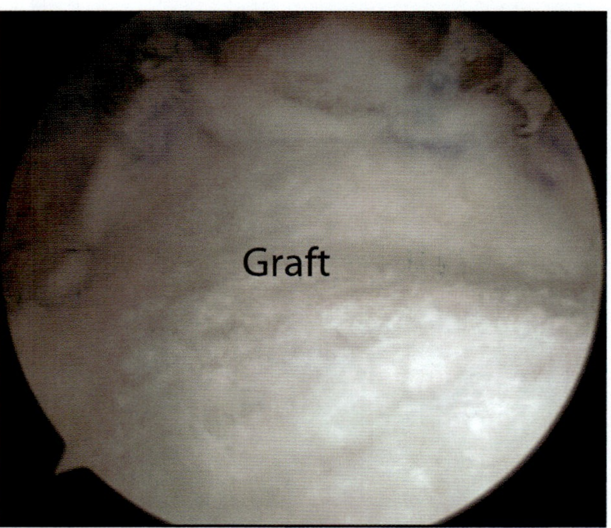

Figure 7.40 Right shoulder, lateral subacroimal viewing portal, demonstrates **(A)** initial appearance of a massive rotator cuff tear, and **(B)** appearance postreplacement with a dermal allograft. G, glenoid; H, humerus; RC, rotator cuff.

ALLOGRAFT AUGMENTATION

We consider allograft reinforcement of reparable rotator cuff tears in young nonsmokers with massive tears, poor tendon mobility, poor inherent tissue quality, or previous failed rotator cuff repair. Significant radiographic evidence of cuff tear arthropathy is a contraindication to allograft augmentation.

In many cases, the tear configuration will be a U- or L-shape, requiring margin convergence sutures, and full footprint coverage will not be obtained. Standard arthroscopic rotator cuff principles are utilized to repair the rotator cuff tear. However, in preparation for the graft, triple-loaded anchors (5.5-mm BioComposite Corkscrew FT) are utilized. From each anchor, two suture limbs are used to secure the rotator cuff with the remaining suture to be used to secure the graft.

Once the rotator cuff repair has been completed, the integrity of the repair, size of the repair area, and footprint coverage are assessed. Generally, the size of the graft required is smaller than that required for a replacement allograft since the graft will essentially cover the repair area only.

Sizing the Graft

Prior to sizing the graft, mattress stitches are placed anteriorly and posteriorly and medially along the medial extent of the repair site. Usually, two stitches are required for medial fixation and are eventually passed as mattress stitches to secure the graft. In larger grafts, a combination of simple stitches and mattress stitches may be used to secure the graft.

While viewing through a lateral subacromial portal, a crescent-shaped SutureLasso is introduced through the posterior portal and penetrates the tendon in a mattress fashion. The Nitinol loop is retrieved through the anterior portal and a #2 FiberWire suture is shuttled through the tendon. The process is repeated for the second suture. These sutures will define the medial extent of the graft (Fig. 7.41)

Using the technique as described previously, the size and shape of the graft required is then estimated using a knotted #1 PDS suture. The size of the graft required is measured anteriorly, posteriorly, medially, and laterally. For example, to measure the medial dimension, the subacromial space is viewed through a lateral portal. A grasper is used to hold the #1 PDS suture over the anterior stitch while a second grasper is used to hold the #1 PDS suture over the posterior stitch. The length of the proposed graft medially can then be measured extracorporeally as described above. The same steps are performed for the anterior, posterior, and lateral margins of the proposed graft with referencing off the medial stitches and anchor sites.

Graft Preparation

The graft is carefully prepared according to its planned suture configuration.

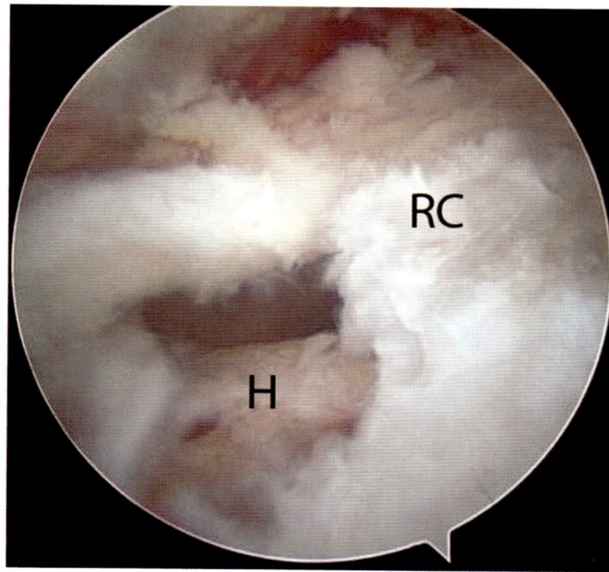

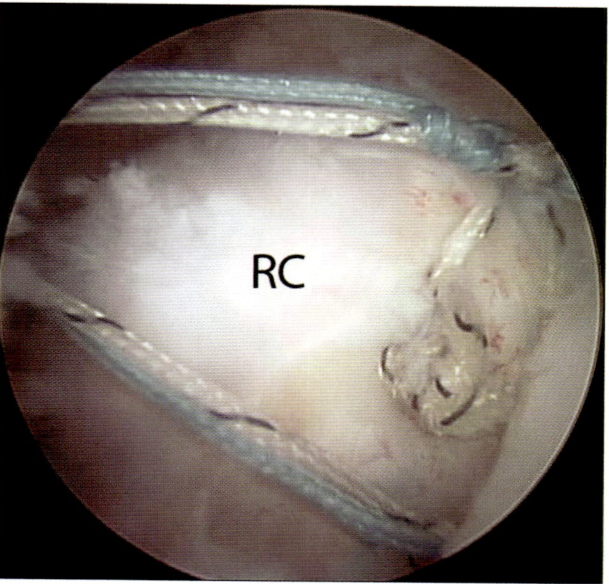

Figure 7.41 **A:** Left shoulder, lateral subacromial viewing portal, demonstrates a rotator cuff tear with poor quality tissue and lateral tendon loss status-post previous attempt at repair. **B:** Same shoulder viewed from a posterior subacromial portal demonstrates medial sutures that have been placed and tied as mattress stitches in preparation for dermal allograft augmentation. H, humerus; RC, rotator cuff.

When preparing the graft laterally, it is important to also determine if simple or mattress sutures will be used to secure the graft. There is usually minimal greater tuberosity available to place further lateral anchors and therefore the residual anchor sutures must be used to secure the graft laterally.

Shuttling the Graft

Unlike the allograft reconstruction for replacement whereby only the medial sutures are retrieved to shuttle the graft into the subacromial space, when performing an augmentation procedure the sutures that will secure the four corners of the graft are sequentially retrieved through a lateral 8.25-mm cannula. The orientation and organization of the sutures is kept in reference to the rotator cuff tear (i.e., anteromedial sutures in the anteromedial aspect of the cannula, etc.). This will help organize the sutures and limit suture tangling.

These sutures are then extracorporeally passed through the graft using a straight needle or a Scorpion suture passer (Fig. 7.42). When passing mattress sutures through the graft, it is critical to ensure that the sutures are not wrapped or twisted. To avoid this, each suture limb should be individually retrieved while maintaining its orientation in order to unravel any twists. A standard knot pusher may also be passed over the suture to confirm that it is not tangled.

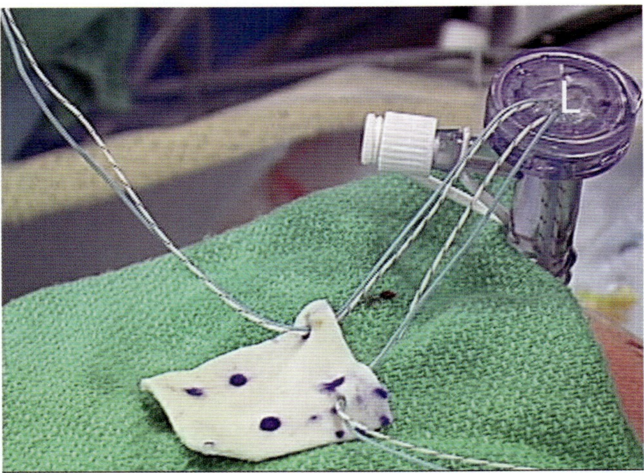

Figure 7.42 External view demonstrates sutures that exit a lateral subacromial portal (L) and have been passed through a dermal allograft in preparation for augmentation of a rotator cuff repair.

Once the four corner stitches have been passed through the graft, the orientation and organization of the graft and sutures is confirmed. A grasper is used to advance the graft down the suture limbs, through the cannula and into the subacromial space. When using mattress stitches, the graft must be "slid" down the sutures reducing it against the rotator cuff repair site (Fig. 7.43).

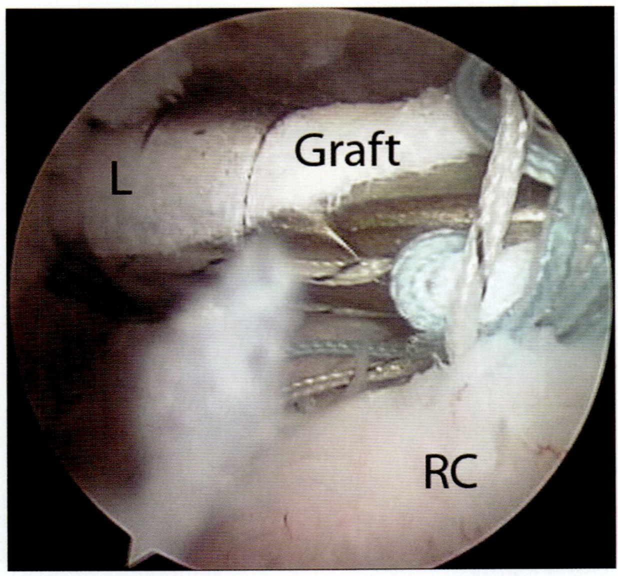

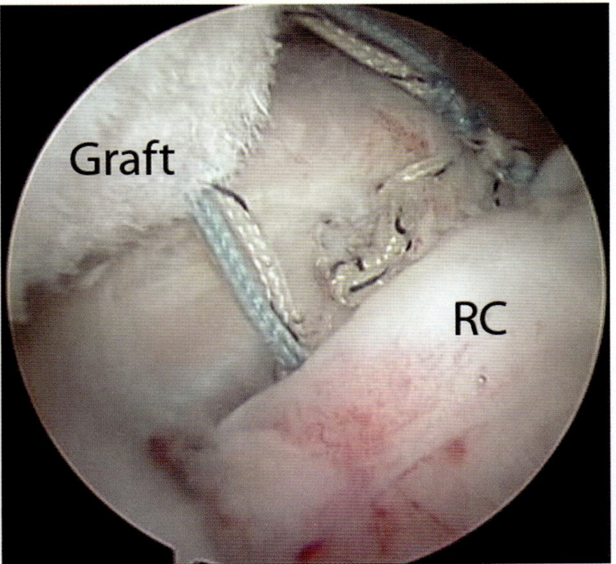

Figure 7.43 Left shoulder, posterior subacromial viewing portal, demonstrates shuttling a dermal allograft for augmentation of a rotator cuff repair. **A:** A grasper is used to push the allograft into the subacromial space via a lateral portal. **B:** The graft is pushed down until it is near the rotator cuff margin.

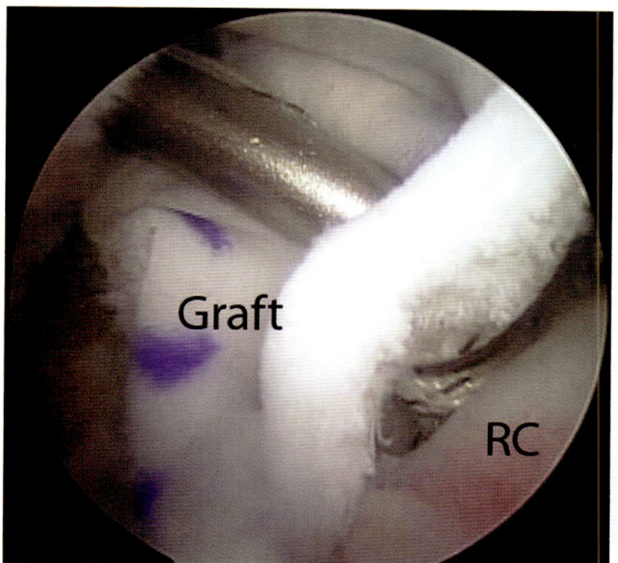

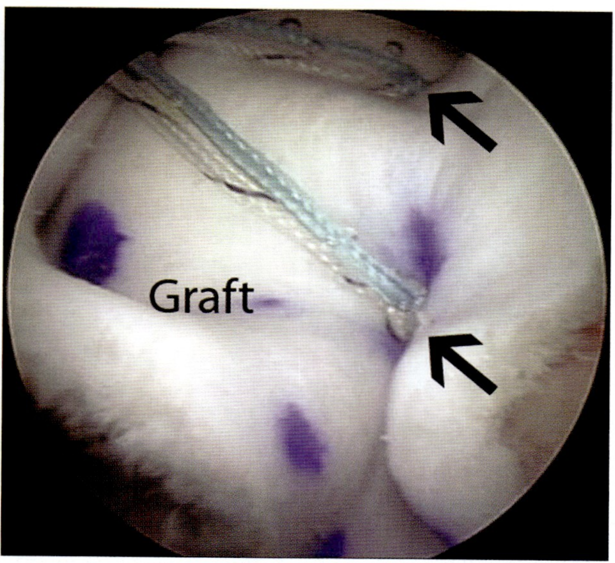

Figure 7.43 *(Continued)* **C:** A knot pusher assists in apposing the graft to the rotator cuff. **D:** The graft has been pushed through previously tied medial mattress knots (*black arrows*) so that the graft rests firmly on the rotator cuff. L, lateral portal; RC, rotator cuff.

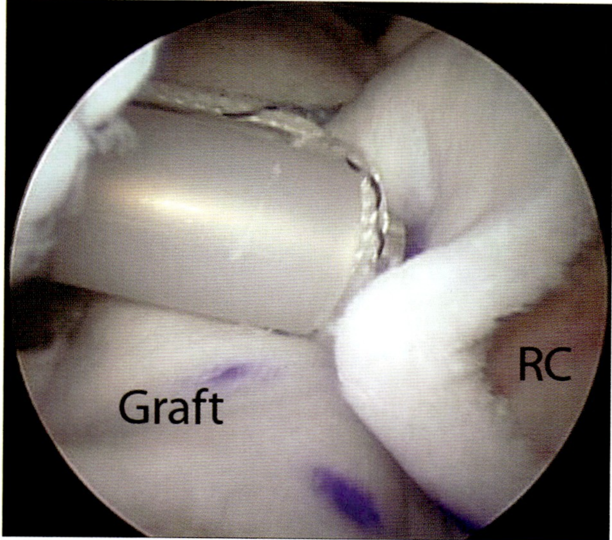

Figure 7.44 Left shoulder, posterior subacromial vieiwng portal. After the graft is opposed to the rotator cuff, suture limbs from the anterior and posterior shuttling sutures are tied together to secure the medial margin of the graft to the lateral rotator cuff margin. RC, rotator cuff.

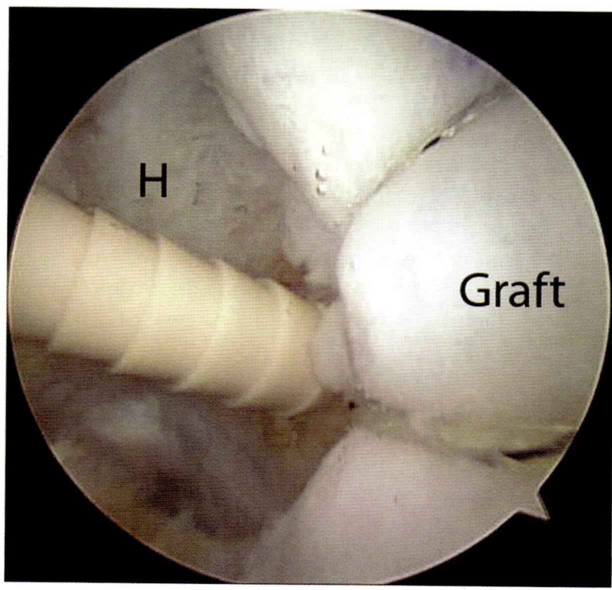

Figure 7.45 Left shoulder, posterior subacromial viewing portal, demonstrates use of PushLock anchor (Arthrex, Inc., Naples, FL) to secure the lateral margin of a dermal allograft. H, humerus.

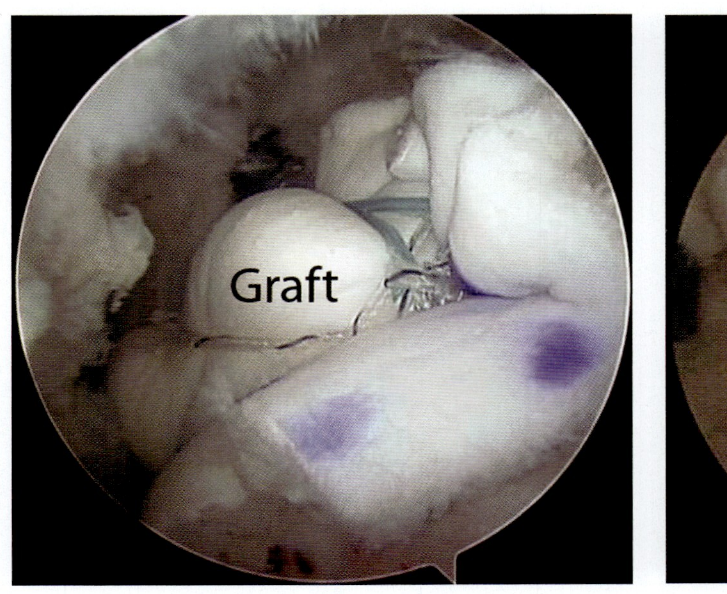

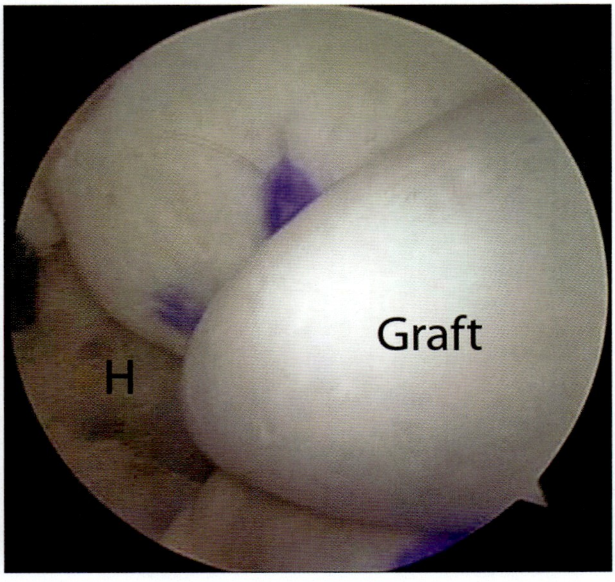

Figure 7.46 **A:** Left shoulder, posterior viewing portal with a 70° arthroscope, demonstrates a profile of the final appearance of a rotator cuff repair with dermal allograft augmenation. **B:** Up-close view demostrates the lateral margin that has been secured to the proximal humerus with knotless anchors. H, humerus.

Securing the Graft

Once the graft has been reduced to the tendon, sutures are sequentially tied. We generally tie sutures starting medially and progressing laterally (Fig. 7.44). The lateral sutures are then tied through the lateral cannula while viewing through a posterior portal. Initial graft fixation is then assessed.

The edges of the graft are then secured. Simple stitches may be used to secure the anterior and posterior margins of the graft. While viewing through the posterior portal, a 45° SutureLasso or Scorpion suture passer is used to penetrate the graft through a prepunctured hole and then passed through the rotator cuff tendon. A #2 FiberWire suture is then shuttled through and tied. The procedure is repeated for the anterior edge. Alternatively, the graft can be secured laterally with knotless anchors similar to a SutureBridge technique (Arthrex, Inc., Naples, FL) (Fig. 7.45).

Prior to closure, bone vents are placed into the footprint to encourage marrow infiltration as described above. Final construct demonstrates coverage of the repair site and fixation of the graft (Fig. 7.46).

REFERENCES

1. Davidson J, Burkhart SS. The geometric classification of rotator cuff tears: a system linking tear pattern to treatment and prognosis. *Arthroscopy*. 2010;26:417–424.
2. Davidson JF, Burkhart SS, Richards DP, Campbell SE. Use of preoperative magnetic resonance imaging to predict rotator cuff tear pattern and method of repair. *Arthroscopy*. 2005;21:1428.
3. Burkhart SS, Barth JR, Richards DP, Zlatkin MB, Larsen M. Arthroscopic repair of massive rotator cuff tears with stage 3 and 4 fatty degeneration. *Arthroscopy*. 2007;23:347–354.

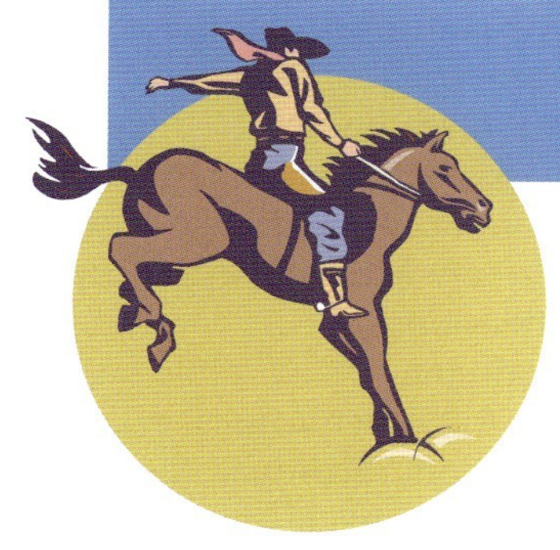

8

Arthroscopic Revision Rotator Cuff Repair

WESTERN WISDOM

A man who looks for easy work goes to bed tired.

In general, the results of open revision rotator cuff repair after failure of the initial surgery have been poor. However, the reports of arthroscopic revision rotator cuff repair have been much better than those of open revision. We first reported our results of arthroscopic revision in 2004 (1), and subsequent authors have reported similarly encouraging results (2,3). We also recently completed a study of 74 revision rotator cuff repairs, the majority of which were massive tears, with a mean follow-up of 63 months (1). Despite the fact that most of these recurrent tears were massive tears, the majority of patients achieved a good or excellent functional outcome and 78% of patients were satisfied with the revision repair. In our opinion, all revision repairs of the rotator cuff should be done arthroscopically.

CAUSES OF FAILURE

There are three broad categories of patients that require a second surgery after the initial rotator cuff repair:

1. Patients with pathology that was missed in the first surgery (e.g., missed subscapularis tear).
2. Patients with postoperative stiffness. These patients almost always have complete healing of the rotator cuff, and they do well with arthroscopic capsular release and subacromial lysis of adhesions (4).
3. Patients with structural failure of the repair. This structural failure occurs for one of three reasons:
    a. Biomechanical failure due to inadequate strength of the repair construct
    b. Biologic failure to heal despite strong fixation
    c. Aggressive postoperative rehabilitation causing structural failure of the repair construct

The rest of this chapter will deal with patients who have structural failure after rotator cuff repair.

CLINICAL EVALUATION

When structural failure occurs, the surgeon must decide if further surgery is indicated. A structural failure does not always result in a clinical failure. Many patients with partial healing of the cuff and a residual defect will be much better after surgery, and in these patients, nothing needs to be done. In general, patients who still have disabling pain and weakness at 9 to 12 months after surgery should be evaluated for possible revision repair.

The clinical examination is important. Active and passive range of motion are measured. We define *pseudoparalysis* as active elevation of <90° in a patient who has full overhead passive elevation in association with an unstable glenohumeral fulcrum; that is, there is a significant discrepancy between active and passive elevation along with the potential for anterosuperior glenohumeral escape. In primary repair cases, we have found that patients with pseudoparalysis will regain overhead motion after repair in 89% of cases (Unpublished Data). However, pseudoparalysis after a failed primary cuff repair is a poor prognostic sign, and many patients in that category with a massive rotator cuff tear will never regain overhead motion with a second surgery. In the setting of revision for massive rotator cuff tears, we have found that 43% of patients with preoperative pseudoparalysis regain active elevation to 90° or greater (Unpublished Data). In our experience, even if a patient does not regain overhead motion after revision cuff repair, function may still be greatly improved below shoulder level if subscapularis function is restored. The subscapularis is very important in personal hygiene, as it is essential for achieving enough internal rotation for independent toileting as well as for obtaining enough horizontal adduction to reach across the body and wash under the opposite axilla. These functions are essential to anyone who lives alone and wishes to be independent. Therefore, evaluation of subscapularis function (bear-hug, belly-press, Napoleon, and lift-off tests) is very important.

Another poor prognostic category is the patient who, after the initial cuff repair, cannot externally rotate to neutral (0°) with the arm at the side. These people will usually have a pseudoparalysis and often will not regain overhead function with a second repair.

If active and passive elevation are limited to the same degree, this is not pseudoparalysis. These patients are typically restricted by capsular contracture and subacromial adhesions and will generally do very well with arthroscopic capsular release and lysis of adhesions.

Imaging studies are important. Plain radiographs should be taken to evaluate for other causes of pain (e.g., chondrolysis, loose anchors, acromial fracture). An MRI scan is important, but the surgeon must not be fooled by the postoperative changes and artifacts that may occur in these patients. For example, an MRI scan taken at 3 months postoperatively can still show large areas of tendon that are undergoing revascularization that can look like a recurrent tear when the tendon is actually intact (Fig. 8.1). Also, we have found that the third-generation high-strength sutures can cause significant artifact that can

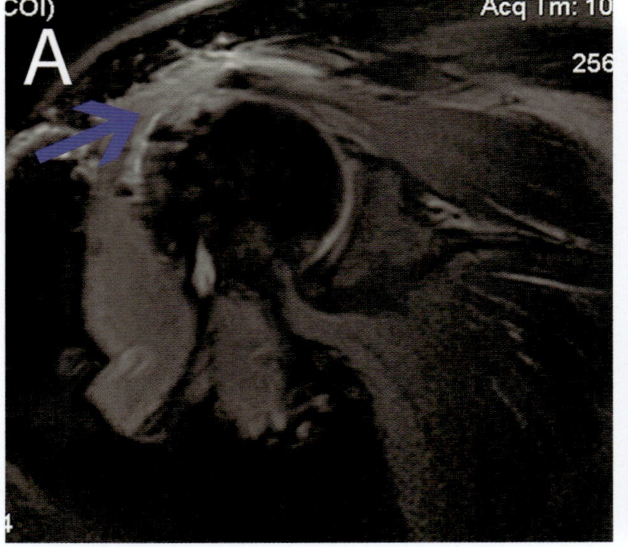

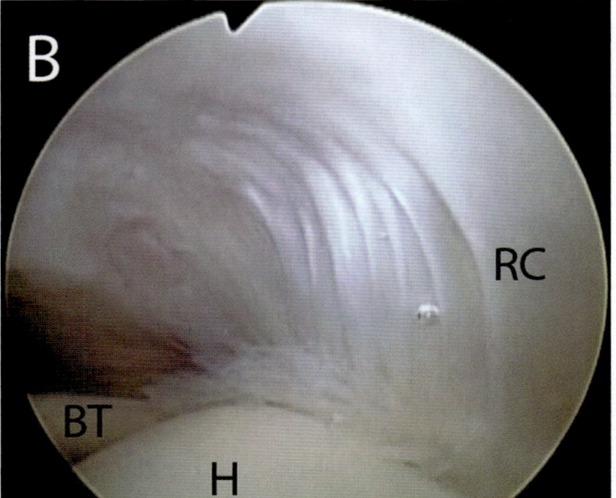

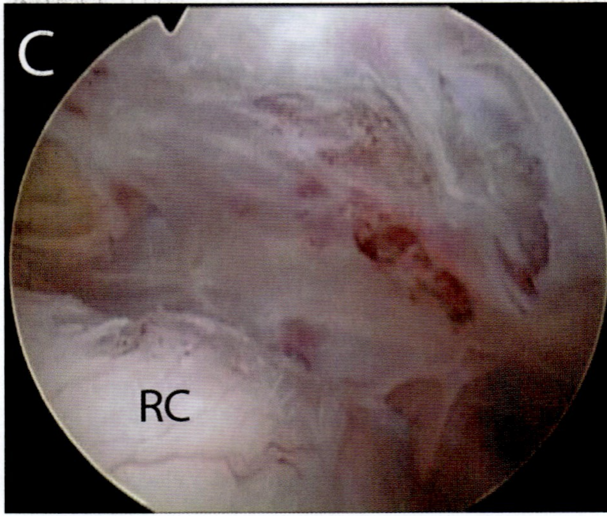

Figure 8.1 **A:** Three-month postoperative coronal magnetic resonance image of a right shoulder demonstrates revascularization (*blue arrow*) that was interpreted as a recurrent rotator cuff tear. Arthroscopic view of the same shoulder from **(B)** posterior glenohumeral and **(C)** posterior subacromial viewing portals, demonstrate a healed rotator cuff. BT, biceps tendon; H, humerus; RC, rotator cuff.

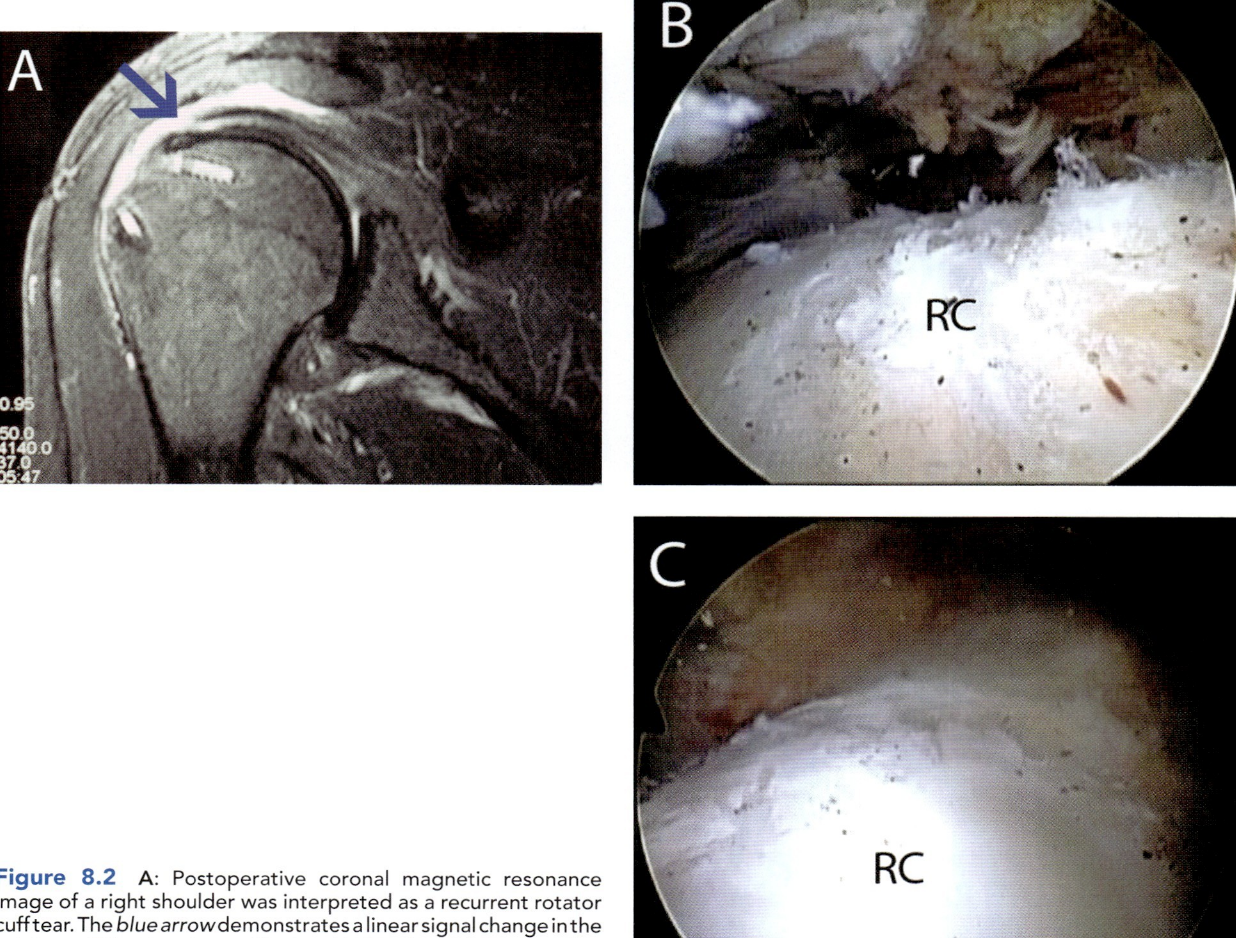

Figure 8.2 A: Postoperative coronal magnetic resonance image of a right shoulder was interpreted as a recurrent rotator cuff tear. The *blue arrow* demonstrates a linear signal change in the rotator cuff that is suture artifact and led to the misinterpretation by a radiologist. Arthroscopic views in the same shoulder from (B) posterior and (C) lateral subacromial portals demonstrate a healed rotator cuff. RC, rotator cuff.

mimic a small recurrent cuff tear, when in fact the cuff is intact (Fig. 8.2).

The T-1 parasagittal MRI cuts are important for evaluating muscle quality, but the cuts must be taken far enough medially to transect the muscle belly, particularly in a retracted tear. Previous authors have recommended that if fatty infiltration is ≥50% of the muscle cross section, then rotator cuff repair should not be done since the patient will not improve with surgery (5). However, our experience has been notably different. We have found that most patients with fatty infiltration of the supraspinatus or infraspinatus of up to 75% will improve at least one grade in strength after cuff repair, so we routinely operate on patients with up to 75% fatty infiltration (6). The subscapularis is an exception to all the rules, as much of its function derives from a tenodesis effect. We have observed complete healing on MRI as well as reversal of pseudoparalysis in patients with 100% fatty infiltration of the subscapularis.

Another consideration in the preoperative imaging studies is to evaluate for the amount of "real estate" in the bone bed of the greater tuberosity that is available for additional suture anchor placement. If large numbers of anchors are already present, or if cystic cavitation has occurred around the anchors, then the surgeon may have to remove some or all of the existing anchors and bone graft the defects (Fig. 8.3). We prefer to do arthroscopic grafting with allograft bone chips packed into an OATS harvester (Arthrex, Inc., Naples, FL). Since it is often difficult to tell how much "good bone" is actually left in the greater tuberosity, we routinely discuss the possible necessity of an allograft bone graft and obtain patient consent to do this in all revision cases.

Finally, the MRI will usually indicate if the supraspinatus and infraspinatus are adhesed to the undersurface of the

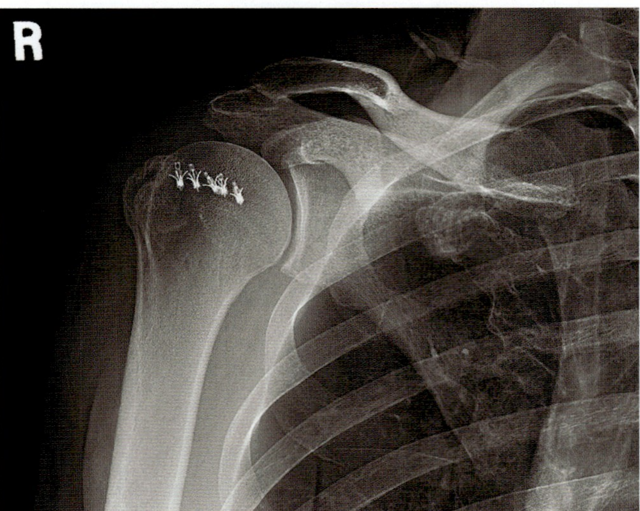

Figure 8.3 Preoperative radiograph of a right shoulder demonstrates multiple metallic anchors from a previous failed repair. In this scenario, bone grafting at the time of revision is often required.

acromion. This is important to determine because we have found that, in the case of extensive tendon adhesion to the acromion, we almost always have to do a modified double-interval slide in order to gain enough lateral excursion of the tendons to reach the bone bed.

ARTHROSCOPIC STEPWISE APPROACH TO REVISION CUFF REPAIR

Overview of Steps

Doing a revision repair of a massive rotator cuff tear can be a daunting undertaking, with hundreds of individual steps involved in the procedure. Therefore it is useful to break down the project into its seven basic components:

1. Biceps tenotomy, or tenotomy plus whipstitch preparation for tenodesis
2. Subscapularis work (dissection and three-sided release, coracoplasty, lesser tuberosity preparation, and repair)
3. Biceps tenodesis
4. Dissection and excavation of bony landmarks (acromion, AC joint, and scapular spine), posterior gutter, and lateral gutter
5. Dissection and excavation of supraspinatus and infraspinatus, if necessary
6. Soft tissue releases (anterior interval slide in-continuity, posterior interval slide), if necessary
7. Repair of posterior and superior rotator cuff

The simplistic way of thinking about revision repair of a massive cuff tear is that we begin our repair anteriorly, with the subscapularis, and gradually work our way posteriorly. Naturally, not all revisions involve massive tears, but since massive tears retear at a higher rate than small tears, the majority of revision repairs will be in massive tears.

If the revision is being done for a small- or a medium-sized retear, the situation is usually much easier. We first do an intra-articular arthroscopy and subacromial bursoscopy and identify the tear. If needed, we do an arthroscopic capsular release and subacromial lysis of adhesions (see technique in Chapter 21, "Shoulder Stiffness"). Then we repair the tear by standard techniques. If possible, we prefer linked double-row footprint reconstruction by SutureBridge or SpeedBridge techniques, but if there is tendon loss or insufficient excursion of the tendon, we do a single-row repair.

For the large and massive revision repairs, it is instructive to take an in-depth step-by-step look at the seven basic components of revision cuff repair.

Addressing the Biceps

A posterior viewing portal is established. In all revision cases that involve the subscapularis, we do an arthroscopic biceps tenotomy or tenodesis. If the patient is low demand, particularly if the arm is fat enough that a "Popeye" deformity would not be noticeable, we do a tenotomy. In the younger patient, the high-demand patient, or the patient in whom cosmesis is important, we do a biceps tenodesis at the top of the bicipital groove with a BioComposite Tenodesis screw (Arthrex, Inc., Naples, FL) and incorporate the suture limbs from that construct into the rotator cuff repair. When a biceps tenodesis is to be done, we first place half-racking sutures in the biceps arthroscopically, then do a biceps tenotomy. The half-racking sutures are then used to deliver the biceps tendon extracorporeally for placement of a whipstitch (Fig. 8.4). The tendon is then allowed to retract back into the shoulder, where it rests out of the way laterally while the subscapularis work is done.

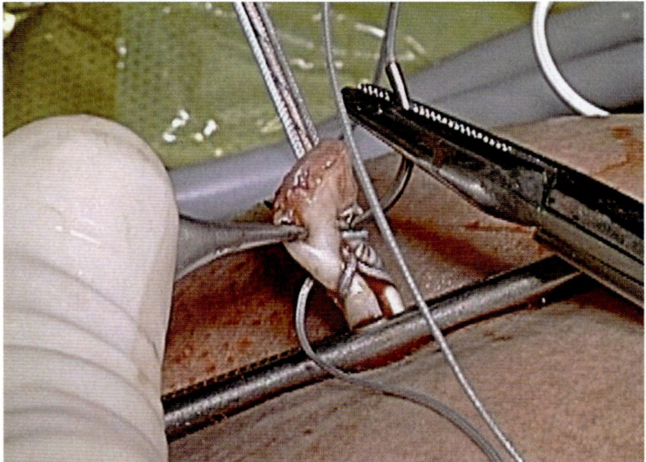

Figure 8.4 External photo demonstrating placement of a whipstitch in preparation for biceps tenodesis.

Addressing the Subscapularis and Related Structures

All of the dissection and preparation of the subscapularis, the coracoid, and the lesser tuberosity are performed through an anterosuperolateral working portal. This portal is established from outside-in while viewing the lesser tuberosity through a posterior viewing portal with a 70° arthroscope. The working portal is established so that its angle of approach into the lesser tuberosity is 5° to 10° (Fig. 8.5).

Then, the arthroscope is switched to a 30° scope while searching for and identifying the subscapularis tendon and the coracoid. Failure to switch to a 30° scope at this juncture can cause the surgeon to wander too far inferiorly while searching for the coracoid tip through a window in the rotator interval.

If the subscapularis tendon is not immediately visible at the front of the joint, it is probably retracted medially to the level of the glenoid margin. It can usually be located by placing the tip of a blunt instrument (e.g., a switching stick introduced through an anterosuperolateral portal) into the soft tissue adjacent to the glenoid rim at the level of the midglenoid notch. The midglenoid notch is the level at which the upper border of the subscapularis tendon usually crosses transversely (Fig. 8.6A). The tip of the switching stick is used to hook into the junction where the superolateral border of the subscapularis tendon joins the *comma tissue* at approximately a right angle (Fig. 8.6B, C). The *comma* is the residual portion of the medial sling that had been attached to the lesser tuberosity adjacent to the subscapularis footprint. In rare circumstances, the comma sign is not identifiable due to significant scarring. In this scenario, a window is created just anterior to the glenoid above the midglenoid notch and dissection is carried medially to the base of the coracoid where the subscapularis can be reliably identified (Fig. 8.7).

The junction of the *comma* with the superolateral subscapularis tendon is an important landmark. Once this junction is identified, we use a Scorpion or a Viper (Arthrex, Inc., Naples, FL) antegrade suture passer to place a traction suture through the superolateral subscapularis tendon just medial to the comma (Fig. 8.8). While pulling laterally on the traction suture, we use the power shaver and electrocautery probe to make a window in the rotator interval, just medial to the comma and just superior to the subscapularis (Fig. 8.9). The coracoid tip and coracoid neck typically are just anterior to the window that is made in the rotator interval, and they will be visible through that window (Fig. 8.10). Until now, the shaver and cautery probe have passed posterior to the comma tissue to create the window and expose the coracoid. However, at this point, we withdraw the shaver and redirect its approach to the coracoid by going anterior to the *comma* (Fig. 8.11). This gives better access to the entire posterolateral coracoid.

Next, we begin our three-sided release of the subscapularis by skeletonizing the posterolateral coracoid. This is the "safe side" of the coracoid. Exposure is maximized by having our second assistant provide a *posterior level push* (Fig. 8.12). The coracoid tip and the lateral portion of the coracoid neck are dissected while viewing with a 30° arthroscope. Then, we switch to a 70° arthroscope for a more panoramic view of the coracoid. If the coracohumeral interval is <7 mm, as judged by the burr diameter of 5 mm, we perform a coracoplasty in the plane of the subscapularis tendon (Fig. 8.13).

For dissection of the coracoid base and the medial portion of the coracoid neck, we always use a 70° arthroscope. This affords a much wider field of view medially for skeletonizing the coracoid neck and coracoid base (Fig. 8.14).

Release of the superior border of subscapularis from the coracoid base is bluntly achieved with a 30° arthroscopic elevator (Fig. 8.15). The length of the blade of this elevator is approximately 8 mm, and this is always long enough because the adhesions between the coracoid and subscapularis tendon are always within the lateral 8 mm of the coracoid neck and base. Therefore, they can always be completely released by sweeping the blade of the 30° elevator from front to back under the coracoid neck and base. There is never a need to dissect any further medially than that, as the adhesions do not occur further medially. Dissection medial to the coracoid is potentially very dangerous due to the proximity of the neurovascular structures, and it is not necessary.

The next step in the three-sided release of the subscapularis is the posterior release. For this step, we switch back to a 30° arthroscope and use a 15° arthroscopic elevator

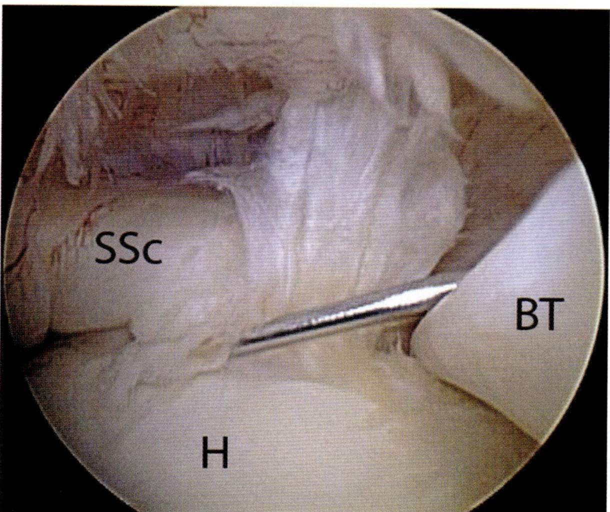

Figure 8.5 Right shoulder, posterior viewing portal with a 70° arthroscope demonstrates use of a spinal needle as a guide to create an anterosuperolateral working portal with a 5° to 10° angle of approach to the lesser tuberosity. BT, biceps tendon; H, humerus; SSc, subscapularis tendon.

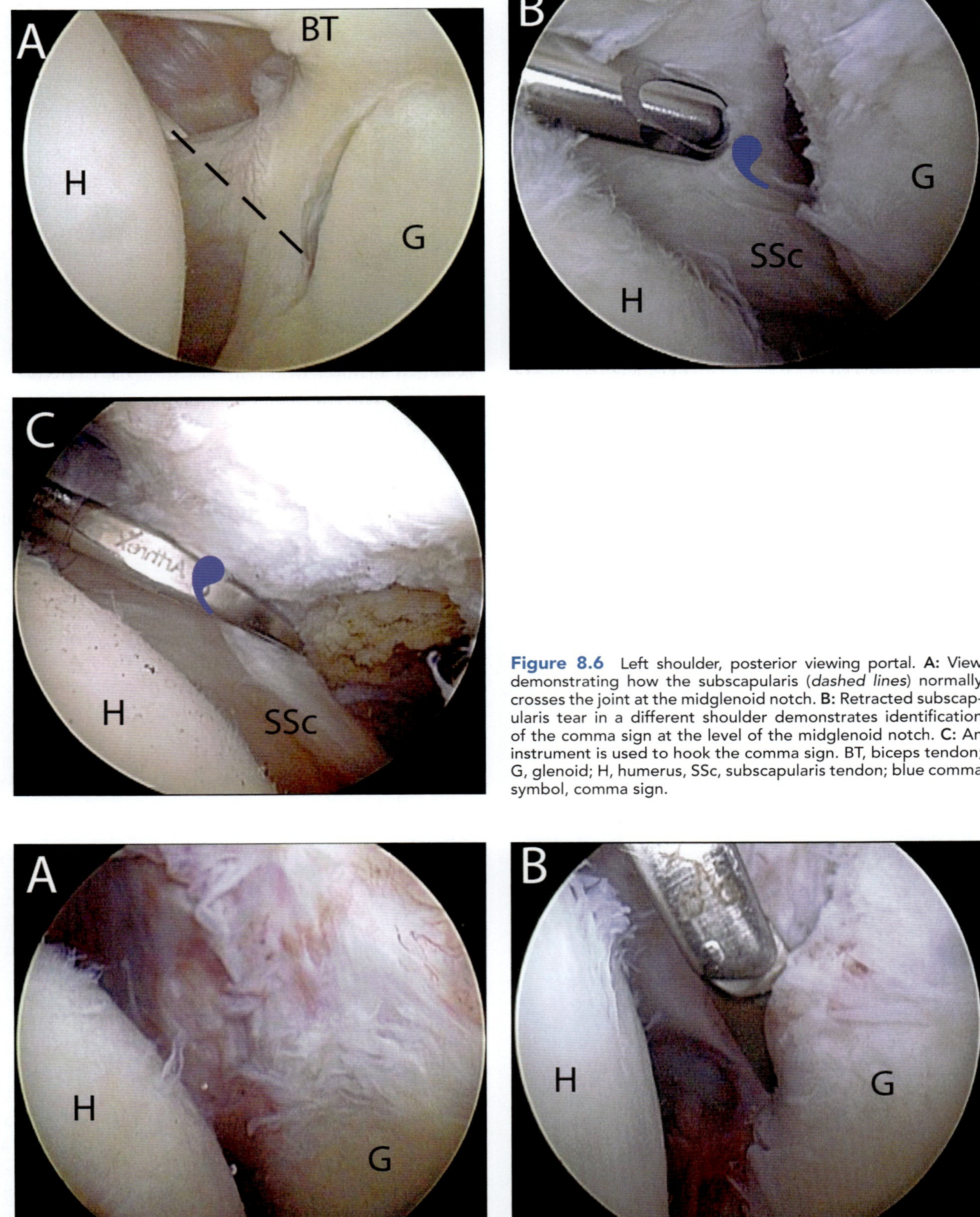

Figure 8.6 Left shoulder, posterior viewing portal. **A:** View demonstrating how the subscapularis (*dashed lines*) normally crosses the joint at the midglenoid notch. **B:** Retracted subscapularis tear in a different shoulder demonstrates identification of the comma sign at the level of the midglenoid notch. **C:** An instrument is used to hook the comma sign. BT, biceps tendon; G, glenoid; H, humerus, SSc, subscapularis tendon; blue comma symbol, comma sign.

Figure 8.7 Left shoulder, posterior viewing portal demonstrates excavation of retracted adhesed subscapularis tendon tear when the comma sign is not readily visible. **A:** In this retracted adhesed tear, the comma sign cannot be visualized. **B:** A window is created anterior to the glenoid above the midglenoid notch.

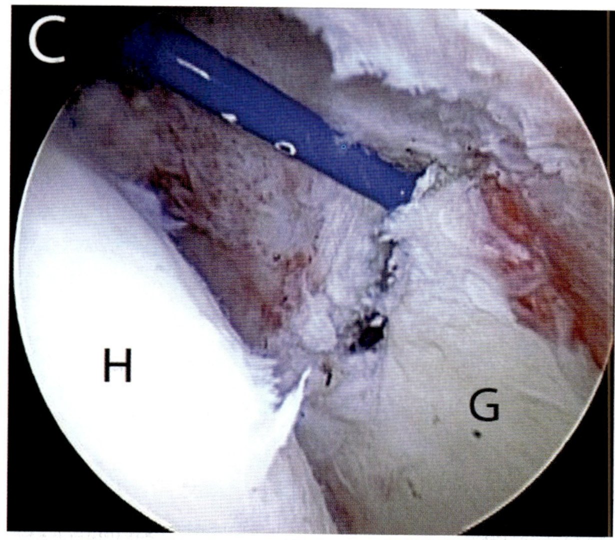

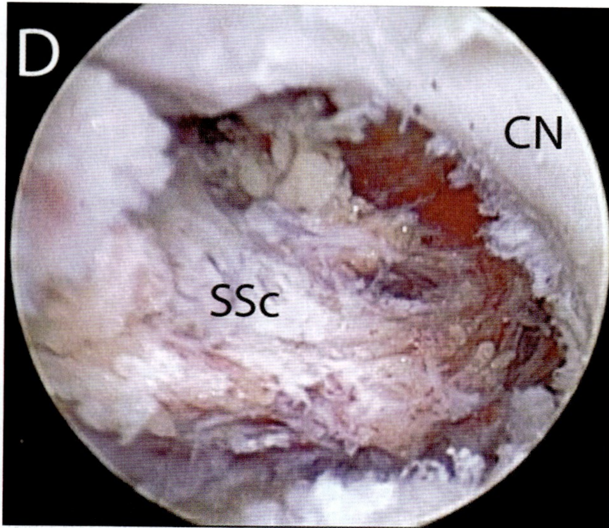

Figure 8.7 *(Continued)* **C:** Dissection is carried medially with an electrocautery device. **D:** View with a 70° arthroscope shows identification of the subscapularis tendon inferior to the coracoid neck. CN, coracoid neck. G, glenoid; H, humerus; SSc, subscapularis tendon.

to lyse the adhesions between the anterior glenoid neck and the posterior surface of the subscapularis. The elevator is introduced between the glenoid and the tendon and is used to blindly and bluntly lyse the adhesions in that plane. This plane is relatively avascular and is devoid of important neurovascular structures, so a blind release of adhesions there is quite safe.

After the three-sided release of the subscapularis has been completed, the surgeon will usually have accomplished the restoration of sufficient lateral excursion of the tendon to reach the bone bed on the lesser tuberosity. Then, the bone bed is prepared with a power shaver, power bur, and ring curettes to a bleeding base. If the tendon does not quite reach the anatomic bone bed, the bone bed can be medialized an additional 5 to 7 mm without adversely affecting function.

Using this technique, we have found that virtually 100% of subscapularis tears are repairable, and we have not found the need for tendon transfers to address the problem of the retracted subscapularis.

The repair of the subscapularis is accomplished with single-row or double-row suture bridge techniques,

(Text continued on page 174)

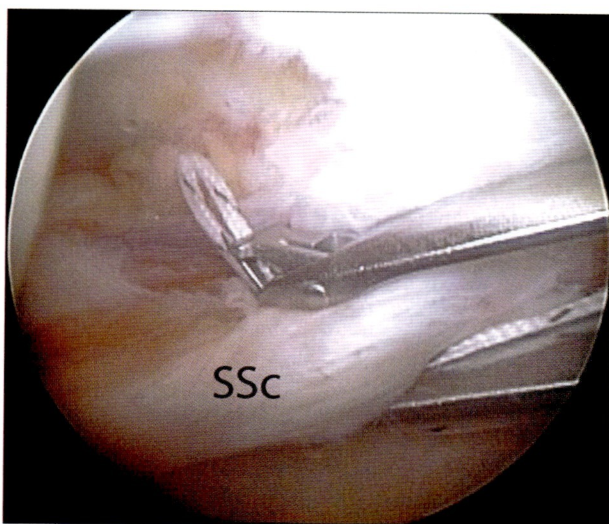

Figure 8.8 Right shoulder, posterior viewing portal demonstrates placement of a traction stitch in a retracted subscapularis tendon tear. SSc, subscapularis tendon.

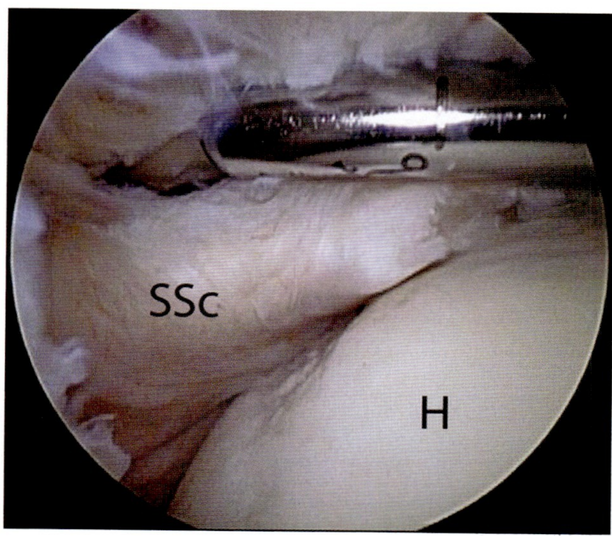

Figure 8.9 Right shoulder, posterior viewing portal demonstrates use of a shaver to create a window in the rotator interval. H, humerus; SSc, subscapularis tendon.

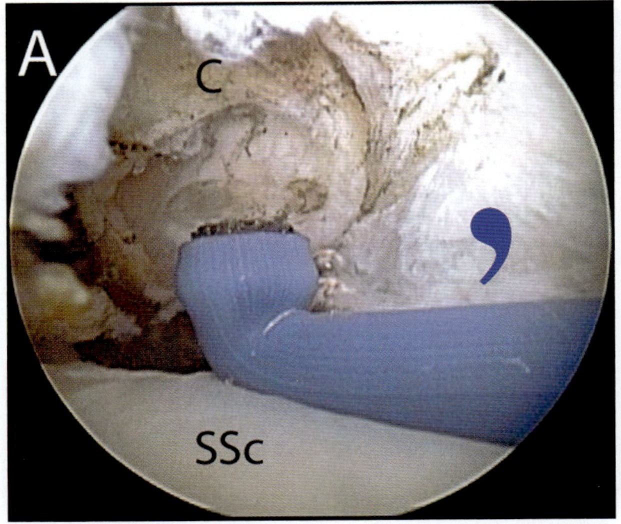

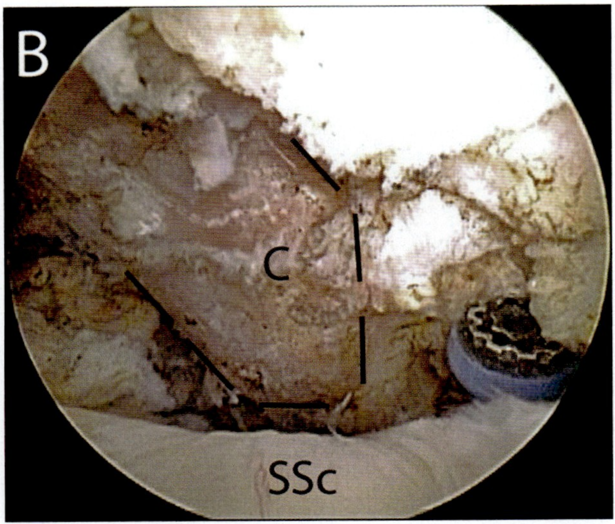

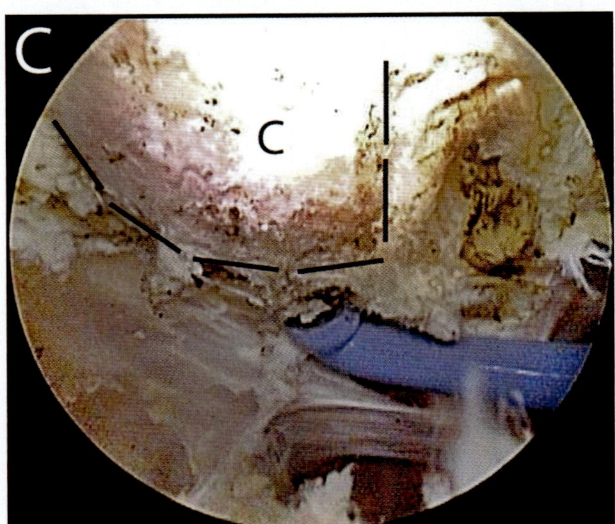

Figure 8.10 Identification of the coracoid tip in a right shoulder viewed from a posterior glenohumeral portal. **A:** With a 30° arthroscope, the coracoid tip is visible through a window that has been created in the rotator interval. **B:** The electrocautery is redirected to work anterior to the comma tissue and is used to skeletonize the posterolateral aspect of the coracoid tip (outlined by *dashed lines*). **C:** View with a 70° arthroscope of the completely skeletonized coracoid tip. C, coracoid tip; SSc, subscapularis tendon; blue comma symbol, comma sign.

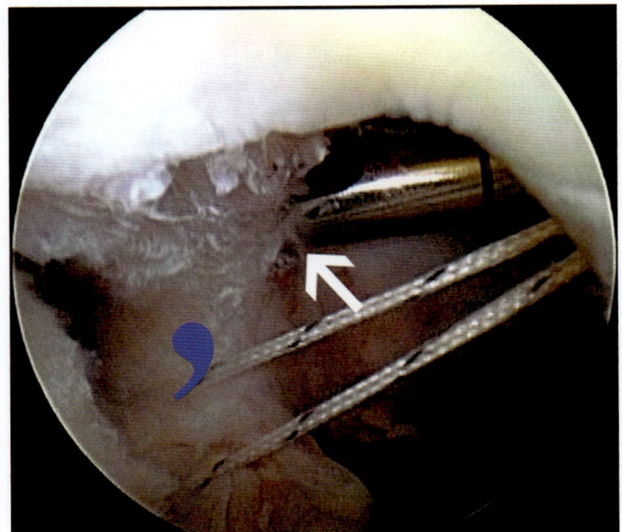

Figure 8.11 Right shoulder, posterior viewing portal. After a window is created in the rotator interval, the approach of an instrument is redirected (*white arrow*) to go anterior to the comma tissue (*blue comma symbol*) to gain better access to the subcoracoid space.

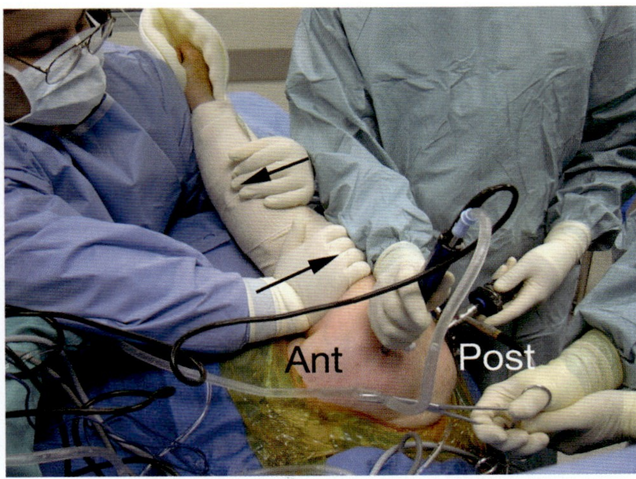

Figure 8.12 Posterior lever push. The second assistant simultaneously pushes the proximal humerus posteriorly and pulls the distal humerus anteriorly. This maneuver effectively increases the working space in the anterior shoulder as the humeral head is subluxed posteriorly.

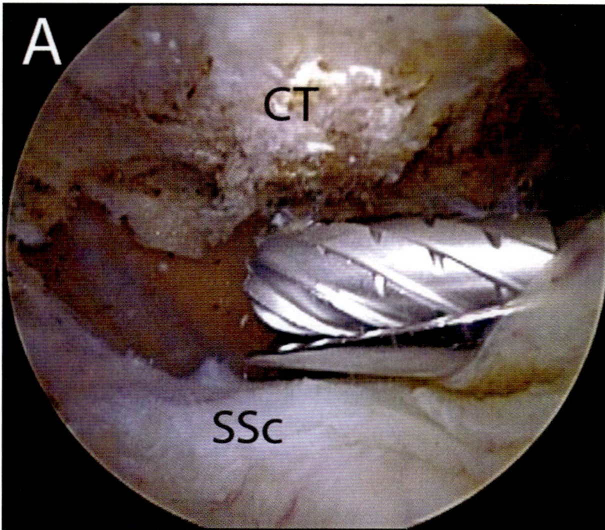

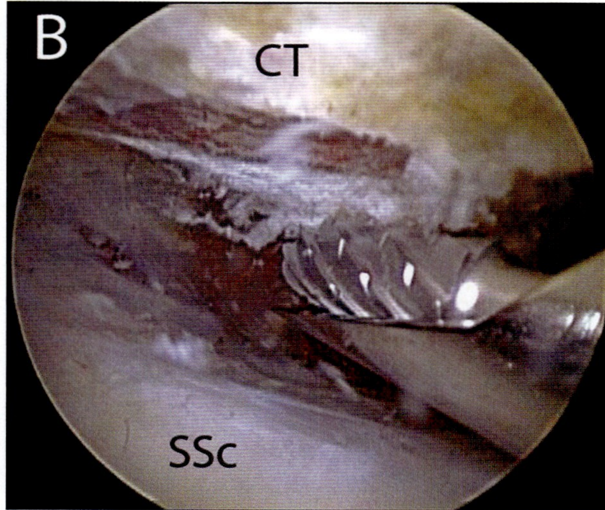

Figure 8.13 Evaluation of the coracohumeral interval in a right shoulder, viewed from a posterior glenohumeral portal. **A:** The native coracohumeral interval is estimated by comparison to the known width of an instrument. In this case, the width of the interval is approximately 6 mm. **B:** A coracoplasty is performed to create a coracohumeral interval of at least 7 mm. CT, coracoid tip; SSc, subscapularis tendon.

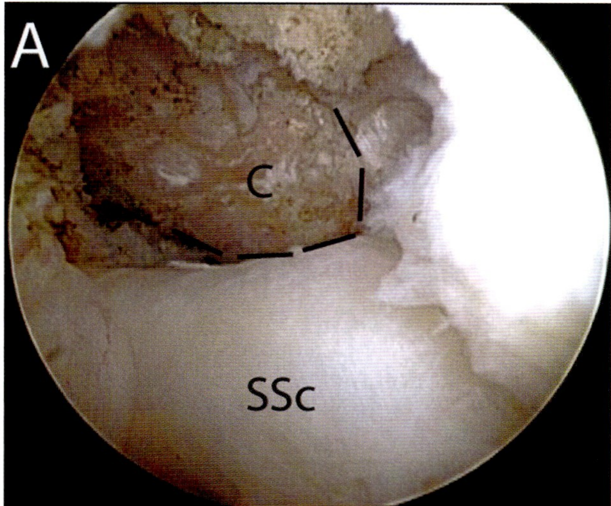

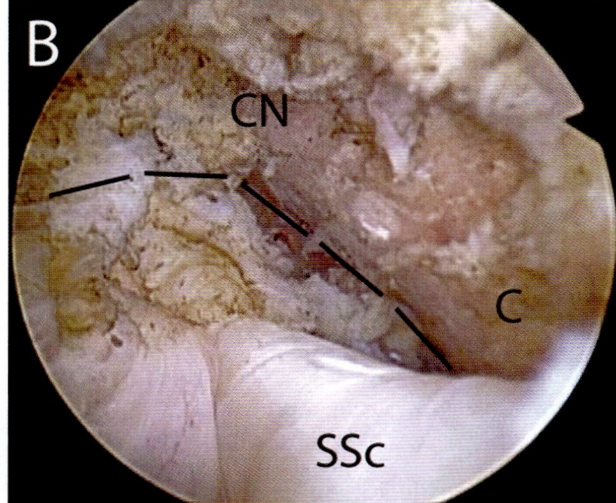

Figure 8.14 Comparative views of the coracoid with 30° and 70° arthroscopes in a right shoulder viewed from a posterior glenohumeral portal. **A:** With a 30° arthroscope, only the coracoid tip (outlined by *dashed lines*) is visible through a window created in the rotator interval. **B:** With a 70° arthroscope, a greater extent of the coracoid (inferior cortex outlined by *dashed lines*) can be seen. The medial border of the subscapularis tendon is also visible as it passes inferior to the coracoid. With this view and further dissection, the base of the coracoid can easily be exposed. C, coracoid tip; CN, coracoid neck; SSc, subscapularis tendon.

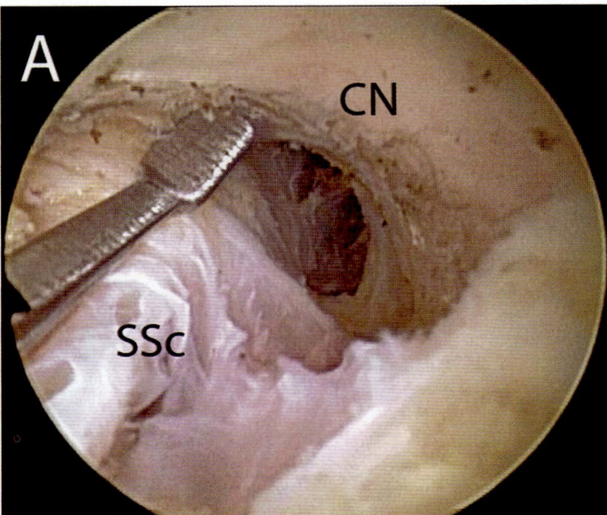

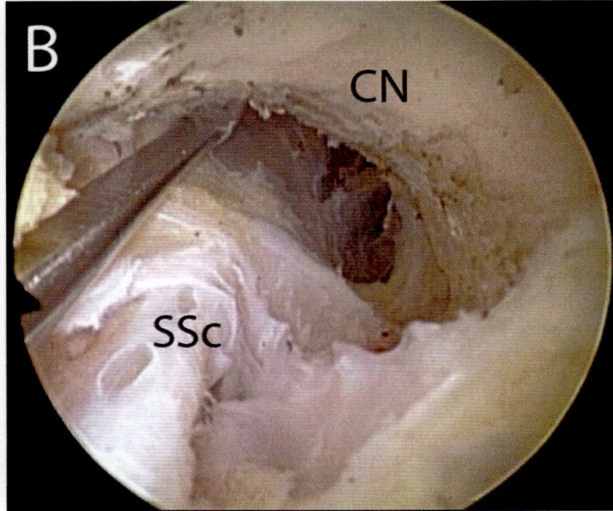

Figure 8.15 Superior release of a retracted adhesed subscapularis tendon tear in a left shoulder viewed from a posterior portal with a 70° arthroscope. **A:** A 30° elevator is introduced from an anterosuperolateral working portal. **B:** Adhesions between the superior subscapularis and the coracoid neck are released. The elevator is inserted only to the base of its blade, which is enough to release the adhesions to the coracoid. CN, coracoid neck; SSc, subscapularis tendon.

depending on the amount of lateral excursion of the tendon (see Chapter 6, "Subscapularis Tendon Tears").

Biceps Tenodesis

After subscapularis repair, we do biceps tenodesis in selected patients who satisfy our criteria for tenodesis rather than tenotomy. The biceps whipstitch has been previously placed, and it is used to retrieve and manipulate the tendon. We typically perform a tendon-to-bone tenodesis at the top of the bicipital groove, fixing the biceps with a BioComposite Tenodesis screw.

Excavation of Bone Landmarks and Posterior and Lateral Gutters

A systematic dissection of the bony landmarks is next carried out. We call this an *excavation* because we carefully preserve any nonfatty fibrous tissue that may contain remnants of rotator cuff.

A lateral subacromial portal is established. Then, the 30° arthroscope is inserted into this portal.

While viewing through the lateral portal, a very important maneuver is carried out, in which a 4.5-mm shaver is placed through the posterior portal, in a plane just below the acromion, and aimed just lateral to the scapular spine. When the scapular spine is palpated with the tip of the shaver, it is swept laterally, maintaining its plane just below the acromion, until the tip of the shaver blade penetrates through the fibrous tissue as it thins out laterally (Fig. 8.16A, B). This maneuver preserves whatever rotator cuff might have been encased within the scar tissue that had become adhesed to the acromion. The shaver blade then completes the dissection of the lateral edge of this soft tissue envelope from the acromion. The electrocautery probe and the power shaver are alternately used to skeletonize the undersurface of the acromion as far medially as the acromioclavicular (AC) joint and the scapular spine. The undersurface of the AC joint is skeletonized as is the scapular spine. The scapular spine is easily located by sweeping the shaver medially from the midacromion. In this location, the surgeon will feel a column of bone projecting inferomedially, and after further dissection will see that it resembles the keel of a boat (Fig. 8.16C). This is the scapular spine. As further verification of this structure, the surgeon may first locate the posterior aspect of the AC joint. The upper flare of the scapular spine can then be located several millimeters posterior to the AC joint (Fig. 8.17).

As mentioned, the scapular spine resembles the keel of a boat. The keel descends to a raphe that divides two muscle bellies: the supraspinatus anteriorly and the infraspinatus posteriorly. This is a useful anatomic relationship in determining tear pattern configuration, because the muscle fibers anterior to the scapular spine will be supraspinatus muscle fibers and those posterior to the scapular spine will be infraspinatus fibers.

After the bony landmarks have been skeletonized and the soft tissue envelope has been dissected off the acromion, there will still be a mass of indistinct soft tissue posteriorly where the infraspinatus is scarred to the posterior and posterolateral deltoid by means of projections of scar tissue that we call *bursal leaders*.

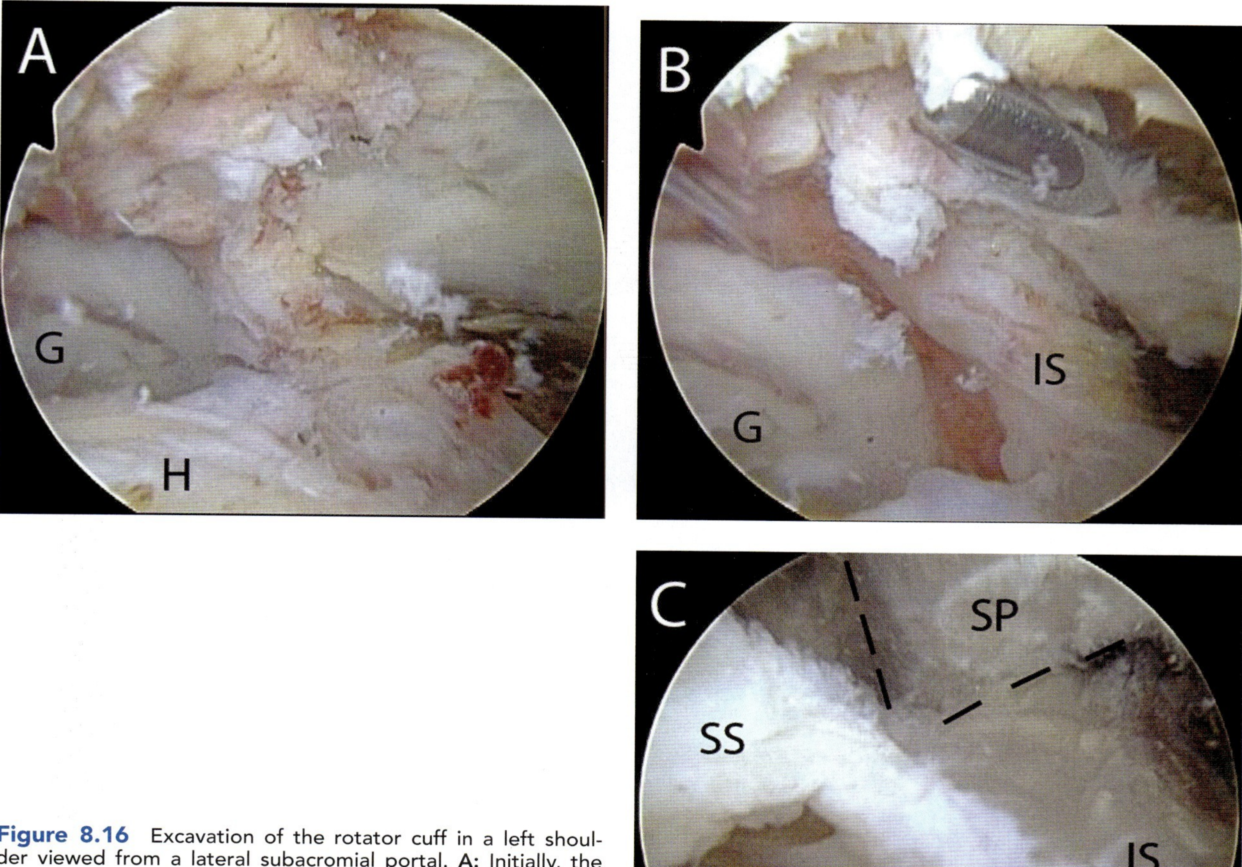

Figure 8.16 Excavation of the rotator cuff in a left shoulder viewed from a lateral subacromial portal. **A:** Initially, the rotator cuff margins are obscured by adhesions. **B:** A shaver introduced from a posterior working portal is used to "bounce off" the scapular spine medially and clear adhesions from the underlying rotator cuff. **C:** Complete dissection with exposure of the scapular spine clearly demonstrates the distinction between the supraspinatus and infraspinatus tendons. G, glenoid; H, humerus; IS, infraspinatus tendon; SP, scapular spine; SS, supraspinatus tendon.

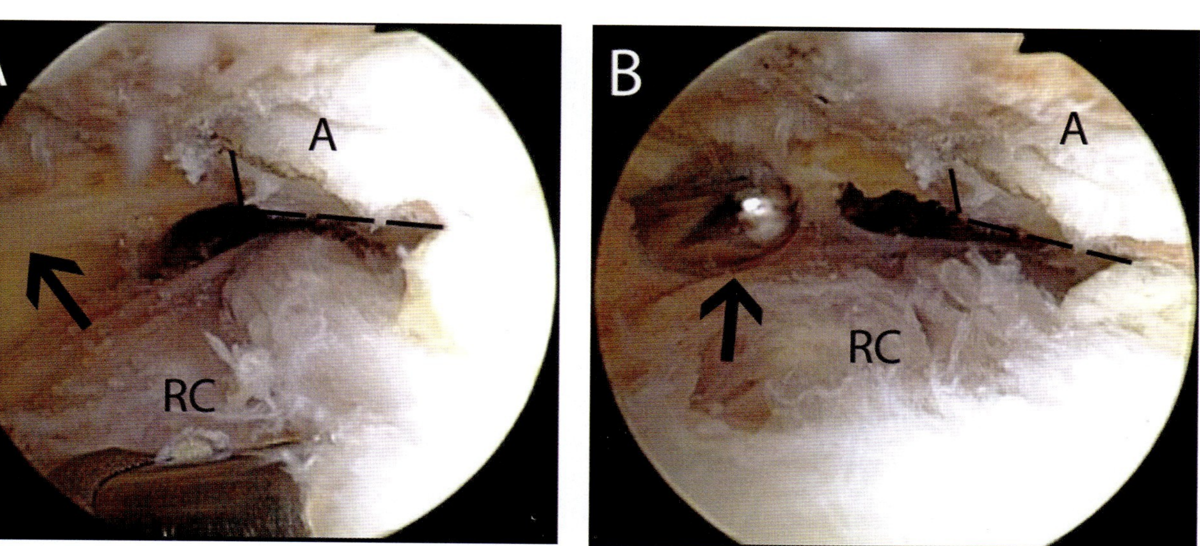

Figure 8.17 Use of the AC joint to identify the scapular spine in a right shoulder viewed from a lateral subacromial portal. **A:** An initial bursectomy has been performed. The inferior border of the distal clavicle is visible as outlined by the *dashed black lines*. The scapular spine is covered with fatty tissue and bursa (*black arrow*) at this point. **B:** Using the AC joint as a landmark, a shaver (*black arrow*) clears tissue posteriorly to uncover the scapular spine.

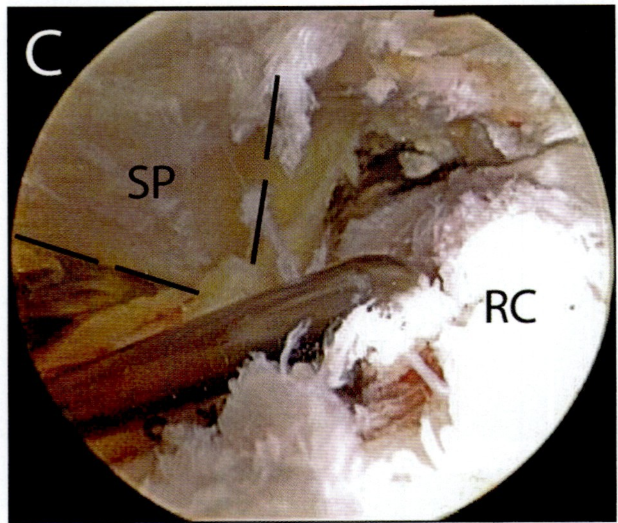

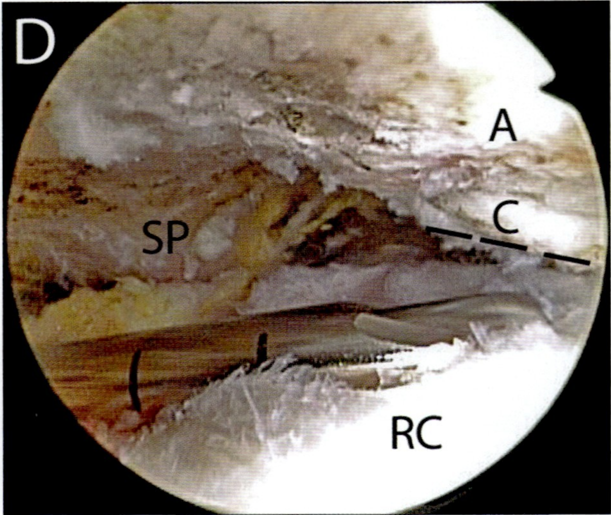

Figure 8.17 *(Continued)* **C:** The scapular spine has been cleared and identified. **D:** Overview shows the relationship between the AC joint (inferior distal clavicle outlined by *dashed black lines*) and the scapular spine. A, acromion; C, distal clavicle; RC, rotator cuff; SP, scapular spine.

It is important to detach the bursal leaders from the deltoid in the proper plane, without destroying deltoid muscle. There is a critical trick that will allow the surgeon to establish the proper plane every time, and the trick is this.

While viewing through a lateral viewing portal, the shoulder is maximally internally rotated by an assistant. This will always bring into view whatever remaining rotator cuff attachments are still intact on the greater tuberosity (Fig. 8.18). At this point, the surgeon can see the proper plane of dissection superiorly, where the soft tissue envelope has been dissected off the acromion, and he can see the proper plane of dissection posteriorly, just superficial to the intact rotator cuff attachments. The surgeon then must visualize a *virtual plane of dissection* connecting the two planes. Then, this virtual plane of dissection is carried out with a combination of electrocautery, arthroscopic scissors, and power shaver. Once this sheet of bursal leaders has been divided, the dissection of the posterior gutter can be completed with a shaver (Fig. 8.19). The dissection of the posterolateral gutter, which is the tightest part of the subacromial space, is facilitated by the use of a 70° arthroscope, alternating it between lateral and posterior viewing portals to afford

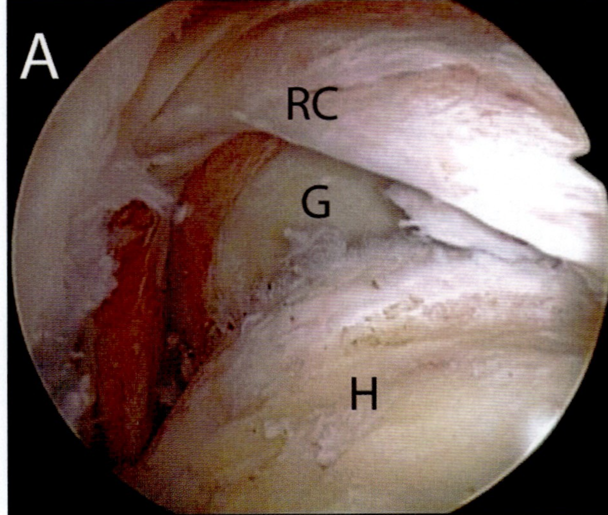

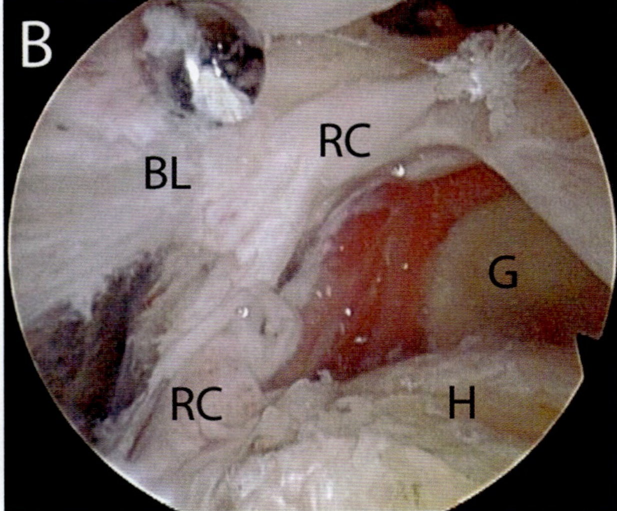

Figure 8.18 **A:** On initial inspection of a right shoulder viewed from a lateral subacromial portal with a 30° arthroscope, it is difficult to delineate the posterior rotator cuff from bursal leader. **B:** Internal rotation of the humerus brings the posterior rotator cuff attachment into view and exposes a posterior bursal leader.

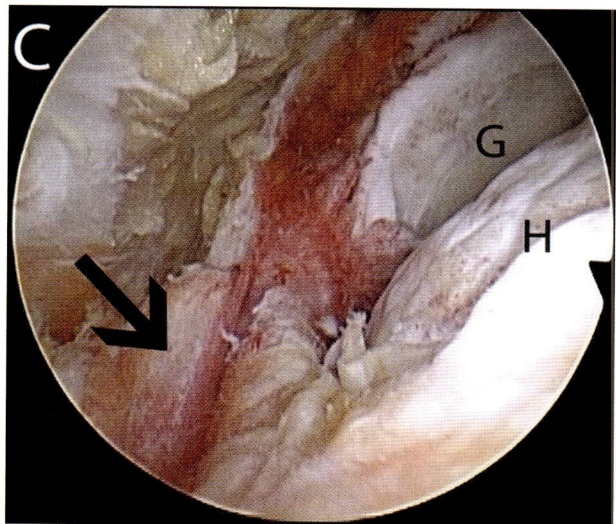

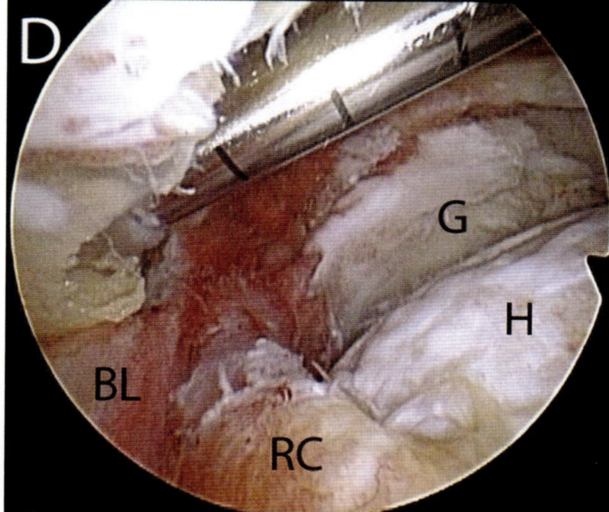

Figure 8.18 *(Continued)* **C:** In another example of a right shoulder viewed from a lateral subacromial portal with a 70° arthroscope, the posterior rotator cuff insertion is difficult to delineate (*black arrow*). **D:** Once again, with internal rotation, the posterior rotator cuff insertion is clearly differentiated from a bursal leader. BL, bursal leader; G, glenoid; H, humerus, RC, rotator cuff.

the best view of that tight space (Fig. 8.20). Finally, while viewing from posteriorly, the lateral gutter is reestablished by dividing any bursal leaders that might be present in the lateral gutter.

Video

Dissection of Supraspinatus and Infraspinatus

After excavating the envelope of soft tissue from the undersurface of the acromion and from the posterior deltoid, one can recognize that this envelope consists of the rotator cuff and a residual bursal leader at the end of the tendon. This residual bursal leader represents a *false cuff* that must be debrided back to tendon. It is usually obvious where the junction of the bursal leader with the tendon is located. A power shaver is used to debride the bursal leader back to the thicker collagen tissue of tendon. We do not try to debride back to well-vascularized tissue. In fact, normal tendon is relatively avascular and the revascularization for rotator cuff healing occurs primarily from the vascularized bone at the bone–tendon interface.

At this point, a grasper is used to pull the tendon laterally toward the bone on the greater tuberosity. If the tendon has adequate excursion to reach the bone bed without undue tension, it is repaired with suture anchors. If the tendon will not reach the bone bed, the surgeon must consider whether to do soft tissue releases.

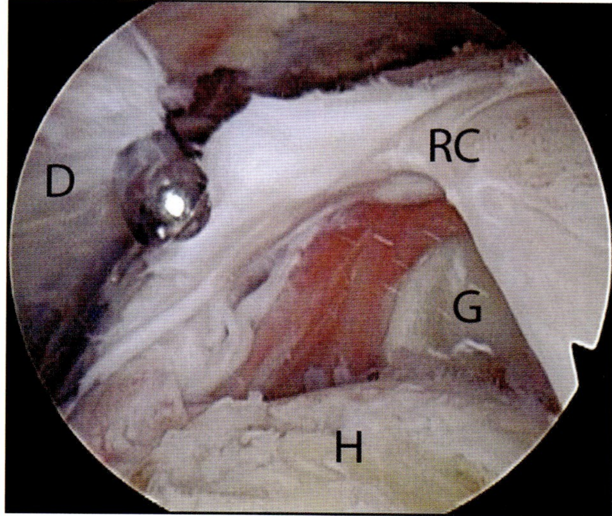

Figure 8.19 Right shoulder viewed from a lateral subacromial portal demonstrates use of a shaver to debride a posterior bursal leader connected to the internal deltoid fascia (compare to Fig. 8.18B). D, internal deltoid fascia; G, glenoid; H, humerus; RC, rotator cuff.

Soft Tissue Releases

The initial soft tissue release that we do is a release of the capsule deep to the tendons that need further excursion. This release is done with an arthroscopic elevator or arthroscopic scissor (Fig. 8.21). One must be careful not to dissect more than 10 to 12 mm medial to the glenoid rim, so as to not injure the suprascapular nerve at the base of the scapular spine. After the capsular release has been done, the excursion is then tested again.

If the tendon will still not reach the bone bed, the arthroscopic grasper is used to test the anterior and posterior mobility of the various portions of the cuff, as well as its medial-to-lateral excursion. By sequentially testing the medial-to-lateral excursion along the entire margin of the cuff tear, the surgeon can tell where the cuff seems to

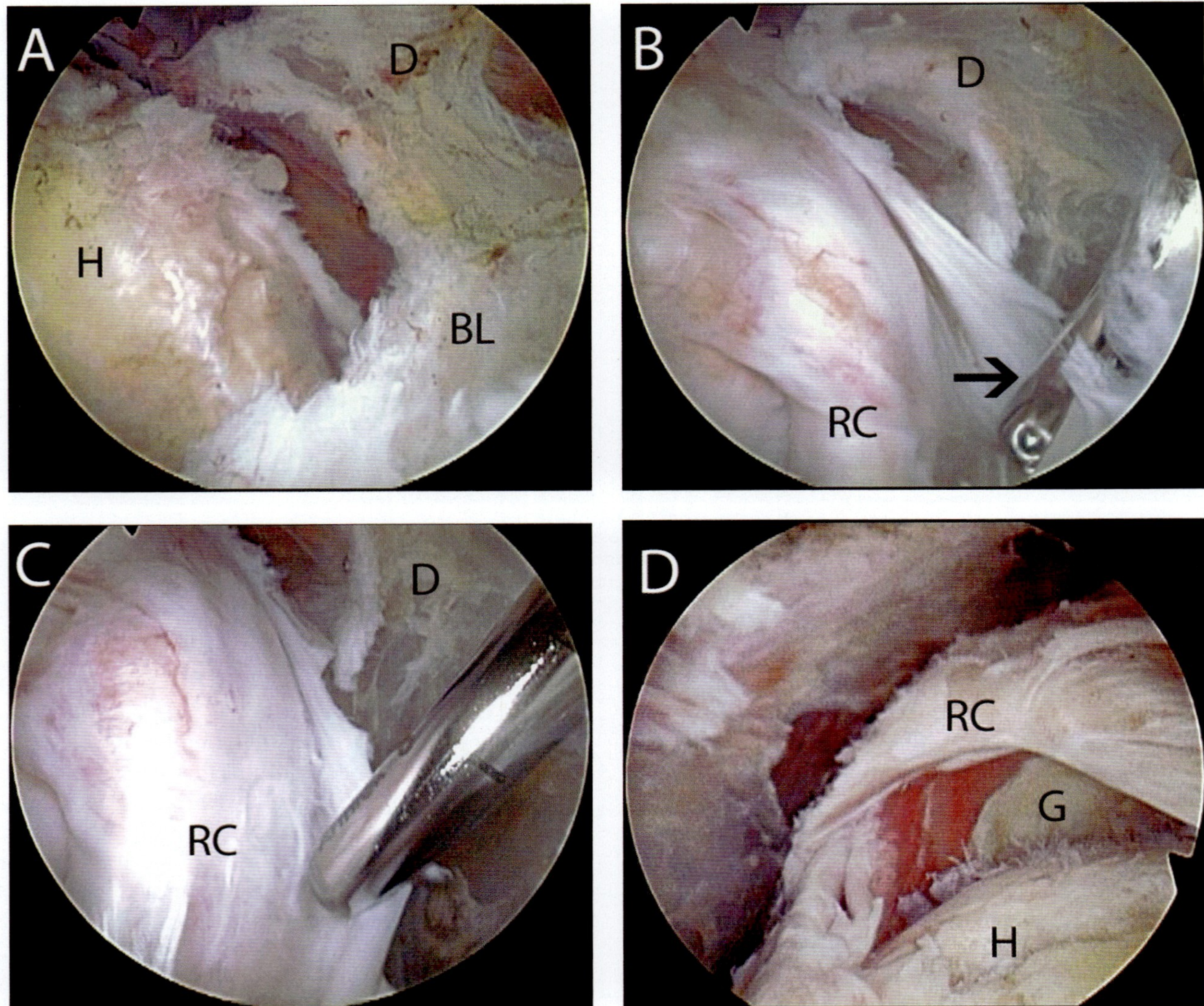

Figure 8.20 **A:** Right shoulder viewed from a posterior subacromial portal with a 70° arthroscope demonstrates a posterolateral bursal leader that attaches to the internal deltoid fascia and obscures visualization of the underlying rotator cuff. **B:** A shaver (*black arrow*) introduced from a lateral working portal is used to debride to the bursal leader. **C:** After debridement of the bursal leader, the posterolateral gutter is restored and the rotator cuff is clearly visible. **D:** View from a lateral subacromial portal demonstrates the completely excavated rotator cuff (compare to Fig. 8.18A). BL, bursal leader; D, internal deltoid fascia; G, glenoid; H, humerus, RC, rotator cuff.

be bound down. If it seems bound down anteriorly, just above the biceps root, one must release the coracohumeral ligament at the base of the coracoid. This is done by introducing the cautery electrode or a 15° elevator or an arthroscopic scissor over the top of the biceps root from a lateral portal, aiming 45° anteromedially, underneath the cuff, toward the base of the coracoid. The soft tissues on that portion of the coracoid base will consist of the coracohumeral ligament, which is then released.

If the cuff margin feels bound down into the region of the scapular spine, then two traction sutures are placed, one at the posterior aspect of the supraspinatus tendon and one at the anterior aspect of the infraspinatus tendon. While pulling laterally on the traction sutures, a posterior interval slide is performed by cutting between the two traction sutures toward the base of the scapular spine with an arthroscopic scissor. The cut continues medially until reaching the perineural fat of the suprascapular nerve, at which point the dissection stops so as to prevent injury to the nerve.

After performing the *modified double-interval slide* (anterior interval slide in-continuity plus posterior interval slide), the surgeon will usually have enough additional lateral excursion of the tendons to perform an arthroscopic repair with suture anchors (see Chapter 7 for a complete description and discussion of interval slides).

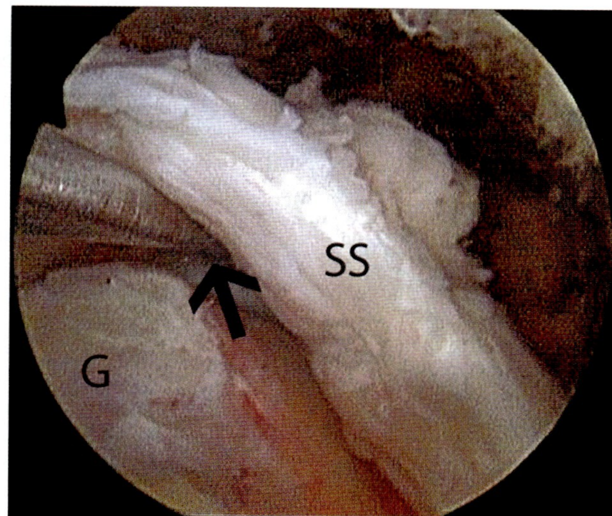

Figure 8.21 Left shoulder, posterior subacromial viewing portal with a 70° arthroscope, demonstrates use of an arthroscopic elevator (*black arrow*) to perform a superior capsular release beneath the supraspinatus tendon. G, glenoid; SS, supraspinatus tendon.

Repair of Posterior and Superior Rotator Cuff

After the modified double-interval slide, the traction sutures are very helpful in stabilizing and manipulating these two floppy tendons. In most cases, suture anchor repair is possible. However, if only partial repair is possible, the surgeon repairs as much of the tendon as he can to bone, and then does a side-to-side repair of supraspinatus to infraspinatus. This side-to-side suture will help to reestablish a crescent-shaped cable that can transmit a distributed load to the anterior and posterior anchor points of the partial repair.

Additional Considerations

In these massive revision cases, we never do a standard acromioplasty. Instead, we do a subacromial smoothing while preserving the coracohumeral arch. If there is a sharp lateral downslope of the acromion, or lateral acromial osteophyte, we do a lateral bevel of the acromion with a high-speed bur.

In many revision situations, there may be deficient tissue involving either the tendon or bone or both. We have some specific tricks that can be useful in dealing with these deficiencies (see Chapter 9, "Managing Poor Tissue or Bone Quality in Rotator Cuff Repair").

REHABILITATION

After revision repair of a massive rotator cuff tear, we go very slowly with rehabilitation. Our overriding goal is to obtain healing after revision cuff repair. We think it is foolish to begin an aggressive early motion regimen, even passive motion, because very few of these shoulders develop postoperative stiffness even with a very slow conservative regimen. Even if they become stiff, we prefer a stiff shoulder with a healed cuff over a supple shoulder with a recurrent cuff tear.

This gets down to the philosophy of a failed shoulder surgery. We would rather have a shoulder surgery fail due to postoperative stiffness than due to mechanical failure of the construct, because the motion can virtually always be restored with an arthroscopic capsular release and lysis of adhesions followed by an immediate aggressive stretching program. However, if the surgery fails because of a recurrent rotator cuff tear, this is a true failure that is depressing to both the patient and the surgeon because they have to start all over again with repair, immobilization, and rehabilitation.

Our protocol following arthroscopic revision repair of a massive cuff tear is to initially immobilize the patient for 6 weeks in a sling. No shoulder motion is allowed during that time.

At the end of 6 weeks, the patient comes out of the sling and begins stretches for overhead elevation and external rotation. Passive internal rotation is delayed until 4 months postoperatively because internal rotation places very high strains on the anterior half of a repaired supraspinatus tendon.

At 4 months postoperatively, we begin strengthening and passive internal rotation. Sonnabend et al. (7) showed in a primate study that Sharpey fibers do not form until 3 months after rotator cuff repair. In first-time cuff repairs, based on this study, we begin strengthening at 3 months. However, for revision cases, we are more cautious and prefer to wait until 4 months to begin strengthening. Strengthening gradually progresses as tolerated, and full activities are allowed at 1 year postoperatively.

REFERENCES

1. Lo IK, Burkhart SS. Arthroscopic revision of failed rotator cuff repairs: technique and results. *Arthroscopy*. 2004;20:250–267.
2. Keener JD, Wei AS, Kim HM, et al. Revision arthroscopic rotator cuff repair: repair integrity and clinical outcome. J Bone Joint Surg Am. 2010;92:590–598.
3. Piasecki DP, Verma NN, Nho SJ, et al. Outcomes after arthroscopic revision rotator cuff repair. Am J Sports Med. 2010;38:40–46.
4. Huberty DP, Schoolfield JD, Brady PC, et al. Incidence and treatment of postoperative stiffness following arthroscopic rotator cuff repair. Arthroscopy. 2009;25:880–890.
5. Goutallier D, Postel JM, Bernageau J, et al. Fatty muscle degeneration in cuff ruptures. Pre- and postoperative evaluation by CT scan. Clin Orthop Relat Res. 1994;(304):78–83.
6. Burkhart SS, Barth JR, Richards DP, et al. Arthroscopic repair of massive rotator cuff tears with stage 3 and 4 fatty degeneration. Arthroscopy. 2007;23:347–354.
7. Sonnabend DH, Howlett CR, Young AA. Histological evaluation of repair of the rotator cuff in a primate model. *J Bone Joint Surg Br* 2010;92:586–594.

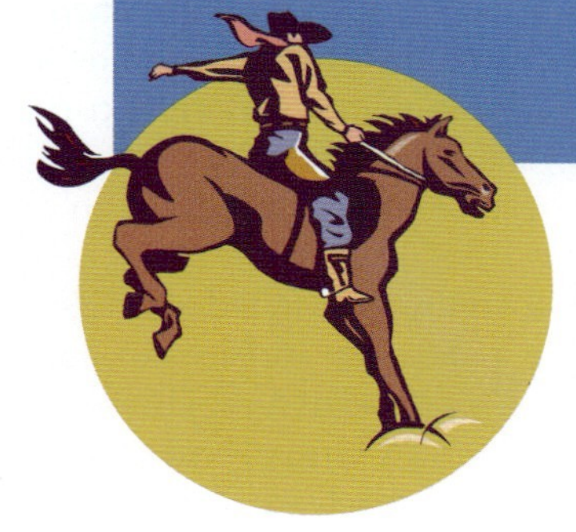

9

Managing Poor Tissue and Bone Quality in Arthroscopic Rotator Cuff Repair

WESTERN WISDOM

A cowchip is paradise for a fly.

The majority of rotator cuff tears occur in individuals over the age of 65. As our population increases in size and advances in age, so too will the number of rotator cuff tears. A growing number of people are remaining active as they age, frequently continuing to place substantial physical demands on their shoulders into their seventh and eighth decades of life. At the same time, the rotator cuff undergoes intrinsic degeneration and the prevalence of osteoporosis increases. Consequently, a significant and growing number of rotator cuff repairs are performed in individuals with poor soft tissue or bone quality. Moreover, while the majority of rotator cuff tears occur at the tendon–bone insertion, fixation quality can be challenged by a tear that occurs more medially, leaving only a small amount of tendon for fixation by suture.

Biologic factors (e.g., poor healing potential) have often been implicated in retearing following rotator cuff repair and have led to attempts to augment healing by means of biologic modalities such as platelet-rich plasma and rotator cuff patches. While retearing certainly increases with advancing age, we believe that biologic explanations (1) for failure of rotator cuff repair have too often been used as excuses for an inadequate repair. We have found that with adherence to basic biomechanical principles, and the occasional use of some advanced tricks, adequate fixation can be achieved in the majority of cases, even in the setting of poor soft tissue quality and osteoporotic bone.

MANAGING POOR SOFT TISSUE QUALITY

Multiple Fixation Points

When soft tissue quality is poor, we prefer to make multiple sutures passes through the rotator cuff and tie as many knots as possible. Increasing the number of points of fixation is one of the simplest ways to improve construct strength. With multiple fixation points, the load per fixation point is decreased, and thus the load the soft tissue must resist to prevent cutout is similarly decreased. Because the number of suture anchors that can be placed in bone is limited by the size of the bone bed, the best way to increase the number of fixation points in the repair construct is to increase the number of sutures by use of double-loaded suture anchors.

For example, based on average cross-sectional areas and muscle contraction, a 4-cm-long rotator cuff tear involving the supraspinatus and infraspinatus will experience a force

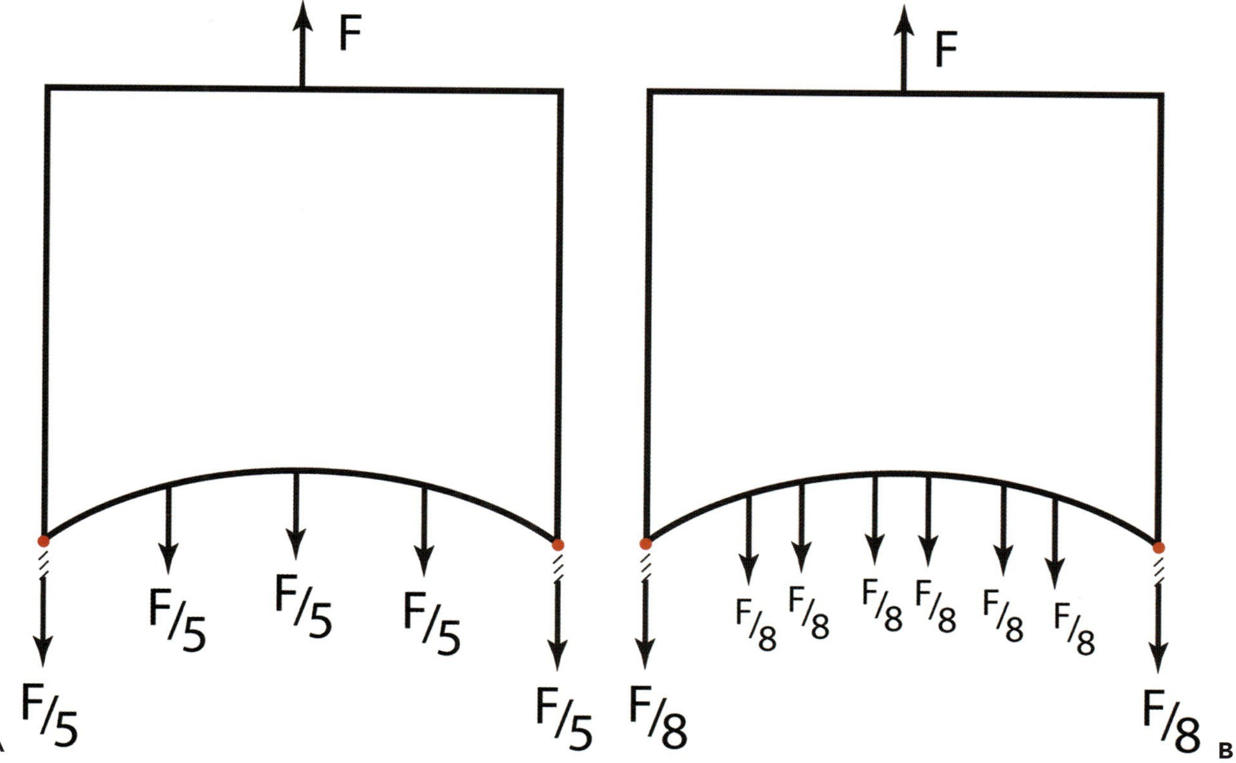

Figure 9.1 Model of three anchor fixation. **A:** With one suture per anchor, there are five fixation points (three by suture, two by tendon-to-bone insertions). **B:** With two sutures per anchor, there are eight fixation points for a three-anchor construct. F, force of rotator cuff.

of 302 N across the rotator cuff (2,3). Suppose that the rotator cuff tear is repaired with three suture anchors, 1 cm apart. If each anchor has one suture, then there are a total of five fixation points (three by suture, two by the tendon-to-bone insertions) that equally share the load of 302 N (Fig. 9.1A). In this case, each suture–rotator cuff interface must resist a load of 60.4 N. If each anchor is double loaded with two sutures, however, eight fixation points exist (six by suture, two by tendon-to-bone insertions) and each suture–rotator cuff interface must now only resist a 37.7-N load (Fig. 9.1B)

It is important to remember that in order to maximize the potential of multiple sutures, the sutures should be passed separately through the rotator cuff and as many knots as possible should be tied. While current suture-bridging double-row repairs may be performed with a knotless technique, a knot increases the resistance to tissue cutout. Therefore, when performing a double-row repair in the setting of impaired tissue quality, it is advantageous to tie knots medially before securing these suture limbs laterally.

Diamondback Repair

The diamondback repair was developed by the senior author (SSB) as an enhanced suture-bridging repair construct that maximizes the concept of multiple fixation points (see Chapter 4, "Complete Rotator Cuff Repair"). This repair configuration provides twice as many linked diagonal compressive sutures with three times the number of intersection points as the standard transosseous equivalent technique (Fig. 9.2). In addition, it provides a compressive bridging mattress suture between the two medial anchors as a means to seal off the footprint from synovial fluid originating in the joint. The theoretical advantages have been borne out in biomechanical testing in which the diamondback repair construct was compared to single- and double-row repairs and demonstrated the highest initial footprint contact area and the lowest decrease in footprint area over time (4). Because footprint restoration is important for healing, this technique is useful for large and massive rotator cuff tears with impaired soft tissue quality.

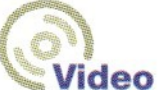

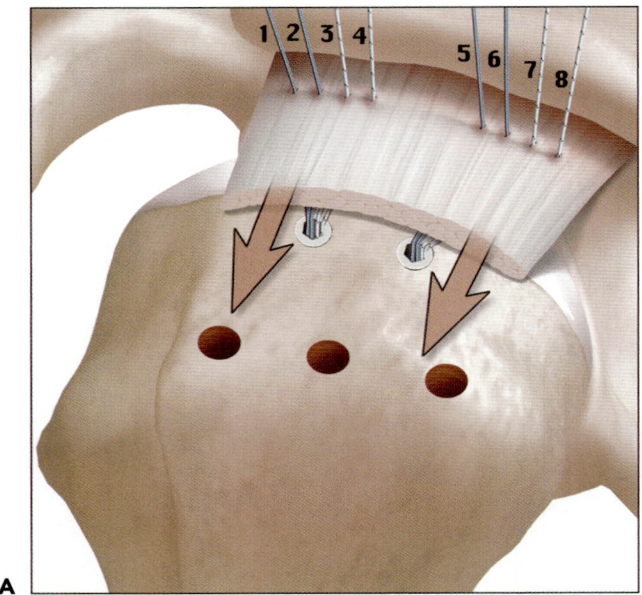

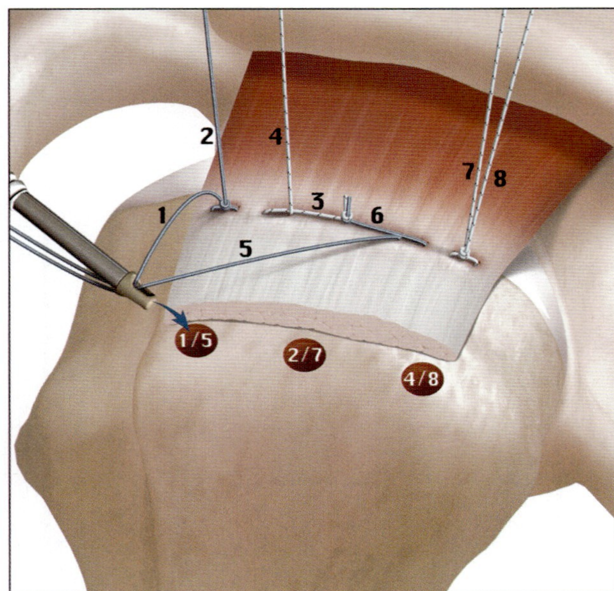

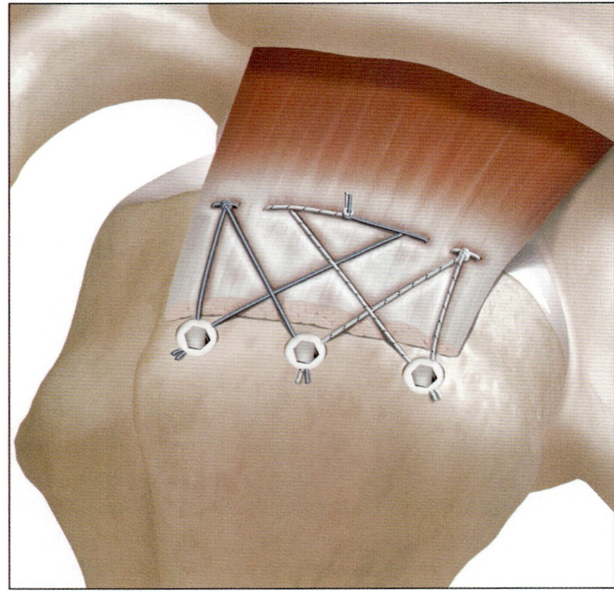

Figure 9.2 Schematic of the diamondback repair. **A:** Two medial screw-in anchors are placed adjacent to the articular margin of the rotator cuff footprint. All sutures are separately passed through the rotator cuff medially. **B:** A mattress stitch is tied between the limb of a suture from the anterior anchor and the limb of a suture from the posterior anchor. The free ends of these knotted sutures are then tensioned, utilizing the eyelets of the two anchors as pulleys to pull the knot down onto the cuff. The remaining sutures are tied as mattress stitches, but the suture tails are not cut. The remaining sutures tails are crisscrossed over the footprint by matching up suture limbs and passing each of these suture pairs through the closed eyelet of three separate knotless screw-in anchors. **C:** Final repair after lateral fixation demonstrates the diamondback pattern of repair.

Stitch Configuration

In order to minimize failure of suture cutting through the tendon, various "grasping-type" suture techniques have been proposed. Gerber et al. (5) reported that a modified Mason-Allen stitch was the strongest of nine different stitch patterns. Unfortunately, the inability to easily perform an arthroscopic Mason-Allen stitch has been used by some authors as justification for open repair. However, weaving suture patterns such as the modified Mason-Allen are prone to early failure by loss of loop security (6). During cyclic loading, the suture weave within the tendon tightens upon itself and the suture loop becomes larger (Fig. 9.3). The result is a loss of loop security, thus a loss of tendon–bone contact. The most efficient way to minimize cinching is to use a single loop of suture—a simple stitch.

A "rip-stop" suture is an effective method of avoiding cinching, while improving resistance to suture cut out. An anterior-to-posterior mattress stitch can be placed in the rotator cuff and tied on itself. Subsequently, simple sutures from an anchor are passed medial to the rip-stop suture that distributes the medial-to-lateral tensile forces and effectively decreases the chance of suture cut out (Fig. 9.4).

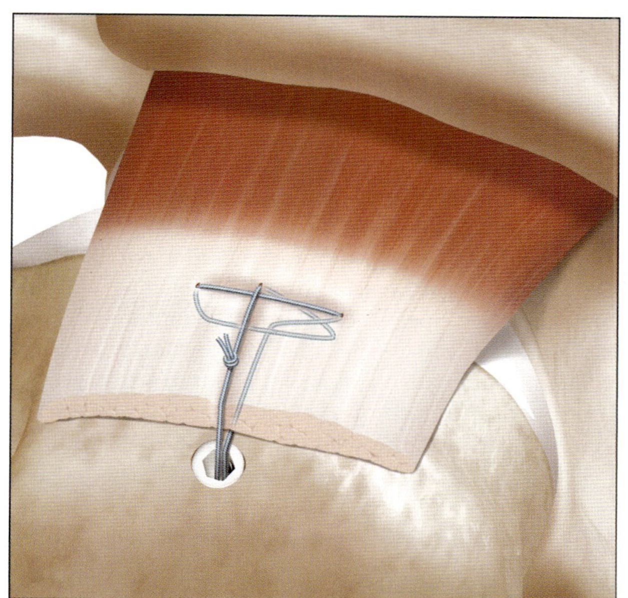

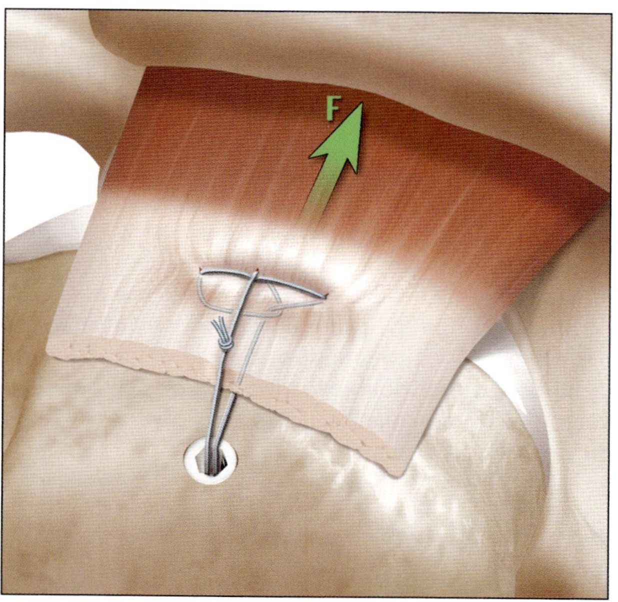

Figure 9.3 Schematic of a modified Mason-Allen stitch. Although this stitch pattern has a high load to failure, it has poor loop security under load. **A:** A modified Mason-Allen stitch based off an anchor has been woven through the rotator cuff. **B:** Under a medial tensile load (*F*), the complex weave cinches upon itself, resulting in loss of loop security and thus medial displacement of the rotator cuff.

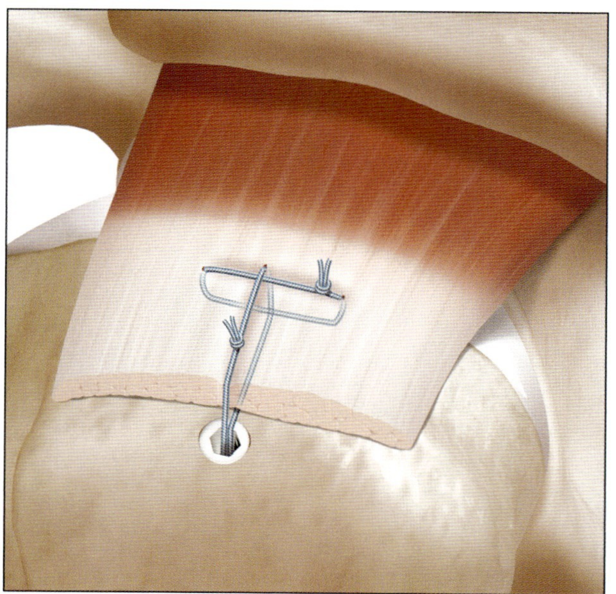

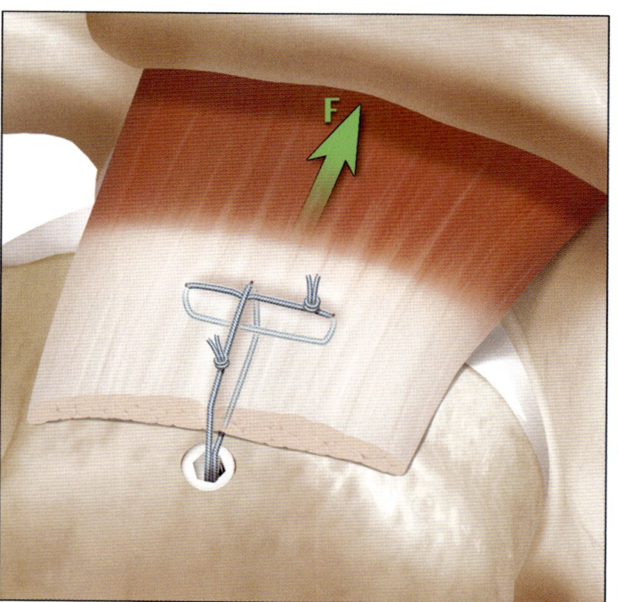

Figure 9.4 Schematic of a rip-stop stitch. This stitch pattern increases pullout and maximizes loop security by using only simple stitch loops. **A:** A simple stitch is placed from anterior to posterior through the rotator cuff perpendicular to the rotator cuff fibers. Then, a simple stitch is passed medial to the rip-stop stitch. This technique can be performed as illustrated or with both sutures based off of the anchor. **B:** Under a tensile load (*F*), the rip-stop stitch resists cutout of the simple stitch.

Such a rip-stop suture may be placed as an isolated suture or with the use of a double- or triple-loaded anchor. In the case of an anchor, the first set of anchor sutures are used to create a mattress stitch and the remaining sutures are passed medial to lateral in a simple pattern. Ma et al. (7) demonstrated that a rip-stop suture with a double-loaded anchor had a load to failure equivalent to a modified Mason-Allen stitch. In a follow-up study, it was reported that a triple-loaded anchor with a horizontal rip-stop stitch and two simple stitches demonstrated even less elongation with cyclic loading (i.e., maintained loop security) and a higher ultimate load to failure compared to the rip-stop configuration with a double-loaded anchor (8). Notably, however, the highest load to failure was observed with a classic double-row repair.

Load-Sharing Rip-stop Double-row Repair

We have developed a rotator cuff repair technique that combines the advantages of a wide rip-stop suture tape and a double-row repair (Figs. 9.5 and 9.6). This technique is particularly useful for cases involving medial tears in which there is limited medial tendon that precludes a standard double-row repair. One or two FiberTape (Arthrex, Inc., Naples, FL) rip-stop sutures are secured to two BioComposite SwiveLock anchors (Arthrex, Inc., Naples, FL) laterally in a modified SpeedFix repair (see Chapter 4, "Complete Rotator Cuff Tears"). The FiberTape rip-stop provides resistance to tissue cut out for simple sutures that are passed from a medial row of two BioComposite Corkscrew FT anchors (Arthrex, Inc., Naples, FL). The FiberTape is also a

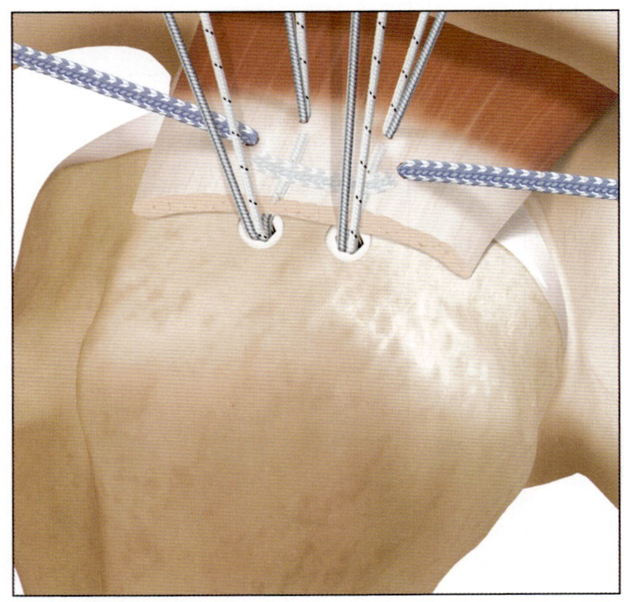

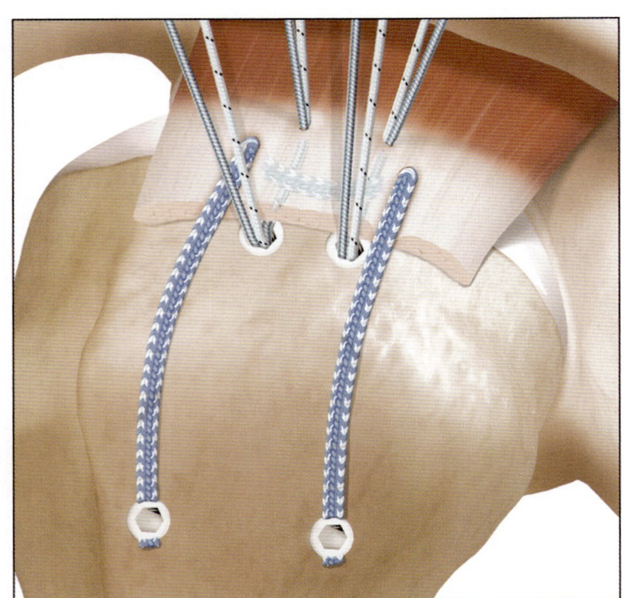

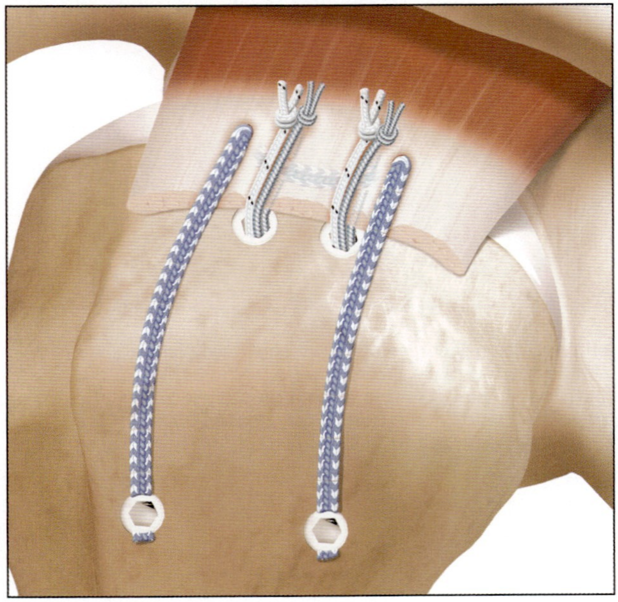

Figure 9.5 Schematic illustration of an anchor-based rip-stop rotator cuff repair for a rotator cuff tear with lateral tendon loss. **A:** A FiberTape (Arthrex, Inc., Naples, FL) suture has been placed as an inverted mattress stitch in the rotator cuff. Two medial anchors (BioComposite Corkscrew FT; Arthrex, Inc., Naples, FL) have also been placed and sutures from these anchors are passed medial to the rip-stop stitch. **B:** Prior to tying sutures from the medial Corkscrew anchors, the rip-stop stitch is secured to bone with two lateral BioComposite SwiveLock C anchors (Arthrex, Inc., Naples, FL). **C:** Tying the suture limbs from the Corkscrew anchors completes the repair.

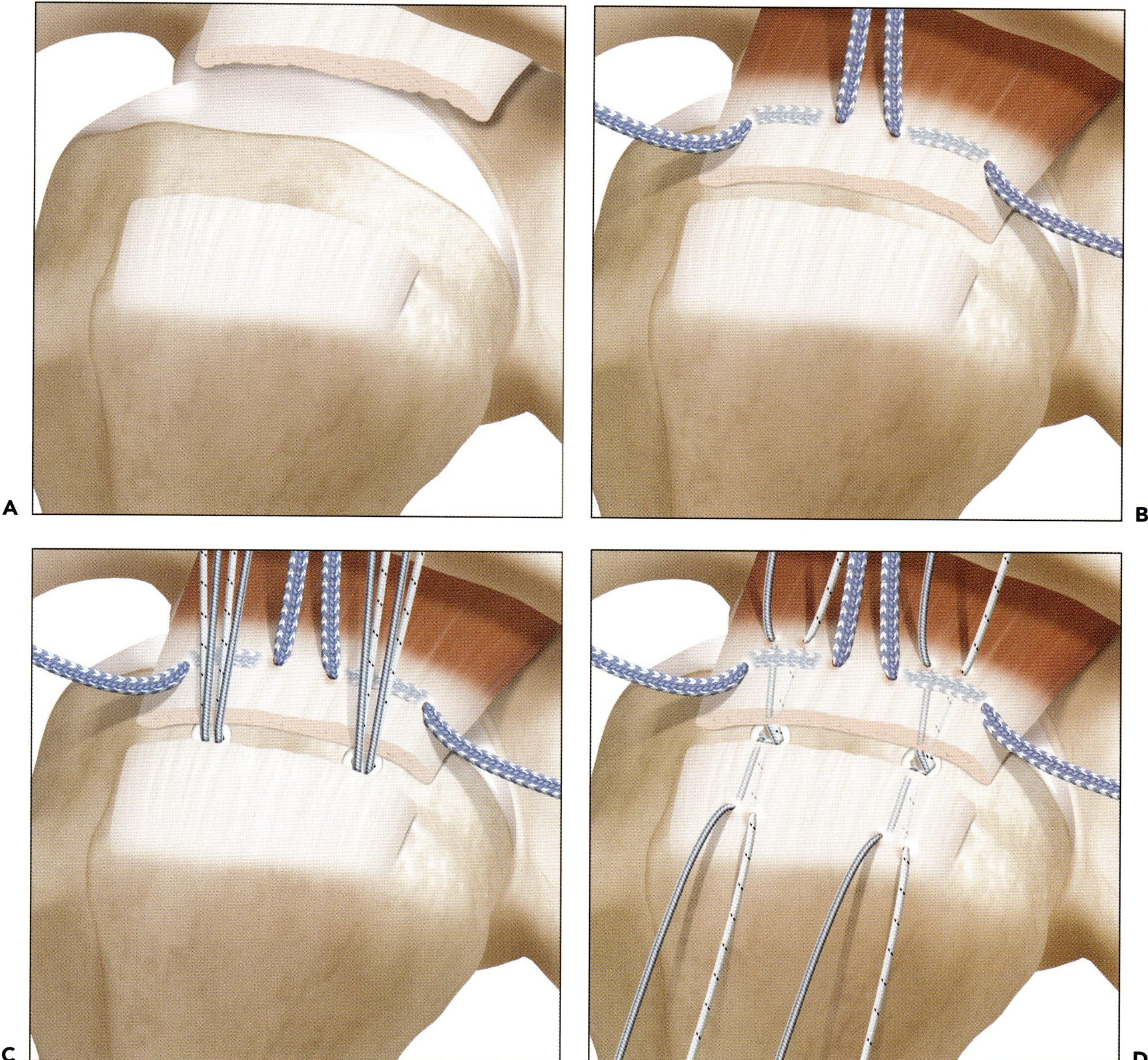

Figure 9.6 Schematic illustration of a dual rip-stop rotator cuff repair. **A:** In this medial rotator cuff tear with a lateral tendon stump, there is limited space to achieve fixation in the medial tendon. **B:** Two FiberTape (Arthrex, Inc., Naples, FL) rip-stop sutures are placed 3 mm lateral to the musculotendinous junction as inverted mattress stitches. **C:** Two BioComposite Corkscrew FT anchors (Arthrex, Inc., Naples, FL) are placed in the greater tuberosity bone bed. **D:** Suture limbs from the Corkscrew anchors are passed medial to the rip-stop stitches. In addition, the opposite suture limbs are passed through the lateral tendon stump.

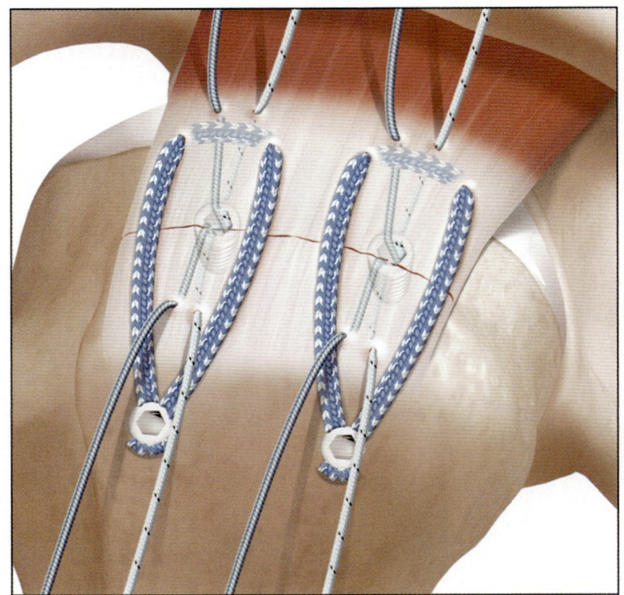

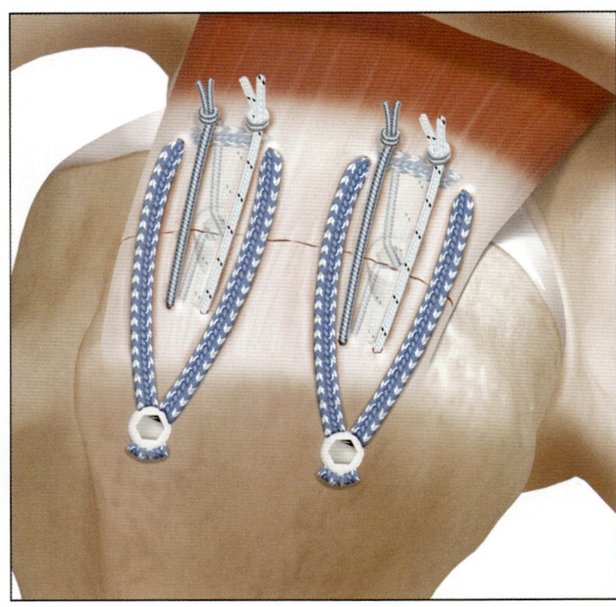

Figure 9.6 *(Continued)* **E:** The FiberTape rip-stop sutures are secured laterally with BioComposite SwiveLock C anchors (Arthrex, Inc., Naples, FL). These rip-stop sutures are load sharing and are secured before the Corkscrew anchor sutures are tied. During this step, it is important to retrieve the rip-stop sutures so that they surround the lateral sutures limbs from the Corkscrew anchors. **F:** The repair is completed by tying the sutures limbs from the Corkscrew anchors.

load-sharing construct that reduces the load that has to be resisted by the simple sutures.

The tear margin is debrided, the bone bed is prepared, and the tear pattern and mobility are assessed (Fig. 9.7). The first step is placement of rip-stop sutures. While viewing from a posterior portal, a FiberTape suture is passed through the rotator cuff as an inverted mattress stitch placed 3 mm lateral to the musculotendinous junction. The FiberTape is passed with either an antegrade technique using a Scorpion FastPass suture passer (Arthrex, Inc., Naples, FL) to directly pass the #2 FiberWire (Arthrex, Inc., Naples, FL) leaders of the FiberTape (Fig. 9.8), or in a retrograde fashion using a hand-off technique. If the tear has a large anterior-to-posterior dimension, a second FiberTape suture may be similarly placed. In either

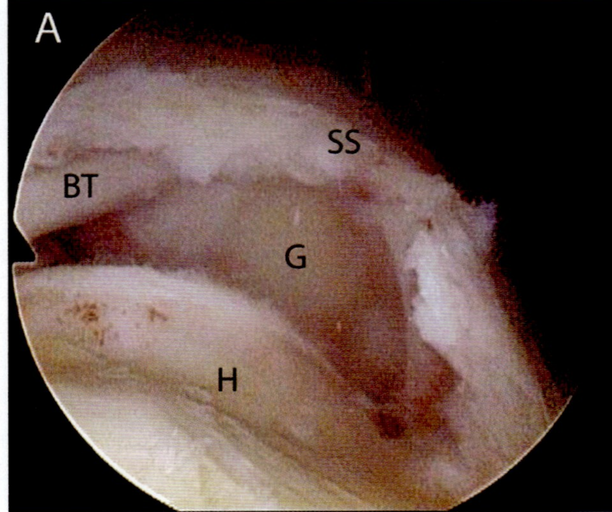

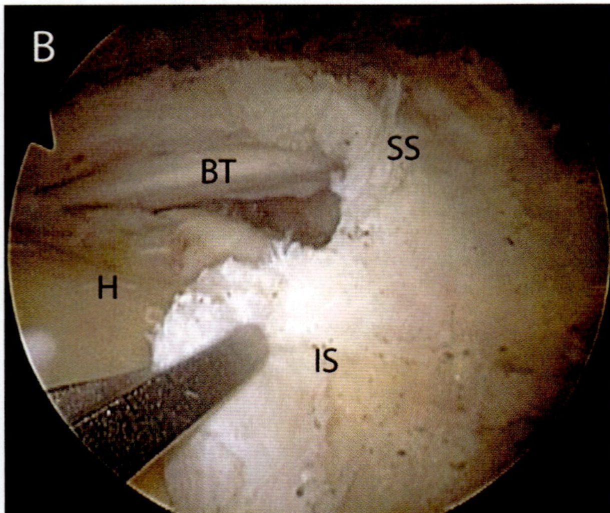

Figure 9.7 **A:** Left shoulder, lateral subacromial viewing demonstrating a large rotator cuff tear involving the supraspinatus and anterior infraspinatus. **B:** Posterior subacromial viewing portal of the same shoulder. The posterior aspect of the tear is mobile, but there is tendon loss of the supraspinatus and the overall quality of the rotator cuff tissue is poor. BT, biceps tendon; G, glenoid; H, proximal humerus; IS, infraspinatus tendon; SS, supraspinatus tendon.

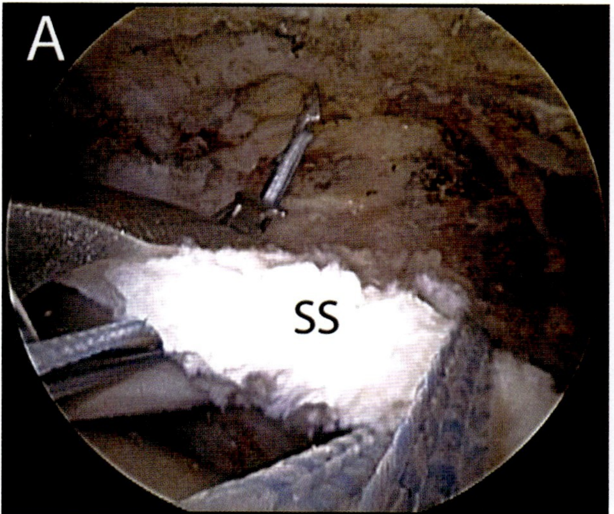

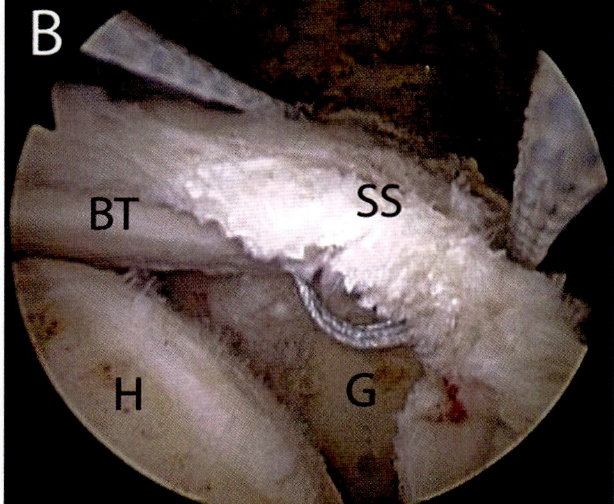

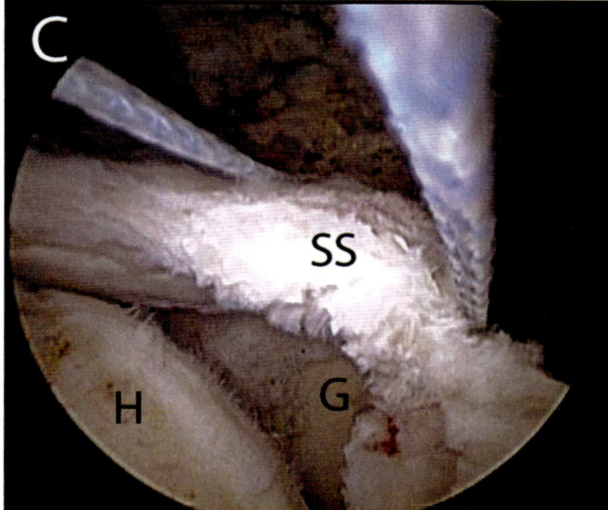

Figure 9.8 Left shoulder, posterior subacromial viewing portal with a 70° arthroscope demonstrates placement of a FiberTape (Arthrex, Inc., Naples, FL) rip-stop stitch. **A:** The posterior limb of the rip-stop suture has been passed (**right**). The anterior limb of the rip-stop stitch is passed antegrade through the supraspinatus (SS) tendon with a Scorpion FastPass (Arthrex, Inc., Naples, FL) **B:** The inverted mattress rip-stop stitch is demonstrated. **C:** Final view after removing slack from the stitch. BT, biceps tendon; G, glenoid; H, proximal humerus.

case, the rip-stop(s) are placed so that they span the entire anterior-to-posterior dimension of the rotator cuff tear. The rip-stop suture limbs are retrieved out an accessory portal and stored for later fixation. These rip-stop suture tapes must not be tensioned and repaired to bone until after the sutures from the medial anchors have been passed circumferentially around them.

Next, two double-loaded BioComposite Corkscrew FT suture anchors are placed anteromedially and posteromedially, adjacent to the articular margin (Fig. 9.9). Beginning posteriorly, the sutures from the medial anchors are retrieved and passed as simple stitches that penetrate the rotator cuff medial to the FiberTape rip-stop suture, 2 to 3 mm lateral to the musculotendinous junction (Fig. 9.10). If there is a significant lateral tendon stump due to a medial tear, the opposite end of each suture limb can be passed through this tendon stump in retrograde fashion with a Penetrator (Arthrex, Inc., Naples, FL) (see *Arthroscopic Rodeo*). Knot tying is delayed at this point and the sutures limbs are held in accessory portals.

Once the medial stitches are passed, the FiberTape rip-stop stitches are retrieved and secured laterally with two SwiveLock anchors (Fig. 9.11). In this step, the FiberTape suture limbs are retrieved so that they encircle the simple sutures from the medial anchors. If only one rip-stop is used, the posterior FiberTape limb is retrieved posterior to the simple stitches and secured with a posterolateral SwiveLock anchor. Then, the anterior FiberTape limb is retrieved anterior to the simple stitches and secured with an anterolateral SwiveLock anchor. If two equally spaced rip-stop sutures have been placed, each must encircle the corresponding medial anchor sutures; for example, the

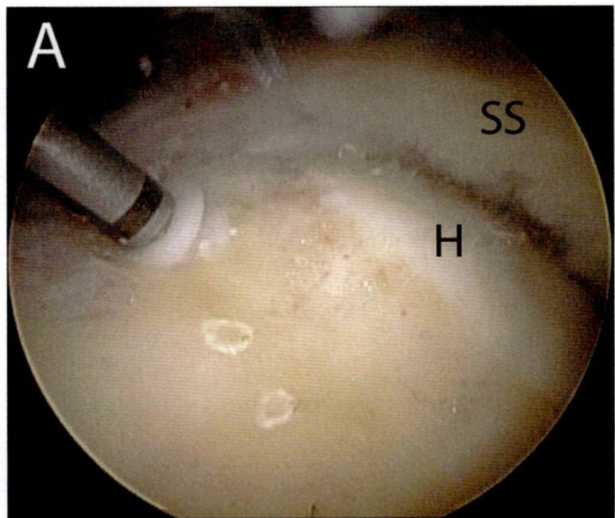

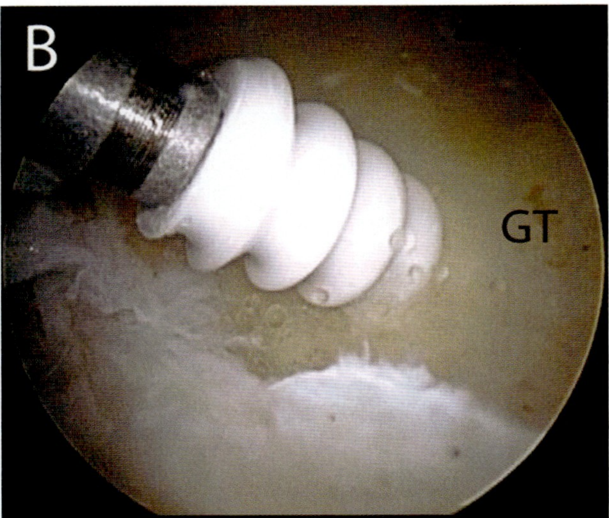

Figure 9.9 Left shoulder, posterior viewing portal. Following placement of a rip-stop suture, an anteromedial **(A)** and a posteromedial **(B)** BioComposite Corkscrew FT anchor (Arthrex, Inc., Naples, FL) are placed in the greater tuberosity (GT) bone bed. H, humeral head; SS, supraspinatus tendon.

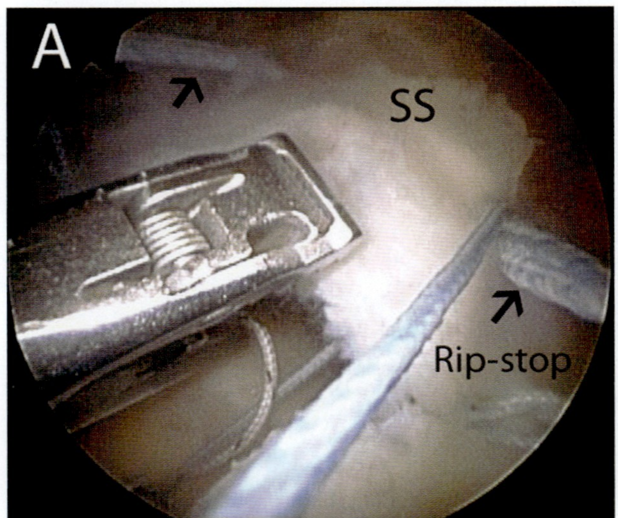

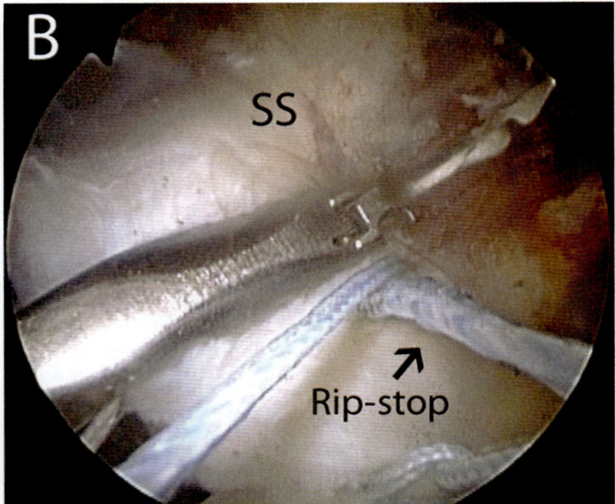

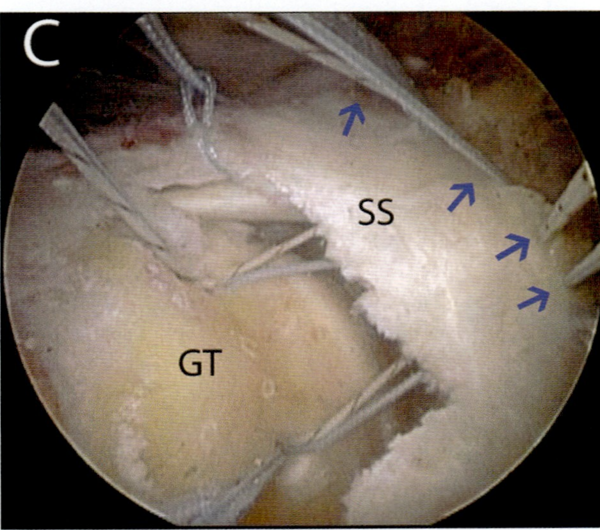

Figure 9.10 Left shoulder, posterior viewing portal. **A:** Sutures from the medial anchors are retrieved and loaded into a Scorpion suture passer (Arthrex, Inc., Naples, FL). The rip-stop suture is also seen (*black arrows*). **B:** Simple stitches are placed medial to a rip-stop stitch (*black arrow*). **C:** View after placing 4 simple stitches (*blue arrows*) (two from the anteromedial anchor, and two from the posteromedial anchor) medial to a rip-stop stitch. GT, greater tuberosity; SS, supraspinatus.

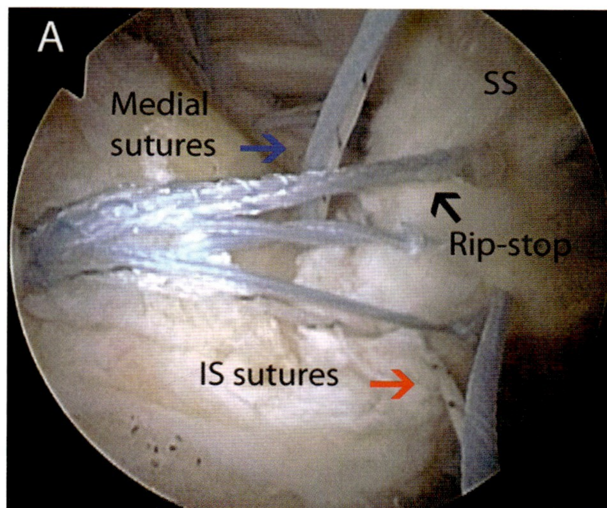

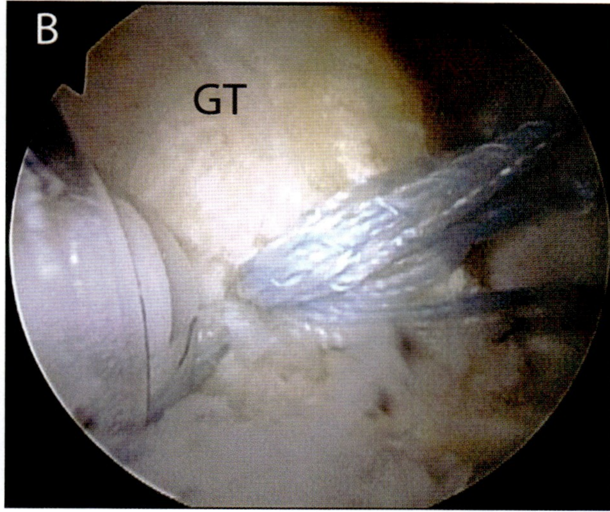

Figure 9.11 Left shoulder, posterior viewing portal. **A:** The posterior limb of the FiberTape (Arthrex, Inc., Naples, FL) rip-stop suture for the supraspinatus (*black arrow*) is retrieved posterior to the suture limbs from the posteromedial anchor (*blue arrow*). The anterior rip-stop FiberTape limb will be retrieved through a lateral portal, passing anterior to the sutures of the anteromedial anchor. In this case, there are also suture limbs visible from fixation of the infraspinatus (*red arrow*). **B:** The FiberTape rip-stop is secured laterally with a SwiveLock anchor (Arthrex, Inc., Naples, FL). In this case, the lateral SwiveLock anchor is used to anchor some sutures for the infraspinatus repair (after they have been tied) in addition to the posterior FiberTape limb for the supraspinatus repair. GT, greater tuberosity; IS, infraspinatus; SS, supraspinatus.

anterior limb of the anterior rip-stop stitch is retrieved so that it passes in front of the sutures from the anteromedial anchor, and the posterior limb of the anterior rip-stop stitch is retrieved so that it passes behind the sutures from the anteromedial anchor. As opposed to the single rip-stop technique in which the anterior and posterior FiberTape limbs are secured with separate SwiveLock anchors, in the case of two rip-stops, the anterior rip-stop is secured with an anterolateral SwiveLock anchor and the posterior rip-stop is secured with a posterolateral SwiveLock anchor.

After the rip-stop stitch or stitches have been secured, the FiberWire simple stitches from the medial anchors are retrieved and static knots are tied with a Surgeon's Sixth Finger Knot Pusher (Arthrex, Inc., Naples, FL) (Fig. 9.12). It is important to delay knot tying until after the rip-stop is secured in order to have a firm, taut rip-stop. The SpeedFix FiberTape rip-stop not only prevents cut out like a standard rip-stop, but also serves to unload the medial sutures since the rip-stop is tensioned laterally to an anchor. Therefore, the medial sutures should not be tied until the rip-stop suture is secured (Figs. 9.13 and 9.14).

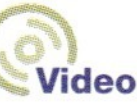
Video

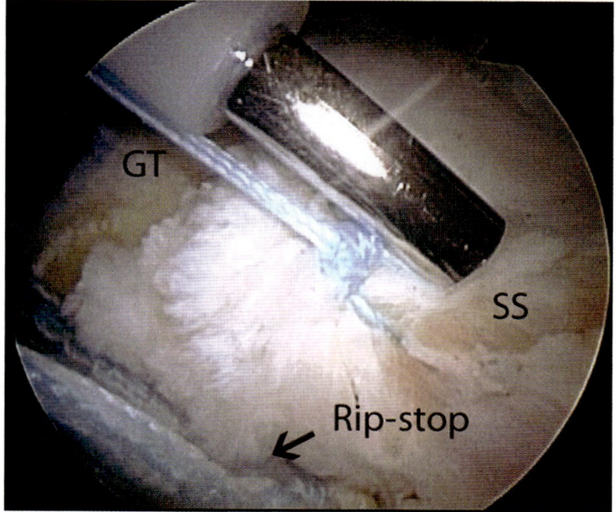

Figure 9.12 Left shoulder, posterior viewing portal. After the rip-stop sutures (*black arrow*) are secured laterally, the simple stitches from the medial anchors are tied as static knots with a Surgeon's Sixth Finger Knot Pusher (Arthrex, Inc., Naples, FL). SS, supraspinatus tendon.

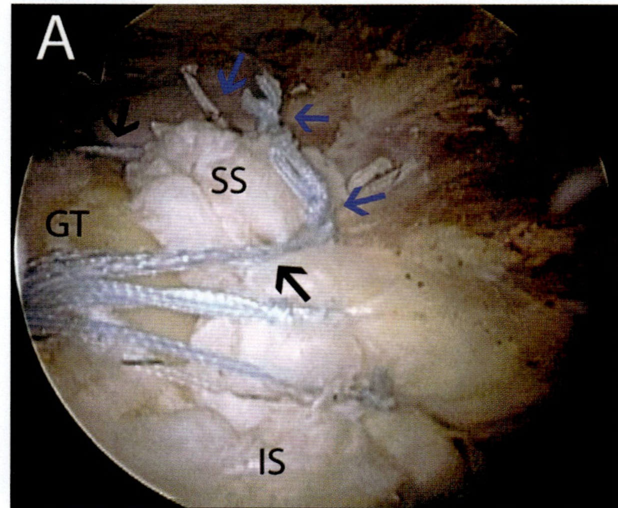

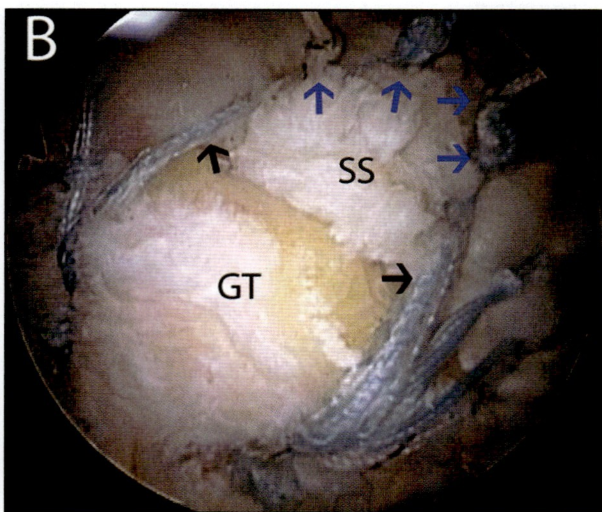

Figure 9.13 Left shoulder, subacromial view from **(A)** posterior and **(B)** lateral viewing portals demonstrates the final SpeedFix rip-stop repair. A FiberTape rip-stop stitch (*black arrows*) has been secured laterally with two anchors and encircles simple stitches (*blue arrows*) that were passed medial to the rip-stop and tied as static knots. The infraspinatus sutures (from the posteromedial anchor) were tied without a rip-stop suture, as the quality of the infraspinatus tendon was much better than that of the supraspinatus tendon. GT, greater tuberosity; IS, infraspinatus tendon; SS, supraspinatus tendon.

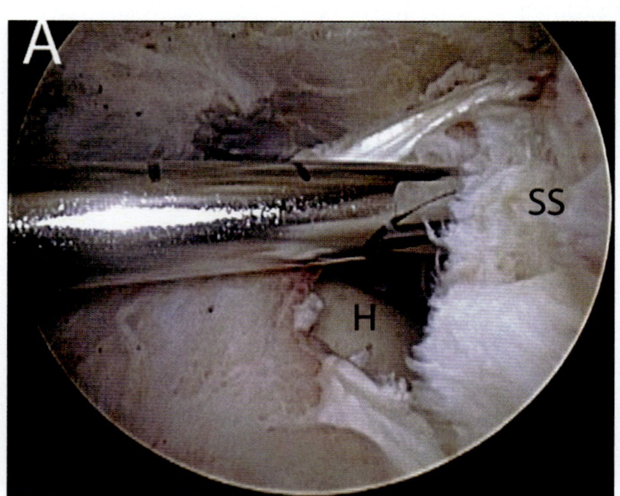

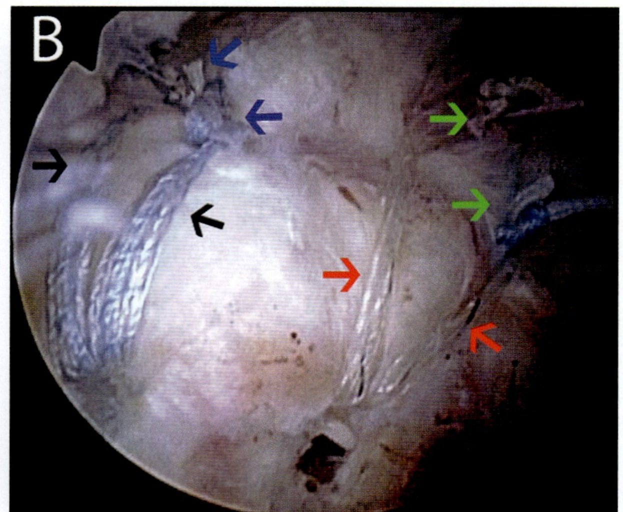

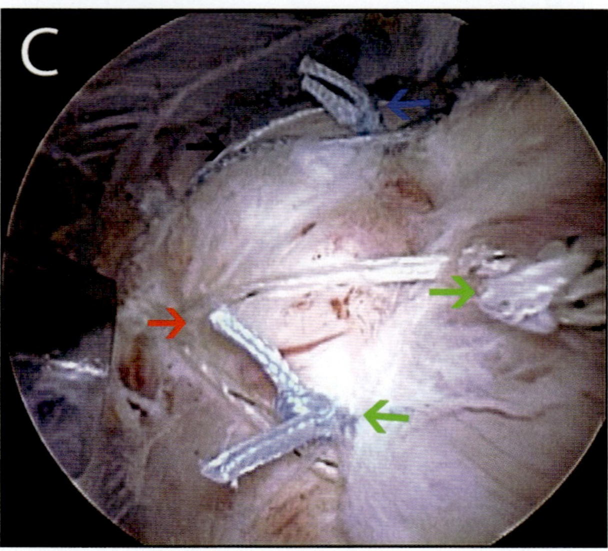

Figure 9.14 Left shoulder demonstrating the final SpeedFix rip-stop double-row repair of rotator cuff tear with two rip-stop sutures. **A:** Posterior subacromial viewing portal demonstrates a medial rotator cuff tear with a lateral tendon stump. **B:** Lateral subacromial viewing portal. When two rip-stop sutures are placed, the anterior FiberTape (Arthrex, Inc., Naples, FL) rip-stop (*black arrows*) encircles simple stitches (*blue arrows*) based from the an anteromedial anchor, and the posterior rip-stop (*red arrows*) encircles simples stitches (*green arrows*) based from the posteromedial anchor. **C:** Posterior subacromial view again demonstrates the rip-stop suture simple stitch construct. H, humeral head; SS, supraspinatus tendon.

MANAGING POOR BONE QUALITY

Principles

For the most part, the use of suture anchors has transferred the weak link in rotator cuff repair from the bone to the rotator cuff tendon. In biomechanical testing, transosseous bone tunnel constructs have demonstrated inferior fixation compared to suture anchor fixation (9). For this reason, we exclusively use suture anchors for fixation of rotator cuff tendon tears. However, in the setting of osteoporotic bone, anchor fixation can still be problematic. Similar to the approach to managing soft tissue quality, secure fixation in osteoporotic bone begins with adherence to biomechanical principles, and if necessary, can be augmented with several arthroscopic technical tricks.

Anchor design and insertion technique are both important in achieving fixation in osteoporotic bone. Biomechanical investigations have shown that fully threaded screw-in anchors provide superior pullout strength in osteoporotic bone compared to hook-type anchors (10). For this reason, we exclusively use fully threaded anchors for fixation when bone quality is a concern (BioComposite Corkscrew FT or SwiveLock; Arthrex, Inc., Naples, FL). To maximize pullout, anchors are inserted at a deadman angle such that the angle the suture makes with the perpendicular to the anchor and the angle the sutures makes with the rotator cuff tendon are both <45° (Fig. 9.15) (11).

Compaction Bone Grafting

Occasionally degenerative cysts are present at the desired location of an anchor. If the cyst involves such a large area that an anchor cannot be inserted adjacently, a compaction bone grafting technique can be used to fill the cyst (12). The cyst contents and any fibrous lining are debrided with an arthroscopic shaver and curettes (Fig. 9.16). Bone grafting is then performed using an osteochondral autograft transfer systems (OATS; Arthrex, Inc., Naples, FL). The size of the cyst is estimated and allograft cancellous bone chips are packed into an OATS harvesting tube of the same diameter (Fig. 9.17). Using a spinal needle as a guide, an accessory lateral portal is created to provide a straight angle of approach to the cyst. The harvester tube is then inserted into the subacromial space via this portal. The harvester tube is placed at the opening of the cyst cavity and the

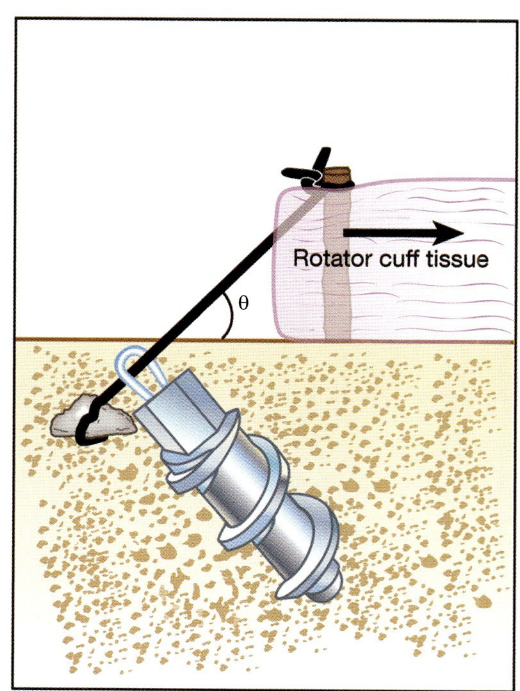

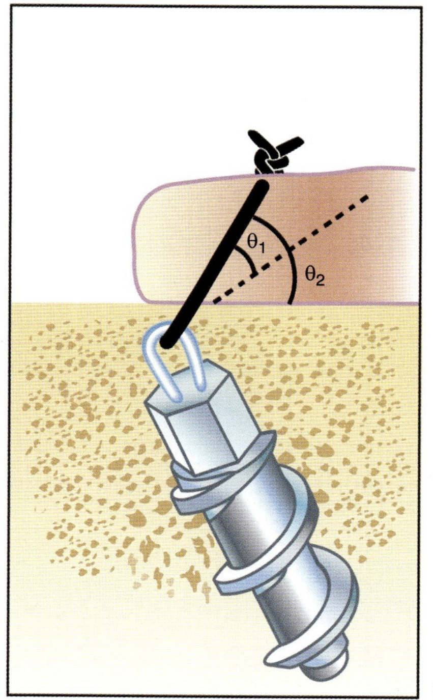

Figure 9.15 Anchor insertion. **A:** The ideal anchor insertion for rotator cuff repair is analogous to the deadman fence post system in which the anchor is analogous to the deadman rock, the deadman wire is analogous to the suture, and the fence post is analogous to the rotator cuff tissue. The ideal deadman angle (θ) is <45°. **B:** Both the pullout angle for the anchor (θ_1; angle the suture makes with the perpendicular to the anchor) and the tension-reduction angle (θ_2; angle the suture makes with the rotator cuff pull direction) for the suture must be considered. Ideally, θ_1 and θ_2 should both be ≤45°.

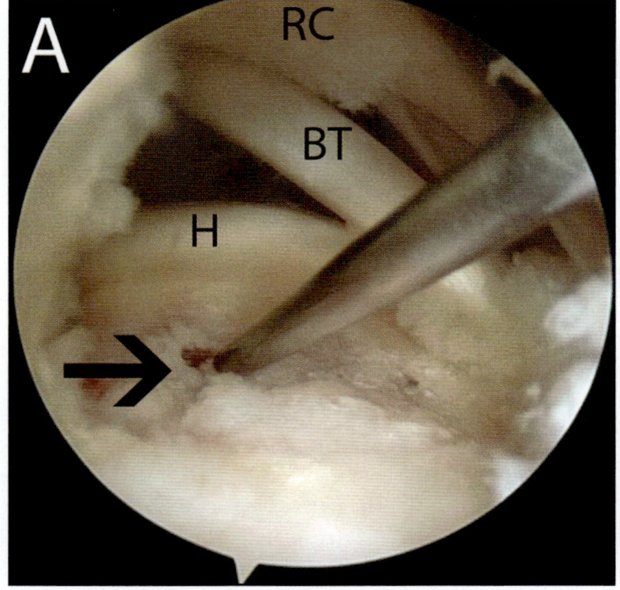

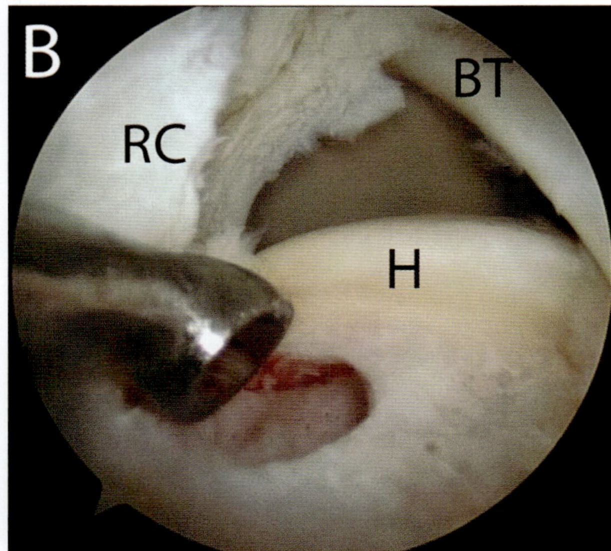

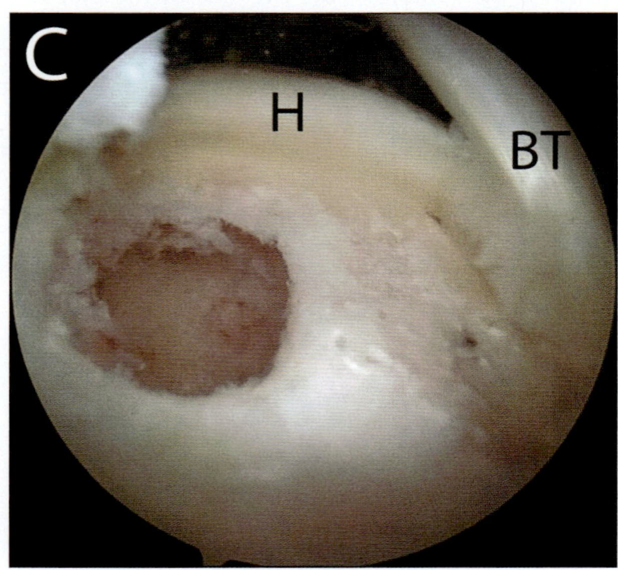

Figure 9.16 Right shoulder, lateral subacromial viewing portal with a 70° arthroscope demonstrates a bone cyst in the proximal humerus. **A:** The tip of a spinal needle has fallen into a bone cyst. **B:** The roof of the cyst has been uncovered and the contents are removed with a curette. **C:** View after complete removal of cyst contents. BT, biceps tendon; H, humerus; RC, rotator cuff.

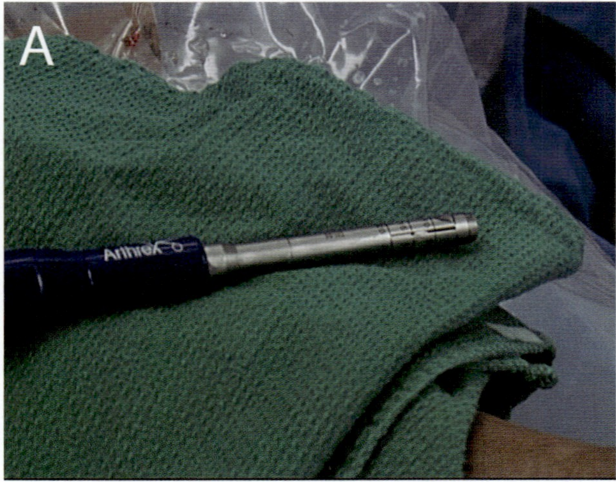

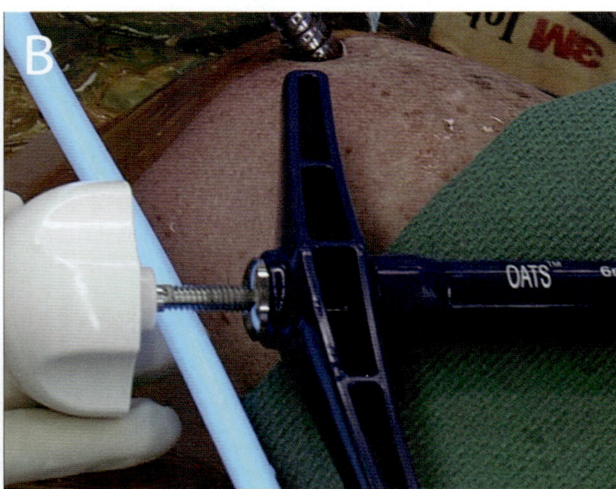

Figure 9.17 **A:** External view of an OATS harvester (Arthrex, Inc., Naples, FL). The metal end of the OATS harvester is packed with cancellous bone graft for arthroscopic cyst grafting. **B:** During cyst grafting, the white handle on the harvester is turned clockwise to advance the bone graft into the defect.

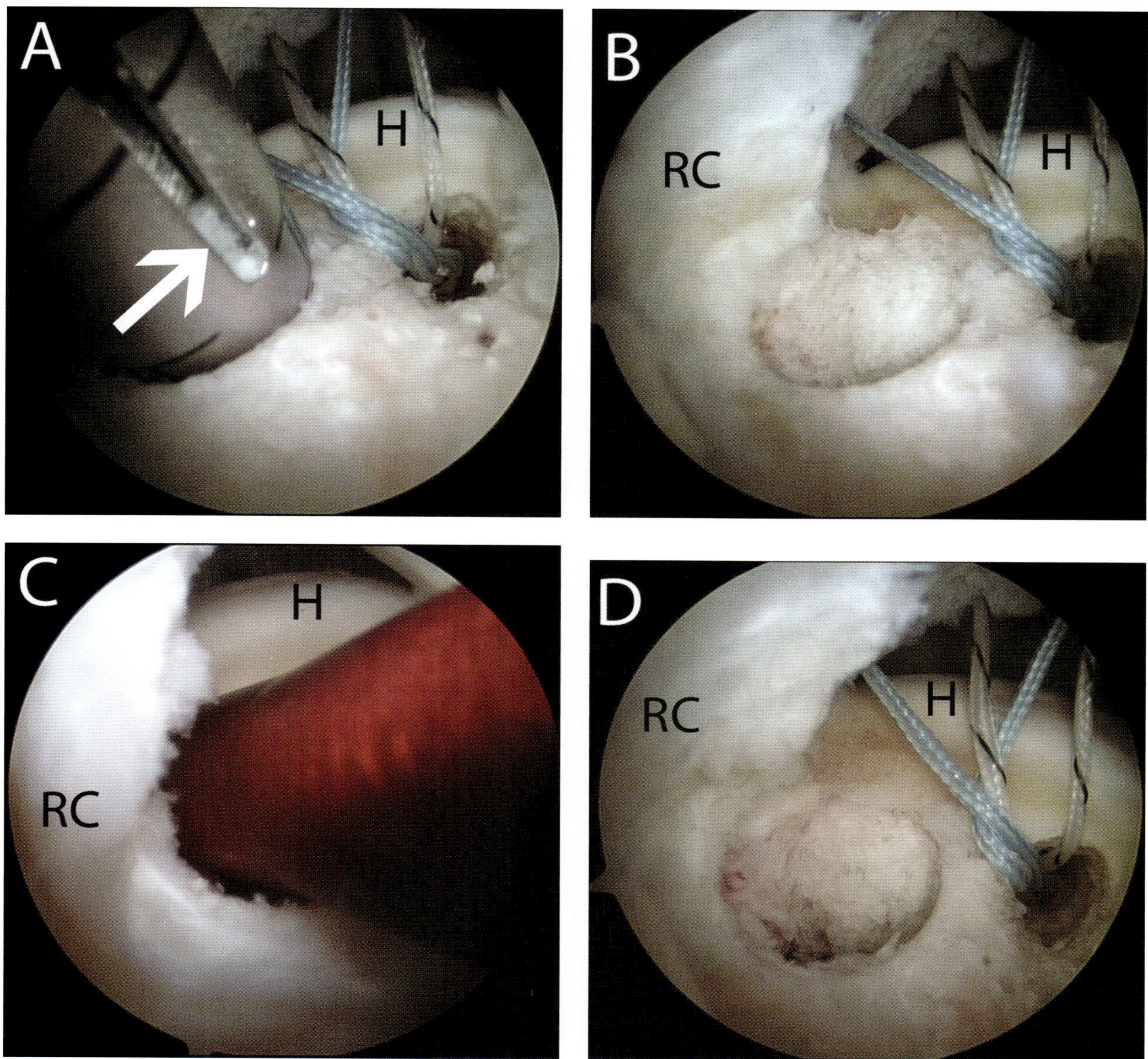

Figure 9.18 Right shoulder, lateral subacromial viewing portal demonstrating compaction grafting technique. **A:** An OATS harvester (Arthrex, Inc., Naples, FL) is seated into a bone cyst and used to fill the cyst with cancellous allograft (*white arrow*). **B:** Appearance after initial placement of bone graft. **C:** A tamp is used to provide additional compression of the allograft. Additional graft may then be added and compressed if needed. **D:** Final appearance after bone compaction grafting. The bone bed is now suitable for anchor placement. H, humerus; RC, rotator cuff.

cancellous bone graft is inserted by means of a screw-in handle that compresses the bone graft into the cyst. The bone graft is further compacted with a tamp. The process is repeated until the cyst is completely filled with well-compacted cancellous bone (Fig. 9.18). Usually, the repair can proceed with standard anchor (5.5- or 6.5-mm BioComposite Corkscrew FT) insertion into the compacted bone graft.

If, however, the cyst is very large, a 7 to 9 mm BioComposite Tenodesis screw (Arthrex, Inc., Naples, FL) can be used for fixation in order to provide additional compaction of the bone as this larger implant is inserted. After grafting the cyst, free #2 FiberWire sutures are passed through the rotator cuff. The tenodesis screwdriver is loaded with a 7 to 9 mm screw and a looped #2 FiberWire suture is threaded through the cannulated screwdriver. Then, the suture limbs previously placed in the rotator cuff are retrieved and extracorporeally passed through the suture loop at the tip of the tenodesis screw. A small punch is used to create a starter hole in the grafted bone cyst. The screwdriver tip is inserted into the starter hole and the tenodesis screw is advanced while tension is maintained both on the rotator cuff suture limbs and the suture loop that was threaded through the screwdriver. The tenodesis screw is advanced until it is flush with the top of the bone graft within the cyst. This technique creates an interference fit between the tenodesis screw, bone, and rotator cuff sutures, similar to that used for fixation with a SwiveLock anchor. Additionally, the free limbs of the rotator cuff sutures as well as the suture loop placed through the screw can be passed back through the rotator cuff and tied together as static knots using a Surgeon's Sixth Finger (Arthrex, Inc., Naples, FL).

Video

Buddy Anchor

The "buddy anchor" technique is used to salvage a loose anchor that has migrated above the surface of the bone after insertion (Fig. 9.19). A punch is used to readvance the anchor to the desired depth. The suture limbs from the loose anchor are retrieved. Then, the punch is used to create a starter hole directly adjacent to the loose anchor. The punch is only inserted halfway in order to create an undersized socket for anchor insertion. A second anchor is inserted into the undersized socket to create an interference fit between the two anchors. While inserting the second anchor, it is important to maintain tension on the suture limbs from the

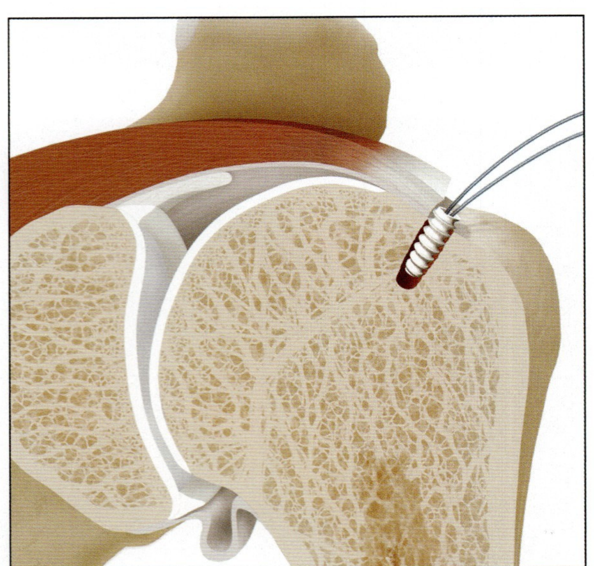

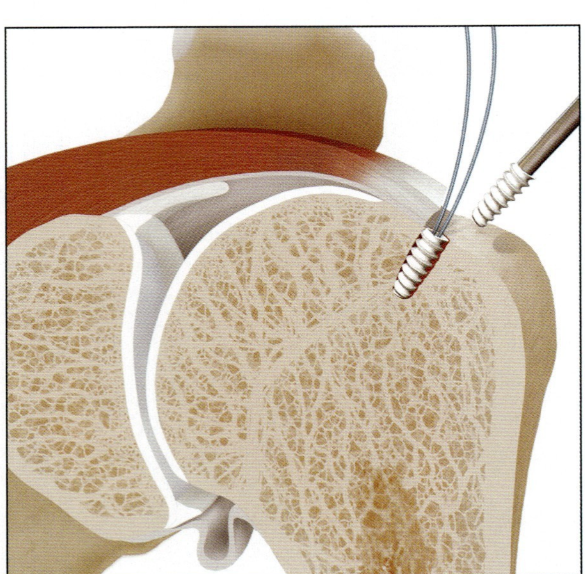

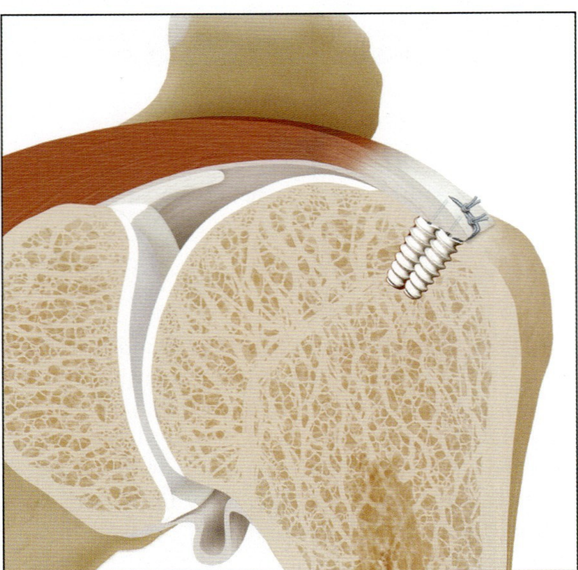

Figure 9.19 Schematic of the "buddy anchor" technique for a loose anchor. **A:** An anchor placed for rotator cuff repair has failed the "tug test" and now sits proud. **B:** The loose anchor is readvanced. Then, a second anchor is inserted adjacently. **C:** An interference fit is achieved between the two anchors that can now be used for rotator cuff repair.

loose anchor in order to avoid driving the loose anchor deep into the bone ahead of the second anchor. In an osteoporotic model, Brady et al. (13) demonstrated that the buddy anchor technique had a higher pullout strength and less displacement during cyclic loading than a single suture anchor.

Rescue Anchor

A final technical trick for managing a loose anchor is to use a "rescue anchor" for load sharing. This technique relies on the fact that fixation in the lateral cortex is biomechanically stronger than fixation in the rotator cuff footprint. For massive contracted tears, it is often only possible to achieve single-row fixation. Occasionally in this scenario, an anchor placed in osteoporotic bone, which originally passes the "tug test," can tilt medially under tension during knot tying (Fig. 9.20A). If this is observed, the construct can still be salvaged by partially distributing the tension forces to a second anchor. After knot tying, the suture limbs are left long and retrieved. A punch is used to create a bone socket in the lateral cortex. The suture limbs from the compromised anchor are threaded through the eyelet of a SwiveLock anchor that is then secured in the lateral bone socket (Fig. 9.20B, C). This technique essentially uses the biomechanical advantage of a double-row technique, although the purpose of the lateral row in this scenario is for load distribution rather than footprint compression.

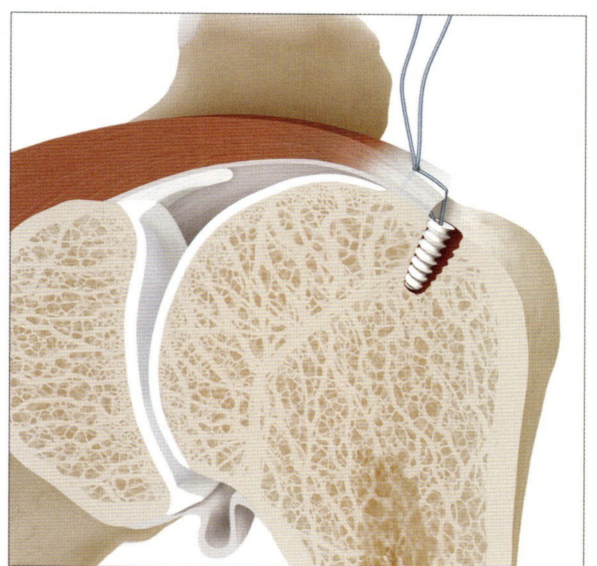

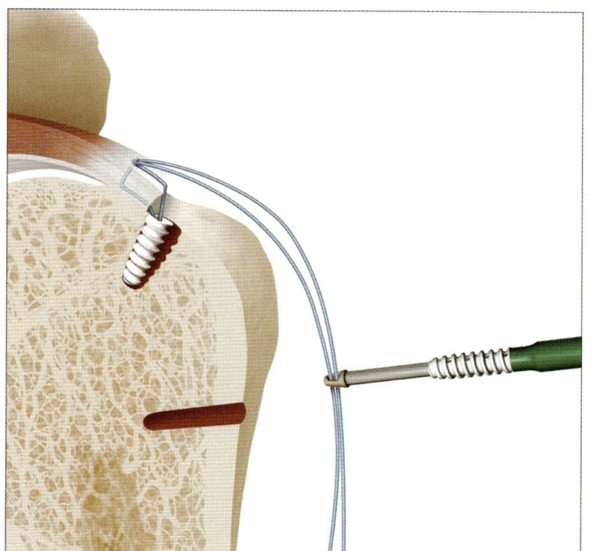

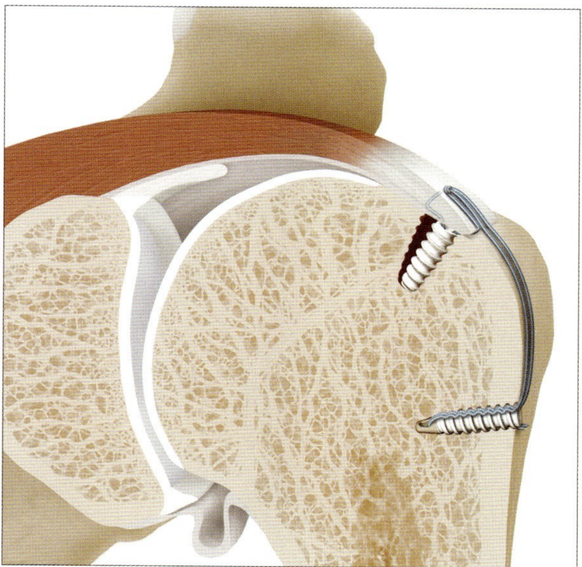

Figure 9.20 Schematic of the "rescue anchor" technique for a loose anchor. **A:** An anchor has been placed in the greater tuberosity for rotator cuff repair. However, while securing the rotator cuff, the anchor has tilted medially under tension in poor quality bone. **B:** Although the tear is not amenable to double-row fixation because of limited mobility, a lateral anchor can be used to salvage the construct. The suture tails passed through the rotator cuff are left long and secured in the lateral greater tuberosity with a knotless SwiveLock anchor (Arthrex, Inc., Naples, FL). **C:** The lateral anchor effectively shares the load of the medial anchor.

Cortical Fixation

A final technical trick for managing poor bone quality is to rely on cortical fixation. We have encountered rare cases in which bone adjacent to the articular margin will not hold an anchor despite compaction grafting, a buddy anchor, or use of a biceps tenodesis screw. In such a scenario, the normal footprint can be bypassed and fixation can usually be reliably obtained laterally in the metaphyseal cortico-cancellous bone.

Bone defects after attempted fixation are first filled using a compaction grafting technique. This provides a biologic substrate for rotator cuff healing. Then, one or two (depending on the width of the tear) FiberTape inverted mattress stitches are placed in the rotator cuff. The suture limbs from a mattress stitch are retrieved out a lateral portal and tensioned using the cannula as a guide to determine the position for a lateral anchor over the lateral corner of the greater tuberosity. The punch for a 4.75 mm BioComposite SwiveLock C is used to create a bone socket in the lateral aspect of the greater tuberosity approximately perpendicular to the bone. Extracorporeally, the FiberTape sutures are fed through the distal eyelet of the BioComposite SwiveLock C anchor and the eyelet is inserted into the bone socket. The FiberTape suture limbs are tensioned, reducing the tendon to its proper position on the bone bed. Then the anchor is inserted to secure the FiberTape in that position.

CONCLUSION

While the majority of rotator cuff tears can be managed with standard repair techniques, poor soft tissue and bone quality can compromise fixation, particularly in elderly patients with degenerative tendon and osteoporotic bone. However, we believe that these factors should not bear the blame deserved by a poor quality repair. Reliable fixation can be achieved in these individuals with adherence to biomechanical principles and the use of advanced arthroscopic reinforcement techniques.

REFERENCES

1. Galatz LM, Ball CM, Teefey SA, et al. The outcome and repair integrity of completely arthroscopically repaired large and massive rotator cuff tears. *J Bone Joint Surg Am.* 2004;86:219–224.
2. Ikai M, Fukunaga T. Calculation of muscle strength per unit cross-sectional area of human muscle by means of ultrasonic measurement. *Int Z Angew Physiol.* 1968;26:26–32.
3. Bassett RW, Browne AO, Morrey BF, et al. Glenohumeral muscle force and moment mechanics in a position of shoulder instability. *J Biomech.* 1990;23:405–415.
4. Burkhart SS, Denard PJ, Obopilwe E, Mazzocca AD. Optimizing pressurized contact area in rotator cuff repair: the diamondback repair. *Arthroscopy.* In press.
5. Gerber C, Schneeberger AG, Beck M, et al. Mechanical strength of repairs of the rotator cuff. *J Bone Joint Surg Br.* 1994;76:371–380.
6. Petit CJ, Boswell R, Mahar A, et al. Biomechanical evaluation of a new technique for rotator cuff repair. *Am J Sports Med.* 2003;31:849–853.
7. Ma CB, MacGillivray JD, Clabeaux J, et al. Biomechanical evaluation of arthroscopic rotator cuff stitches. *J Bone Joint Surg Am.* 2004;86-A:1211–1216.
8. Ma CB, Comerford L, Wilson J, et al. Biomechanical evaluation of arthroscopic rotator cuff repairs: double-row compared with single-row fixation. *J Bone Joint Surg Am.* 2006;88:403–410.
9. Burkhart SS, Diaz Pagan JL, Wirth MA, et al. Cyclic loading of anchor-based rotator cuff repairs: confirmation of the tension overload phenomenon and comparison of suture anchor fixation with transosseous fixation. *Arthroscopy.* 1997;13:720–724.
10. Tingart MJ, Apreleva M, Lehtinen J, et al. Anchor design and bone mineral density affect the pull-out strength of suture anchors in rotator cuff repair: which anchors are best to use in patients with low bone quality? *Am J Sports Med.* 2004;32:1466–1473.
11. Burkhart SS. The deadman theory of suture anchors: observations along a south Texas fence line. *Arthroscopy.* 1995;11:119–123.
12. Burkhart SS, Klein JR. Arthroscopic repair of rotator cuff tears associated with large bone cysts of the proximal humerus: compaction bone grafting technique. *Arthroscopy.* 2005;21:1149.
13. Brady PC, Arrigoni P, Burkhart SS. What do you do when you have a loose screw? *Arthroscopy.* 2006;22:925–930.

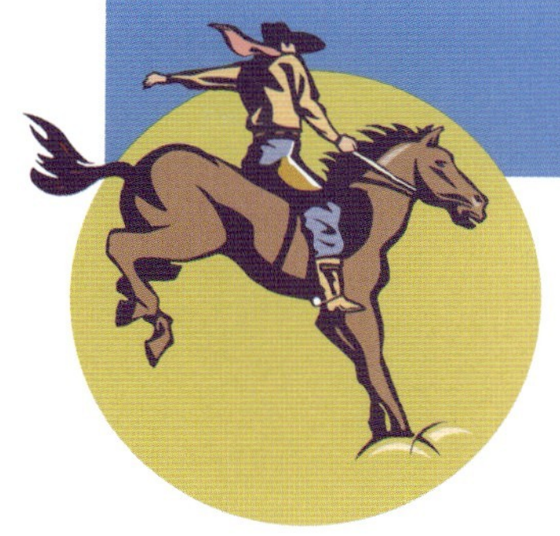

10

The Biceps Tendon

WESTERN WISDOM

Some folks can't see no higher than the steam from their own pot of stew.

The biceps tendon has long been considered a potential cause of pain in the shoulder. However, despite its long history of treatment, the diagnosis, management, and surgical treatment of disorders of the long head of the biceps (LHB) remain controversial. Because of the poor sensitivity and specificity of the majority of physical examination tests for biceps pathology, the arthroscopist must carefully evaluate the LHB tendon with a high index of clinical suspicion.

The spectrum of pathology related to the LHB may include inflammation, various degrees of degeneration, partial tearing, subluxation, and dislocation (Fig. 10.1). While the indications for debridement, tenotomy, and tenodesis are controversial, much of the treatment is tailored to the patient's age, symptoms, associated pathology, and expectations. In the vast majority of cases, patients with subluxation, dislocation, or partial tearing >30% are treated with tenotomy or tenodesis. In addition, in patients with concomitant subscapularis tendon repair, formal treatment (i.e., by tenotomy or tenodesis) of the biceps tendon is associated with improved outcomes.

We generally perform a biceps tenodesis rather than tenotomy in patients who are <70 years of age, males, laborers, or where preservation of biceps is important. In addition, if cosmesis is a concern (e.g., bodybuilders, females with thin arms), then a biceps tenodesis is performed. We reserve biceps tenotomy for patients over the age of 70, particularly if the arm is fat enough to conceal a potential distal biceps lump. In addition, in patients where the treatment of the biceps pathology will dictate the rehabilitation process, then a biceps tenotomy may be a consideration if a prolonged rehabilitation program is undesirable.

Our preferred technique for biceps tenodesis is tendon-to-bone interference fixation with a BioComposite Tenodesis Screw (Arthrex, Inc., Naples, FL). This provides much greater fixation strength than standard suture anchor or soft tissue techniques. This technique allows maintenance of the biceps length–tension relationship while achieving strong fixation. Although the exact preferred location of tenodesis is still controversial, we generally perform the tenodesis intra-articularly near the top of the bicipital groove, unless the extent of pathology warrants a more distal tenodesis. We have not found residual anterior shoulder pain, as reported by some authors, to be a significant problem. In fact we do not think that this is a valid concern, as the biceps that is tenodesed high in the bicipital groove will not have any contractile or elastic elements within the bicipital groove and therefore cannot have any excursion of the tendon over any osteophytes that might cause inflammation (Fig. 10.2).

We generally perform a biceps tenodesis close to the footprint of the supraspinatus in patients with a concomitant supraspinatus (+/− infraspinatus) tendon tear in patients where the bicipital groove portion of the biceps tendon appears normal. In this scenario, the biceps tenodesis is performed at the periphery of the supraspinatus tendon footprint and is used for securing the biceps tendon and part of the supraspinatus tendon. In patients with intact supraspinatus tendons, the tenodesis may still be performed high in the groove where visualization is easier and the technique simpler.

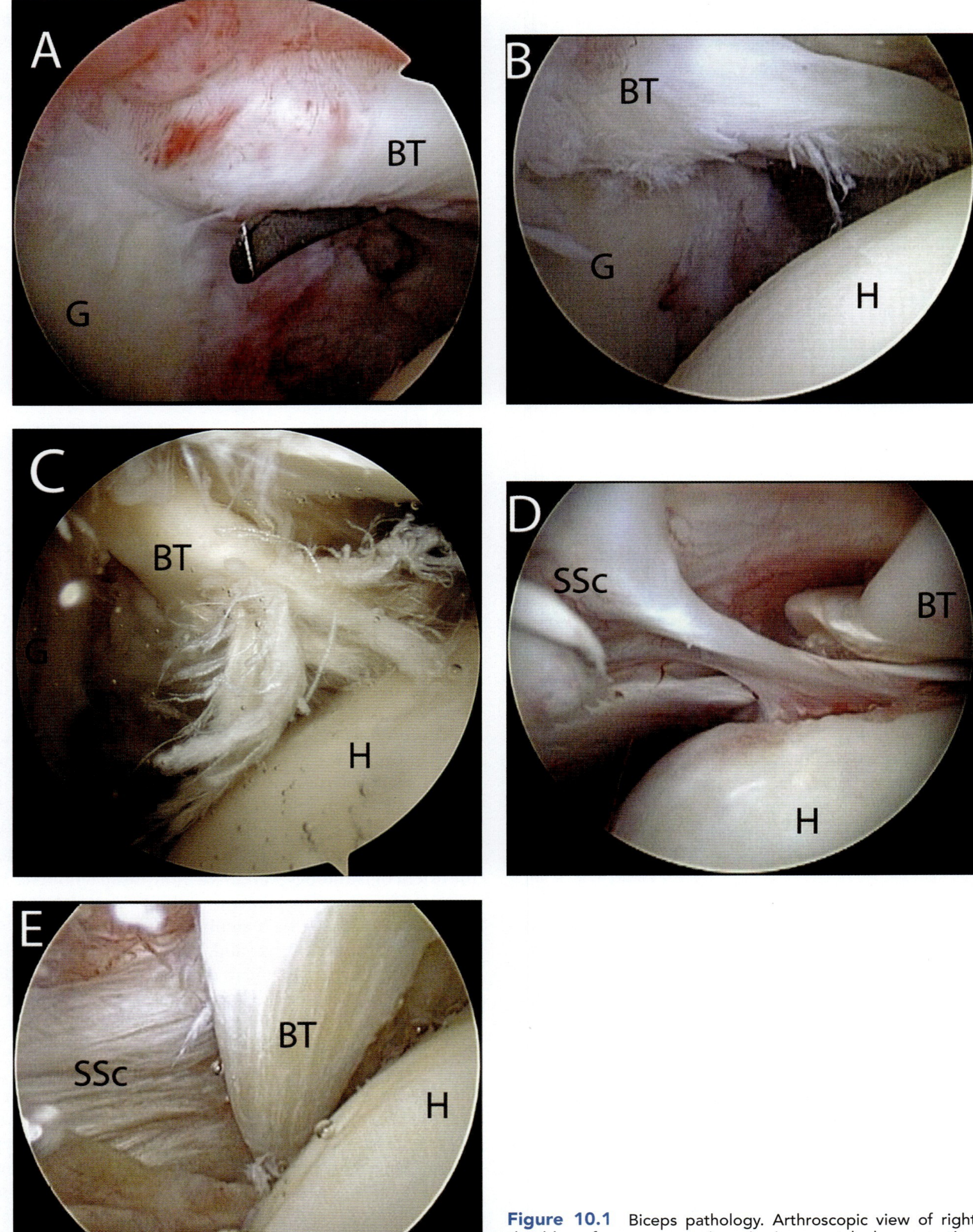

Figure 10.1 Biceps pathology. Arthroscopic view of right shoulders from a posterior viewing portal demonstrating **(A)** inflammation of the biceps; **(B)** degeneration; **(C)** partial tearing; **(D)** medial subluxation; and **(E)** dislocation. BT, biceps tendon; G, glenoid; H, humerus; SSc, subscapularis tendon.

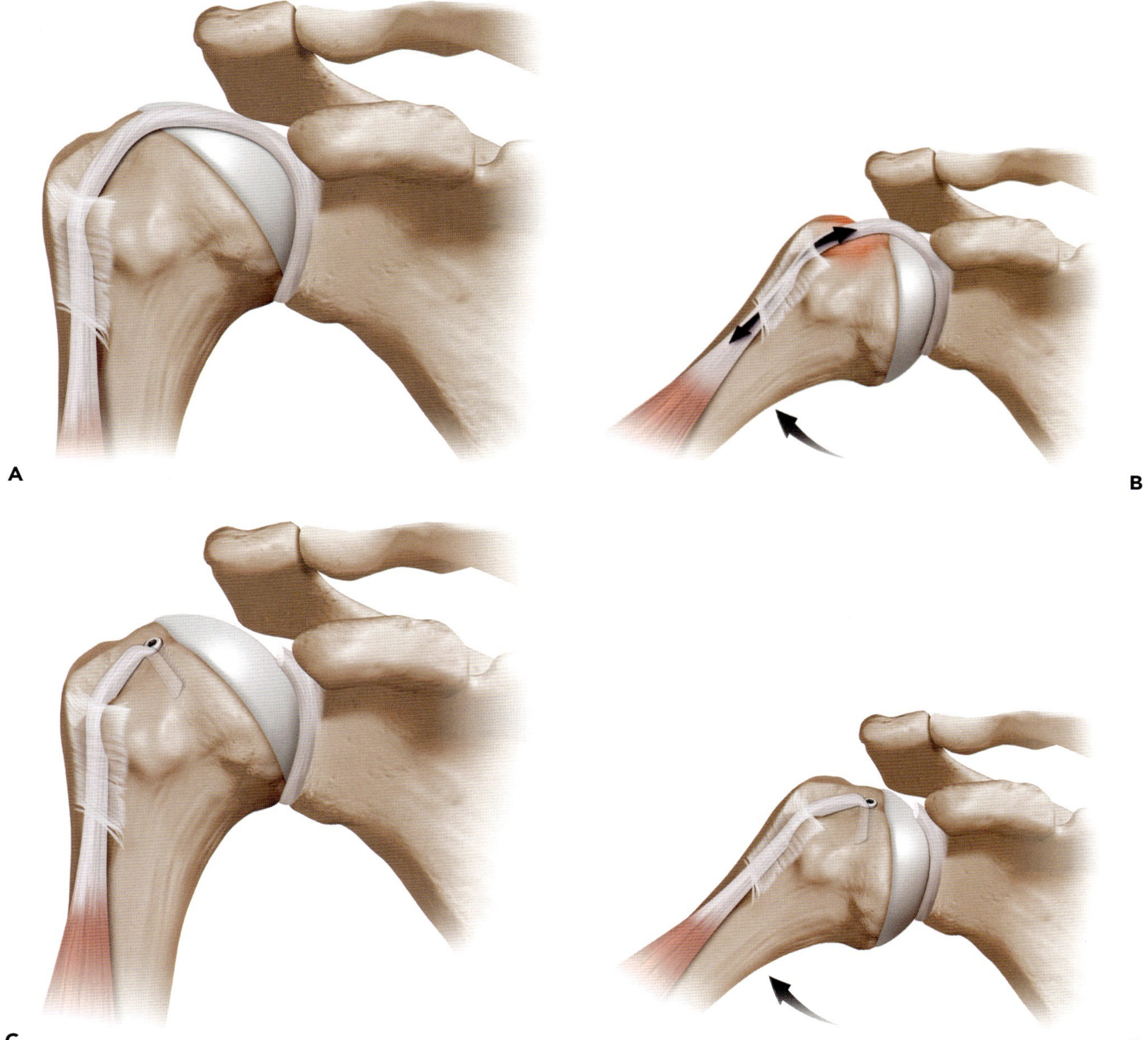

Figure 10.2 Schematic of a biceps tenodesis high in the bicipital groove. **A:** Prior to tenodesis, the biceps tendon crosses the glenohumeral joint. **B:** Movement of the glenohumeral joint results in relative motion of the biceps tendon within the bicipital groove. **C:** Following a biceps tenodesis high in the bicipital groove, the tendon no longer crosses the glenohumeral joint. **D:** Because the tendon no longer crosses the glenohumeral joint, movement of the joint does not result in any relative motion within the bicipital groove. Therefore, pain generation by movement of an inflamed tendon in the groove is eliminated.

In patients with a concomitant subscapularis tendon tear, visualization of the bicipital groove and anterior structures is facilitated by rupture of the subscapularis. In this scenario, we may perform biceps tenodesis lower in the groove near its distal extent, particularly if disease is demonstrated in the bicipital groove portion of the LHB. In small patients with limited footprint area for fixation, we sometimes medialize the tenodesis site to the superolateral aspect of the lesser tuberosity, then use the sutures from the biceps tenodesis construct to fix the superolateral subscapularis tendon to its footprint.

Video

The Cobra technique is reserved for ruptures of the LHB tendon. In this technique, the LHB is retrieved through a distal skin incision on the arm and the tendon is retensioned and reduced back through the bicipital groove and into the shoulder. This technique is used when sufficient length and quality of the LHB tendon is present for reduction and fixation. However, in patients who have poor-quality tissue or insufficient tendon length, but desire reduction of deformity, a mini-open subpectoral biceps tenodesis is performed for tendon fixation to bone.

When performing biceps tenodesis, the major technical pitfalls are related to visualization, maintenance of the biceps tendon length–tension relationship, reduction of the tendon into the bone socket, final tensioning of the tendon, and securing fixation. Each scenario is addressed below with its specific technique.

ISOLATED BICEPS TENODESIS WITH TENODESIS SCREW FIXATION (HIGH IN THE FOOTPRINT OR GROOVE)

Biceps tenodesis performed in the anteromedial supraspinatus footprint or high in the intertubercular groove is the least difficult method of tenodesis. In this method, visualization is maximized because of the proximal location of the tenodesis. Visualization may be improved by using a 70° arthroscope or by positioning the arm in external rotation and abduction. All procedures are begun by diagnostic arthroscopy through a posterior glenohumeral portal. An anterior portal is established and the LHB tendon is evaluated (Fig. 10.3). By placing traction on the intra-articular portion and drawing the tendon into the joint, the bicipital groove portion of the biceps may be evaluated. However, with a 70° arthroscope, a significant amount of the intertubercular groove portion of the biceps (approximately 2.5 cm) can be visualized without the need to pull the biceps into the joint (Fig. 10.4). If the LHB tendon demonstrates significant intra-articular disease but minimal bicipital groove disease, then a tenodesis high in the groove may be performed, particularly in the presence of an intact supraspinatus tendon. However, even when there is mild-to-moderate degeneration of the tendon in the proximal groove, tenodesis in that area will eliminate relative motion between the tendon and the bone, and we have noted excellent clinical results in such patients.

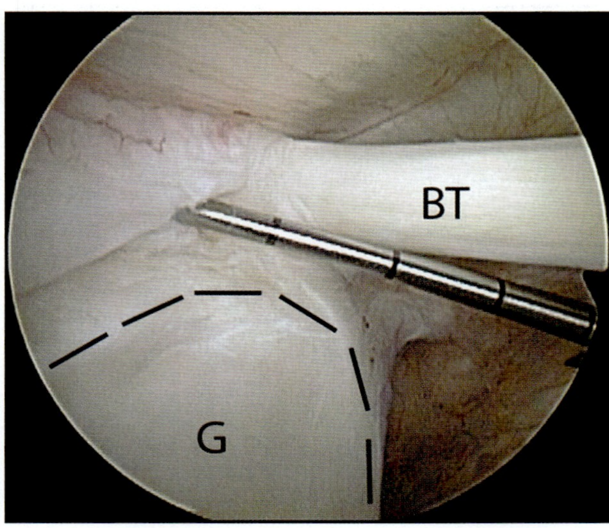

Figure 10.3 Right shoulder, posterior viewing portal. A probe introduced through an anterior portal is used to assess the biceps root. In this case, there is a displaceable biceps root. The glenoid rim is outline by *dashed black lines*. BT, biceps tendon; G, glenoid.

An anterosuperolateral portal is then established with an 8.25-mm clear threaded cannula (Arthrex, Inc., Naples, FL) perpendicular to the bicipital groove just as the tendon exits into the bicipital groove. Two half-racking traction stitches (#2 FiberWire; Arthrex, Inc., Naples, FL) are then placed through the biceps tendon. To place a half-racking stitch, the middle of a #2 FiberWire suture

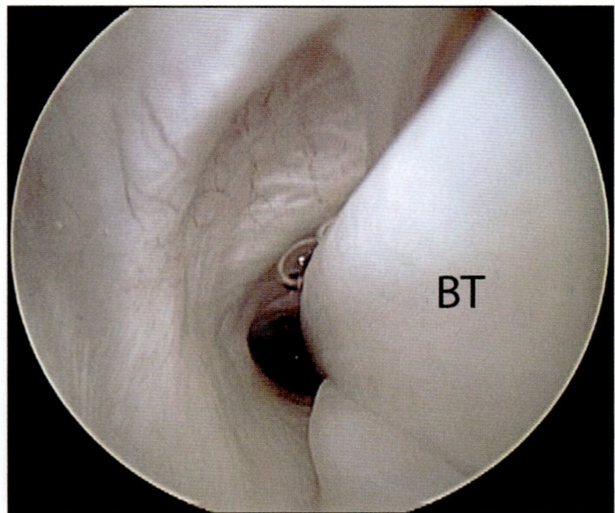

Figure 10.4 Right shoulder, posterior viewing portal. With a 70° arthroscope, a significant amount of the intertubercular groove portion of the biceps (approximately 2.5 cm) can be visualized. BT, biceps tendon

is loaded onto a Penetrator (Arthrex, Inc., Naples, FL) (Fig. 10.5). The Penetrator is inserted through the anterosuperolateral portal and is used to pass through the middle of the biceps tendon (Fig. 10.6A), advancing about 2 cm past the tendon in order to leave a loop of suture in the joint (Fig. 10.6B.). The suture is released and the Penetrator is withdrawn and passed posterior to the biceps tendon to grasp the suture loop that is retrieved out the anterosuperolateral portal (Fig. 10.6C). Extracorporeally, the free ends of the suture are threaded through the looped end to create a half-racking stitch. Pulling on the free suture limbs cinches the knot down on the biceps tendon (Fig. 10.7). Alternating traction on the suture limbs can be used to tighten the knot. A second half-racking stitch is similarly placed just distal to the first stitch (Fig. 10.8). The tendon is released from its origin at the superior labrum and retrieved into the cannula (Fig. 10.9). While maintaining traction on the biceps tendon, the cannula is pulled out of the skin, and traction is removed so that the shoulder

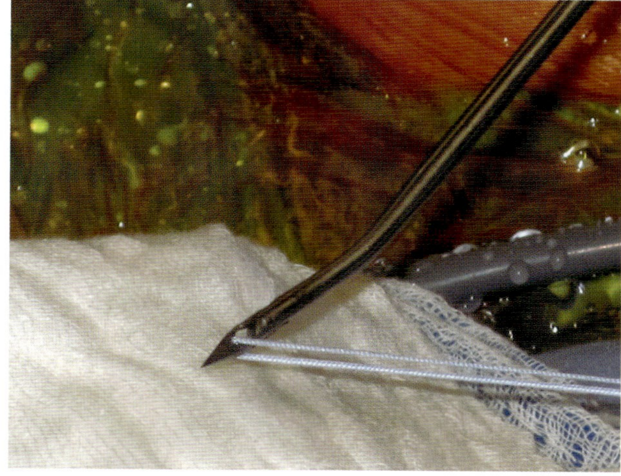

Figure 10.5 External photo demonstrates a #2 FiberWire (Arthrex, Inc., Naples, FL) that has been loaded in the middle onto a Penetrator (Arthrex, Inc., Naples, FL) in preparation for placement of a half-racking stitch in the biceps tendon.

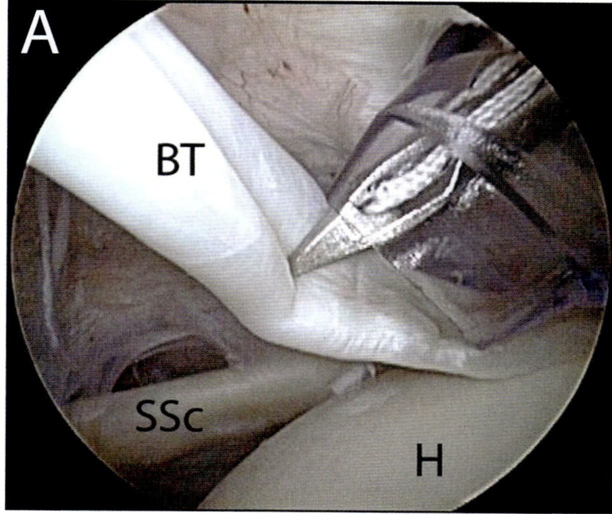

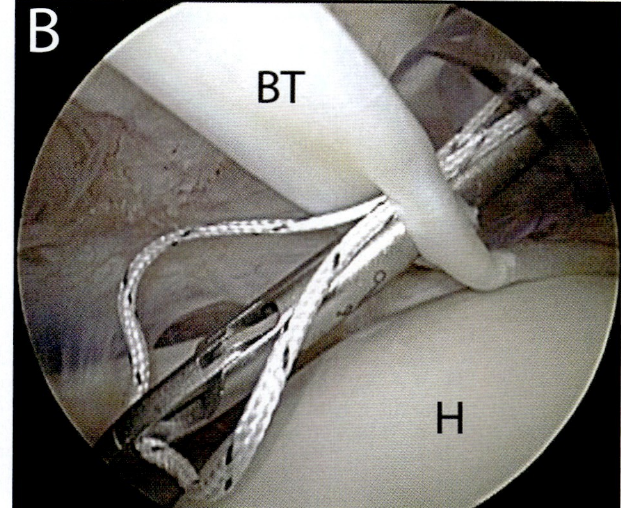

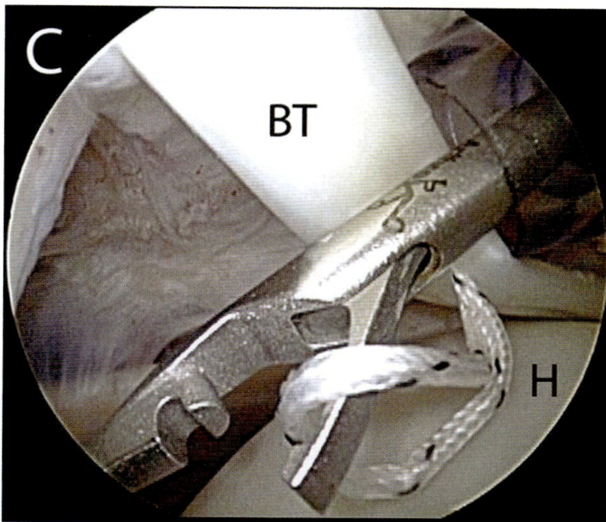

Figure 10.6 Half-racking stitch placement in the biceps prior to tenotomy in right shoulder viewed from a posterior portal. **A:** The middle of a #2 FiberWire suture (Arthrex, Inc., Naples, FL) has been loaded onto a Penetrator (Arthrex, Inc., Naples, FL). The Penetrator is inserted through an anterosuperolateral portal and used to pass through the center of the biceps tendon. **B:** The Penetrator is advanced about 2 cm beyond the biceps tendon where it will release the suture. **C:** Then, the Penetrator is withdrawn and passes posterior to the tendon to retrieve the suture loop. BT, biceps tendon; H, humerus; SSc, subscapularis tendon.

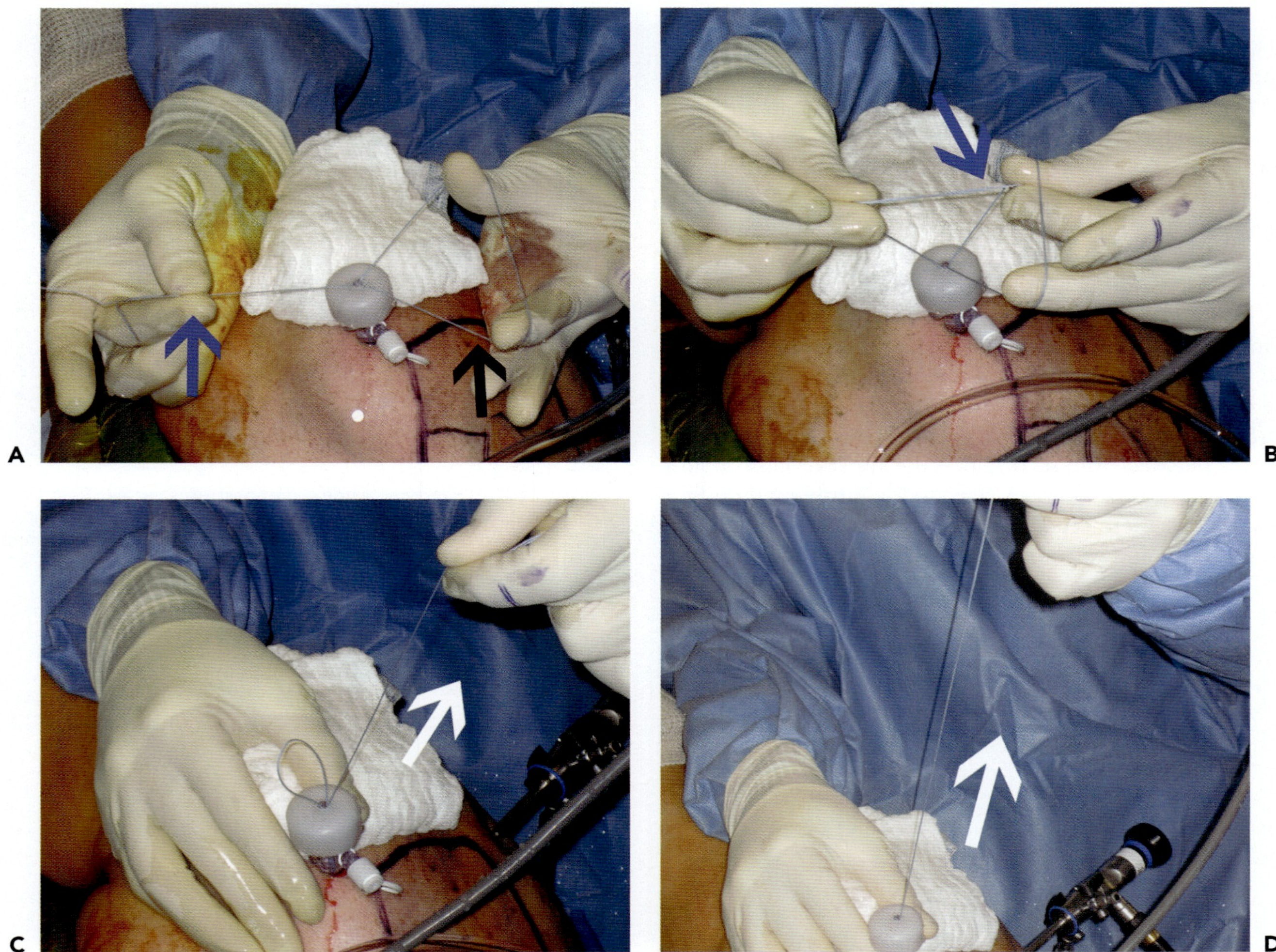

FIGURE 10.7 External view of steps for completing a half-racking stitch. **A:** The looped end of a suture (*black arrow*), which has been passed through the biceps tendon, and the free ends of the suture (*blue arrow*) are grasped. **B:** The free suture ends (*blue arrow*) are passed through the loop. **C:** Pulling tension (*white arrow*) on the free ends of the suture cinches the loop. **D:** Tension is applied (*white arrow*) until the knot rests on the biceps tendon.

and elbow can be flexed to relax the biceps and improve exposure (Fig. 10.10).

Extracorporeally, a small portion of the LHB is sometimes removed based upon the amount of disease but also on the position of tenodesis. When estimating the amount of tendon to remove, it is important to remember that the intra-articular portion of the LHB tendon is approximately 2.5 cm and that the bone socket drilled is approximately 25 mm in depth to accommodate a 23-mm BioComposite Tenodesis screw. Furthermore, the whipstitch in the biceps tendon is begun about 5 mm from the end of the tendon. Therefore, if the tenodesis is performed high in the groove, we do not typically remove any tendon length.

A #2 FiberWire whipstitch is used to secure a 2- to 2.5-cm portion of the proximal end of the biceps tendon (Fig. 10.11A). It is important that the whipstitch enters and exits the tendon on the superior aspect of the biceps, approximately 5 mm from the end of the tendon, so that the driver can push the tendon into the bone socket during insertion while the anatomical orientation of the biceps is preserved. Shaping the tip like a bullet is also important for easing reduction of the tendon into the bone socket (Fig. 10.11B). One of the previously placed half-racking stitches is removed after the whipstitch has been placed. Using the thumb pad from the tenodesis driver, the tendon is sized and usually measures 7 or 8 mm (Fig. 10.11C). Then, the tendon is allowed to retract back into the shoulder. The anterosuperolateral portal is reestablished, but the sutures in the biceps are left outside the cannula.

In rare cases, the biceps tendon may be larger than 8 mm in diameter and will be too large to secure with an 8-mm tenodesis screw. In such cases, prior to placing the whipstitch, the tendon is easily downsized by sharply excising a

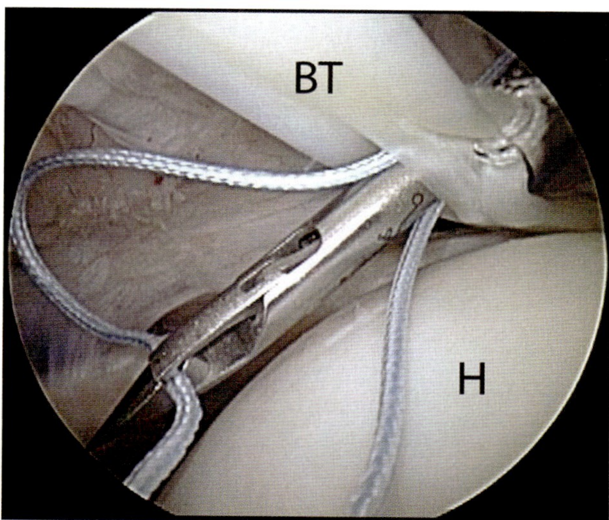

Figure 10.8 Right shoulder, posterior viewing portal, demonstrates placement of a second half-racking suture in the biceps tendon. This suture is placed just distal to the first suture for added security. BT, biceps tendon; H, humerus.

small section of the proximal tendon for a length of about 3 cm (Fig. 10.12)

While viewing through a posterior glenohumeral portal, a guide pin is placed at the proximal aspect of the bicipital groove (Fig. 10.13A, B). Since the anterosuperolateral cannula was established with reference to the proximal aspect of the groove, the guide pin may usually be appropriately placed through this cannula and a separate portal is not required. Care is taken to ensure the guide pin is placed perpendicular to the groove.

A headed reamer of the same diameter as the tendon is then used to prepare a bone socket to a depth of 25 mm (to accommodate a 23-mm screw length plus the minor width of the tendon) (Fig. 10.13C). Generally speaking, if the tendon is between sizes, we will drill one size larger. This is because too tight a bone socket will make reduction of the tendon into the bottom of the hole extremely difficult and frustrating. Therefore, if the tendon measures approximately 6.5 mm, we will drill a 7-mm hole and place a 7-mm screw. Drilling and overstuffing the bone socket with a similar sized screw and tendon is possible due to the relatively soft cancellous bone of the proximal humerus.

Preparation of the bone socket is completed by removing soft tissue that may impede reduction of the tendon-screw unit (Fig. 10.14). The distal edge of the bone socket may also be beveled with a burr to minimize abrasion of the LHB. The sutures from the biceps whipstitch are then retrieved and passed through the cannulation of the tenodesis driver so that the tip of the screwdriver is against the biceps tendon. The screwdriver tip can be used to directly manipulate the end of the tendon (Fig. 10.15). Under direct vision, the screwdriver tip is then placed into the bottom of the bone socket, thereby reducing the tendon. Reduction of the tendon is confirmed by visualization of the whipstitch disappearing into the bone socket.

While holding the thumb pad on the screwdriver and maintaining tension on the biceps whipstitch sutures, the screw is advanced into the bone socket, securing tendon fixation to bone (Fig 10.16). The reduction of the tendon and screw depth can be confirmed by holding the screwdriver handle in place and turning the thumb pad clockwise to withdraw the screwdriver sleeve (Fig. 10.17). A suture from the whipstitch in the biceps (passing now through

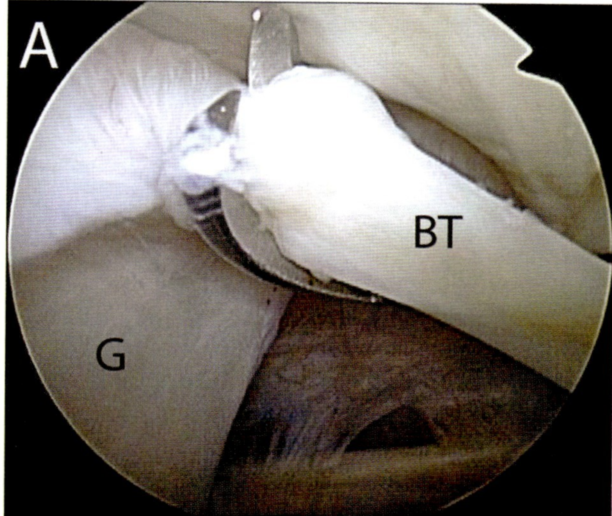

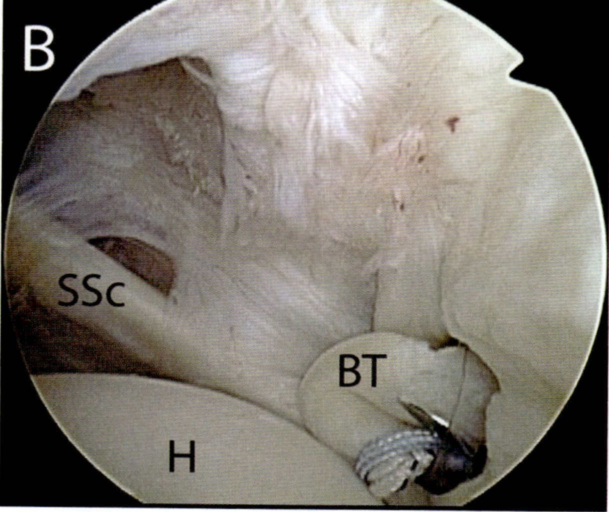

Figure 10.9 **A:** Right shoulder, posterior viewing portal demonstrating tenotomy of the biceps tendon, **(B)** followed by retrieval through the anterosuperolateral portal with a Kingfisher retriever (Arthrex, Inc., Naples, FL). BT, biceps tendon; G, glenoid; H, humerus; SSc, subscapularis tendon.

A

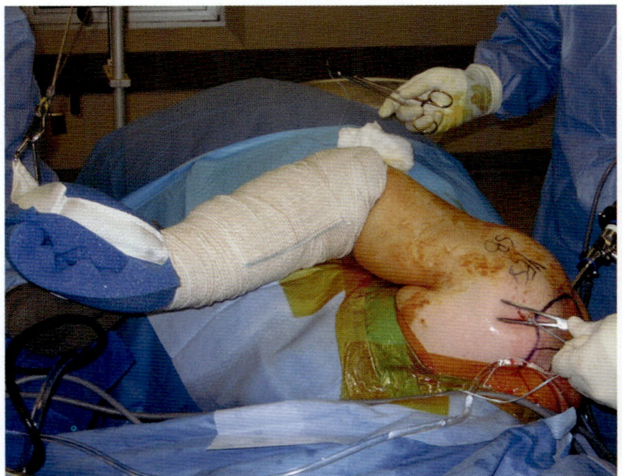

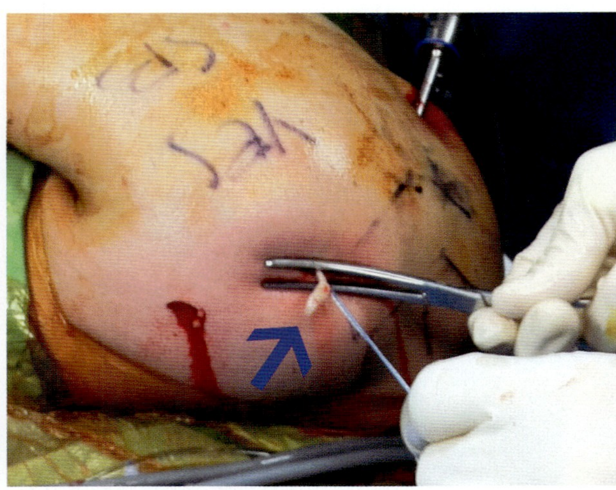

B

Figure 10.10 **A:** External view of a right shoulder. Access to the exteriorized biceps tendon is increased by removing the arm from traction and flexing the elbow. **B:** Pushing down on the skin with an instrument and pulling traction on the half-racking stitches also helps provide access to the biceps tendon (*blue arrow*) for placement of a whipstitch.

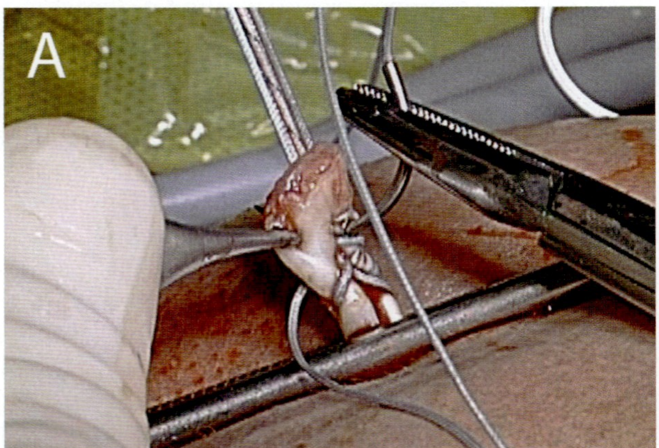

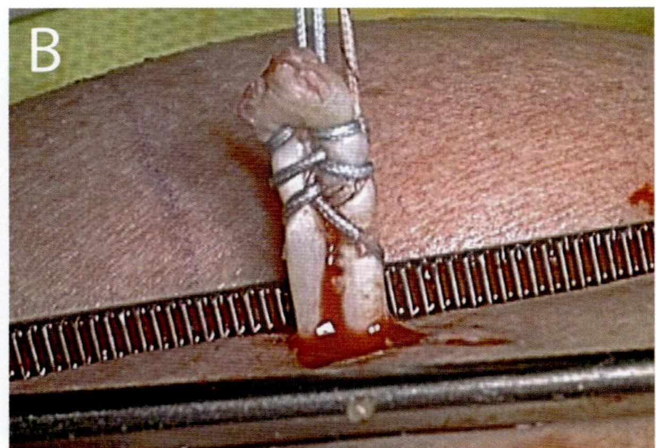

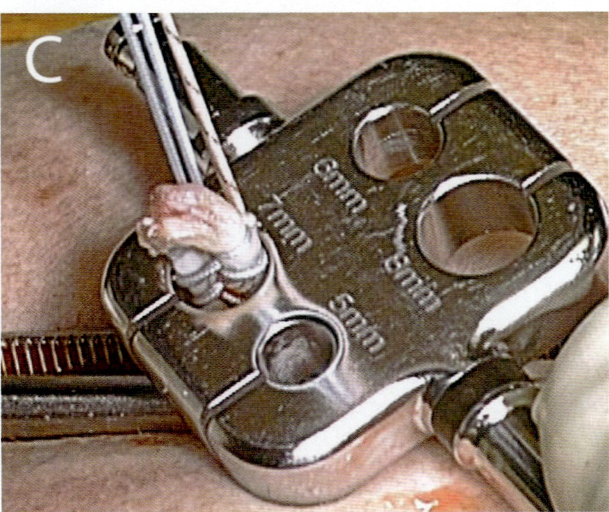

Figure 10.11 Preparation of the biceps tendon. **A:** A FiberWire whipstitch is placed in the biceps tendon and exits the tendon 5 mm from its proximal end. **B:** The leading edge of the tendon is trimmed so that it is shaped like a bullet. Note that overlapping the two rows of the whipstitch as in this case is useful when tissue quality is poor. **C:** The tendon is sized; in this case, a 7-mm screw will be selected.

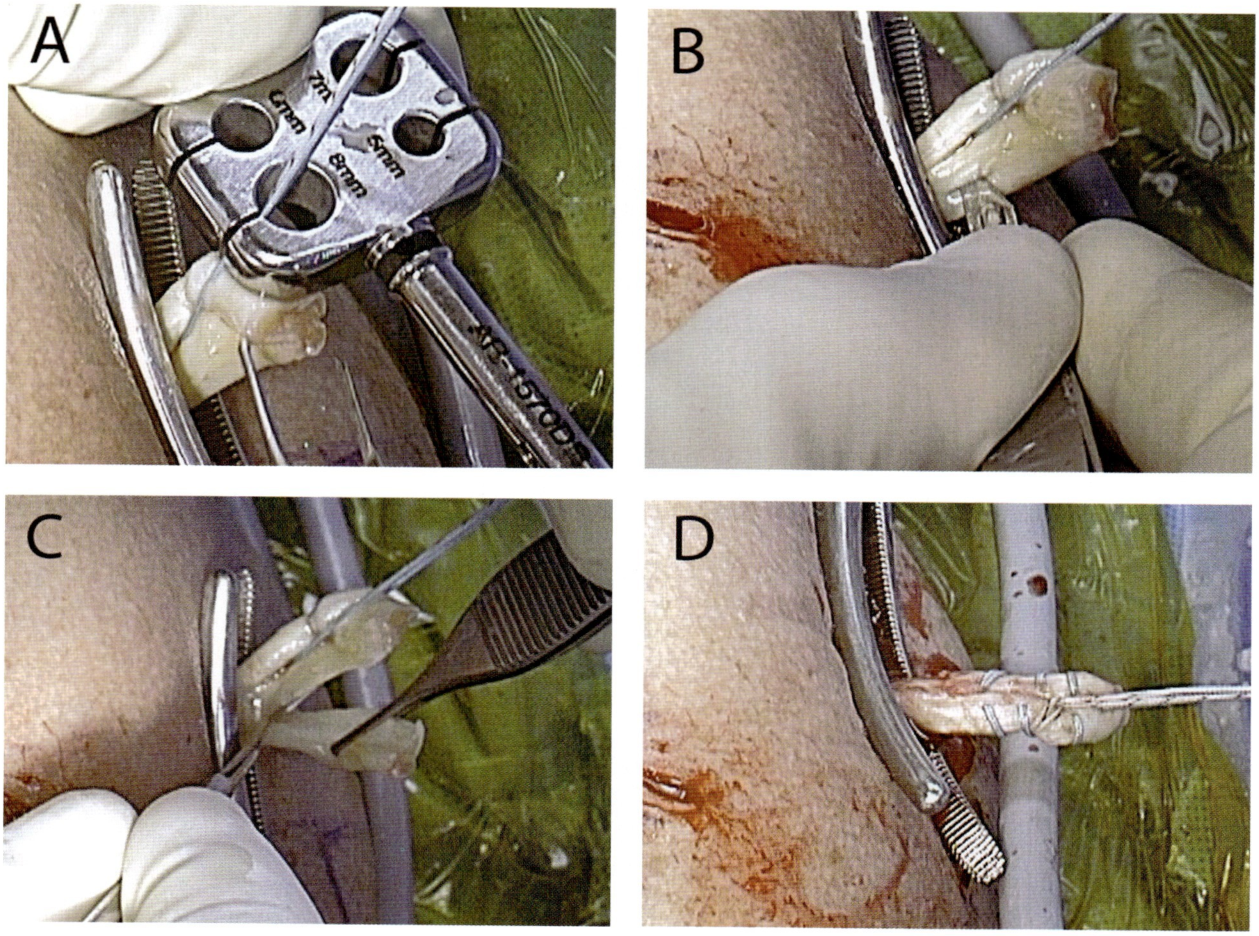

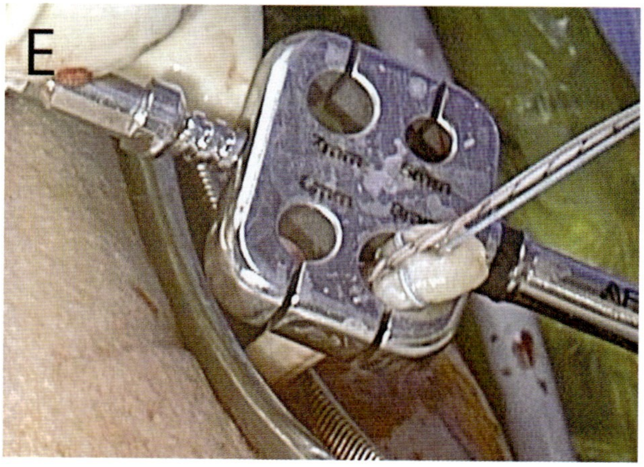

Figure 10.12 Downsizing a large biceps tendon to accommodate an 8-mm tenodesis screw. **A:** In rare cases, the biceps tendon is larger than 8 mm in diameter. **B, C:** In such a case, the tendon can be downsized by sharply excising a thin longitudinal section of tendon. **D:** The tendon is then prepared with a whipstitch in the usual manner. **E:** After downsizing, the tendon is 8 mm in diameter and can now be secured with an 8-mm tenodesis screw.

the center of the screw), and a suture from the retained half-racking stitch are then tied together, and repeated with the second set of sutures, so that the sutures completely encircle the screw from its inner cannulation to its outer threads (Fig. 10.18). This maximizes fixation by ensuring that the entire construct would have to fail for the tendon to lose fixation. Alternatively, the sutures from the biceps tenodesis construct may be used to repair the defect in the roof of the bicipital groove, repairing this tissue directly over the top of the biceps tenodesis.

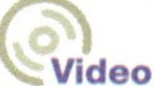

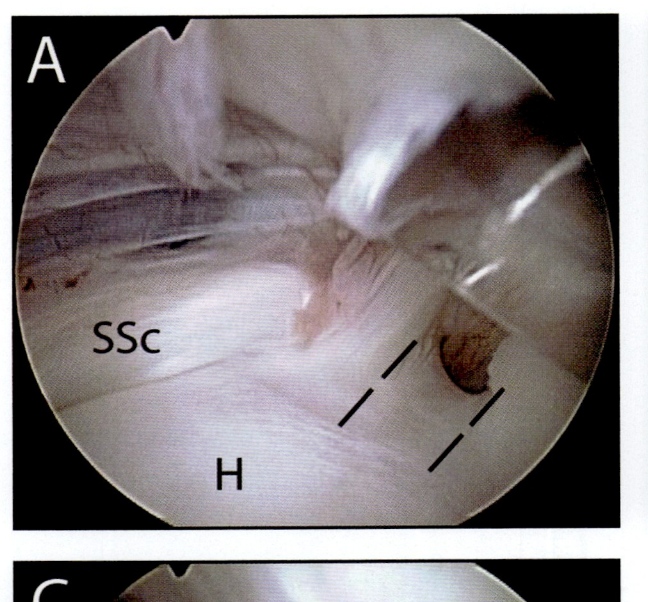

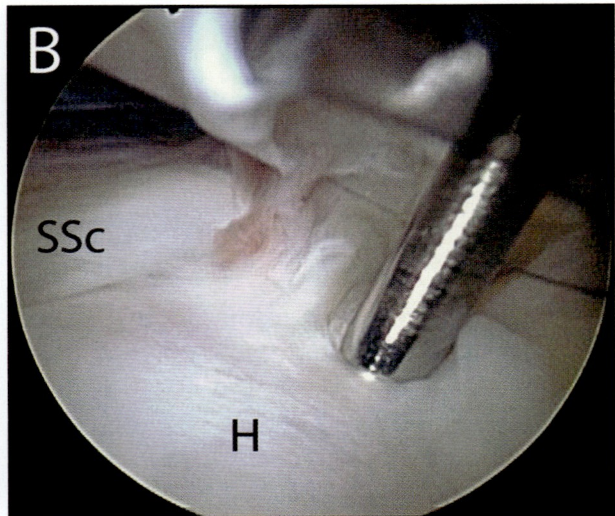

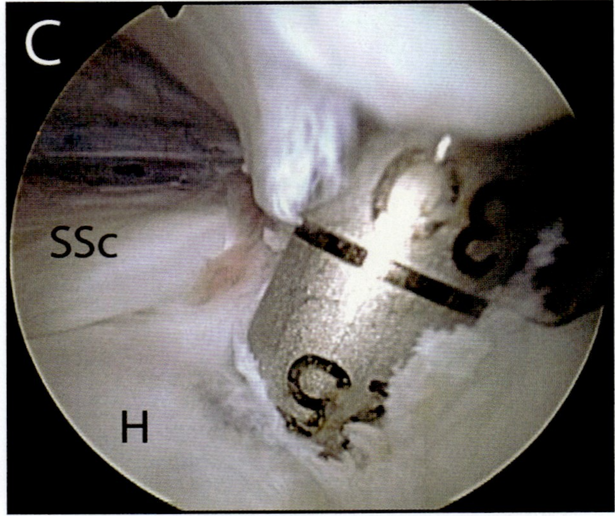

Figure 10.13 Location for biceps tenodesis in a right shoulder viewed from a posterior portal. **A:** The bicipital groove (*dashed blacked lines*) is visualized. **B:** A guide pin is inserted through an anterosuperolateral portal at the top of the bicipital groove. **C:** A reamer is then inserted over the guide pin and advanced to 25 mm to accommodate the 23-mm-long screw. H, humerus; SSc, subscapularis tendon.

BICEPS TENODESIS TECHNIQUE WITH SWIVELOCK C SUTURE ANCHOR FOR INTERFERENCE FIXATION

We have recently begun using a new fixation technique for biceps tenodesis in the proximal portion of the bicipital groove. This technique utilizes a SwiveLock C suture anchor (Arthrex, Inc., Naples, FL) rather than a BioComposite Tenodesis screw for interference fixation of the tendon. The technique is particularly useful for cases in which the biceps tendon is <7 mm in diameter. It is a little less cumbersome in its execution because the suture ends from the whipstitch in the biceps tendon simply have to be threaded and tensioned through the eyelet of the anchor rather than being threaded and tensioned through the entire length of a cannulated inserter (as is done with the Tenodesis screw technique).

The technique is as follows. Two half-racking sutures are arthroscopically placed in the biceps. The biceps is tenotomized at its root, and then exteriorized so that a whipstitch can be placed.

The whipstitch differs in one critical way from the whipstitch that is used in the Tenodesis screw technique. With the latter technique, the free ends of the whipstitch exit 5 mm from the cut end of the tendon, so that the Tenodesis driver can be used to push the tendon into the bone socket. With the SwiveLock technique, the free ends of the whipstitch exit the very end of the tendon (Fig. 10.19). This allows the end of the tendon to be pulled snugly against the eyelet of the anchor so that the tendon can be pulled (rather than pushed) to the base of the bone socket. This is an important distinction because the sutures must be side loaded (rather than end loaded) into the eyelet of the anchor, and therefore the tendon must be pulled (rather

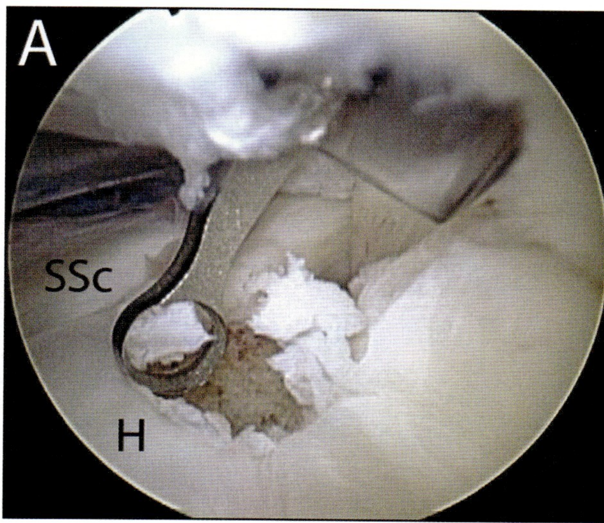

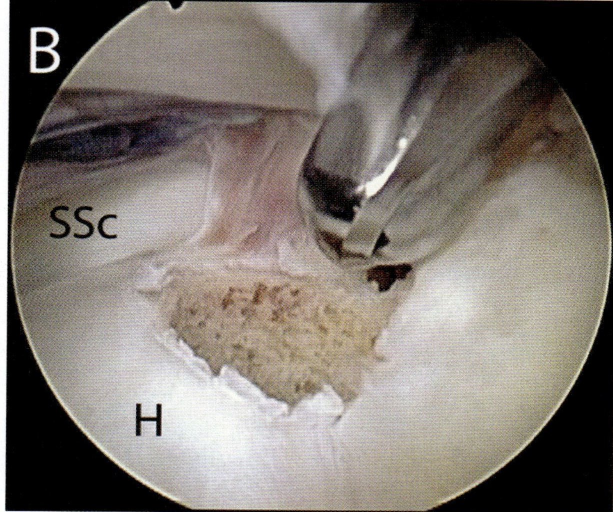

Figure 10.14 Right shoulder, posterior viewing portal. To provide unobstructed access for tenodesis, the margins of the bone socket are cleared with **(A)** a ring curette and **(B)** shaver. H, humerus; SSc, subscapularis tendon.

than pushed) into the bone socket. By having the suture limbs exit the end of the tendon, the smallest possible profile of the tendon is being presented into the bone socket, thereby facilitating insertion of the tendon into the bone socket.

After the whipstitch has been placed and the subscapularis has been repaired, the bone socket is made with a special noncannulated, headed reamer that has a small point on the end to gain purchase in the bone so that the drill does not "walk" on the bone (Fig. 10.20). This drill-tipped reamer obviates the need for a guide pin, thereby saving a step. The bone socket is created at the top of the bicipital groove to a depth of 20 mm. Prior to drilling the bone socket, we size the diameter of the biceps tendon, to be sure that it will fit in the bone socket; if it is too large, we drill to the measured diameter of the tendon to a depth of 20 mm. Most often, we drill a 7-mm bone socket in women, and an 8-mm socket in men. Soft tissues are cleared from the mouth of the bone socket with a combination of power shaver, electrocautery, and ring curette.

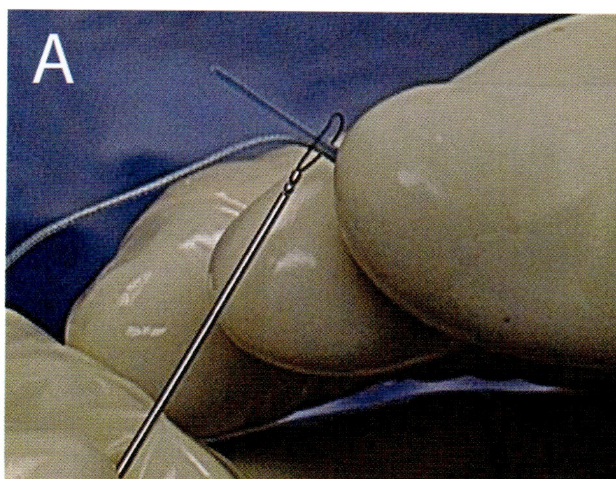

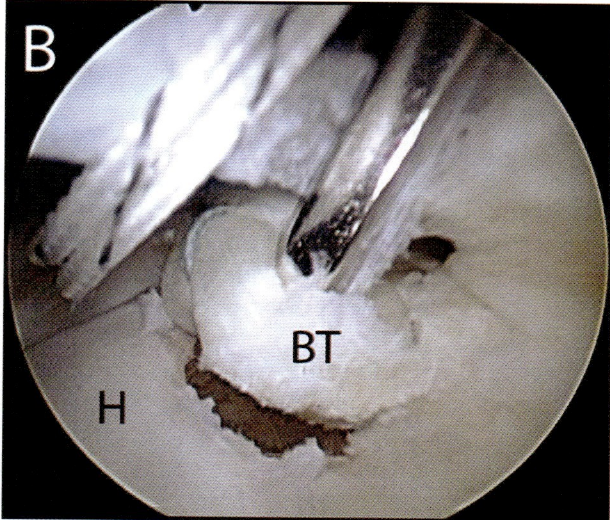

Figure 10.15 Insertion of the biceps tendon. **A**: Externally, the whipstitch tails are passed through a wire loop used to bring the end of the tendon to the tip of the tenodesis screwdriver. **B**: Arthroscopic view in a right shoulder, viewed from posterior. The tendon is adjacent to the tip of the tenodesis screwdriver that is then used to seat the biceps tendon into a bone socket. BT, biceps tendon; H, humerus.

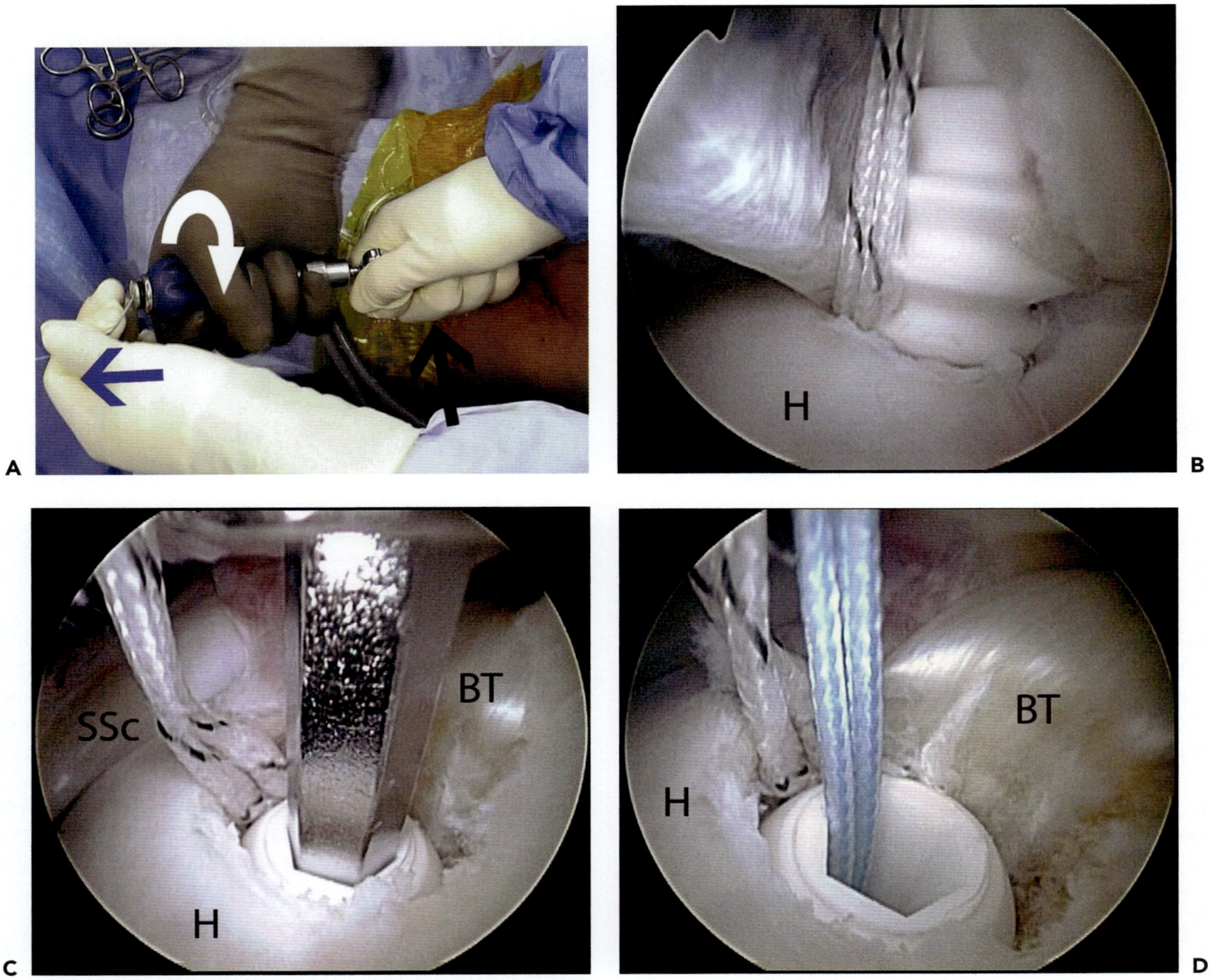

Figure 10.16 Biceps tenodesis screw placement in a right shoulder viewed from a posterior portal. **A:** External view of a right shoulder. While maintaining tension (*blue arrow*) on the sutures, the thumb pad is held (*black arrow*) and the screwdriver handle is turned (*white arrow*) to advance the tenodesis screw. **B:** Arthroscopic view of a right shoulder viewed from a posterior portal with a 70° arthroscope. The tenodesis screw is advanced until (**C**) the screw is just below the level of the articular margin. **D:** Tendon-bone fixation is achieved. BT, biceps tendon; H, humerus; SSc, subscapularis tendon.

The free ends of the whipstitch are then threaded through the eyelet of the SwiveLock C anchor. The suture ends are tensioned and the eyelet is pushed along the sutures until the end of the biceps tendon abuts firmly against the eyelet. While maintaining tension on the sutures, the eyelet is used like a joystick to maneuver the tendon to the base of the bone socket (Fig. 10.21). The body of the anchor is then screwed into place to achieve interference fixation (Fig. 10.22). The sutures from the whipstitch may then be sutured together to strengthen the construct (Fig. 10.23), or they may be incorporated into the repair of the rotator cuff or repair of the portal defect in the roof of the bicipital groove.

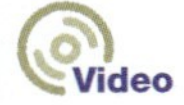

BICEPS TENODESIS HIGH IN THE FOOTPRINT IN COMBINATION WITH SUPRASPINATUS ROTATOR CUFF REPAIR

The keys to biceps tenodesis high in the footprint with rotator cuff repair are proper screw positioning and suture setup. Essentially the same procedures and principles are used to tag and release the tendon. However, since the tenodesis is now being performed in the supraspinatus footprint, the tendon should not be shortened at all. Depending on the anticipated suture anchor configuration, the anchor may be placed in the anteromedial or anterolateral portion of the footprint. To accommodate the position

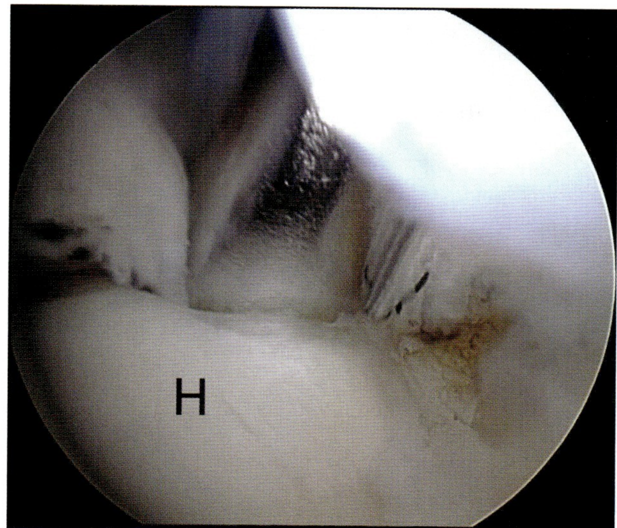

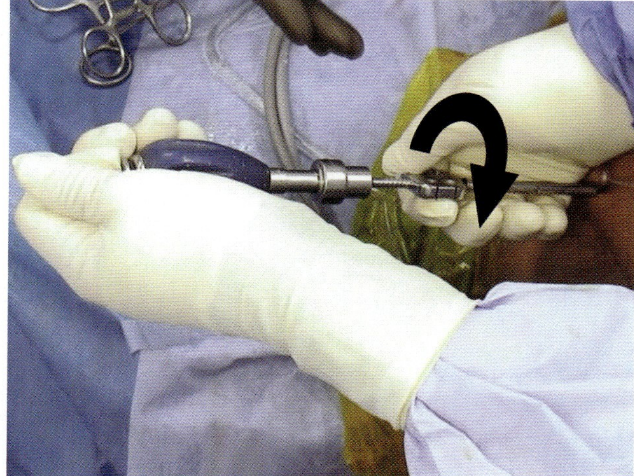

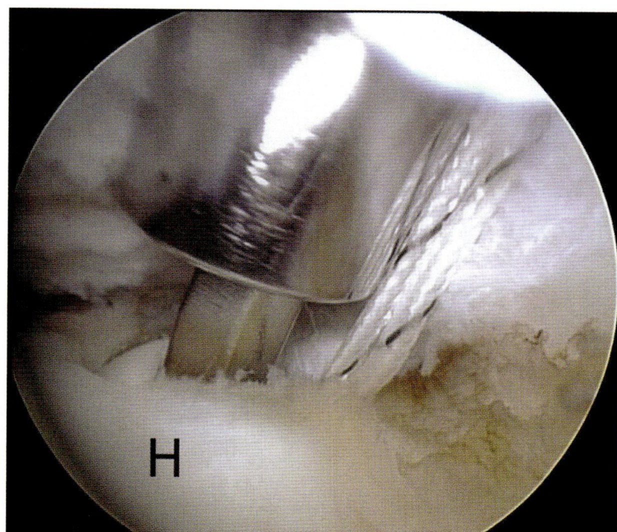

Figure 10.17 Right shoulder demonstrates confirming the depth of a tenodesis screw. **A:** Posterior viewing portal with a 70° arthroscope demonstrates a completely seated tenodesis screw. **B:** External view. The screwdriver handle is held in place while the thumb pad is turned clockwise (*black arrow*) to back off the driver sleeve. **C:** Arthroscopic view demonstrates the sleeve that has been slightly backed off to confirm that the tenodesis screw is seated just below the bone. H, humerus.

of the tenodesis, the proximal transverse ligament may be released to increase excursion.

Once the position of the biceps tenodesis has been determined (Fig. 10.24), a bone socket is prepared as previously described. Depending on bone quality, the drill may be downsized to maximize fixation in softer greater tuberosity bone. To provide additional sutures for rotator cuff tear fixation, a free suture may be passed up through the cannulated screwdriver (tails first) so that a loop of suture is at the distal end of the screwdriver tip. The loop of suture is then used to capture the whipstitch sutures as the screwdriver is slid down to control the proximal end of the LHB tendon. Alternatively, the whipstitch sutures may be threaded directly into the cannulation of the screwdriver for better control of the tendon.

The biceps tendon is then similarly tenodesed into the bone socket leaving the two pairs of sutures for rotator cuff repair. These sutures may be used to assist with arthroscopic rotator cuff repair (Fig. 10.25).

ISOLATED BICEPS TENODESIS (LOW IN THE GROOVE) WITH INTACT ROTATOR CUFF

An arthroscopic biceps tenodesis may also be performed lower in the groove. This is particularly relevant in cases where the bicipital groove portion of the tendon is significantly diseased and weakened, and needs to be removed (Fig. 10.26).

If tendon quality is sufficient, the biceps tendon is tagged with traction stitches and released from the superior labrum as previously described. However, in this situation since the tenodesis is now to be performed low in the

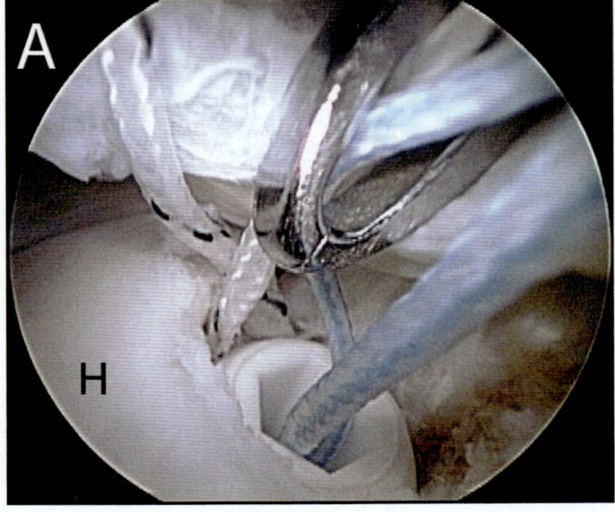

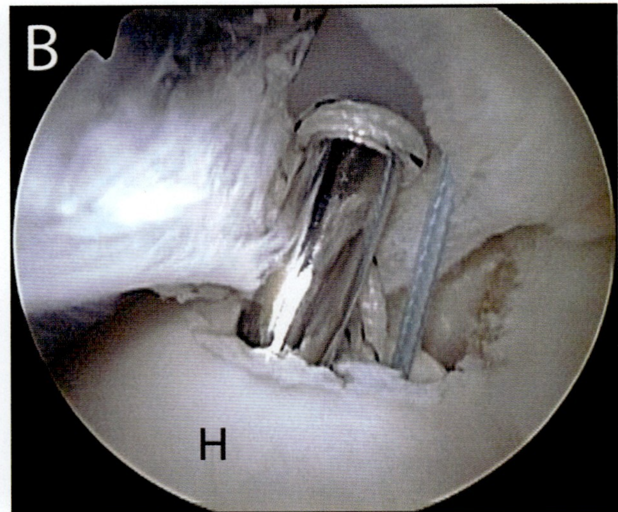

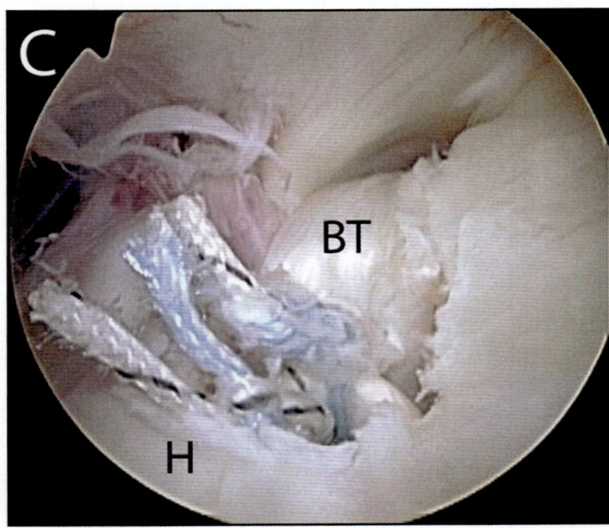

Figure 10.18 Reinforcement of a biceps tenodesis in a right shoulder viewed from a posterior portal with a 70° arthroscope. **A:** A suture from the whipstitch (*blue*) and suture from the retained half-racking stitch (*white*) are retrieved. **B:** The sutures are tied. **C:** Final repair demonstrating secure tendon–bone fixation. BT, biceps tendon; H, humerus.

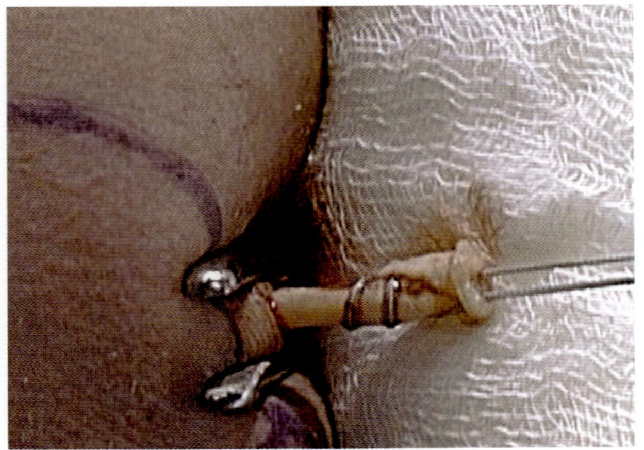

Figure 10.19 External view of a whipstitch placed in the biceps tendon in preparation for tenodesis with a 6.5-mm BioComposite SwiveLock anchor. A SwiveLock anchor is chosen because the tendon in this patient is only 6 mm in diameter. Note that the whipstitch exits the biceps tendon directly at the edge as opposed to 5 mm distal to the edge as is used for a standard tenodesis.

groove, approximately 3 to 4 cm of the tendon should be excised to accommodate for the extra length provided by the bicipital groove portion.

In cases of an intact cuff, the biceps tendon and bicipital groove must be identified in the subacromial space in order to do the tenodesis low in the groove. The arthroscope is placed through a posterior subacromial portal and a lateral portal is established. A brief subacromial bursectomy is performed just to identify the subacromial space. Poor visualization is the most common problem encountered, but it can be improved by keeping in mind several tips. Usually the biceps tendon is anteriorly located and extrabursal. To access this region, the anterior wall of the bursa must be excised and unfortunately this area commonly collapses with swelling. To maximize the space available, the arm is positioned in flexion to relax the overlying deltoid muscle. A 70° arthroscope is routinely used through the posterior or lateral portal to look down onto the anterior structures. Furthermore, release of the

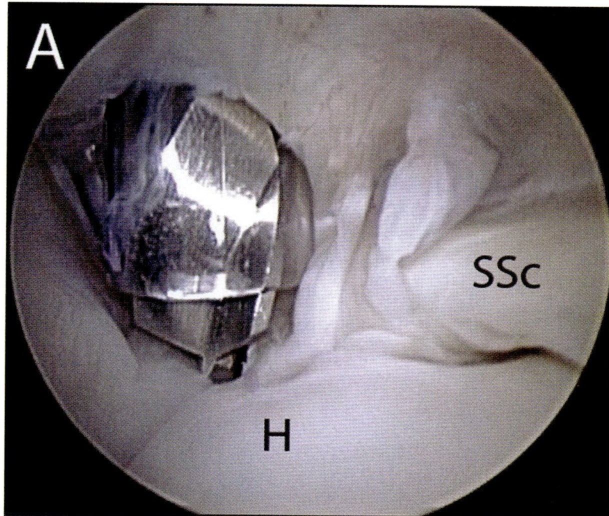

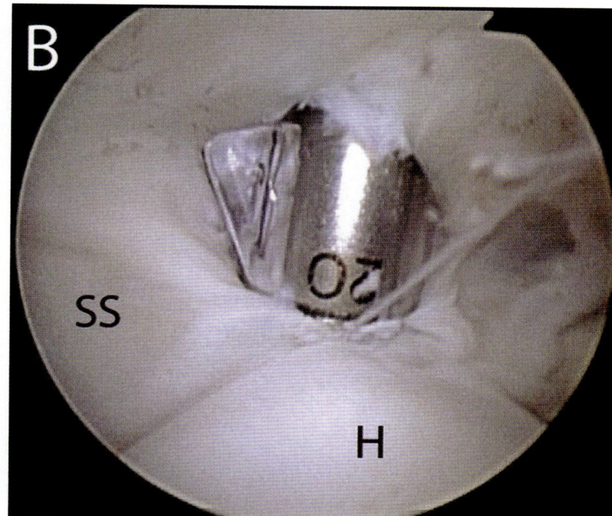

Figure 10.20 Left shoulder, posterior viewing portal demonstrating preparation of a bone socket for biceps tenodesis with a 6.25-mm BioComposite SwiveLock anchor. **A:** A headed reamer prepares the bone socket that is different from the tapered punch used to insert a standard SwiveLock anchor. **B:** The reamer is advanced to 20 mm to create a bone socket for the 19-mm-long anchor. H, humerus; SS, supraspinatus tendon; SSc, subscapularis tendon.

coracoacromial ligament is delayed until the tenodesis is performed since early release of the ligament allows the deltoid to collapse into the anterior working space. If additional working space is required, a switching stick may be placed through the lateral or accessory lateral portal to retract the anterior deltoid.

In the anterior subdeltoid space, the biceps tendon is carefully identified at its exit through the bicipital groove. The transverse ligament is then incised using an electrocautery device or arthroscopic scissors (Fig. 10.27). Care is taken to ensure that the medial subscapularis tendon is not inadvertently damaged. A complete release is confirmed by unobstructed mobility of the tendon. It is important to remember that the ascending branch of the anterior humeral circumflex lies adjacent to the biceps tendon in the groove and is a source of potential bleeding.

Using needle localization, an accessory anterior portal is created in the lower part of the bicipital groove perpendicular to the groove and the lowest extent of the groove is confirmed using a switching stick. The remainder of the procedure is as described above with the tendon preparation, bone socket preparation, reduction of the tendon into the bone socket, and screw fixation (Fig. 10.28).

If it is possible to place intra-articular traction stitches and exteriorize the biceps tendon, identification of the groove in the subacromial space will be relatively easy following

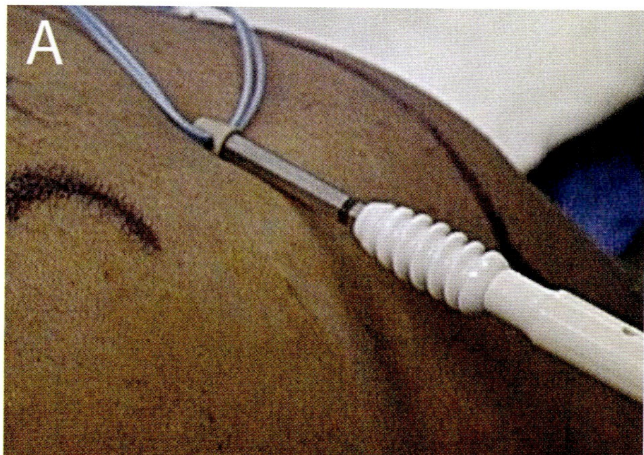

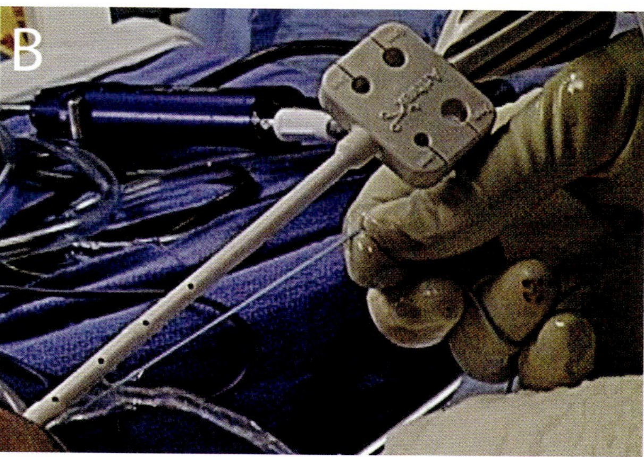

Figure 10.21 External view of insertion of biceps-SwiveLock construct. **A:** The biceps whipstitch sutures are passed through the eyelet of the SwiveLock anchor. **B:** The construct is inserted. Note that the surgeon's hand must maintain tension on the whipstitch sutures during insertion.

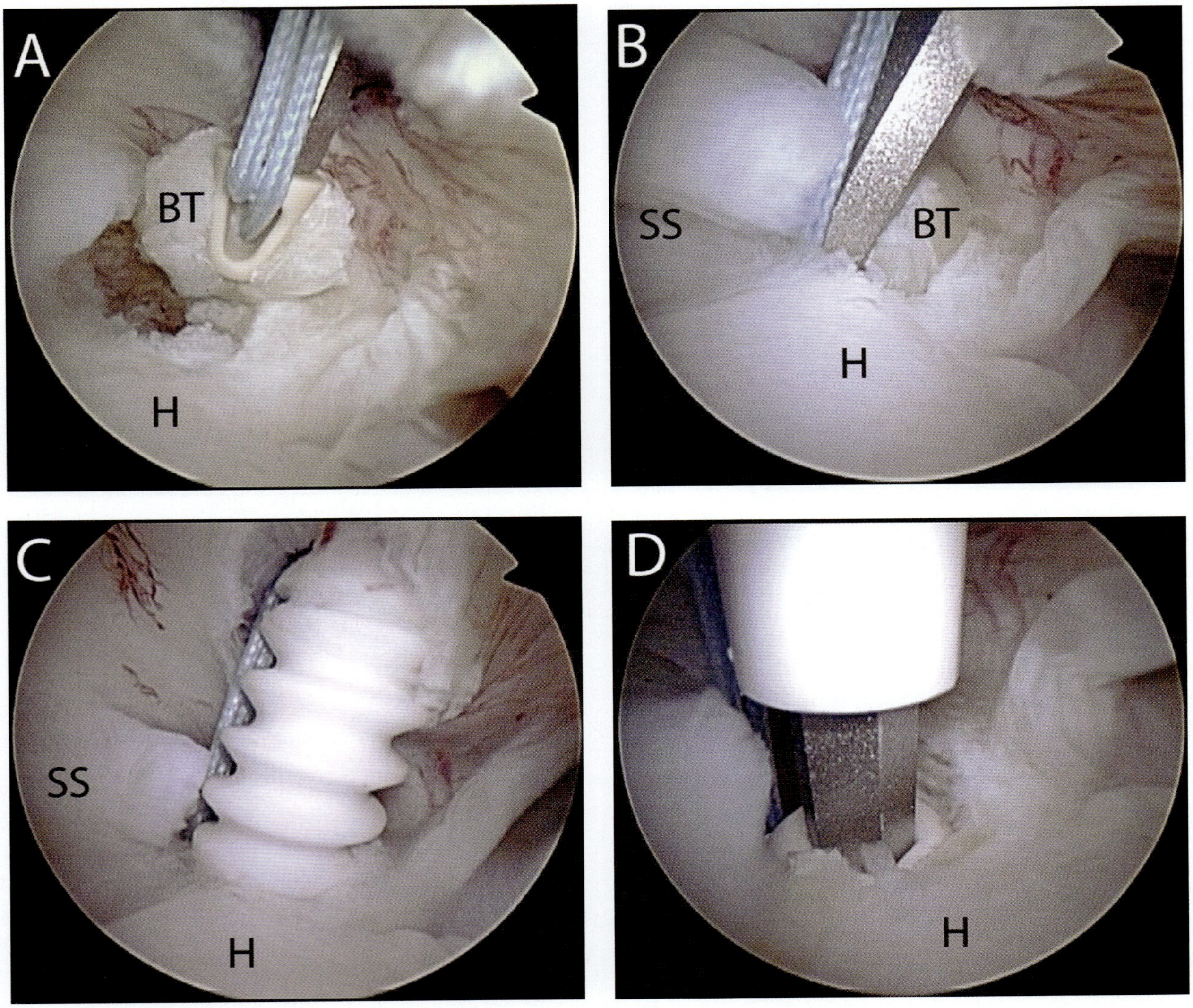

Figure 10.22 Arthroscopic view of insertion of biceps-SwiveLock construct in a left shoulder viewed from a posterior portal. **A:** The biceps edge is adjacent to the SwiveLock anchor eyelet, **(B)** that guides the tendon into the bone socket. **C:** The SwiveLock anchor is advanced, until **(D)** it is seated just below the bone surface. BT, biceps tendon; H, humerus; SS, supraspinatus tendon.

the above description. In some cases, however, the proximal biceps tendon quality may be so poor that traction stitches cannot be placed in the tendon. In such cases, identification of the bicipital groove is much more difficult. It is helpful to first mark the path of the bicipital groove with spinal needles while viewing intra-articularly (Fig. 10.29). It is important when working in the anterior subdeltoid space not to stray medial and distal so as to avoid inadvertent injury to the major neurovascular structures of the arm. By marking the bicipital groove, the spinal needles help one maintain orientation and will prevent iatrogenic injury.

After marking the groove, the arthroscope is moved to a posterior subacromial viewing portal and a bursectomy is performed to identify the spinal needles (Fig. 10.30). Working between the spinal needles, the bicipital groove is unroofed with electrocautery and arthroscopic scissors (Fig. 10.31). Then, traction stitches are placed in the tendon and the procedure proceeds as described above with tendon preparation, bone socket preparation, and fixation with a tenodesis screw low in the groove.

BICEPS TENODESIS (LOW IN THE GROOVE) ASSOCIATED WITH ROTATOR CUFF REPAIR

In patients with significant biceps disease particularly along the bicipital groove, biceps tenodesis may be performed arthroscopically low in the groove. This is particularly relevant in patients with complete subscapularis tendon tears,

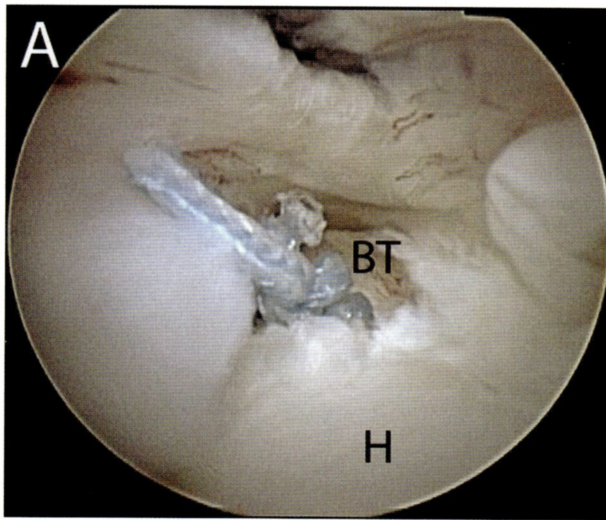

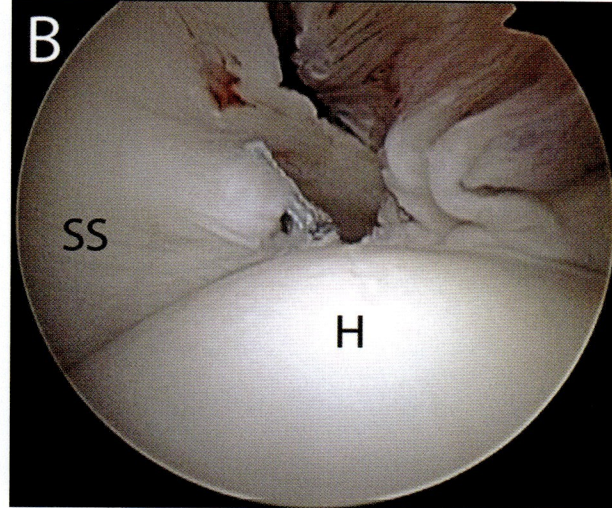

Figure 10.23 Final arthroscopic view of a biceps tenodesis performed with a SwiveLock anchor in a left shoulder viewed from a posterior portal. **A:** The whipstitch sutures passing through the cannulation of the screw are tied together. **B:** Overview shows a low-profile tenodesis performed just lateral to the articular margin. BT, biceps tendon; H, humerus; SS, supraspinatus tendon.

where the tendon may be dislocated medially out of the bicipital groove. However, in these cases with complete subscapularis tendon tearing, visualization of the anterior structures (i.e., distal bicipital groove) is facilitated by subscapularis tendon rupture.

In this situation, following diagnostic arthroscopy an anterosuperolateral portal is established for subscapularis tendon repair (see Chapter 6, "Subscapularis Tendon Tears," for a complete discussion). The LHB tendon is similarly secured and tenotomized early in the procedure to improve visualization of the subscapularis tendon. In this case, 2 to 3 cm of tendon is removed prior to placing the #2 FiberWire whipstitch.

In cases where the subscapularis tendon is torn, identification of the bicipital groove is not difficult. Following tenotomy of the biceps tendon in preparation for tenodesis, the subscapularis tendon is approached and a three-sided release is performed to improve mobility.

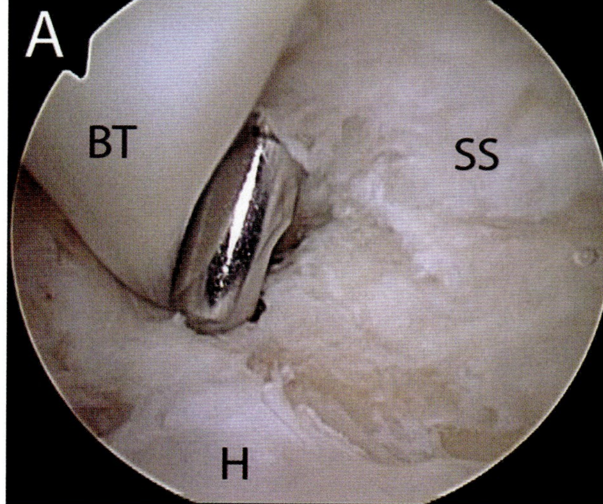

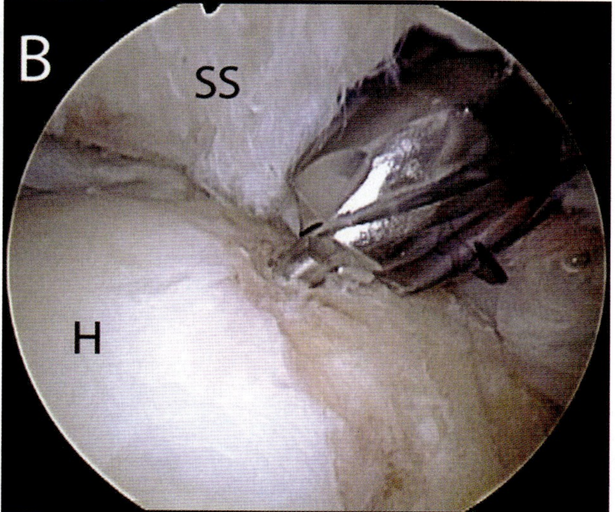

Figure 10.24 Incorporating biceps tenodesis into rotator cuff repair in a right shoulder viewed from a posterior portal. **A:** The normal preferred location for biceps tenodesis is at the top of the bicipital groove. **B:** For incorporation of a tenodesis into rotator cuff repair, a bone socket is created at the anteromedial footprint of the supraspinatus tendon, in this case by working through the defect in the rotator cuff. BT, biceps tendon; H, humerus; SS, supraspinatus tendon.

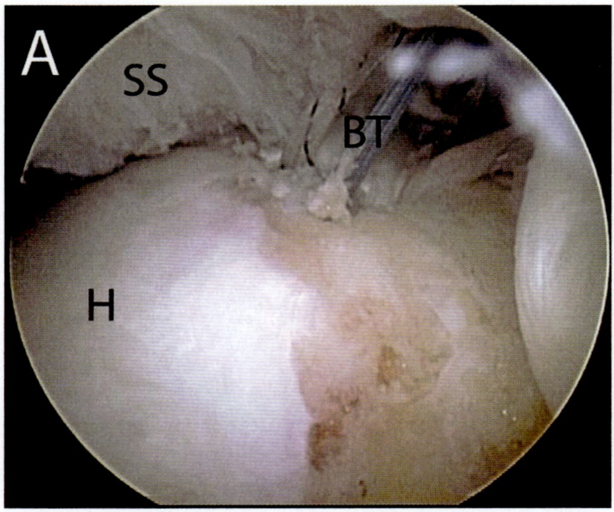

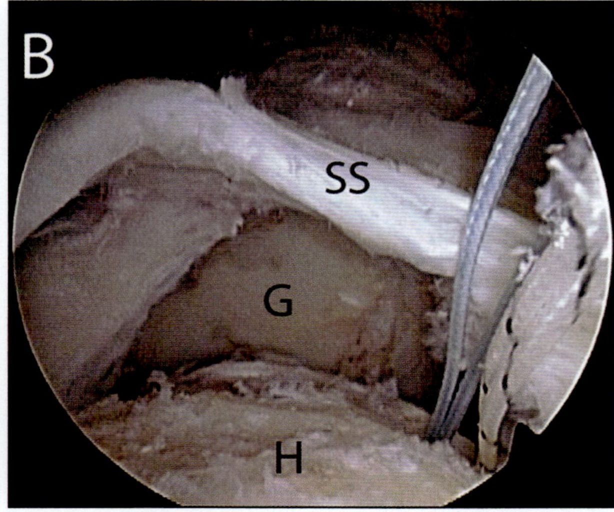

Figure 10.25 **A:** Right shoulder, posterior viewing portal demonstrates completed tenodesis in the anteromedial supraspinatus footprint. **B:** Subacromial view from a lateral portal demonstrating sutures that may be incorporated into the rotator cuff repair. BT, biceps tendon; G, glenoid; H, humerus; SS, supraspinatus tendon.

Once mobility of the subscapularis tendon has been achieved, the biceps tenodesis may be performed either before or after fixation of the subscapularis tendon. An accessory anterior portal is therefore created at the lower border of the bicipital groove and an 8.25-mm threaded clear cannula is established. A bone socket is prepared as previously described (Fig. 10.32). The biceps tendon is reduced in the bone socket and secured with a tenodesis screw (Fig. 10.33). The sutures are then tied to form a single screw–tendon construct.

COBRA TECHNIQUE

Treatment of spontaneous ruptures of the LHB has typically been nonoperative consisting of observation and symptomatic treatment. Outcomes with such nonoperative management have generally been reported as good to excellent (1–3). However, distal retraction of the LHB frequently leads to a "Popeye" deformity that may be cosmetically unappealing to some patients. Additionally, nonoperatively managed patients demonstrate diminished strength in both

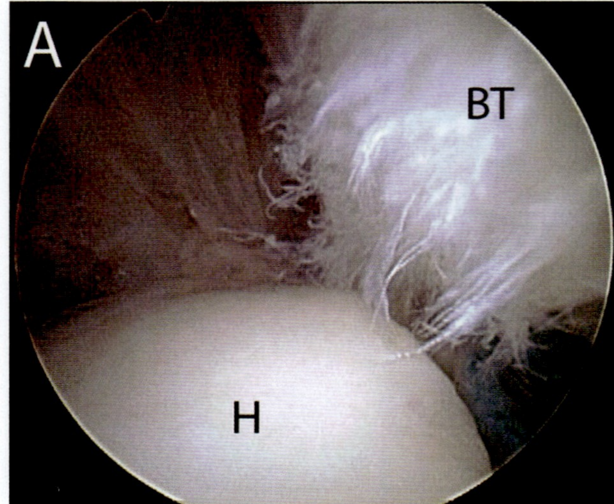

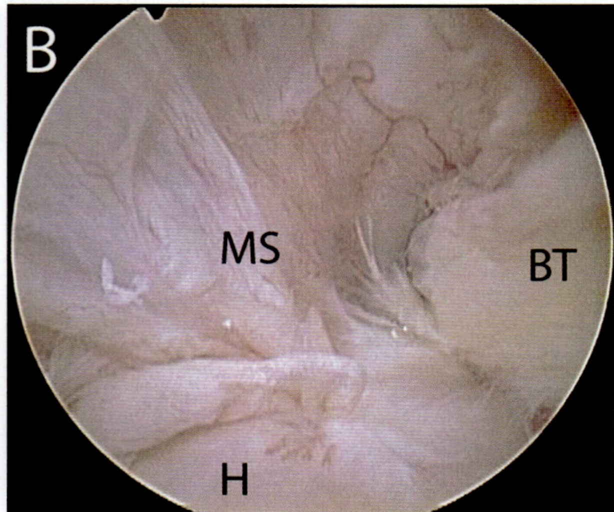

Figure 10.26 Right shoulder, posterior viewing portal with a 70° arthroscope demonstrates **(A)** a biceps tendon with degenerative changes which **(B)** extend distally into the bicipital groove. Significant biceps pathology in the bicipital groove is our primary indication for a tenodesis low in the groove. BT, biceps tendon; H, humerus; MS, medial sling of the biceps tendon.

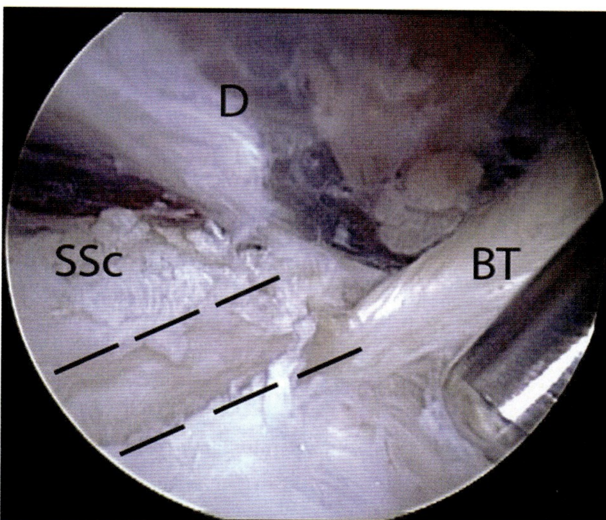

Figure 10.27 Right shoulder, posterior subacromial viewing portal with a 70° arthroscope. The bicipital groove (outlined by *black dashed lines*) has been unroofed and the biceps tendon is exteriorized through an accessory anterior portal. BT, biceps tendon; D, internal deltoid fascia. SSc, subscapularis tendon.

flexion and supination after LHB rupture ranging between 8% and 21% (1,3). While such strength loss is well tolerated and may even go unnoticed in the majority of patients, a subset of patients find this amount of deficit unacceptable. In our experience, strength loss following LHB rupture is particularly problematic in body builders, heavy manual laborers, and other individuals who engage in frequent forced flexion and supination activities (e.g., bowlers).

When evaluating a patient with an LHB rupture, it is important to establish an understanding of each patient's symptoms and functional demands. In general, LHB ruptures either occur as an acute traumatic event (with no preceding pathology) or as an element of chronic impingement syndrome causing biceps tendinopathy followed by an eventual rupture event. In the former category, patients often give a history of a significant eccentric force to a flexed arm with an audible "pop." Pain and ecchymosis often accompany this type of an event. This scenario is typical for younger patients with no prior shoulder problems. More commonly, patients give a history of ongoing shoulder and/or arm pain followed by a rupture event. This type of LHB rupture event usually results from a relatively benign activity and may or may not be accompanied by a noticeable "pop" or ecchymosis. Often, these patients report an improvement in their impingement symptoms and sometimes substantial pain relief.

Recently, the popularity of open subpectoral biceps tenodesis has increased. While we agree that this option is preferable to leaving the LHB ruptured and retracted, there are several downsides to this approach. First, with tendon to bone fixation in this region, there is potential for producing a stress riser in the proximal humeral diaphysis. Due to the width of the biceps tendon at this location, tenodesis in bone often requires a minimum of an 8-mm bone socket. A weakened proximal humeral diaphysis may be particularly susceptible to fatigue fracture because of the large opposing muscles of the pectoralis major and latissimus dorsi that insert in this region. A second concern is the potential for soft tissue irritation underneath the pectoralis major. If an anchor is not well seated, or if the bone edges are rough, active patients may experience chronic persistent symptoms. We have personally seen patients who have had an open subpectoral biceps tenodesis by other surgeons who complain of persistent anterior shoulder

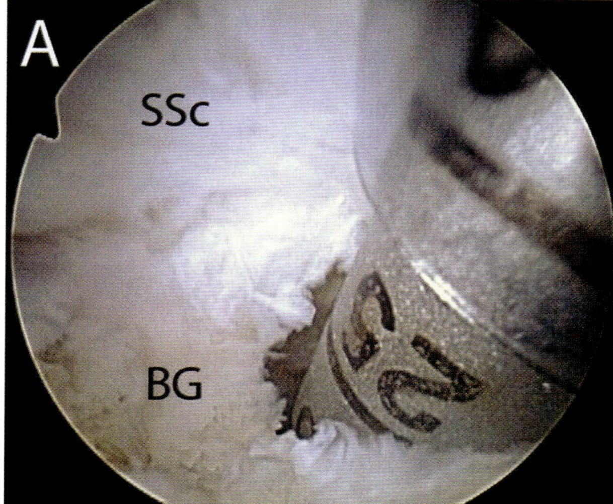

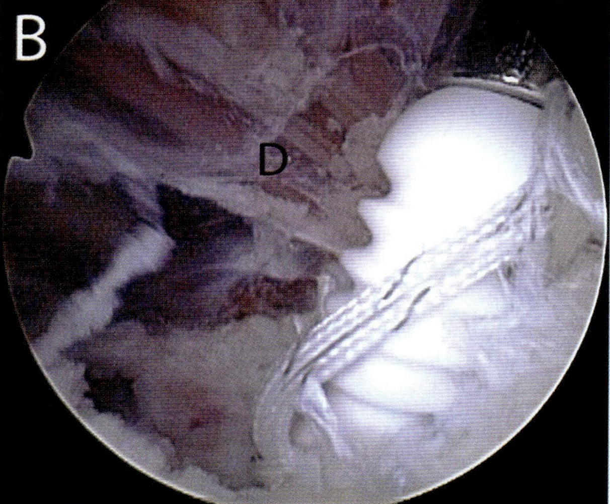

Figure 10.28 Right shoulder, posterior subacromial viewing portal with a 70° arthroscope. **A:** A bone socket is prepared low in the bicipital groove (BG). **B:** Tendon to bone fixation of the biceps tendon is performed with a biceps tenodesis screw. BG, bicipital groove; D, internal deltoid fascia; SSc, subscapularis tendon.

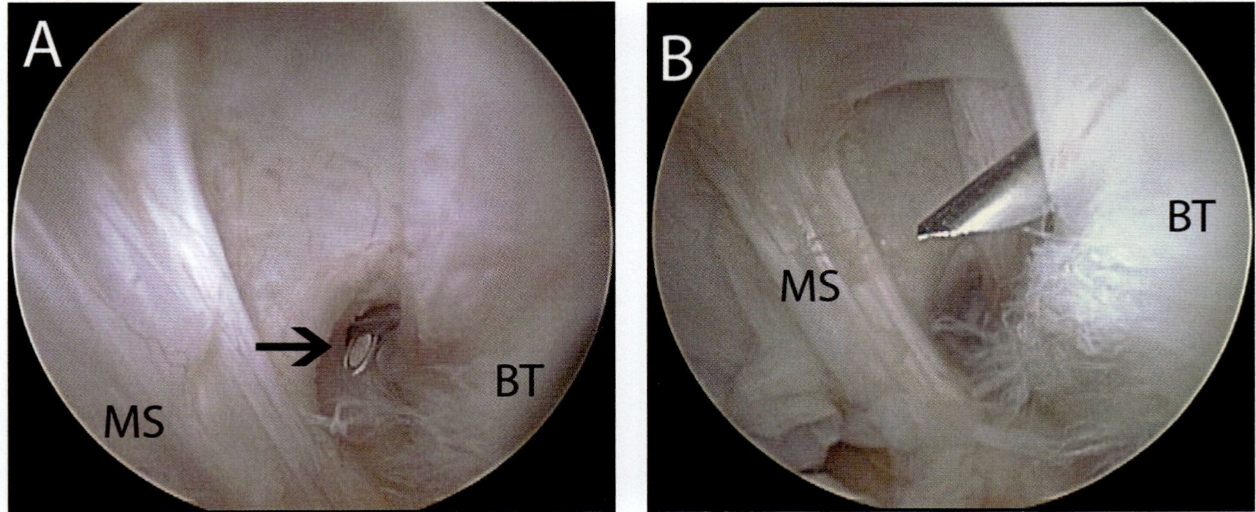

Figure 10.29 Right shoulder, posterior viewing portal with a 70° arthroscope. **A:** In preparation for subacromial identification of the bicipital intraarticular groove, the distal extent of the bicipital groove is marked with a spinal needle (*black arrow*). **B:** Then, the proximal extent of the bicipital groove is also marked. This technique is important if proximal biceps tendon disease prevents placement of traction stitches in the intra-articular portion of the tendon. BT, biceps tendon. MS, medial sling of the biceps.

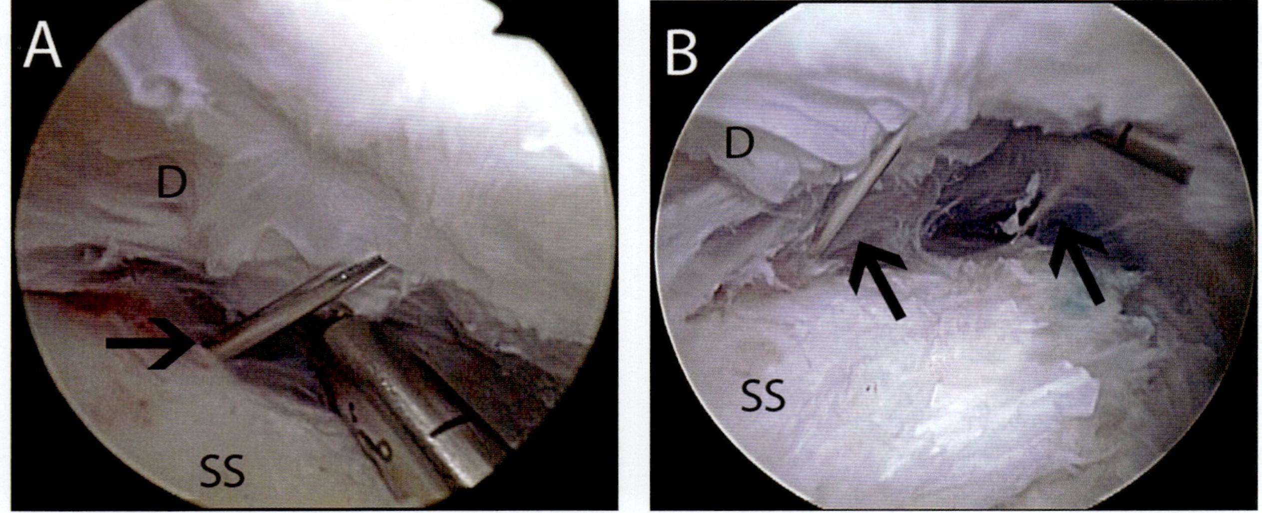

Figure 10.30 Right shoulder, posterior subacromial viewing portal with a 70° arthroscope. **A:** A bursectomy is performed in the anterior subdeltoid space to identify previously placed proximal and (**B**) distal spinal needles (*black arrows*) that mark the bicipital groove. D, internal deltoid fascia; SS, supraspinatus tendon.

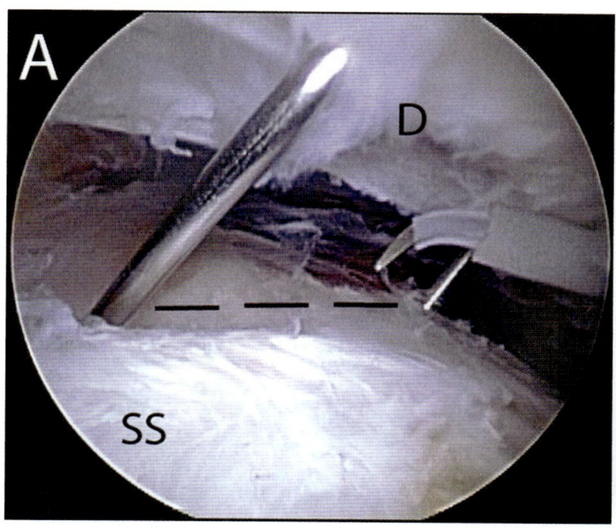

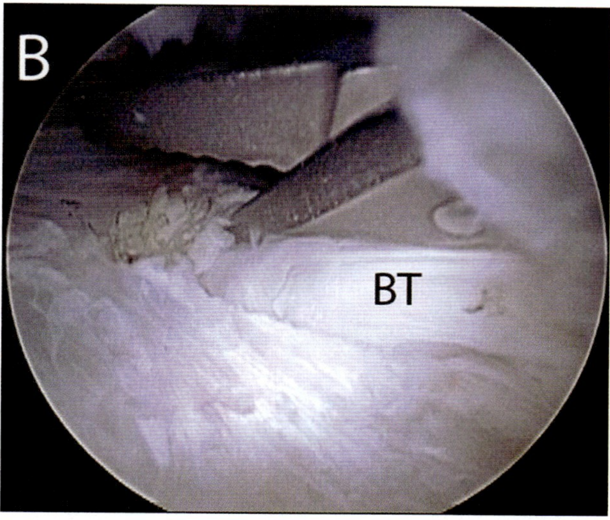

Figure 10.31 Right shoulder, posterior subacromial viewing portal with a 70° arthroscope. **A:** The bicipital groove (*dashed black lines*) is unroofed with a pencil-tip electrocautery and **(B)** arthroscopic scissors. BT, biceps tendon; D, internal deltoid fascia; SS, supraspinatus tendon.

pain. Following removal of hardware, these patients have improved significantly and have been satisfied with their final outcomes.

Because of these potential issues, we prefer to perform a biceps tenodesis high within the bicipital groove of the humerus. Therefore, while we make a small open subpectoral incision to locate the ruptured LHB, we then tunnel the tendon back up into the bicipital groove for tenodesis.

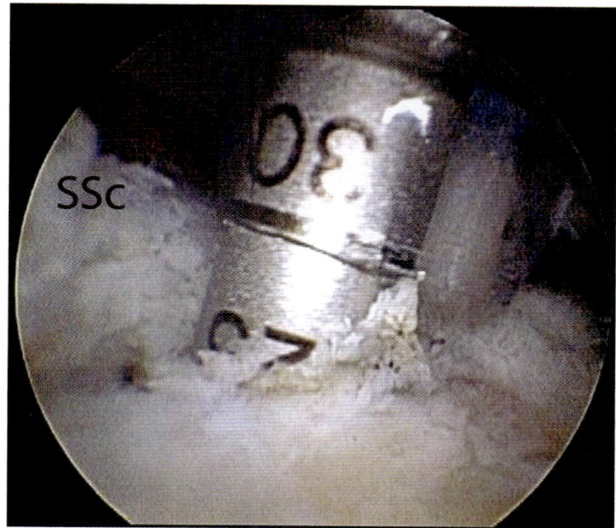

Figure 10.32 Right shoulder, posterior subacromial viewing portal with a 70° arthroscope demonstrates preparation of a bone socket low in the bicipital groove. SSc, subscapularis tendon.

We have termed this technique the "cobra procedure" in reference to the large tattoo of a cobra on the arm of the first patient to undergo the procedure (Fig. 10.34). While we do not advocate this procedure for the majority of LHB ruptures, with proper indications the technique is quite effective and gratifying for both the surgeon and the patient.

The procedure begins with a diagnostic arthroscopy to confirm the LHB rupture (Fig. 10.35) and identify any associated intra-articular pathology. If additional pathology is identified, it is important to perform the Cobra procedure first as fluid extravasation will limit visualization in the anterior shoulder. An anterosuperolateral portal is established within the ceiling of the bicipital groove such that it will allow a good angle of approach to perform the tenodesis in the groove, and also be in line with the bicipital groove to allow for instruments to be passed distally underneath the pectoralis major tendon.

The subacromial space is accessed and a thorough bursectomy is performed. The anterior and lateral gutters should be thoroughly cleared as visualization in this area will be critical during the biceps tenodesis procedure.

The arm is taken out of traction and the inferior border of the pectoralis major is palpated; abduction and external rotation can help identify this inferior border. A small oblique 2-cm subpectoral incision is created near the inferior pectoralis major border (Fig. 10.36). Typically, the ruptured biceps tendon can be palpated near the bottom of the incision, just superficial to the humeral shaft. The ruptured LHB tendon is delivered from the wound and the quality and length of the tendon is inspected to confirm

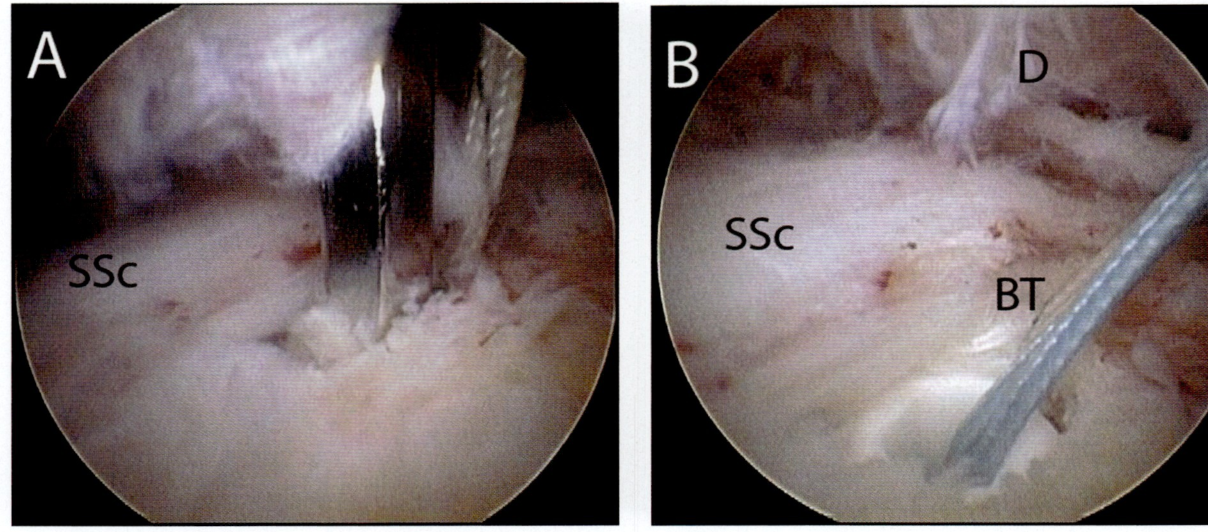

Figure 10.33 Right shoulder, posterior subacromial viewing portal with a 70° arthroscope. **A:** The biceps tendon is reduced into a bone socket low in the bicipital groove and secured with **(B)** a tenodesis screw. BT, biceps tendon; D, internal deltoid fascia. SSc, subscapularis tendon.

that it is adequate for tenodesis in the bicipital groove (Fig. 10.37). The tendon is secured with a #2 FiberWire suture beginning approximately 5 to 10 mm from the proximal end of the tendon. The tendon suture can be placed as a whipstitch or by using a FiberLoop (Arthrex, Inc., Naples, FL) (Fig. 10.38). After the tendon is prepared, it is sized as previously described (Fig. 10.39).

Attention is returned to the arthroscopic view. Under arthroscopic visualization, the blunt end of the ACL TransFix femoral guide pin (Arthrex, Inc., Naples, FL) is passed through the anterosuperolateral portal down the bicipital groove to the level of the pectoralis major tendon (Fig. 10.40). Usually, the bicipital groove can be well palpated during passage of the guide pin. To see the pin pass distally, it may be necessary to establish a lateral subacromial portal and view the bicipital groove with a 70° arthroscope.

Utilizing digital palpation in the subpectoral incision, the location of the TransFix pin underneath the pectoralis

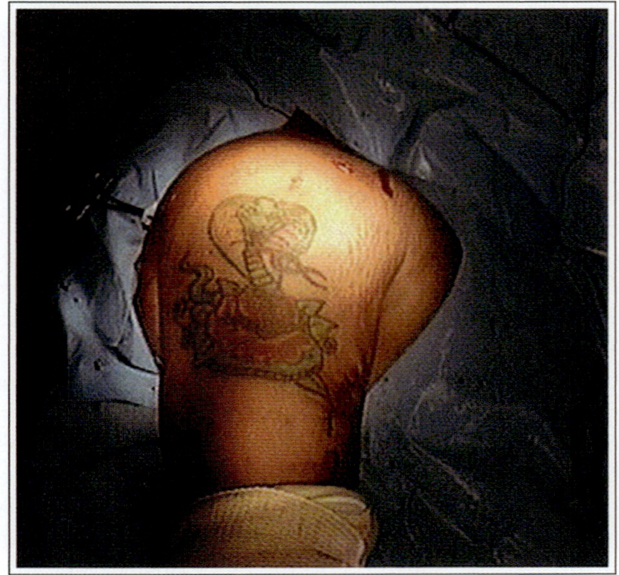

Figure 10.34 Intraoperative photo of patient's arm from which the cobra procedure derives its name.

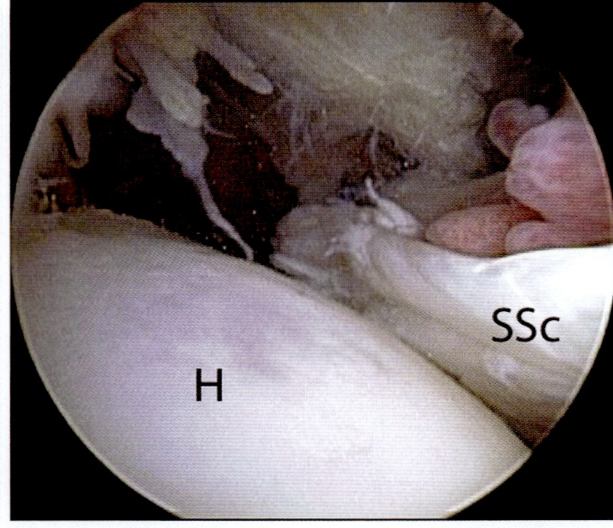

Figure 10.35 Left shoulder, posterior glenohumeral viewing portal, demonstrates an absent biceps in an individual with an acute proximal biceps rupture. H, humerus; SSc, subscapularis tendon.

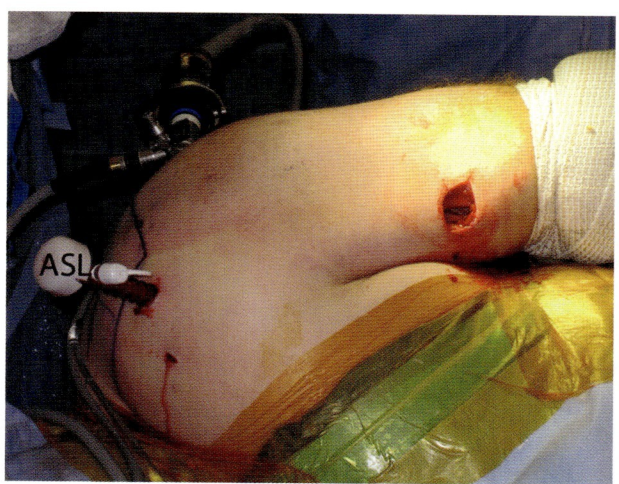

Figure 10.36 External view of a left shoulder demonstrates a subpectoral incision which has been made to identify the biceps tendon. ASL, anterosuperolateral portal.

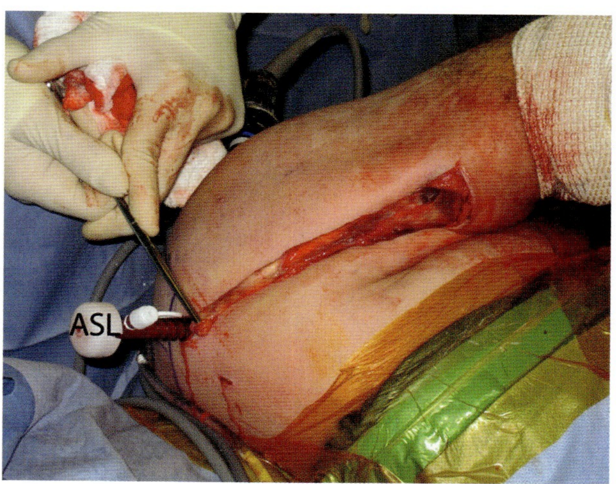

Figure 10.37 External view of a left shoulder demonstrates a retrieved biceps tendon with sufficient length to perform a Cobra procedure. ASL, anterosuperolateral portal.

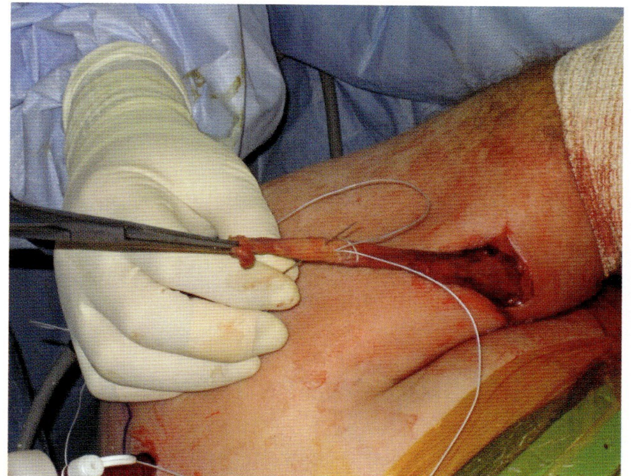

A

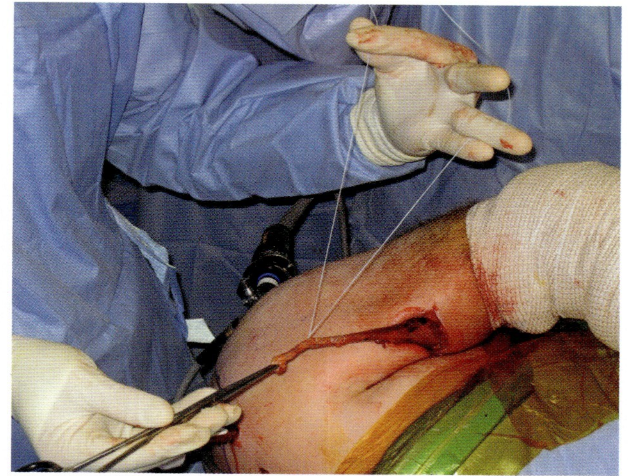

B

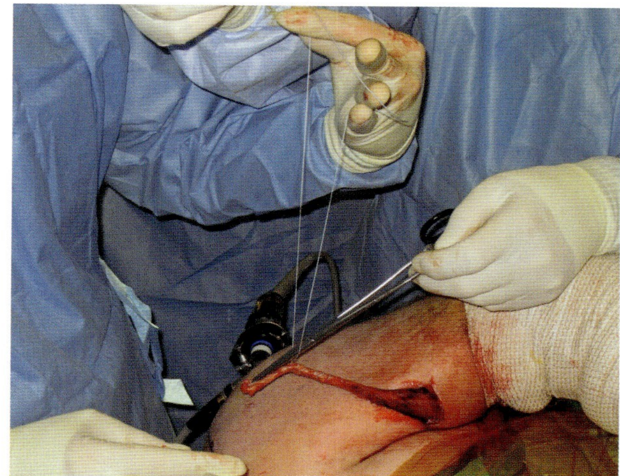

C

Figure 10.38 External views of a left shoulder demonstrating the use of a FiberLoop (Arthrex, Inc., Naples, FL) to prepare a biceps tendon for tenodesis. **A:** Beginning distally, a FiberLoop is passed through the tendon with a straight needle. **B:** After each pass of the needle, the suture loop is opened and **(C)** the tendon is passed through the loop.

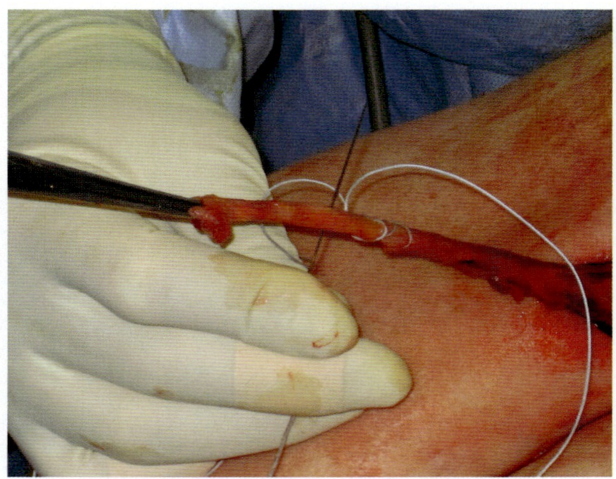

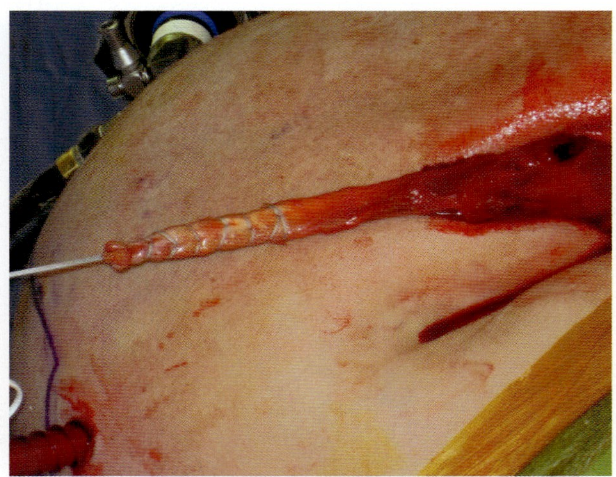

Figure 10.38 *(Continued)* **D:** A subsequent pass is then made. The steps are repeated until **(E)** the suture exits the proximal tendon.

is confirmed to follow the normal tract of the LHB. The pin is then advanced distally and out the arm incision (Fig. 10.41A). The suture tails from the whipstitch suture are passed through the eyelet in the TransFix pin (Fig. 10.41B). The TransFix pin is then pulled proximally and removed out of the ASL portal so that the whipstitch sutures exit through the ASL portal. Pulling the whipstitch suture ends delivers the biceps tendon out the ASL portal (Fig. 10.41C). The shuttled biceps tendon is then viewed arthroscopically (Fig. 10.42). Once this is achieved, a typical arthroscopic biceps tenodesis is performed as previously described (Fig. 10.43).

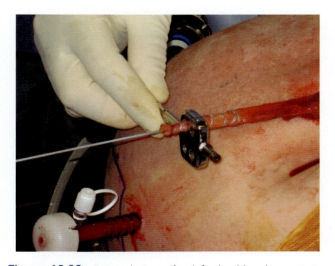

Figure 10.39 External view of a left shoulder demonstrates sizing a biceps tendon for tenodesis.

The Cobra procedure must be performed within the first 6 weeks after rupture of the LHB. After that, tendon shortening (from fixed retraction and tendon loss) may preclude this procedure, leaving subpectoral tenodesis as the only option.

This procedure has allowed for a minimally invasive reconstruction of a ruptured and retracted LHB tendon. Once again, this procedure is DEFINITELY not indicated for the majority of LHB ruptures. However, in the select patient, this procedure is quite effective and gratifying for both the surgeon and the patient.

SUBPECTORAL BICEPS TENODESIS

Although some surgeons may choose to perform a subpectoral biceps tenodesis as their primary biceps tenodesis, we generally reserve subpectoral biceps tenodesis for patients with a ruptured LHB tendon that is not amenable to a Cobra procedure due to insufficient length or poor-quality tissue. Usually in this situation, the biceps tendon rupture is chronic and degenerative but the stump may still be palpable in the proximal or midarm. An incision is made at the inferior border of the pectoralis major tendon extending 3 to 4 cm distally depending on the amount of distal retraction (Fig. 10.44). Soft tissue dissection is taken down to the fascia where the biceps and coracobrachialis are identified along with the lower border of the pectoralis major. The fascia is incised just below the pectoralis major muscle and the biceps tendon is usually identifiable just under the inferior edge of the pectoralis major. The pectoralis major tendon is retracted superiorly and the coracobrachialis and short head of the biceps are carefully retracted medially avoiding injury to the medial musculocutaneous nerve.

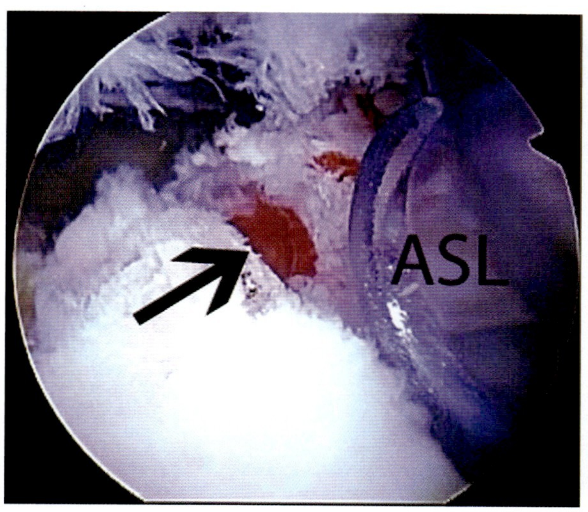

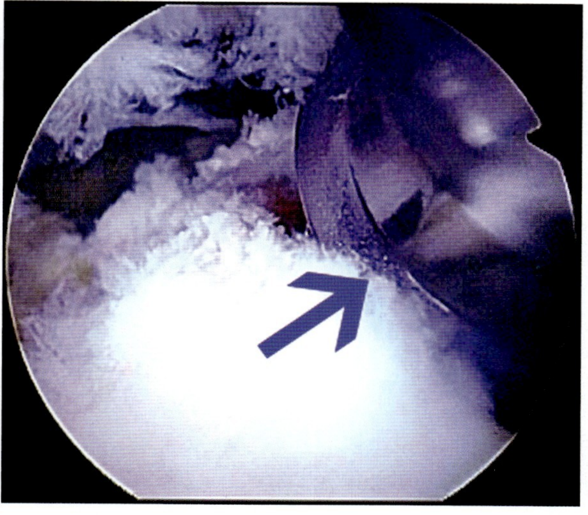

Figure 10.40 Left shoulder, lateral subacromial viewing portal with a 70° arthroscope. **A:** The location of the bicipital groove (*black arrow*). **B:** Then, a TransFix pin (*blue arrow*) (Arthrex, Inc., Naples, FL) is introduced through an anterosuperolateral portal and advanced down the bicipital groove under direct visualization. ASL, anterosuperolateral portal.

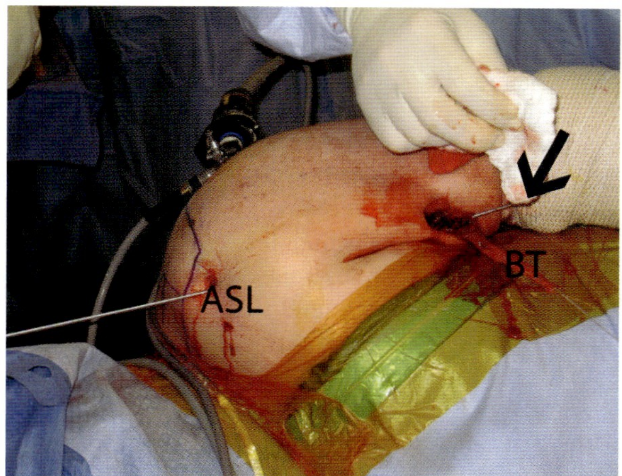

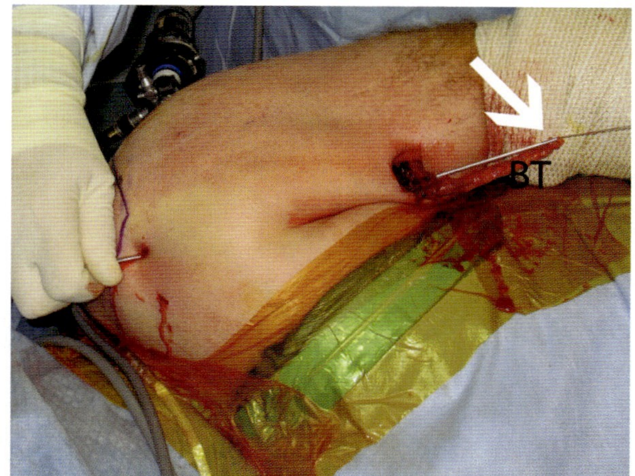

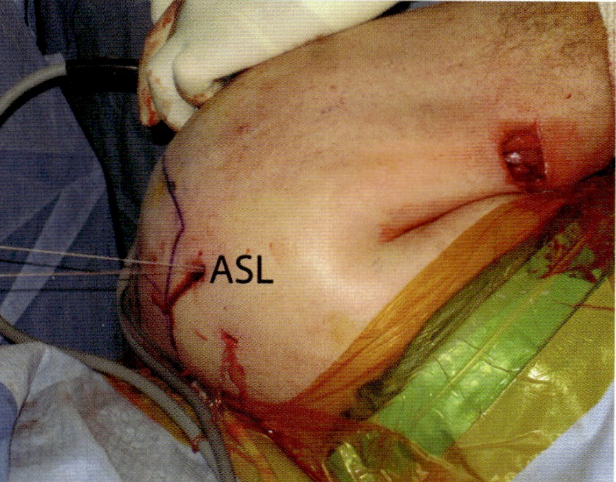

Figure 10.41 **A:** External view of a left shoulder demonstrates a TransFix pin (Arthrex, Inc., Naples, FL) that has been passed down the bicipital groove and retrieved out a subpectoral incision (*black arrow*). **B:** The biceps sutures have been passed through the slotted end of the TransFix pin (*white arrow*). **C:** The biceps tendon has been delivered proximally by pulling the TransFix pin out the anterosuperolateral portal. BT, biceps tendon; ASL, anterosuperolateral portal.

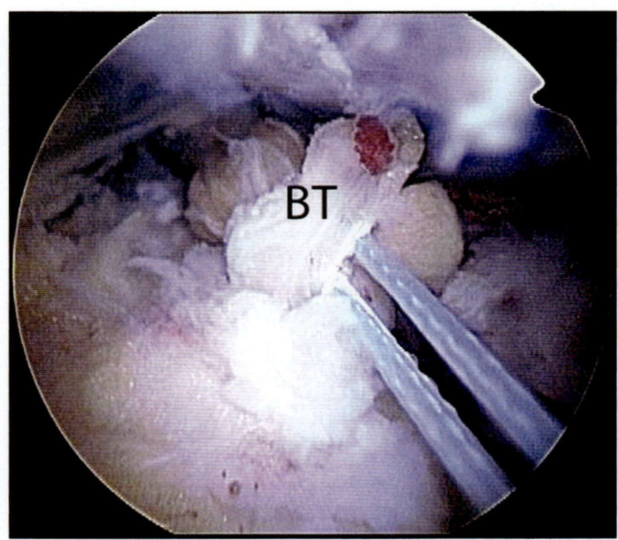

Figure 10.42 Left shoulder, lateral subacromial viewing portal with a 70° arthroscope confirms a properly proximally shuttled biceps tendon. BT, biceps tendon.

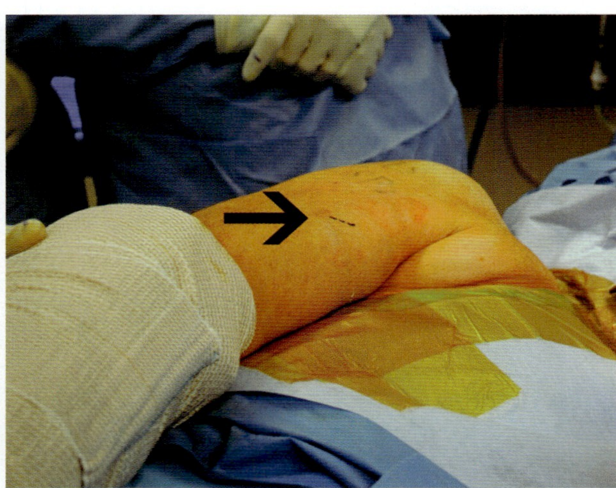

Figure 10.44 External photo of a right shoulder demonstrates the incision (*black arrow*) for a subpectoral tenodesis.

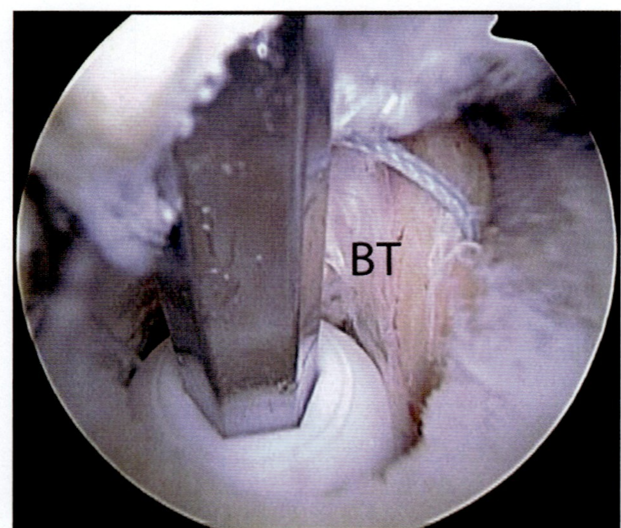

Figure 10.43 Left shoulder, lateral subacromial viewing portal with a 70° arthroscope demonstrates tenodesis of the biceps tendon within the bicipital groove. BT, biceps tendon

The biceps tendon is then retrieved out of the wound using a tendon hook or hemostat (Fig. 10.45). It is important to remember that the musculotendinous junction of the biceps rests at approximately 2 cm above the inferior border of the pectoralis major. The LHB should be resected until there is only approximately 1.5 to 1.7 cm of tendon proximal to the musculotendinous junction, since the short Bio-Composite Tenodesis screws (10 or 12 mm in length) will need to be used in the diaphysis of the humerus, which has a much smaller diameter than the metaphysis. A #2 FiberWire stitch is then used to secure the proximal end of the tendon (Fig. 10.46).

The periosteum is then reflected just proximal to the pectoralis major tendon and a guidewire and reamer are used (Fig. 10.47). In this hard, cortical bone, it is important to upsize if the tendon is between sizes. However, we prefer not to create large holes in the humerus. Usually, a 7- or 8-mm drill hole is made to the appropriate depth (10 mm deep for a 7-mm screw; 12 mm deep for an 8-mm screw). Then, the tendon is similarly reduced

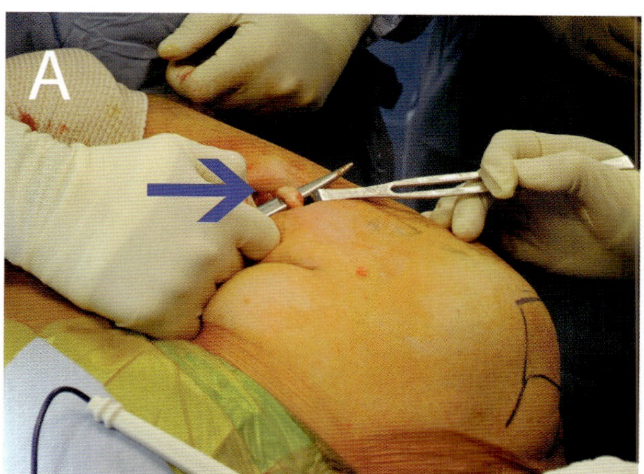

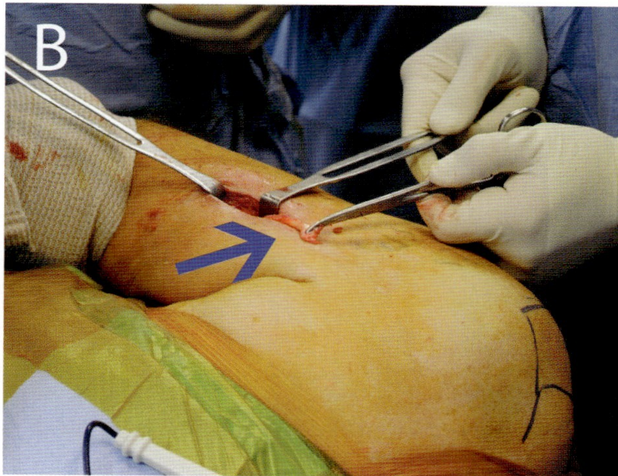

Figure 10.45 **A:** External photo of a right shoulder. The biceps tendon (*blue arrow*) has been hooked with an instrument. **B:** The biceps tendon (*blue arrow*) has been extracted from the incision.

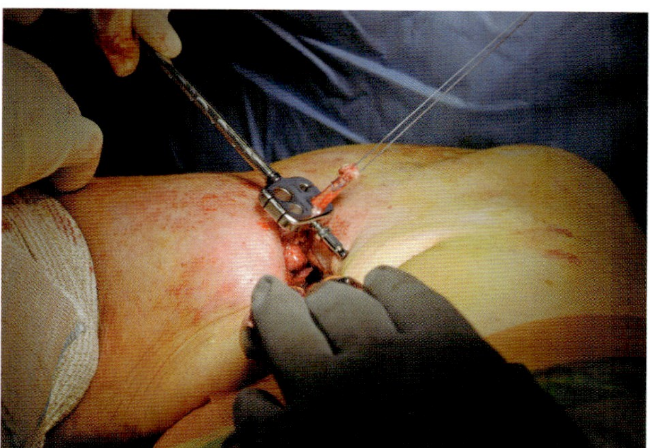

Figure 10.46 External photo of a right shoulder. After exposing the biceps tendon, the tendon is prepared with a whipstitch and sized in preparation for subpectoral tenodesis.

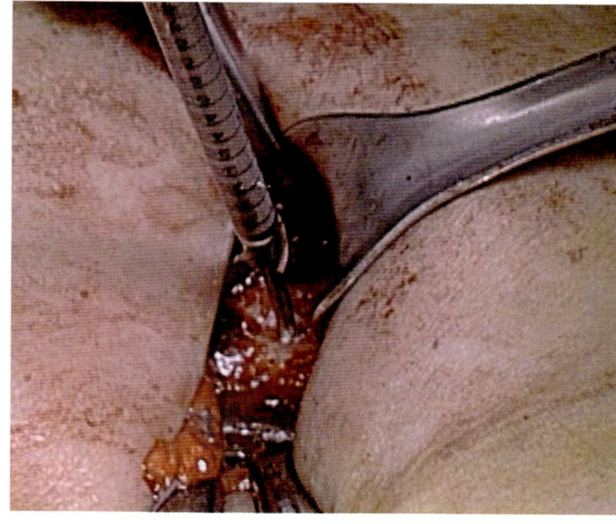

Figure 10.47 External photo of a right shoulder. A reamer is placed over a guide pin to create a bone socket for a subpectoral biceps tenodesis.

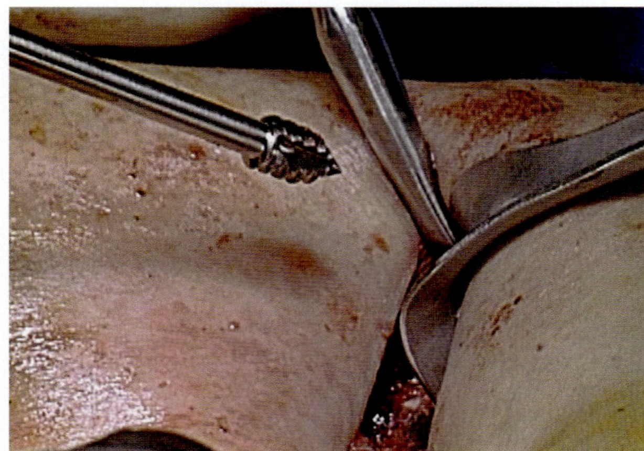

Figure 10.48 External photo of a right shoulder. A metal tap is used to prepare a bone socket for a BioComposite Tenodesis screw (Arthrex, Inc., Naples, FL). The tap is essential when one is placing a BioComposite screw in cortical bone.

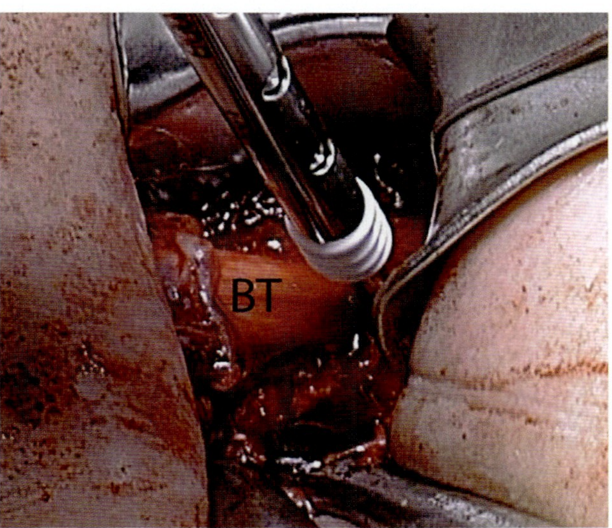

Figure 10.49 External photo of a right shoulder demonstrating subpectoral tenodesis of the biceps tendon (BT) with a BioComposite Tenodesis Screw (Arthrex, Inc., Naples, FL).

and the screw advanced. It is our preference to use a short (10 to 12 mm) BioComposite Tenodesis screw (Arthrex, Inc., Naples, FL). Unlike with their use in metaphyseal bone (e.g., intra-articular tenodesis high in the groove), these screws require the use of a tap in this region due to the hard cortical bone (Figs. 10.48 and 10.49). If the biceps tendon has been appropriately tensioned, then its musculotendinous junction should lie 2 cm above the inferior border of the pectoralis major tendon at the end of the procedure.

REFERENCES

1. Mariani EM, Cofield RH, Askew LJ, et al. Rupture of the tendon of the long head of the biceps brachii. Surgical versus nonsurgical treatment. *Clin Orthop Relat Res*. 1988;(228):233–239.
2. Warren RF. Lesions of the long head of the biceps tendon. *Instr Course Lect*. 1985;34:204–209.
3. Sturzenegger M, Beguin D, Grunig B, et al. Muscular strength after rupture of the long head of the biceps. *Arch Orthop Trauma Surg*. 1986;105:18–23.

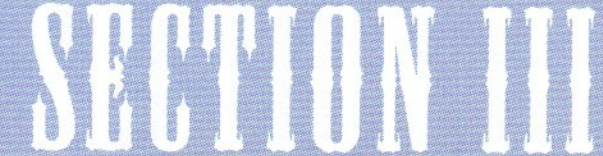

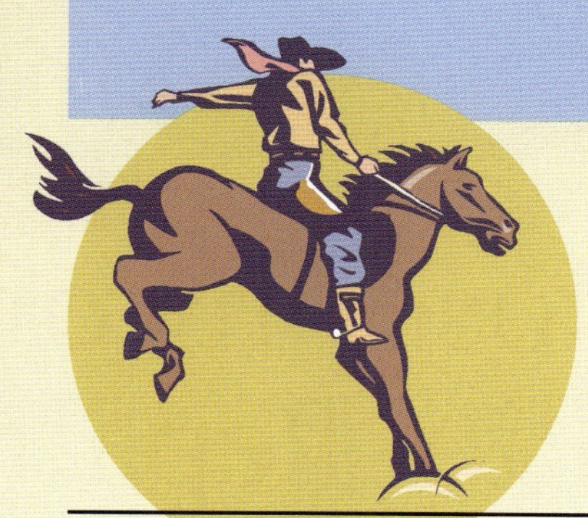

SECTION III

INSTABILITY AND RELATED TOPICS

COWBOY PRINCIPLE 5

Never approach a bull from the front, a horse from the rear, or a fool from any direction.

A sense of direction is a mighty handy thing to have. If you know what and where the problem is, you'll know how to approach it.

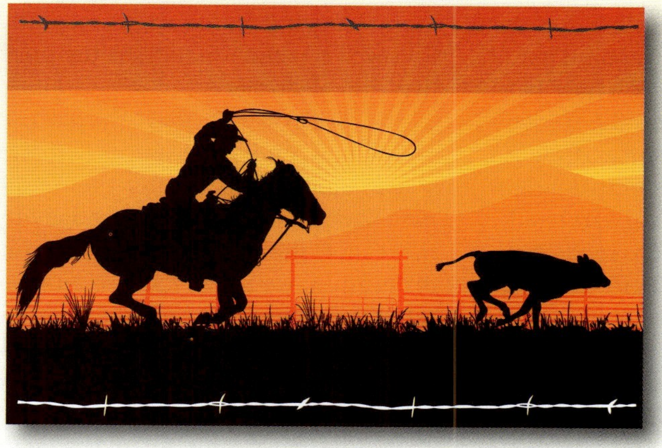

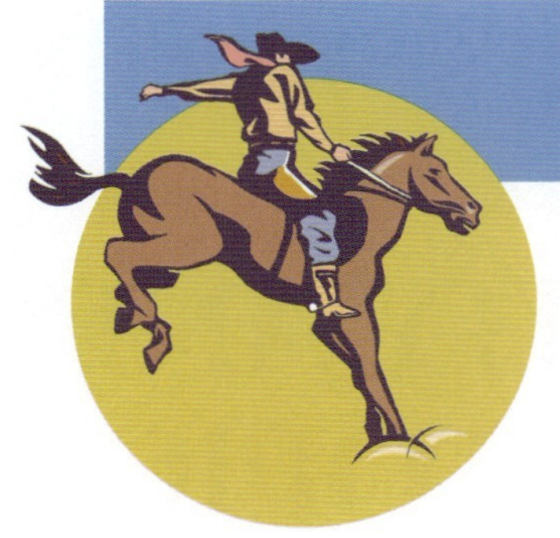

11

Philosophy of Instability Repair

WESTERN WISDOM

When two play, one wins.

We have come a long way since the 1990s, when "experts" would openly debate whether arthroscopic instability repairs should even be done because of their high failure rate. Today, there is no question that most instability repairs can be successfully performed arthroscopically with a failure rate that is approximately the same as that of open instability repairs.

Two things have primarily been responsible for our improved results in arthroscopic instability repair. First of all, the techniques of arthroscopic Bankart repair have been greatly refined over the past decade. Second, the recognition that significant bone defects require bone grafting for successful results has largely eliminated the bone-deficient patient as a cause of failure of arthroscopic Bankart repair.

The senior author (SSB) recalls that, prior to incorporating the Latarjet reconstruction into his practice for cases of bone loss, the biggest unsolved problem in his shoulder practice was how to treat the unstable shoulder that had bone loss. Through the end of the 20th century, the conventional wisdom in the United States was that all shoulder instability could be addressed with soft tissue repairs. However, it was obvious that most of our failures of arthroscopic Bankart repair in the 1980s and 1990s were in patients with significant amounts of bone loss.

Dr. Joe DeBeer, after visiting Dr. Gilles Walch in Lyon, France, and seeing his success with the Latarjet procedure and its coracoid bone graft, convinced the senior author (SSB) that this procedure was the answer to the great unsolved problem in his practice. Over time, after adopting the Burkhart–DeBeer modification of the original Latarjet, the proof of its efficacy was clear. We owe a great debt of gratitude to Dr. Gilles Walch for preserving the nearly lost art of the Latarjet procedure and to Dr. Joe DeBeer for introducing this procedure to us.

WHEN TO OPERATE

Despite the incredibly high recurrence rates with nonoperative treatment of instability in athletic young people, many surgeons continue to recommend immobilization followed by rehabilitation as the preferred treatment in all first-time dislocators.

We disagree with that approach. For all active athletic individuals under the age of 30, we recommend arthroscopic Bankart repair after the first dislocation. In active patients over the age of 30, we may try nonoperative treatment after the first dislocation, but if they have a second dislocation, we usually advise arthroscopic Bankart repair. It has been our experience that, with repeated dislocations, bone loss and articular cartilage damage are rapidly cumulative. In fact, we have found that most people with recurrent dislocations whose total time with the shoulder "out of joint" (i.e., the total cumulative time between dislocation and reduction of all episodes of instability) is >5 hours will have significant bone loss that will require bone grafting. Our philosophy is that we would prefer to treat these patients with a less invasive arthroscopic procedure before their bone loss reaches a significant level, so we generally recommend arthroscopic repair after the first or second episode.

PHILOSOPHY OF ARTHROSCOPIC FIXATION

We believe that specific technical criteria must be satisfied in order to achieve successful arthroscopic instability repairs. These criteria have both mechanical and biologic components, and they include

1. Bone loss criteria
2. Soft tissue preparation
3. Bone bed preparation
4. Mechanical fixation
5. Ancillary fixation (plication sutures, rotator interval closure, remplissage)
6. Rehabilitation criteria

Bone Loss Criteria

We have previously defined significant bone loss as

1. Loss of ≥ 25% of the inferior glenoid diameter or
2. A deep Hill-Sachs lesion that engages the anterior glenoid rim in the 90-90 position (90° abduction plus 90° external rotation)

We found that arthroscopic Bankart repair in the face of one or both of these significant bone lesions led to an unacceptable recurrence rate of 67% (1). Therefore, we typically perform open Latarjet reconstructions in patients with significant bone loss. This procedure achieves stability in almost all patients by means of extending the articular arc of the glenoid so far that the Hill-Sachs lesion cannot engage, as well as by utilizing the sling effect of the conjoined tendon to augment the anterior stabilizing structures.

For small acute bony Bankart lesions, we typically repair the glenoid bone fragment with suture anchors. For large acute bony Bankart lesions (i.e., glenoid fractures), we perform arthroscopic reduction and internal fixation (ARIF) with cannulated screws.

As with most things in life, there is a "gray zone" where the criteria are not so clear. The "gray zone" is the category of patients that have a relatively normal inferior glenoid diameter (i.e., <25% bone loss) with an accompanying deep Hill-Sachs lesion (≥4 mm deep). Dr. Phillippe Hardy found that patients with this combination of pathology had a high failure rate after arthroscopic Bankart repair, with a 61% rate of recurrent subluxation or dislocation (personal communication, 2009). In this clinical situation, we now augment our arthroscopic Bankart repair with an arthroscopic remplissage in which we inset the infraspinatus tendon into the humeral head defect and secure it with suture anchors (Fig. 11.1). In this way, we exclude the Hill-Sachs lesion from the humeral articular arc, changing it from an intra-articular bone defect to an extra-articular defect that can no longer engage the anterior glenoid rim. In addition to the obvious advantages for stability enhancement, we believe that this procedure repairs some of the footprint disruption of the infraspinatus that occurs with repeated dislocations (i.e., PASTA lesions of the infraspinatus that we see commonly in association with large Hill-Sachs lesions).

Soft Tissue Preparation

Soft tissue preparation revolves around the principle of optimal tension at the bone-soft tissue interface. The capsulolabral sleeve must be repaired in such a way that it is not too tight and not too loose. In cases with medialized soft tissue healing on the glenoid neck (anterior labral periosteal sleeve avulsion [ALPSA] lesions), the capsule and labrum must be dissected from the glenoid neck so that the underlying subscapularis muscle belly can clearly be seen deep to the capsule. Once the capsule has been adequately mobilized, it will "float up" to the level of the glenoid rim where it can be repaired to bone without tension.

On the other hand, if there is excessive laxity to the capsule, the laxity must be reduced by means of plication sutures. Some surgeons recommend capsular plication directly to the labrum if the labrum is intact, as in cases of multidirectional instability (MDI). However, most patients with MDI have hypoplastic, hyperelastic labra that do not provide firm anchorage points for plication. Therefore, in cases of MDI, we prefer to plicate using suture anchors in the glenoid, as the anchors will provide the firm fixation points we need. Also, in dealing with MDI, we pay special attention to plicating the axillary recess, which is always redundant in such cases.

For traumatic instability cases, we try to recreate a "bumper" of tissue at the glenoid rim. This visual "bumper" is usually attained only by achieving physiologic tensioning of the capsule. Our end point is to achieve centering of the humeral head on the bare spot of the glenoid (Fig. 11.2). When we see this centering, as viewed from an anterosuperolateral portal, we know that we have correctly retensioned the capsule.

The arthroscope offers the advantage of seeing all the pathology, but the surgeon must be sure to look at all the areas where pathology can occur. We have seen several cases where there was a Bankart lesion and a HAGL lesion in the same patient, requiring fixation on both the glenoid side and the humeral side. Furthermore, we have seen quite a few triple labral lesions (combined anterior Bankart, posterior Bankart, and superior labrum anterior and posterior [SLAP] lesion) in patients suspected of having only anterior instability. These lesions must all be recognized and fixed.

In the case of a triple labral lesion, the order of steps is very important. Our first area for anchor placement is for the SLAP lesion, where the supralabral recess tends to swell and close off early. Therefore, we place the SLAP anchors and pass the SLAP sutures early, but do not tie them until the final step of the procedure. Tying them early can close down the remaining capsular space, making it very difficult

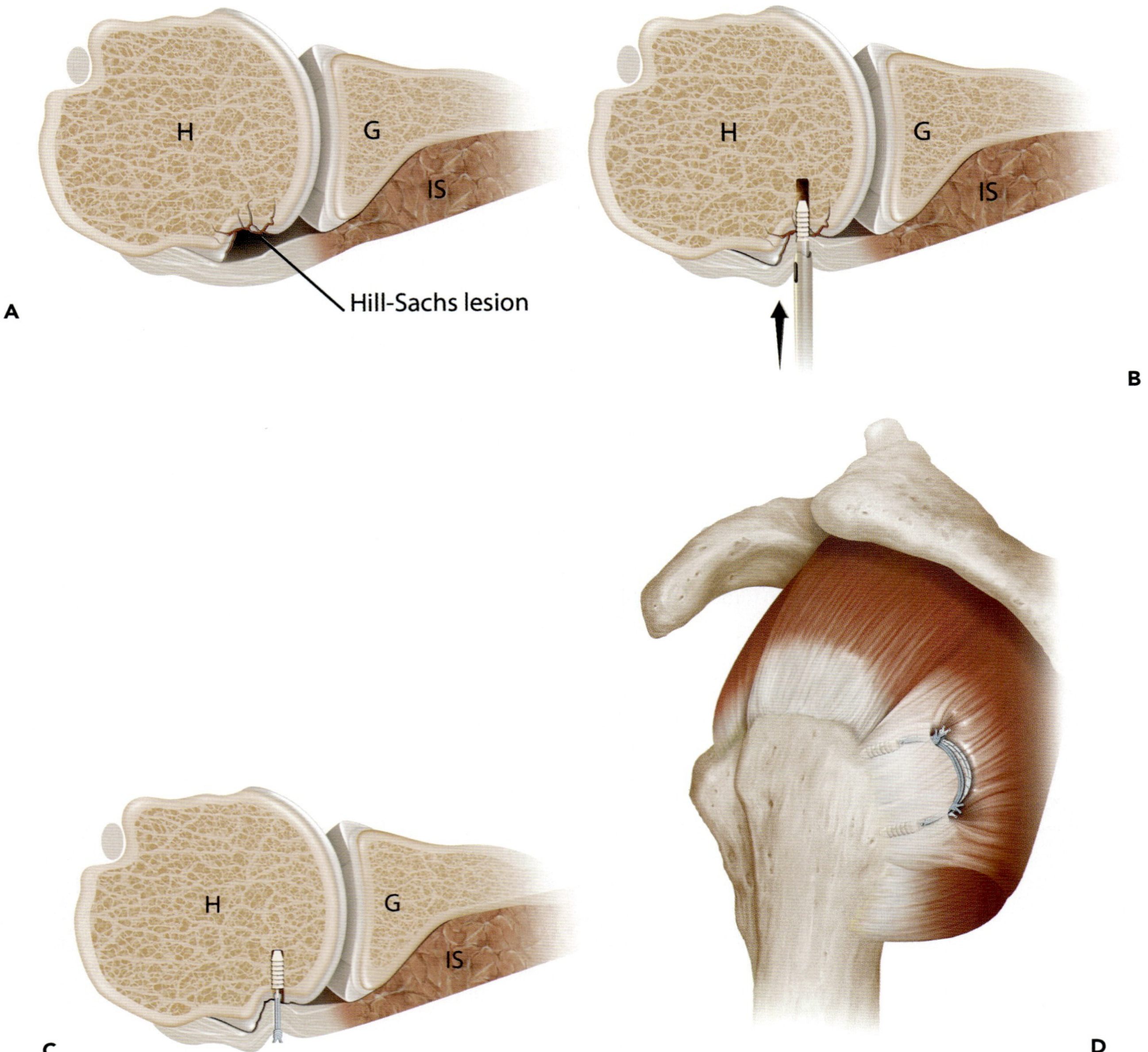

Figure 11.1 Schematic of remplissage for a Hill-Sachs lesion. **A:** Axial schematic of a Hill-Sachs lesion. **B:** Anchors are placed into the Hill-Sachs defect. **C:** Sutures are passed through the infraspinatus tendon and tied to inset the tendon into the defect. Insetting of the infraspinatus into the defect converts the Hill-Sachs lesion to an extra-articular defect. **D:** Sagittal oblique view demonstrates the mattress stitches between the two anchors that have been tied using a double-pulley technique. G, glenoid; H, humerus; IS, infraspinatus tendon.

to do the Bankart repair. The next step is to place the most inferior anchors at the 5 o'clock, 6 o'clock, and 7 o'clock positions, to pass their sutures, and to tie them. The principle here is to perform the repair in the tightest working space first. After that, we place anchors anteriorly, pass their sutures, and tie those knots for an anterior Bankart repair. Then we do the posterior Bankart repair. The posterior repair is done last because visualization is easier posteroinferiorly, even after a Bankart repair has been done. Finally, we tie the SLAP sutures, completing the repair.

Bone Bed Preparation

We believe that bone bed preparation to a base of bleeding bone is critical to the success of the instability repair. The bone bed must actually be seen as it is prepared, either with a 30° arthroscope through an anterosuperolateral viewing portal or a 70° arthroscope through a posterior viewing portal. The indirect view afforded by a 30° scope through a posterior viewing portal is not adequate (Fig. 11.3). We prefer ring curettes and power shaver for preparing the

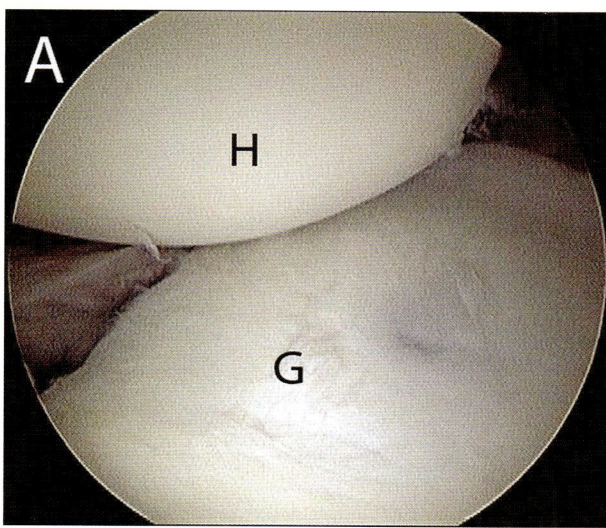

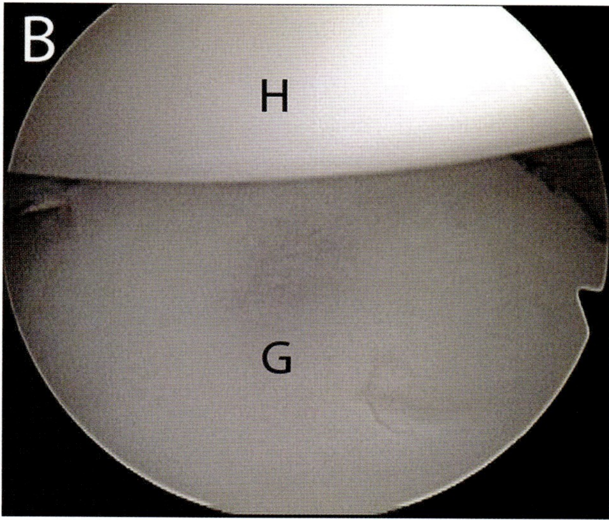

Figure 11.2 Right shoulder, anterosuperolateral viewing portal demonstrating completed Bankart repair. **A:** Initial view prior to repair demonstrates anterior subluxation of the humeral head. **B:** A well-performed repair is confirmed when the humeral head is centered over the bare spot of the glenoid. G, glenoid; H, humerus.

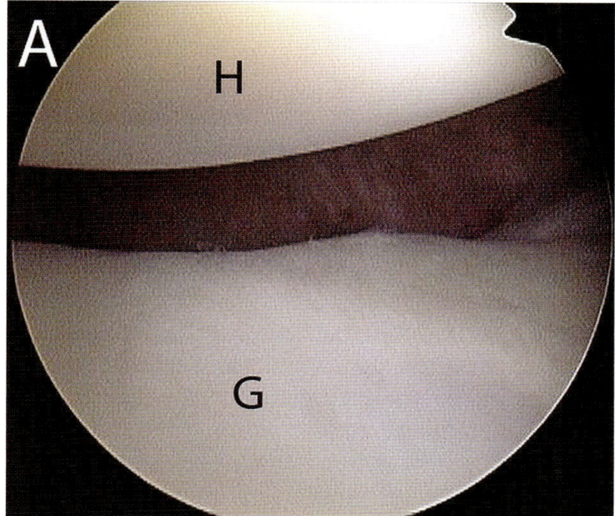

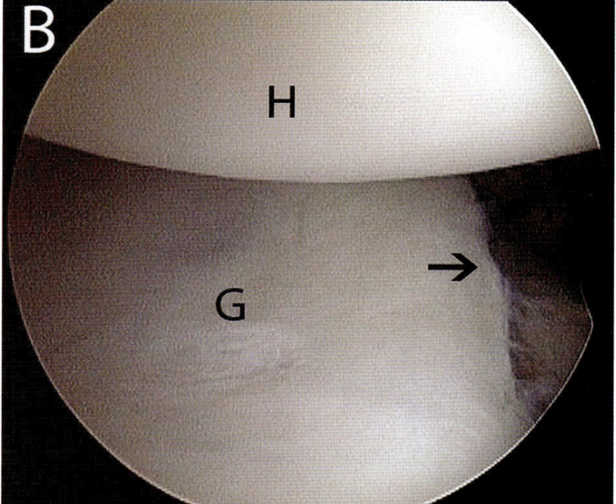

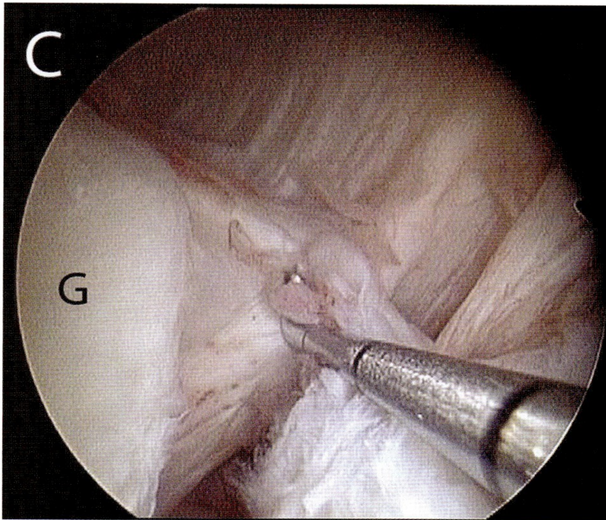

Figure 11.3 Left shoulder, demonstrating comparing visualization of the anterior labrum through the posterior and anterosuperolateral portals. **A:** Viewing with a 30° arthroscope from a posterior portal the labrum is not well seen. **B:** From an anterosuperolateral viewing portal in the same shoulder, it is clear that the labrum has medialized (ALPSA) (*black arrow*) and the humeral head is subluxed anteriorly. **C:** A close-up view from the anterosuperolateral viewing portal further demonstrates the medialized labrum. G, glenoid; H, humerus.

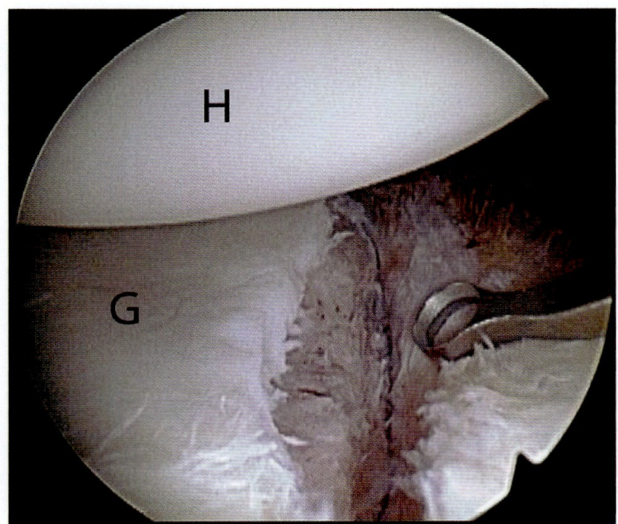

Figure 11.4 Left shoulder, anterosuperolateral viewing portal demonstrates a glenoid rim with a 2-mm strip of articular cartilage that has been removed with a curette in preparation for Bankart repair. G, glenoid; H, humerus.

glenoid neck. We seldom use a high-speed bur for this part of the case because we feel that the bur is too aggressive and could remove some important glenoid bone.

We believe that it is critically important to remove a 2-mm strip of articular cartilage along the damaged glenoid rim. This is done with a small ring curette (Fig. 11.4). It provides some additional bleeding bone for capsular healing, and it positions the capsule in such a way that it will never heal in a medialized position.

Mechanical Fixation

As with all repairs at a bone–soft tissue interface, we strive for knot security and loop security. We also try to reduce capsular redundancy when necessary, by means of plication sutures.

Significant bone loss has its own set of mechanical deficiencies that must be addressed, and we shall discuss this shortly.

Ancillary Fixation (Plication Sutures, Rotator Interval Closure, and Remplissage)

The only time we do rotator interval closure is in very loose jointed patients with MDI. Some authors have recommended the routine use of posterior plication sutures in addition to anterior anchors for treatment of traumatic anterior instability. We do not believe in that approach, so we do not place posterior sutures unless there has been damage to the posterior capsule. However, we believe there is often a component of axillary recess redundancy, so we frequently place a double-loaded 6 o'clock anchor and then secure axillary recess plication sutures to that anchor.

As outlined above, we reserve remplissage for patients with near-normal width of the inferior glenoid diameter coupled with a deep (>4 mm) Hill-Sachs lesion.

When to Open the Shoulder: Significant Bone Defects

Since we have been doing the Latarjet procedure, we have found that there is never a need to bone graft the Hill-Sachs lesion in an instability patient. Even with a very large Hill-Sachs lesion, it will not engage after Latarjet reconstruction.

We do a Latarjet reconstruction with coracoid bone graft if the patient has anterior instability associated with a significant bone defect (≥25% loss of the inferior glenoid diameter; deep, ≥4 mm, Hill-Sachs lesion that engages with the arm in a 90-90 position; or both). After fixing the coracoid bone graft to the glenoid with two screws, we try to forcefully dislocate the shoulder on the table and we find that we can virtually never dislocate it, even before we repair the capsule. We consider that our capsular repair to the native glenoid simply serves to create a smooth covering over the coracoid graft so that it becomes an extra-articular structure that cannot abrade the articular cartilage of the humerus.

Rehabilitation Principles

After arthroscopic instability repair, we immobilize the arm in a sling for 6 weeks, allowing no more than 0° external rotation. The one exception to this rule is the overhead athlete whose dominant shoulder has undergone an arthroscopic instability repair. In this case, we allow up to 30° external rotation during the first 6 weeks. In nonoverhead athletes, we prefer the shoulder to be slightly stiff at 3 months post-op, with about half the external rotation as the normal side (with the arm at the side).

In a straightforward Bankart repair, we allow both stretching and strengthening to begin at 6 weeks postoperatively. However, if a remplissage has also been done, we delay strengthening until 3 months post-op. The rationale for this delay is that the remplissage (insetting of the infraspinatus into the Hill-Sachs defect) has the same biologic healing requirements as a rotator cuff repair. Since Sharpey fibers do not form until 3 months after rotator cuff repair, we delay strengthening until 3 months post-op after remplissage.

Full activities are allowed at 6 months post-op, after arthroscopic Bankart repair, whether remplissage was done or not. Once again, the exception to this rule is the throwing athlete, who is not allowed to begin an interval throwing program until 9 months post-op. Furthermore, MDI patients are not allowed to return to athletic activities until one year postoperatively.

Rehabilitation after Latarjet reconstruction is as follows:

- Sling for 6 weeks
- At 6 weeks post-op, begin stretching
- At 3 months post-op, begin Theraband strengthening
- At 6 months post-op, begin weight lifting in the gym
- Full activities are allowed when the consolidation of the bone graft is apparent on x-rays, or at one year post-op.

Special Situations

Patients with a history of dislocation and grand mal seizures comprise a challenging category. We insist that they must be on a regimen of medication that allows them to be seizure free for at least 3 months prior to surgery. If patients cannot be medically managed to remain seizure free for at least 3 months, we do not operate on them as the surgery would be doomed to failure by a seizure in the early postoperative period.

CONCLUSION

Attention to the technical criteria in this chapter should yield very successful results, with well under a 10% recurrence rate. As they say, the devil is in the details. But in arthroscopic shoulder surgery, every detail is important. It's all about the details.

REFERENCE

1. Burkhart SS, De Beer JF. Traumatic glenohumeral bone defects and their relationship to failure of arthroscopic Bankart repairs: significance of the inverted-pear glenoid and the humeral engaging Hill-Sachs lesion. *Arthroscopy* 2000;16:677–694.

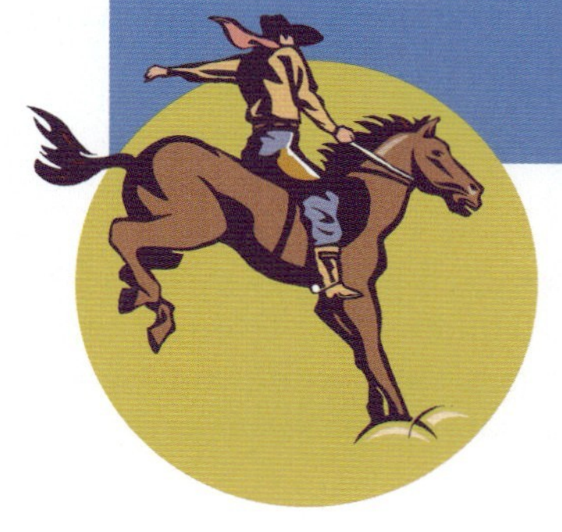

12

Repair of Anterior Instability without Significant Bone Loss

WESTERN WISDOM

The man who can't make a choice makes a choice.

Anterior instability repair, or Bankart repair, is one of the most common surgeries performed by the shoulder arthroscopist. Although arthroscopic Bankart repair is commonly perceived as a technically easier procedure than arthroscopic rotator cuff repair, the construction of a secure, anatomic, effective Bankart repair is very complex. This is due to challenges in visualization and angle of approach, as well as the diverse pathology that may be encountered in instability repair. Furthermore, while most cases are effectively managed arthroscopically, it is important to evaluate each case for substantial bone loss that requires open reconstruction.

THE SETUP

Like all shoulder arthroscopies, we perform arthroscopic instability repair in the lateral decubitus position. In instability cases, the lateral decubitus position has many distinct advantages over the beach chair position. These include the ability to exert translational loads to the shoulder via traction to improve visualization and the use of the anterosuperolateral portal. This portal is created approximately 5 to 10 mm lateral to the anterolateral corner of the acromion, superior to the biceps and anterior to the supraspinatus tendon with a 45° angle of approach to the superior glenoid (Fig. 12.1). This portal is one of the major reasons patients should have arthroscopic instability surgery in the lateral decubitus position. The anterosuperolateral portal, which is used mostly as a viewing portal during arthroscopic Bankart repair, provides optimal visualization of the anterior, inferior, and posterior aspect of the glenoid, and it frees the right and/or left hands for easy and ergonomic approaches to these regions. Although a similar portal may be established in the beach chair position, the awkward stance required when visualizing through this portal makes it extremely difficult to use and minimizes its benefit.

In general, we use a three-portal technique for almost all instability repairs (i.e., anterior, SLAP, or posterior repairs). These include a standard posterior portal, created 3 to 4 cm medial and 3 to 4 cm inferior to the posterolateral corner of the acromion and a low anterior portal created just above the lateral half of subscapularis tendon (Fig. 12.2). With this routine setup, the vast majority of pathologies may be identified and further portals may be created when necessary.

ACCESSORY PORTALS FOR ANTERIOR BANKART REPAIR

In some cases, access to the inferior aspect of the glenoid requires accessory portals for anchor insertion only. These portals are established to provide a 45° angle of approach to the 5 o'clock and 7 o'clock positions.

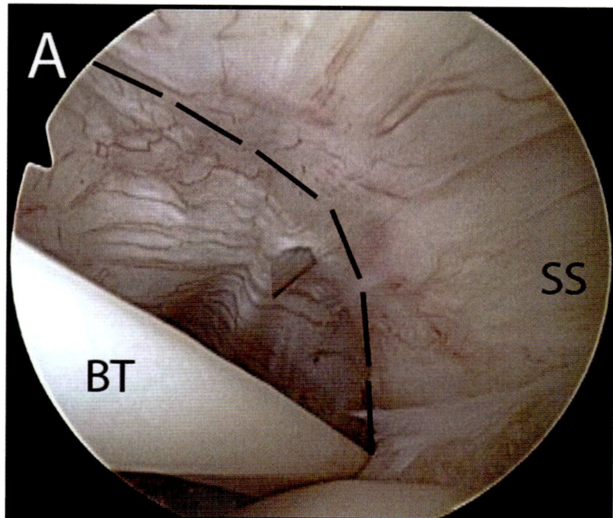

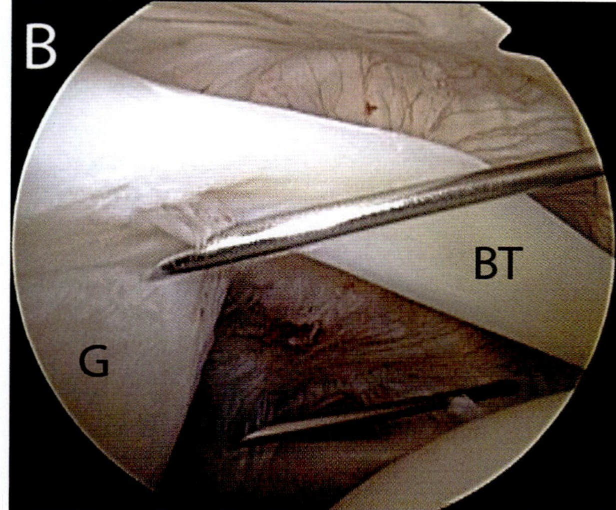

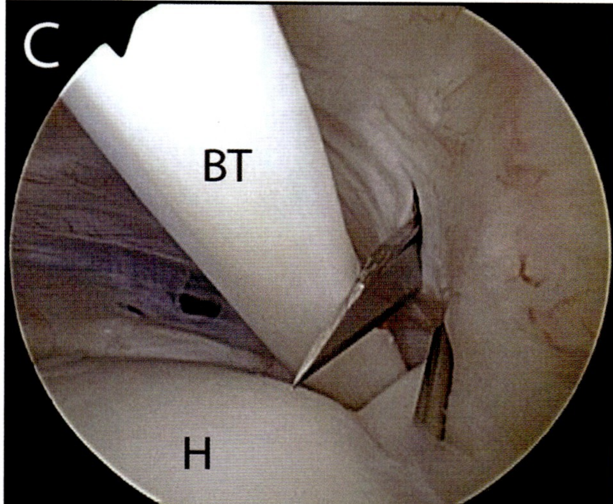

Figure 12.1 Right shoulder, posterior viewing portal, demonstrating establishment of an anterosuperolateral portal. **A:** A spinal needle is placed 5 to 10 mm lateral to the anterolateral acromion and enters the joint just anterior the supraspinatus (anterior ridge outlined by dashed lines). **B:** The portal should provide approximately a 45° angle of approach to the superior glenoid rim. A spinal needle from an anterior portal is seen in the background. **C:** A knife is walked down the spinal needle to incise the capsule. BT, biceps tendon; G, glenoid; H, humerus; SS, supraspinatus tendon.

5 O'clock Portal

This portal is created approximately 1 to 2 cm inferior to the standard anterior portal and is created transtendon through the subscapularis. A cannula is not required since the 5 o-clock trans-subscapularis portal is generally used for anchor insertion only. While viewing through a posterior portal, a spinal needle is used to localize the correct angle of approach transtendon through the subscapularis (Fig. 12.3). A small skin incision is created and a switching stick is inserted following the direct line of the spinal needle. The spear guide for a BioComposite SutureTak anchor is then slid over the switching stick. Alternatively, the spear guide may be "walked down" the spinal needle to enter the joint alongside the needle. With this more direct angle of approach, anchor insertion may now be performed at a less oblique angle to the anteroinferior glenoid.

Posterolateral Portal (7 O'clock)

In patients with labral tears that extend beyond the 6 o'clock position posteriorly, an anchor in the posterior inferior corner of the glenoid may be required to secure the posterior inferior labrum. However, the standard posterior portal usually does not provide the correct angle of approach to the posterior inferior glenoid. A separate low posterolateral portal or 7 o'clock portal is required that is created usually 4 to 5 cm inferior to the posterolateral corner of the acromion and approximately 4 to 5 cm lateral to the standard posterior portal. This portal is created to provide a 45° of approach to the posterior inferior glenoid and is used for anchor insertion (Fig. 12.4). The spear guide for a BioComposite SutureTak anchor is inserted using a switching stick technique as described above.

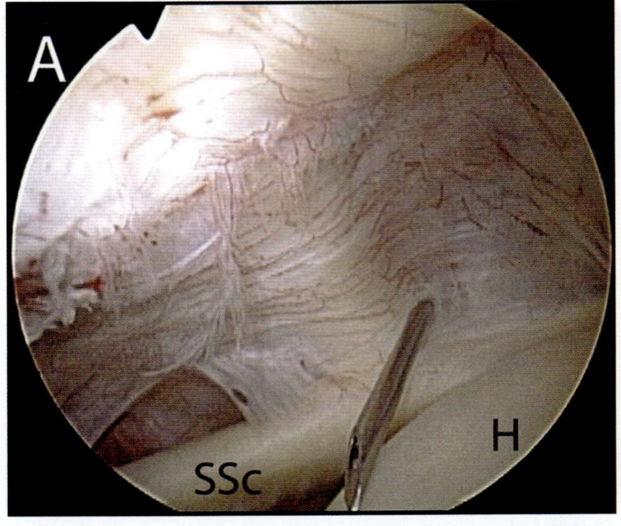

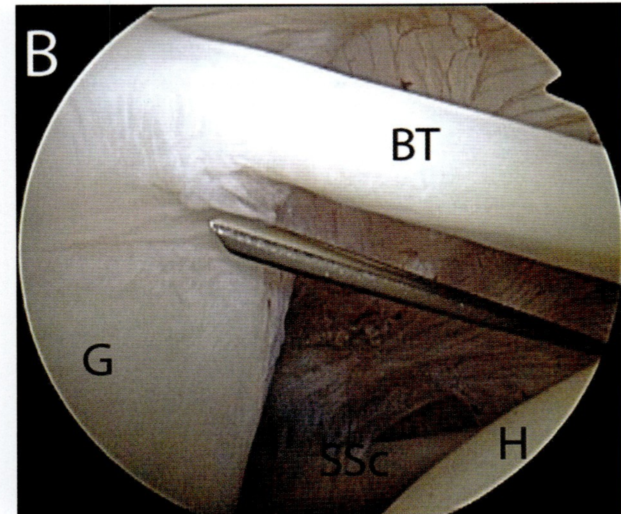

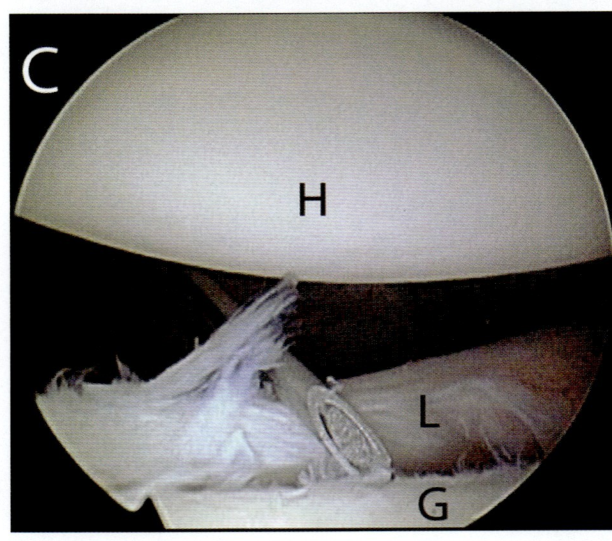

Figure 12.2 Right shoulder, posterior viewing portal demonstrating establishment of an anterior portal for Bankart repair. **A:** A spinal needle enters the glenohumeral joint just superior to the lateral half of the subscapularis tendon. **B:** The angle of approach allows access to the anterosuperior glenoid. **C:** This portal also provides a 45° angle of approach to the inferior glenoid for anchor placement. BT, biceps tendon; G, glenoid; H, humerus; L, labrum; SSc, subscapularis tendon.

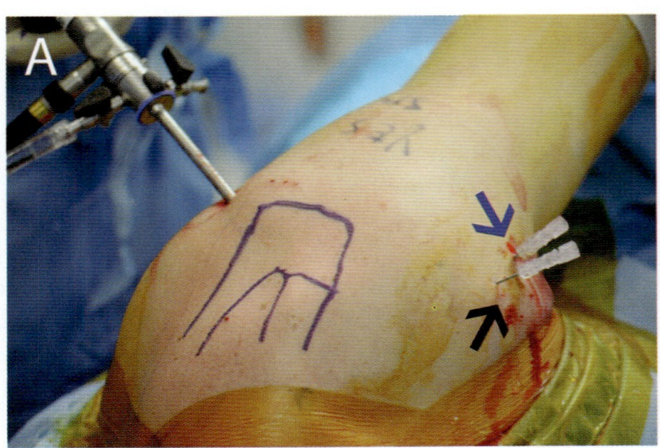

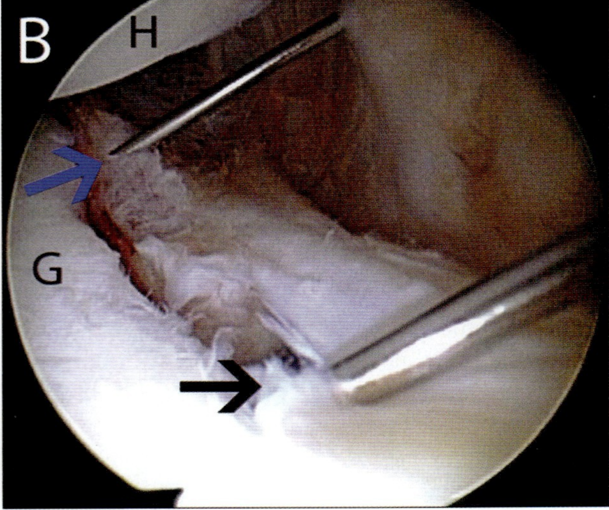

Figure 12.3 The 5 o'clock portal in a left shoulder. **A:** External view demonstrates spinal needle localization for a 5 o'clock portal (*blue arrow*) that is 1 to 2 cm inferior to our standard anterior portal (*black arrow*). **B:** Anterosuperolateral viewing portal demonstrates use of a spinal needle to determine an adequate angle of approach to the anteroinferior glenoid (*blue arrow*). A spinal needle from the anterior portal is seen in foreground (*black arrow*).

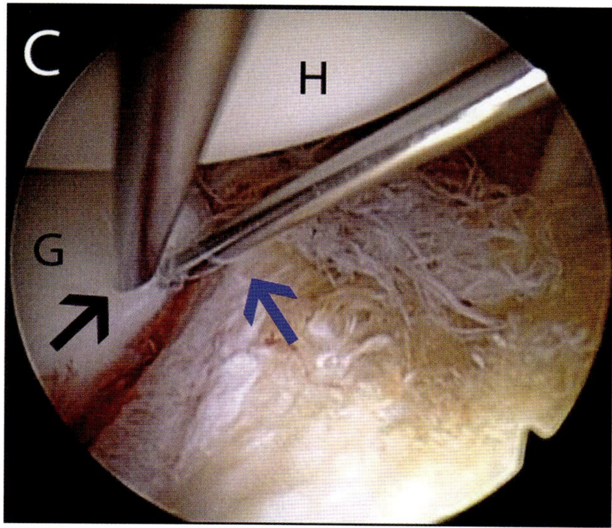

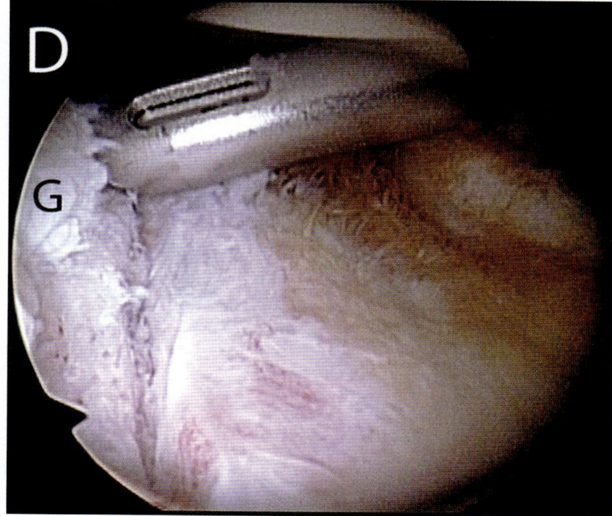

Figure 12.3 *(Continued)* **C:** Same shoulder demonstrates the improved angle of approach to the anteroinferior glenoid achieved with the 5 o'clock portal (*blue arrow*) compared to a standard anterior portal (*black arrow*). **D:** Following spinal needle localization, a spear guide can be walked down the spinal needle for anchor placement. G, glenoid; H, humerus.

MAXIMIZING VISUALIZATION

While viewing through the anterosuperolateral portal the anterior, posterior, and inferior aspects of the glenohumeral joint may be accessed. To maximize visualization and access of the anterior inferior glenohumeral joint, two techniques are commonly utilized. To provide temporary visualization and facilitate the angle of approach to the anterior inferior glenoid, an assistant standing behind the patient can provide lateral traction, abduction, and posterior translation to the glenohumeral joint. This technique will maximize the anterior inferior working space. To increase the working space inferiorly, a roll of towels or gowns may be placed in the patient's axilla. Adduction of the arm over this roll (Fig. 12.5) places a lateral distraction force on the glenohumeral joint and increases the working space inferiorly (Fig. 12.6).

BANKART REPAIR SUTURE ANCHOR TECHNIQUE

After establishing the standard three portals for instability repair, a diagnostic arthroscopy is performed to identify all pathologies. This includes measurement of bone loss, documentation of all labral pathology, and an assessment of the rotator cuff and any cartilage damage. Standard Bankart lesions +/– SLAP lesions with minimal bone loss may be approached using a three-portal technique. We establish 8.25 mm × 7 cm threaded clear cannulas (Arthrex, Inc., Naples, FL) in the anterior and anterosuperolateral portals to facilitate glenohumeral access. An 8.25 mm × 9 cm cannula is usually required for the posterior portal due

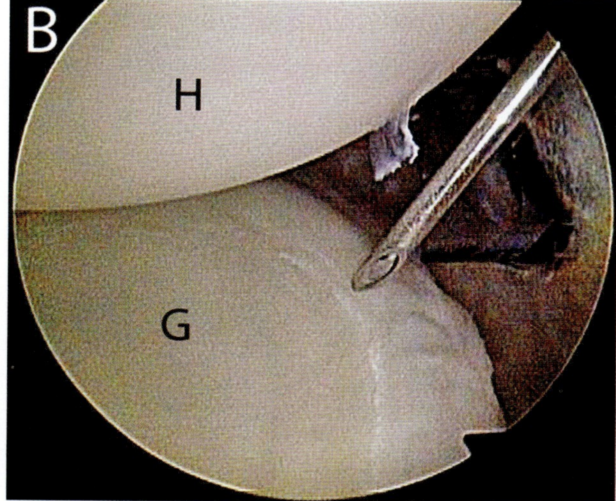

Figure 12.4 Right shoulder, demonstrating placement of the posterolateral portal. **A:** External view showing spinal needle placement (*white arrow*) for the posterolateral portal. **B:** Anterosuperolateral portal demonstrating that the spinal needle provides a 45° angle of approach to the posteroinferior glenoid. G, glenoid; H, humerus.

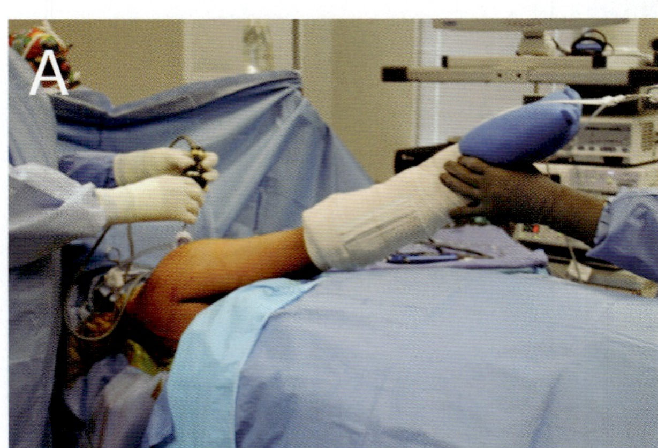

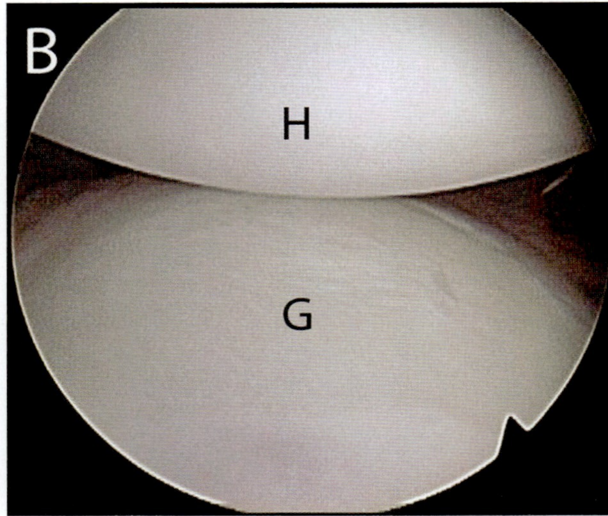

Figure 12.5 Right shoulder, anterosuperolateral viewing portal demonstrating standard view of the inferior glenoid. **A:** Patient positioned in the lateral decubitus position. **B:** View of the inferior glenoid prior to placement of an axillary bump. G, glenoid; H, humerus.

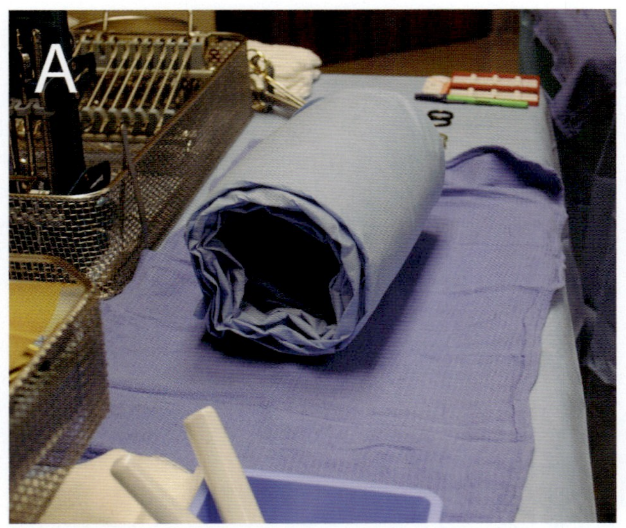

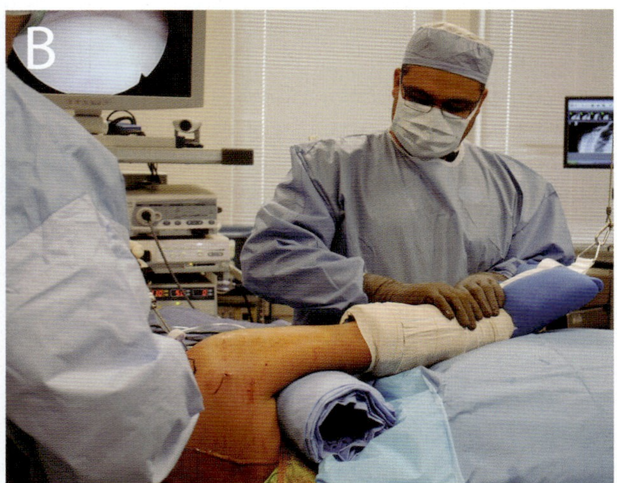

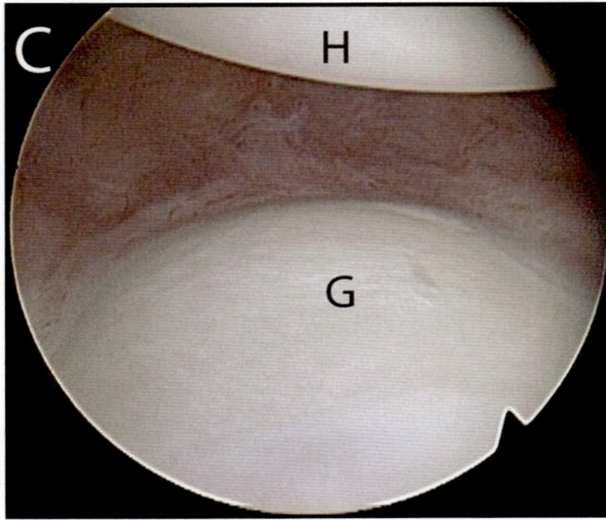

Figure 12.6 Augmenting visualization of the inferior glenoid. **A:** An axillary roll is created. **B:** The axillary roll is placed and an assistant provides distraction and a varus force to the operative arm. **C:** Right shoulder, anterosuperolateral viewing portal demonstrating improved visualization with the axillary roll compared to the previous visualization (Fig. 12.5). G, glenoid; H, humerus.

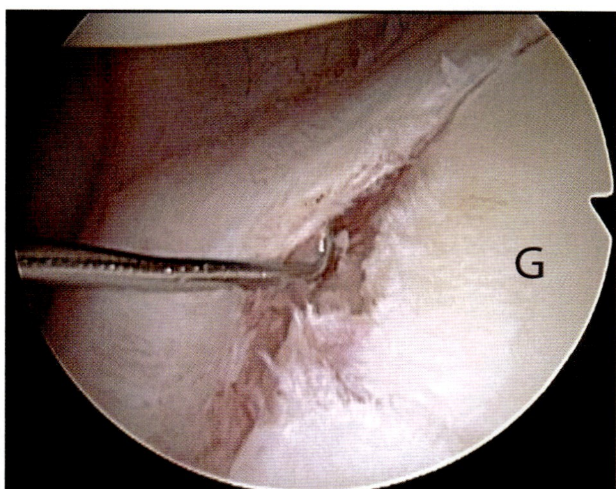

Figure 12.7 Right shoulder, anterosuperolateral viewing portal demonstrates a Bankart lesion. G, glenoid.

to the increased distance from the skin to the glenohumeral joint posteriorly.

If a concomitant type II SLAP lesion is identified during instability repair, this should be repaired to augment repair of the Bankart lesion and to enhance stability of the glenohumeral joint. In general, the SLAP lesion is approached as the first stage of the procedure with bone preparation, anchor insertion, and suture passage. The reason for this is because soft tissue swelling as the case progresses will make suture passage superiorly more difficult. However, knot tying is delayed until the conclusion of the procedure. Early knot tying can prematurely constrict the glenohumeral joint, limiting the effect of traction/translation, and obstructing visualization. In atypical cases of type III or type IV SLAP repair in association with Bankart repair, one may choose to tie sutures early in the procedure to reduce the displaced bucket-handle tear and to provide a stable base for subsequent Bankart repair.

While viewing through the anterosuperolateral portal, the Bankart lesion is identified (Fig. 12.7). The extent of the lesion, displacement of the labrum, and quality of the tissue are all assessed. Using a combination of an arthroscopic elevator, arthroscopic scissors, and a shaver, the Bankart lesion is meticulously mobilized off the anterior and anteroinferior glenoid neck (Fig. 12.8A). In lesions that approach but do not extend beyond the 6 o'clock position, an arthroscopic scissor and elevator are commonly used to extend the lesion to just beyond the 6 o'clock position. This ensures adequate mobilization of the labrum and anterior inferior glenohumeral ligaments, facilitating an inferior to superior shift.

The entire anterior inferior glenoid labrum is mobilized until the underlying muscular fibers of the subscapularis are identified (Fig. 12.8B). Adequate mobilization is achieved when the glenoid labrum naturally floats to or above the level of the glenoid. This ensures that an anatomic, tension-free repair of the labrum may be obtained.

Mobilization is particularly important in ALPSA lesions (anterior labroligamentous periosteal sleeve avulsion), where the anterior inferior labrum is displaced medially and is scarred along the medial neck of the glenoid (Fig. 12.9). Aggressive mobilization is required for these lesions to ensure that a tension-free repair is obtained.

Once the labrum has been mobilized, the anterior glenoid neck is debrided to a bleeding bone surface. Care is taken to debride the glenoid neck, removing soft tissue without removing bone. A soft tissue shaver or burr may be used. Since the labrum is repaired back up onto the edge of the face of the glenoid, a small, thin strip of bone is exposed on the anterior glenoid rim to enhance healing. A sharp ring curette is used to create a narrow strip of bare bone on the articular surface of the glenoid rim, along the proposed bone–labrum interface (Fig. 12.10).

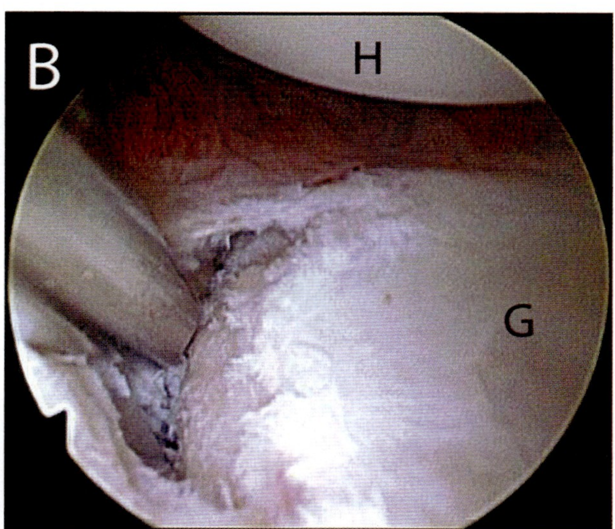

Figure 12.8 Right shoulder, anterosuperolateral portal demonstrating mobilization of a Bankart lesion. **A:** A 15° arthroscopic elevator is introduced through an anterior portal to mobilize the labrum. **B:** A shaver assists in the mobilization. Mobilization is complete when subscapularis muscle fibers are visualized medially, deep to the capsule. G, glenoid; H, humerus.

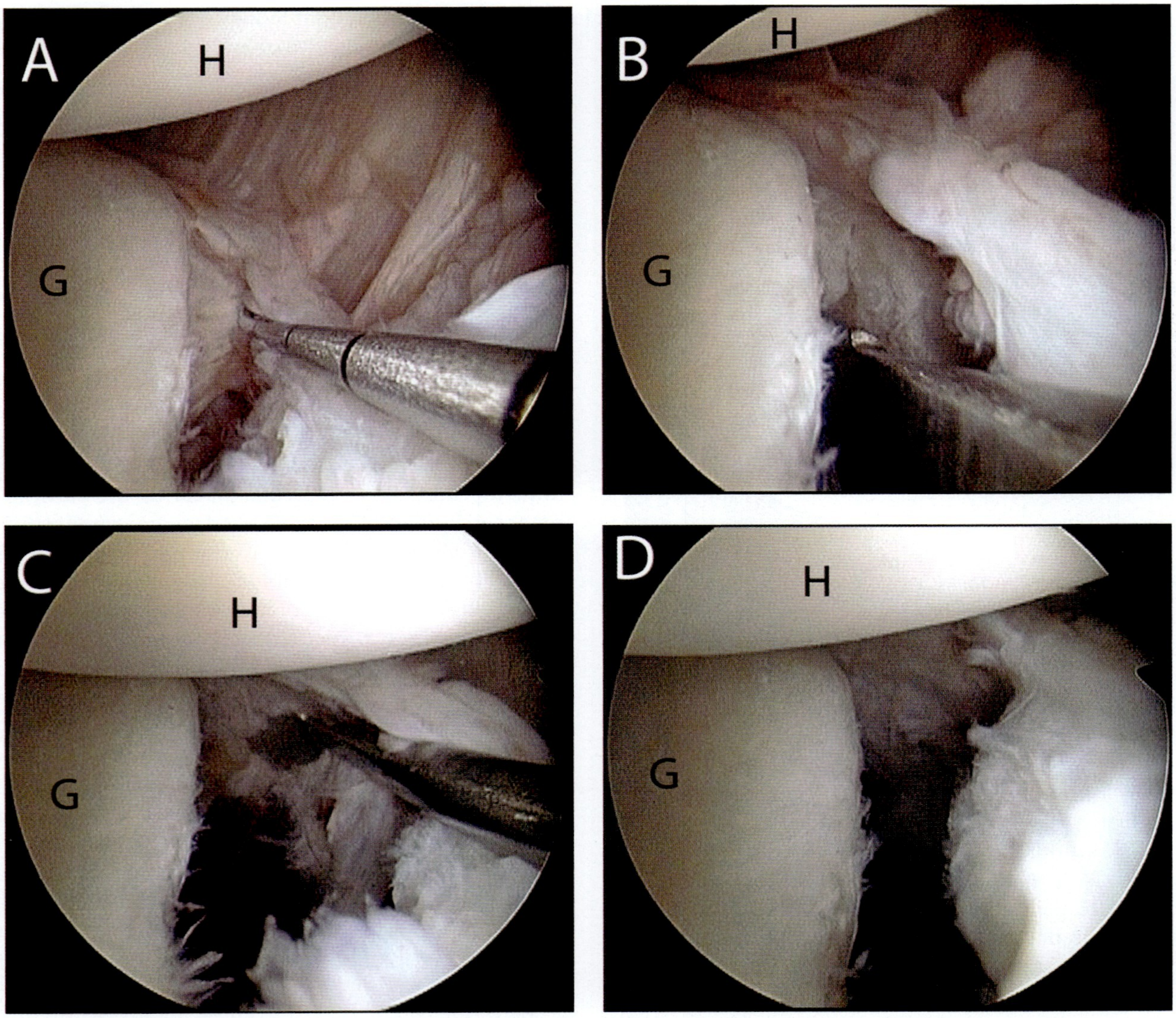

Figure 12.9 Left shoulder, anterosuperolateral viewing portal demonstrating **(A)** an anterior labroligamentous periosteal sleeve avulsion (ALPSA) that has resulted in a medialized labrum. **B:** An arthroscopic elevator introduced through an anterior portal is used to mobilize the ALPSA lesion. **C:** Mobilization is complete when the subscapularis muscle is visualized. **D:** Following complete mobilization the labrum "floats up" above the level of the glenoid. G, glenoid; H, humerus

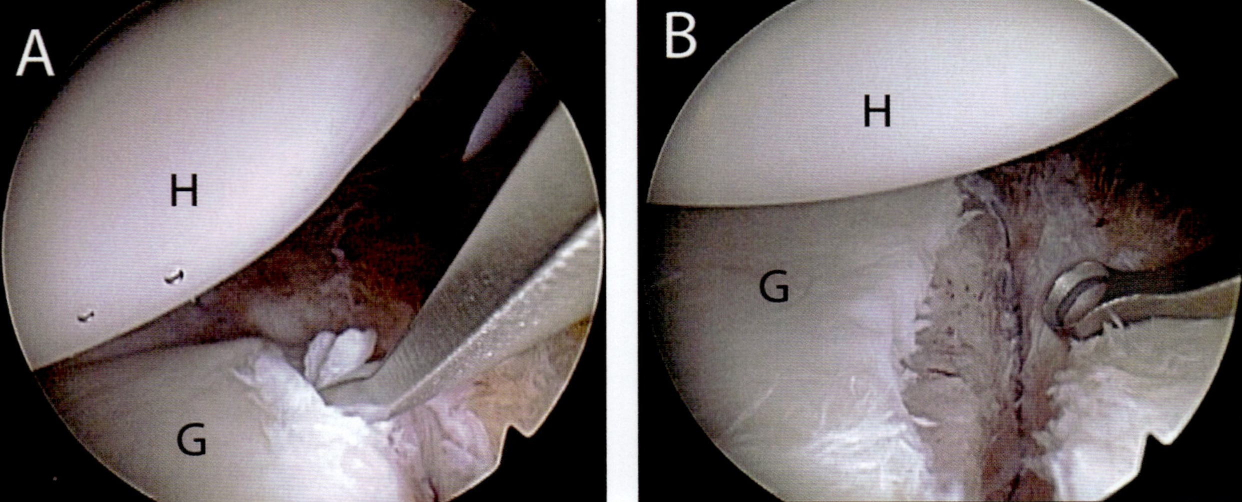

Figure 12.10 Left shoulder, anterosuperolateral viewing portal demonstrating bone bed preparation for an anterior Bankart repair. **A:** A ring curette is used to define a small strip of bare bone on the anterior glenoid to facilitate labrum to bone healing. **B:** View after complete preparation. G, glenoid; H, humerus.

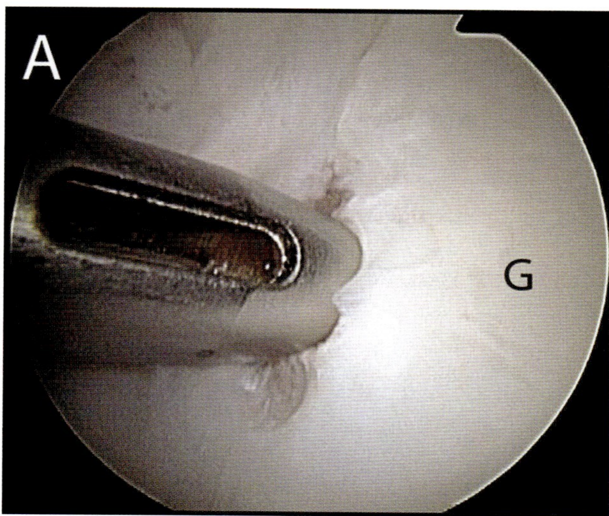

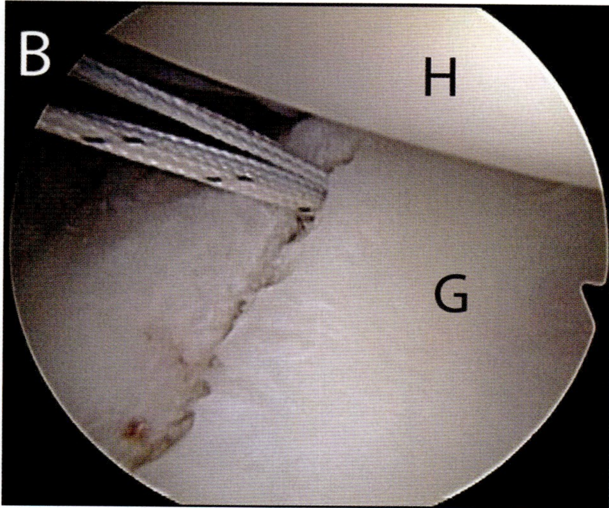

Figure 12.11 Right shoulder, anterosuperolateral viewing portal demonstrating anchor placement for a Bankart repair. **A:** A BioComposite SutureTak Spear Guide (Arthrex, Inc., Naples, FL) is placed through the anterior portal and is seated on the glenoid. **B:** View after placement of a double-loaded anchor. G, glenoid; H, humerus

Anchors are then inserted just onto the face of the glenoid along the strip of prepared bare bone, starting from inferior to superior. It is important to plan and space anchors appropriately for anchor insertion. On average, we use three 3.0-mm BioComposite SutureTak anchors double loaded with No. 2 FiberWire (Arthrex, Inc., Naples, FL). All anchors are inserted so that they are at or below the midglenoid notch. When the patient's anatomy allows, anchors may be inserted through the standard anterior portal. The BioComposite SutureTak Spear is placed just onto the articular surface and is used to lever the humeral head posteriorly to improve the angle of approach to the glenoid rim. A mallet may be used to gently tap the spear into the glenoid bone that will fix the spear onto the glenoid and prevent slippage during subsequent drilling and anchor insertion (Fig. 12.11). Without moving the spear, the bone is then drilled and the anchor is inserted through the cannulated spear.

Suture passage may be performed in one of three ways: antegrade (Scorpion; Arthrex, Inc., Naples, FL), shuttling (SutureLasso; Arthrex, Inc., Naples, FL), or retrograde (BirdBeak; Arthrex, Inc., Naples, FL) techniques. We have

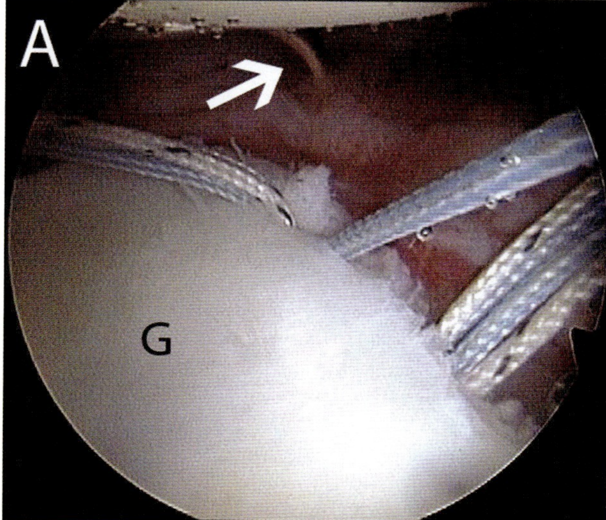

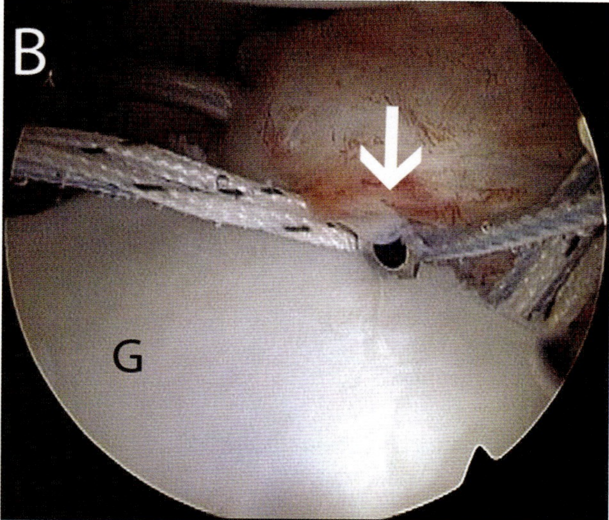

Figure 12.12 Left shoulder, anterosuperolateral portal demonstrates shuttling technique for suture passage during Bankart repair. In some cases, the most anteroinferior suture is easiest to pass from a posterior portal. **A:** A SutureLasso (*white arrow*) (Arthrex, Inc., Naples, FL) curved opposite the operative shoulder is introduced from a posterior portal. **B:** The SutureLasso (*white arrow*) is used to perform a pass through the anteroinferior capsule and labrum.

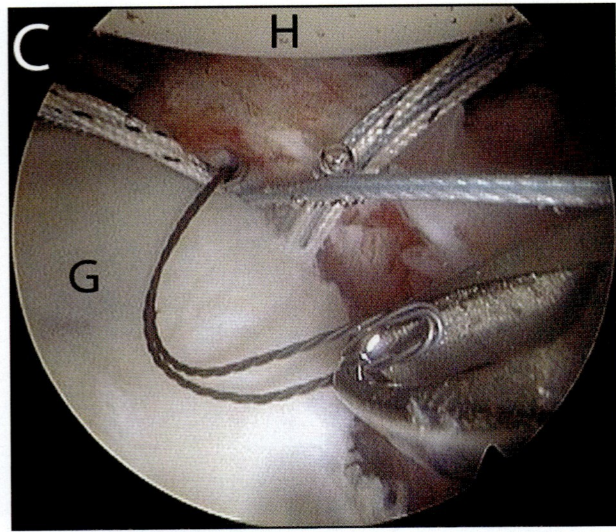

Figure 12.12 *(Continued)* **C:** A Nitinol loop is retrieved from an anterior portal. A *blue suture* has previously been retrieved through this anterior portal and will be passed through the Nitinol loop to shuttle it through the labrum and capsule. G, glenoid; H, humerus.

found that antegrade suture passage is only possible in large patients, where there is adequate room for opening the jaws of the Scorpion suture passer. It is more important, however, to place the stitch appropriately and accurately through the labrum than to use one specific technique. Of critical importance are the sutures for the most inferior anchor, which will capture the inferior axillary recess and anterior inferior glenohumeral ligament. These sutures are critical in retensioning the "hammock" and effectively shifting the capsule superiorly.

Shuttling is our preferred technique for suture passage in most cases. Often, it is easiest to pass the most inferior stitch by shuttling from the posterior cannula with an opposite 25° Tight Curve SutureLasso (i.e., left curved for a right shoulder). Three of the four sutures are retrieved out the posterior portal and the SutureLasso, inserted through the posterior portal, penetrates the inferior capsule exiting the labrum just anteriorly and inferiorly (Fig. 12.12). The suture shuttle wire is then retrieved through the anterior portal and the suture limb remaining in this portal is shuttled out the posterior cannula. To pass the second more anterior suture, usually the standard SutureLasso is used (25° right angled hook for a right shoulder) through the anterior portal (Fig. 12.13). To follow the same

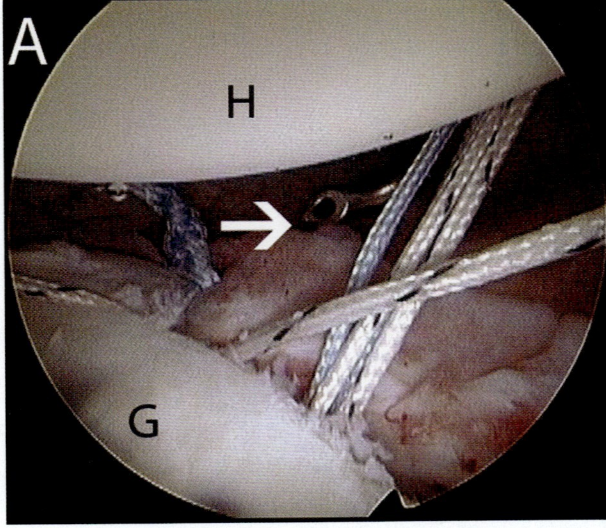

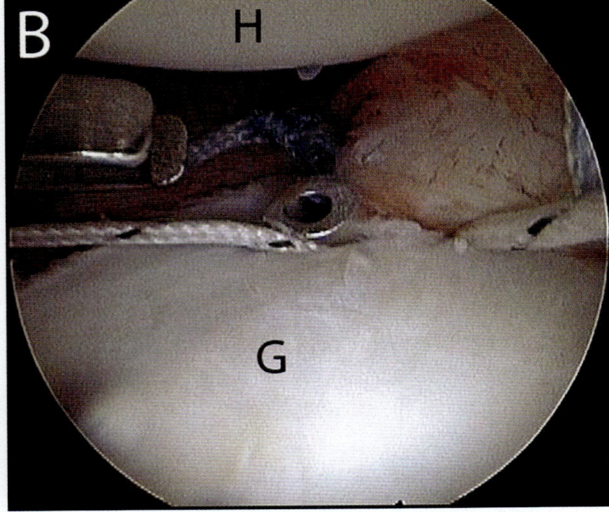

Figure 12.13 Left shoulder, anterosuperolateral viewing portal. After the most anteroinferior suture has been passed (Fig. 12.12), it is easiest to pass the remaining sutures from an anterior portal. **A:** A SutureLasso (*white arrow*) (Arthrex, Inc., Naples, FL) curved to the same side of the operative shoulder is introduced from an anterior portal. **B:** The SutureLasso is passed through the capsule and labrum.

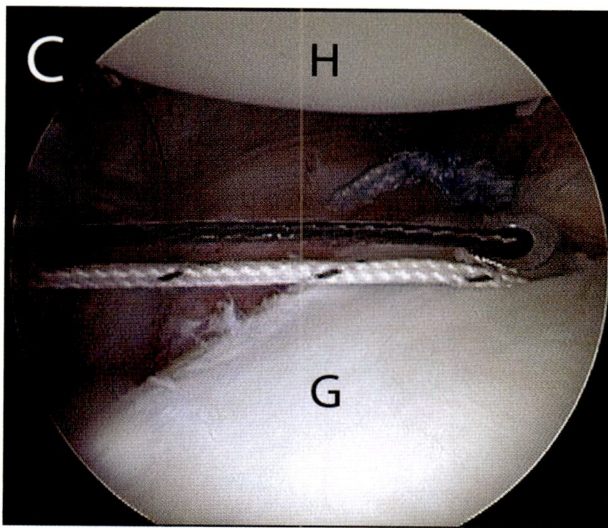

Figure 12.13 *(Continued)* **C:** A Nitinol loop is retrieved out the posterior portal and will be used to shuttle a suture previously retrieved out this portal. G, glenoid; H, humerus.

sequence for shuttling, a suture limb is retrieved out the posterior portal prior to passing the SutureLasso. This step ensures that the sutures do not tangle as they are shuttled under the labrum and through the capsule. Alternatively, a "single-step" approach may be used by retrieving a suture and the suture shuttle wire at the same time. Retrograde instruments are usually difficult to use low in the glenohumeral joint due to the relatively acute angle of approach.

The second anchor is inserted just onto the face of the glenoid and sutures are passed in a similar fashion. When the approach is more directly in line with the cannula, usually with the third anchor from the bottom, retrograde suture passage is possible (Fig. 12.14), but may create a larger hole through the labrum when compared to a SutureLasso shuttling technique. Usually, sutures are passed approximately 1 to 1.5 cm inferior to the anchor, effectively shifting the labrum/capsule superiorly. The same sequence is repeated for each anchor. We routinely use three double-loaded anchors for a standard Bankart repair.

In patients with standard traumatic unidirectional instability, a formal capsular plication is rarely performed anteriorly or posteriorly. While posterior capsular plication has recently been advocated by some surgeons as a method of closing the inferior capsular recess, we have found that this is rarely required when using the above technique since the inferior sutures capture the inferior axillary recess and advance them superiorly and anteriorly effectively retensioning the axillary recess.

To simplify suture management, sutures are "tied as you go" using standard knot tying techniques through the anterior portal (Fig. 12.15). Although early labrum fixation to bone can limit anchor insertion and suture passage, multiple double-loaded anchors in a tight glenohumeral joint can also make suture management difficult and frustrating. As a balance, a "keep ahead" by one anchor approach may be used. That is, the inferior two anchors are inserted and sutures passed, then the first anchor sutures

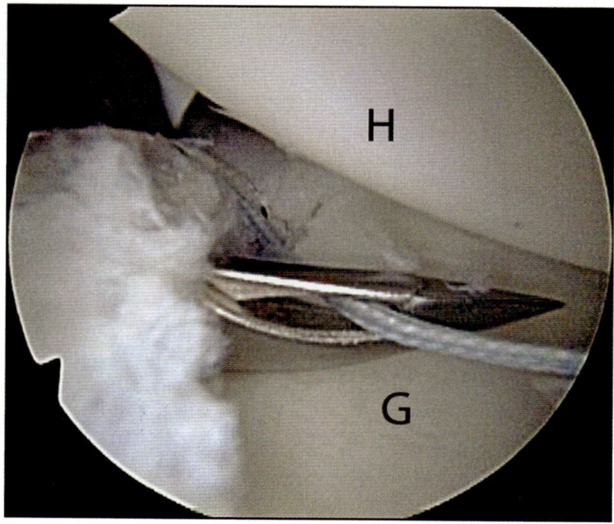

Figure 12.14 Right shoulder, anterosuperolateral viewing portal demonstrating retrograde suture passage with a BirdBeak (Arthrex, Inc., Naples, FL). This technique may be used when the portal is directly in line with the suture to be passed. G, glenoid; H, humerus.

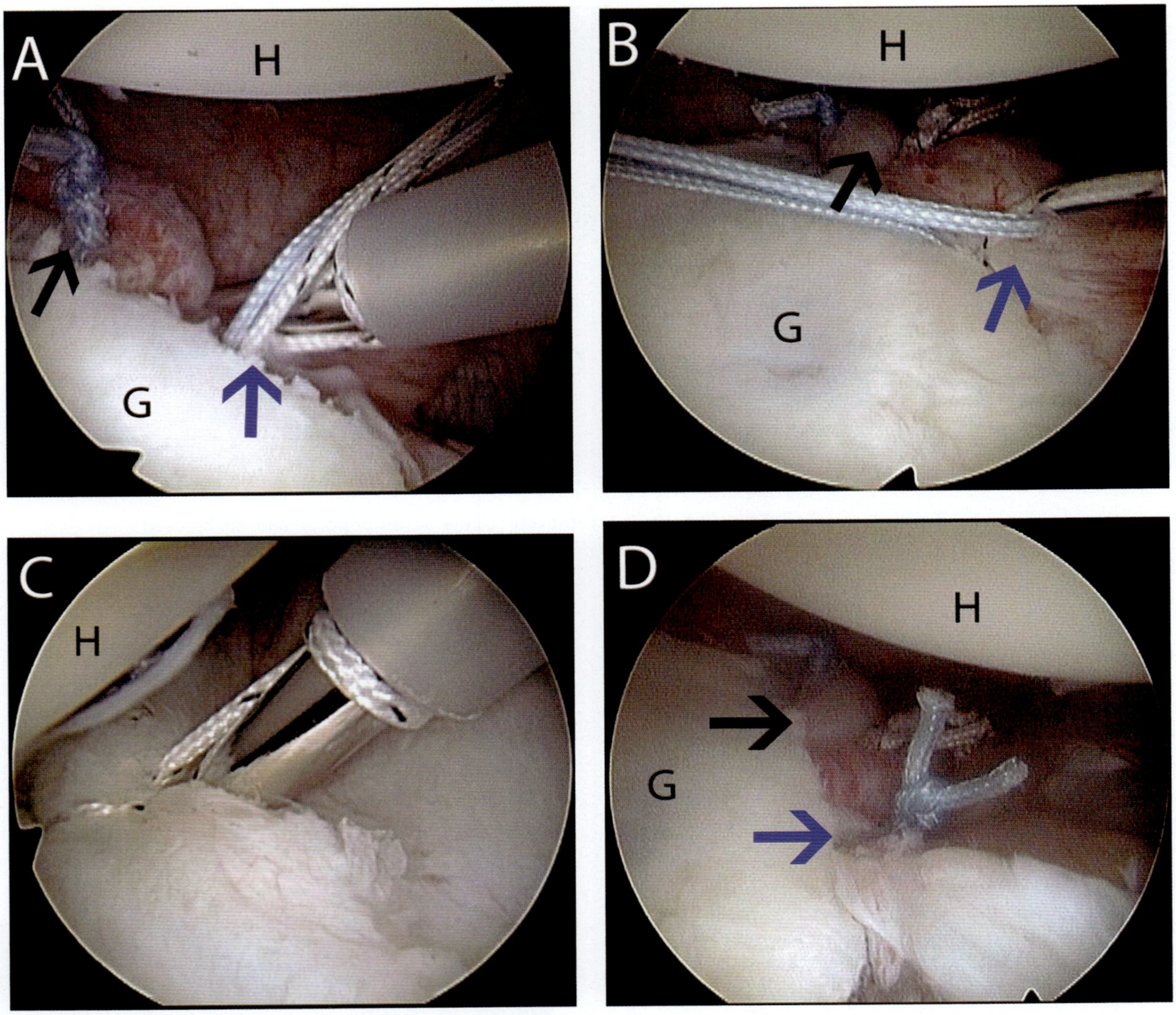

Figure 12.15 Left shoulder, anterosuperolateral viewing portal, demonstrates the "tie as go" sequence for Bankart repair. **A:** Two anteroinferior anchors have been placed via a 5 o'clock portal (see Fig. 12.20). Sutures from the 1st anchor are passed and tied as static knots using a Surgeon's Sixth Finger Knot Pusher (Arthrex, Inc., Naples, FL). The *black arrow* points to a knot that has been tied with a suture from the 1st anchor. The *blue arrow* points to sutures from the 2nd anchor that have not yet been passed. **B:** After the sutures from the 1st anchor have been tied (*black arrow*), the sutures from the 2nd anchor (*blue arrow*) are passed. **C:** Sutures from the 2nd anchor are tied. **D:** Appearance after sutures from the 1st (*black arrow*) and 2nd (*blue arrow*) anchor have been tied. Note: In this case, a 3rd anchor will be placed as well. G, glenoid; H, humerus.

are tied. The third anchor is inserted and sutures passed, and the second anchor sutures are tied. The process is continued as necessary, "keeping ahead" by one anchor so that there are no more than two anchors in the joint at once that have untied sutures, and suture passage is never limited by tying of an adjacent suture (Fig. 12.16). In contrast, "tying as you go" can bind the capsule so tightly to the glenoid rim that passing the sutures through the tightly bound capsule is very difficult.

At the completion of the repair, the final construct is evaluated for recreation of the anterior labrum bumper, restoration of the tension of the inferior glenohumeral ligament and axillary recess, and centering of the humeral head over the glenoid (Fig. 12.17).

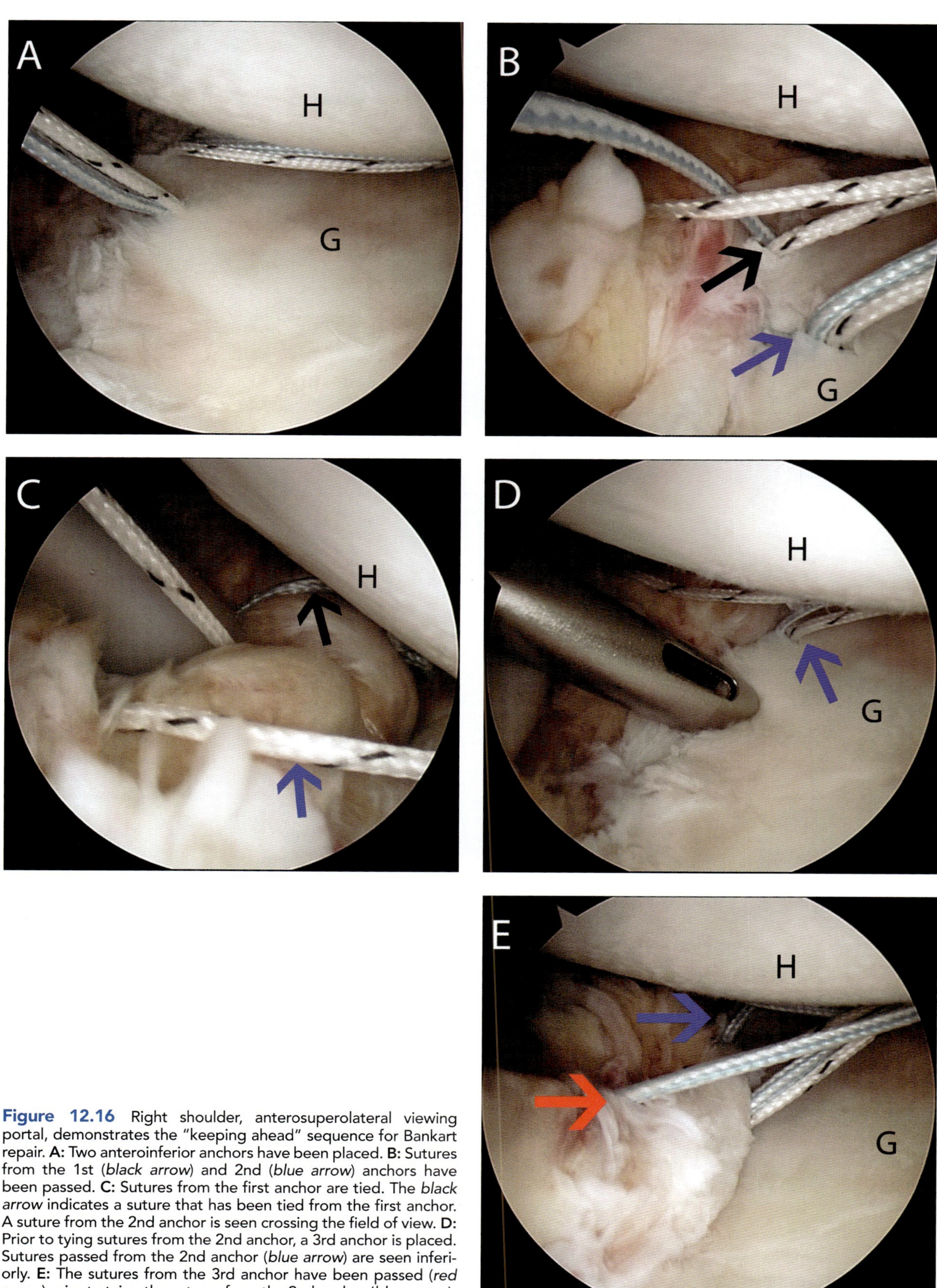

Figure 12.16 Right shoulder, anterosuperolateral viewing portal, demonstrates the "keeping ahead" sequence for Bankart repair. **A:** Two anteroinferior anchors have been placed. **B:** Sutures from the 1st (*black arrow*) and 2nd (*blue arrow*) anchors have been passed. **C:** Sutures from the first anchor are tied. The *black arrow* indicates a suture that has been tied from the first anchor. A suture from the 2nd anchor is seen crossing the field of view. **D:** Prior to tying sutures from the 2nd anchor, a 3rd anchor is placed. Sutures passed from the 2nd anchor (*blue arrow*) are seen inferiorly. **E:** The sutures from the 3rd anchor have been passed (*red arrow*) prior to tying the sutures from the 2nd anchor (*blue arrow*). G, glenoid; H, humerus.

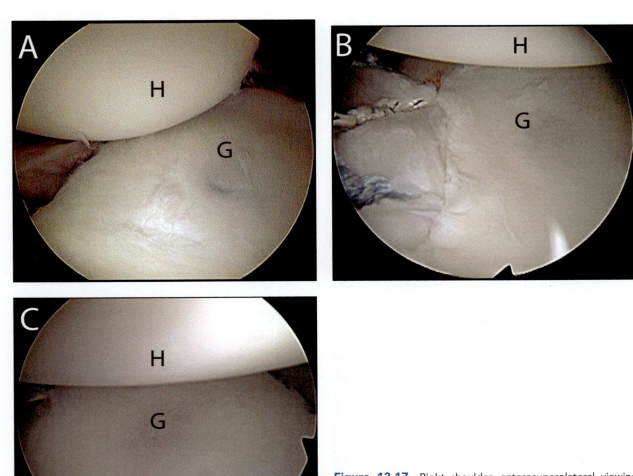

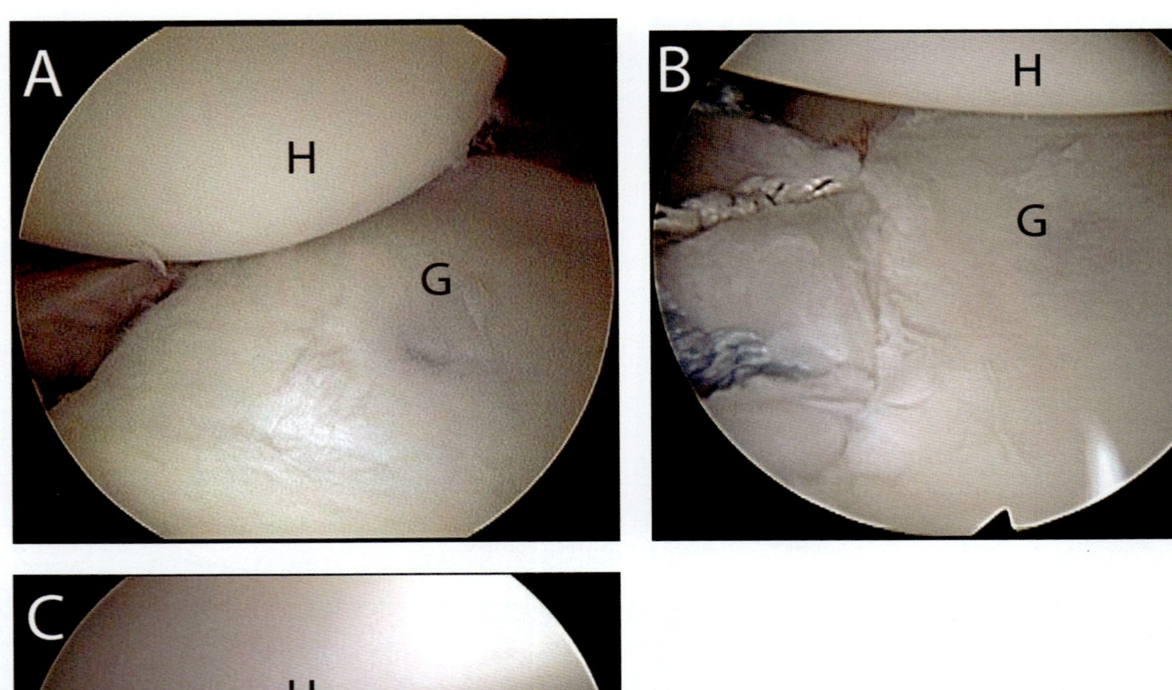

Figure 12.17 Right shoulder, anterosuperolateral viewing portal demonstrating completed Bankart repair. **A:** Initial view prior to repair demonstrates anterior subluxation of the humeral head. **B:** The anterior labrum has been repaired to the glenoid with multiple anchors. **C:** A well-performed repair is confirmed when the humeral head is centered over the glenoid bare spot. G, glenoid; H, humerus.

BANKART REPAIR UTILIZING THE 5 O'CLOCK PORTAL

In some patients, the angle of approach for anchor insertion through the standard anterior portal is too oblique to the inferior aspect of the anterior glenoid. In this scenario, suture anchor insertion will either be so oblique that the anchor slips off the rim of the glenoid, or to improve the angle, anchor insertion is forced too superior or medial on the glenoid. In such cases, anchor insertion through the 5 o'clock portal will provide the correct angle of approach.

Standard anterior, posterior, and anterosuperolateral portals are created and the labrum is mobilized. If the angle of approach for anchor insertion is assessed and confirmed to be inadequate (Fig. 12.18), a 5 o'clock portal is then established as described above. The glenohumeral joint is viewed through the posterior portal and a spinal needle is used to determine the correct angle of approach. It penetrates the subscapularis tendon 1.5 to 2.0 cm inferior to the upper subscapularis border. Then, the spear guide is "walked" alongside the spinal needle for transtendon insertion (Fig. 12.19).

The glenohumeral joint is then viewed through the anterosuperolateral portal and the angle of approach is again assessed. We often insert two or three anchors through the 5 o'clock portal to maximize its utility. The lowest anchor is inserted first. However, without removing the spear guide from the body, the tip is lifted away from the glenoid exposing the sutures. A suture retriever is inserted through the posterior portal and retrieves the sutures out the posterior portal. The spear guide is then used again to

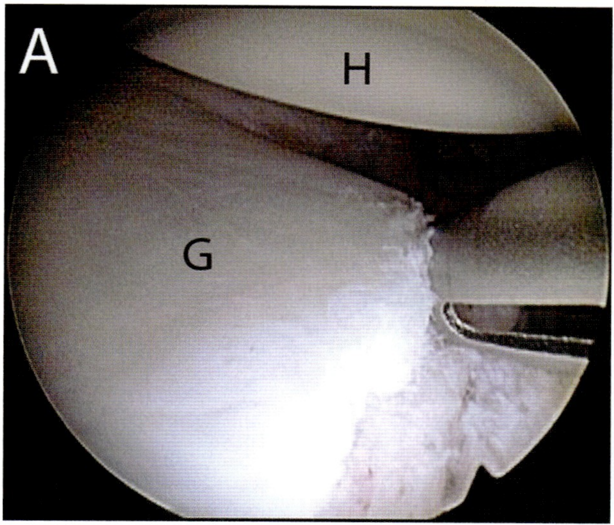

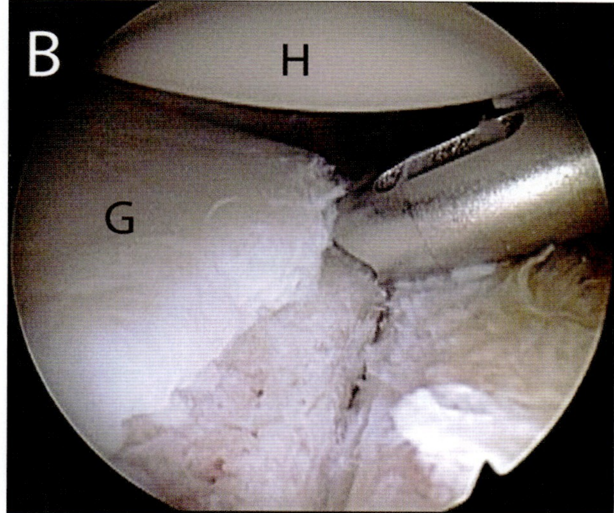

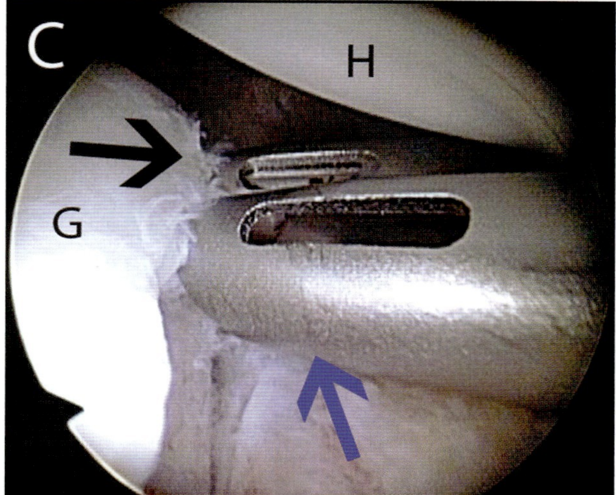

Figure 12.18 Left shoulder, anterosuperolateral viewing portal. **A:** The angle of approach for anchor placement is assessed and in this case the angle achieved through the anterior portal is too steep to place an anteroinferior anchor. **B:** The angle of approach is improved with a 5 o'clock portal. **C:** View with two spear guides in place, comparing the angle of approach to the anteroinferior glenoid achieved with the anterior portal (*blue arrow*) and the 5 o'clock portal (*black arrow*). G, glenoid; H, humerus.

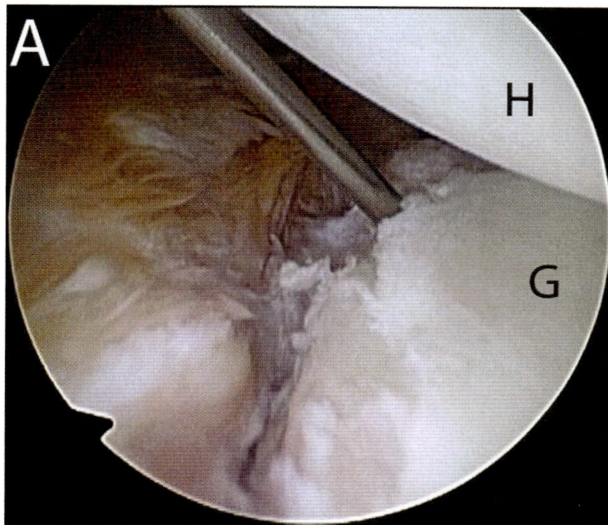

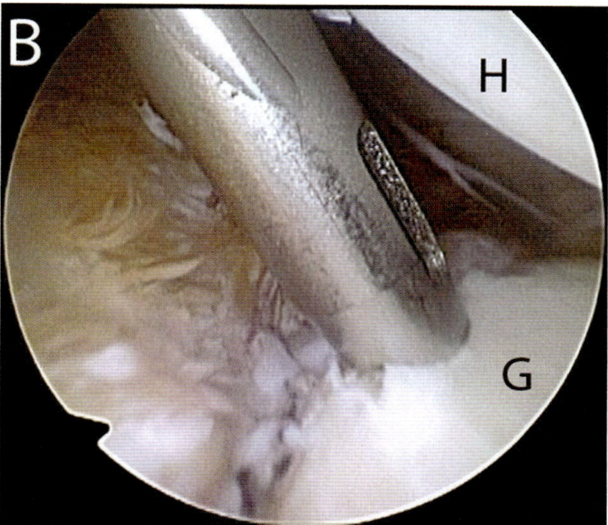

Figure 12.19 Right shoulder, anterosuperolateral viewing portal demonstrating use of the 5 o'clock portal for anchor placement in Bankart repair. **A:** A spinal needle confirms a proper angle of approach to the anteroinferior glenoid with the use of a 5 o'clock portal. **B:** A spear guide is inserted percutaneously alongside the spinal needle to place an anteroinferior anchor. G, glenoid; H, humerus.

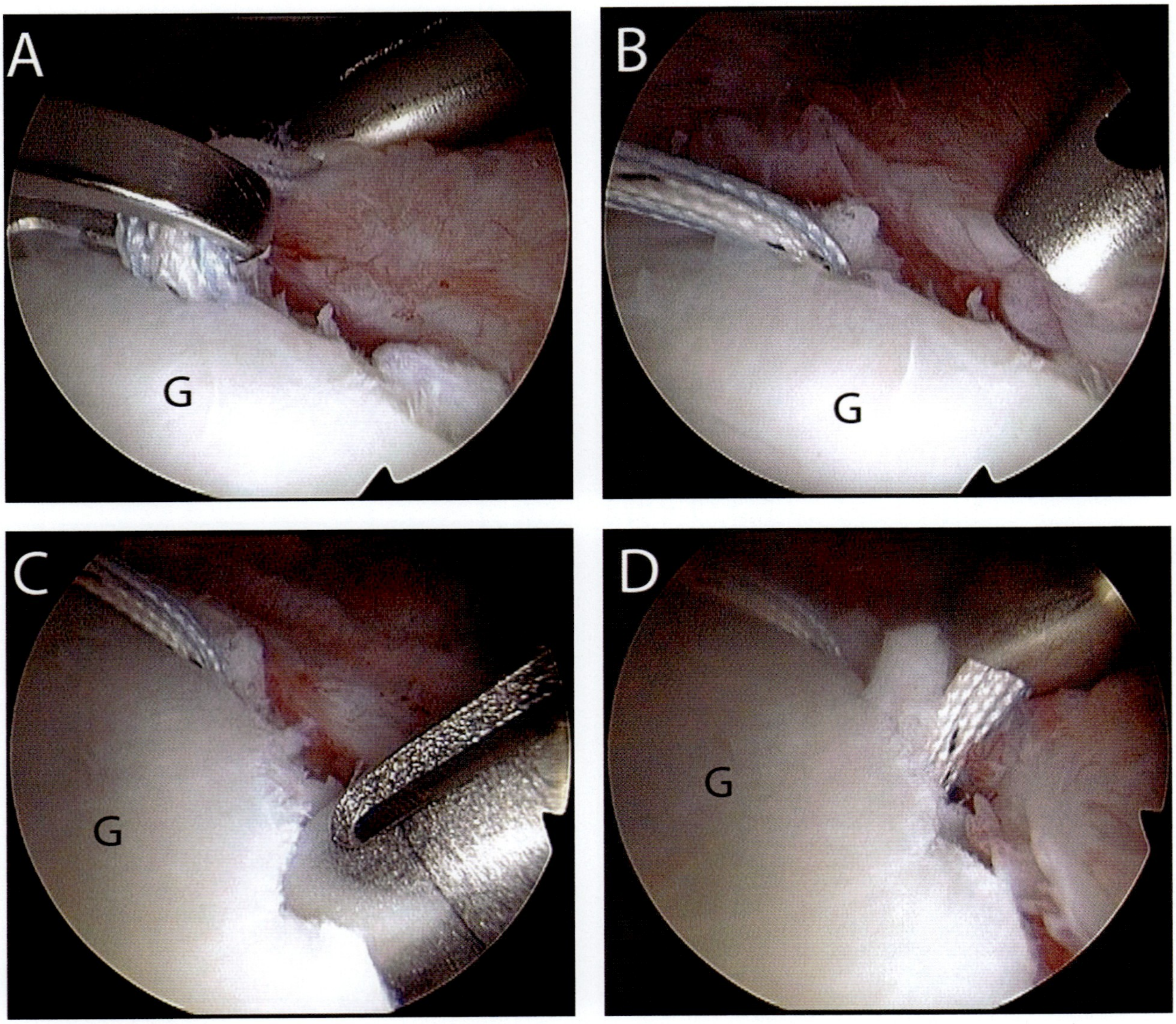

Figure 12.20 Left shoulder, anterosuperolateral viewing portal demonstrating technique for placing multiple anchors through a 5 o'clock portal. This technique is useful for the 5 o'clock portal because a transtendon cannula is not established. **A:** After placing the most inferior anchor through a 5 o'clock portal, the spear guide is withdrawn slightly to expose the sutures from the suture anchor for retrieval out the posterior portal. **B:** Sutures are seen exiting at posterior portal and the spear guide has not been removed from the joint. **C:** The guide is seated for placement of a second suture anchor. **D:** When all anchors are placed, the spear guide is removed from the joint. If desired, a third anchor could be placed using the same technique. G, glenoid.

direct the approach for the second anchor (Fig. 12.20). The process may be repeated a third time if necessary. The spear is removed once all anchors have been inserted.

Even in situations with larger patients and awkward angles of approach, anchors may be inserted through the 5 o'clock portal, at the level of the bare spot and below, maximizing fixation at the critical anterior inferior glenoid.

Once the anchors have been inserted, the sutures are passed from inferior to superior and progressively tied using the techniques as described above. The final construct is then evaluated for recreation of the anterior labrum bumper, restoration of the tension of the inferior glenohumeral ligament and axillary recess, and centering of the humeral head over the glenoid bare spot.

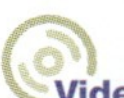

BANKART REPAIR UTILIZING THE POSTEROLATERAL PORTAL

In patients whose Bankart lesion extends posteriorly across the 6 o'clock position, particularly to and beyond the 7 o'clock position, formal repair of the posterior inferior labrum is required. In this situation, the posterior inferior labrum must be prepared prior to Bankart repair.

Standard anterior, posterior, and anterosuperolateral portals are created. The Bankart lesion is mobilized and its extension across the 6 o'clock position is evaluated (Fig. 12.21). Often, the posterior inferior labrum may be mobilized with a 30° elevator through the anterior portal (while viewing through the anterosuperolateral portal) or through the anterosuperolateral portal (while viewing through the anterior portal) (Fig. 12.22).

The posterolateral portal is then established. This portal is created to provide a 45° angle of approach to the posterior inferior glenoid and is used for anchor insertion. A spinal needle is used to determine the proper angle of approach. A switching stick is used and parallels the spinal needle. In most cases, if the posterior inferior labrum and bone have been adequately prepared through the anterior or anterosuperolateral portals, a standard cannula is not required and the BioComposite SutureTak Spear may be inserted directly over the switching stick. However, if the preparation of the posterior inferior labrum is inadequate, an 8.25 mm × 9 cm cannula may be established to allow preparation through this angle of approach. Care is taken to ensure that preparation and mobilization of the inferior labrum (particularly at the 6 o'clock position) is complete.

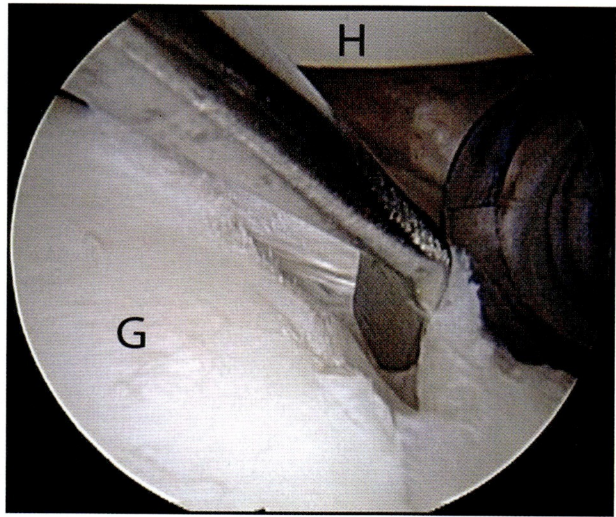

Figure 12.22 Right shoulder, anterosuperolateral viewing portal. A 30° arthroscopic elevator introduced from an anterior working portal is used to mobilize the posterior labrum of a Bankart tear with posterior extension. G, glenoid; H, humerus.

Once the entire labral tear is prepared, a "J-shaped" tear is observed (Fig. 12.23). Progression of the labral repair proceeds from posterior to anterior. A 3.0-mm BioComposite SutureTak anchor is inserted through the low posterolateral

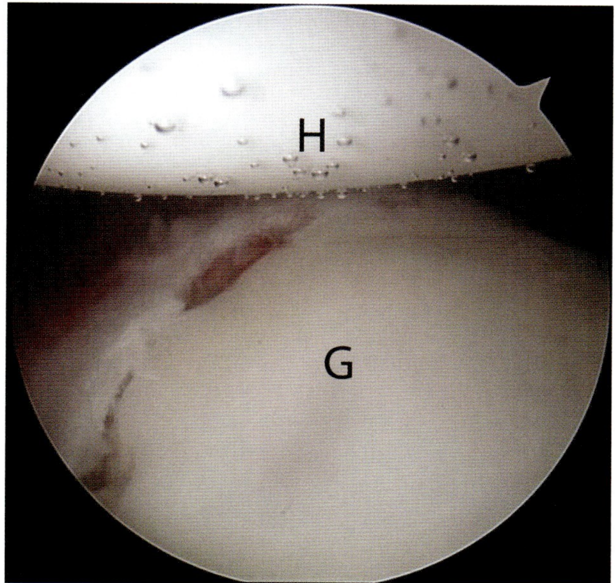

Figure 12.21 Right shoulder, anterosuperolateral portal demonstrating Bankart lesion with posterior extension past the 6 o'clock position.

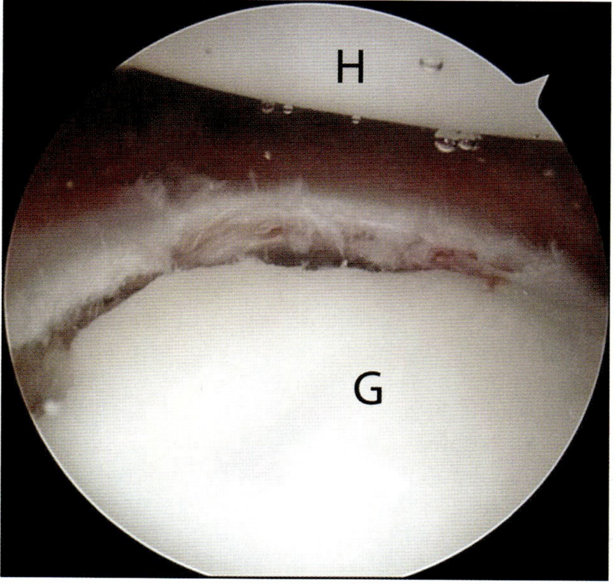

Figure 12.23 Right shoulder, anterosuperolateral viewing portal, demonstrates a Bankart tear with posterior extension that has been mobilized for repair. G, glenoid; H, humerus.

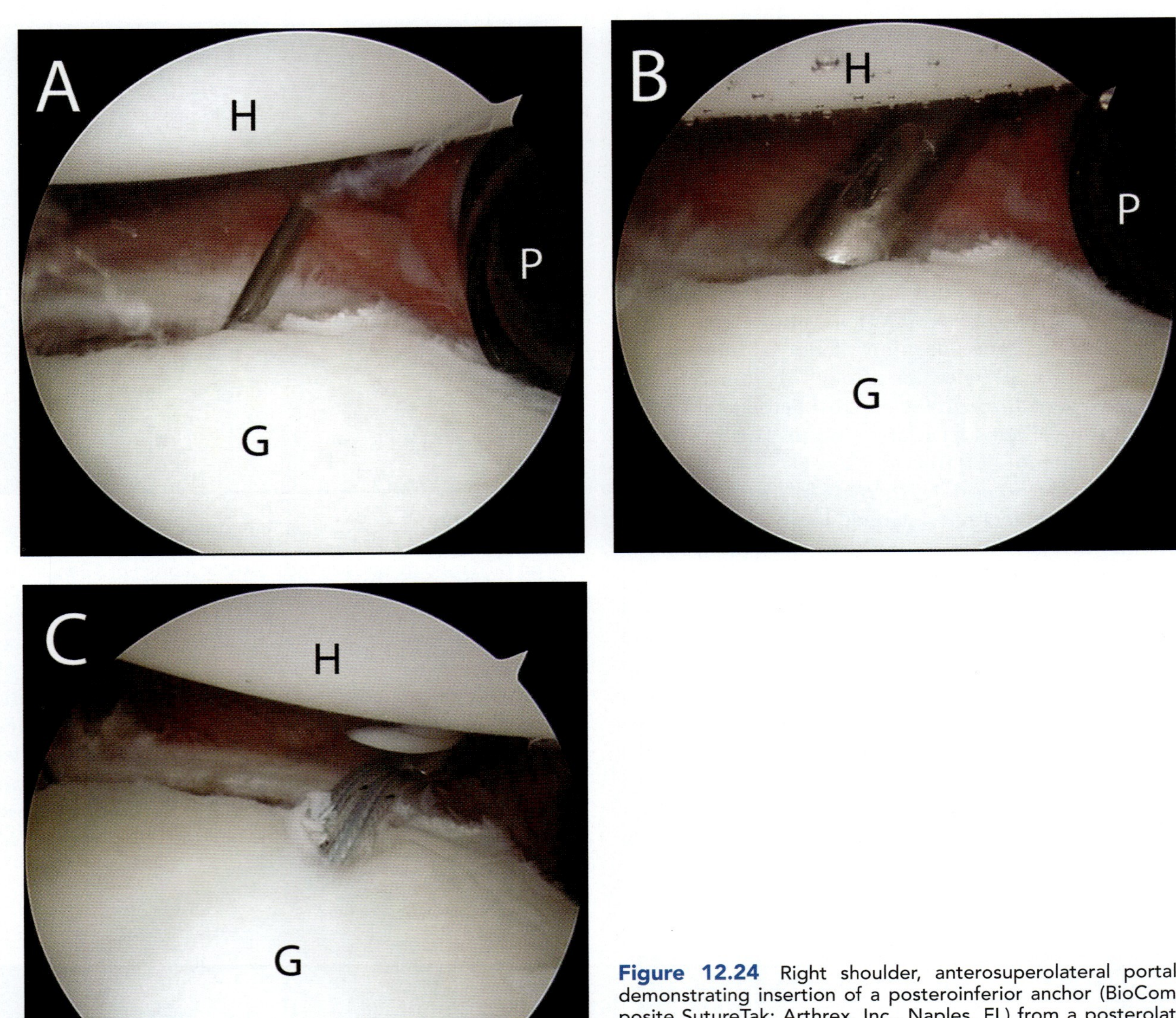

Figure 12.24 Right shoulder, anterosuperolateral portal, demonstrating insertion of a posteroinferior anchor (BioComposite SutureTak; Arthrex, Inc., Naples, FL) from a posterolateral portal. **A:** A spinal needle is used as a guide to obtain an adequate angle of approach. **B:** A spear guide is inserted. **C:** View after anchor insertion at the 6:30 position. G, glenoid; H, humerus; P, posterior portal.

portal at the posterior inferior aspect of the glenoid (Fig. 12.24). Usually, one anchor is required for fixation of the posterior portion of a J-shaped tear. Sutures are then passed. Depending on the angle of approach, the 25° Tight Curve SutureLasso may be inserted through the posterior or the posterolateral portal. If the posterolateral portal is utilized for suture passage, the sutures should be retrieved through the posterior portal for suture shuttling. The SutureLasso is used to penetrate the labrum, and the suture is shuttled utilizing the posterior portal. The second suture is passed in a similar fashion. The posterior sutures are not tied until after the anterior Bankart repair has been completed. Tying the posterior sutures first can prematurely compromise the already tight anteroinferior working space.

Once the posterior inferior sutures have been passed, the repair proceeds toward the anterior Bankart lesion. The first anterior inferior anchor is inserted through the anterior cannula. As described above, the sutures are passed to shift the labrum superiorly. It is important to ensure that the sutures from the anterior inferior anchor do not crisscross the sutures from the posterior inferior anchor, but rather shift the entire axillary recess superior on the glenoid. Once the sutures from the anterior inferior anchor have been passed (Fig. 12.25), they are tied to secure the anteroinferior labrum.

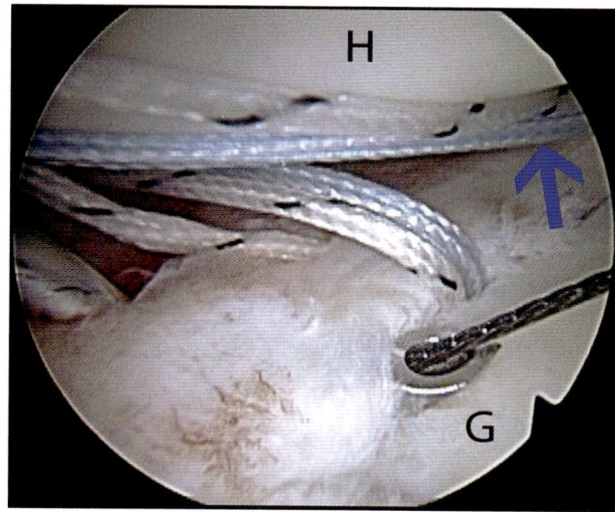

Figure 12.25 Right shoulder, anterosuperolateral viewing portal. After posterior anchor placement and suture passage, anterior anchors are placed and shuttled with a SutureLasso (Arthrex, Inc., Naples, FL) through the anteroinferior labrum. Note: The posterior sutures (*blue arrow*) have not yet been tied and cross the field of view. G, glenoid; H, humerus.

The Bankart repair may now proceed as described above with insertion of the second anchor and third anchor and suture passage. After the knots have been tied for the anterior Bankart repair, the posterior knots are tied. The final repair is again assessed and the J-shaped repair evaluated (Fig. 12.26).

BANKART REPAIR KNOTLESS TECHNIQUE

Arthroscopic Bankart repair may also be performed using a knotless technique. In most cases, we prefer to tie knots when repairing a Bankart lesion. Our main indication for a completely knotless technique is an older, less active individual, with a nondisplaced Bankart lesion. Knotless anchors may also be mixed with knotted anchors in a hybrid construct. For nondisplaced Bankart lesions, we sometimes use knotted anchors as the two lower anchors, then use a knotless anchor as our superior anchor to facilitate the speed of the surgery. This is our most common indication for a knotless anchor in an instability repair.

All of our usual principles are utilized for repair including mobilization of the labrum, preparation of the bone bed, and repair and retensioning of the anterior inferior labrum, inferior glenohumeral ligament and axillary recess. When performing a knotless technique, sutures (No. 2 FiberWire; Arthrex, Inc., Naples, FL) are passed first, prior to insertion of the anchor (3.5-mm BioComposite PushLock; Arthrex, Inc., Naples, FL).

If multiple knotless anchors are to be placed, sutures may be passed sequentially with anchor insertion or all at once, prior to insertion of any of the anchors. We generally pass sutures as simple stitches. However, a cinching stitch that loops and captures the labrum may also be utilized. To pass a cinching stitch, a SutureLasso is used to pass a Nitinol loop through the labrum, which is retrieved through the posterior portal. A No. 2 FiberWire suture is

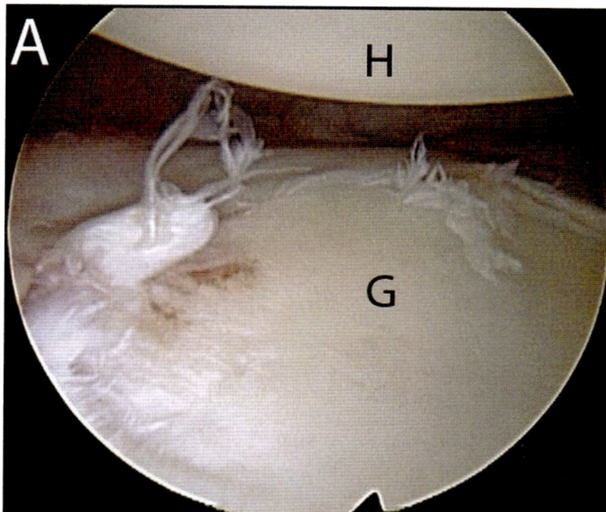

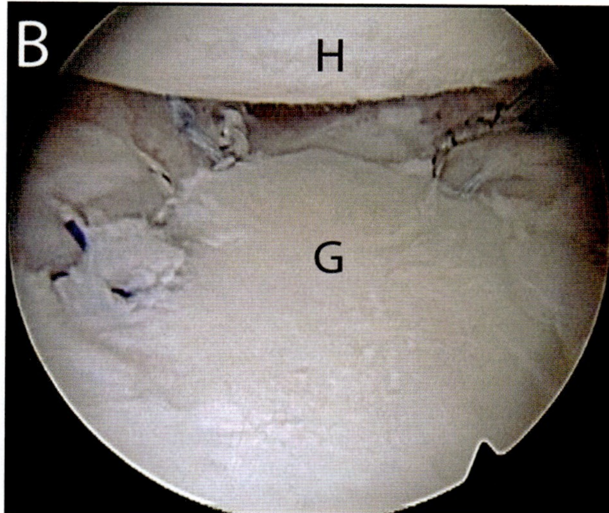

Figure 12.26 **A:** Right shoulder, anterosuperolateral viewing portal, demonstrating a Bankart lesion with posterior extension. **B:** Final repair of the same lesion. Note: The posterior extension has been repaired with a posteroinferior anchor (**right**) and the humeral head is well centered over the glenoid. G, glenoid; H, humerus.

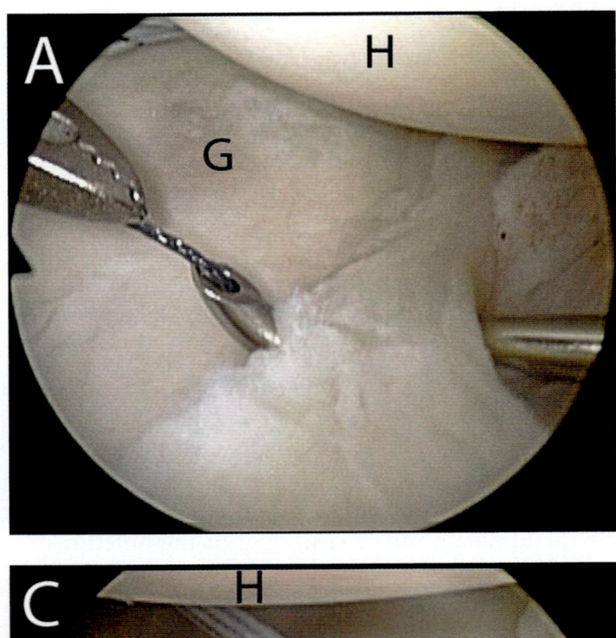

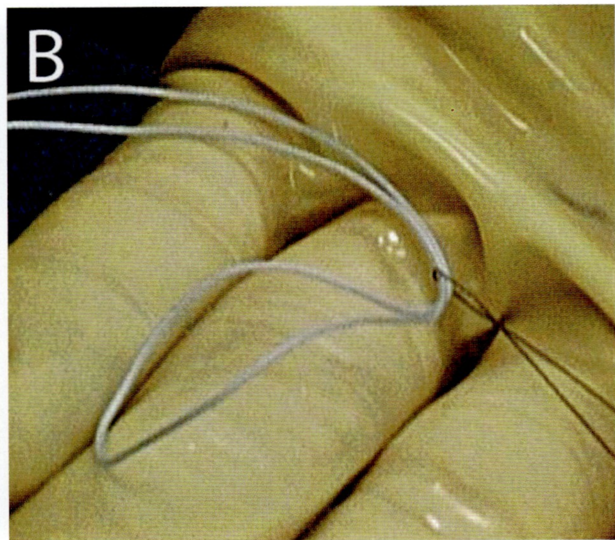

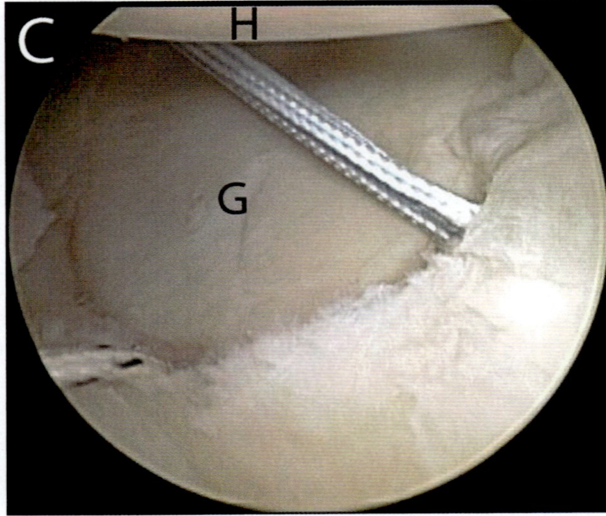

Figure 12.27 Passing a cinch loop for a knotless Bankart repair. **A:** Left shoulder, anterosuperolateral viewing portal. A Nitinol loop is passed through the labrum and retrieved out a posterior portal. **B:** Extracorporeally, a free No. 2 FiberWire suture (Arthrex, Inc., Naples, FL) is folded in half on itself and the looped end is passed through the Nitinol loop. **C:** Retrieving the Nitinol wire shuttles looped suture through the labrum. G, glenoid; H, humerus.

folded on itself and the looped end is threaded through the Nitinol loop and then shuttled through the labrum (Fig. 12.27). The free suture ends are then retrieved out the anterior portal and passed through the previously shuttled suture loop. Pulling the free ends of the sutures creates a cinch loop that is delivered to the labrum by alternating tension on the free suture ends (Fig. 12.28). Alternatively, the looped end of a FiberLink suture (Arthrex, Inc., Naples, FL) may be used create a cinch loop. The only difference is that this suture has a prelooped end.

Once the sutures have been passed, anchor insertion proceeds to secure the labrum from inferior to superior. It is important to again plan the positioning of the anchors to shift the labrum/capsule from inferior to superior. When placing knotless anchors, a number of technical factors should be considered. Since the labrum is pulled to the bone socket, rather than being pushed toward the anchor (as in knot tying), the anchor must be placed slightly more on the face of the glenoid to recreate a similar bumper effect. In addition, when placing anchors low on the glenoid face, if the trocar has been used to push the humeral head posteriorly to gain a favorable angle of approach during drilling, the slotted guide (Shoehorn Cannula; Arthrex, Inc., Naples, FL) must be similarly used when the anchor is inserted. Attempting to translate the humeral head using the PushLock handle may bend the inserter, dislodge the implant from the inserter, or lead to off-axis insertion of the anchor.

The PushLock Spear is inserted through the anterior portal and a bone socket is drilled (Fig. 12.29). Care is

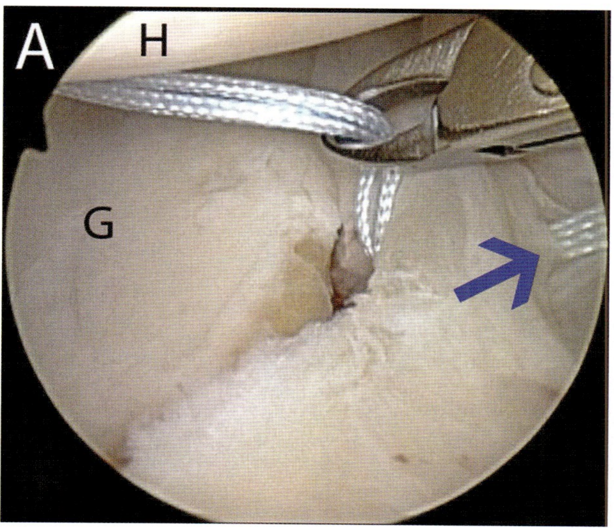

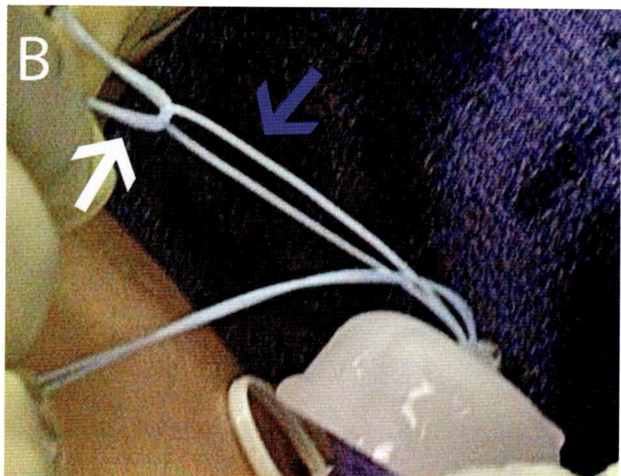

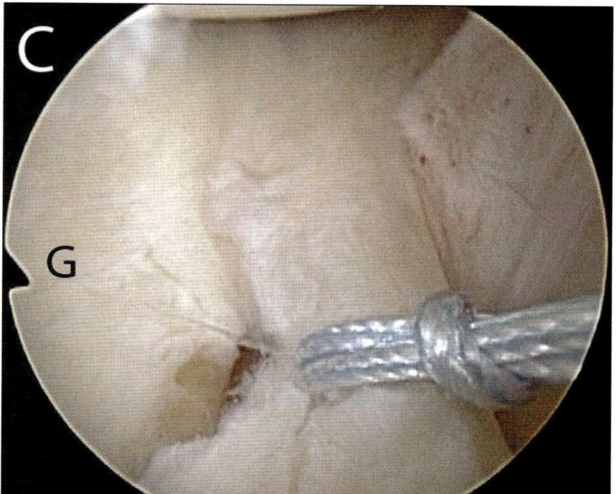

Figure 12.28 Completion of a cinch loop for a knotless Bankart repair. **A:** Left shoulder, anterosuperolateral viewing portal. After a looped No. 2 FiberWire (Arthrex, Inc., Naples, FL) has been passed through the labrum (*blue arrow*), the free ends of the suture are retrieved. **B:** Extracorporeally, the free ends of the No. 2 FiberWire suture (*white arrow*) are passed through the looped end (*blue arrow*) to create a cinch loop. **C:** Arthroscopic view demonstrates the completed cinch loop encircling the labrum. G, glenoid; H, humerus.

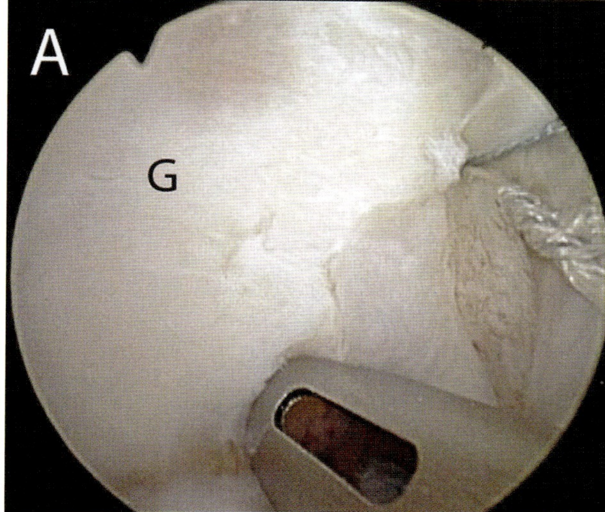

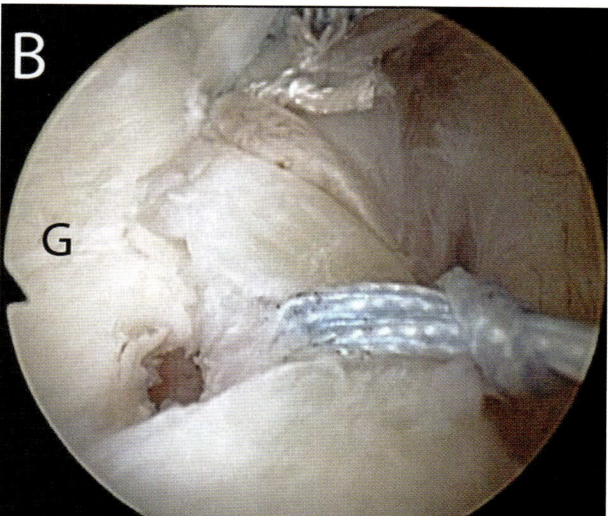

Figure 12.29 Left shoulder, anterosuperolateral viewing portal. **A:** A spear guide is inserted through an anterior working portal to create a bone socket for a PushLock anchor (Arthrex, Inc., Naples, FL). **B:** View of the bone socket and previously placed cinch loop (**right**). G, glenoid.

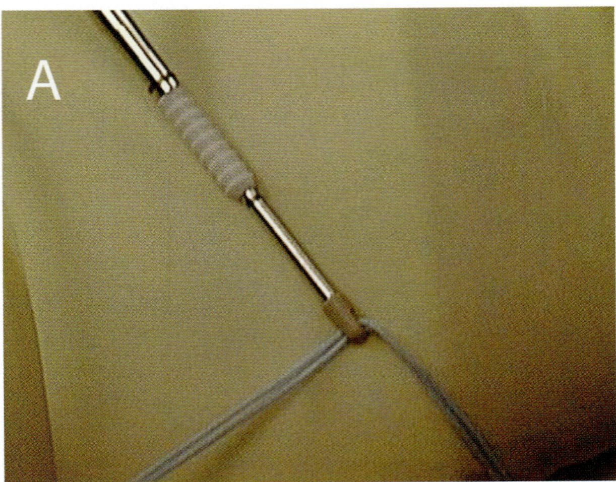

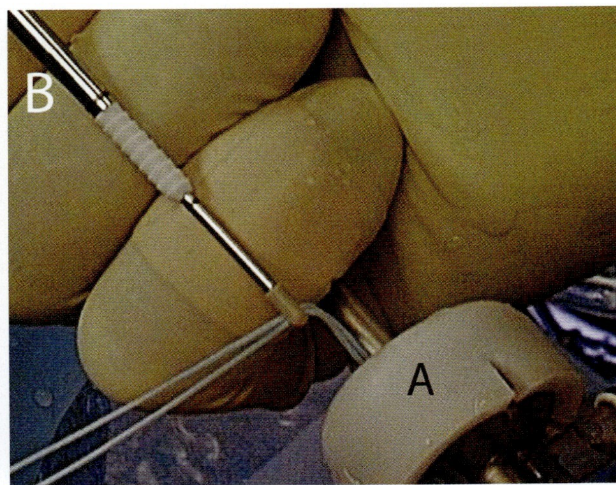

Figure 12.30 **A:** Sutures previously passed through the labrum are threaded through the eyelet of a PushLock anchor (Arthrex, Inc., Naples, FL), and then **(B)** the anchor is slid down the sutures to be seated intra-articularly in a bone socket. A, anterior portal.

taken to protect the sutures while drilling. The sutures are retrieved through the anterior portal (if they are not already in this portal) and fed through the distal eyelet of the PushLock anchor (Fig. 12.30A). The anchor is inserted through the anterior cannula and slid down the sutures (Fig. 12.30B). Prior to anchor insertion, the anchor and eyelet are oriented to remove any twists within the suture. The sutures are then tensioned so that when the PushLock eyelet is inserted into the base of the bone socket this will lead to reduction of the labrum, tensioning of the ligaments, and recreation of the anterior bumper. With the eyelet at the bottom of the bone socket, and the sutures tensioned, the PushLock anchor is impacted into place securing the labrum (Fig. 12.31).

If additional knotless anchors are planned, the same steps can be repeated. The final construct is evaluated for recreation of the anterior labrum bumper, restoration of the tension of the inferior glenohumeral ligament and axillary recess, and centering of the humeral head over the glenoid (Fig. 12.32).

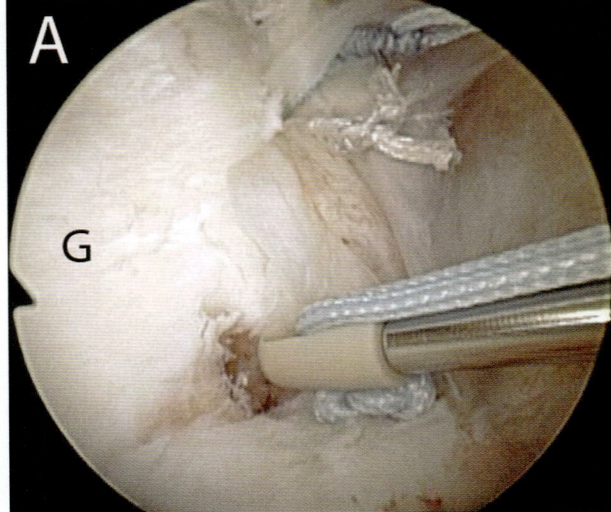

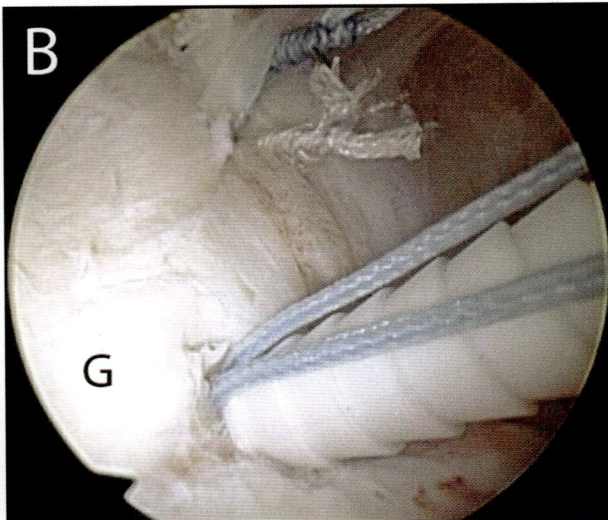

Figure 12.31 Left shoulder, anterosuperolateral viewing portal, demonstrates placement of a PushLock anchor (Arthrex, Inc., Naples, FL) for a knotless component to a labral repair. **A:** The eyelet of the anchor is seated in a previously prepared bone socket. **B:** After the sutures are tensioned, the anchor is impacted into the bone socket.

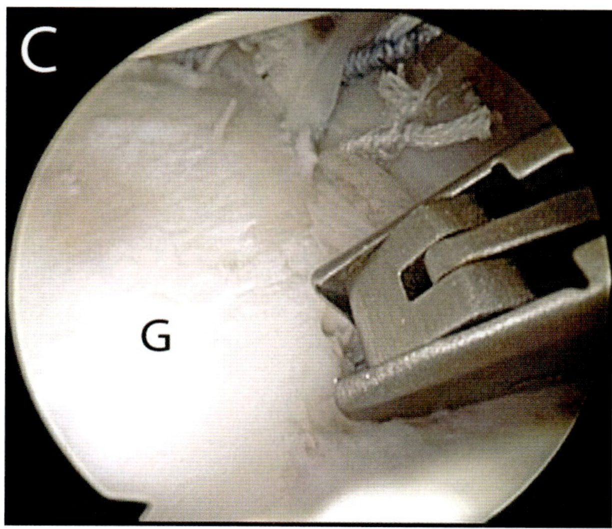

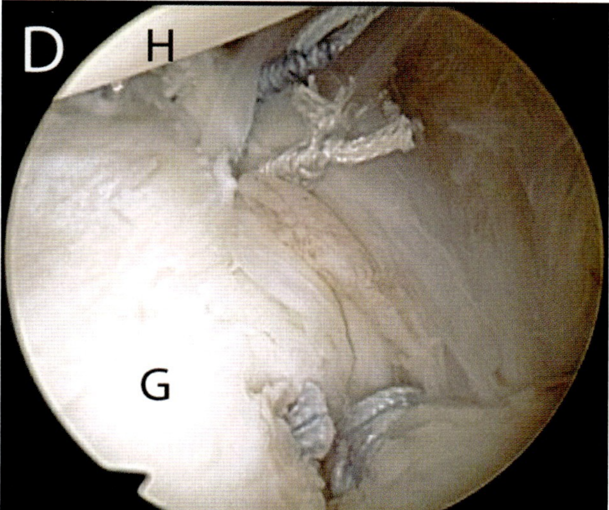

Figure 12.31 *(Continued)* **C:** Sutures are cut flush with the anchor. **D:** The final knotless construct is seen in the lower portion of the figure. G, glenoid; H, humerus.

BONY BANKART REPAIR (SUTURE ANCHOR BASED)

Bony Bankart lesions are extremely common. It is estimated that approximately 90% of patients with traumatic anterior instability have some degree of glenoid bone loss and in approximately 50% of these cases a bony Bankart lesion is present (as opposed to bony erosion) (1). Fortunately, the majority of cases involve a bony Bankart lesion <25% of the inferior diameter of the glenoid and a suture anchor based technique may still be utilized incorporating the bony fragment within the repair.

In most cases, the residual bony Bankart fragment is smaller than the amount of glenoid bone loss. This is pertinent in patients with recurrent anterior instability where subsequent instability episodes likely further erode the anterior inferior glenoid bone stock. Even in patients where the bone fragment is smaller than the glenoid defect, incorporating the bony fragment within the repair improves the surgical outcome and postoperative

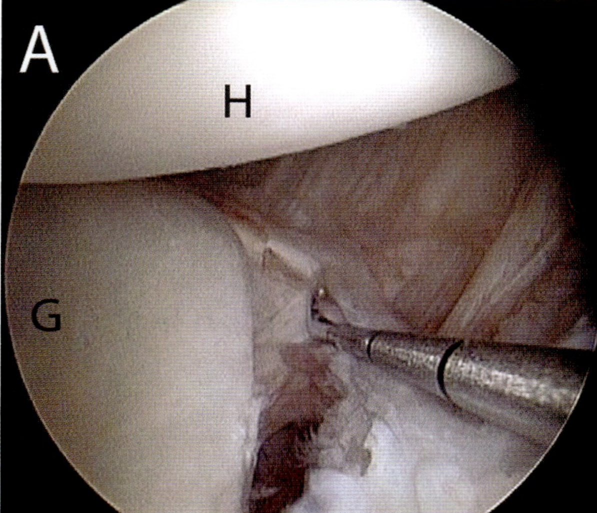

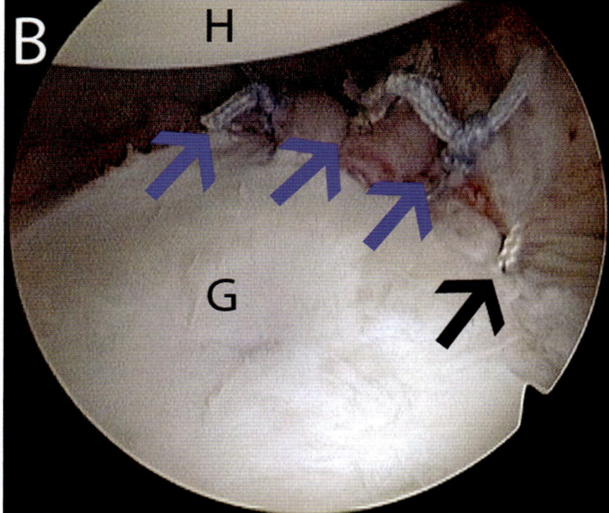

Figure 12.32 **A:** Left shoulder, anterosuperolateral viewing portal, demonstrates a minimally displaced Bankart lesion. Note: The humeral head is subluxed anteriorly relative to the glenoid. **B:** A hybrid repair was performed using two knotted anchors inferiorly (*blue arrows*) and a knotless anchor (*black arrow*) at the superior aspect of the lesion. The humeral head has been recentered over the glenoid. G, glenoid; H, humerus.

stability. This is particularly relevant in patients where the incorporation of the bony fragment can restore bone loss to <25%.

In patients with bony Bankart lesions, the standard anterior, posterior, and anterosuperolateral portals are established. A standard diagnostic arthroscopy is performed, evaluating for concomitant lesions including SLAP lesions and Hill-Sachs lesions. It is not uncommon for patients with bony Bankart lesions to have significant Hill-Sachs lesions that may require treatment (e.g., remplissage procedure).

While viewing through the anterosuperolateral portal, the bony Bankart lesion is identified, and glenoid bone loss and its relationship to the Hill-Sachs lesion are documented (Fig. 12.33). If a remplissage procedure is required, preparation of the Hill-Sachs lesion and anchor insertion into the Hill-Sachs are performed prior to bony Bankart repair. However, these sutures are not tied until the after the Bankart repair is completed as tying these sutures limits the working space. Furthermore, the force used in placing the remplissage anchors into the Hill-Sachs lesion after the Bankart repair has been completed can disrupt the Bankart repair. So, one can see that the order of steps is critically important.

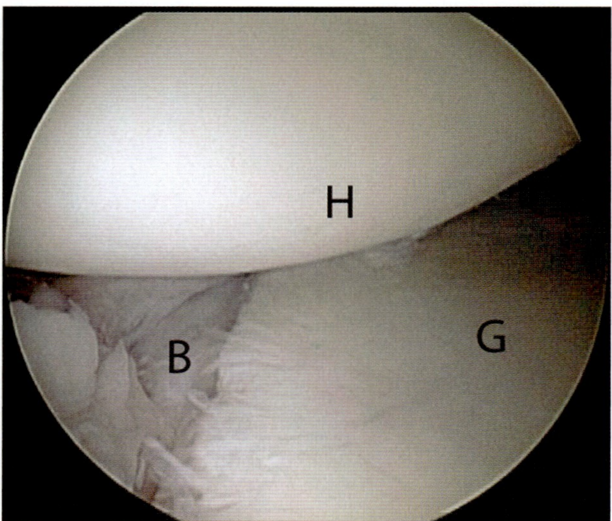

Figure 12.33 Right shoulder, anterosuperolateral viewing portal, demonstrates a small bony Bankart lesion amenable to suture-based fixation. B, bony Bankart lesion; G, glenoid; H, humerus.

The labrum and bony Bankart lesion are next mobilized. Using an arthroscopic elevator, the bony Bankart lesion is carefully mobilized off the anterior glenoid neck (Fig. 12.34A). When encountered, the bony Bankart lesion is usually slightly more difficult to mobilize due to fibrous/bony union to the glenoid neck. In rare cases, an osteotome may be required to mobilize a medially healed bony Bankart lesion if bone union is significant. To facilitate eventual repair, it is important when mobilizing the bony Bankart lesion to maintain the continuity of the bony Bankart lesion to the labrum. Just as in Bankart/ALPSA lesions, the bony Bankart fragment and labrum must be mobilized until the subscapularis muscle belly is observed and the labrum and bone naturally float up to the level of the glenoid face (Fig. 12.34B).

The bony Bankart fragment is then evaluated for its size and quality. If the fragment is small and comminuted into several fragments, the arthroscopist may choose to excise the fragment. However, in the vast majority of cases,

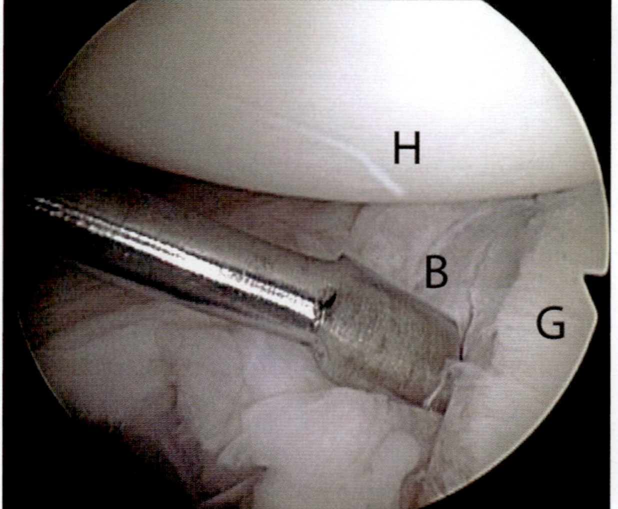

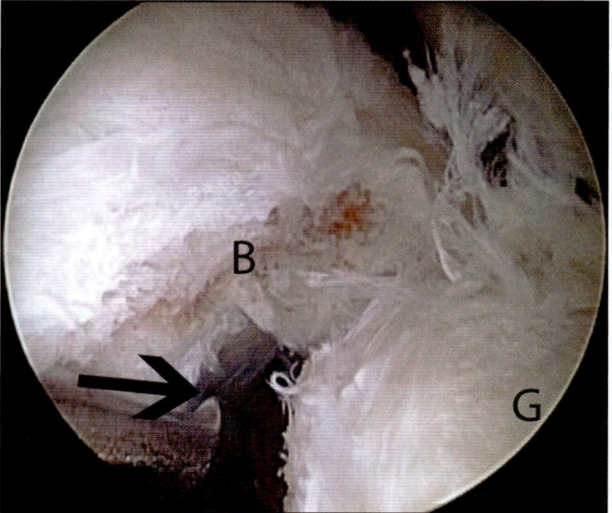

Figure 12.34 **A:** Right shoulder, anterosuperolateral viewing portal, demonstrates use of an arthroscopic elevator to mobilize a bony Bankart fragment. **B:** Mobilization is complete when the subscapularis muscle is visible (*black arrow*) between the bony fragment and the glenoid. B, bony Bankart fragment; G, glenoid; H, humerus.

incorporating the fragment is not difficult and improves outcome. The bony Bankart fragment is lightly debrided to exposed bone and the apposing glenoid neck similarly prepared. In some cases, there may be a periosteal sleeve extending from the medial aspect of the bony Bankart fragment. This can obscure the medial margin of the bone fragment and make suture passage around the fragment difficult. In this situation, a narrow punch or elevator is introduced through the anterior portal to release the fragment from the periosteal sleeve facilitating suture passage and improving fragment mobility as well.

We often use four anchors for arthroscopic bony Bankart repair. The most inferior and superior anchors are used to repair the labrum and stabilize the fragment, while the middle two anchors are used to capture the bony Bankart fragment. However, the exact number of anchors used will vary, depending on the size of the fragment. Additionally, while we always tie knots above and below the bony Bankart fragment, a cinch loop with knotless fixation as discussed below often facilitates encircling the bony Bankart.

When placing anchors for bony Bankart repair, the position of the anchor is altered compared to a standard Bankart repair. Because sutures will encircle the bony fragment, the anchors are placed at the bone–articular cartilage junction (as opposed to on the glenoid face) to anatomically reduce the fragment and avoid an overreduction. Therefore, in general, we place the superior and inferior anchors (used for labral repair) up onto the face of the glenoid, whereas the middle two anchors (used to capture the bony fragment) are placed at the bone–articular cartilage junction.

The most inferior anchor is placed first, at the 5 o'clock position, slightly onto the face of the glenoid (Fig. 12.35A). In many cases, a 5 o'clock portal will be required to place the lowest anchor. Sutures are passed distal to the fragment, capturing the labrum and capsule inferior to the bony Bankart fragment. Usually antegrade suture passage (Scorpion) or shuttling suture passage (SutureLasso) through an anterior or posterior portal will provide the correct angle of approach to the inferior labrum.

Sutures are passed but not tied since premature knot tying will bind the labrum to the glenoid and make subsequent suture passage extremely difficult (Fig. 12.35B). This is especially relevant in bony Bankart repairs since more excursion of the bone–capsule–labrum is required to encircle the bone fragment that for standard capsulolabral repair.

The second anchor is then inserted at the bone–articular cartilage junction (since it will be used for fragment fixation) using a similar technique. When passing sutures to secure the bony Bankart fragment, two techniques are commonly utilized: encircling sutures and transosseous sutures. Encircling sutures are passed as simple sutures that capture the bony Bankart fragment within the suture loop (Figs. 12.36 and 12.37). This suture configuration is the easiest to perform and is our first choice for suture passage. Transosseous sutures (Fig. 12.38) are more difficult to pass and are only performed if encircling the fragment is not possible due to its size. This is particularly useful in fragments that are large (in a medial-to-lateral direction) but thin. Sutures are usually passed as mattress sutures to compress the fragment against the glenoid neck.

To pass an encircling suture, a SutureLasso (right curved for a right shoulder) is used to capture the fragment similar to a labral repair. However, it is important when capturing the suture that the hook penetrates the capsule adjacent to the fragment and encircles the medial aspect of the fragment. If the fragment is mobile (and small), the hook may be brought to the edge of the glenoid face and the shuttle advanced (Fig. 12.39). If the fragment is large however, the

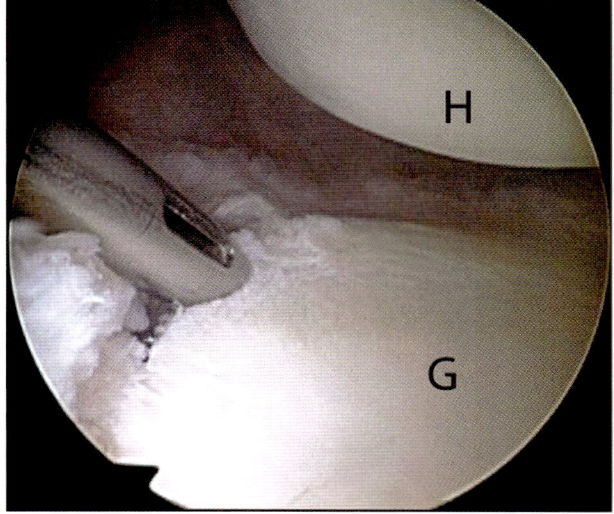

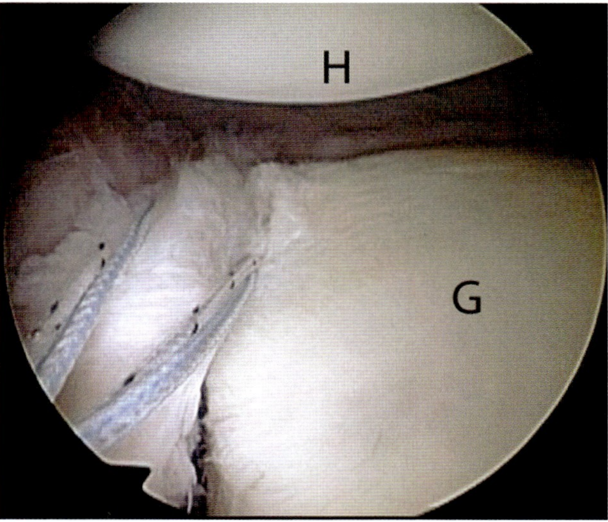

Figure 12.35 Right shoulder, anterosuperolateral viewing portal. **A:** Following mobilization of a bony Bankart fragment, an anchor is placed inferior to the fragment. **B:** Sutures from this anchor have been passed through the labrum inferior to the bony Bankart fragment, but knot tying is delayed until after the bony fragment sutures are passed. G, glenoid; H, humerus.

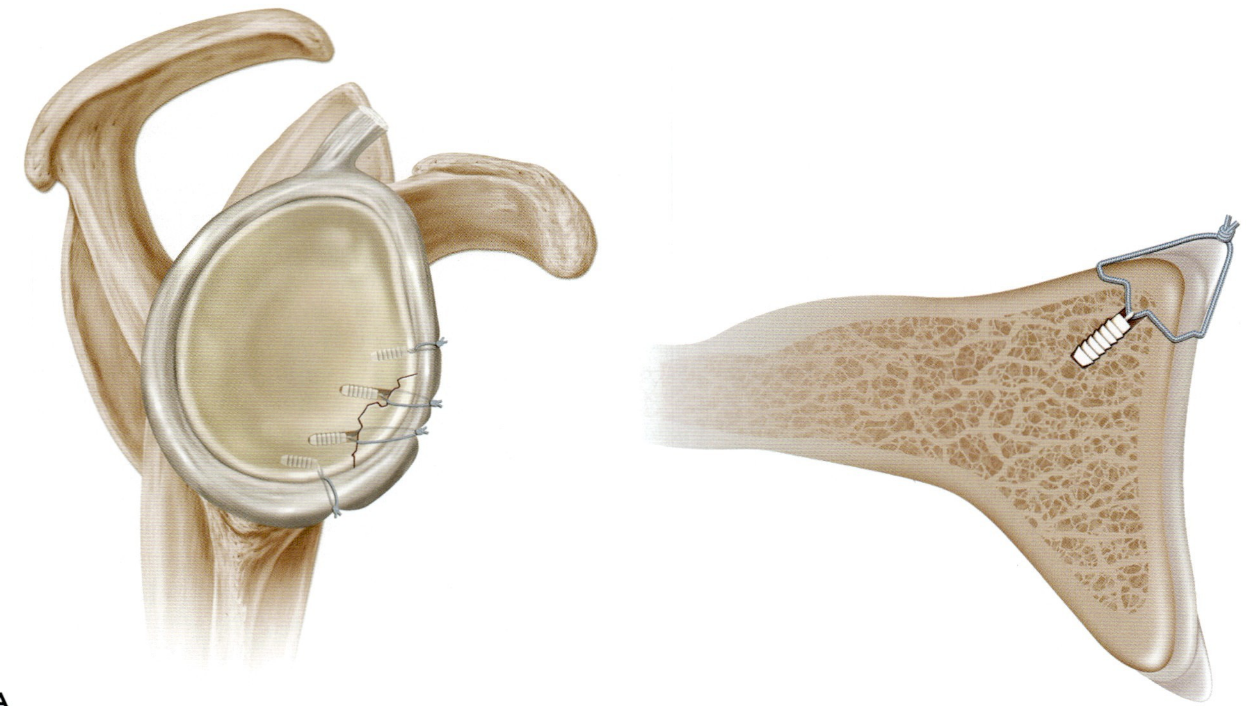

Figure 12.36 Schematic of an encircling suture technique for an anchor-based repair of a bony Bankart lesion. **A:** Sagittal view of a four anchor repair. Two BioComposite SutureTak (Arthrex, Inc., Naples, FL) anchors are placed in the glenoid and the sutures from these are passed to encircle the bony Bankart fragment. Additionally, an anchor is placed above and below the fragment and the sutures from these anchors are passed through the labrum. **B:** Axial cross section demonstrates the encircling suture technique.

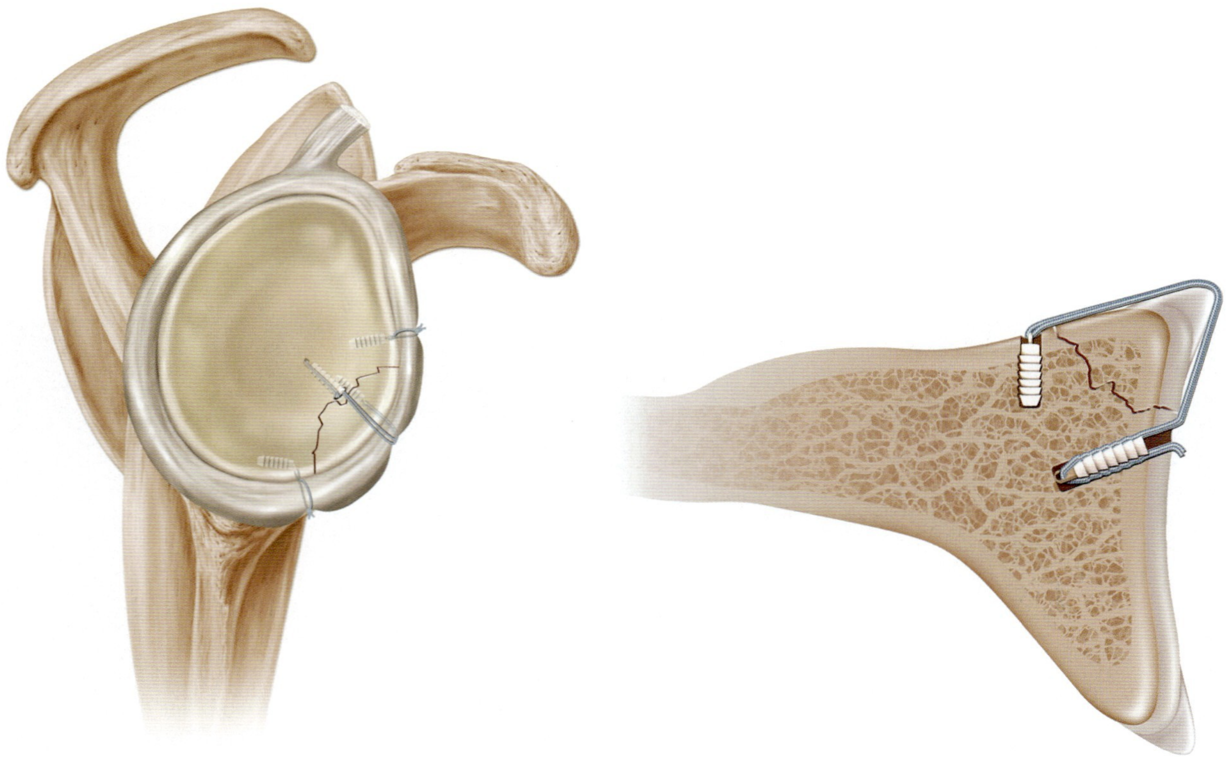

Figure 12.37 Schematic of a two-anchor encircling suture technique (Millett technique) for an anchor-based repair of a bony Bankart lesion. **A:** Sagittal view. BioComposite SutureTak anchors (Arthrex, Inc., Naples, FL) are placed above and below the bony fragment and sutures from these anchors are passed through the labrum. To encircle the bony Bankart fragment, a BioComposite SutureTak anchor is placed in the glenoid neck, medial to the fragment. Then, the sutures from this anchor are passed to encircle the bony Bankart fragment and they are secured at the fracture margin with a BioComposite PushLock (Arthrex, Inc., Naples, FL). **B:** Axial view of this encircling technique.

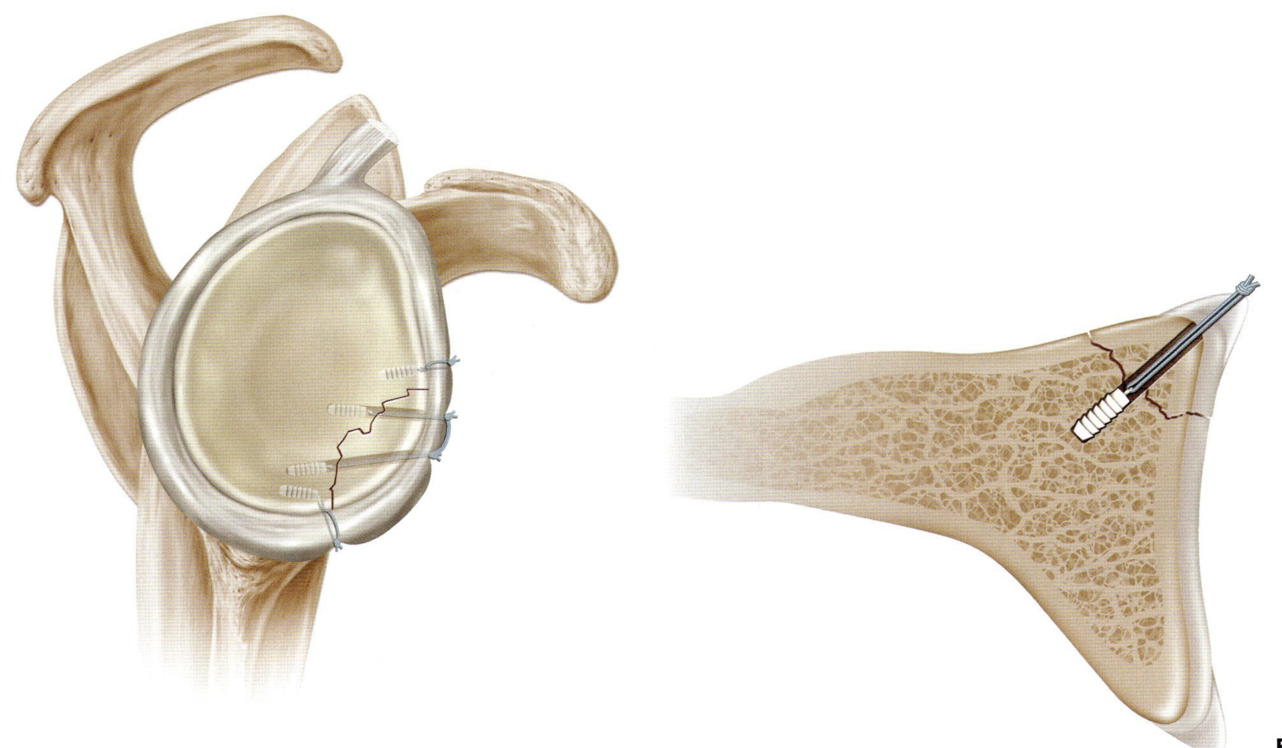

Figure 12.38 Schematic of transosseous suture technique for an anchor-based repair of a bony Bankart lesion. **A:** Sagittal view of a four anchor repair. Two BioComposite SutureTak (Arthrex, Inc., Naples, FL) anchors are placed in the glenoid and the sutures from these are passed through the bony Bankart fragment. Additionally, an anchor is placed above and below the fragment and the sutures from these anchors are passed through the labrum. **B:** Axial cross section demonstrates the transosseous suture technique.

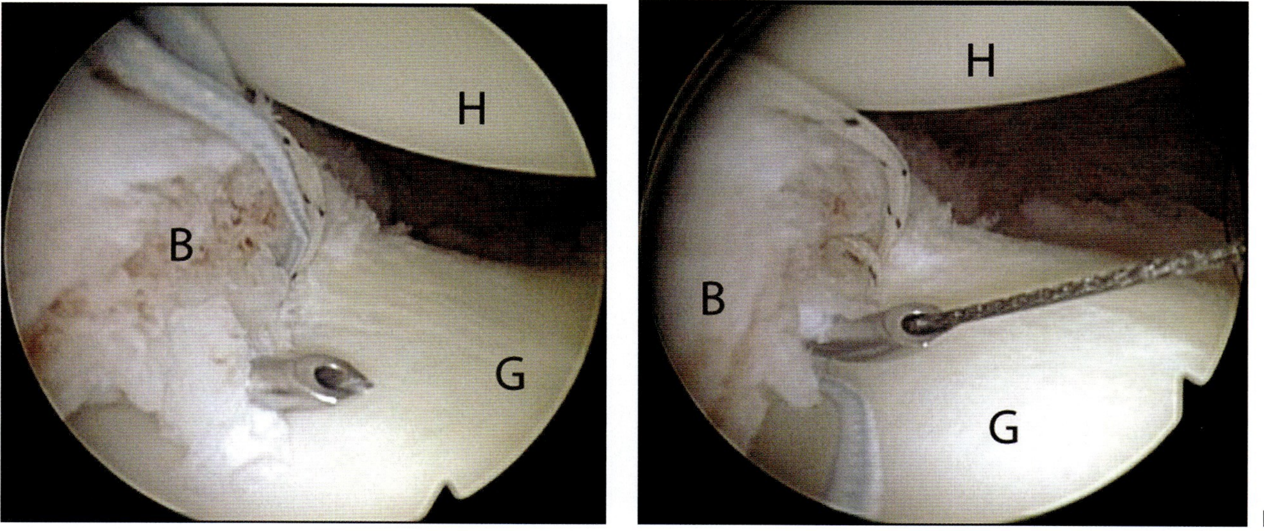

Figure 12.39 **A:** Right shoulder, anterosuperolateral view portal, demonstrates a SutureLasso (Arthrex, Inc., Naples, FL) that has been passed around a bony Bankart fragment. In this case, the fragment is small and mobile, allowing the instrument to be delivered to the glenoid rim. **B:** A Nitinol loop has been passed and retrieved out a posterior portal in order to shuttle a suture to encircle the bony fragment. B, bony Bankart fragment; G, glenoid; H, humerus.

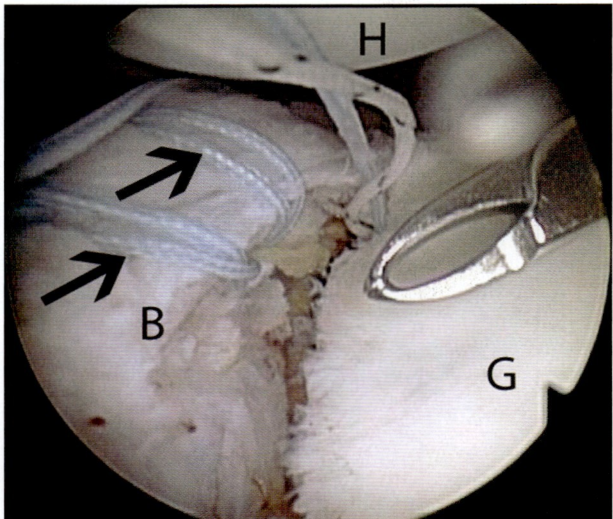

Figure 12.40 Right shoulder, anterosuperolateral viewing portal. Two cinch-loop stitches (*black arrows*) have been placed to encircle a bony Bankart fragment. Note: These sutures have been placed prior to tying sutures based off an inferior anchor that capture the labrum. B, bony Bankart fragment; G, glenoid; H, humerus.

shuttle will usually have to be retrieved between the fragment and the glenoid. The suture shuttle is retrieved and a No. 2 FiberWire suture from an anchor is shuttled around the fragment. Alternatively, in a knotless technique, a FiberLink can be shuttled around the fragment to create a cinch loop.

When an encircling suture is not possible, a transosseous suture is passed. A BirdBeak (45° or 22.5°) or SideWinder suture passer (Arthrex, Inc., Naples, FL) is introduced through the anterior cannula and is used to penetrate the fragment. It is important when performing this that the instrument is used to slowly "bore" through the fragment to avoid comminuting the fragment and is inserted through only enough to pass the suture. Usually, a hand-off technique is required to deliver the suture to the BirdBeak or SideWinder.

If the fragment is too thick to penetrate with these instruments, another transosseous technique may be utilized, where a tunnel is created in the fragment with a K-wire. While viewing through the anterosuperolateral portal, the fragment is held with a Kingfisher (Arthrex, Inc., Naples, FL) from the anterior cannula. A K-wire is introduced through the posterior cannula, traversing the glenohumeral joint, drilling the fragment in the proposed suture location. A SutureLasso is then used to penetrate the fragment through the drilled tunnel and the Nitinol suture shuttle is passed. A No. 2 FiberWire suture is then shuttled through the fragment.

The subsequent anchors and/or sutures are passed in a similar fashion (Fig. 12.40). We generally wait until all sutures capturing the bony Bankart fragment, are passed prior to tying the inferior sutures. Early knot tying will significantly restrict the mobility of the bony Bankart fragment making suture passage difficult. It is important to reduce the fragment anatomically while still creating a bumper effect (Figs. 12.41 and 12.42). It is important to avoid overreducing the fragment, particularly if encircling suture configurations have been passed. Overreduction can be avoided by introducing a switching stick or grasper through the posterior portal to hold the fragment into place.

The final suture anchor is placed superior to the margin of the fragment and sutures are passed with a shuttling technique as previously described to secure the adjacent labrum (Fig. 12.43). The final construct is assessed for fragment stability, creation of a soft tissue bumper, and centering of the glenohumeral joint (Fig. 12.44).

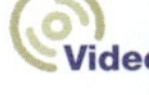

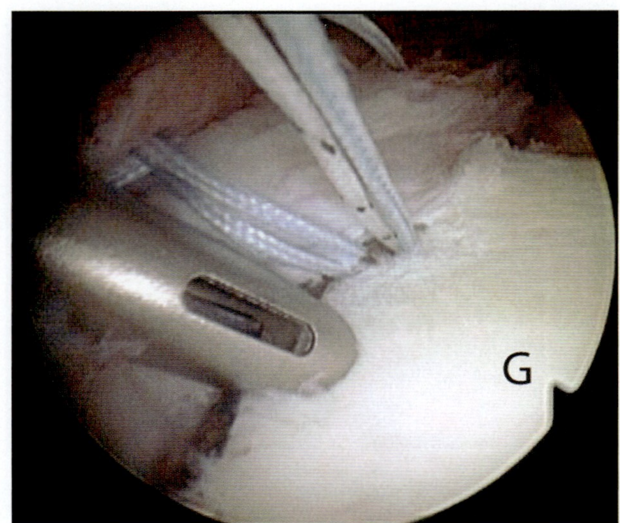

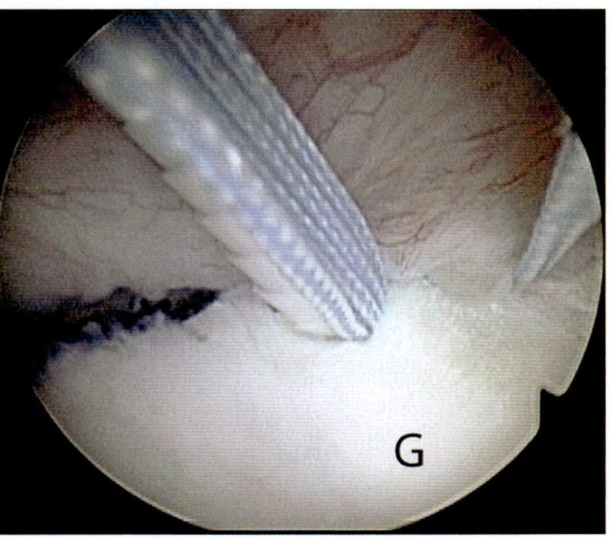

Figure 12.41 **A:** Right shoulder, anterosuperolateral viewing portal. A bone socket is created for **(B)** a BioComposite PushLock anchor (Arthrex, Inc., Naples, FL) that is used to secure cinch loops that encircle a bony Bankart Fragment.

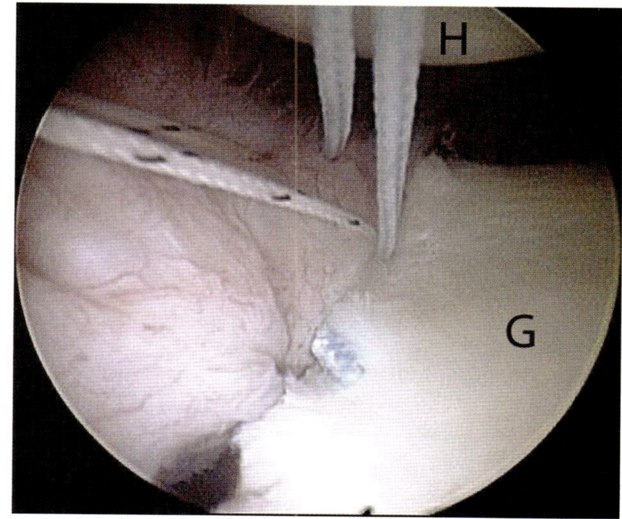

Figure 12.41 *(Continued)* **C:** Appearance after knotless fixation of the bony Bankart fragment. G, glenoid; H, humerus.

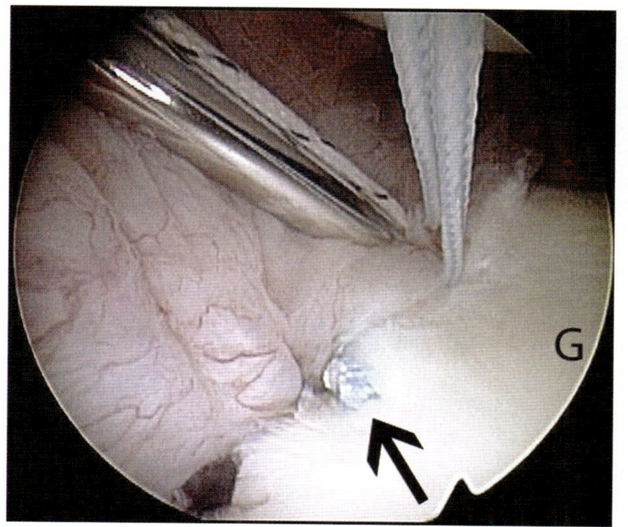

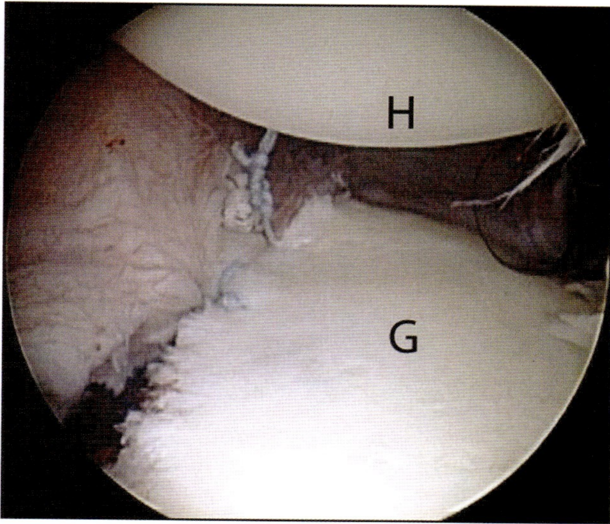

Figure 12.42 **A:** Right shoulder, anterosuperolateral viewing portal. Sutures previously passed inferior to a bony Bankart fragment are tied. A knotless technique (*black arrow*) has been used to secure the bony Bankart fragment. **B:** Appearance after securing the bony Bankart fragment and tying inferior labral sutures. An anchor will be placed above the bony Bankart fragment. G, glenoid; H, humerus.

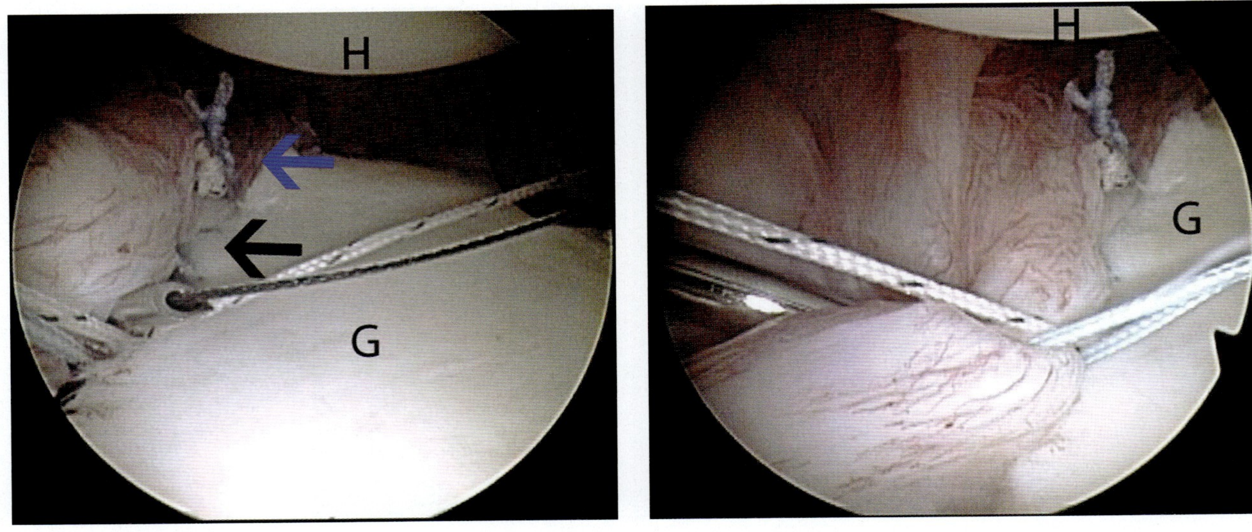

Figure 12.43 **A:** Right shoulder, anterosuperolateral viewing portal, demonstrates suture shuttling for an anchor placed superior to a knotless (*black arrow*) and standard suture anchor (*blue arrow*) that were used to secure a bony Bankart fragment and inferior labrum. **B:** Sutures for anchors superior to a bony Bankart fragment are "tied as you go." G, glenoid; H, humerus.

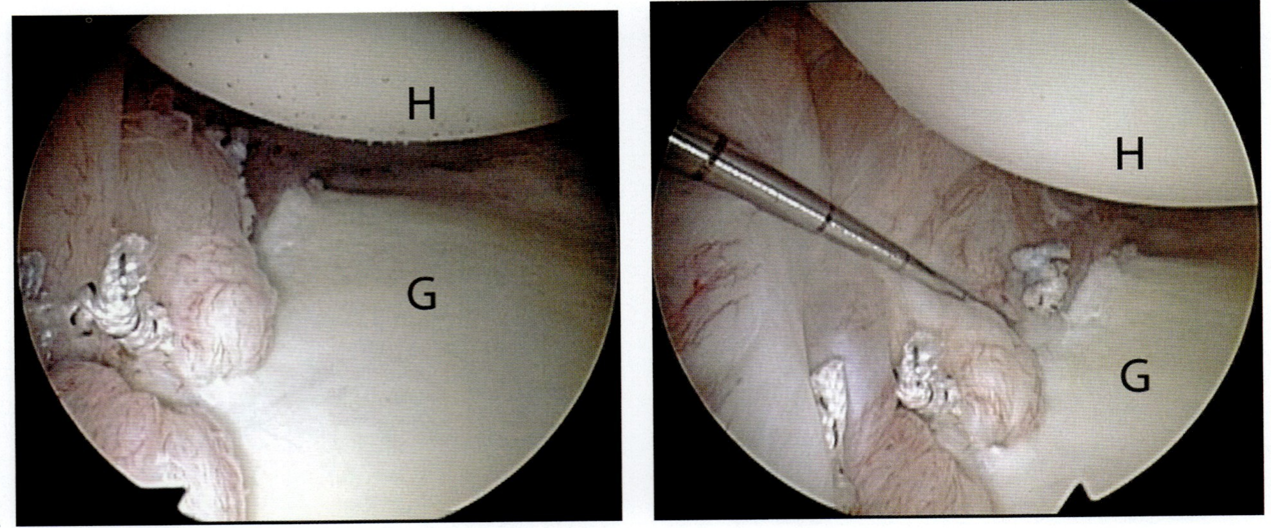

Figure 12.44 **A:** Right shoulder, anterosuperolateral viewing portal, demonstrates a bony Bankart fragment that has been repaired with suture anchors. The humeral head is centered over the glenoid. **B:** A probe marks the site of knotless fixation of the bony Bankart fragment. Knots were tied above and below the fragment. G, glenoid; H, humerus.

BONY BANKART REPAIR (SCREW FIXATION)

When the bony Bankart fragment is large (>20% to 25% of the diameter of the inferior glenoid) and of significant quality, arthroscopic screw fixation may provide superior fixation to suture anchor repair. This is particularly relevant in acute fractures of the anteroinferior glenoid, with minimal comminution where intercalation of the fracture margins is less demanding. Furthermore, when the actual fragment is very large (in contrast to the amount of glenoid bone loss), suture passage methods can be extremely difficult. These lesions essentially represent glenoid fractures and should be treated as such. For a full description of the surgical technique, refer to Chapter 19 "Arthroscopic Treatment of Fractures about the Shoulder."

SPLIT SUBSCAPULARIS TENDON FLAP FOR CAPSULOLABRAL DEFICIENCY

The importance of identifying bone lesions of the glenoid or humeral head has been recognized and treatment algorithms for this are well defined. Inadequate soft tissue characteristics such as a thin ligament–labrum complex or capsular deficiency also predispose to recurrent instability. While soft tissue quality is usually adequate in first-time dislocations, multiple dislocations can stretch and thin the anterior capsule. More commonly, capsulolabral deficiency occurs postsurgically after multiple failed surgical stabilizations or after thermal capsulorrhaphy. In these cases, a traditional arthroscopic Bankart repair is not possible. We have described a technique of arthroscopic Bankart augmentation of capsulolabral deficiency using a split subscapularis tendon flap to reinforce a deficient capsule and labrum (2). Candidates for this procedure will have capsulolabral deficiency without bone loss.

A diagnostic arthroscopy is performed to assess the quality of the capsulolabral tissue and confirm the absence of bone loss (Fig. 12.45). The remaining capsulolabral sleeve is dissected from the glenoid neck with an arthroscopic elevator until the subscapularis muscle is visible deep to the cleft and the glenoid rim is prepared as previously described. A capsulolabral repair is performed inferiorly with whatever good tissue remains (Fig. 12.46). Following placement of anchors, if there is insufficient capsulolabral tissue to create the desired "bumper" along the anterior glenoid rim, the surgeon must consider various reconstructive options, including a split subscapularis tendon flap.

To augment the capsulolabral deficiency, a flap of the posterior portion of the superior half of the subscapularis tendon is mobilized and tenodesed to the anterior glenoid. This flap is created in a "trap-door" fashion such that the capsular surface of the subscapularis tendon is reflected from medial to lateral as a separate lamina while the outer surface in left unaltered (Fig. 12.47). Using arthroscopic scissors introduced through the anterior

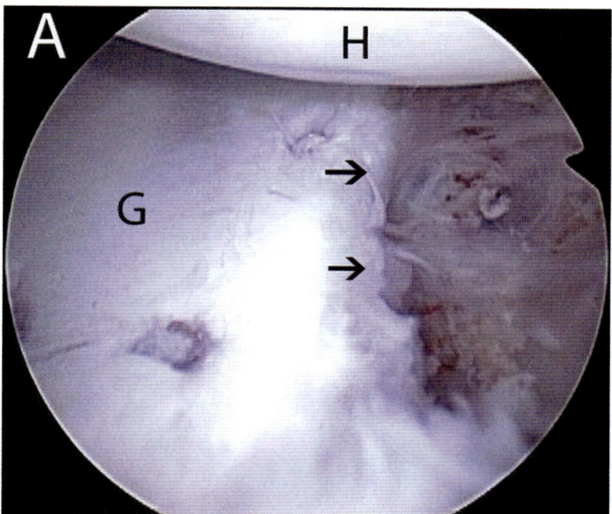

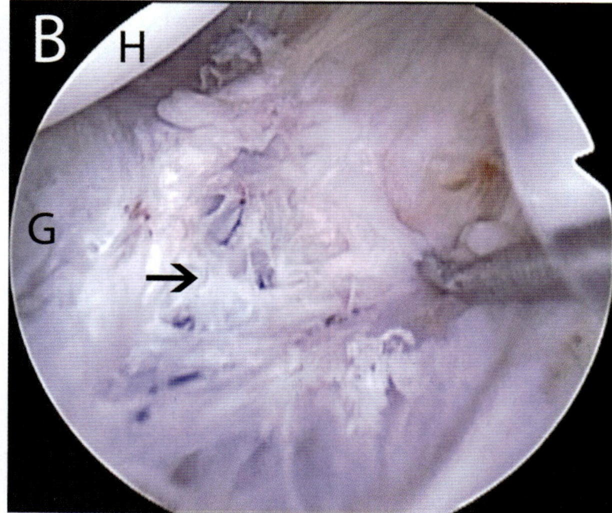

Figure 12.45 Left shoulder, anterosuperolateral viewing portal. **A,B:** Severe capsulolabral deficiency (*black arrows*) is observed in this patient who has had multiple previous failed attempts at instability repair.

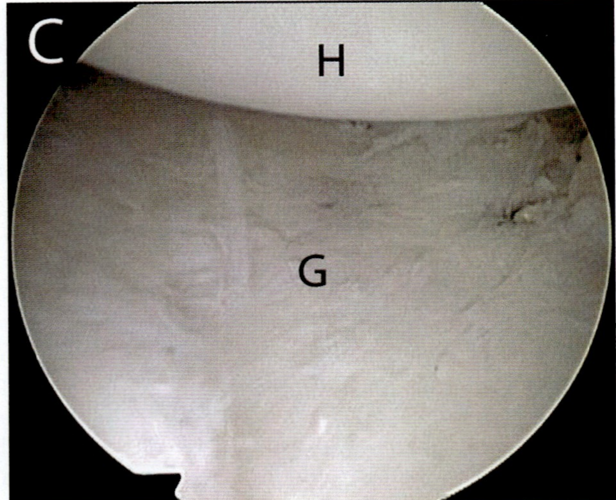

Figure 12.45 *(Continued)* **C:** The absence of a significant bone defect is confirmed arthroscopically. G, glenoid; H, humeral head.

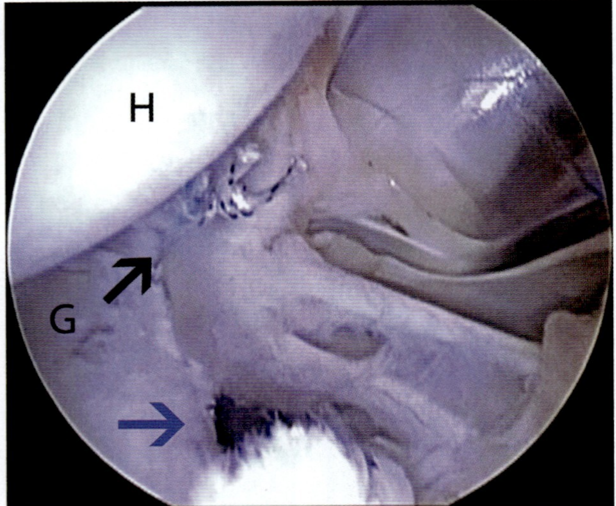

Figure 12.46 Left shoulder, anterosuperolateral viewing portal. Following placement of a 7 o'clock anchor (*black arrow*) in a patient with capsulolabral deficiency, there is inadequate capsulolabral tissue superiorly (*blue arrow*) to continue a traditional arthroscopic Bankart procedure. G, glenoid; H, humeral head.

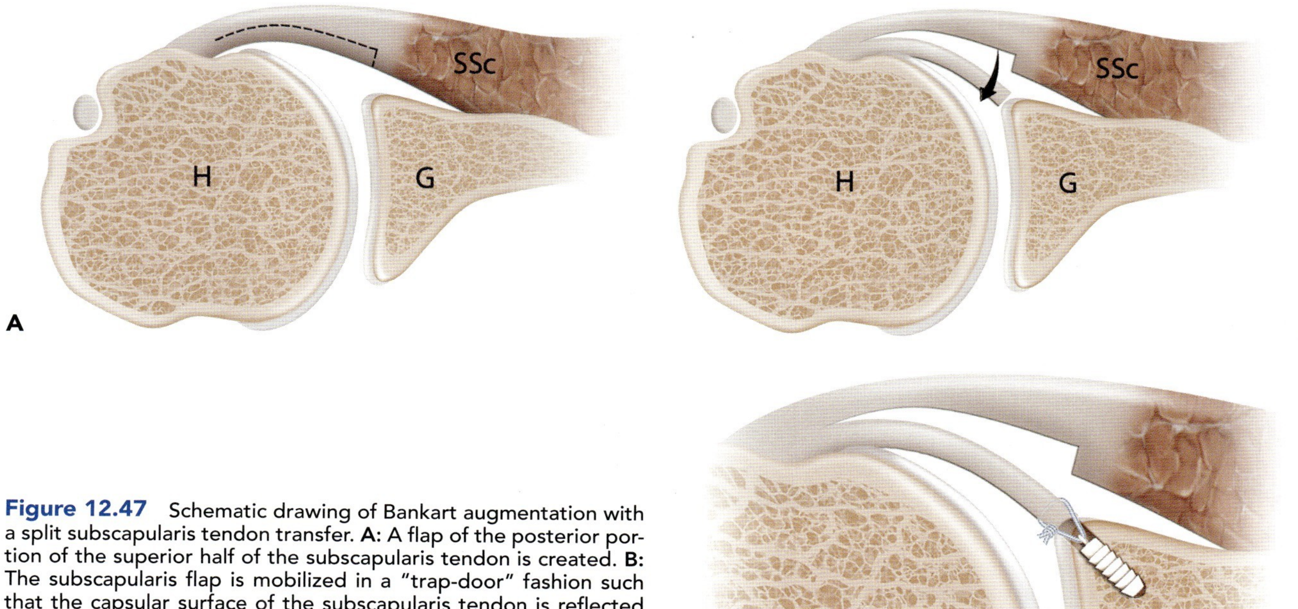

Figure 12.47 Schematic drawing of Bankart augmentation with a split subscapularis tendon transfer. **A:** A flap of the posterior portion of the superior half of the subscapularis tendon is created. **B:** The subscapularis flap is mobilized in a "trap-door" fashion such that the capsular surface of the subscapularis tendon is reflected from medial to lateral as a separate lamina while the outer surface in left unaltered. **C:** The subscapularis flap is tenodesed to the anterior glenoid suture anchors in order to augment capsulolabral deficiency. G, glenoid; H, humeral head; SSc, subscapularis tendon.

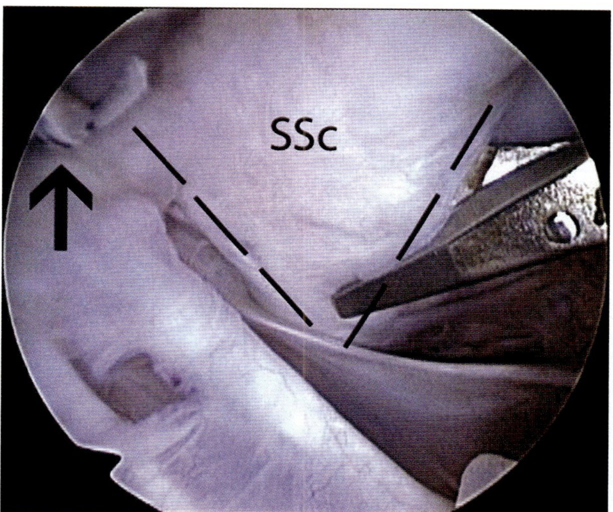

Figure 12.48 Left shoulder, anterosuperolateral viewing portal, demonstrates creation of a split subscapularis flap to augment a Bankart repair in the setting of capsulolabral deficiency. The flap (*outlined by dashed black lines*) is created with arthroscopic scissors introduced through an anterior portal. Suture is also seen from an inferior glenoid suture anchor (*black arrow*). SSc, subscapularis tendon.

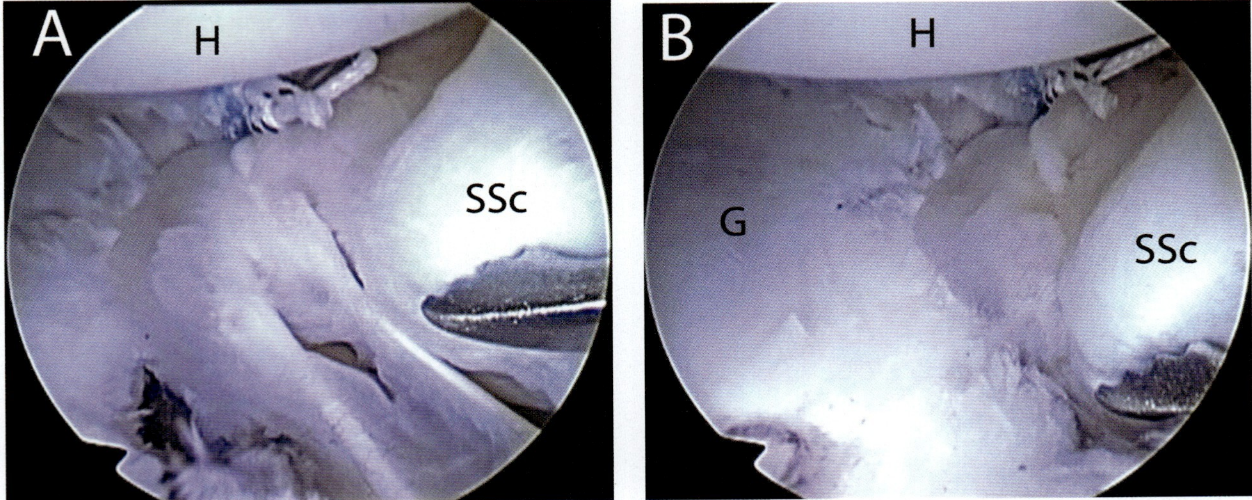

Figure 12.49 Left shoulder, anterosuperolateral viewing portal. **A:** Mobilization of a subscapularis (SSc) flap is assessed with tissue grasper. **B:** Adequate mobilization is confirmed when the subscapularis flap reaches the anterior glenoid without excessive tension. G, glenoid; H, humeral head.

portal, a longitudinal incision through one-half the thickness of the subscapularis is created in the superior half of the tendon (Fig. 12.48). Care is taken not to violate the full thickness of the subscapularis. The subscapularis flap dissection progresses from medial to lateral until the leading medial edge of the flap is mobile enough to reach the anterior glenoid (Fig. 12.49).

Following mobilization of the subscapularis tendon flap, additional suture anchors are placed on the previously prepared glenoid strip at the 8 o'clock and 9 o'clock positions. Sutures from the anchors are passed through the subscapularis flap and tied as described above (Fig. 12.50). This completes the augmentation with a split subscapularis tendon flap (Fig. 12.51).

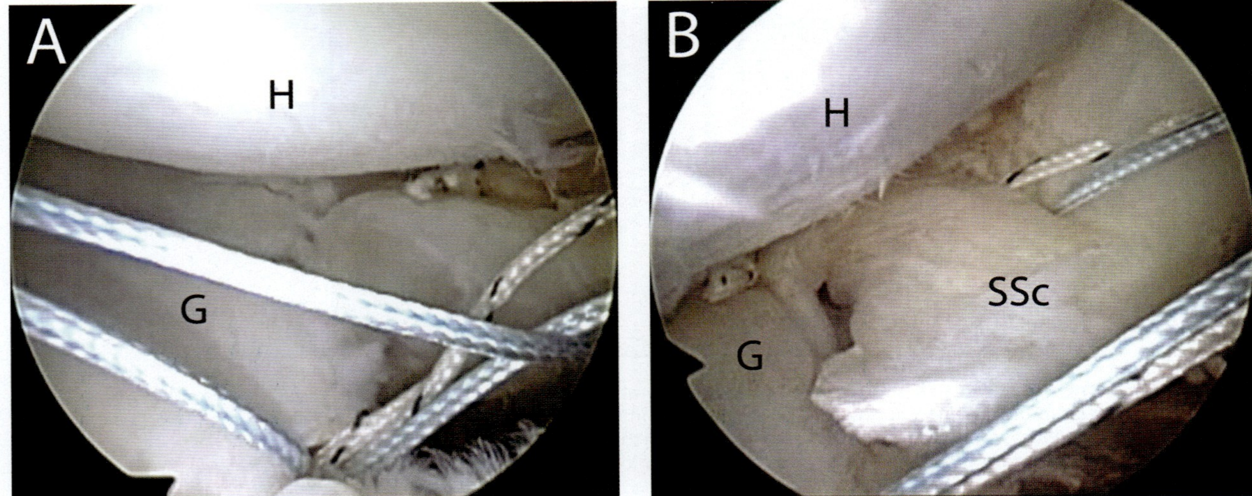

Figure 12.50 Left shoulder, anterosuperolateral viewing portal. **A:** Anchors have been placed in the glenoid in preparation for tenodesis of a split subscapularis flap. **B:** Sutures are passed through the split subscapularis (SSc) flap to allow advancement to the anterior glenoid. G, glenoid; H, humeral head.

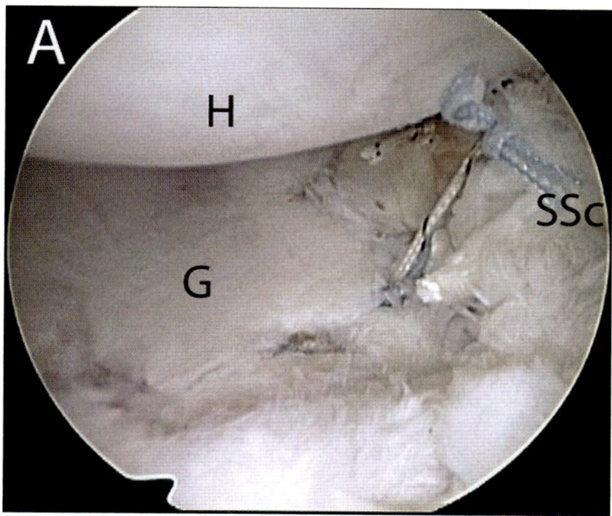

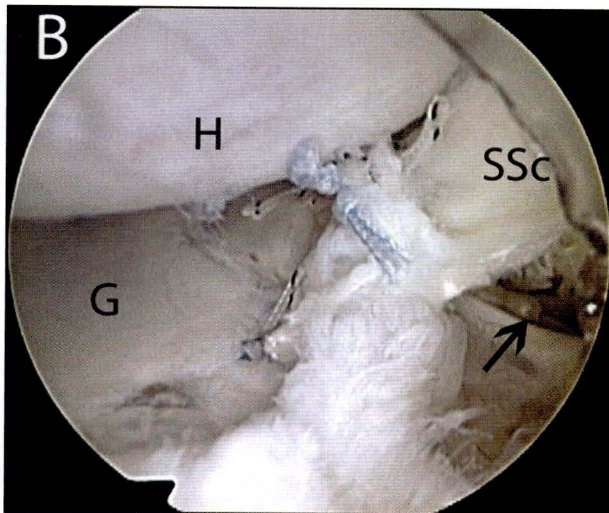

Figure 12.51 Left shoulder, anterosuperolateral viewing portal demonstrating completed arthroscopic Bankart repair augmented with a split subscapularis flap in the setting of capsulolabral deficiency **A:** Completed repair showing restoration of anterior soft tissue using the split subscapularis tendon flap. **B:** The split in the subscapularis (*black arrow*) is visualized anterior to the tenodesed flap. G, glenoid; H, humeral head; SSc, subscapularis tendon.

REFERENCES

1. Sugaya H, Moriishi J, Dohi M, et al. Glenoid rim morphology in recurrent anterior glenohumeral instability. *J Bone Joint Surg Am* 2003;85:878–884.
2. Denard PJ, Narbona P, Lädermann A, Burkhart SS. Bankart augmentation for capsulolabral deficiency using a split subscapularis tendon flap. *Arthroscopy* 2011;27:1135–1141.

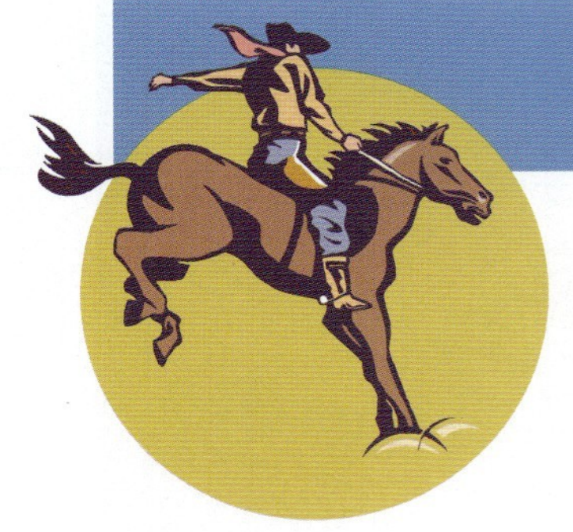

13

Instability Associated with Bone Loss

WESTERN WISDOM

If you ain't got a choice, be brave.

Recognizing and properly addressing bone defects is crucial to achieving good surgical outcomes in shoulder instability. One of the most important requirements for glenohumeral stability is a long congruent articular arc in which the humerus and glenoid remain in contact throughout motion. Loss of this congruent arc can occur from glenoid bone loss or defects in the posterior humeral head (i.e., Hill-Sachs lesions) (Figs. 13.1 and 13.2). Such lesions are present in up to 95% of patients with recurrent shoulder instability (1). Examining the glenoid alone, Sugaya et al. (2) reported that 90% of patients with recurrent instability have glenoid bone abnormalities (including bone loss or abnormal contour). Glenoid bone loss was seen in 50% of cases, in over half of which the defect was >5% of the glenoid width. Thus, while many of these bone defect are small, a substantial number of patients will have lesions that are large enough to compromise glenohumeral stability by altering the congruent arc.

In 2000 Burkhart and DeBeer demonstrated a 67% recurrence rate following arthroscopic capsulolabral repair in patients with an inverted-pear glenoid (i.e., loss of ≥25% of the inferior glenoid diameter) or an engaging Hill-Sachs defect (3). By comparison, individuals without significant bone loss had a 4% recurrence rate with arthroscopic repair. Similar findings were reported by Boileau et al. who noted a 75% rate of recurrence with arthroscopic Bankart repair in the setting of >25% glenoid bone loss (4).

In 2007, Burkhart et al. reported on the use of Latarjet in 102 individuals with significant bone loss (5). At a mean follow-up of over 4 years, the recurrence rate was only 4.9%. These studies demonstrate that recognizing significant bone loss and altering the treatment approach accordingly is the most important factor in preventing recurrent instability following surgical stabilization.

EVALUATION FOR BONE LOSS

Our evaluation for bone loss is based on preoperative and intraoperative assessments. We routinely obtain AP, transscapular lateral, and axillary radiographs of the glenohumeral joint. Radiographs are evaluated on all patients for the presence of glenoid bone loss or a Hill-Sachs lesion (Fig. 13.3). While plain radiographs can grossly demonstrate bone defects, the severity is often underestimated. We therefore obtain a computed tomography (CT) scan with three-dimensional (3D) reconstructions on all individuals with suspected bone loss. Additionally, we have a low threshold for obtaining a CT in patients without plain radiographic evidence of bone loss but otherwise having risk factors for recurrence (e.g., young patients, multiple dislocations). To estimate glenoid bone loss, bilateral 3D CTs are obtained. Assuming a normal contralateral shoulder, the percentage of bone loss is easily estimated by comparing the width of the glenoid on the affected side to the width of the glenoid on the normal shoulder in the *en face* view (Fig. 13.4). We previously reported that in 96% of cases, this technique accurately stratified glenoid bone loss as less than or greater than >25% of glenoid width (6).

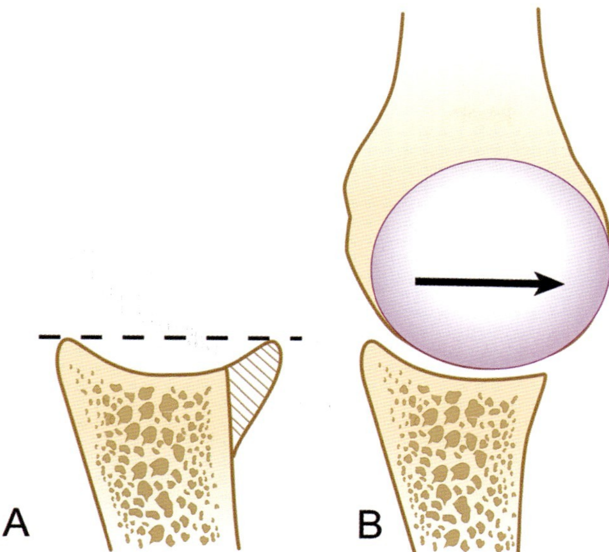

Figure 13.1 A: The anterior glenoid rim serves to "deepen the dish" of the glenoid and acts as a buttress to resist dislocation. B: A glenoid with bone loss has a decreased congruent arc with less resistance to shear forces and less resistance to obliquely applied off-axis loads.

We perform an arthroscopic assessment of bone loss in all patients with instability who are managed surgically. The patient is placed in the lateral decubitus position. Through an anterosuperolateral viewing portal the width of the inferior glenoid is assessed with a calibrated probe inserted through the posterior portal (Fig. 13.5) (7). The bare spot of the glenoid marks the center of the inferior glenoid and is used to compare the posterior glenoid diameter to the anterior diameter. The posterior proximal humerus is assessed for the presence and severity of a Hill-Sachs lesion. A calibrated probe can be used to estimate the depth of the lesion (Fig. 13.6A). The arm is then removed from traction and placed in a position of 90° of abduction and 90° of external rotation to assess for an engaging Hill-Sachs lesion (Fig. 13.6B). If either glenoid bone loss of >25% or an engaging Hill-Sachs lesion in the 90-90 position is noted, we next address any associated pathology that is amenable to arthroscopic repair (e.g., superior labrum anterior and posterior [SLAP] tear), close the wounds, then reposition and redrape in a modified beach-chair position and perform a Latarjet.

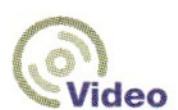

One might ask, why perform an arthroscopic evaluation in patients with a 3D CT indicating >25% bone loss? First, although it is highly predictive, the 3D CT is not 100% accurate. Second, utilizing arthroscopy prior to Latarjet, we have shown that 73% of patients have associated intra-articular

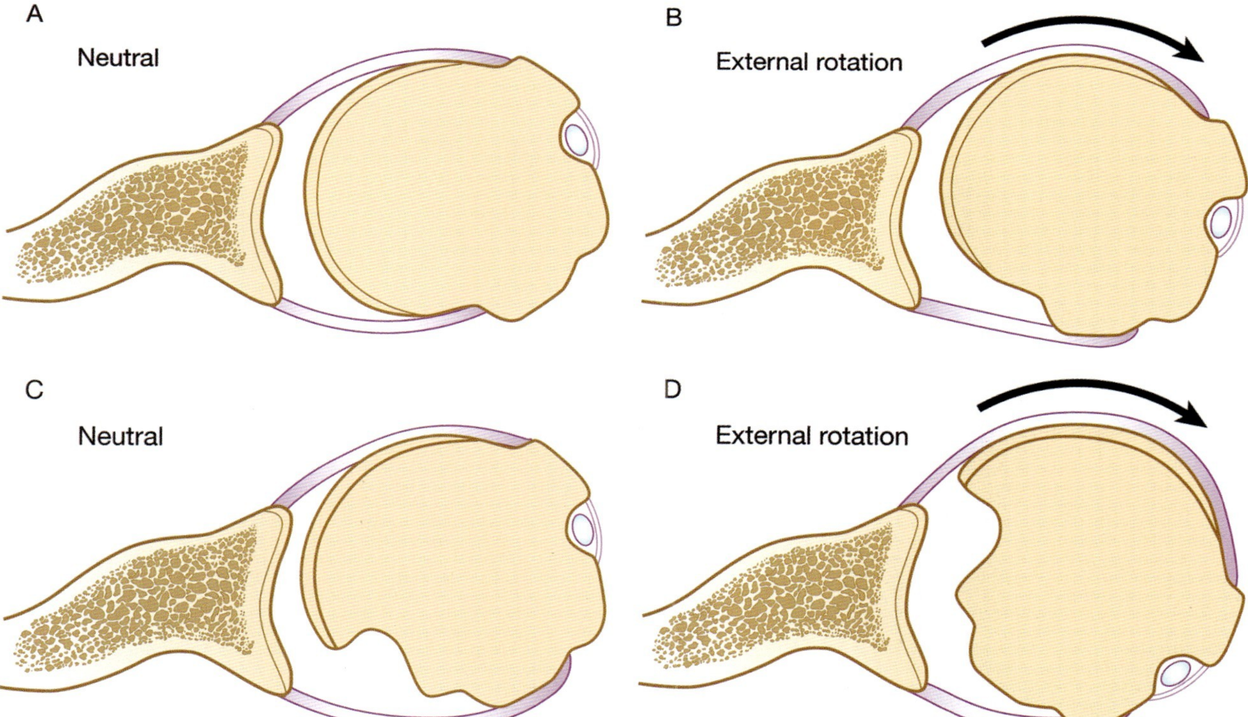

Figure 13.2 A: Normal relationship of the glenoid and humeral articular surfaces. B: Full external rotation still maintains contact between the humeral and glenoid articular surfaces. C: Large Hill-Sachs lesion creates an articular arc length mismatch. D: A small amount of external rotation will cause the Hill-Sachs lesion to engage the anterior corner of the glenoid.

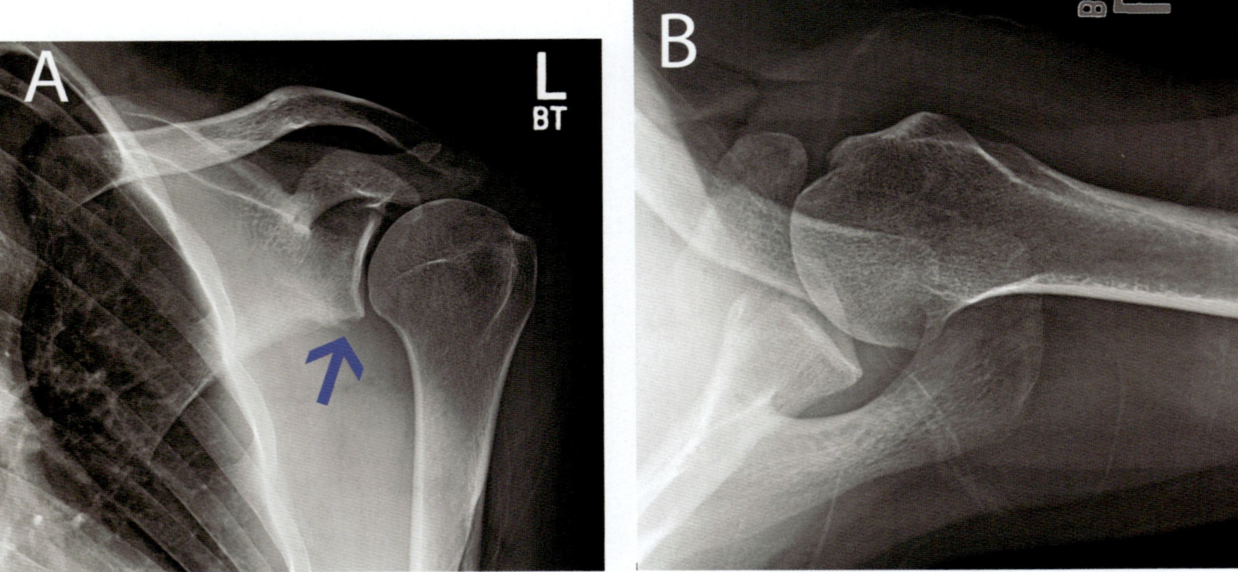

Figure 13.3 **A:** AP with a radiograph of a left shoulder in a patient with recurrent instability. There is loss of the inferior glenoid cortical rim (*blue arrow*) suggesting glenoid bone loss. **B:** An axillary radiograph is also suggestive of anterior glenoid bone loss, but the amount cannot be well quantified.

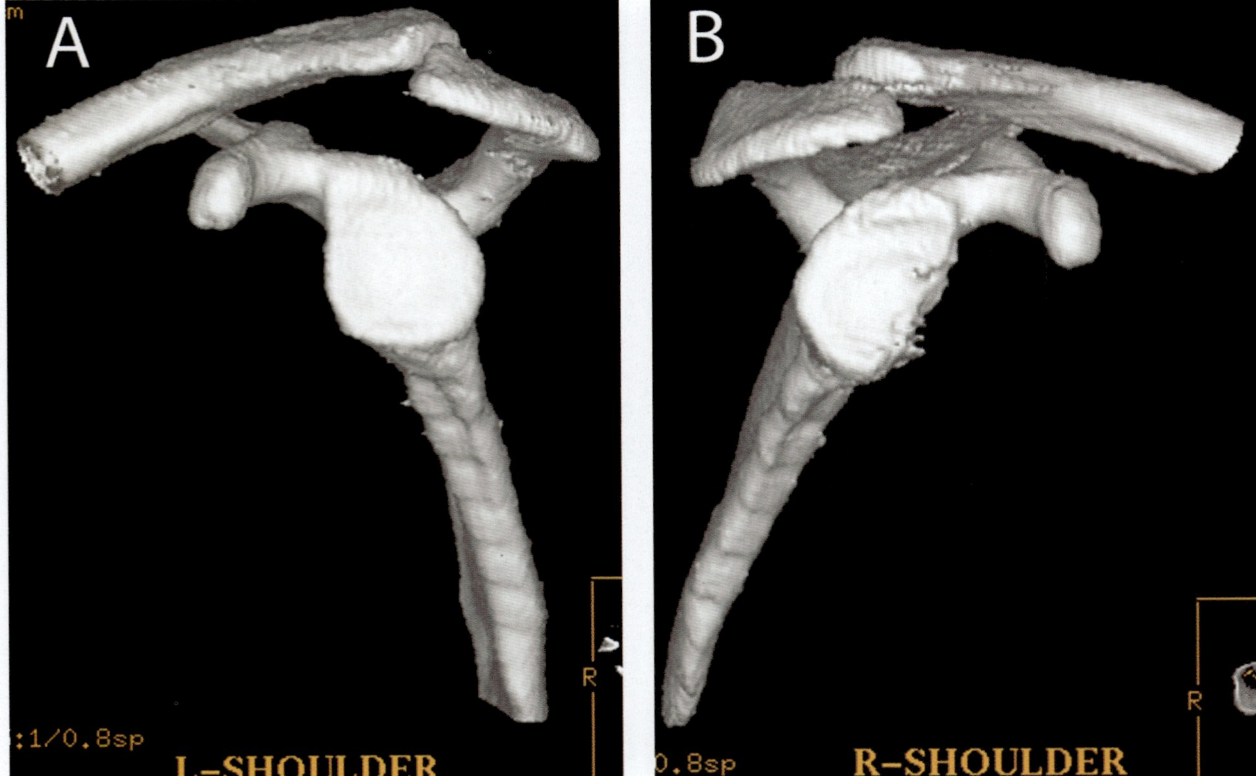

Figure 13.4 Glenoid bone loss can be quantified with a three-dimensional CT of the **(A)** normal and **(B)** affected extremities. The percentage of glenoid bone loss can be easily calculated on the *en face* view by comparing the inferior glenoid diameter of the normal side to that of the affected side.

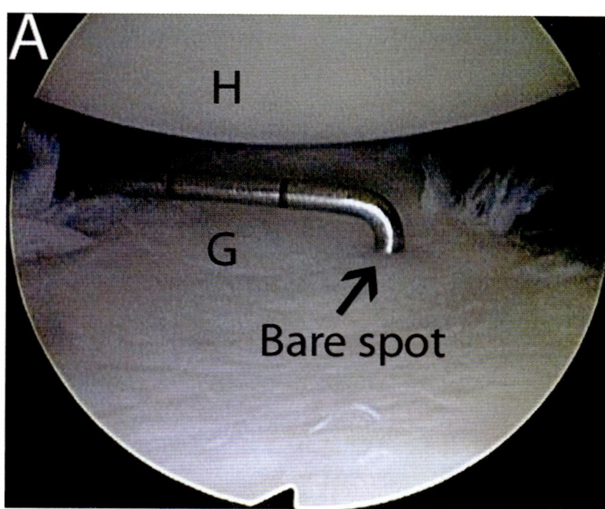

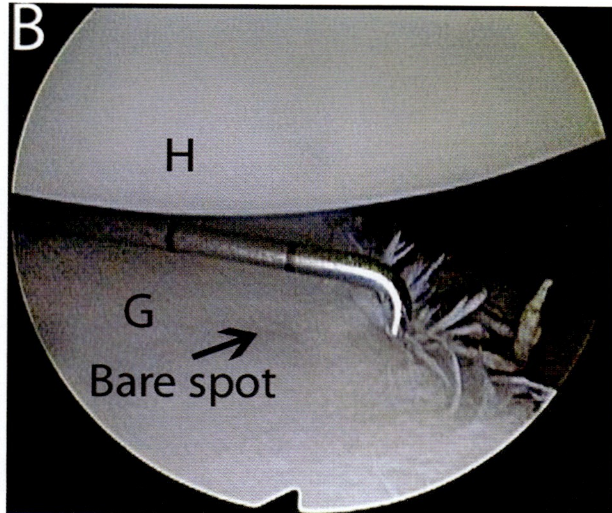

Figure 13.5 Measuring glenoid bone loss arthroscopically from an anterosuperolateral viewing portal in a left shoulder. **A:** A calibrated probe introduced from a posterior portal marks the distance from the glenoid bare spot to the posterior rim. In this case, the posterior distance is approximately 12 mm. **B:** The probe is used to measure the distance from the remaining anterior glenoid rim to the glenoid bare spot. In this case, the distance is 6 mm. Thus, there is 6 mm of bone loss anteriorly, or 25% loss of the inferior glenoid diameter. G, glenoid; H, humerus.

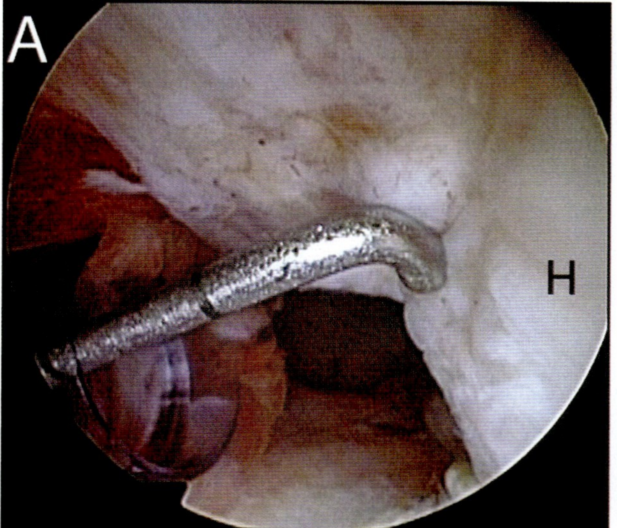

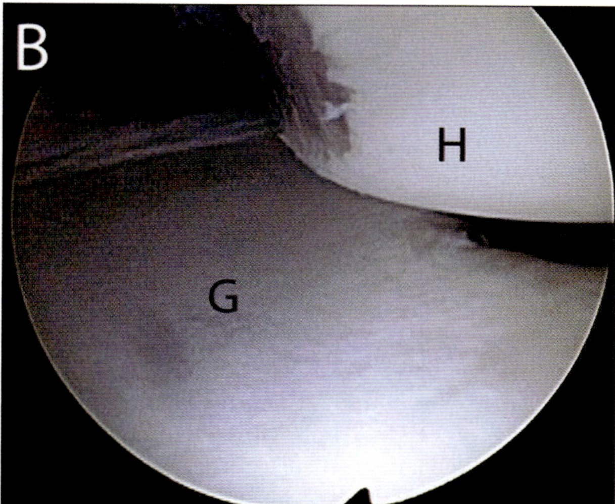

Figure 13.6 Evaluation of a Hill-Sachs lesion from an anterosuperolateral portal in a left shoulder. **A:** A calibrated probe introduced from a posterior portal is used to estimate the depth of the lesion. In this case, the defect is 5 mm deep. **B:** The arm is removed from traction and placed in abduction and external rotation to determine whether the lesion engages the anterior glenoid. In this case, the Hill-Sachs lesion engages the glenoid rim. G, glenoid; H, humerus.

pathology including a SLAP tear in 64% of cases (8). Given the contribution of the superior labrum to glenoid stability, we feel that it is important to repair a SLAP tear in all cases of glenohumeral instability, and this is best done arthroscopically.

Others have asked, why perform the arthroscopy in the lateral decubitus position when the patient has to be repositioned and redraped in the beach-chair position to perform a Latarjet? First, we perform all shoulder arthroscopy in the lateral decubitus position and do not want to compromise our technique. Second, the addition of the arthroscopic remplissage, as discussed below, has increased our armamentarium of surgical options and blurred the lines between which patients require an open Latarjet and which patients can be managed arthroscopically. For example, a patient may have borderline bone loss of 23% on a preoperative CT. If arthroscopy reveals that the bone loss is actually 26%, we would perform a Latarjet. On the other hand, if arthroscopic bone loss is measured to be 20% and the patient is otherwise in a lower category of risk for recurrence, we would perform an arthroscopic Bankart repair and remplissage of the Hill-Sachs, which we strongly believe is best performed in the lateral decubitus position.

LATARJET RECONSTRUCTION

Indications

Since 1996, our indications for performing an open Latarjet procedure have remained the same. They are

1. Glenoid bone loss of >25% of the inferior glenoid diameter (inverted-pear glenoid)
   or
2. Deep Hill-Sachs lesion that engages in a position of 90° abduction plus 90° external rotation (position of athletic function)
   or
3. A combination of 1 and 2

In general, we have found that a large engaging Hill-Sachs lesion usually occurs in combination with an *inverted-pear glenoid*, so such a case satisfies both indications. Also, when there is a large Hill-Sachs lesion, the coracoid bone graft in the Latarjet procedure will lengthen the articular arc to such an extent that the Hill-Sachs lesion will not be able to engage the glenoid rim. In this way, the Latarjet procedure effectively addresses the Hill-Sachs lesion without the need for an additional bone graft to the humeral defect.

One relative indication for the Latarjet reconstruction is in the patient with severe soft tissue loss involving the anterior labroligamentous complex. Such soft tissue deficiency can occur due to thermal capsular necrosis, or due to multiple failed soft tissue procedures for instability. Although some authors have recommended soft-tissue allografts, we have preferentially done the Latarjet reconstruction without soft tissue augmentation. In this way, we prevent recurrent anterior dislocation by lengthening the glenoid articular arc, as well as providing the "sling effect" of the conjoined tendon, which resists anterior translational forces as the arm goes into abduction and external rotation. The idea for utilizing the Latarjet procedure to address soft tissue loss came from the intraoperative observation that after the coracoid bone graft was secured in place, the shoulder could not be manually dislocated with a significant anteriorly directed force applied by the surgeon, even though the capsule had not yet been repaired. That is, the stability of the Latarjet construct was not at all related to the integrity of the anterior capsule.

Alternatively, we have noted that there are occasional cases with partial loss of the capsule (thermal capsular necrosis; multiple failed surgeries) without any significant bone loss. We have found that such cases may be amenable to arthroscopic repair utilizing a flap of the deep surface of the subscapularis to augment or to substitute for the anterior capsule (see Chapter 12, "Repair of Anterior Instability without Bone Loss").

Evolution of the Coracoid Bone Graft Technique

Coracoid bone grafting for anterior instability has a long history among French orthopaedic surgeons. We are grateful to our French colleagues, Dr. Gilles Walch and Dr. Johannes Barth, for communicating its history to us, because this story is not readily available in the English-language orthopaedic literature.

Trillat was the first to treat anterior instability with coracoid reinforcement. He did a partial coracoid osteotomy, leaving the inferior cortex intact and then levering the coracoid with an osteotome to create a greenstick fracture through the inferior cortex. A screw then secured the coracoid as an anterior buttress against the subscapularis, tensioning the subscapularis to provide resistance to anterior translation of the humerus.

Latarjet further developed this concept by detaching the pectoralis minor from the coracoid and incising the coracoacromial ligament, leaving a stump of the coracoacromial ligament attached to the coracoid, and then completing the osteotomy at the base of the coracoid so that it could be placed as a bone graft against the anterior glenoid neck. The coracoid was passed through a split in the subscapularis and positioned so that its inferior surface was in contact with the anterior glenoid neck, where it was secured with two screws (Fig. 13.7). In doing so, the posterolateral surface of the coracoid was placed adjacent to the glenoid joint surface.

Patte attributed the success of the Latarjet procedure to a so-called *triple effect* composed of

1. Lengthening of the articular arc by the bone graft
2. The sling effect of the conjoined tendon
3. Tensioning of the lower subscapularis by means of the conjoined tendon in its new position (draped over the lower subscapularis)

Allain et al. (9) looked at the effect of the position of the coracoid graft on long-term results. They found that the best results were in the group of patients in which the lateral edge of the coracoid graft was placed flush with the articular surface of the glenoid. If the coracoid was placed medial to this ideal location, there was an increase in the rate of recurrent dislocation and subluxation; if it was laterally placed, there was a high rate of late degenerative change in the glenohumeral joint.

Burkhart and DeBeer further modified the Latarjet technique, developing the "Congruent-arc Latarjet Procedure," and they first reported on it in 2000 (3). This technique incorporated two important modifications:

1. The coracoid graft was rotated 90° around its long axis so that the concave inferior surface of the coracoid became the extension to the glenoid concavity, providing a much more anatomic articular arc to the reconstructed glenoid surface (Fig. 13.8) (10).
2. The capsule was reattached to the native glenoid by means of suture anchors so that the coracoid graft was extra-articular, thereby preventing abrasion of the humeral articular surface against the coracoid graft.

The original congruent-arc technique required freehand positioning of the coracoid graft. We now use an instrumented Latarjet guide system (Arthrex, Inc., Naples, FL) to assure accurate and reproducible positioning of the coracoid graft.

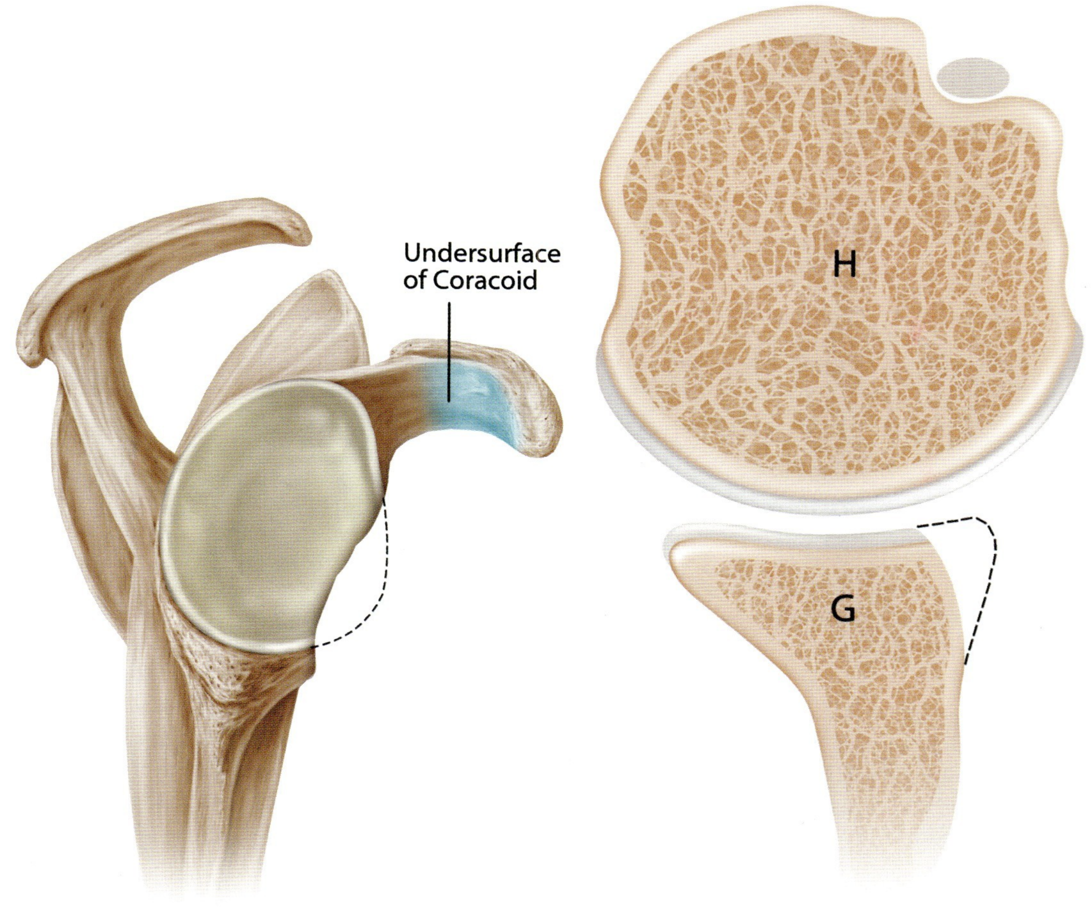

Figure 13.7 Schematic of the French technique for Latarjet reconstruction. Sagittal **(A)** and axial **(B)** schematics prior to latarjet reconstruction.

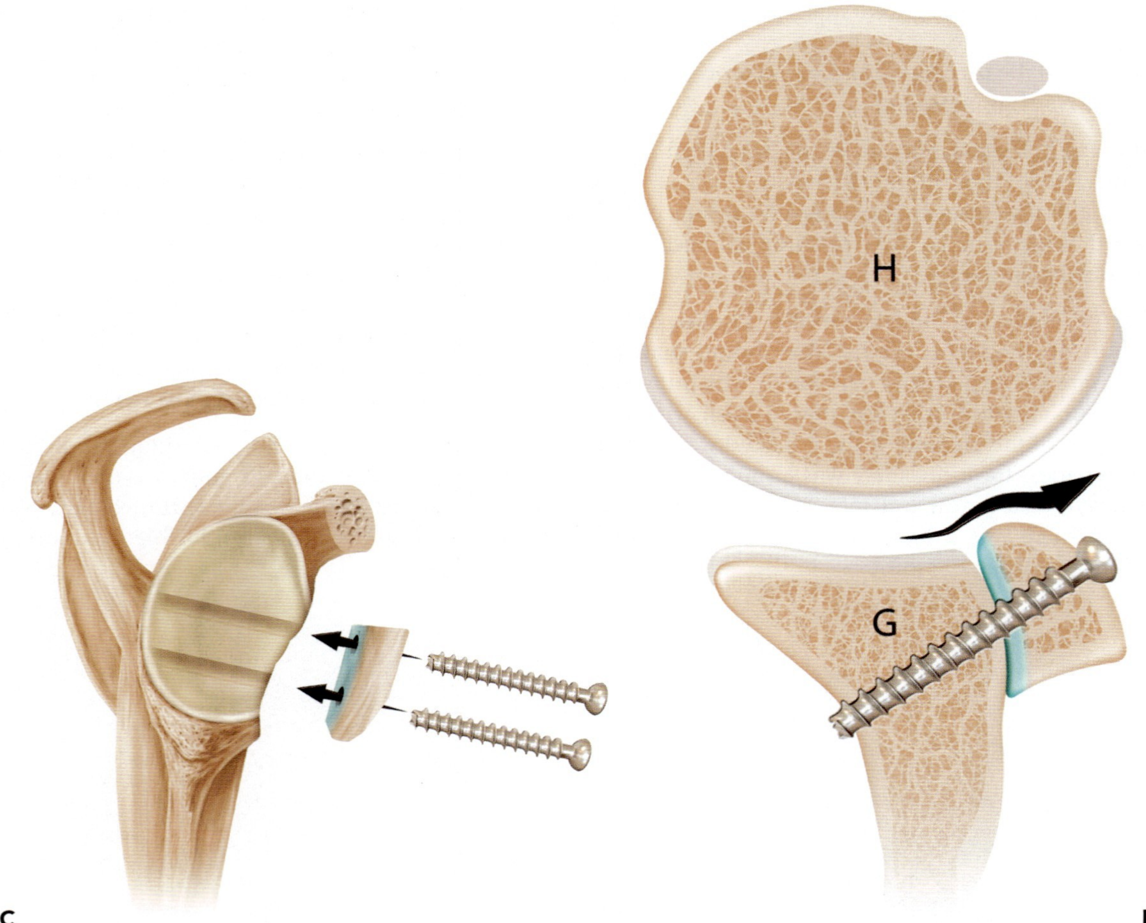

Figure 13.7 *(Continued)* **C,D:** The coracoid is osteotomized and the undersurface of the coracoid is fixed directly to the glenoid. The contour of the coracoid graft does not match the contour of the native glenoid. G, glenoid; H, humerus.

Surgical Technique of Congruent-arc Latarjet Reconstruction

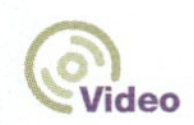

We call our surgical technique the *congruent-arc* technique because we place the coracoid graft in an orientation such that the arc of its inferior surface is a congruent extension to the glenoid articular arc.

We always perform diagnostic arthroscopy just prior to the Latarjet in order to accurately measure the amount of glenoid bone loss, to assess the Hill-Sachs lesion, and also to evaluate the joint for additional pathology, particularly SLAP lesions. We have found an a 64% incidence of SLAP lesions in our patients who are undergoing Latarjet reconstruction (8). In these cases, we perform an arthroscopic SLAP repair with the patient in the lateral decubitus position. Then, we turn the patient supine and adjust the table to a modified beach-chair position, then re-prep and redrape for the open Latarjet.

Coracoid Osteotomy

In performing the congruent-arc Latarjet, a standard deltopectoral incision is used. The cephalic vein is preserved and retracted laterally with the deltoid muscle. The coracoid is exposed from its tip to the insertion of the coracoclavicular ligaments at the base of the coracoid. The coracoacromial ligament is sharply dissected from the lateral aspect of the coracoid, and the pectoralis minor tendon insertion on the medial side of the coracoid is also sharply dissected from the bone (Fig. 13.9). The medial surface of the coracoid, from which the pectoralis minor is detached, is the surface that will later be in contact with

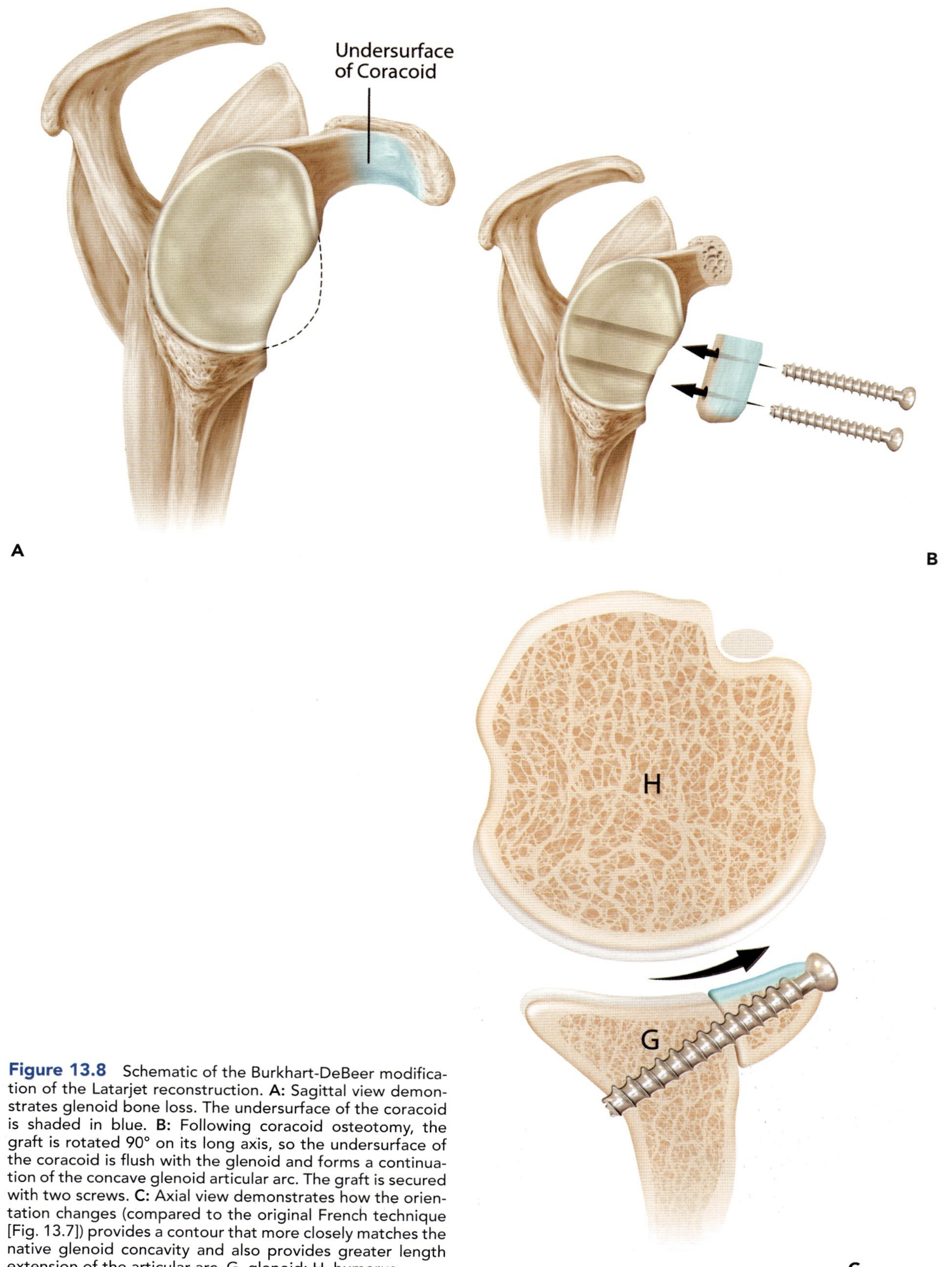

Figure 13.8 Schematic of the Burkhart-DeBeer modification of the Latarjet reconstruction. **A:** Sagittal view demonstrates glenoid bone loss. The undersurface of the coracoid is shaded in blue. **B:** Following coracoid osteotomy, the graft is rotated 90° on its long axis, so the undersurface of the coracoid is flush with the glenoid and forms a continuation of the concave glenoid articular arc. The graft is secured with two screws. **C:** Axial view demonstrates how the orientation changes (compared to the original French technique [Fig. 13.7]) provides a contour that more closely matches the native glenoid concavity and also provides greater length extension of the articular arc. G, glenoid; H, humerus.

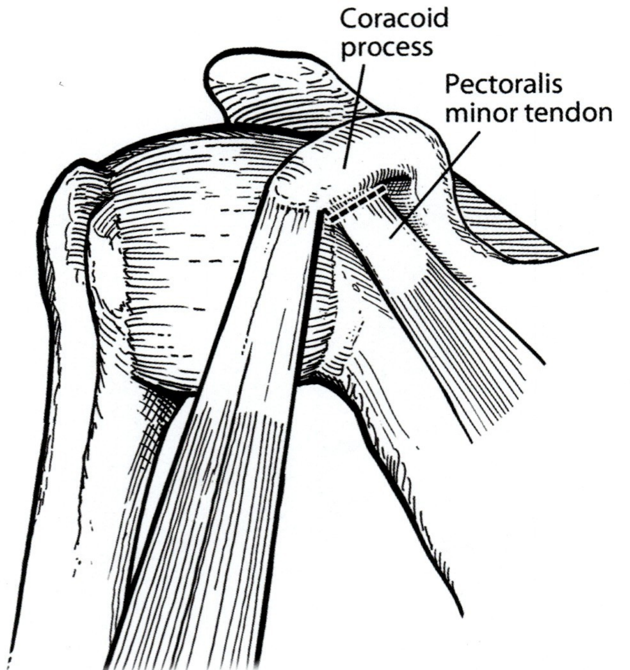

Figure 13.9 In preparation for coracoid osteotomy, the pectoralis minor tendon is sharply dissected off the medial edge of the coracoid.

the anterior glenoid neck when the graft is secured by screws.

For the coracoid osteotomy, two options are available. Option 1 involves the use of an osteotome to create the osteotomy (Fig. 13.10A). We believe that an osteotome should be used only in thin patients. In a muscular patient with a large deltoid and pectoralis major, the bulk of these muscles may prevent a proper angle of approach anterior to the glenoid, resulting in the possibility of intra-articular glenoid fracture. Option 2, for muscular patients, involves the use of an angled saw blade to create the osteotomy (Fig. 13.10B). Neurovascular structures are protected by retractors medial and inferior to the saw blade. With either technique, the osteotomy is made just anterior to the coracoclavicular ligaments in order to obtain as much length to the coracoid graft as possible. A graft measuring 2.5 to 3.0 cm in length is ideal, though in small patients a graft of 2.0 cm is adequate for fixation with two screws.

The conjoined tendon is left attached to the coracoid graft to maintain vascularity of the graft and to augment stability of the glenohumeral joint by providing a *sling effect* upon completion of the procedure. After mobilization of the coracoid and conjoined tendon, the musculocutaneous nerve is protected by retracting the coracoid medially, thereby preventing any stretch injury to the nerve.

Glenohumeral Joint Exposure

Once the coracoid has been osteotomized, there is a clear view of the anterior shoulder. The upper half of the subscapularis tendon is detached distally and reflected medially (Fig. 3.11). The insertion of the lower half of the subscapularis is preserved. After detachment of the upper subscapularis tendon, the plane between lower subscapularis tendon and anterior joint capsule is developed.

Alternatively, the glenoid may be exposed by using a subscapularis split approach. A deep Gelpi retractor is used

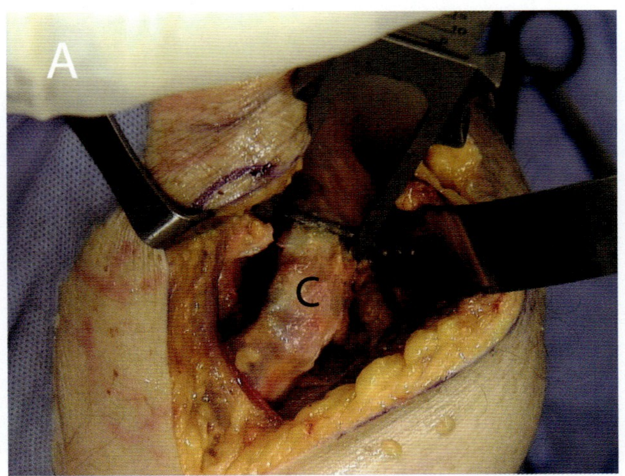

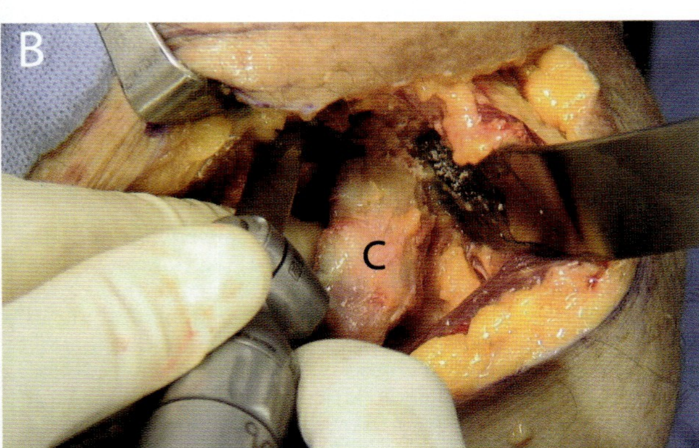

Figure 13.10 Coracoid osteotomy may be performed with **(A)** an osteotome, or **(B)** an angled saw blade. C, coracoid.

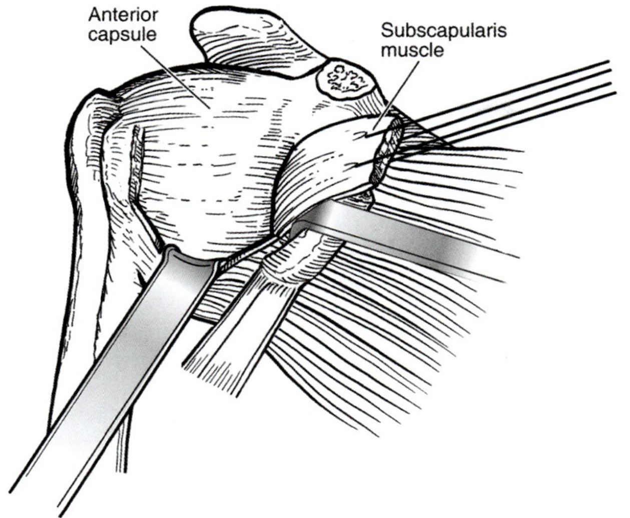

Figure 13.11 Management of the subscapularis tendon. Detach the superior half of the tendon, then develop a plane between the inferior half of the subscapularis and the capsule.

to spread the split in the muscle. The subscapularis split is made through the muscular fibers at the junction of the superior and middle thirds of the muscle. The capsule is bluntly dissected from the subscapularis, and then the capsular incision is made. We prefer not to use the subscapularis-splitting approach because visualization can be quite limited, and the position of the split severely limits the surgeon's ability to change the position of the graft on the glenoid if needed.

The capsular incision is begun 1 cm medial to the rim of the glenoid by subperiosteal sharp dissection to preserve enough capsular length for later reattachment (Fig. 3.12). The anterior glenoid neck is prepared as the recipient bed for the coracoid bone graft by means of a curette or a burr, being careful to preserve as much native glenoid bone as possible. "Dusting" of the anterior glenoid neck to a bleeding surface is performed with a high-speed burr without actually removing bone.

Coracoid Preparation

While stabilizing the coracoid with a Kocher grasper, use an oscillating saw to remove a thin sliver of bone from the medial coracoid surface where the pectoralis minor had been inserted. This is the surface that will be in contact with the anterior glenoid neck (Fig. 13.13).

Grasp the coracoid graft with the grasping Coracoid Drill Guide (Arthrex, Inc., Naples, FL) (Fig. 13.14). Position the guide on the graft so that the elongated clearance slots are on the freshened surface of the coracoid that will eventually be in contact with the glenoid.

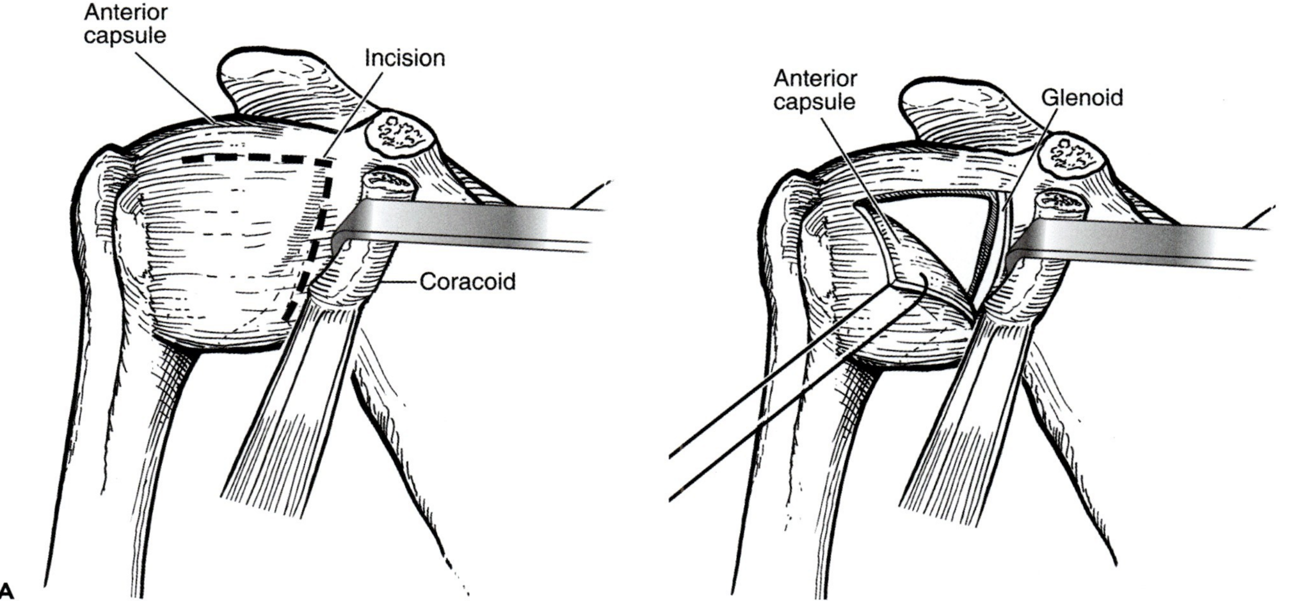

Figure 13.12 **A:** Outline of capsulotomy. **B:** Dissect the capsule 1 cm medial to the glenoid rim before detaching it from the glenoid neck to preserve as much capsular length as possible for later reattachment.

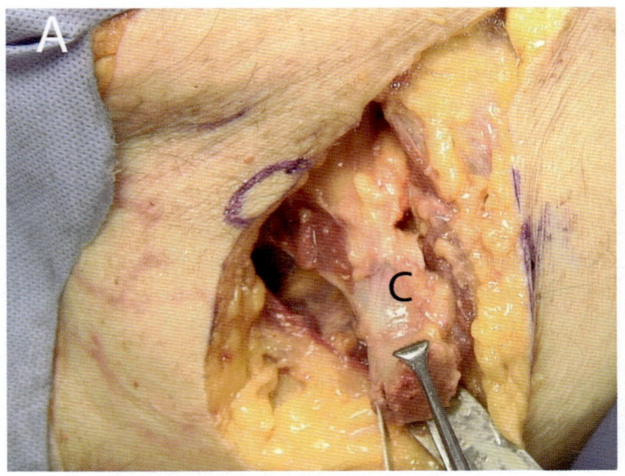

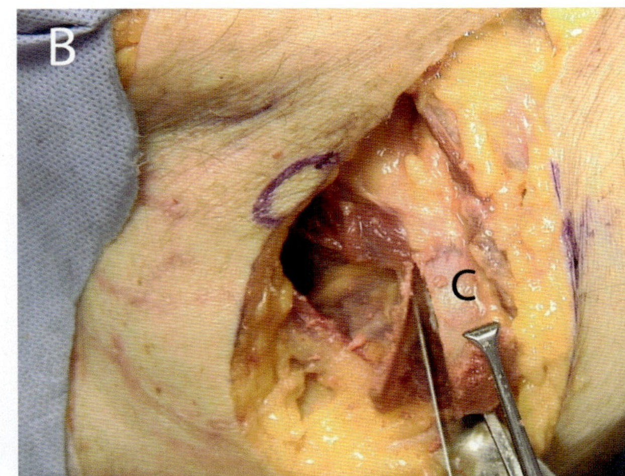

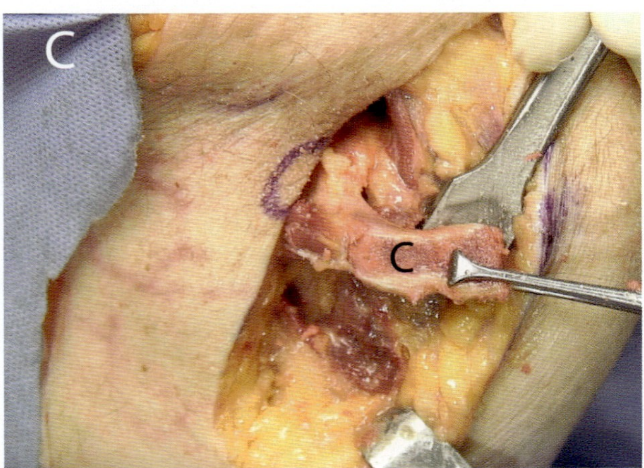

Figure 13.13 Coracoid graft preparation. **A:** The coracoid is grasped with an instrument. **B:** A straight saw blade is used to remove a thin sliver of bone from the medial surface. **C:** The medial surface has been cut and will be secured to the glenoid rim. C, coracoid graft.

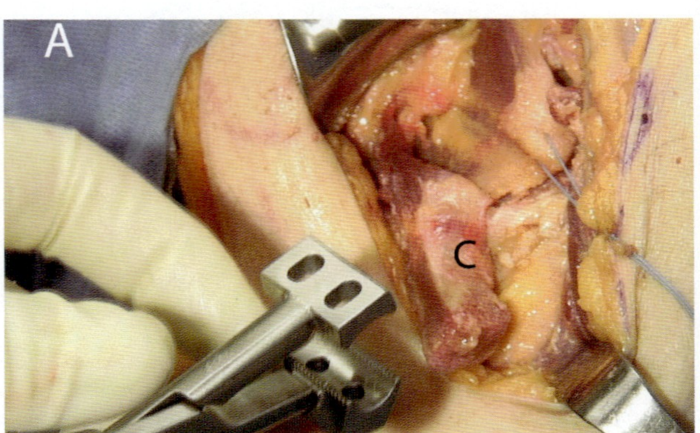

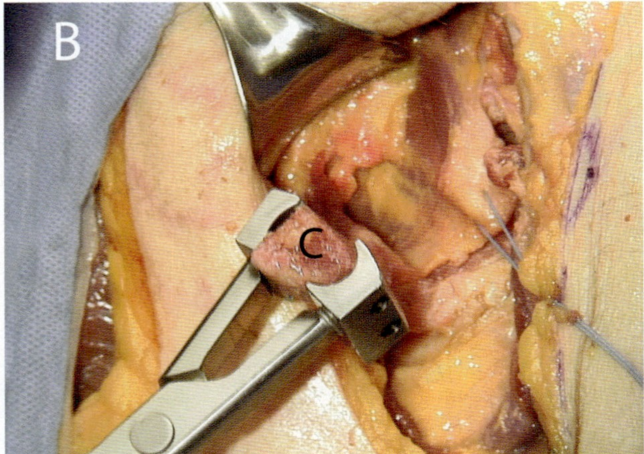

Figure 13.14 Coracoid Drill Guide. **A:** The Coracoid Drill Guide (Arthrex, Inc., Naples, FL) has slots for drilling the coracoid in preparation for Latarjet. **B:** The elongated slots are placed on the medial surface of the coracoid graft (the side that will rest against the glenoid). The guide facilitates placement of two 4-mm parallel drill holes. C, coracoid graft.

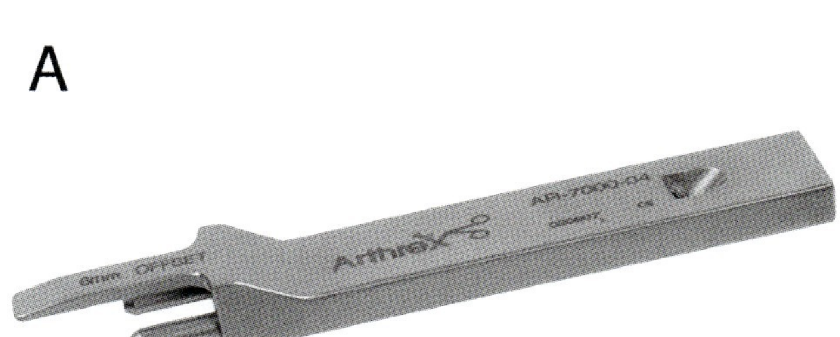

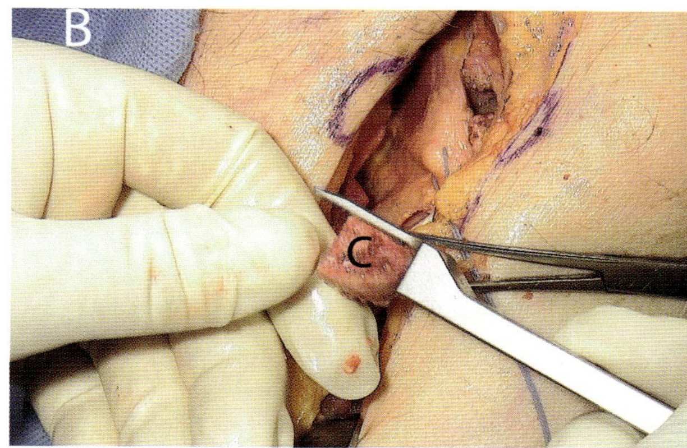

Figure 13.15 The Parallel Drill Guide (Arthrex, Inc., Naples, FL). **A:** Pegs on the guide mate with the predrilled holes in the coracoid graft. Different offsets are available to accommodate grafts of varying thickness. A 6-mm offset guide is pictured. **B:** An optimal fit occurs when the overhanging fin is flush with the coracoid graft. C, coracoid graft.

The Coracoid Drill Guide allows the surgeon to drill two parallel 4-mm holes through the graft. Care is taken to ensure that the holes are centered on the graft and are perpendicular to the prepared bone surface.

Positioning the Parallel Drill Guide on the Graft

Prior to the development of the Glenoid Bone Loss Set (Arthrex, Inc., Naples, FL), the coracoid graft had to manually be positioned on the glenoid in a freehand manner. This was technically very difficult and was not easily reproducible. The Parallel Drill Guide (Arthrex, Inc., Naples, FL) has greatly simplified this part of the procedure and has also made it very reproducible.

The pegs on the Parallel Drill Guide mate with the predrilled holes on the coracoid graft (i.e., those that were created with the Coracoid Drill Guide) to allow for easy control and positioning of the coracoid graft onto the glenoid (Fig. 13.15A).

Three offset sizes are available (4, 6, and 8 mm) to adapt to various graft diameters. Some additional shaping of the graft with a rongeur or a power burr may be required to obtain the best possible fit of the guide against the graft. An optimal fit occurs when the coracoid is flush under the overhanging offset fin once the pegs are fully engaged (Fig. 13.15B).

Positioning the Coracoid Graft on the Glenoid and Securing the Graft

The glenoid is optimally exposed by placing a Fukuda retractor to lever the humeral head posteriorly and by placing a 2-pronged Hohmann retractor medially to retract the medial soft tissues.

Proper position of the coracoid bone graft relative to the glenoid is critical. The graft must be placed so that it serves as an extension of the articular arc of the glenoid (Fig. 13.16). The Parallel Drill Guide is invaluable in placing the graft flush with the articular surface of the glenoid so that it is neither too far medial nor too far lateral (Fig. 13.17). It is important to be sure that the guide is angled slightly medially, toward the face of the glenoid, to achieve the proper screw insertion angle and to avoid any potential screw penetration into the articular cartilage.

Use a pin driver to advance the shorter (6 in) of the two guide wires directly through the lower hole of the guide and graft, and then into the glenoid neck. The guide wires are not terminally threaded to allow for better feel when the posterior glenoid cortex is penetrated. Next, advance the longer (7-in) guide wire through the second guide cannulation (Fig. 13.18A).

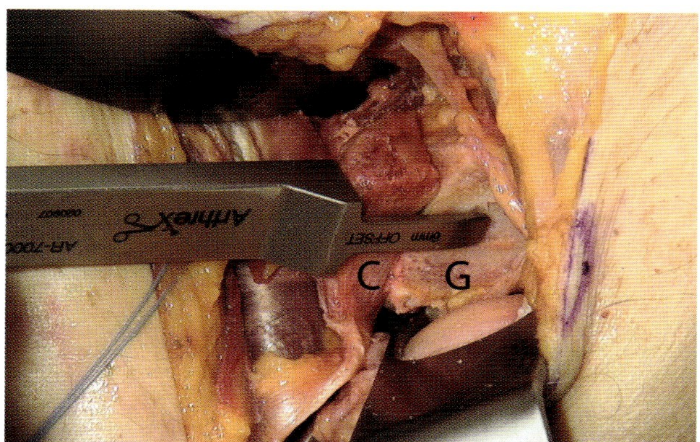

Figure 13.16 Correct placement of the coracoid bone graft occurs when the graft is flush with the glenoid surface so that the arc of the glenoid is effectively extended. The Parallel Drill Guide (Arthrex, Inc., Naples, FL) facilitates proper placement of the graft. C, coracoid graft; G, glenoid.

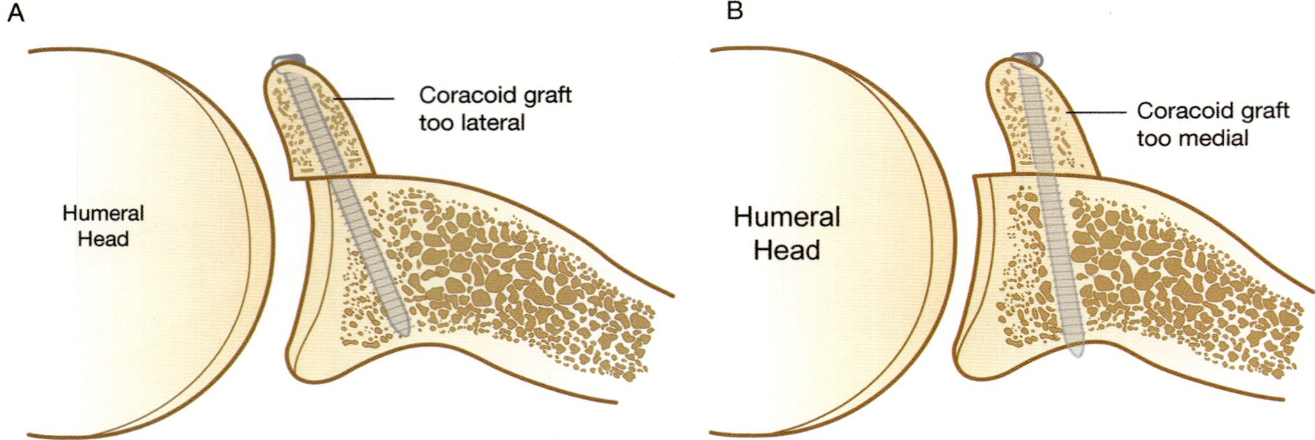

Figure 13.17 Incorrect placement of coracoid bone graft. **A:** The graft must not be placed so that it protrudes lateral to the joint surface and acts as a bone block. Such placement produces a high incidence of late osteoarthritis. **B:** Conversely, it is important also to avoid medial placement of the graft because this can predispose to recurrent dislocation or subluxation.

Next, remove the Parallel Drill Guide. Hold the graft firmly against the glenoid with an instrument (as the pegs may be tightly wedged into the coracoid drill holes) while the Parallel Drill Guide is withdrawn, leaving both guide wires in place (Fig. 13.18B). Although the 3.75-mm, fully threaded, cannulated titanium screws are self-drilling and self-tapping, it is recommended to use the 2.75-mm cannulated drill to penetrate only the near cortex of the native glenoid prior to screw insertion. Due to the potential proximity of the screws to the suprascapular nerve posteriorly, it is advisable to rely on the self-drilling and self-tapping nature of the screws to penetrate the posterior glenoid cortex.

The screw-length depth gauge can then be used to help determine the proper screw length. Screw length is read directly from the back end of the shorter 6-in guide wire, and from the laser line of the longer 7-in guide wire. We have found that the most common screw lengths are 34 mm for the more inferiorly positioned screw, and 36 mm for the superior screw.

Each screw is inserted over its guide wire using a cannulated hex driver. One must be careful not to overtighten the screws as this may crack or damage the graft. Once the screws are almost fully seated, the surgeon double-checks the position of the coracoid graft. If the position

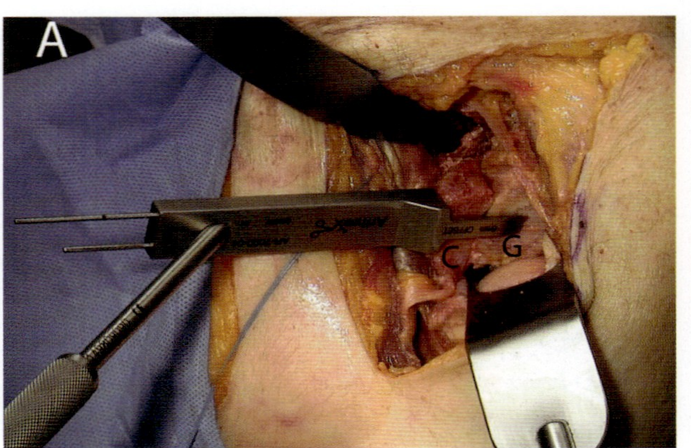

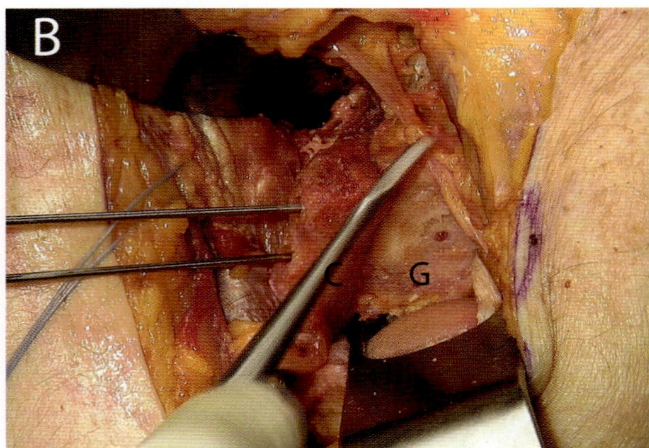

Figure 13.18 Securing the coracoid bone graft. **A:** Guide wires are inserted through the Parallel Drill Guide (Arthrex, Inc., Naples, FL) to temporarily hold the graft in place. **B:** The drill guide is removed and the appropriate screw length can be measured.

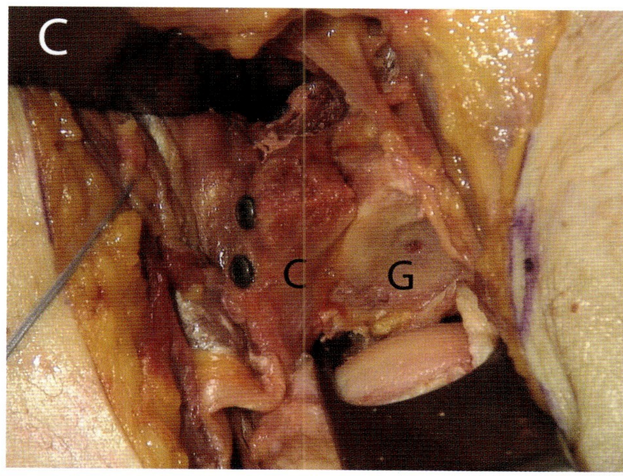

Figure 13.18 *(Continued)* **C:** Final appearance of secured graft after placement of two cannulated 3.75-mm screws. The graft is flush with the glenoid articular surface and extends the native glenoid arc. C, coracoid graft; G, glenoid.

is satisfactory, the guide pins are removed and the screws are advanced to their fully seated position (Fig. 13.18C). Intraoperative AP and axillary x-rays are taken to confirm satisfactory position of the screws and graft.

At this point, the surgeon assesses the stability of the Latarjet construct. One of the most amazing things about this construct is that, with the arm in abduction and external rotation and with a manually applied anteriorly directed force, the shoulder cannot be dislocated, even though the capsule has not yet been repaired.

Capsular Reattachment

Place 3 BioComposite SutureTak anchors (Arthrex, Inc., Naples, FL) into the native glenoid above, between, and below the cannulated screws to repair the capsule. This makes the graft an extra-articular structure and prevents its articulation directly against the humeral head, eliminating any abrasive potential of the graft against the articular cartilage of the humerus (Fig. 13.19).

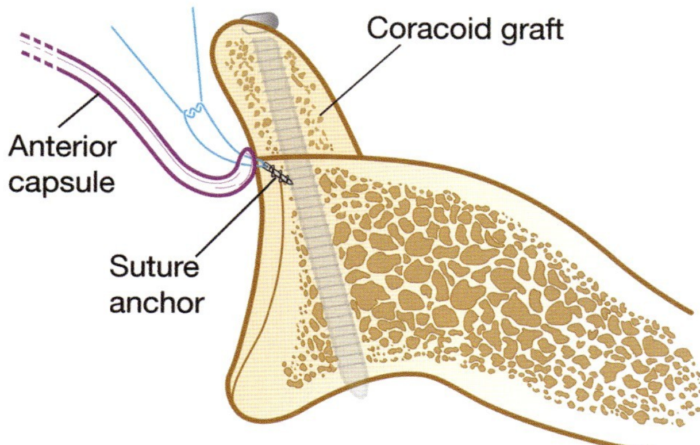

Figure 13.19 Suture anchors are placed at the interface of the graft and the native glenoid arc and are used to repair the anterior capsule so that the coracoid graft remains extra-articular.

Subscapularis Repair

If a subscapularis split has been used, the upper and lower subscapularis muscle segments will reapproximate themselves once the retractors have been removed, and no sutures are necessary. When the upper subscapularis has been detached and retracted medially during the exposure, it is usually repaired back to its stump with No. 2 FiberWire suture (Arthrex, Inc., Naples, FL). If the tendon stump is of poor quality, then BioComposite Cork-Screw FT suture anchors (Arthrex, Inc., Naples, FL) are used.

It is not necessary to reattach the pectoralis minor to the residual coracoid base or adjacent soft tissues because it does not retract. We have not observed any residual symptoms or cosmetic deformity relative to the unrepaired pectoralis minor.

After subscapularis repair, a standard skin closure is performed.

Postoperative Rehabilitation

The patient uses a sling for 6 weeks, with external rotation restricted to 0°. After 6 weeks, the sling is discontinued and overhead motion is encouraged. Gentle external rotation stretching is begun at 6 weeks postoperative, with the goal that at 3 months postoperative external rotation on the operated shoulder will be half that on the opposite shoulder. At 3 months postoperative, the patient begins strengthening with Therabands. At 6 months, he progresses to weight lifting in the gym if the graft remains in good position and shows early signs of consolidation. Contact sports or heavy labor is generally allowed when the bone graft appears radiographically healed, which is usually 9 to 12 months postoperative.

ARTHROSCOPIC REMPLISSAGE

Hill-Sachs defects definitely play a role in recurrent instability, but the treatment parameters for addressing the Hill-Sachs lesion surgically have not been well elucidated. In this section, we describe our treatment paradigm for Hill-Sachs lesions.

In 2000, Burkhart and DeBeer reported an unacceptably high recurrence rate (67%) after arthroscopic Bankart repair in patients that had "significant bone defects" (3). Significant bone defects on the glenoid side were defined as "inverted-pear" glenoids, in which there was a loss of ≥25% of the inferior glenoid diameter. On the humeral side, significant bone defects were found to be "engaging Hill-Sachs lesions," which were defined as those lesions that engaged the anterior glenoid rim in a position of athletic function (90° abduction combined with 90° external rotation).

In the 2000 paper, we did not specify the depth of the engaging Hill-Sachs lesions, though they were all >5 mm deep. With these deep engaging Hill-Sachs lesions, we found that arthroscopic Bankart repair alone was not adequate, and in subsequent patients we chose to address these lesions with open Latarjet reconstructions. This procedure was effective because, by lengthening the articular arc of the glenoid, we would prevent engagement of even the largest and deepest Hill-Sachs lesions (Fig. 13.20).

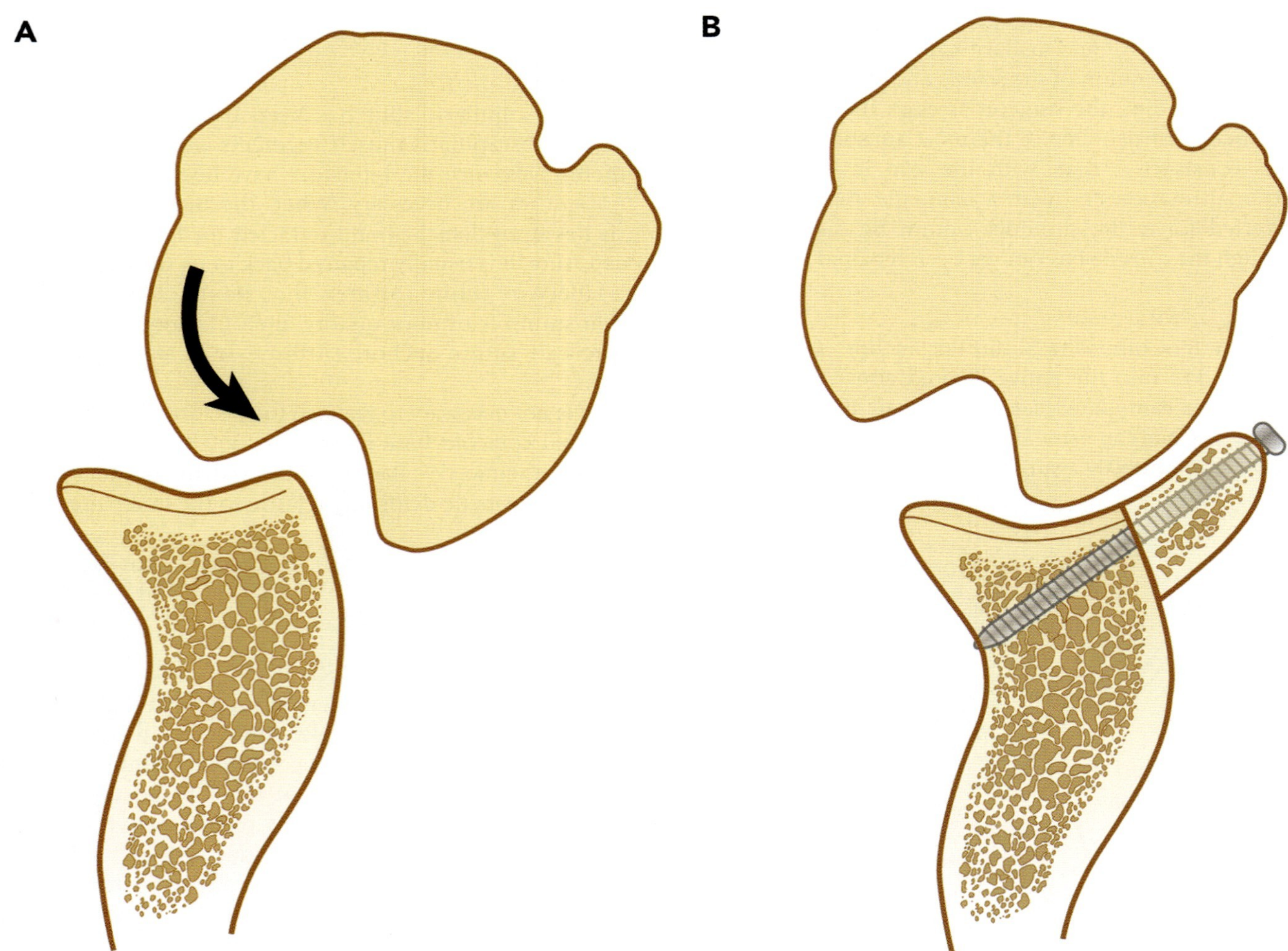

Figure 13.20 Schematic drawing demonstrating the use of a modified Latarjet procedure to lengthen the glenoid articular arc to prevent engagement of an engaging Hill-Sachs lesion. **A:** Engagement of Hill-Sachs lesion. **B:** Prevention of engagement by lengthening the glenoid articular arc.

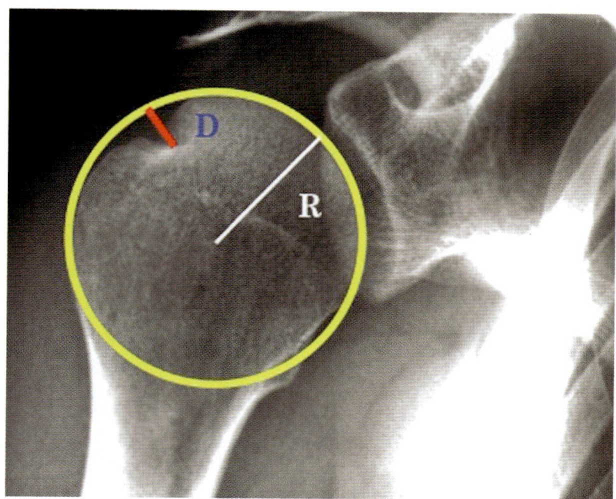

Figure 13.21 Hill-Sachs defect measured on an anterior–posterior plain radiograph with the arm in internal rotation (photo courtesy of Phillippe Hardy, MD). R, radius of humeral head; D, depth of Hill-Sachs defect.

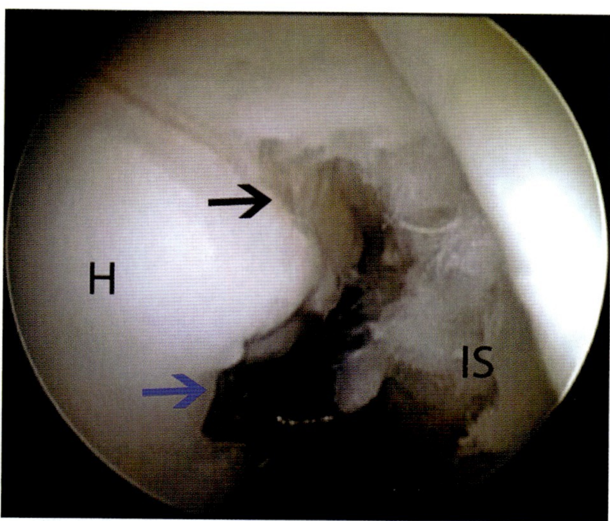

Figure 13.22 Right shoulder, anterosuperolateral viewing portal demonstrates a partial articular surface tendon tear (PASTA) of the infraspinatus (*black arrow*) in association with a Hill-Sachs lesion (*blue arrow*) in an individual with anterior instability. H, humerus; IS, infraspinatus tendon.

Hardy reported in 2009 that the depth of the Hill-Sachs lesion is important (Personal Communication). Using a standard AP x-ray taken in full internal rotation, he measured the depth of the Hill-Sachs lesion, and also determined the radius of the humeral head (Fig. 13.21). He did these measurements in 100 patients that had undergone arthroscopic Bankart repair. What he found was that in patients that had an isolated Hill-Sachs lesion with a depth >15% of the radius of the humeral head, there was a 62% failure rate (recurrent dislocation or subluxation) after arthroscopic Bankart repair. This study highlighted the fact that patients with normal glenoids and isolated Hill-Sachs lesions beyond a threshold depth of approximately 3.5 mm (15% of the radius of the average humeral head) need more than a simple arthroscopic Bankart repair. But would an adjunctive arthroscopic procedure addressing the Hill-Sachs lesion be enough? And at what point of bone loss would this combined arthroscopic approach be insufficient, and a Latarjet procedure be required?

Wolf coined the term "remplissage" (French for "filling a defect") to designate an arthroscopic procedure to fill the Hill-Sachs defect with the infraspinatus. He reported on his technique of remplissage in 2008 (11). We published our modified technique of remplissage in 2009 (12).

We developed our technique in response to a couple of observations. First of all, we noted that many Hill-Sachs lesions were associated with PASTA lesions of the infraspinatus (Fig. 13.22). Therefore, it made sense to repair this PASTA lesion by insetting the infraspinatus into the Hill-Sachs defect to restore its function in addition to providing a mechanical block to engagement of the Hill-Sachs lesion. By means of remplissage, the Hill-Sachs lesion was converted to an extra-articular bone defect that could no longer engage the intra-articular corner of the glenoid.

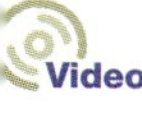

Secondly, we noted that the dramatically large and deep (>1 cm deep) Hill-Sachs lesions were virtually always accompanied by inverted-pear glenoids. Therefore, based on our glenoid bone loss criteria, we always treated these combined deep Hill-Sachs lesions and glenoid lesions with open Latarjet procedures. However, the moderately deep Hill-Sachs lesions (3 to 7 mm in depth) sometimes did not coexist with inverted-pear glenoids.

Based on these observations, we began doing our remplissage technique in selected patients. Our indications for a combined arthroscopic Bankart repair and arthroscopic remplissage are in patients that have

1. *No* significant glenoid bone loss (i.e., *no* inverted pear)
2. Hill-Sachs lesion between 3 and 7 mm in depth (these may be either engaging or nonengaging Hill-Sachs lesions)

Technique of Arthroscopic Remplissage

This procedure, like all of our arthroscopic shoulder procedures, is done with the patient in the lateral decubitus position. We begin with three standard portals: posterior, anterior, and anterosuperolateral.

Viewing from an anterosuperolateral portal, the glenoid is visualized and evaluated for bone loss (Fig. 13.23). If there is >25% loss of the inferior glenoid diameter, the procedure is converted to an open Latarjet reconstruction. Next, arthroscopic evaluation is continued as the arm is removed from its

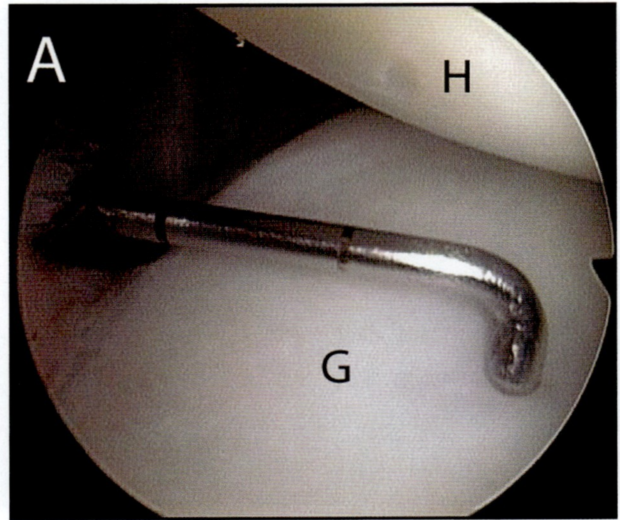

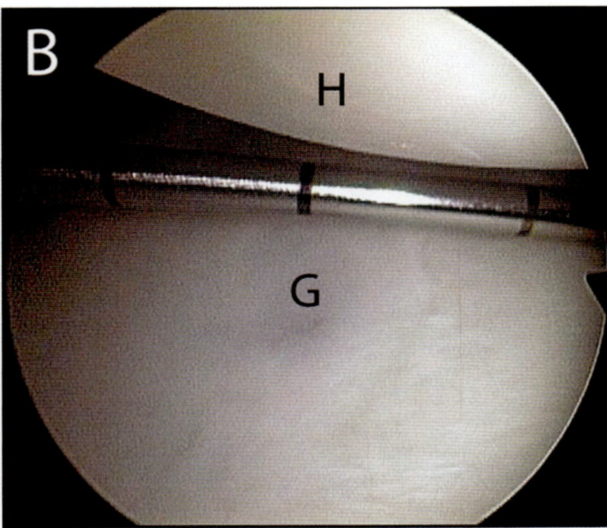

Figure 13.23 Left shoulder anterosuperolateral portal demonstrating absence of glenoid bone loss in an individual with anterior glenohumeral instability. **A:** A calibrated probe inserted from a posterior portal measures a distance of 10 mm from the bare area to the posterior glenoid rim. **B:** The distance from the anterior glenoid rim to the bare area is also 10 mm. G, glenoid; H, humerus.

balanced suspension and is rotated as it is brought through a range of abduction. This allows assessment of the position of engagement of the Hill-Sachs lesion as well as its depth (Fig. 13.24). If there is no significant glenoid bone loss and if the Hill-Sachs lesion is between 3 and 7 mm deep, we proceed with an arthroscopic Bankart repair and remplissage.

The Bankart lesion is addressed first, with anchor placement and suture passage, but the knots are not tied until after the remplissage anchors have been placed. The reason for this sequence is that the anteriorly directed forces associated with placing suture anchors in the back of the humerus can disrupt the suture fixation of the labrum if the Bankart knots are tied before placing the Hill-Sachs anchors.

For the remplissage, the bone bed in the Hill-Sachs lesion is prepared by means of ring curettes placed through

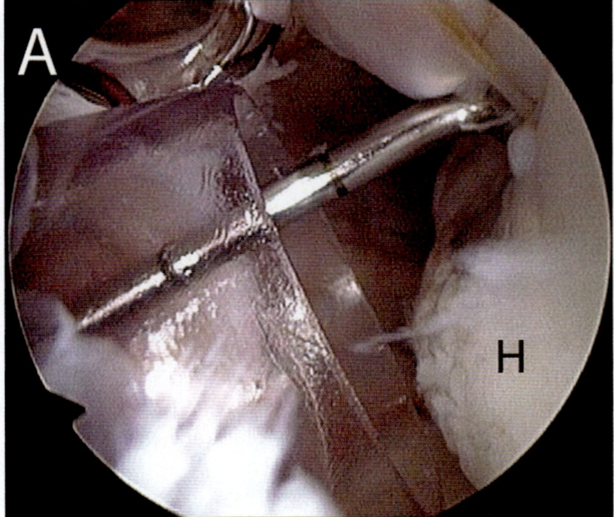

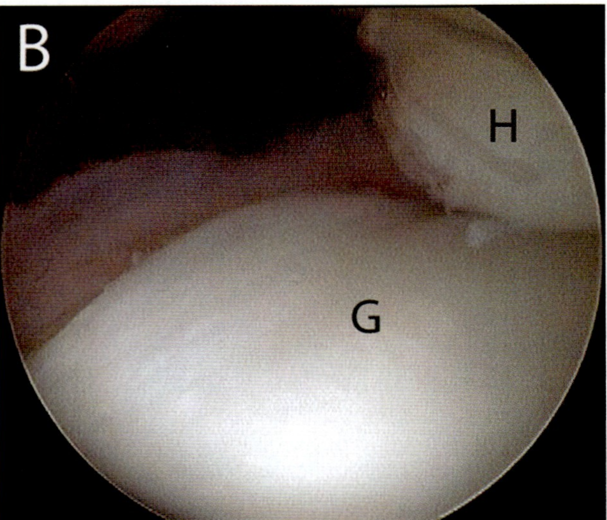

Figure 13.24 Left shoulder, anterosuperolateral viewing portal demonstrates a Hill-Sachs lesion amenable to remplissage. **A:** A calibrated probe inserted from a posterior portal estimates the depth of the lesion to be 5 mm. **B:** Removing the arm from traction and placing it in the 90-90 position demonstrates that the Hill-Sachs lesion does not engage the anterior glenoid. G, glenoid; H, humerus.

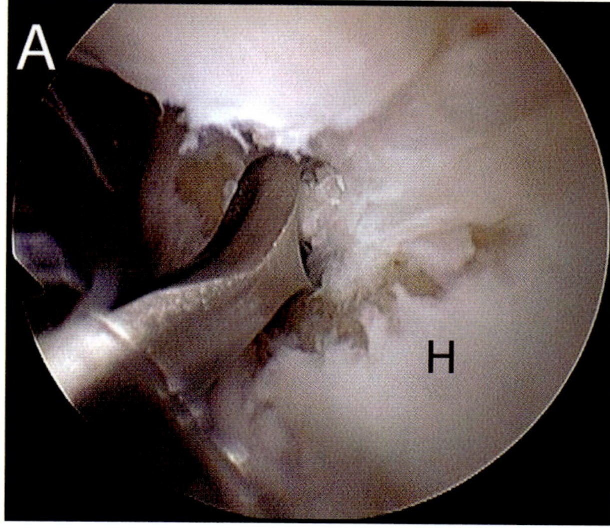

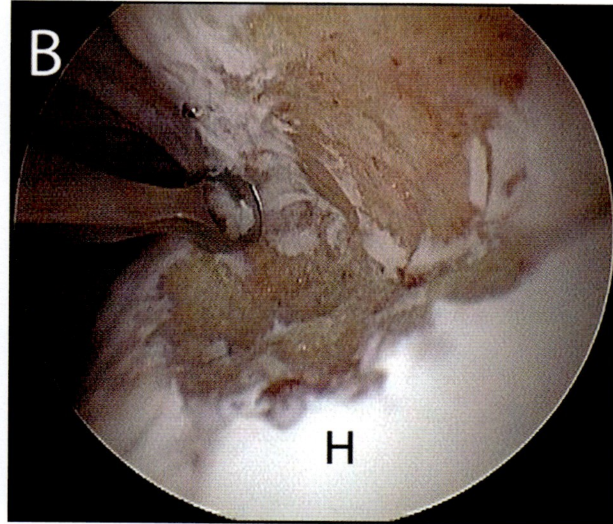

Figure 13.25 Left shoulder, anterosuperolateral viewing portal demonstrating bone bed preparation of the Hill-Sachs lesion **A:** A ring curette is introduced from a posterior portal and used to remove soft tissue. **B:** Completely prepared bone bed of a Hill-Sachs lesion. H, humerus.

a posterior working portal while viewing from the anterosuperolateral portal (Fig. 13.25).

Next, the subacromial space is prepared. Bursa and fibrofatty tissue are removed by alternating between posterior and lateral portals for viewing and working. Care is taken to clear out the posterior gutter so that the entire infraspinatus tendon can be visualized.

The arthroscope is then reinserted intra-articularly through the anterosuperolateral viewing portal. The concept of our technique of remplissage is to inset the infraspinatus *tendon* into the Hill-Sachs defect, in contradistinction to other methods that insert capsule and muscle into the defect. This means that our sutures must obtain fixation more laterally than these other techniques, in order to ensure capture of the tendon rather than muscle.

Continuing to view through an anterosuperolateral portal, we next place two spinal needles percutaneously through the infraspinatus tendon, at a 30° to 45° angle to the Hill-Sachs lesion. The humerus may be internally or externally rotated to provide a better angle of approach to the bone (Fig. 13.26A). We then use a 5-mm transtendon metal cannula (Arthrex, Inc., Naples, FL) parallel to each of

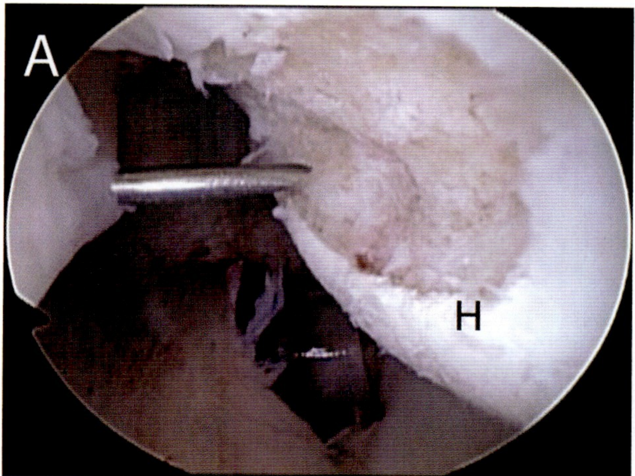

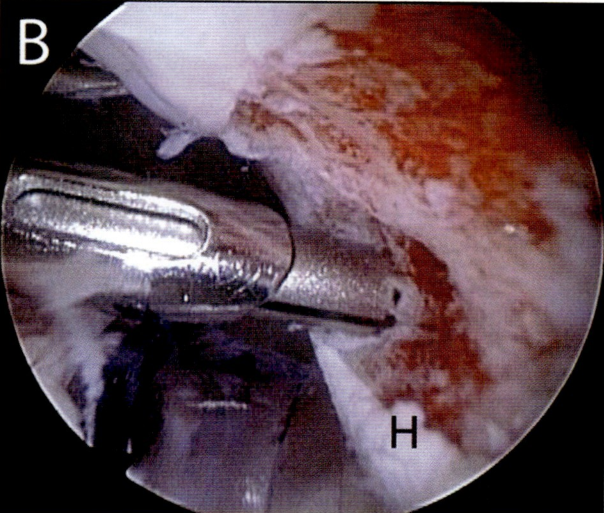

Figure 13.26 Left shoulder, anterosuperolateral viewing portal demonstrating percutaneous placement of suture anchors for remplissage. **A:** A spinal needle is used as a guide to establish the proper angle of approach to the Hill-Sachs lesion. **B:** An inferior anchor is placed transtendon with the use of a metal cannula.

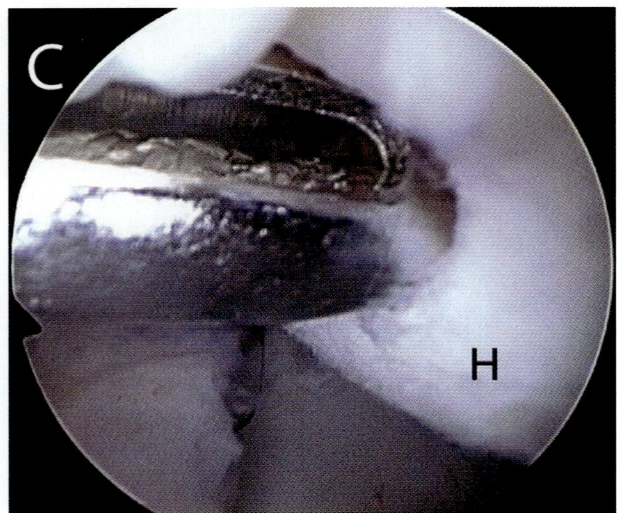

Figure 13.26 *(Continued)* **C:** Using the same technique, a second anchor is placed in the bone bed superior to the first anchor. H, humerus.

the two spinal needles to place two suture anchors, one at the top of the Hill-Sachs lesion and the other at the bottom (Fig. 13.26B, C). A Spear drill-guide (Arthrex, Inc., Naples, FL) is used to stabilize the drill for creating the sockets for insertion of double-loaded BioComposite SutureTak suture anchors (Arthrex, Inc., Naples, FL). In some cases, anchor placement requires an angle of approach that begins too far lateral for the anchors to be placed transtendon. In this case, the solution is to place the anchors through the posterior portal, then perform retrograde retrieval of the sutures of each anchor through two separate transtendon passes with a Penetrator (Arthrex, Inc., Naples, FL) (Fig. 13.27). In either case, by placing the anchors transtendon or retrieving the sutures transtendon in this way, all four suture limbs from a given anchor will exit the same point in the tendon. Then, the *double-pulley* repair technique is used to complete the remplissage. However, prior to completing the remplissage, one should tie the knots for the Bankart repair so that subacromial fluid extravasation during the remplissage will not compromise the space required for Bankart repair.

To inset the infraspinatus tendon into the Hill-Sachs lesion, we use the same double-pulley technique that we

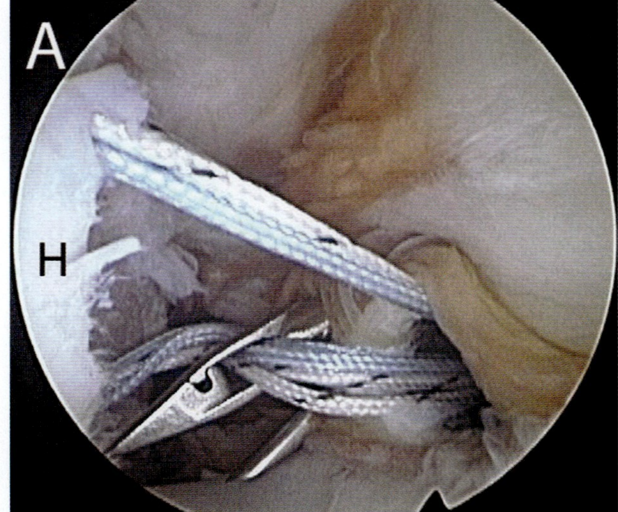

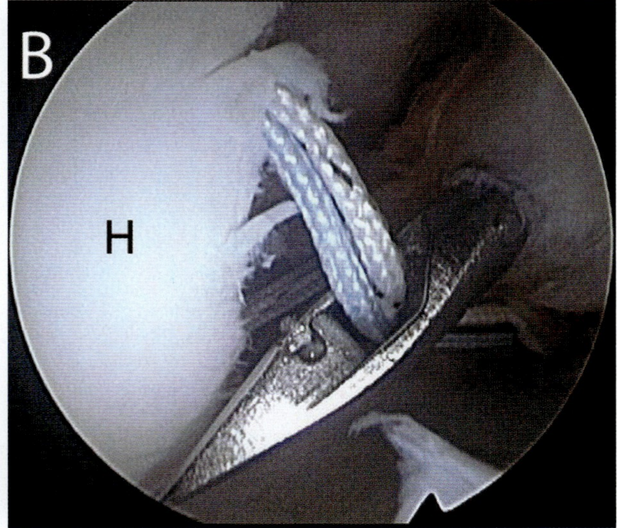

Figure 13.27 Right shoulder, anterosuperolateral portal demonstrating suture passage for remplissage using a retrograde technique. **A:** Sutures are seen exiting a posterior portal following anchor placement via the posterior portal. Using a spinal needle as a guide, the inferior sutures are passed through the infraspinatus tendon with a Penetrator (Arthrex, Inc., Naples, FL). **B:** The superior sutures are passed. H, humerus.

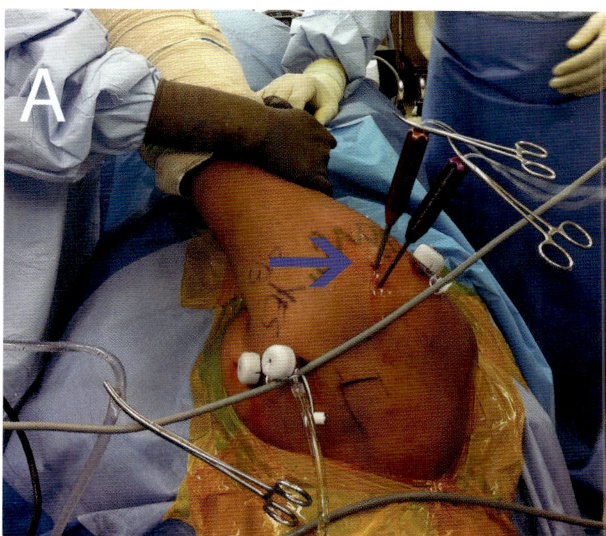

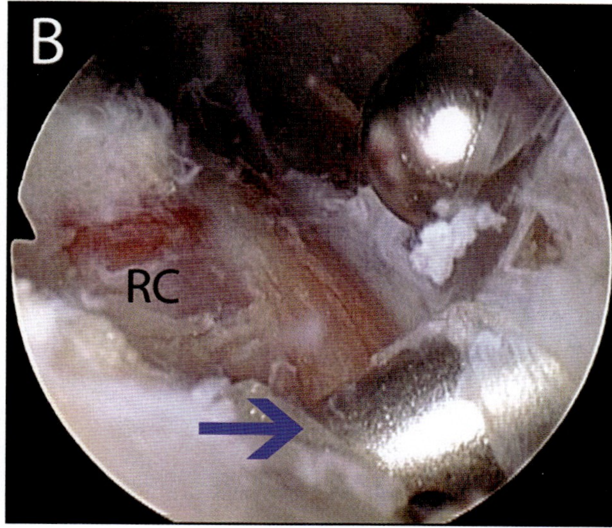

Figure 13.28 Right shoulder demonstrating use of Spear guides to locate and protect remplissage sutures. **A:** External view shows Spear guides (*blue arrow*) in place over sutures passed through the infraspinatus tendon. **B:** Lateral subacromial view in the same shoulder. The Spear guide (*blue arrow*) protects the sutures as a shaver clears the bursa overlying the muscle and tendon. RC, rotator cuff.

use for PASTA repairs (see Chapter 5, "Partial Thickness Rotator Cuff Tears"). This technique entails creating two double-mattress sutures between the two anchors by tying the sutures of one anchor to those of the other anchor. Subacromial viewing is done either through a posterior or a lateral subacromial portal, depending on which one gives the best view. Although a bursectomy has been previously performed in order to aid in visualizing the sutures, placing Spear guides over the sutures is helpful for protecting and locating the sutures (Fig. 13.28).

One suture limb of a given color from each anchor is retrieved through the working cannula. Then, outside the patient's body, these two suture limbs are tied to each other over the top of a rigid instrument by means of a six-throw surgeon's knot. Next, the two corresponding "free" limbs are tensioned and pulled, using the suture anchors' eyelets like pulleys, to pull the knot into the subacromial space and onto the top of the infraspinatus tendon (Fig. 13.29). Then, the two "free" limbs are tied together with a static six-throw surgeon's knot using the Surgeon's Sixth Finger Knot Pusher

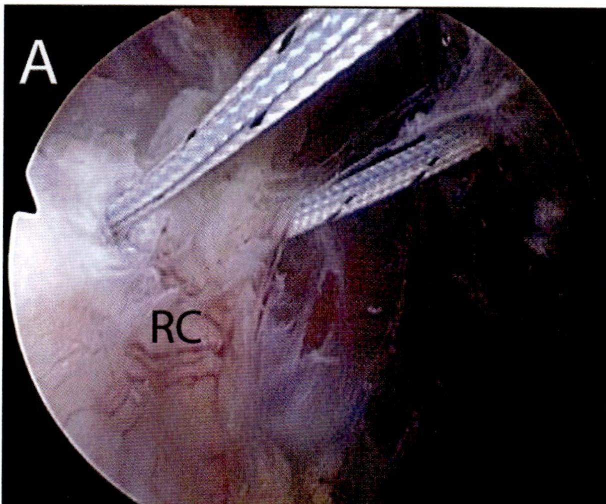

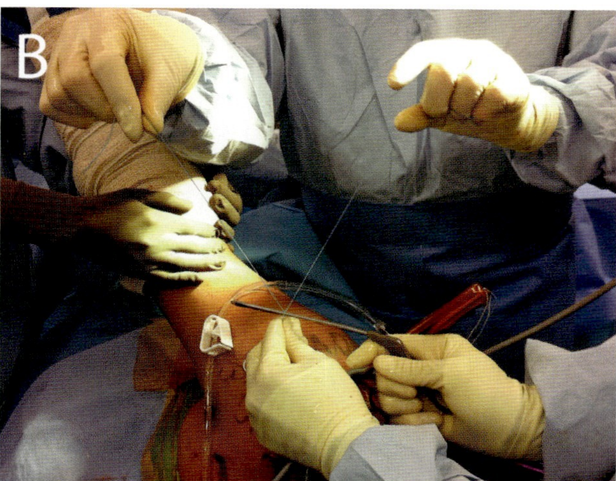

Figure 13.29 The double-pulley technique for remplissage in a right shoulder. **A:** Lateral subacromial viewing portal. Sutures from two anchors placed in a Hill-Sachs lesion are visualized in the subacromial space passing through the infraspinatus. **B:** A single blue suture limb from each anchor is retrieved and extracorporeally tied over an instrument.

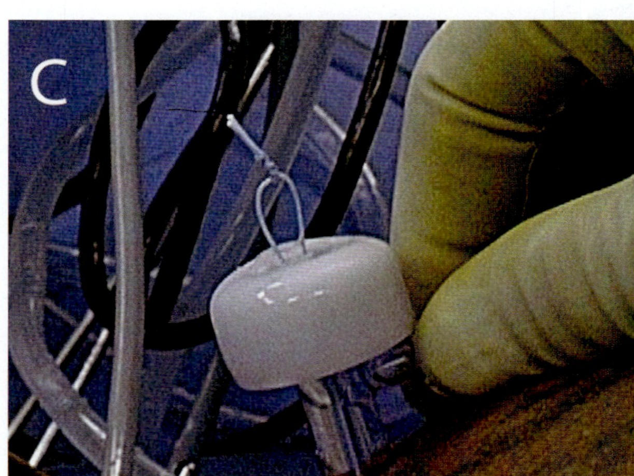

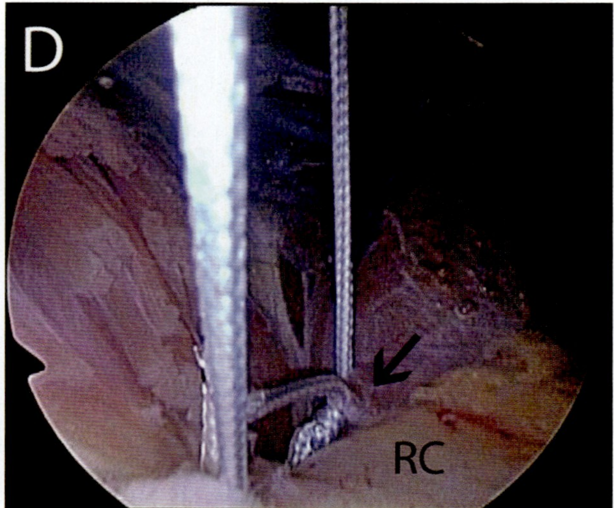

Figure 13.29 *(Continued)* **C:** The suture limbs are cut and the knot is delivered back into the subacromial space by pulling on the opposite blue suture limbs. **D:** The first knot now rests on the infraspinatus. The remaining suture limbs may be retrieved and tied as a static knot to complete the double pulley. RC, rotator cuff.

(Arthrex, Inc., Naples, FL). It should be noted that this second knot must be a static knot; a sliding knot cannot be tied here because the other two suture limbs of this pair have already been fixed with a knot that will prevent sliding. Finally, the two other suture pairs are tied with the *double-pulley* technique in the same way as the first two suture pairs, creating another double-mattress configuration. Then, we again look intra-articularly to be sure that the tendon has inset all the way into the Hill-Sachs lesion (Fig. 13.30B).

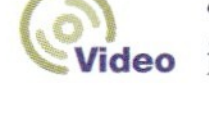

Postoperatively, we keep the patient in a sling for 6 weeks and then begin a stretching program. We do not start strengthening until 12 weeks post-op. The rationale for the delayed strengthening is that for rehabilitation considerations, we view remplissage in the same way as an infraspinatus tendon repair, and for rotator cuff repairs we do not allow strengthening until 12 weeks post-op with this regimen. We have not observed clinically significant loss of internal or external rotation after remplissage. However, we have not done remplissage in an overhead athlete, and we suspect it would affect the amount of combined abduction-external rotation that could be achieved in the late cocking phase of throwing.

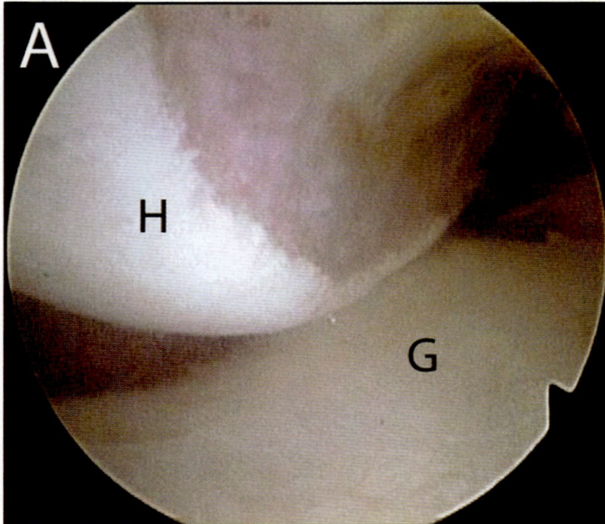

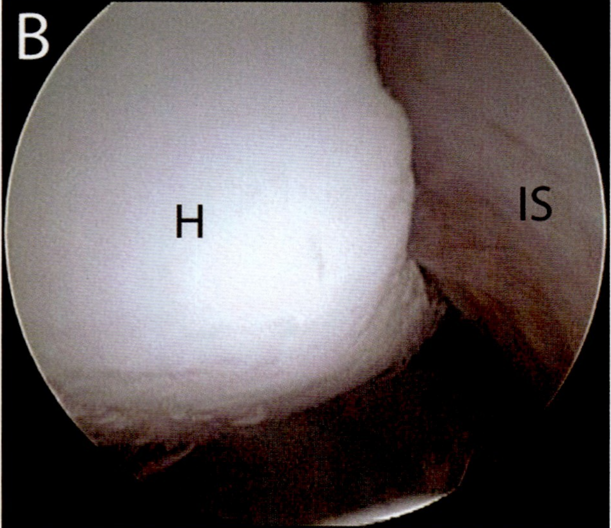

Figure 13.30 **A:** Right shoulder, anterosuperolateral portal demonstrating a Hill-Sachs lesion. **B:** Following a remplissage, the infraspinatus fills the defect so that the lesion is now extra-articular.

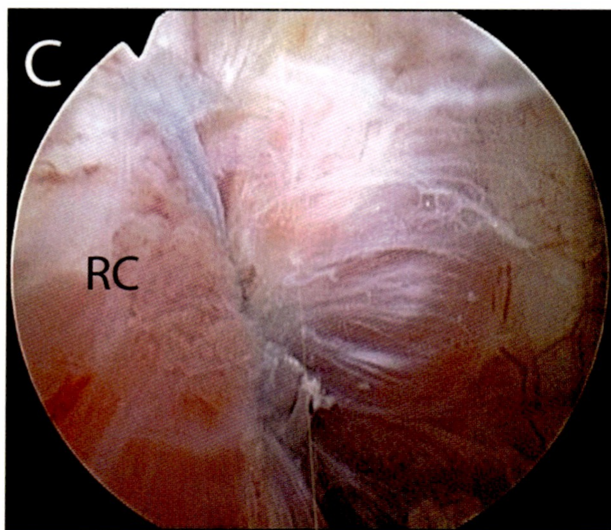

Figure 13.30 *(Continued)* **C:** Posterior subacromial viewing portal in the same shoulder after remplissage showing the mattress sutures tied with a double-pulley technique. G, glenoid; H, humerus; IS, infraspinatus tendon; RC, rotator cuff.

ARTHROSCOPIC ILIAC CREST BONE GRAFT

In some situations (e.g., coracoid fracture or failed Latarjet) when restoration of glenoid bone stock is required, a graft from a source other than the coracoid must be used. In this scenario, an arthroscopic bone grafting procedure can be performed. Graft options include an iliac crest autograft or fresh frozen distal tibia allograft. Although distal tibia allograft has demonstrated a similar contour to the glenoid, we prefer an iliac crest autograft because of the higher reported healing rate with autograft. This is particularly important in light of the fact that our indication for either is most often a revision. In our experience, the most common indications for a graft source other than the coracoid are when the coracoid is not available (e.g., coracoid fracture, previous Bristow or Latarjet procedure), or if a massive amount of bone is required (i.e., >15 mm) and there is concern that the coracoid will not provide sufficient bone stock. However, in the latter scenario, due to the large size of the graft, arthroscopic placement is more difficult. Other considerations include the ability to preserve the subscapularis tendon (particularly in revision of previous open cases) and the minimal distortion of local anatomy. We do not currently recommend arthroscopic bone grafting as a primary procedure. First, the procedure is technically challenging. Second, graft site morbidity from an iliac crest bone graft is a significant disadvantage and may be unacceptable in some patients. Third, and most importantly, while biomechanical studies have demonstrated that a coracoid graft, iliac crest graft, and distal tibia allograft all restore contact area and contact pressure, it is our strong opinion that the addition of the conjoined tendon (i.e., Latarjet) improves graft site healing and dynamic stability of the glenohumeral joint.

Technique of Iliac Crest Bone Graft

Bone Graft Harvest

Due to swelling that may occur during initial diagnostic arthroscopy and debridement, we prefer to harvest the iliac crest bone graft prior to arthroscopy. If, however, there is any question as to the amount of bone loss or the indication for a bone grafting procedure, an expedient diagnostic arthroscopy can be performed initially. Patients are placed in the standard lateral decubitus position. Using a standard incision parallel to the crest of the iliac wing and approximately 2 cm posterior to the anterior superior iliac spine, the iliac crest is exposed. A bicortical bone graft of approximately 20 mm × 15 mm × 15 mm is harvested. The graft is harvested from the area of the iliac crest to provide the optimal thickness of the graft. The iliac crest graft is then contoured to the appropriate size and No. 2 FiberWire sutures (Arthrex, Inc., Naples, FL) are passed through the leading and trailing edges of the graft (Fig. 13.31).

Glenohumeral Arthroscopy

Glenohumeral arthroscopy is then performed and the standard three glenohumeral portals are established (anterior, posterior, anterosuperolateral). The glenohumeral

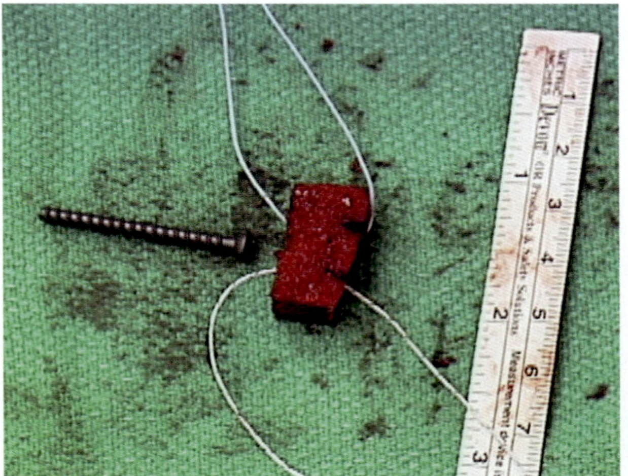

Figure 13.31 An iliac crest bone graft is harvested and free sutures are passed through it after predrilling.

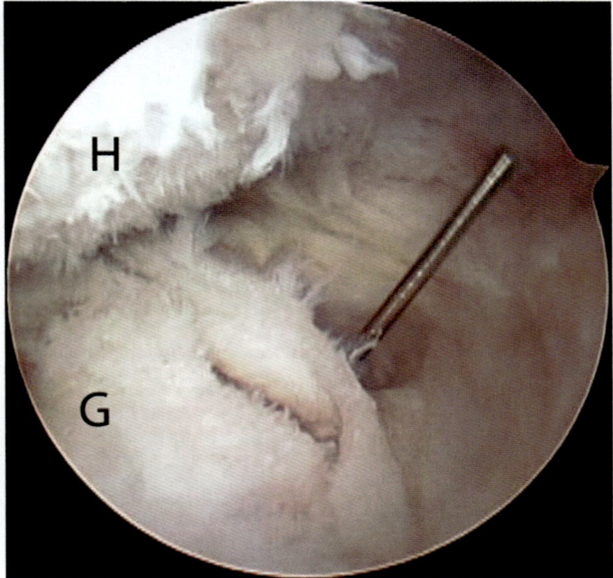

Figure 13.33 Arthroscopic photo of a left shoulder from an anterosuperolateral portal. A spinal needle is used to locate the approximate angle of approach for eventual cannulated screw fixation. G, glenoid; H, humerus.

joint is viewed through the anterosuperolateral portal, and the amount of bone loss and the need for a bone restoring procedure are confirmed. Any concomitant lesions are treated. In the revision setting, prominent bone anchors from previous reconstruction may require removal (Fig. 13.32).

Prior to mobilization of the Bankart lesion, the approximate angle of approach for eventual percutaneous fixation using cannulated screws is determined. While viewing through the anterosuperolateral portal, an 18-gauge spinal needle or 1.6-mm guide wire is placed percutaneously into the glenohumeral joint in the appropriate position for fixation of the graft (Fig. 13.33). This is performed first since swelling of the capsule and shoulder can make locating the angle of approach and percutaneous fixation difficult.

The Bankart lesion is then mobilized using an arthroscopic elevator and shaver. It is important to widely mobilize the labrum beyond the 6 o'clock position and expose the subscapularis muscle beneath the labrum (Fig. 13.34). When mobilizing the labrum for a grafting procedure the

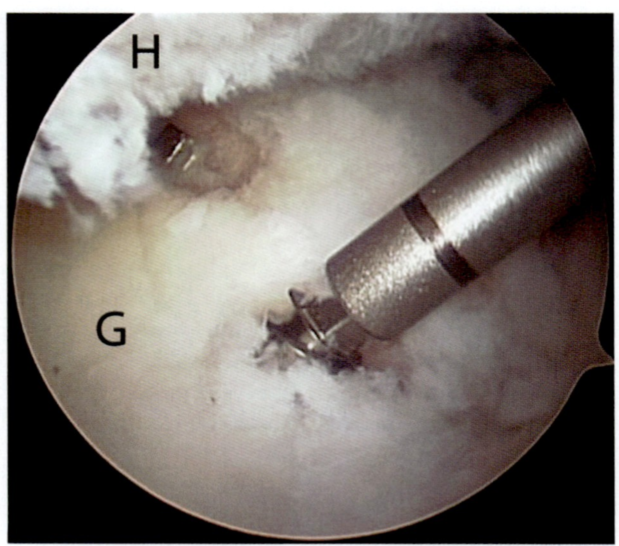

Figure 13.32 Arthroscopic photo of a left shoulder from an anterosuperolateral portal. Prominent metallic bone anchors from a previous surgery are removed. G, glenoid; H, humerus.

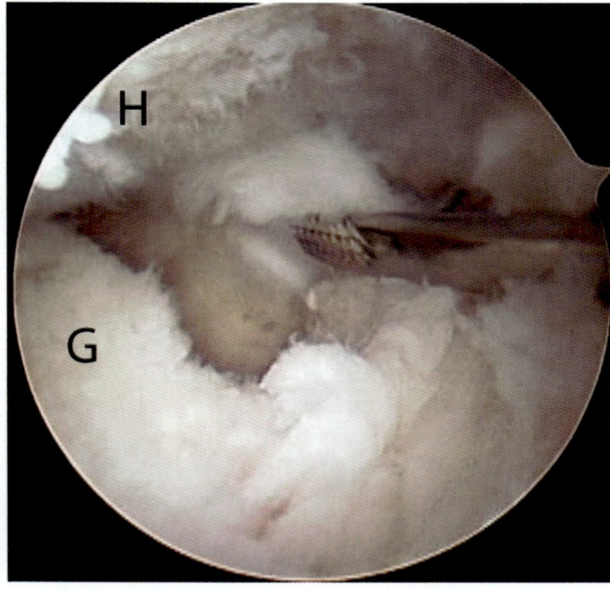

Figure 13.34 Arthroscopic photo of a left shoulder from an anterosuperolateral portal. The anteroinferior labrum is widely mobilized to accommodate an iliac crest bone graft. G, glenoid; H, humerus.

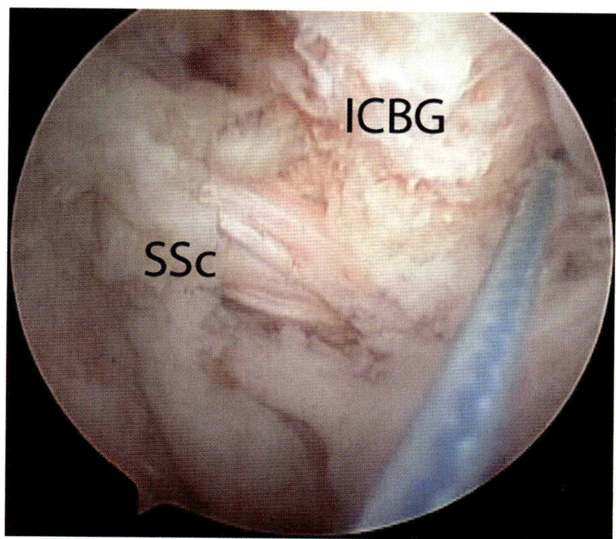

Figure 13.35 Arthroscopic photo of a left shoulder from the posterior portal demonstrating the iliac crest graft passing through the rotator interval. ICBG, iliac crest bone graft; SSc, subscapularis tendon.

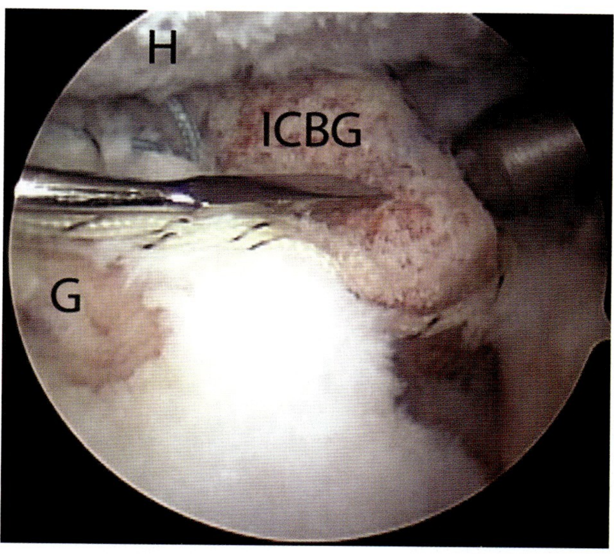

Figure 13.37 Arthroscopic photo of a left shoulder from an anterosuperolateral portal. The graft is held in place with an instrument introduced from the posterior portal. Then, a guide wire secures the graft to the glenoid neck using a nested drill guide introduced anteriorly alongside the previously placed spinal needle (see Fig. 13.33).

labrum must be mobilized to provide a tension-free repair but also to accommodate the size of the graft. The anterior glenoid is debrided to provide a flat surface for bone-to-bone apposition.

The iliac crest graft is then shuttled into the glenohumeral joint. The arthroscope is reintroduced into the posterior portal and a shaver and electrocautery are utilized to resect the rotator interval widely to accommodate insertion of the graft. Care is taken to preserve the upper border of the subscapularis tendon, the medial sling of the biceps tendon and the middle glenohumeral ligament. A Kelly clamp is then used to dilate the passage through the skin, subcutaneous tissue, and deltoid. The arthroscope is returned to the anterosuperolateral portal. The leading graft sutures are passed into the joint and retrieved through the posterior portal. Using

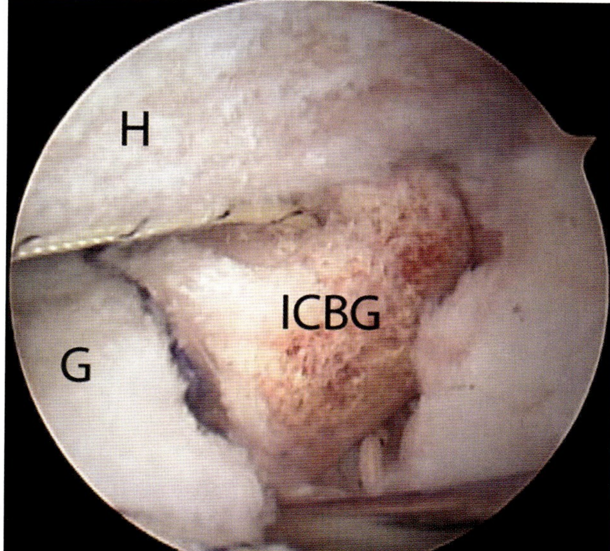

Figure 13.36 Arthroscopic photo of a left shoulder from an anterosuperolateral portal. The iliac crest bone graft is manipulated into place against the anterior inferior glenoid neck. G, glenoid; H, humerus; ICBG, iliac crest bone graft.

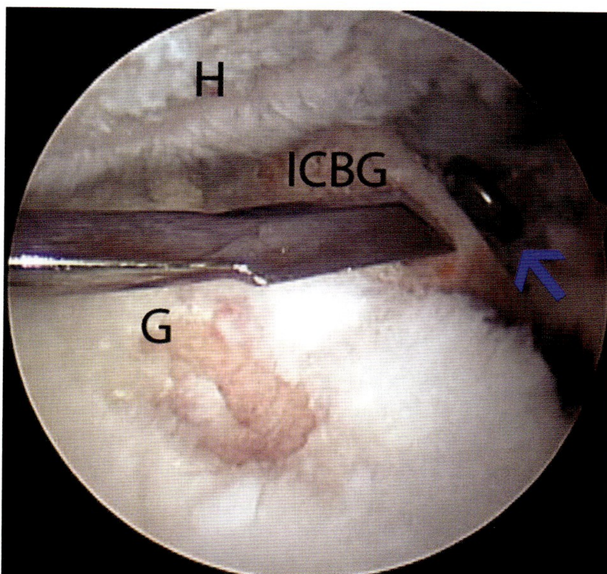

Figure 13.38 Arthroscopic photo of a left shoulder from an anterosuperolateral portal. A cannulated screw (*blue arrow*) has been placed over a guide wire to secure the iliac crest bone graft to the anterior glenoid. G, glenoid; H, humerus; ICBG, iliac crest bone graft.

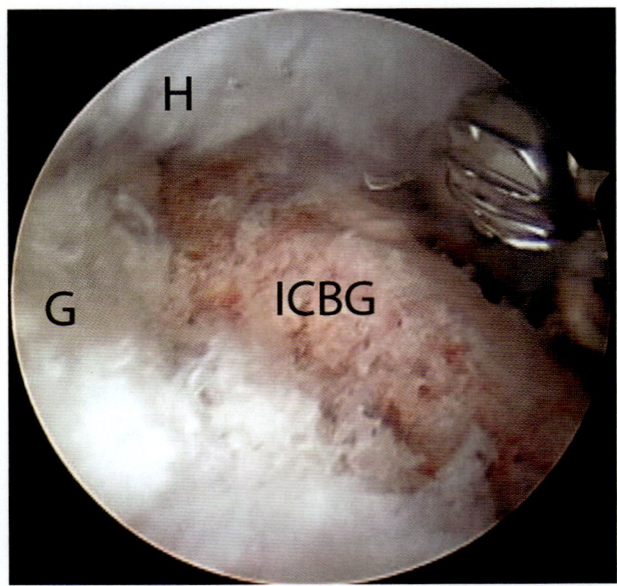

Figure 13.39 Arthroscopic photo of a left shoulder from an anterosuperolateral portal. After the iliac crest graft is secured, final contouring may be performed with a burr to eliminate any lateral overhang and create a congruent arc. G, glenoid; H, humerus; ICBG, iliac crest bone graft.

Figure 13.40 Arthroscopic photo of a left shoulder from an anterosuperolateral portal demonstrating final appearance after arthroscopic placement of an iliac bone graft. G, glenoid; H, humerus; ICBG, iliac crest bone graft.

a combination of traction on the leading sutures, and a Kelly clamp, the graft is introduced into the glenohumeral joint (Fig. 13.35). A Shoehorn cannula (Arthrex, Inc., Naples, FL) may also be used to assist passage of the bone graft through the soft tissues.

Once inside the joint, the iliac crest graft is manipulated into place using a switching stick or a grasper (Fig. 13.36). Correct orientation and placement of the graft is confirmed from posterior, anterior, and anterosuperolateral views. It is important to ensure that the graft is not prominent.

While viewing through the anterosuperolateral portal, two 1.6-mm guide wires are placed into the correct orientation. Nested Drill Guides (Bone Loss Set; Arthrex, Inc., Naples, FL) are then used to dilate the soft tissue passage (Fig. 13.37) and the 1.6-mm guide wires are passed through the graft and glenoid neck. The screw length is then measured using the screw sizer. Then a 2.75-mm drill is used to drill the graft and the near cortex of the anterior glenoid, and a 3.75-mm screw of the appropriate length is inserted. To assist in visualization, the inferior screw is placed first followed by the superior screw (Fig. 13.38).

Final graft alignment is then assessed. A switching stick introduced from the posterior portal and tangential to the glenoid face may be used to assess whether the graft is prominent (Fig. 13.39). Final contouring may be achieved using a burr from the anterior portal (Fig. 13.40).

Two or three BioComposite SutureTak anchors (Arthrex, Inc., Naples, FL) are then inserted into the native glenoid rim and used to repair the Bankart lesion to the native glenoid rim creating an extra-articular graft.

REFERENCES

1. Edwards TB, Boulahia A, Walch G. Radiographic analysis of bone defects in chronic anterior shoulder instability. *Arthroscopy* 2003;19:732–739.
2. Sugaya H, Moriishi J, Dohi M, et al. Glenoid rim morphology in recurrent anterior glenohumeral instability. *J Bone Joint Surg Am* 2003;85:878–884.
3. Burkhart SS, De Beer JF. Traumatic glenohumeral bone defects and their relationship to failure of arthroscopic Bankart repairs: significance of the inverted-pear glenoid and the humeral engaging Hill-Sachs lesion. *Arthroscopy* 2000;16:677–694.
4. Boileau P, Villalba M, Hery JY, et al. Risk factors for recurrence of shoulder instability after arthroscopic Bankart repair. *J Bone Joint Surg Am* 2006;88:1755–1763.
5. Burkhart SS, De Beer JF, Barth JR, et al. Results of modified Latarjet reconstruction in patients with anteroinferior instability and significant bone loss. *Arthroscopy* 2007;23:1033–1041.
6. Chuang TY, Adams CR, Burkhart SS. Use of preoperative three-dimensional computed tomography to quantify glenoid bone loss in shoulder instability. *Arthroscopy* 2008;24:376–382.
7. Burkhart SS, DeBeer JF, Tehrany AM, et al. Quantifying glenoid bone loss arthroscopically in shoulder instability. *Arthroscopy* 2002;18:488–491.
8. Arrigoni P, Huberty D, Brady PC, et al. The value of arthroscopy before an open modified latarjet reconstruction. *Arthroscopy* 2008;24:514–519.
9. Allain J, Goutallier D, Glorion C. Long-term results of the Latarjet procedure for the treatment of anterior instability of the shoulder. *J Bone Joint Surg Am* 1998;80:841–852.
10. Ghodadra N, Gupta A, Romeo AA, et al. Normalization of glenohumeral articular contact pressures after Latarjet or iliac crest bone-grafting. *J Bone Joint Surg Am* 2010;92:1478–1489.
11. Purchase RJ, Wolf EM, Hobgood ER, et al. Hill-sachs "remplissage": an arthroscopic solution for the engaging hill-sachs lesion. *Arthroscopy* 2008;24:723–726.
12. Koo SS, Burkhart SS, Ochoa E. Arthroscopic double-pulley remplissage technique for engaging Hill-Sachs lesions in anterior shoulder instability repairs. *Arthroscopy* 2009;25:1343–1348.

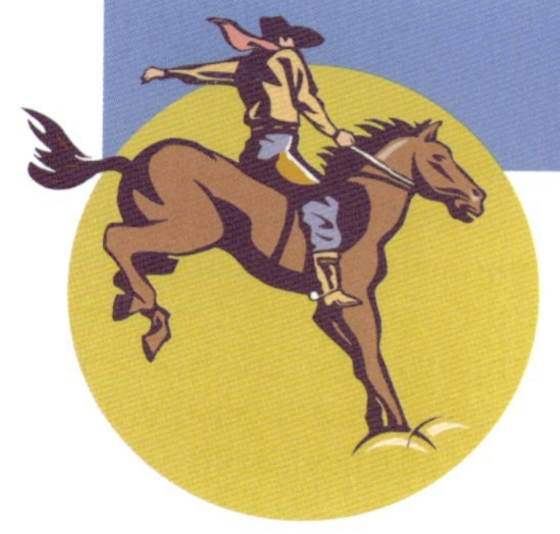

14

Unusual Instability Patterns

WESTERN WISDOM

Waitin' to climb a hill don't make it smaller.

While the majority of glenohumeral instability is anterior, the arthroscopist must also be adept at recognizing and treating unusual patterns of instability including posterior instability, triple labral lesions, humeral-sided capsuloligamentous disruption, and multidirectional instability. Because these patterns are less common, they can often go unrecognized or be misdiagnosed. Furthermore, their repair techniques are less familiar to surgeons than techniques for standard Bankart repair. Each pattern presents unique technical challenges that are discussed below.

POSTERIOR INSTABILITY REPAIR

Patients with posterior instability commonly present with one or both of two major complaints: posterior pain and posterior instability. These two symptoms should be clearly delineated and may assist the surgeon in making the appropriate preoperative and intraoperative treatment decisions. Furthermore, many patients may present with similar symptoms but with diverse pathologies (e.g., nonlabral tear instability, osteochondral defects, and glenoid version abnormalities). Although the vast majority of patients with posterior instability may be treated arthroscopically, certain patients may not be reliably treated arthroscopically and may require open posterior bone grafting (e.g., glenoid version abnormality).

Patients with posterior pain commonly present with a history of an acute traumatic injury (e.g., defensive lineman with posterior translational load), complaints of pain along the posterior joint line with activities (e.g., bench press, overhead press, dips), a positive relocation sign for pain (i.e., similar to a posterior SLAP lesion), pain with posterior load and shift, and a tear of the posterior labrum but with minimal signs of true instability. In contrast, many patients with true posterior instability will demonstrate pain and general soreness, but with the predominant complaint of instability, generalized ligamentous laxity, a positive sulcus sign, a positive Jerk test, and the ability to demonstrate their instability. In many cases, the instability is voluntary but positional; that is, the patient's shoulder is dislocated/subluxed in the position of forward flexion, pronation, and internal rotation but relocates with the arm brought into abduction and extension (circumduction sign).

In this scenario, it is critical to obtain a high-quality MR arthrogram to determine if a true posterior labral tear is present. Despite having voluntary, positional posterior instability, patients with concomitant posterior labral tears may benefit from posterior labral repair and capsular shift. In contrast, in patients with voluntary, habitual, positional posterior instability, without a labral tear, the arthroscopist should reemphasize the importance of nonoperative treatment and the regaining of dynamic muscular stability and control.

MR arthrogram and radiographs should also be evaluated for the presence of a posterior bony Bankart or degenerative changes of the glenoid. Posterior bony Bankart lesions are commonly associated with an acute instability episode. However, patients with pure cartilage damage and decreased glenohumeral joint space, particularly if associated with symptoms of pain and minimal history of trauma, may present with a degenerative posterior labral tear and early osteoarthritic symptoms. Management of arthritic posterior lesions with arthroscopic repair may not provide long-term relief of symptoms. Like all labral tears, posterior labral tears may also have associated paralabral cysts, which may be decompressed appropriately through the lesion. Unlike spinoglenoid cysts, posterior or posteroinferior labral cysts do not result in compression of the suprascapular nerve with suprascapular neuropathy.

Finally, patients who have experienced a true posterior dislocation episode will commonly present with pain and symptoms of instability. In this situation, careful evaluation of the MR arthrogram will usually demonstrate the presence of a reverse Hill-Sachs lesion indicative of a true instability episode. Chronic locked posterior dislocations or posterior dislocations associated with major traumatic injury (e.g., epilepsy, electrical shocks) may have large reverse Hill-Sachs lesions that require treatment (e.g., reverse remplissage).

Posterior Labral Repair (Knotted Suture Anchor Technique)

In patients with a pure posterior labral tear with minimal complaints of instability and without the presence of a major reverse Hill-Sachs lesion, a standard posterior labral repair is indicated. In this situation, because ligamentous laxity is usually not present, large capsular plication stitches in conjunction with posterior labral repair are not indicated.

Standard three-portal access to the glenohumeral joint is initially established including anterior, anterosuperolateral, and posterior portals. A diagnostic arthroscopy is performed and the glenohumeral joint is viewed through the anterosuperolateral portal to identify the posterior labral tear (Fig. 14.1). Since the standard posterior portal is tangential to the face of the glenoid, this portal does not provide an adequate angle of approach to the posterior glenoid for labral mobilization, glenoid neck preparation, and anchor insertion. A separate posterolateral portal is created approximately 4 cm inferior to the posterolateral corner of the acromion at approximately a 45° angle of approach toward the posterior inferior glenoid rim (Fig. 14.2).

The posterior labrum is mobilized off the glenoid neck using an elevator or arthroscopic scissor. The correct angle of approach for mobilization of the posterior labrum is commonly and surprisingly through the anterior portal (Fig. 14.3). This portal is especially helpful for the initial release of the labrum off the rim of the glenoid followed

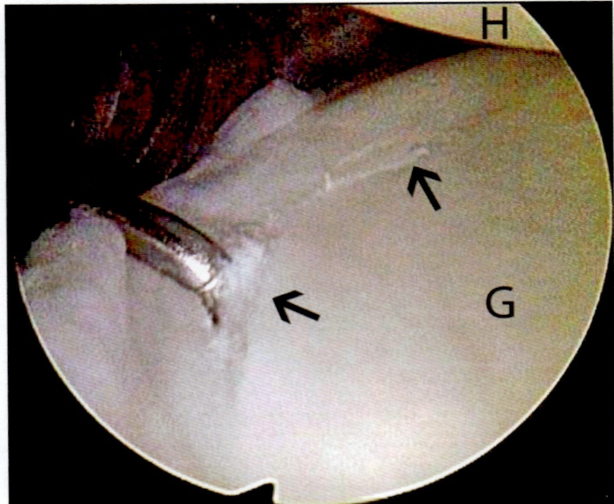

Figure 14.1 Left shoulder, anterosuperolateral viewing portal demonstrates a posterior Bankart lesion (*black arrows*). G, glenoid; H, humerus.

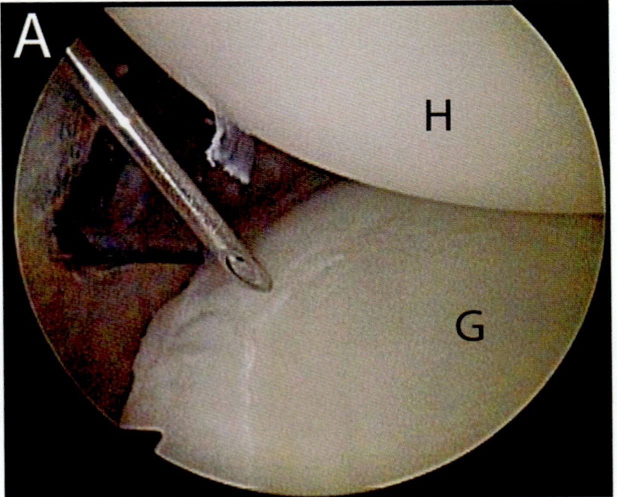

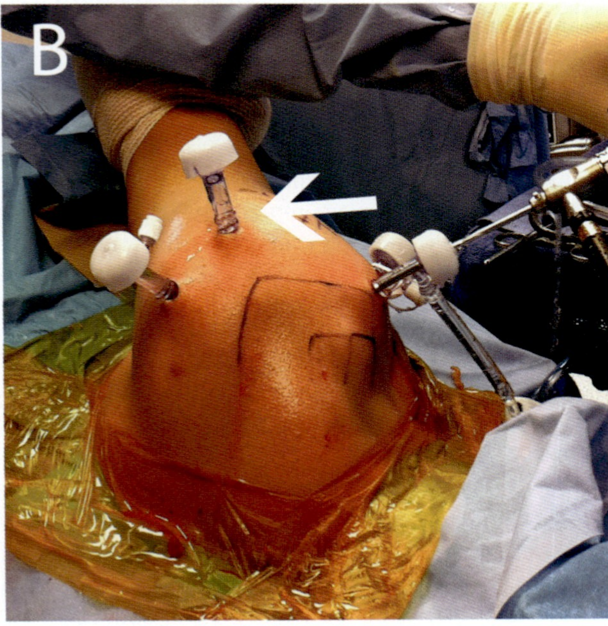

Figure 14.2 Left shoulder demonstrates placement of a posterolateral portal. **A:** Arthroscopic view from an anterosuperolateral portal shows the use of a spinal needle to determine an appropriate angle of approach to the posteroinferior glenoid. The cannula of the standard posterior portal is seen in the background. **B:** External view shows the location of the posterolateral portal (*white arrow*) relative to the posterior portal and the posterolateral acromion. G, glenoid; H, humerus.

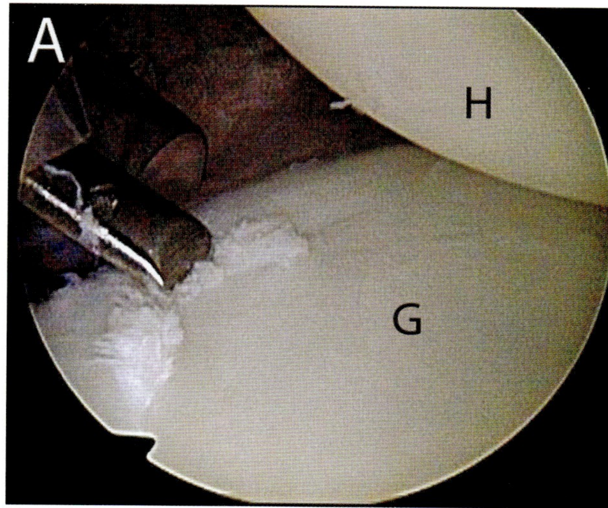

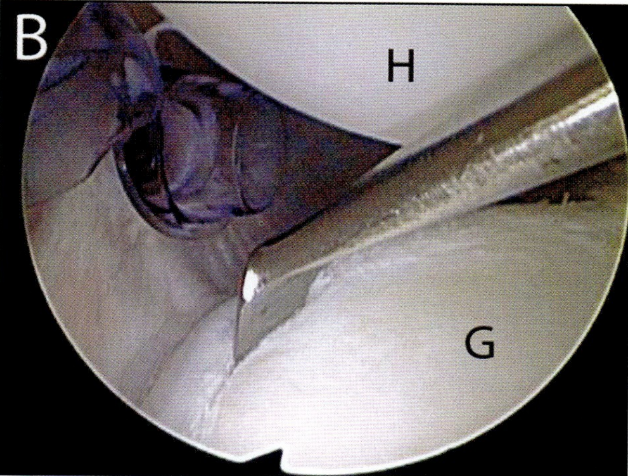

Figure 14.3 Left shoulder, anterosuperolateral viewing portal demonstrates mobilization of a posterior Bankart lesion. **A:** In this case, the angle of approach through the posterior portal is too acute to properly mobilize the labrum. **B:** A 30° elevator introduced from an anterior working portal provides a proper angle of approach to mobilize the posterior labrum. G, glenoid; H, humerus.

by further mobilization through a posterior or posterolateral working portal. In some cases, initial evaluation of the posterior glenoid labrum may only reveal a small crack or fissuring within the posterior labrum. This usually represents a hidden lesion and subsequent evaluation of the lesion with an elevator usually results in easy stripping of the labrum off the posterior glenoid neck (Fig. 14.4).

If the anterior portal does not provide a correct angle of approach, the posterolateral portal may provide the correct angle of approach while viewing through an anterosuperolateral portal (Fig. 14.5). The labrum is elevated off the posterior glenoid neck and the posterior neck is debrided with a shaver and curette (Fig. 14.6).

Anchors are then inserted along the posterior glenoid rim starting from inferior to superior. Anchors are inserted through the posterolateral portal just onto the articular surface of the glenoid. Usually two or three anchors are required and may be sequentially placed (Fig. 14.7). We prefer 3.0-mm BioComposite SutureTak anchors double loaded with No. 2 FiberWire (Arthrex, Inc., Naples, FL). In patients with chondral damage leaving exposed glenoid bone, the anchors may be placed slightly further onto the

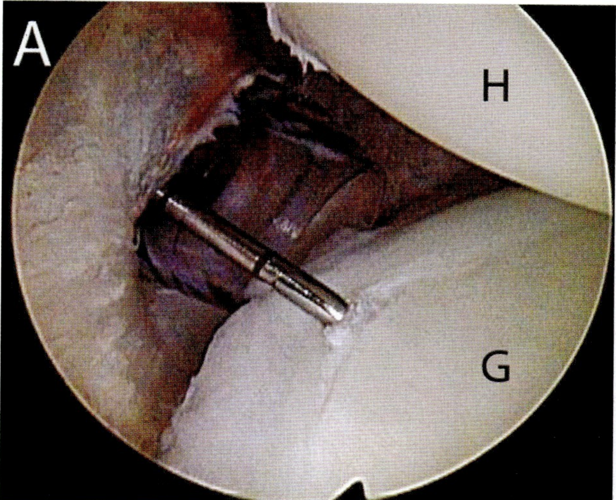

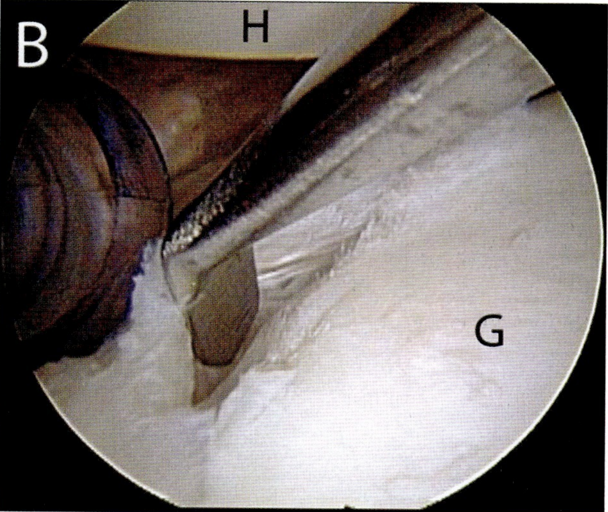

Figure 14.4 Left shoulder, anterosuperolateral viewing portal demonstrates **(A)** a hidden posterior Bankart lesion that is revealed with a probe. **B:** An elevator introduced from an anterior working portal shows that the labrum is not firmly attached to the posterior glenoid. When a posterior Bankart lesion is suspected, it is important to probe for hidden lesions that can be missed with a cursory examination. G, glenoid; H, humerus.

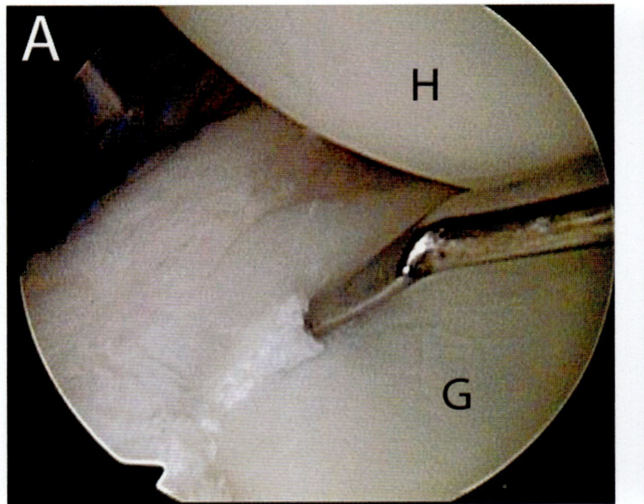

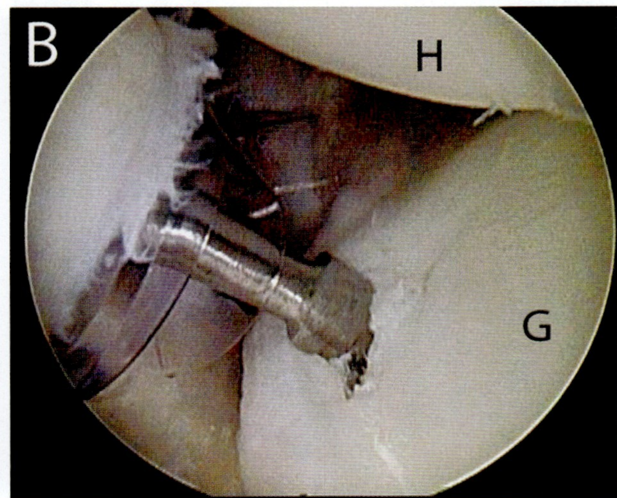

Figure 14.5 Left shoulder, anterosuperolateral viewing portal demonstrates mobilization of a posterior Bankart lesion. **A:** In this case, the angle of approach through the anterior portal is too acute to properly mobilize the labrum. **B:** A 15° elevator introduced from a posterolateral working portal provides a proper angle of approach to mobilize the posterior labrum. G, glenoid; H, humerus.

glenoid face to advance the labrum over the chondral defect and provide a soft tissue interposition while repairing the labrum (see Chapter 22, "Glenohumeral Arthritis").

Once anchors are placed, sutures are passed through the labrum. In patients with pain but with minimal complaints of instability, a standard labral repair may be performed without major capsular shift or plication. Similar to anterior labral repair, multiple options are available to pass sutures including antegrade suture passage (Scorpion; Arthrex, Inc., Naples, FL), a shuttling technique (SutureLasso; Arthrex, Inc., Naples, FL) and retrograde suture passage (BirdBeak; Arthrex, Inc, Naples, FL).

Antegrade suture passage does not require an extra step of shuttling and makes a small puncture hole through the capsule or labrum. If labral mobilization was performed through an anterior portal, this usually indicates that antegrade suture passage may be performed with a Scorpion suture passer in the anterior portal while viewing through the anterosuperolateral portal. Alternatively, if the anterosuperolateral portal was used for labral mobilization while viewing through the anterior portal, the Scorpion may be placed through the anterosuperolateral portal. Using either approach, the Scorpion can sometimes be used for suture passage in the posterior labrum (Fig. 14.8).

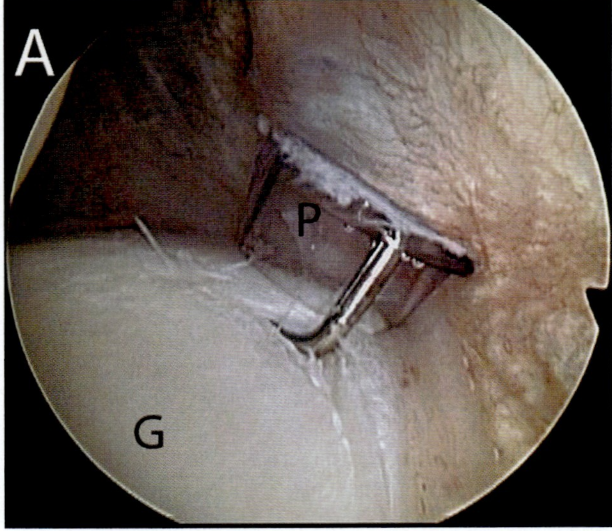

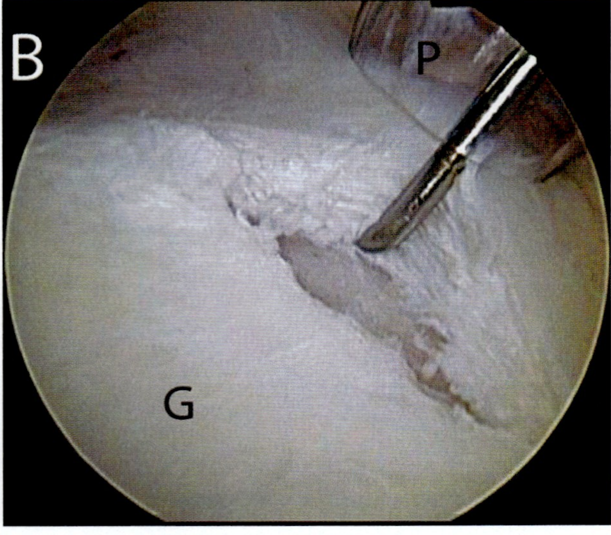

Figure 14.6 **A:** Right shoulder, anterosuperolateral viewing portal demonstrates a hidden posterior labral lesion. **B:** Same shoulder following completed preparation for repair of the posterior Bankart lesion. A strip of bare bone has been prepared to facilitate healing of the labrum to bone. G, glenoid; P, posterior portal.

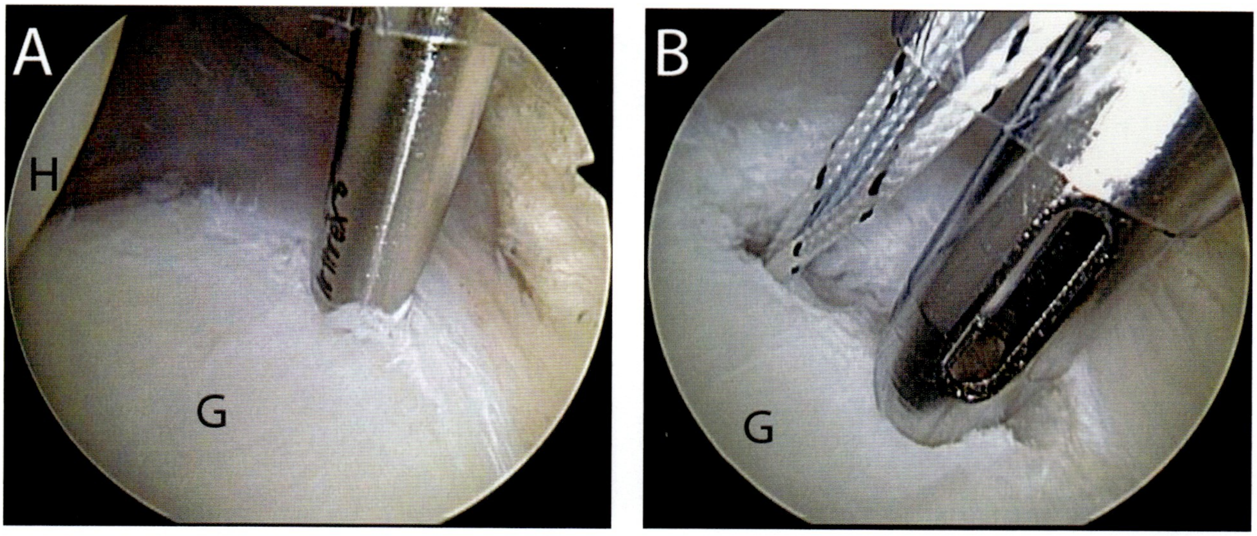

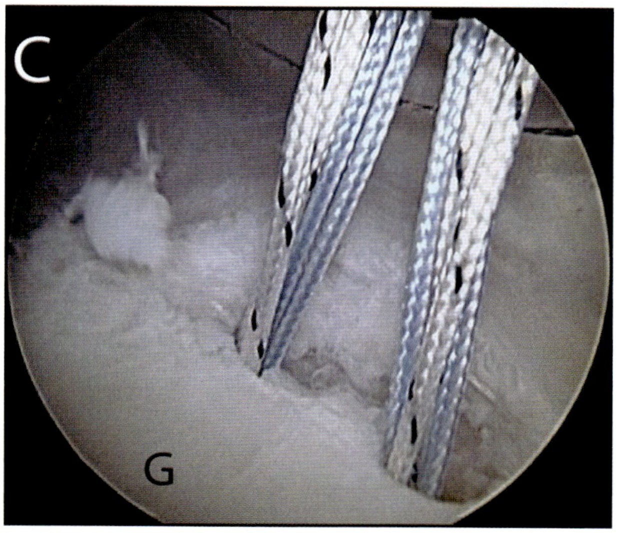

Figure 14.7 Right shoulder, anterosuperolateral viewing portal demonstrates anchor placement for a posterior Bankart repair. **A:** An inferior anchor is placed slightly onto the face of the glenoid via a posterolateral portal. **B:** A second anchor is placed prior to passing sutures. **C:** Appearance after placement of both anchors. G, glenoid; H, humerus.

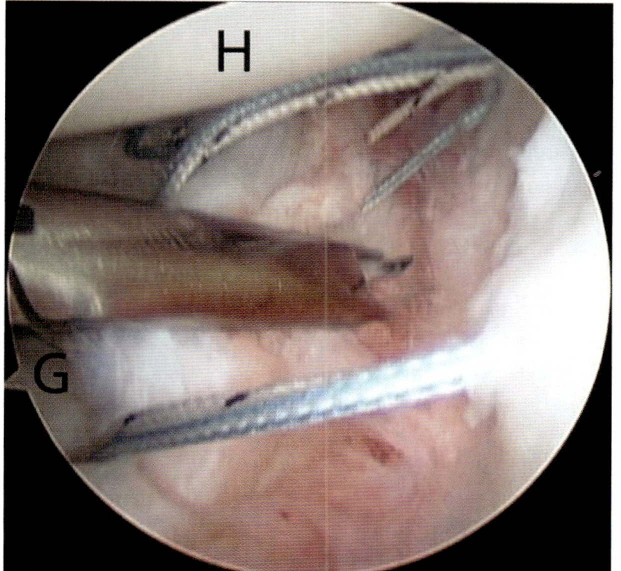

Figure 14.8 Right shoulder, anterosuperolateral viewing portal. A Scorpion (Arthrex, Inc., Naples, FL) is introduced from an anterior working portal and used to pass a suture through the posterior labrum. G, glenoid; H, humerus.

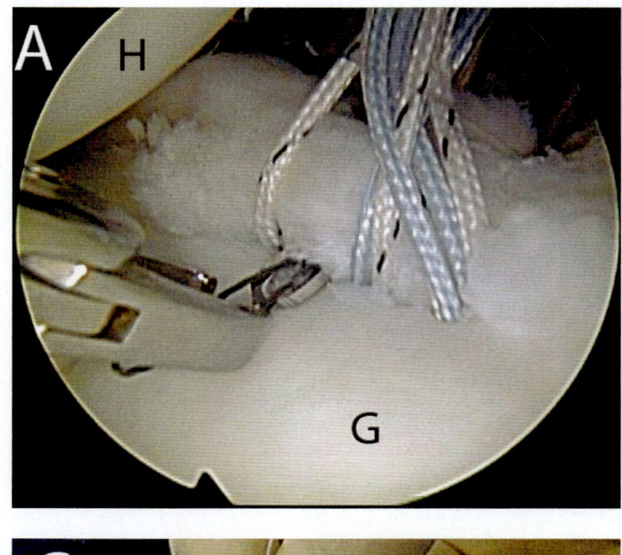

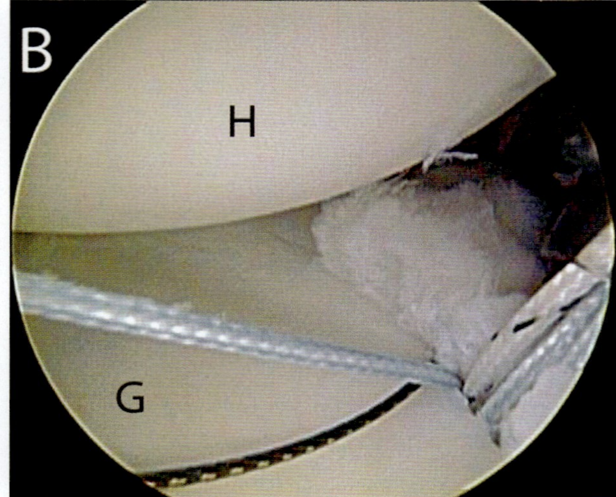

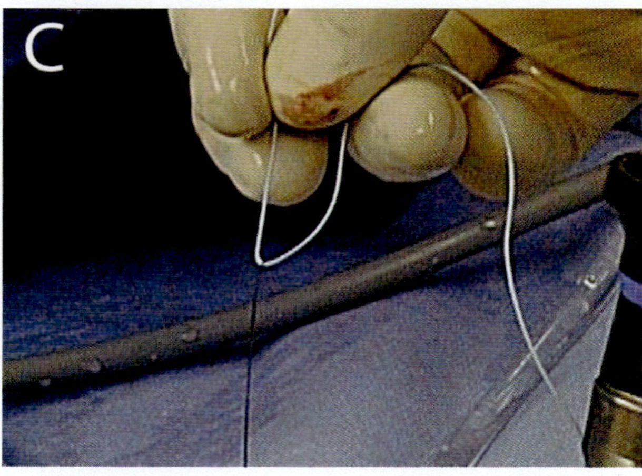

Figure 14.9 Right shoulder demonstrates suture shuttling for a posterior Bankart repair. **A:** A SutureLasso (Arthrex, Inc., Naples, FL) is passed through the posterior labrum and **(B)** retrieved out an anterior working portal along with one of the sutures. **C:** Externally, the suture limb is threaded through the loop in the Nitinol wire so that it may be shuttled through the labrum. G, glenoid; H, humerus.

A shuttling technique is used when the angle of approach does not allow antegrade suture passage. In addition, the shuttling technique is useful when previous fixation (i.e., suture passage and fixation with knot tying) has bound the labrum and prevents the use of larger instruments (e.g., Scorpion). Shuttling is usually performed while viewing through an anterosuperolateral portal with instruments inserted through a posterior portal or posterolateral portal. The remaining portal is used as a suture management and suture shuttling portal.

The correct angle of approach for suture passage is usually obtained with a 25° Tight Curve SutureLasso (left curved for a right shoulder) in the posterior inferior quadrant, a Straight SutureLasso directly posterior, and an opposite25° Tight Curve SutureLasso (right curve for a right shoulder) in the posterior superior quadrant. After passing the SutureLasso, the suture and suture shuttle are retrieved through another portal and then relayed through the labrum (Fig. 14.9).

Retrograde suture passage using BirdBeak suture passers may also be used for labral repair. Retrograde suture passage is usually most valuable for suture passage directly

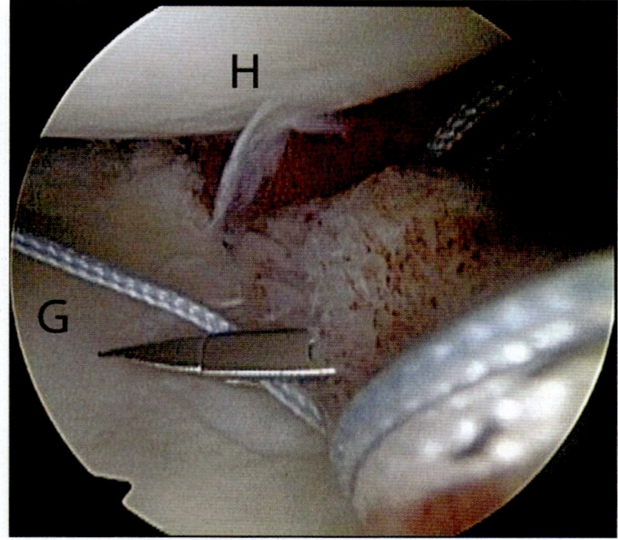

Figure 14.10 Right shoulder, anterosuperolateral viewing portal, demonstrates use a BirdBeak (Arthrex, Inc., Naples, FL) to pass sutures for a posterior labral repair. The BirdBeak is useful when the angle of approach to the sutures is in line with the posterior portal. G, glenoid; H, humerus.

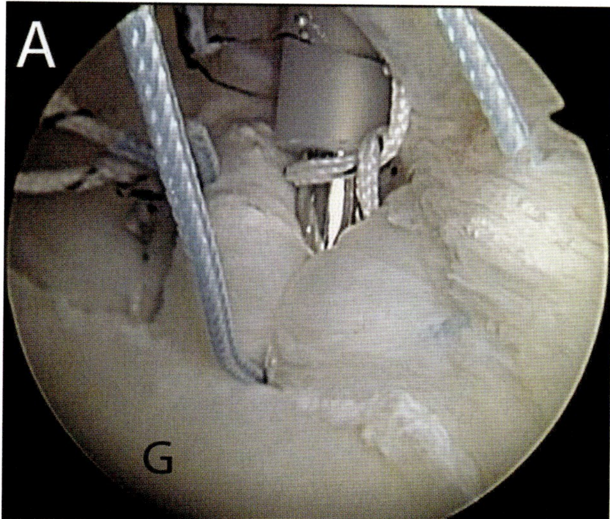

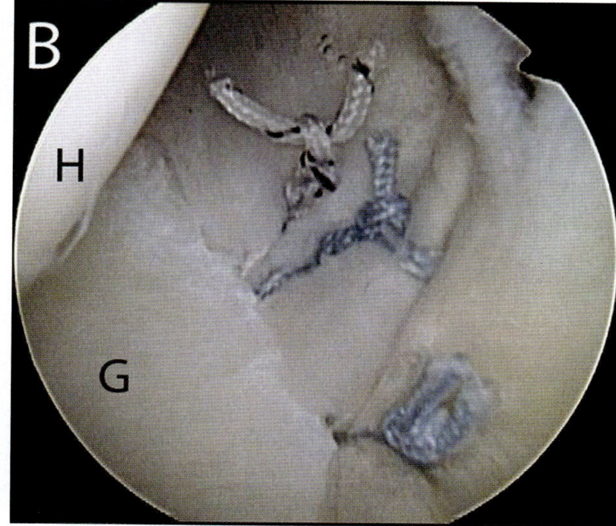

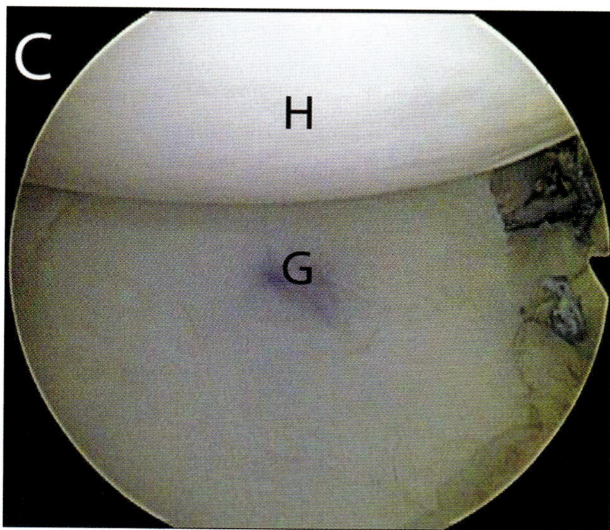

Figure 14.11 Right shoulder, anterosuperolateral viewing portal. **A:** After suture passage knots are tied for a posterior Bankart repair using a Surgeon's Sixth Finger Knot Pusher (Arthrex, Inc., Naples, FL). **B:** Close-up view of the final repair shows restoration of the posterior labral bumper. **C:** Profile view of the final repair demonstrates that the humeral head is centered over the glenoid. G, glenoid; H, humerus.

posteriorly or for an anchor within close proximity of the utilized portal (Fig. 14.10). This is due to the limited angular change permitted by retrograde suture passing instruments. Furthermore, if significant capsular plication is indicated, the larger BirdBeak instrumentation may be contraindicated because it creates a significant hole through soft tissue, potentially damaging the more fragile capsule.

A "tie as you go" technique is used to sequentially pass and tie sutures from inferior to superior, securing the final repair construct (Fig. 14.11). Video

Combined Posterior Labral Tear and SLAP Lesion

A combined posterior labral tear and superior labrum anterior and posterior (SLAP) lesion is commonly encountered in patients with posterior pain following a traumatic injury. Essentially the same repair technique may be performed as above. A standard four portal approach is again established. Both the superior labrum and posterior labrum are mobilized and the glenoid bone is prepared.

Usually the posterior labral tear is contiguous with the superior labral tear and the entire posterior half of the glenoid labrum is prepared (Fig. 14.12). In some cases, a small portion of posterior superior labrum may be intact. In this scenario, we will commonly complete the tear, making it contiguous to ensure adequate mobilization and repair.

In combined cases, the SLAP lesion anchors and sutures are passed first. Usually, this progresses with anchor insertion through the anterosuperolateral portal followed by passage through the labrum just posterior to the biceps root, followed by posterolateral anchor insertion through a percutaneous Port of Wilmington portal (Fig. 14.13). Usually, we delay passing the second suture from this posterior anchor until the posterior labral repair is completed. In this way, suture passage may be performed with reference to the final suture passed during the posterior labral repair.

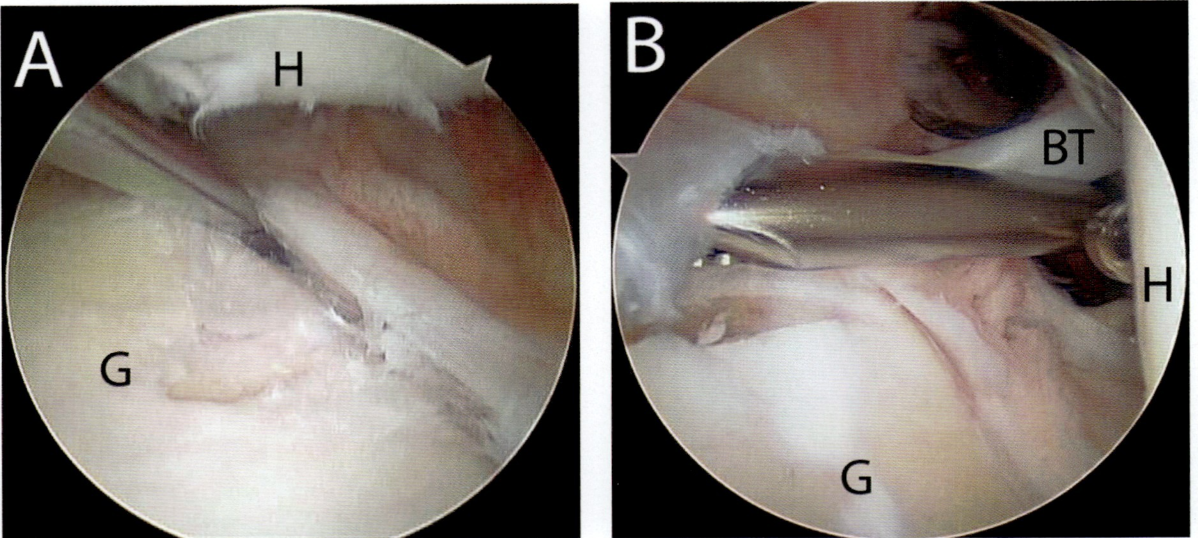

Figure 14.12 **A:** Right shoulder, anterosuperolateral viewing portal, demonstrates a large posterior Bankart lesion that is mobilized for repair. **B:** Posterior viewing portal in the same shoulder demonstrates a SLAP lesion that extends posteriorly. BT, biceps tendon; G, glenoid; H, humerus.

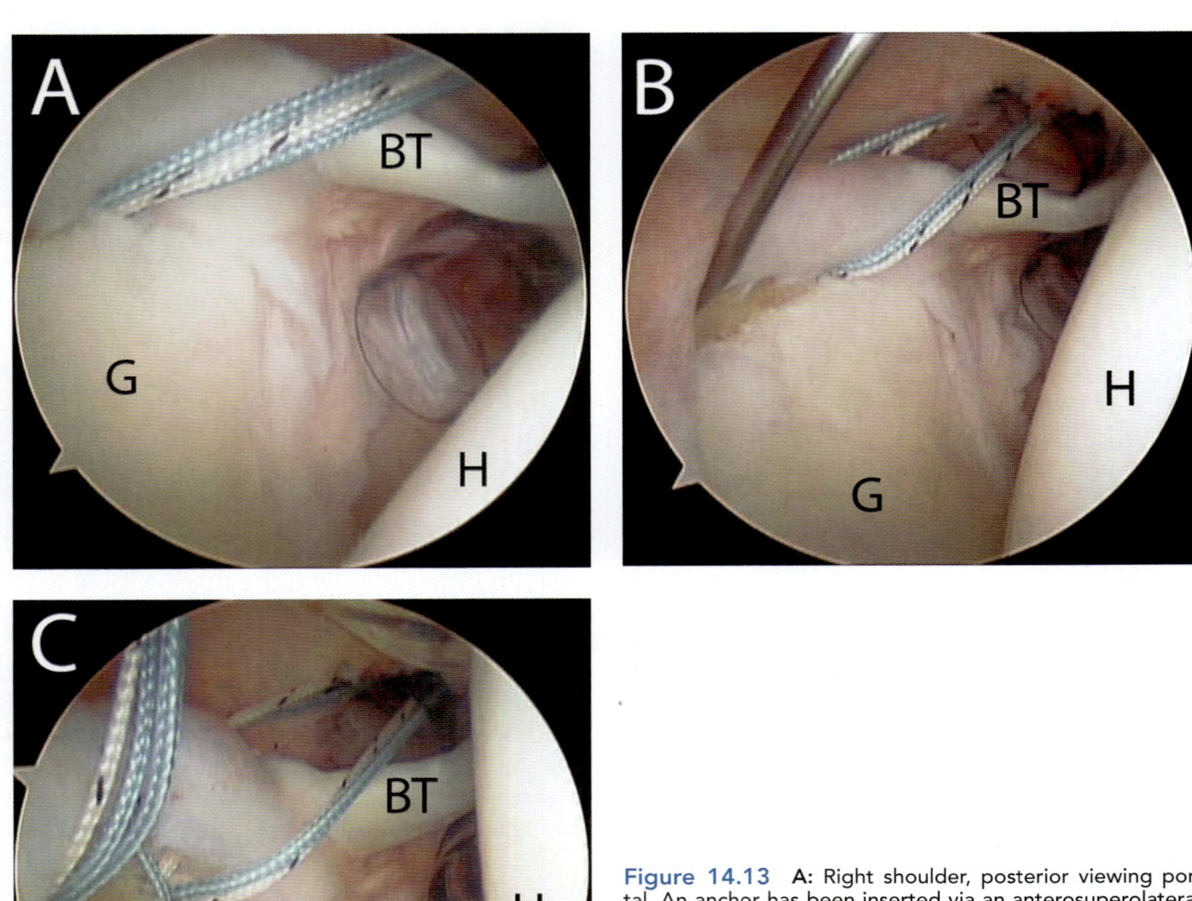

Figure 14.13 **A:** Right shoulder, posterior viewing portal. An anchor has been inserted via an anterosuperolateral portal for a superior labral repair. **B:** In this case, the lesion extends posteriorly and there is also a posterior Bankart lesion (not seen). Thus, a Port of Wilmington portal is established using a spinal needle as a guide. **C:** View after placement of both anchors. Note: The three sutures have been passed, but not tied at this point because there is also a posterior Bankart lesion. The final suture is not passed until the posterior Bankart lesion is repaired because the location of the pass will be influenced by the posterior repair. BT, biceps tendon; G, glenoid; H, humerus.

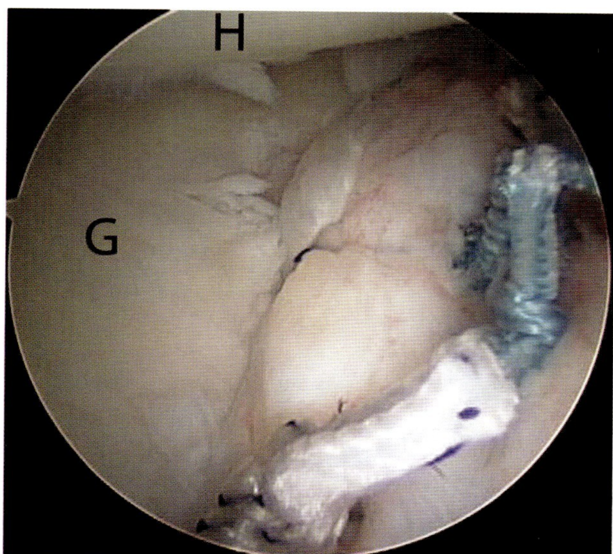

Figure 14.14 Right shoulder, anterosuperolateral viewing portal, demonstrates a posterior Bankart lesion that was repaired with three anchors (compare to Fig. 4.12A). G, glenoid; H, humerus.

Additionally, in order to maintain working space in the glenohumeral joint, the SLAP lesion sutures are not tied until the posterior labrum is repaired.

The posterior labrum is then repaired using the techniques as described above (Fig. 14.14). After the final posterior labrum suture is passed and tied, the final SLAP lesion suture from the anchor inserted through the Port of Wilmington portal is passed. The SLAP lesion sutures are then progressively tied, progressing from posterior to anterior (Fig. 14.15).

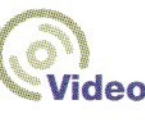

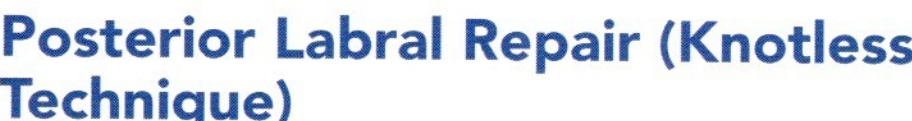

Posterior Labral Repair (Knotless Technique)

Any labral repair may be performed with a knotted or knotless technique, and thus may be performed for posterior labrum repair as well. The principles of labral repair are similar with mobilization, bone preparation, subsequent suture passage and anchor insertion. The steps for a knotless anchor were previously described in Chapter 12, "Repair of Anterior Instability without Bone Loss." In the vast majority of cases, our preference is to tie knots during repair of a posterior labral tear.

Posterior Labral Repair with Reverse Remplissage

In some cases of posterior instability, a large reverse Hill-Sachs lesion may be encountered. This is usually present in patients with chronic locked posterior dislocations or in cases with a significant traumatic history (e.g., seizure disorder, electrical injury). Patients with positional posterior instability with ligamentous laxity usually do not present with significant reverse Hill-Sachs lesions.

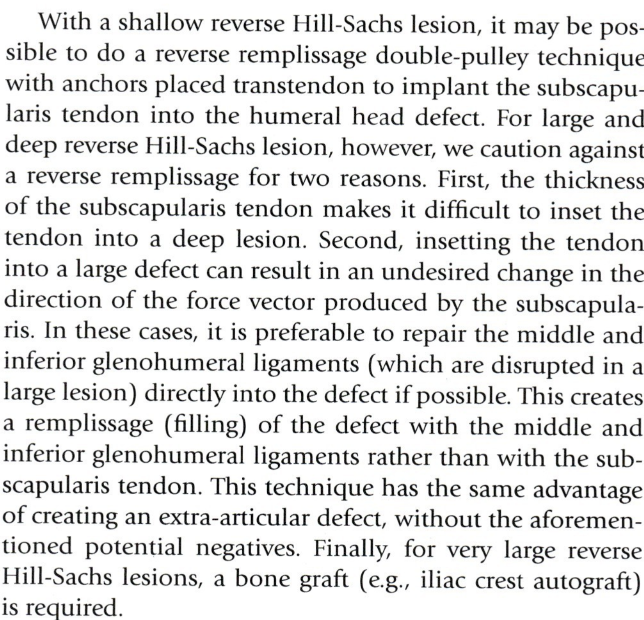

With a shallow reverse Hill-Sachs lesion, it may be possible to do a reverse remplissage double-pulley technique with anchors placed transtendon to implant the subscapularis tendon into the humeral head defect. For large and deep reverse Hill-Sachs lesion, however, we caution against a reverse remplissage for two reasons. First, the thickness of the subscapularis tendon makes it difficult to inset the tendon into a deep lesion. Second, insetting the tendon into a large defect can result in an undesired change in the direction of the force vector produced by the subscapularis. In these cases, it is preferable to repair the middle and inferior glenohumeral ligaments (which are disrupted in a large lesion) directly into the defect if possible. This creates a remplissage (filling) of the defect with the middle and inferior glenohumeral ligaments rather than with the subscapularis tendon. This technique has the same advantage of creating an extra-articular defect, without the aforementioned potential negatives. Finally, for very large reverse Hill-Sachs lesions, a bone graft (e.g., iliac crest autograft) is required.

The decision as to which procedure to perform is guided by preoperative imaging and is ultimately based on arthroscopic appearance. Similar to our protocol for evaluating bone loss in anterior instability, we recommend a preoperative computed tomography scan with three-dimensional reconstructions. In addition, the posterior labral and the reverse Hill-Sachs lesions are evaluated arthroscopically before deciding on the definitive treatment. Unlike traditional Hill-Sachs lesions, reverse Hill-Sachs lesions are usually not accompanied by significant glenoid bone loss. Since these cases are rare, the pathology and position of reverse Hill-Sachs lesions are not as well defined as engaging Hill-Sachs lesions. Recommendations for implantation of the subscapularis tendon have been largely based on trauma literature regarding chronic locked posterior dislocations and may not be appropriate with today's arthroscopic technology.

Using a 70° arthroscope from a posterior portal (after arthroscopic-assisted reduction of the posterior dislocation), an aerial view of the subscapularis tendon and the reverse Hill-Sachs lesion is obtained (Fig. 14.16). This view may be further enhanced by internal rotation, traction, and a posterior lever push similar to that used for subscapularis tendon repairs.

The bone bed in the reverse Hill-Sachs lesion is prepared in the same way as during subscapularis tendon repair, although in this scenario the upper border of the subscapularis tendon commonly obstructs direct access. Internal rotation will improve access, particularly to the inferior part of the reverse Hill-Sachs lesion.

Two anchors (5.5-mm BioComposite Corkscrew FT; Arthrex, Inc., Naples, FL) are inserted in the inferior and superior aspects of the reverse Hill-Sachs lesion (Fig. 14.17). If a reverse remplissage is planned, both anchors are inserted percutaneously through the subscapularis tendon. For insetting of the glenohumeral ligaments, usually the superior anchor can be placed above the subscapularis

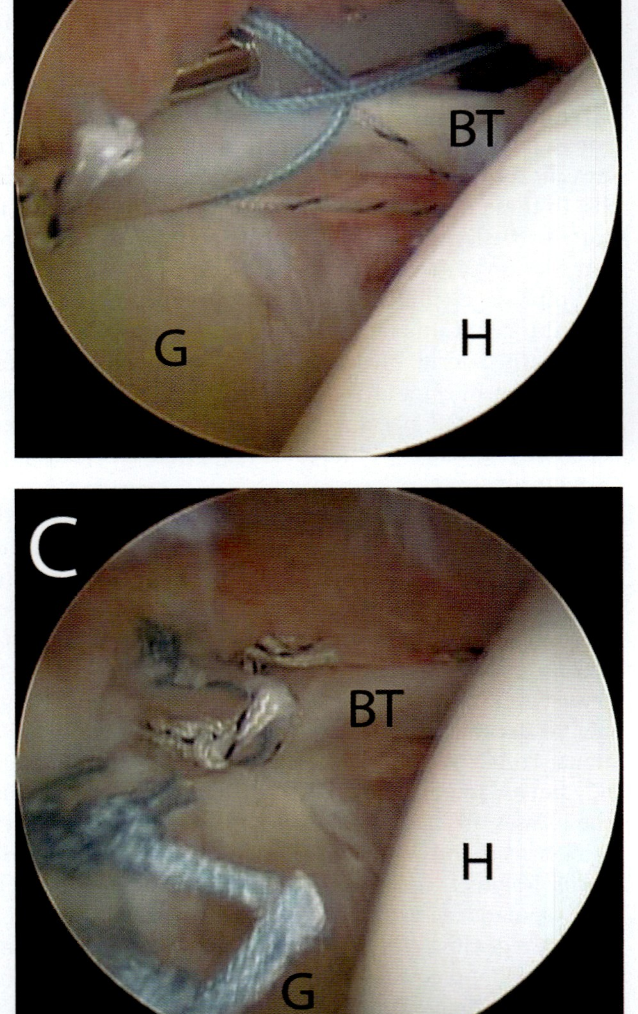

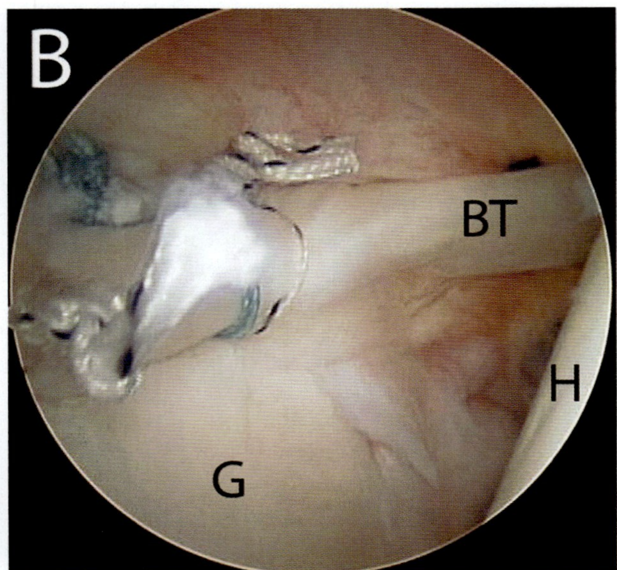

Figure 14.15 **A:** Right shoulder, posterior viewing portal. After a posterior Bankart lesion has been repaired, previously placed sutures for a superior labral repair are tied. Note: Soft tissue swelling above the superior labrum at this point in the procedure can be appreciated as well; this is why these sutures were placed at the beginning of the procedure. **B:** Final repair of the superior labrum. **C:** Profile view demonstrates the posterior extension. BT, biceps tendon; G, glenoid; H, humerus.

tendon without a transtendon portal, but the inferior anchor always requires transtendon placement.

For reverse remplissage cases, knot tying is delayed at this point and attention is turned to the posterior labrum that is repaired using the previously described techniques. Then, attention is returned to the reverse remplissage. Using a double-pulley technique (see Chapter 4, "Complete Rotator Cuff Tears"), one suture from each anchor (of the same color) is then retrieved through the anterior portal. The sutures are then tied extracorporeally over an instrument and pulled into the joint using the anchors as pulleys. The matching suture limbs are then retrieved and a static knot is tied with a Surgeon's Sixth Finger. The steps are repeated for the other suture pairs.

If an insetting of the inferior and middle glenohumeral ligaments is planned, we prefer to pass and tie these sutures immediately since swelling with subsequent surgery commonly limits visualization in the subcoracoid space. Sutures are passed through the inferior and middle glenohumeral ligaments with retrograde instruments. Static knots are then tied with a Surgeon's Sixth Finger Knot Pusher (Fig. 14.18). After the insetting is complete, the posterior labrum is repaired using the techniques previously described.

TRIPLE LABRAL LESIONS

Triple labral lesions are combined tears of the labrum involving the anterior, posterior, and superior labrum.

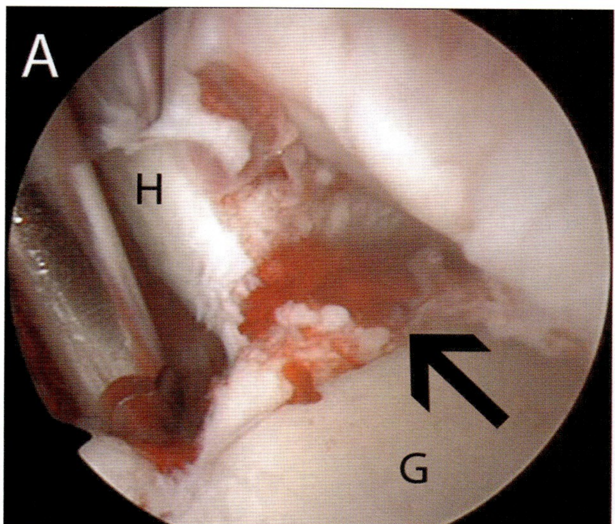

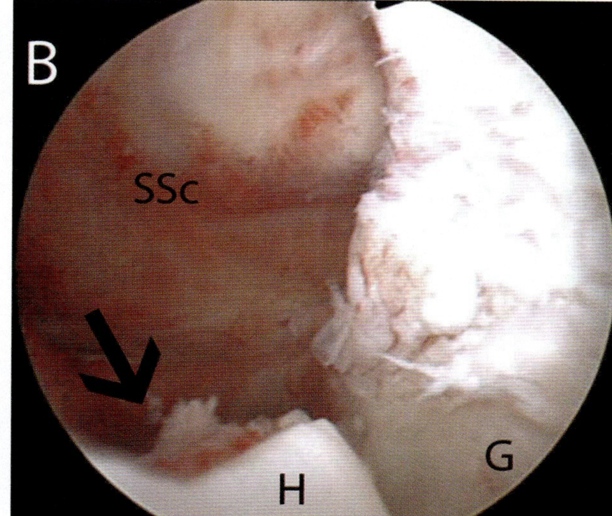

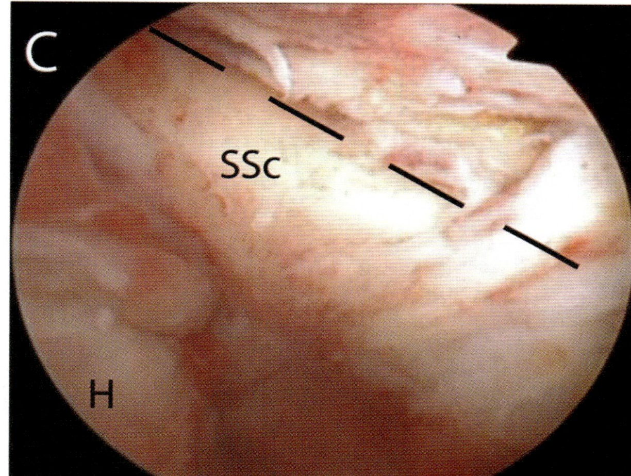

Figure 14.16 **A:** Left shoulder, anterosuperolateral viewing portal, demonstrates a locked posterior glenohumeral dislocation with a large reverse Hill-Sachs lesion (*black arrow*). **B:** Posterior viewing portal in the same shoulder following arthroscopic-assisted reduction shows a large reverse Hill-Sachs lesion (*black arrow*). **C:** Up-close view demonstrates an intact subscapularis (superior border outlined by *dashed black lines*) insertion. Note: There is a large distance between the subscapularis tendon and the remaining humeral head. In this case, the reverse Hill-Sachs lesion is too large for a reverse remplissage. G, glenoid; H, humerus; SSc, subscapularis tendon.

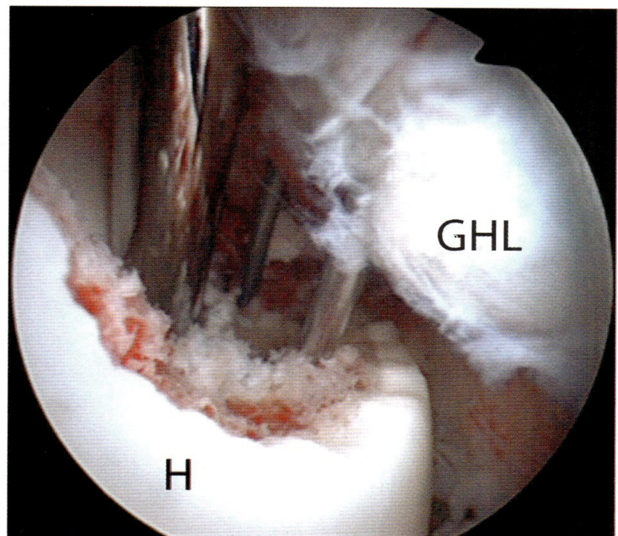

Figure 14.17 Left shoulder, posterior viewing portal with a 70° arthroscope. Spinal needles are used to determine an adequate angle of approach for an anchor in the humeral head. Then, a punch (left in image) is walked down the spinal needle and used to create a bone socket for an anchor. H, humerus; GHL, glenohumeral ligaments.

Loosely defined, tears of the anterior labrum are located from the 2 o'clock to 6 o'clock positions (Bankart lesion), tears of the posterior labrum (reverse Bankart lesion) are located from the 6 o'clock to 10 o'clock positions, and SLAP tears are located from the 10 o'clock to 2 o'clock positions. Although the principles of repair are relatively similar to isolated lesions, these complex tears require special consideration due to the extensive damage to the labrum circumferentially around the glenoid.

Most patients with triple labral lesions will present with a primary complaint of anterior instability and a prolonged history of recurrent instability (>5 instability episodes) following a significant trauma. However, unlike patients with isolated Bankart lesions, patients with triple labral lesions will commonly complain of chronic pain and discomfort between instability episodes. Thus, patients with triple labral lesions may present with complaints of both instability and pain.

On physical exam, patients with triple labral lesions will commonly demonstrate positive tests for anterior instability (e.g., apprehension test, relocation test), posterior instability (e.g., jerk test, push-pull test, posterior load and shift), and superior labral pathology (e.g., O'Brien test,

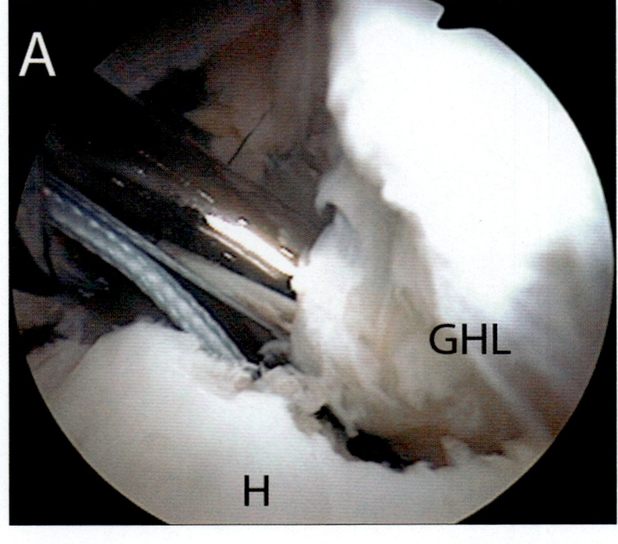

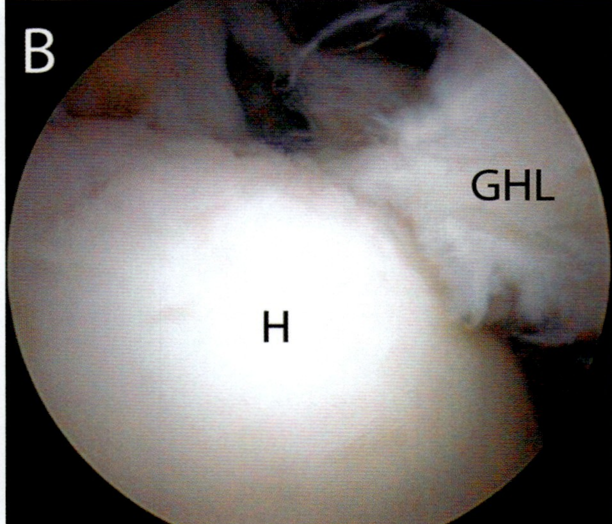

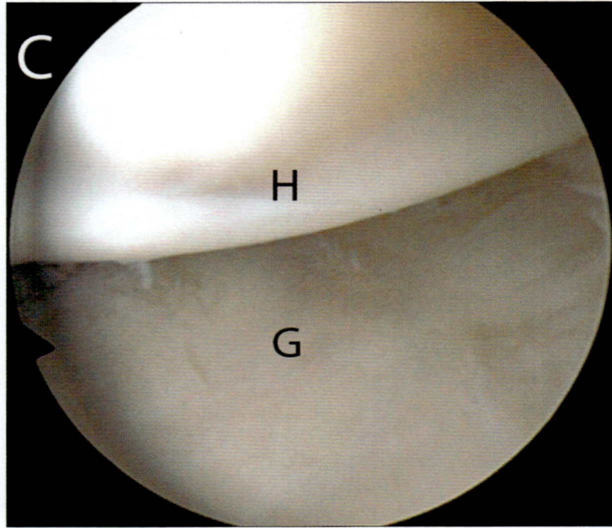

Figure 14.18 **A:** Right shoulder, posterior viewing portal with a 70° arthroscope. Knots are tied from an anterosuperolateral working portal to inset the glenohumeral ligaments into a reverse Hill-Sachs defect. **B:** Same view following completion of the insetting. The insetting has made the defect an extra-articular lesion. **C:** Anterosuperolateral viewing portal demonstrates that the humeral head has been centered over the glenoid. G, glenoid; H, humerus; GHL, glenohumeral ligaments.

O'Driscoll sign), raising the suspicion for complex labral pathology. However, there is no specific test that has been described for triple labral lesions.

Most patients with triple labral tears will have relatively preserved passive range of motion. However, patients with true restriction of passive range of motion, particularly globally, should raise the suspicion of glenohumeral arthritis. Although glenohumeral arthritis may present with circumferential or near circumferential labral tears, these degenerative lesions should not be confused with complex labral lesions. Inadvertent repair of these degenerative lesions may lead to increased pain, stiffness, and potential progression of osteoarthritis. Careful evaluation of radiographic and magnetic resonance imaging studies can help differentiate these lesions (e.g., chondromalacia changes on glenoid or humeral side, labral detachment without displacement, humeral head osteophytes, absence of Hill-Sachs lesion).

The indications for repair of triple labral lesions are similar to the indications for isolated lesions. Similarly, the major contraindication to arthroscopic repair is substantial bone loss.

Technique for Triple Labral Repair

Due to their complexity, the surgical planning and sequence of repair of triple labral lesions requires special consideration. Early repair of some lesions can lead to constriction of the joint and limitation of visualization. The sequence for repair of triple labral lesions is

1. Preparation, anchor insertion, suture passage for SLAP lesion
2. Preparation of anterior and posterior labral tears
3. Anchor insertion and suture passage for the anterior labral tear
4. Tie anterior sutures

5. Anchor insertion and suture passage for the posterior labral tear
6. Tie posterior sutures
7. Tie superior sutures

While this is the most common sequence, tear-specific considerations may change the sequence repair in individual cases. For example, in patients with a type III SLAP lesion, tying the SLAP lesion sutures first reduces the bucket handle tear, improving visualization of the inferior aspect of the glenohumeral joint, and subsequently providing a stable base for repair of the anterior and posterior labrum.

Standard anterior, posterior, and anterosuperolateral portals are established and a diagnostic arthroscopy is performed confirming a SLAP lesion (Fig. 14.19A), Bankart lesion (Fig. 14.19B), and reverse Bankart lesion (Fig. 14.19C). The amount of bone loss on the glenoid and the humeral side is documented to confirm that an arthroscopic repair is indicated.

The tear of the superior labrum is addressed first and is carefully evaluated for its extension anteriorly and posteriorly. It is not uncommon in patients with triple labral lesions to have a small portion of the labrum still attached between the 9 o'clock and 10 o'clock positions. Depending on the robustness of the residual attachment, this small area is commonly released to ensure a complete release and mobilization of the labrum (Fig. 14.20).

The bone bed is debrided and 3.0-mm BioComposite SutureTak anchors are inserted just under the biceps root (through the anterosuperolateral portal), just anterior to the biceps (through the anterosuperolateral portal), and at the posterosuperior glenoid rim (through the Port of Wilmington). These anchors are advantageous for triple labral lesion repair when glenoid "real estate" is at a premium due to their small size and multiple sutures. Progressing anterior to posterior, sutures are passed using a shuttling technique (Micro SutureLasso) anterior and posterior to the biceps tendon, and through the posterior superior labrum. The anterosuperior sutures are used to repair the superior glenohumeral

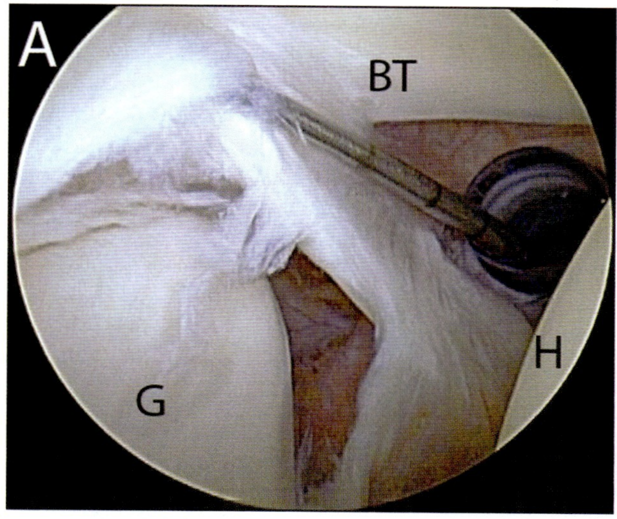

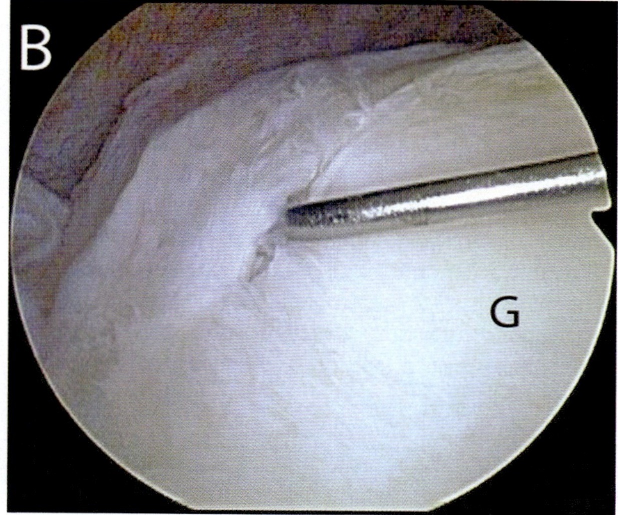

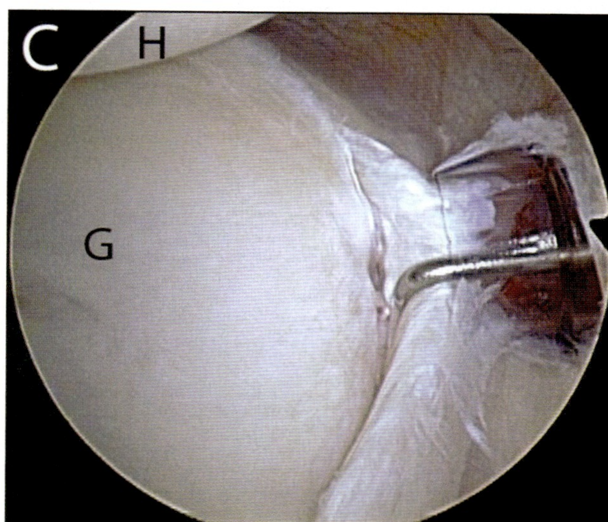

Figure 14.19 Triple labral lesion in a right shoulder. **A:** Posterior viewing portal demonstrates a SLAP lesion. **B:** Anterosuperolateral viewing portal demonstrates a Bankart lesion and **(C)** posterior Bankart lesion. BT, biceps tendon; G, glenoid; H, humerus.

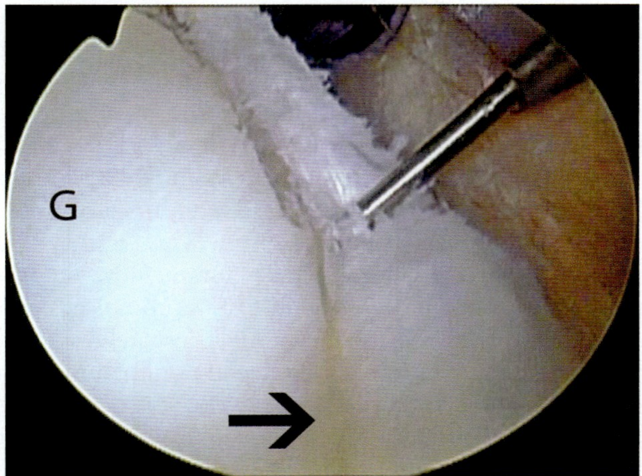

Figure 14.20 Right shoulder, anterosuperolateral viewing portal, demonstrates inspection of the posterosuperior labrum in a triple labral lesion. In this case, the posterosuperior labrum is robust (*black arrow*) above the posterior Bankart lesion. If there is only a minimal attachment, this area should be mobilized and repaired. G, glenoid.

ligament. The superior sutures are provisionally held in the anterosuperolateral portal and not tied until the end of the procedure since tying the sutures early can limit visualization and access to the inferior joint (Fig. 14.21). For a complete discussion of SLAP lesion repair, refer to Chapter 16.

The inferior labral tears are addressed next. While viewing through the anterosuperolateral portal, the anterior and posterior labra are mobilized similar to the technique for isolated lesions. A separate posterolateral portal may be required for posterior mobilization. If a small portion of the labrum at the 6 o'clock position is still intact, the tear is completed to connect the anterior and posterior lesions, creating a horseshoe tear. This ensures that an adequate inferior to superior shift can be performed both anteriorly and posteriorly.

Anchors for the anterior labrum are inserted next. Swelling of the shoulder will compromise the anteroinferior working space before it compromises the posteroinferior working space. Usually three anchors are required for anterior repair. In some cases, if one notices that visualization is becoming obscured, Bankart lesion sutures may be "tied as you go" or in a "leap frog fashion" (i.e., placing second anchor sutures first and then tying first anchor sutures, etc.), which can also assist in suture management (Fig. 14.22A). For a complete discussion of Bankart repair, see Chapter 12.

Similarly, the most superior suture from the posterior labrum anchor should account for the position of the most posterior SLAP suture. In this region where capsular shifting is less of a concern, sutures are merely spaced equally to provide uniform fixation. Again, the sutures are not tied until after the anterior labrum is addressed.

The posterior Bankart lesion anchors are inserted next followed by standard suture passage. Usually, three anchors are required to ensure complete repair of the posterior labrum. Sutures are passed using the techniques (i.e., antegrade, shuttling, retrograde) previously described (Fig. 14.22B). It is important when passing the most inferior and most superior sutures to account for the position of the Bankart and SLAP sutures, respectively. Generally, if the patient's primary direction of instability is anterior, the most inferior suture for the posterior labrum repair is placed at the 7 o'clock position. This is to ensure that adequate capsulolabral tissue is available for Bankart repair, which is usually passed directly inferiorly at the 6 o'clock position. The posterior sutures are then tied, followed by superior sutures, to complete the repair (Fig. 14.23).

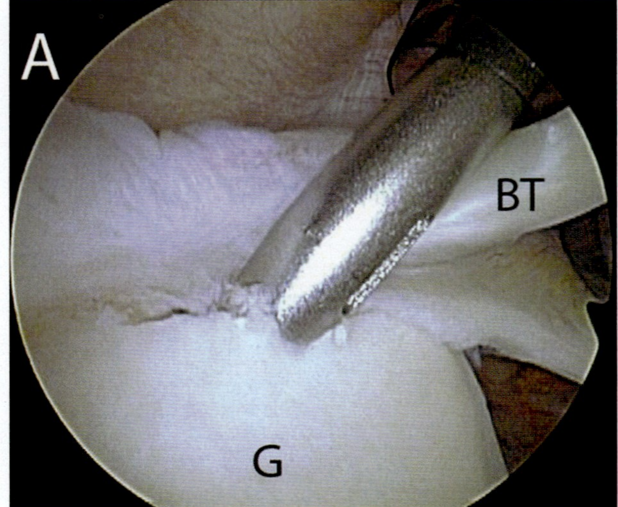

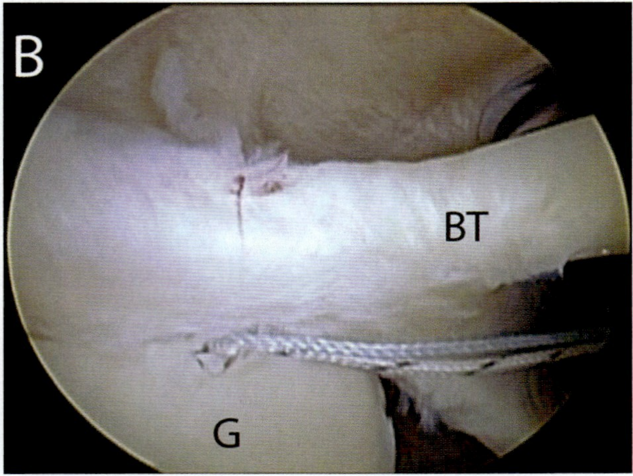

Figure 14.21 **A:** Right shoulder, posterior viewing portal, demonstrates anchor placement for a SLAP lesion. **B:** Because this lesion is accompanied by a Bankart lesion and posterior Bankart lesion (triple labral lesion), the sutures are passed, but not tied. This is our first step for repair of a triple labral lesion. BT, biceps tendon; G, glenoid.

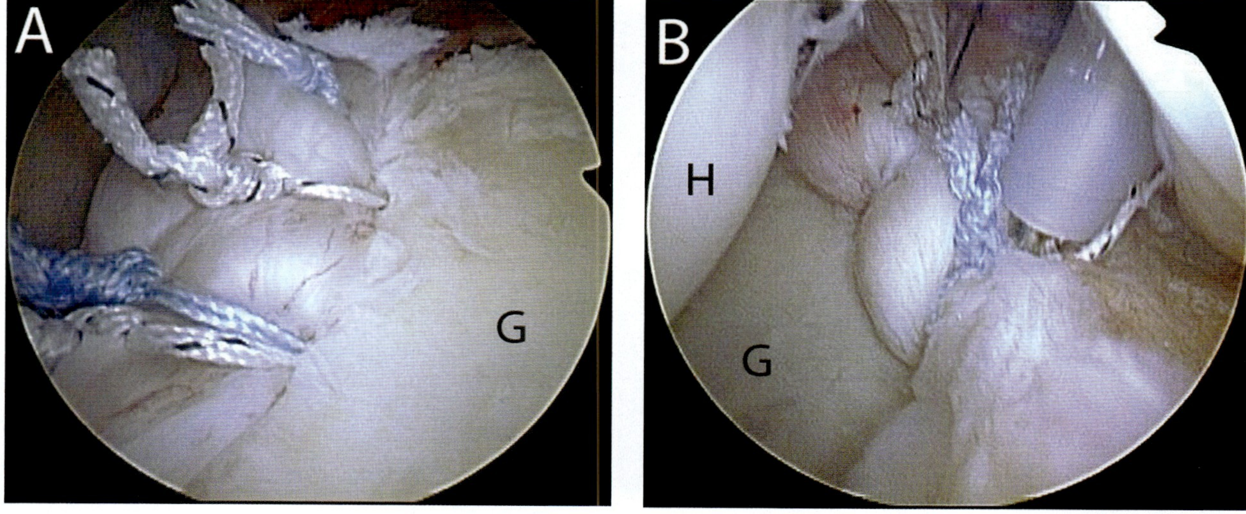

Figure 14.22 **A:** Right shoulder, anterosuperolateral viewing portal. After placing sutures for the superior labral repair, the Bankart lesion is repaired. **B:** Then, the posterior Bankart lesion is repaired. G, glenoid; H, humerus.

INSTABILITY DUE TO HUMERAL-SIDED CAPSULOLIGAMENTOUS DISRUPTION

HAGL (Humeral Avulsion of the Glenohumeral Ligaments) Lesion

HAGL lesions, in our experience, are uncommon causes of anterior instability. The surgeon must be very suspicious of a HAGL lesion in a patient who presents with a history of documented anterior dislocation, yet does not have a Bankart lesion. Conversely, the presence of a Bankart lesion does not preclude a HAGL lesion, and we have seen both lesions in the same patient.

The HAGL lesion can be missed while viewing from a posterior portal with a 30° arthroscope. HAGL lesions are best seen from a posterior portal with a 70° arthroscope or, even better, from an anterosuperolateral portal with a 30° arthroscope.

There are three variants of HAGL lesions:

1. Avulsion from bone
2. Capsular split
3. Combined bone avulsion and capsular split

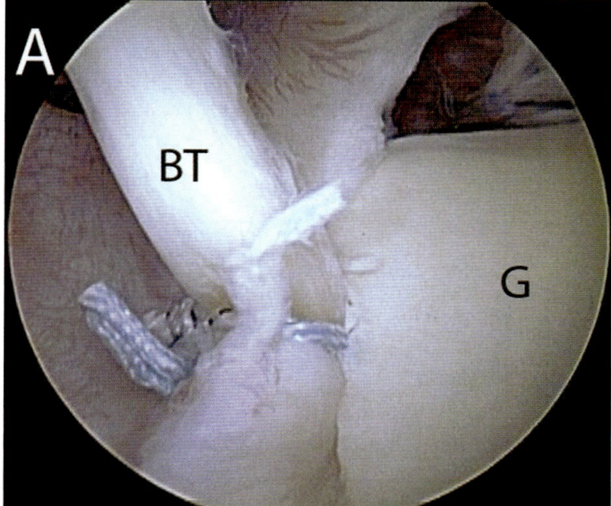

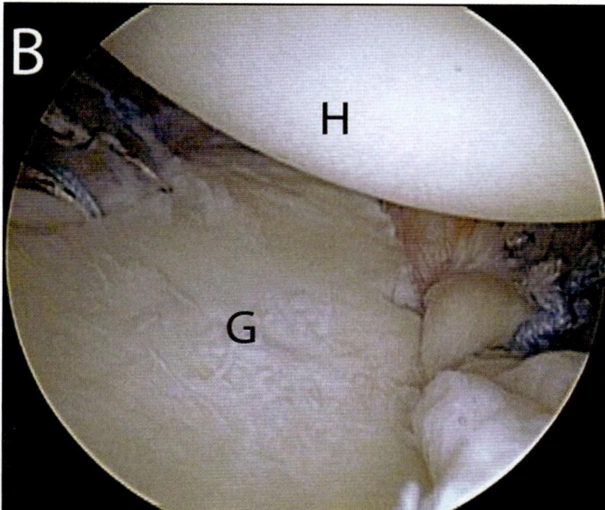

Figure 14.23 **A:** Right shoulder, posterior viewing portal, demonstrates a repaired SLAP lesion in an individual with a triple labral lesion. Note: Sutures for the SLAP lesion were not tied until after the anterior and posterior labrum were repaired. **B:** Anterosuperolateral portal in the same shoulder demonstrates the final repair of the Bankart lesion and posterior Bankart lesion. G, glenoid; H, humerus.

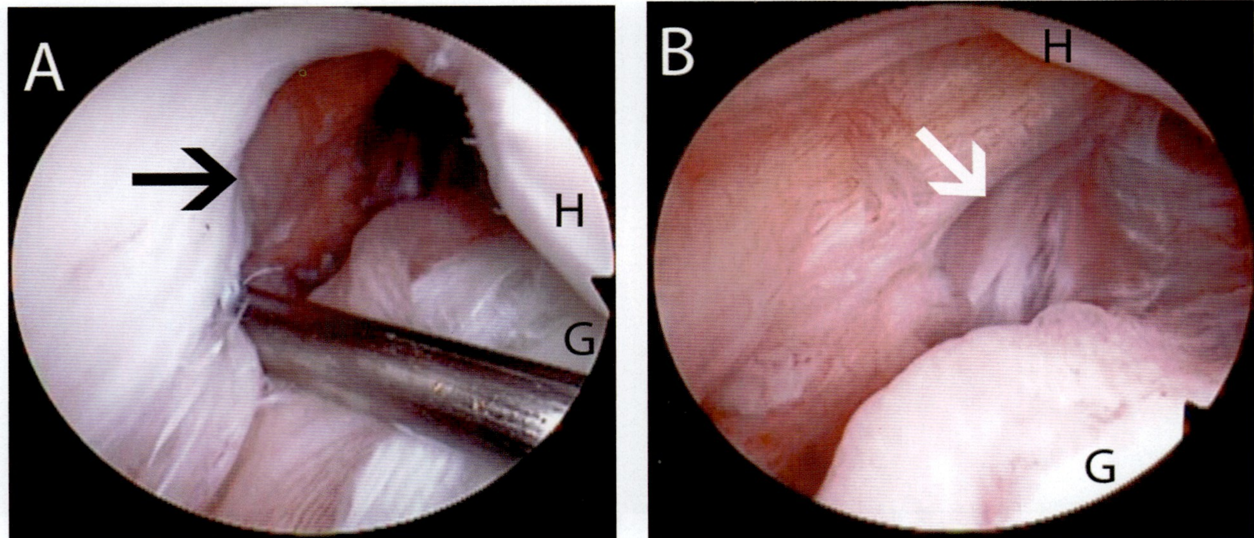

Figure 14.24 **A:** Left shoulder, anterosuperolateral viewing portal, demonstrates a capsular split variant of a reverse humeral avulsion of the glenohumeral ligaments (*black arrow*). **B:** Up-close view demonstrates muscle visible (*white arrow*) underlying the capsular split. G, glenoid; H, humerus.

Capsular splits are the least common type, and can be easily addressed by side-to-side repair (Fig. 14.24). We prefer the Suture Lasso or the BirdBeak for passing No. 2 FiberWire to accomplish the repair (Fig. 14.25).

Capsular avulsion from the humerus is considerably more problematic. The capsular avulsion commonly extends quite low on the humerus, usually to the 5 o'clock position or beyond. In cases with significant inferior extension of the capsular rent, the angle of approach to insert a suture anchor is quite oblique relative to the bone bed. This angle can be very difficult to recreate, and if the surgeon is off by 5° or 10°, the angle may be too oblique for anchor placement. For this reason, we call this the "killer angle," and we have found that placement of the inferior anchor for HAGL repair is one of the most difficult maneuvers in arthroscopic surgery. Furthermore, because of the retroversion of the humeral neck, the proper angle of approach often requires that the accessory anterior portal be located somewhat more medially than the standard 5 o'clock portal (Fig. 14.26). The surgeon must be careful not to stray

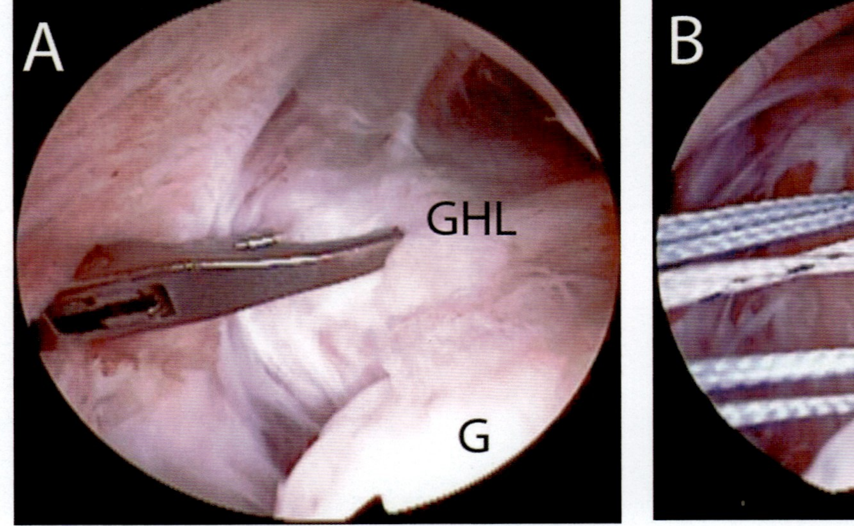

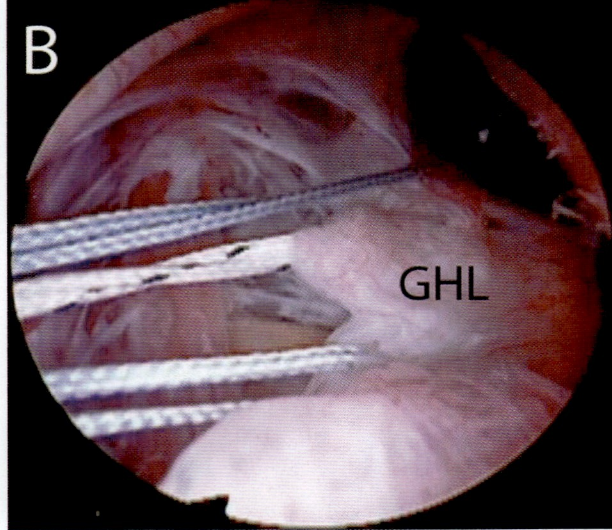

Figure 14.25 Left shoulder, anterosuperolateral viewing portal with a 70° arthroscope, demonstrates repair of a capsular split variant of a reverse humeral avulsion of the glenohumeral ligaments. **A:** A grasper is introduced to assess the mobility of the capsular split. **B:** Three sutures have been placed in the inferior leaf of the capsular split.

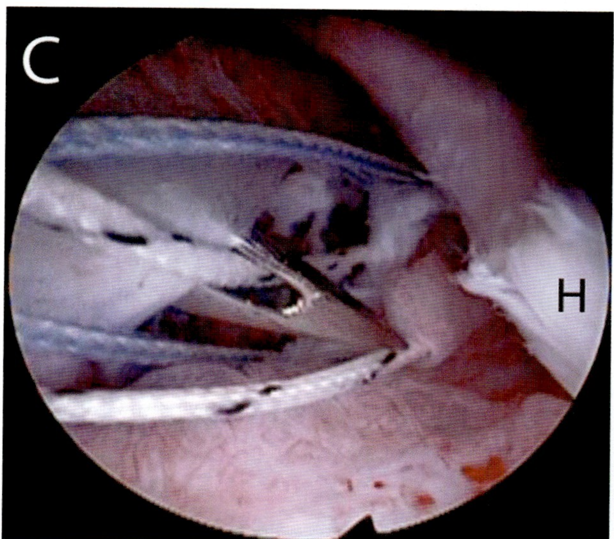

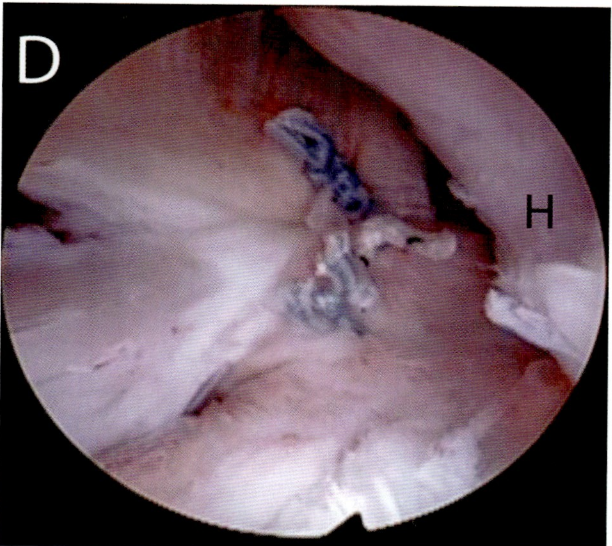

Figure 14.25 *(Continued)* **C:** Sutures are retrieved with a BirdBeak (Arthrex, Inc., Naples, FL) to pass them through the superior leaf of the capsular split. **D:** Final repair following knot tying. G, glenoid; GHL, glenohumeral ligaments; H, humerus.

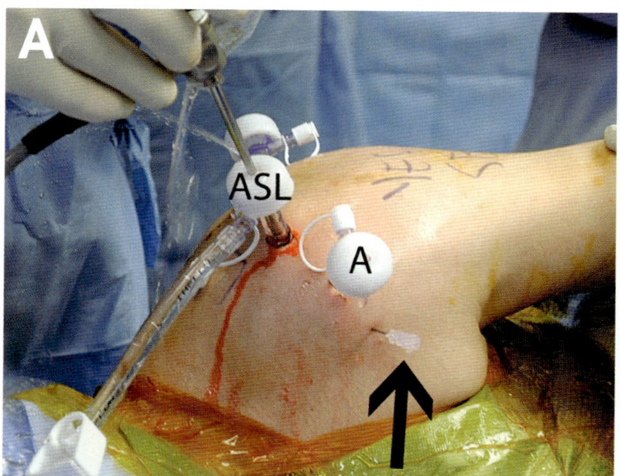

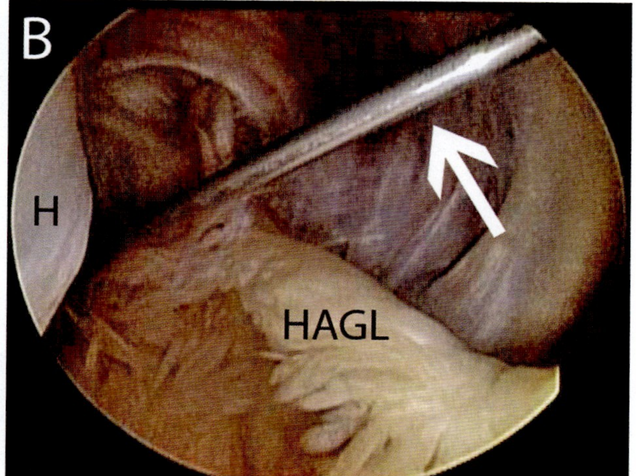

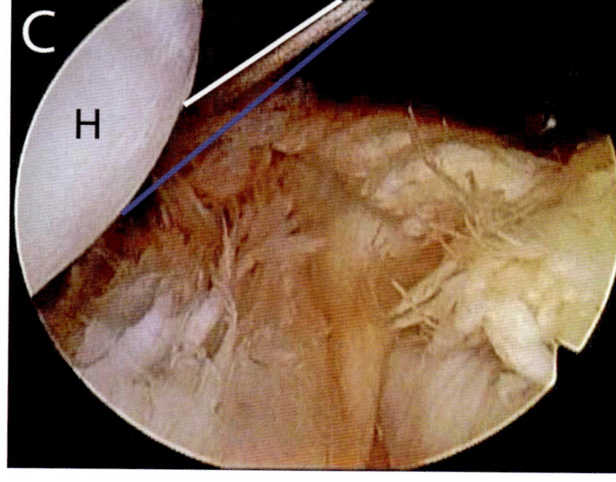

Figure 14.26 The killer angle. **A:** External view in a left shoulder demonstrates the location of the medial low anterior portal (*black arrow*). Note: This portal begins medial to the 5 o'clock portal, which is normally directly inferior to the anterior portal. **B:** Anterosuperolateral viewing portal demonstrates spinal needle (*white arrow*) location in the glenohumeral joint. **C:** Up-close view shows the killer angle. The *white line* parallels the trajectory of the spinal needle. The *blue line* parallels the humeral head. The angle between these two lines is acute with little room for error. Thus, the phrase "killer angle." A, anterior portal; ASL, anterosuperolateral portal; H, humerus; HAGL, humeral avulsion of the glenohumeral ligaments.

medial to the conjoined tendon in order to avoid neurovascular injury. External rotation of the humerus will lateralize the appropriate trajectory for instrumentation, but it will close off the intra-articular working space.

Initially, a spinal needle is used to determine the proper angle of approach, which passes through the subscapularis. Then, portal dilators (Arthrex, Inc., Naples, FL) are sequentially used to enlarge the portal so that a 4-mm Spear Guide can be used as a delivery cannula for a 3.0-mm double-loaded BioComposite SutureTak anchor. Sometimes a single anchor is sufficient, but for larger lesions a second suture anchor can be placed through the same modified 5 o'clock portal. Sutures are then passed through the capsule with either retrograde (SutureLasso or BirdBeak) or antegrade (Scorpion or Viper) instrumentation. We then tie the sutures as static six-throw surgeon's knots using the Surgeon's Sixth Finger Knot Pusher (Fig. 14.27).

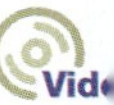

Postoperatively, the arm is held in a pillow sling for 6 weeks. Then, active and active-assisted motion is begun, along with progressive strengthening. Full activities are allowed at 6 months after repair.

Reverse HAGL (RHAGL) Lesion

The RHAGL lesion is the mirror image of the HAGL lesion, in that it occurs posteriorly and involves avulsion of the posterior capsuloligamentous tissue from the humerus.

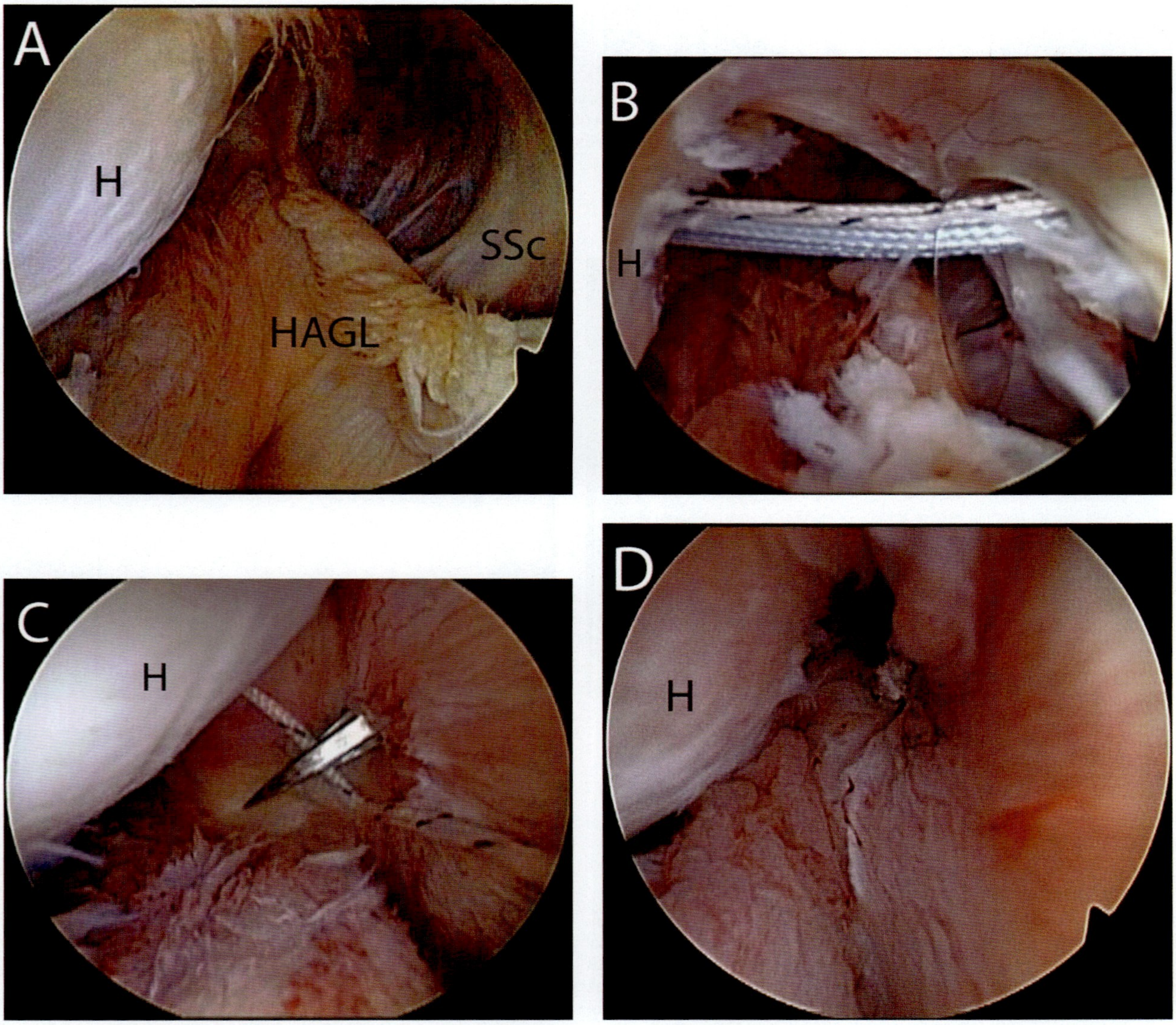

Figure 14.27 Left shoulder, viewed from an anterosuperolateral portal with a 70° arthroscope, demonstrates repair of a HAGL lesion. **A:** View of the HAGL lesion. Note: The muscle of the subscapularis tendon is visible anteriorly (right in the image). **B:** An anchor has been placed in the humeral head. **C:** Sutures are passed retrograde through the avulsed ligaments. **D:** Final repair demonstrates restoration of the glenohumeral ligament insertion. H, humerus; HAGL, humeral avulsion of the glenohumeral ligament; SSc, subscapularis tendon.

Like the HAGL lesion, it may involve a capsular split, avulsion from the bone, or a combination of the two.

Repair of a RHAGL lesion is much easier than repair of a HAGL lesion because the neurovascular structures are not at such risk with a posterior approach. Furthermore, anchor placement is much easier because the humeral neck retroversion is advantageous for posterior anchor placement, and because there is no posterior bone structure equivalent to the coracoid that must be "dodged" during anchor placement.

Recognition of this unusual entity is key. If one views only through a posterior viewing portal, the lesion may be missed. It is essential to view the posterior capsule from an anterosuperolateral viewing portal (Fig. 14.28). In addition, we believe that the lateral decubitus position affords a much better view with more posterior working space than the beach-chair position.

Suture anchors are placed through a posterior portal while viewing through an anterosuperolateral portal. Then, the posterior cannula is withdrawn slightly so that its mouth is just outside the joint capsule. Then, a retrograde passer (BirdBeak or Penetrator) can be used to pass the sutures through capsule. The mouth of the cannula is held just outside (superficial to) the capsule while a blind static or sliding knot is tied. This is repeated for each suture pair of each anchor (Fig. 14.29).

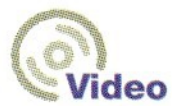

Postoperatively, the patient wears a pillow sling for 6 weeks, with the thicker end of the wedged pillow placed anteriorly in order to prevent excessive tension on the posterior sutures. At the end of 6 weeks, the sling is removed and active motion is allowed, along with progressive strengthening. We avoid passive stretching due to the thin nature of the posterior capsule in most patients.

Combined Humeral and Glenoid Lesions

We have seen cases of combined HAGL and Bankart lesions, as well as combined RHAGL and reverse Bankart lesions. As a general principle, when this occurs, we first

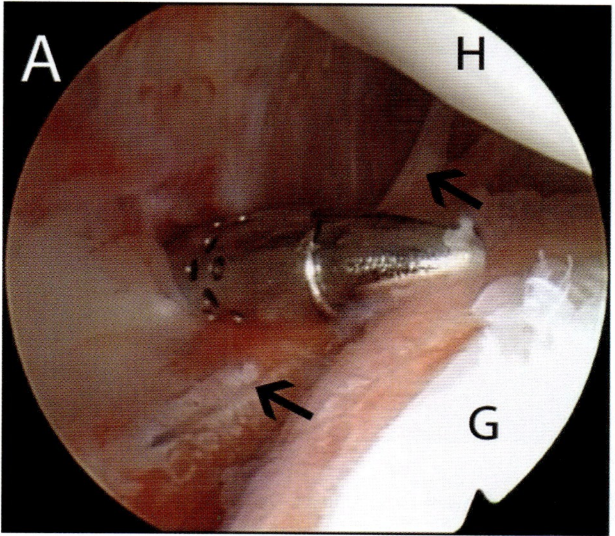

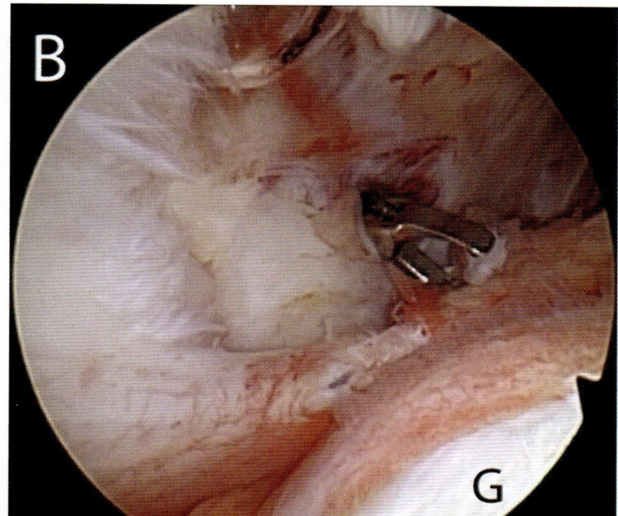

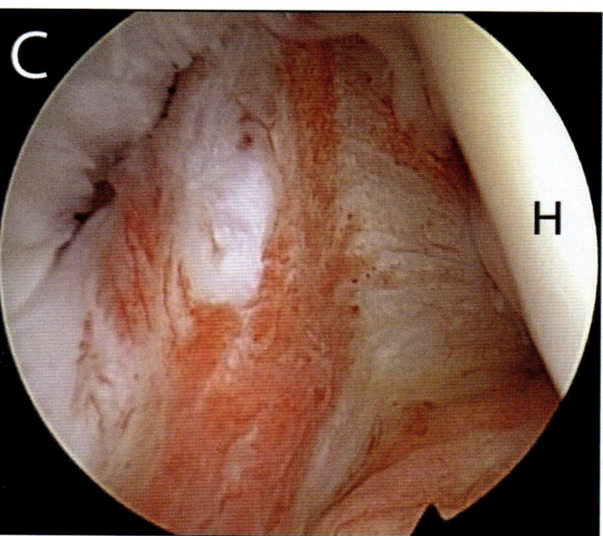

Figure 14.28 Left shoulder, anterosuperolateral viewing portal demonstrates **(A)** a reverse humeral avulsion of the glenohumeral ligaments (RHAGL lesion) (*black arrows*). **B:** A grasper is introduced from a posterior portal to assess capsular mobility. **C:** View demonstrating sufficient mobility of the RHAGL lesion to reach the posterior humerus. G, glenoid; H, humerus.

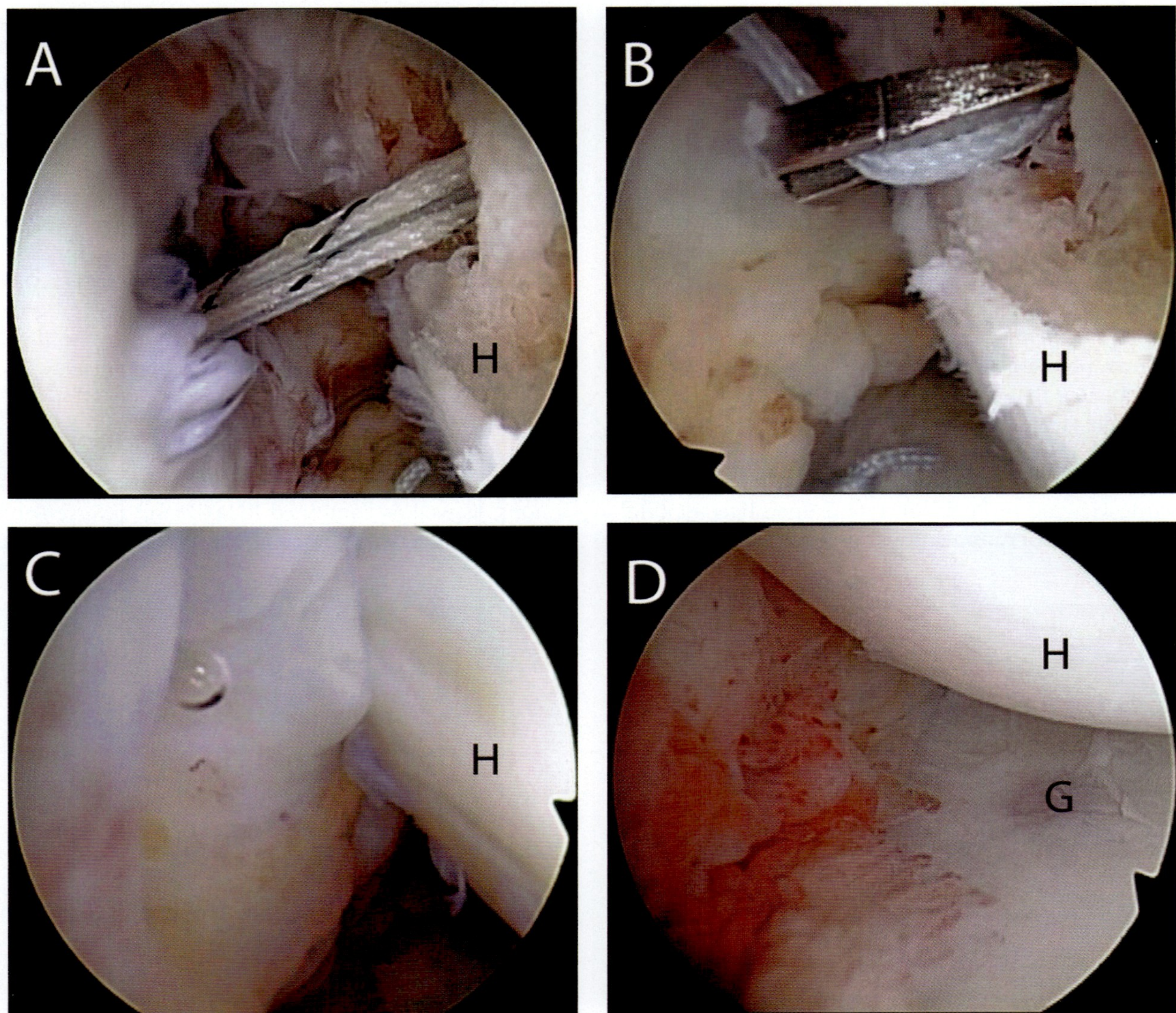

Figure 14.29 Left shoulder, anterosuperolateral viewing portal, demonstrating repair of a reverse humeral avulsion of the glenohumeral ligaments (RHAGL). **A:** View with a 70° arthroscope shows anchors placed in the posterior humeral head. **B:** The posterior cannula is withdrawn and a retrograde instrument (BirdBeak; Arthrex, Inc., Naples, FL) is used to pass sutures through the posterior glenohumeral ligaments. **C:** Final view of the repair shows repair of the posterior glenohumeral ligaments to the humerus. **D:** Profile view with a 30° arthroscope through an anterosuperolateral viewing portal demonstrates restoration of the posterior glenohumeral ligaments (compare to Fig. 14.28A). G, glenoid; H, humerus.

repair the glenoid disruption in order to stabilize one end of the unstable capsular sheet, and then repair the humeral side after that.

MULTIDIRECTIONAL INSTABILITY

Multidirectional instability is an uncommon surgical disorder compared to other instability patterns. The vast majority of patients with multidirectional instability may be treated nonoperatively through retraining and rehabilitation of the dynamic muscular stabilizers of the glenohumeral and scapulothoracic joints. This section considers only surgical treatment of non-Bankart (i.e., nonlabral tear) multidirectional instability. Patients with traumatic multidirectional instability (e.g., triple labral lesion) are distinct and were previously addressed in this chapter.

The surgical goal of multidirectional instability is to shorten the ligaments and decrease the volume of the glenohumeral joint. The most reliable method to surgically reduce the volume of the glenohumeral joint is through multiple suture plications. In this fashion, precise shortening of the ligaments can lead to direction-specific changes in ligament tension and reduction of joint volume.

Furthermore, a number of technical variables may be altered depending on the desired surgical outcome. These include the amount of plication, suture configuration, and suture type. Obviously the amount of plication is the most important surgically modifiable factor. In addition, many different suture configurations have been described to plicate the capsule and augment the labrum (e.g., simple, mattress [or box], figure-of-8).

Although some stitches may plicate and augment the labrum in different fashions, we prefer simple stitches (passed in a pinch-tuck fashion), which provide the tightest loop configuration.

In patients with a predominant direction of instability, we always use permanent suture (No. 2 FiberWire) for capsular plication in the predominant direction of instability and occasionally use absorbable suture (No. 1 PDS; Ethicon, Somerville, NJ) for plication of the rest of the glenohumeral joint. However, in patients with global instability, No. 2 FiberWire is used universally for capsular plication. In this fashion, suture type is used to titrate the surgical outcome.

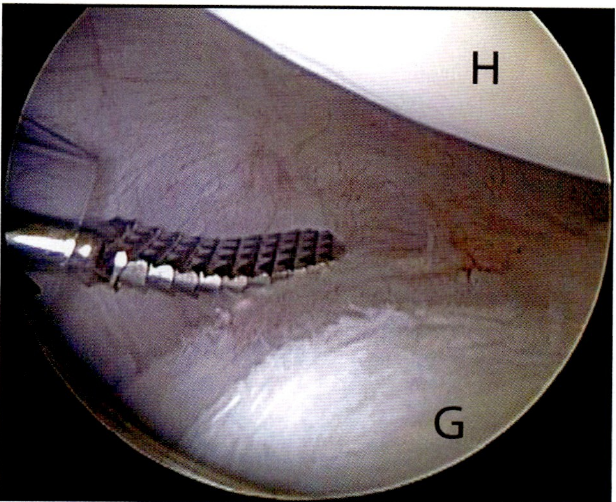

Figure 14.30 Left shoulder, anterosuperolateral viewing portal. A rasp has been introduced through a posterior working portal to lightly excoriate the capsule in a patient with multidirectional instability. G, glenoid; H, humerus.

Arthroscopic Capsular Plication

An examination under anesthesia is performed to confirm glenohumeral joint laxity in the anterior, posterior, and inferior directions. Comparison to the opposite shoulder and consideration of preoperative symptoms are critical to determine the surgical goals of treatment (e.g., global and equal capsular plication, global capsular plication anterior predominant).

Standard anterior, posterior, and anterosuperolateral cannulas are established and a complete diagnostic arthroscopy is performed. In all cases of multidirectional instability, it is important to evaluate the joint carefully for signs of instability including chondral injury, labral fraying or fissuring, capsular lesions (thinning, tears, avulsions), and bone lesions (Hill-Sachs, reverse Hill-Sachs, and bone defects of the glenoid). These findings are supportive of the suspected predominant direction of instability and may alter the surgical procedure. However, in most cases, patients with atraumatic multidirectional instability will have no clear pathology indicating a significant translational episode.

The glenohumeral joint is viewed through the anterosuperolateral portal, and adequate anterior and posterior access to the inferior capsule is confirmed. A Slotted Whisker Shaver Blade (Arthrex, Inc., Naples, FL) or rasp is introduced through the anterior and posterior portals to lightly excoriate the capsule and created a healing surface for capsular plication (Fig. 14.30). Suction is avoided on the shaver and care is taken to ensure that damage to the fragile capsule does not occur.

The quality and integrity of the labrum is then evaluated. In patients without labral tearing and with robust labral tissue, direct capsular plication to the labrum may be utilized and has been shown to have a similar strength to anchor-based repairs. However, we have found that in most patients with multidirectional instability, the labrum is hypoplastic and quite elastic, so we usually prefer to place suture anchors in order to have a firm fixation point to which we can plicate. If there is a predominant direction of instability, the surgical procedure begins and focuses on this region first. However, in patients with global instability, we generally pass posteroinferior sutures first, and progress to anteroinferior, then midanterior, and then midposterior.

While viewing through the anterosuperolateral portal, a 25° Tight Curve SutureLasso (left curved for a right shoulder) is introduced through the posterior portal and a "pinch-tuck" technique is used to plicate the capsule to the labrum. In this technique, the SutureLasso is first used to capture a fold of capsular tissue (Fig. 14.31A), completely penetrating the capsular fold. While maintaining the capsular fold within the SutureLasso, the hook is used to penetrate the labrum in the proposed capsular plication location (Fig. 14.31B).

The SutureLasso is only advanced enough through the labrum to allow passage of the shuttling suture (PDS suture). Care is taken to ensure minimal damage to the labrum. The shuttling suture is retrieved through the anterior portal (Fig. 14.31C) and a No. 2 FiberWire suture is shuttled through the labrum and capsule completing the capsular plication stitch (Fig. 14.31D). Using a similar technique, second and/or third sutures are passed through the posteroinferior capsule and labrum as required. Sutures are held provisionally in the anterior portal for suture management.

In some cases, the access and angle of approach to the capsule and labrum are awkward and the "pinch-tuck" technique cannot be performed in a single pass. When this occurs, separate passes are used for the capsular tuck and

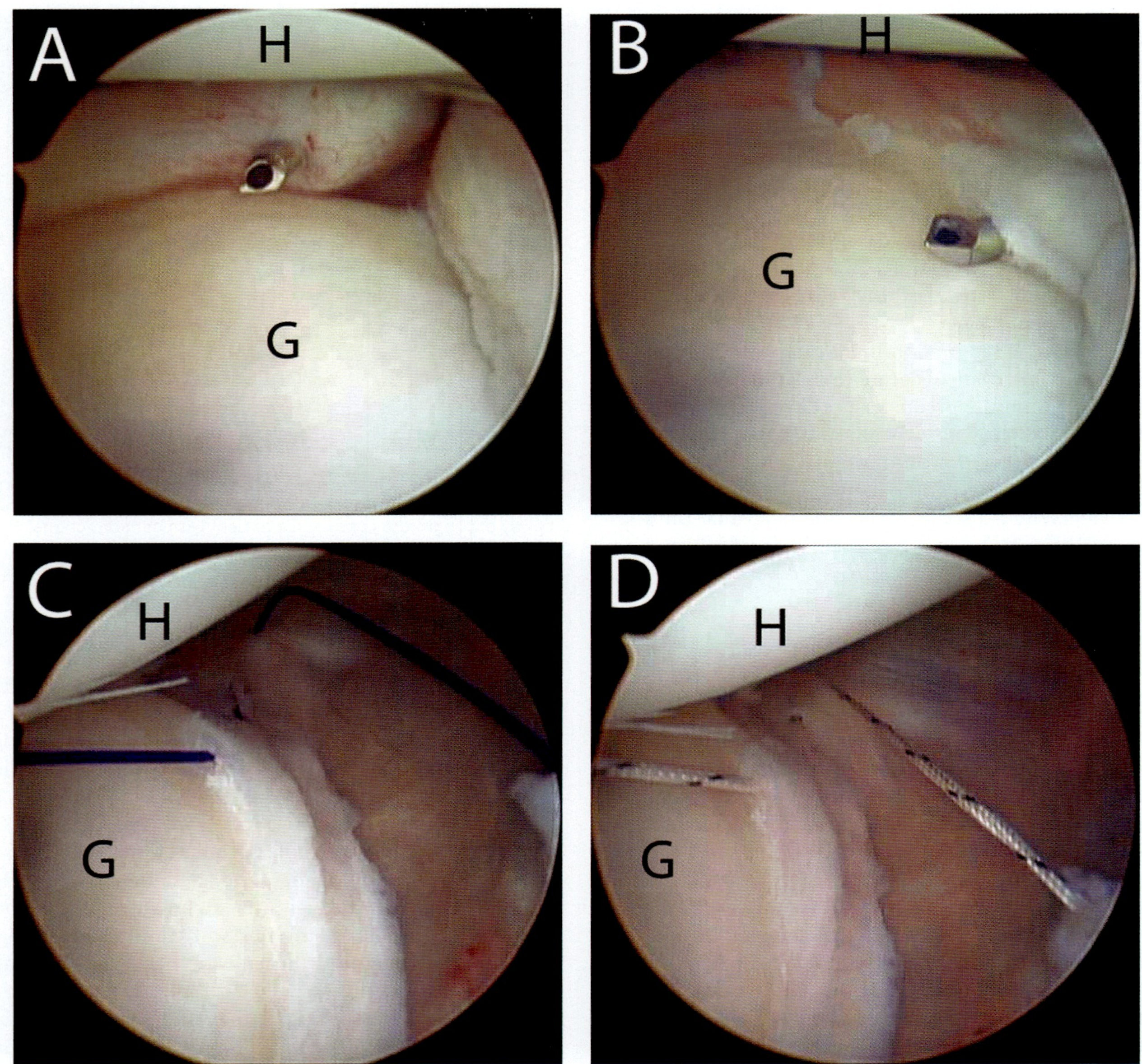

Figure 14.31 Right shoulder, anterosuperolateral viewing portal, demonstrates suture passage for a capsular-based plication. **A:** A SutureLasso (Arthrex, Inc., Naples, FL) is introduced from a posterior working portal and is used to capture posteroinferior capsule. **B:** Without withdrawing the SutureLasso, a second pass is made more superior to advance the capsule. **C:** A shuttling suture has been passed through the capsule and labrum. **D:** A No. 2 FiberWire suture (Arthrex, Inc., Naples, FL) is then shuttled through the capsule and labrum. G, glenoid; H, humerus.

labral stitches, shuttling the No. 2 FiberWire suture after each pass.

Once the posteroinferior sutures have been passed, the anteroinferior capsule is approached. The previously placed posteroinferior sutures are retrieved through the posterior portal for suture management. Using the same technique, a 25° Tight Curve SutureLasso (right curved for a right shoulder) is used to plicate the anteroinferior capsule to the labrum. The suture shuttle is retrieved through the posterior portal and a No. 2 FiberWire is shuttled through the capsule and labrum. It is critical that the most inferior two stitches from the anterior and posterior plications capture the inferior capsule and labrum to reduce inferior laxity and volume. Failure to do so will create a "funnel-shaped" repair with persistent inferior instability. Usually, two or three sutures are required for the anteroinferior capsular plication (Fig. 14.32).

Once the inferior sutures (posterior and anterior) have been passed, static knots are tied with a Surgeon's Sixth Finger to reduce the inferior capsule to the labrum or suture

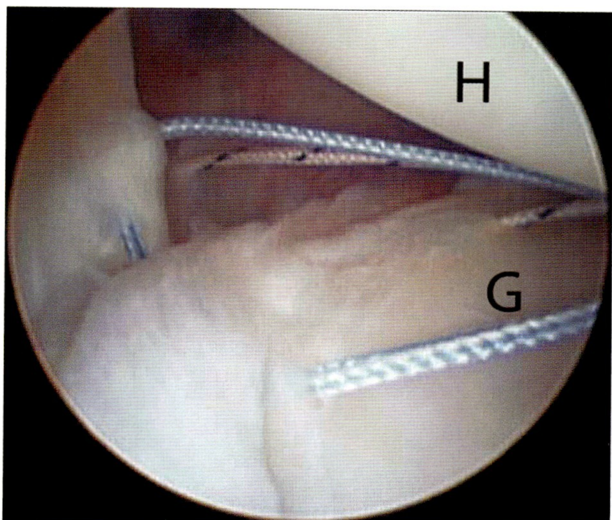

Figure 14.32 Right shoulder, anterosuperolateral viewing portal, demonstrates sutures that have been passed anteroinferiorly for a capsular-based plication. Note: The sutures pass through both the capsule and the labrum in two separate passes. G, glenoid; H, humerus.

anchors (Fig. 14.33). We prefer static knots when performing capsular plications since sliding knots can cut through the capsule and labrum when sliding the knot down the post limb.

Next, sutures are placed to plicate the midanterior capsule and middle glenohumeral ligament to the labrum (Fig. 14.34). Care is taken to avoid overconstraining the joint by aggressive middle glenohumeral ligament plication. Instead, the capsule is plicated to augment the labrum rather than shorten the ligament. In this region, visualization is usually excellent and sutures may be tied immediately following suture passage. Plication is continued to the superior border of the subscapularis tendon (Fig. 14.35).

Finally, the midposterior and posterosuperior capsule are similarly plicated. However, when passing sutures superior to the posterior cannula, we often prefer to view through the anterior portal. The SutureLasso is introduced through the anterosuperolateral portal and provides an excellent angle of approach to the midposterior and posterosuperior capsule and labrum. Suture plication is continued to the posterior aspect of the biceps tendon (Fig. 14.36). In this region, sutures may be tied immediately following suture passage.

Once suture plication has been completed, the glenohumeral joint is reevaluated for centering of the humeral head, reduction of the drive through sign, augmentation of the labrum, reduction of joint volume, and shortening of the capsule/ligaments. If further plication is required, then it is performed now, otherwise attention is turned toward closure of the posterior portal and the rotator interval.

While viewing through the anterosuperolateral portal, the posterior portal closing suture is passed. The cannula is retracted out of the glenohumeral joint until it is just superficial to the capsule without any interposed rotator cuff musculature. A Straight SutureLasso is introduced through the posterior cannula, penetrating the capsule adjacent to the posterior portal, and a No. 1 PDS or No. 2 FiberWire suture is retrieved through the anterior portal. To complete the stitch, a Penetrator is introduced through the posterior capsule opposite to the previous puncture and retrieves the

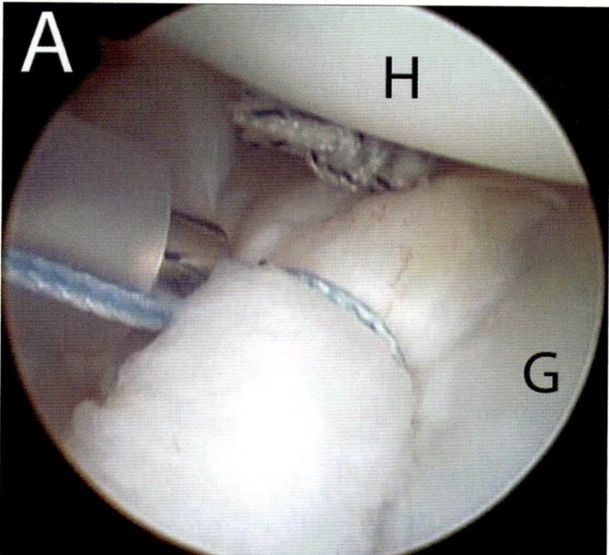

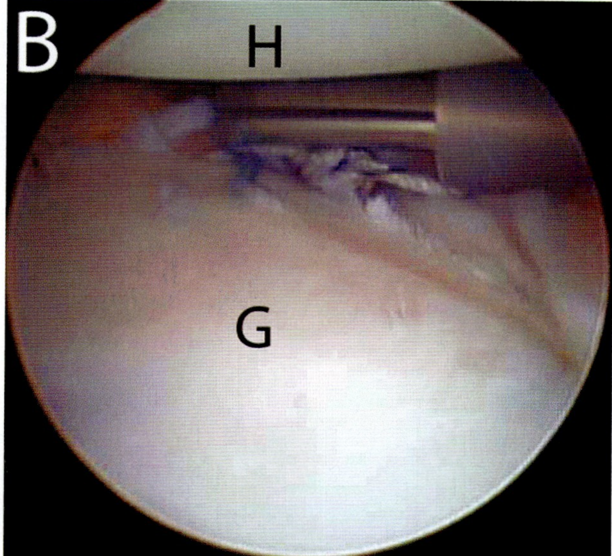

Figure 14.33 Right shoulder, anterosuperolateral viewing portal. After posteroinferior and anteroinferior sutures are placed for a capsular plication, the **(A)** anterior and **(B)** posterior sutures are tied with a Surgeon's Sixth Finger Knot Pusher (Arthrex, Inc., Naples, FL) G, glenoid; H, humerus.

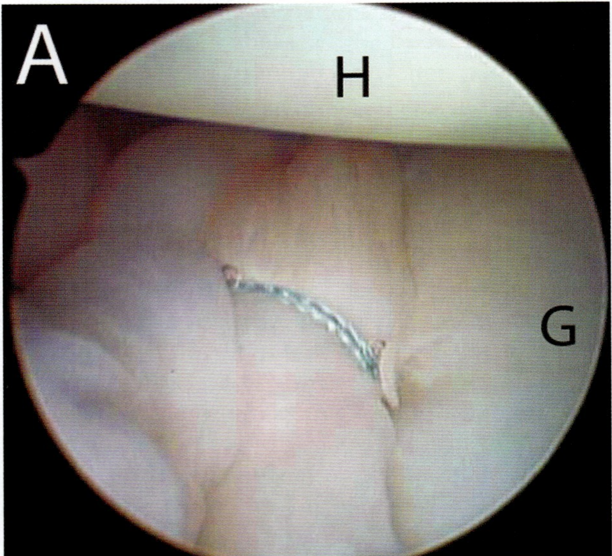

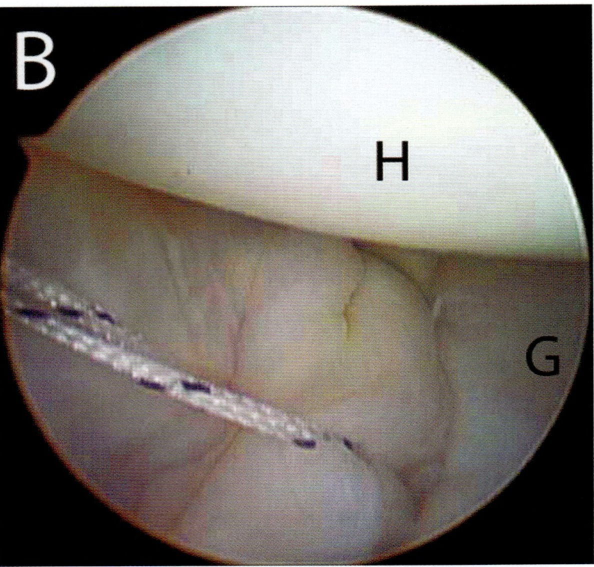

Figure 14.34 **A,B:** Right shoulder, anterosuperolateral viewing portal. Once inferior sutures have been tied, plication is continued anteriorly by passing additional sutures through the middle glenohumeral ligament and midlabrum. G, glenoid; H, humerus.

suture through the posterior cannula (Fig. 14.37). The posterior portal closing suture is not tied until all other sutures have been tied, at the end of the case.

For rotator interval closure, the glenohumeral joint is viewed through the posterior portal. However, to avoid creating a second defect through the posterior capsule, a switching stick is first used to reestablish the posterior portal for the 4.5-mm diameter arthroscope sheath while viewing through the anterosuperolateral portal. The rotator interval is viewed through the posterior portal and the subscapularis, middle glenohumeral ligament, and superior glenohumeral ligament are identified.

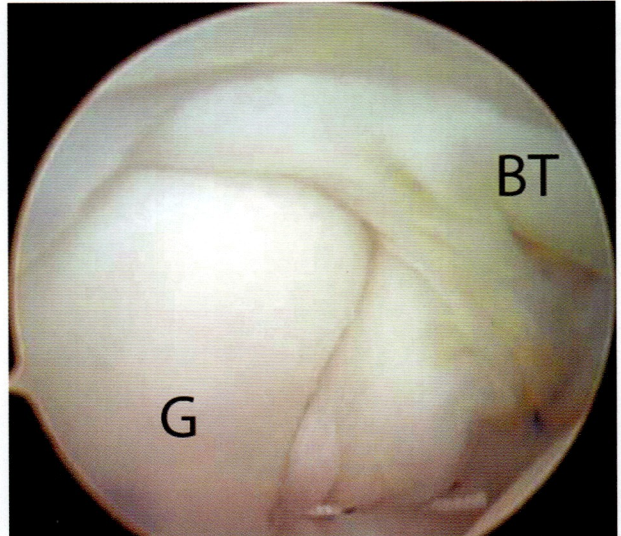

Figure 14.35 Right shoulder, posterior viewing portal, demonstrates extent of anterior plication for multidirectional instability. The plication is performed up to the superior border of the subscapularis tendon that is at about the midglenoid level. BT, biceps tendon; G, glenoid.

Our preference is to plicate the superior glenohumeral ligament to the middle glenohumeral ligament and avoid overconstraint that occurs by suturing to the supraspinatus or subscapularis tendons. Using a similar technique to closure of the posterior portal, the cannula is retracted out of the glenohumeral joint until it is just superficial to the capsule. A Straight SutureLasso is used to penetrate the middle glenohumeral ligament and a PDS suture or No. 2 FiberStick (Arthrex, Inc., Naples, FL) is passed into the glenohumeral joint. The SutureLasso is retracted, leaving the suture in the glenohumeral joint. A Penetrator is then passed from the anterior cannula through superior glenohumeral ligament to retrieve the suture. If a PDS suture is used, a No. 2 FiberWire is then shuttled into place; this step can be avoided by using a No. 2 FiberStick (Fig. 14.38). The steps are repeated if a second suture if required.

Keeping the cannula extracapsular, the sutures are tied blind in the cannula to close the rotator interval. Alternatively, the sutures may be retrieved in the subacromial space and tied under direct vision. Finally, the arthroscope is removed and the posterior sutures are tied to close the posterior portal.

Pancapsular Plication (Anchor Based)

When the quality of labral tissue is poor, an anchor-based capsular plication is the best alternative. The same principles of repair are respected and the sequence of plication is identical to that above. The decision as to whether to plicate to the labrum or anchor is based upon the arthroscopist's

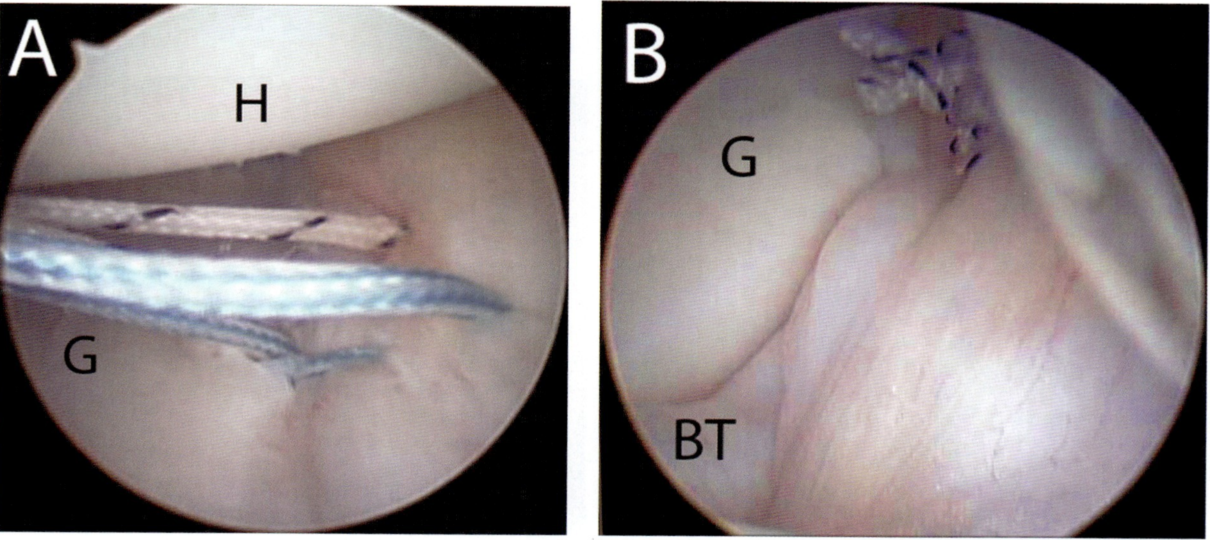

Figure 14.36 **A:** Right shoulder, anterosuperolateral viewing portal. Once anterior plication is completed, additional posterior sutures are placed and tied. **B:** The posterior plication continues superiorly to the biceps tendon. BT, biceps tendon; G, glenoid; H, humerus.

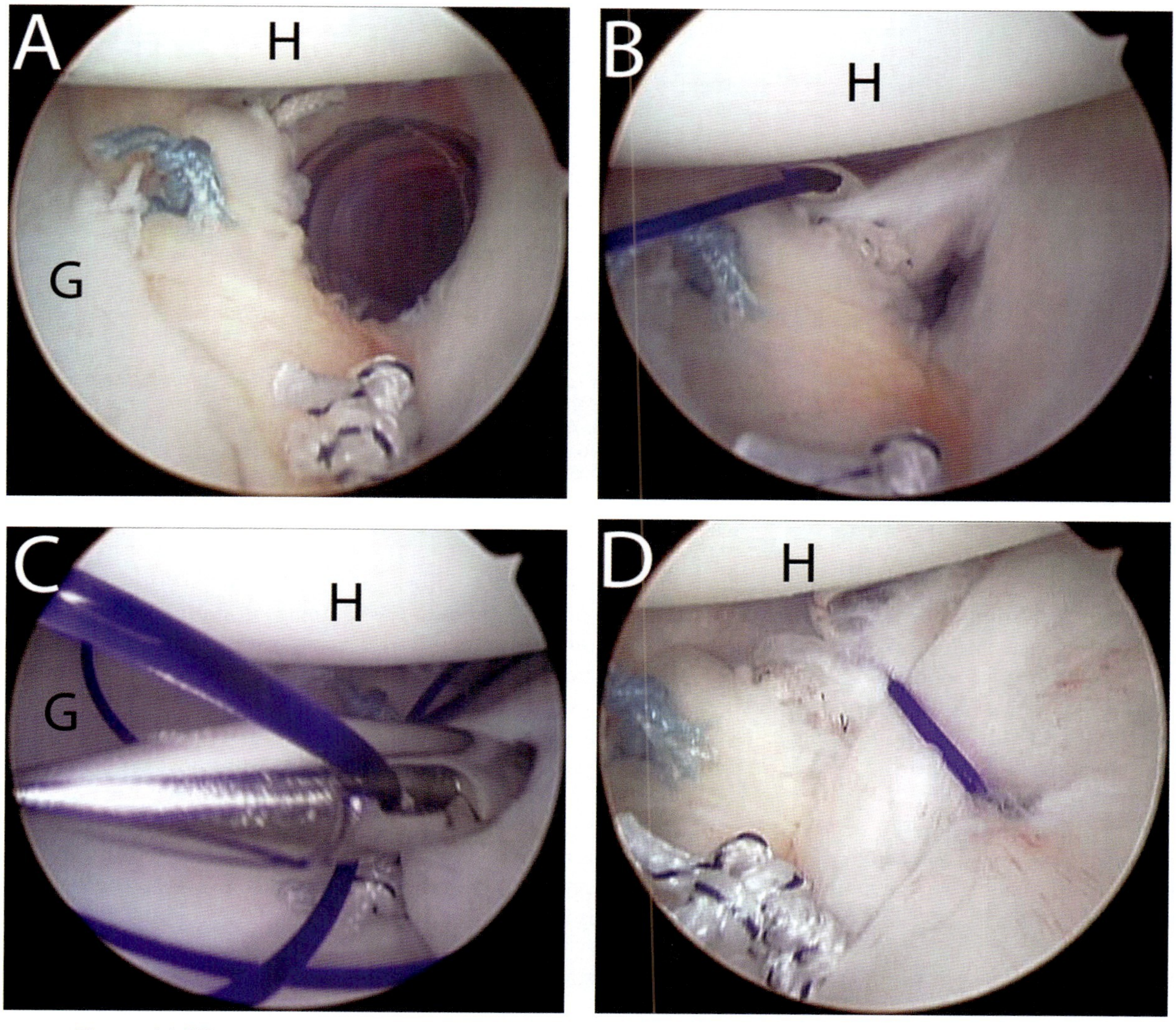

Figure 14.37 Right shoulder, anterosuperolateral viewing portal, demonstrates posterior portal closure. **A:** View prior to portal closure. **B:** The cannula is withdrawn and a SutureLasso (Arthrex, Inc., Naples, FL) is used to pass a suture through the posterior capsule on one side of the portal defect. **C:** A retrograde suture retriever penetrates the capsule on the opposite side of the portal defect and retrieves the other end of the suture. **D:** View after closure of the posterior portal. G, glenoid; H, humerus.

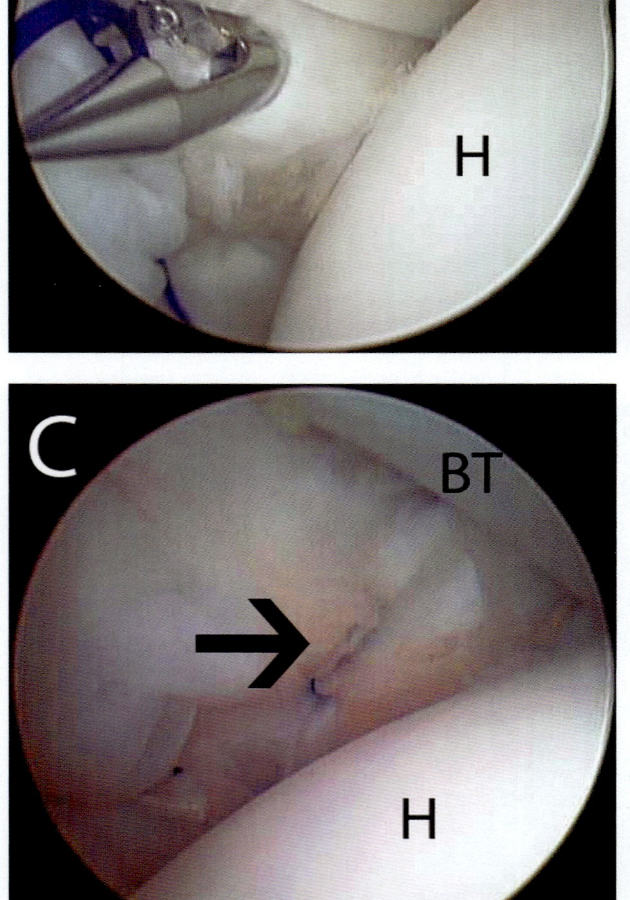

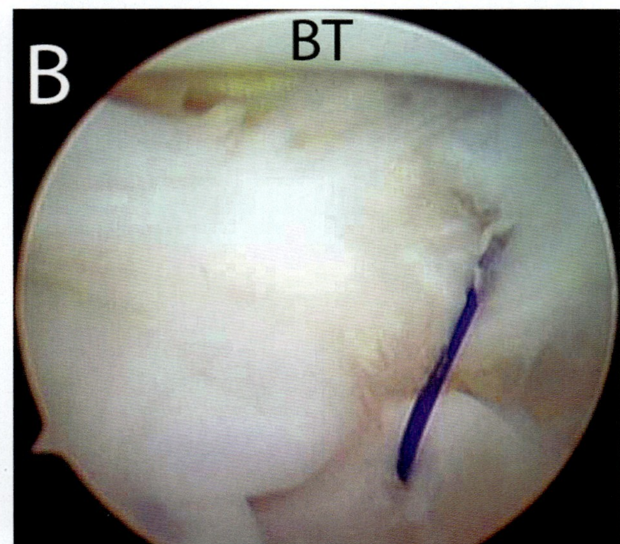

Figure 14.38 Right shoulder, posterior viewing portal, demonstrates rotator interval closure. **A:** A suture shuttle has previously been passed through the middle glenohumeral ligament. A retrograde suture passer is advanced through the superior glenohumeral ligament and used to retrieve the suture shuttle. **B:** Appearance after the suture shuttle has been placed. **C:** A No. 2 FiberWire suture (Arthrex, Inc., Naples, FL) is shuttled into place (*black arrow*) and tied to close the rotator interval. BT, biceps tendon; H, humerus.

judgment of the ability of the labrum to hold sutures and withstand the forces of early rehabilitation. Generally, patients with hypoplastic, diminutive labra are candidates for anchor-based capsular plications. Alternatively, the arthroscopist may choose to place anchors in the predominant direction of instability to provide secure fixation to bone, while plicating directly to the labrum in the nondominant directions of instability.

Standard anterior, posterior, and anterosuperolateral portals are created and the labral quality is assessed. The capsule is lightly excoriated to create a healing interface. In this scenario, the labrum is also debrided since the capsule will be advanced up on top of labrum and glenoid face. For anchor-based pancapsular plication, usually four or five 3.0-mm BioComposite SutureTak anchors double loaded with No. 2 FiberWire will be used.

While viewing through the anterosuperolateral portal, anchors are inserted into the posteroinferior glenoid. A separate low posterolateral portal is created approximately 4 to 5 cm inferior to the posterolateral corner of the acromion to provide a 45° angle of approach to the posteroinferior glenoid. It is usually easier to place an inferior glenoid anchor via a posterior portal, rather than from anterior where the subscapularis tendon and axillary nerve restrict inferior placement. A small skin puncture incision is created after a spinal needle determines the correct angle of approach, and a switching stick is then used to parallel the angle of approach. The BioComposite SutureTak Spear is then slid over the switching stick and placed at the chondrolabral junction. A bone socket is drilled, and the anchor is inserted (Fig. 14.39).

Using standard suture passing techniques, capsular tissue is plicated and advanced to the labrum (Fig. 14.40). In contrast to suture plication to the labrum where the capsule is advanced to the labrum, suture plication to an anchor causes the capsule to advance further up onto and over the labrum. Therefore, in general, the "bite" of capsule is slightly less when plicating to an anchor. The suture

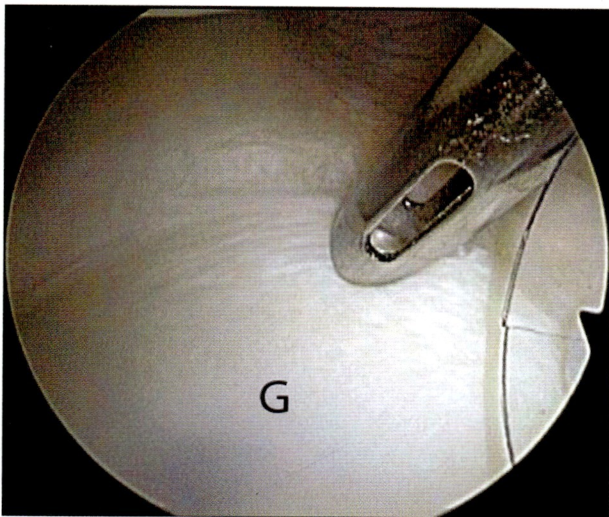

Figure 14.39 Right shoulder, posterior viewing portal, demonstrates placement of a posteroinferior anchor for anchor-based capsular plication. G, glenoid.

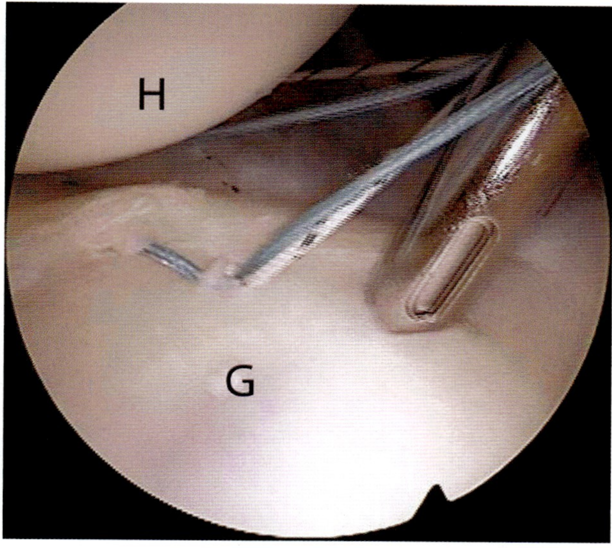

Figure 14.41 Right shoulder, posterior viewing portal, after sutures are passed for the posteroinferior anchor, a second anchor is placed posteriorly. G, glenoid; H, humerus.

shuttle is retrieved through the anterior portal with the No. 2 FiberWire suture and the suture is shuttled through the tissue. The second suture is then passed.

A second posterior anchor is inserted and sutures are passed advancing the capsule superiorly and shortening the glenohumeral ligaments (Fig. 14.41).

Attention is now turned to the anteroinferior glenohumeral joint. The previously placed posterior sutures are retrieved through the posterior portal for holding. An anchor is placed in the anteroinferior aspect of the glenoid (Fig. 14.42) and a 25° Tight Curve SutureLasso (right curved for a right shoulder) is used to superiorly advance the inferior capsule and close the axillary recess. It is again important to ensure that the inferior stitches completely and equally close the inferior glenohumeral joint to ensure that a "funnel-shaped" repair does not result. Once the anteroinferior sutures have been passed, the anterior and posterior sutures may be tied (Fig. 14.43).

The steps are repeated for the second anterior anchor and third posterior anchor. The final construct is assessed for centering of the humeral head, reduction of the drive through sign, augmentation of the labrum, reduction of joint volume, and shortening of the capsule/ligaments (Fig. 14.44). The posterior portal and rotator interval may be closed as desired and indicated.

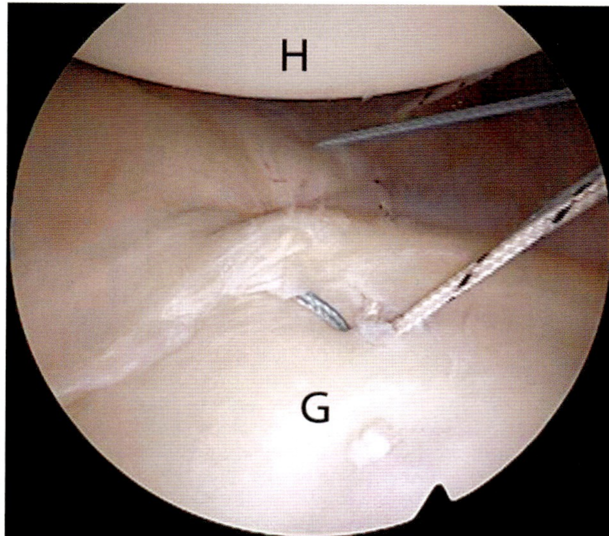

Figure 14.40 Right shoulder, posterior viewing portal, demonstrates sutures that have been passed from a posteroinferior anchor for anchor-based capsular plication. G, glenoid.

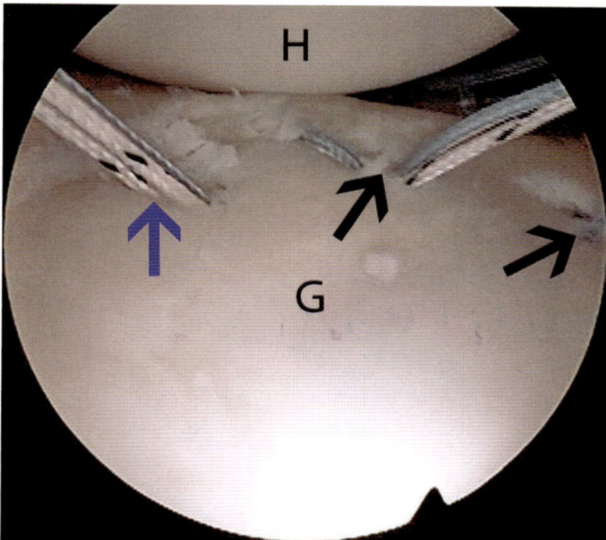

Figure 14.42 Right shoulder, posterior viewing portal. Two posterior anchors (*black arrows*) have been placed and sutures have been passed. Prior to tying these sutures, an anterior anchor (*blue arrow*) is placed and sutures from this anchor will be passed through the capsule and labrum. G, glenoid; H, humerus.

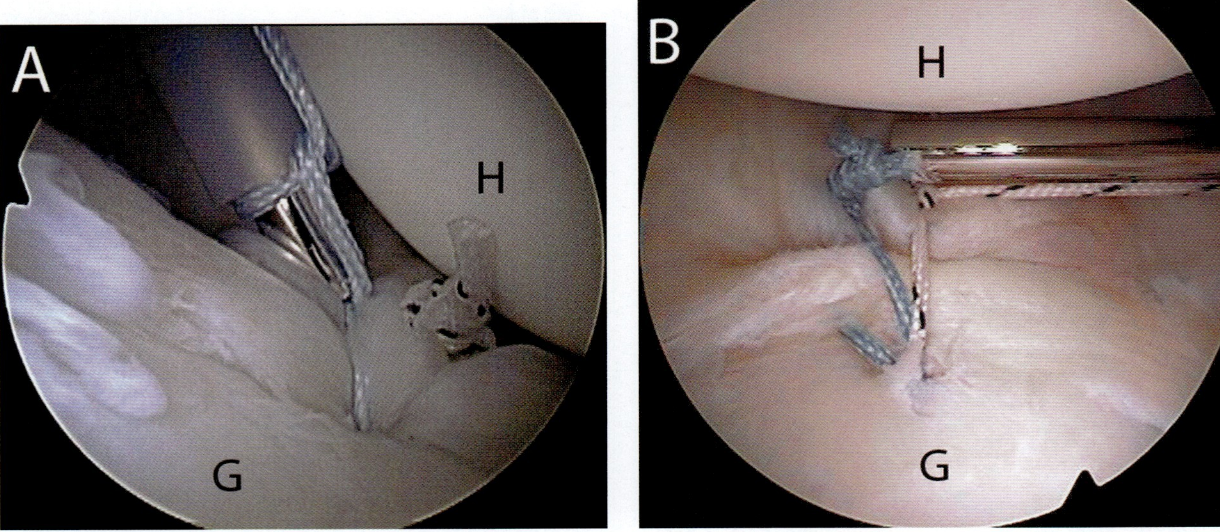

Figure 14.43 Right shoulder. After the anteroinferior and posteroinferior sutures are passed, the (**A**) anterior sutures (viewed from a posterior portal in this case), and (**B**) posterior sutures (viewed from an anterosuperolateral portal in this case) are tied with a Surgeon's Sixth Finger Knot Pusher (Arthrex, Inc., Naples, FL) G, glenoid; H, humerus.

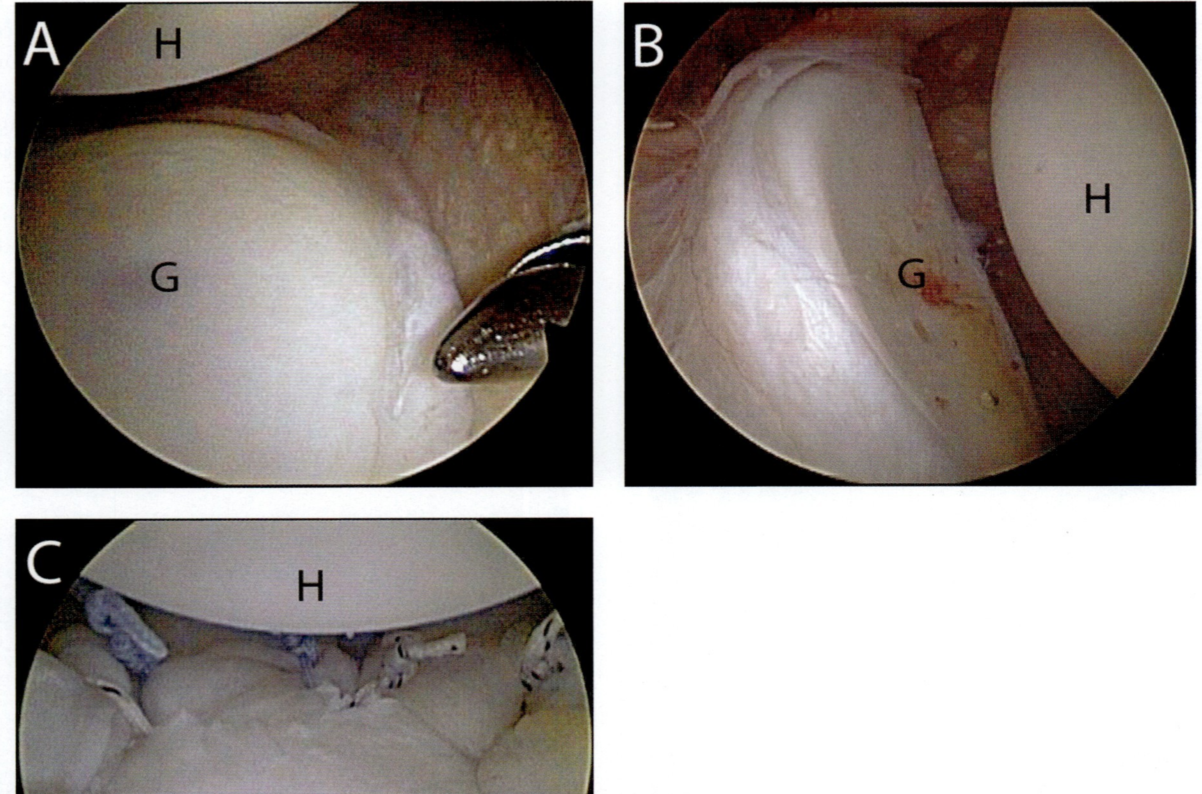

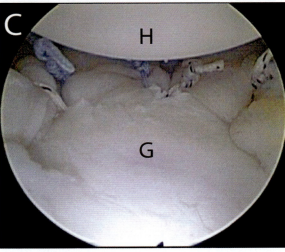

Figure 14.44 **A:** Right shoulder, anterosuperolateral viewing portal, demonstrates a patulous capsule and hypoplastic labrum in an individual with multidirectional instability. **B:** Posterior viewing portal in the same shoulder. **C:** Anterosuperolateral viewing portal in the same shoulder demonstrates anchor-based capsular plication. The humeral head is centered on the glenoid and the capsule has been advanced to the glenoid rim with multiple anchors. G, glenoid; H, humerus.

MULTIDIRECTIONAL INSTABILITY WITH A LABRAL TEAR

Although instability has classically been separated into the categories of (a) multidirectional and atraumatic versus (b) unidirectional and traumatic, several variants can exist. A patient with multidirectional instability can present with a labral tear and a primary direction of instability. In patients with positional posterior instability with an associated posterior labral tear, for instance, surgical repair can eliminate posterior instability and restore function. In addition to having a labral tear with a corresponding primary direction of instability, some individuals present with generalized hyperlaxity signs, external rotation of >80°, a sulcus sign >2 cm, hyperabduction, and translation with load and shift to at least the rim of the glenoid. In such patients, a more aggressive and global approach to the shoulder instability should be considered, including capsular plication in conjunction with labral repair for the primary direction of instability, and consideration of capsular plication opposite the labral tear, closure of the rotator interval, and closure of the posterior portal. Each case is unique and the decision to perform these latter procedures is based on the surgeon's judgment of the extent of pathology.

The order of the steps must be considered for visualization and for ease of suture passage and anchor insertion such that all areas may be addressed without prematurely tightening the joint or limiting visualization. Our standard progression following labral mobilization is the following:

1. Insert all anchors (both for labral repair and for capsular plication)
2. Pass sutures for SLAP repair
3. Pass and tie sutures for an anchor-based labral repair
4. Pass and tie capsular plication sutures for an anchor-based plication
5. Tie SLAP sutures
6. Place posterior portal closure sutures
7. Close the rotator interval
8. Tie posterior portal closure sutures

In patients with SLAP lesions, anchors (BioComposite SutureTak) are placed through the anterosuperolateral portal and Port of Wilmington portal if the tear extends to the posterosuperior quadrant (see Chapter 16, "SLAP lesions," for a complete discussion). Sutures are passed using a Micro SutureLasso (Arthrex, Inc., Naples, FL) to encircle the labrum and provide secure fixation. Although sutures are passed, they are not tied until later in the procedure. Sutures are provisionally held through the anterosuperolateral portal for suture management.

The labral repair is then performed as described previously. However, in these cases, capsular plication is performed in conjunction with anchor-based labral repair (Fig. 14.45). Usually, a 25° Tight Curve SutureLasso is the primary instrument of choice to perform the capsular plication. In most cases, approximately 1 cm of capsule is plicated to the labrum although the exact amount of capsular plication must be individualized to the patient's degree of laxity. Anchor placement and suture passage are performed progressively from inferior to superior.

The capsular plication is performed next. In patients with generalized ligamentous laxity and a positive sulcus sign (>2 cm), a capsular plication can be important to ensure balancing of the glenohumeral joint. Plication is performed

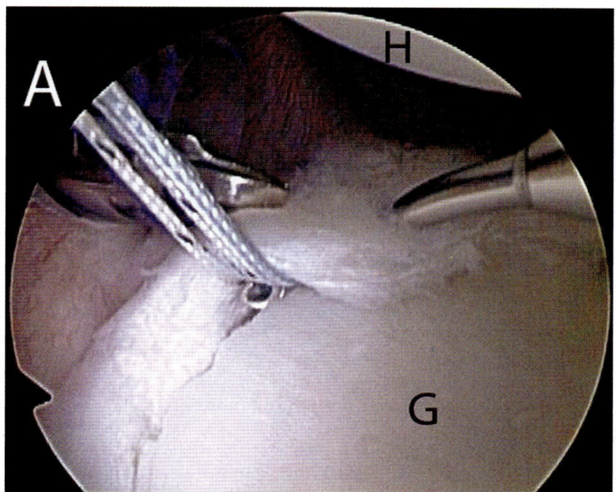

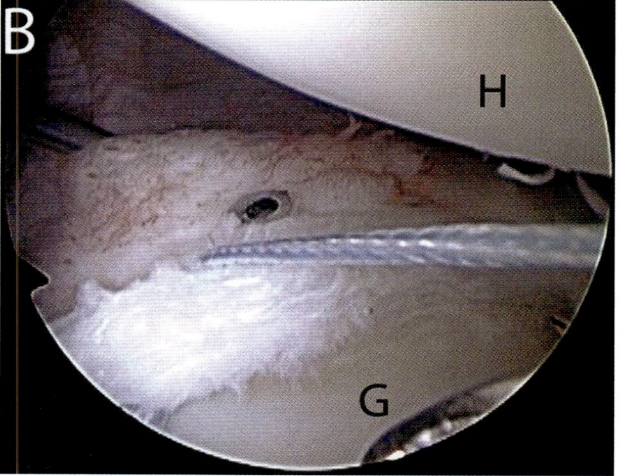

Figure 14.45 Left shoulder, anterosuperolateral viewing portal, demonstrates labral repair and capsular plication in an individual with a posterior Bankart lesion and hyperlaxity. **A:** Following anchor placement, a SutureLasso (Arthrex, Inc., Naples, FL) is used to shuttle a suture through the labrum. **B:** A second and separate pass with the SutureLasso is made through the capsule. **C:** Appearance after placement of the capsulolabral stitch. **D:** A second suture has similarly been passed. G, glenoid; H, humerus.

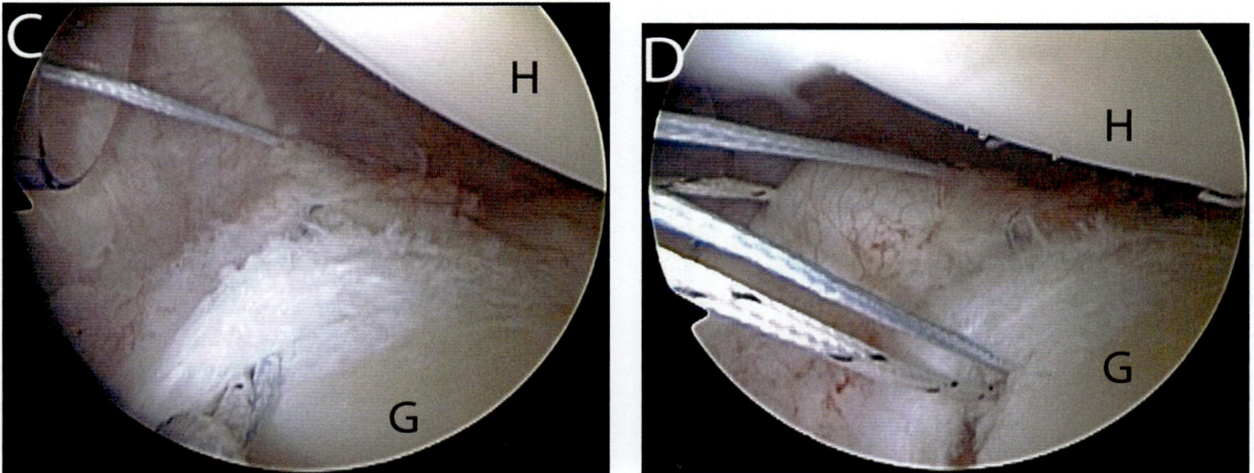

Figure 14.45 (*Continued*) **C:** Appearance after placement of the capsulolabral stitch. **D:** A second suture has similarly been passed. G, glenoid; H, humerus.

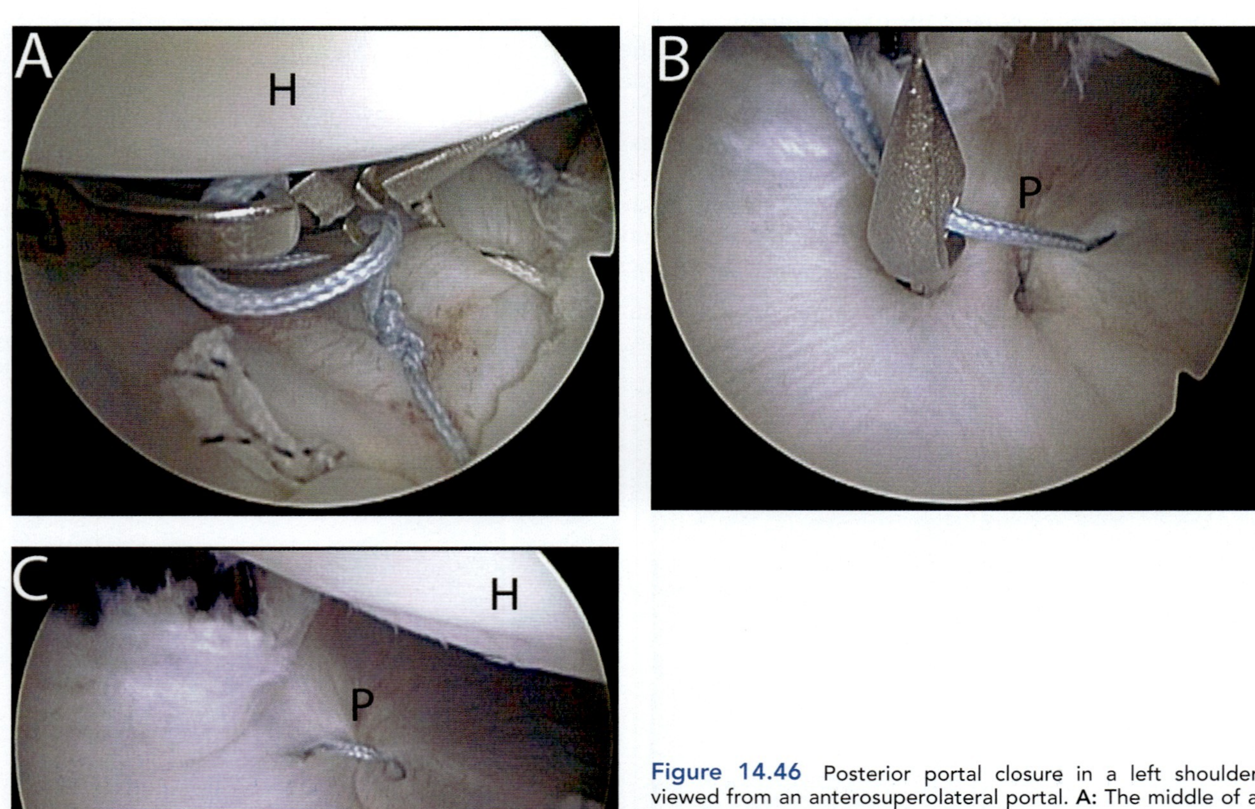

Figure 14.46 Posterior portal closure in a left shoulder viewed from an anterosuperolateral portal. **A:** The middle of a suture has been loaded onto a Penetrator (Arthrex, Inc., Naples, FL) that is advanced into the glenohumeral joint adjacent to a posterior portal defect. The suture loop is released by means of a hand off to a suture retriever in the glenohumeral joint and the Penetrator is withdrawn. **B:** The Penetrator is advanced through the opposite side of the posterior portal defect and retrieves the suture. **C:** Tensioning the sutures demonstrates closure of the posterior portal. Sutures are not tied at this point if further intra-articular work will be performed. H, humerus; P, posterior portal.

opposite the labral tear using the previously described techniques. Because the labrum is usually hypoplastic in these very lax individuals, we usually plicate by using No. 2 FiberWire sutures from an anchor (BioComposite Suture-Tak) in order to plicate to a firm fixation point (the anchor).

Following the capsular plication, attention is returned to the SLAP lesion and the previously placed sutures are tied. With these sutures tied, the humeral head should be centered over the glenoid.

In patients with a posterior labral tear and hyperlaxity, we routinely perform a closure of the posterior portal as previously described (Fig. 14.46). We have not routinely performed posterior portal closure in the setting of a Bankart lesion, with or without hyperlaxity. We reserve rotator interval closure only for very severe cases of hyperlaxity.

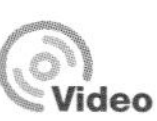

If the quality of the capsule is poor, some authors have recommended plicating the subscapularis tendon to the supraspinatus tendon. We caution against this due to the possibility of significantly restricting motion. If both a posterior portal and rotator interval closure are performed, two sequences can be used. The first is to place the posterior portal sutures, but not tie the sutures. Then, the rotator interval closure is performed and afterward the posterior portal sutures are tied blind. The second option is to perform the rotator interval closure first while viewing from the posterior portal. Then, the posterior portal is closed while viewing from an anterosuperolateral portal.

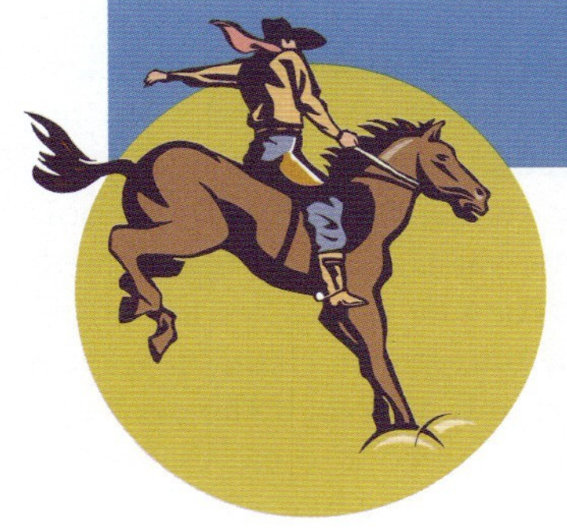

15

Philosophy of Managing SLAP Lesions

WESTERN WISDOM

A wink is as good as a nod to a blind mule.

The role of the biceps/superior labral complex in overhead athletics as well as in daily activities remains an enigma. An intact biceps root appears to be essential for high-level performance in throwing a baseball. That is why SLAP repair is essential in returning a baseball pitcher to his previous level of function. We are not aware of any professional or college baseball pitchers who have returned to their prior level of performance after having their biceps root disrupted by tenodesis, tenotomy, or rupture of the long head of the biceps.

In contrast, we have had college tennis players return successfully after a biceps tenodesis. We know of professional football quarterbacks who have had biceps rupture or tenotomy without any loss of speed, accuracy, or distance in throwing a football.

We have found that, in general, the younger high-performance baseball players that ultimately come to surgery will have one or more of the following 3 surgical lesions:

Video

1. SLAP lesion, requiring arthroscopic suture anchor repair

Video

2. Glenohumeral internal rotation deficit (GIRD) of >40°, requiring posterior capsular release
3. Hyperexternal rotation >130°, which is confirmed arthroscopically by observing the thrower's internal impingement "contact point" (between the glenoid labrum and the greater tuberosity of the humerus with combined abduction and external rotation) to occur in the posteroinferior quadrant of the glenoid rather than the posterosuperior quadrant. This is most easily observed while viewing from an anterosuperolateral portal while the arm is brought back into the cocked position, with the shoulder in 90° abduction and maximal external rotation. In some cases of hyperexternal rotation, a posteroinferior labral lesion (diffuse abrasive labral wear) may be visualized at the contact point of internal impingement. Such a posteroinferior labral lesion should not be "repaired," as this could further exacerbate posterior capsular tightness (GIRD).

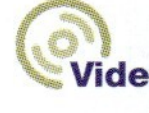

We believe that, over time, hyperexternal rotation causes symptomatic undersurface fiber failure of the rotator cuff due to repetitive torsional overload. In young throwers who are confirmed arthroscopically to meet the hyperexternal rotation criterion of reaching the contact point of internal impingement in the posteroinferior quadrant, we recommend anterior mini-plication to restrict external rotation by 10° to 15°. Our mini-plication consists of placing 2 sutures to plicate the middle glenohumeral ligament (MGHL) to the anterior band of the inferior glenohumeral ligament (IGHL). We do not use suture anchors to plicate in overhead athletes.

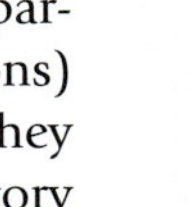

In older baseball pitchers (usually >30 years old), partial articular surface rotator cuff tears (PASTA lesions) may develop over time. These do reasonably well if they are arthroscopically debrided. This is the only category of patient in which we debride rather than repair PASTA lesions, since repair will typically reduce external rotation to such an extent that the pitcher cannot be effective in throwing a fastball.

There seems to be something unique about throwing a baseball at high speeds that requires an intact biceps root.

This probably has to do with the extremely high angular accelerations that occur in throwing a fastball. These accelerations produce angular velocities of up to 7,000 degrees per second, which is by far the fastest movement in all of sports. Throwing a football and serving a tennis ball both require totally different kinematics with significantly lower angular velocities than those required to throw a baseball.

One consideration in managing SLAP lesions is the anticipated level of future performance and demand when the patient returns to his or her sport. For example, a 40-year-old man with a SLAP lesion treated with a biceps tenodesis can perform quite well on his recreational softball team or pitching batting practice to his son's Little League baseball team.

All of the above observations and considerations have influenced our algorithm for the management of SLAP lesions. The one category of patient that absolutely requires repair of a SLAP lesion is the high-performing baseball player who wishes to continue to complete at his current level. In addition, we believe in SLAP repair for all young (<35 years old) overhead athletes (volleyball, tennis, football) who have not had previous surgery.

For virtually all other categories of patients, we usually recommend biceps tenodesis by the technique of tendon-to-bone interference fixation. This recommendation also holds for nonbaseball overhead athletes who have had failure of a previous SLAP repair. In these overhead athletes, biceps tenodesis can return them to high levels of performance. However, in baseball players with failed SLAP repairs, we recommend revision repair of the SLAP lesion.

The only other exceptions are individuals with an unstable shoulder (i.e. Bankart tear and SLAP tear) where repair may improve stability, and a symptomatic spinoglenoid cyst where repair will prevent recurrence of the cyst.

Although SLAP lesions can be disabling to young overhead athletes, we have found that middle-aged and older patients can have symptomatic disruptions of the biceps root attachment, which we call *degenerative SLAP lesions*. Arthroscopically, these patients do not have a positive peel-back sign, but they do have a displaceable biceps root when palpating it with a hook probe, as if the biceps does not have a firm attachment into bone (Fig. 15.1). These patients display positive *biceps tension signs* on physical exam and with daily activities, where there is pain when the biceps is placed under tension. The most reliable biceps tension sign in our hands is the O'Driscoll sign, or Mayo Shear sign, as originally described by Dr. Shawn O'Driscoll (Fig. 15.2).

Once patients are beyond the age of competitive high-level sports, usually about 35 years of age, we recommend biceps tenodesis routinely as the treatment for SLAP lesions.

In our experience advancing age and worker's compensation claims are associated with a poorer outcome following SLAP repair. We recently reported on 55 isloated SLAP repairs at a mean of 77 months (1). Overall, we observed 87% good or excellent results. However, the percentage of good and excellent results among patients >40 years of age (81%) was lower than among patients <40 years of age (97%). The difference was more dramatic with regard to worker's compensation status where cases without a claim had 95% good or excellent results, compared to only 65% when there was a work claim. Moreover, we recently retrospectively compared primary biceps tenodesis to SLAP repair in individuals over the age of 35 and noted more predictable results following a primary biceps tenodesis (Unpublished Data).

In general, we do not combine the tenodesis with superior labral repair, and we have found that the function usually returns to near-normal levels without the added risk of postoperative stiffness that accompanies labral

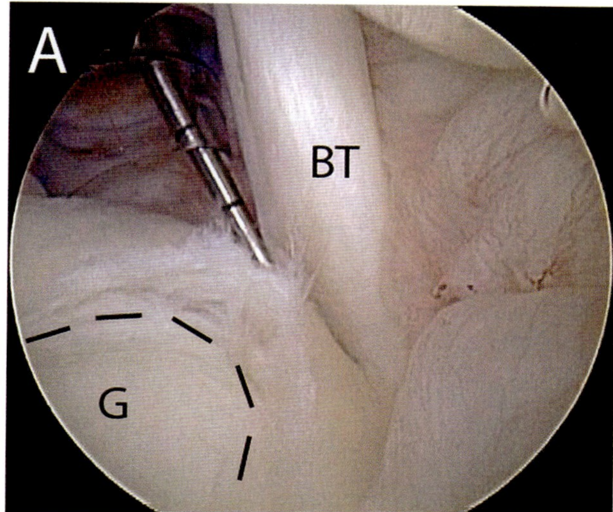

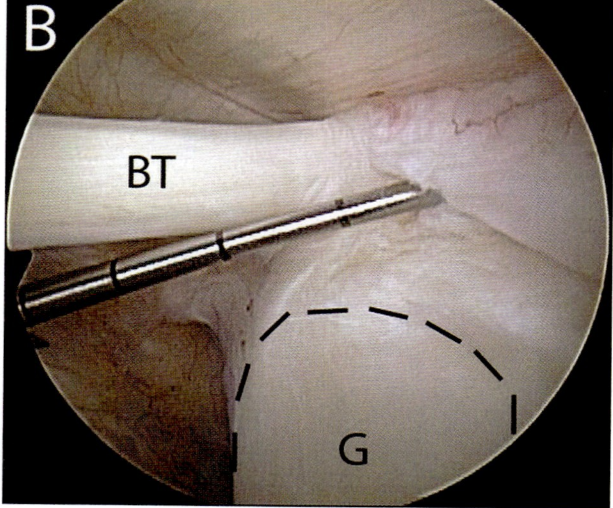

Figure 15.1 Left shoulder, posterior glenohumeral viewing portal. **A, B:** A probe introduced from an anterior portal is used to demonstrate two different examples of a displaceable biceps root. The *dashed black lines* outline the glenoid. BT, biceps tendon; G, glenoid.

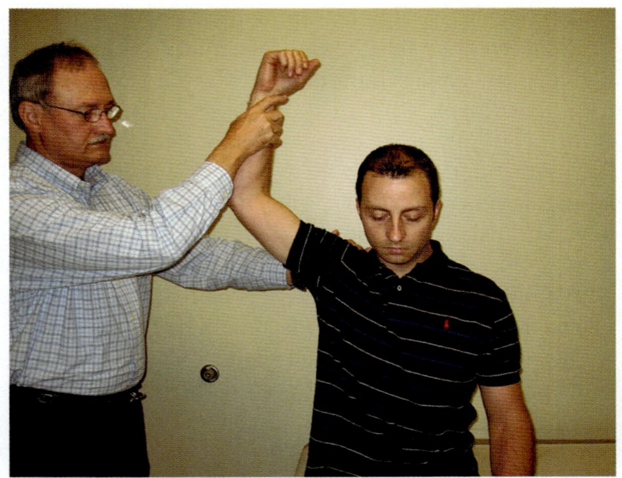

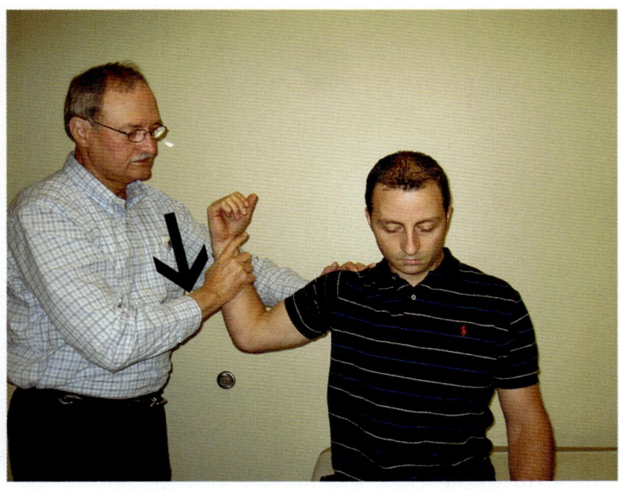

Figure 15.2 O'Driscoll sign (Mayo Shear sign). **A:** Starting position. The arm is placed in 90° of external rotation and approximately 120° of abduction with the elbow positioned slightly behind the plane of the scapula. **B:** Ending position. While stabilizing the shoulder, the arm is adducted (*black arrow*) to approximately 60°. Pain during this maneuver is considered a positive O'Driscoll sign for a proximal biceps lesion.

repair. The only time we combine a tenodesis with a superior labrum repair is when there is a concomitant spinoglenoid cyst that needs to be sealed off with a labral repair or when the superior labral disruption extends so far posteriorly that it creates the possibility of posterior instability.

We usually perform the biceps tenodesis with an interference screw (BioComposite Tenodesis Screw; Arthrex, Inc., Naples, FL) at the top of the bicipital groove. Although some authors have warned that osteophytes in the bicipital groove can be a lingering source of pain by causing irritation of the tendon if it is tenodesed high in the groove, we have not seen that occur. In fact we do not think that this is a valid concern, as the biceps that is tenodesed at that level will not have any contractile or elastic elements within the bicipital groove and therefore cannot have any excursion of the tendon over the osteophytes that might cause inflammation (Fig. 15.3). The only time we do a distal or subpectoral tenodesis is when there is a ruptured and retracted long head of the biceps. As a routine, we do not like to put a bone socket or drill hole through the cortical bone

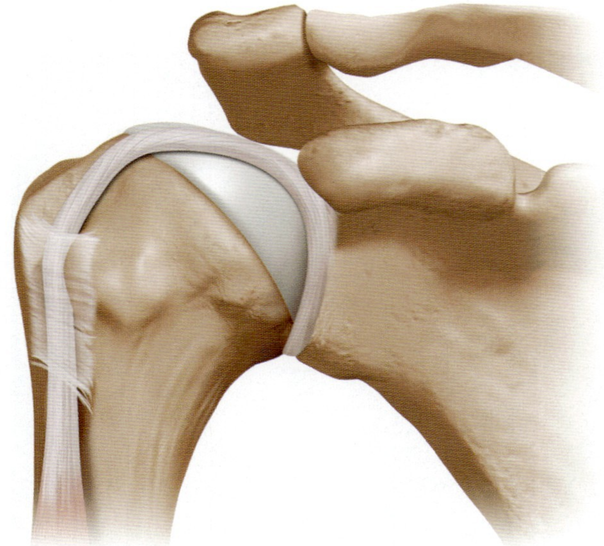

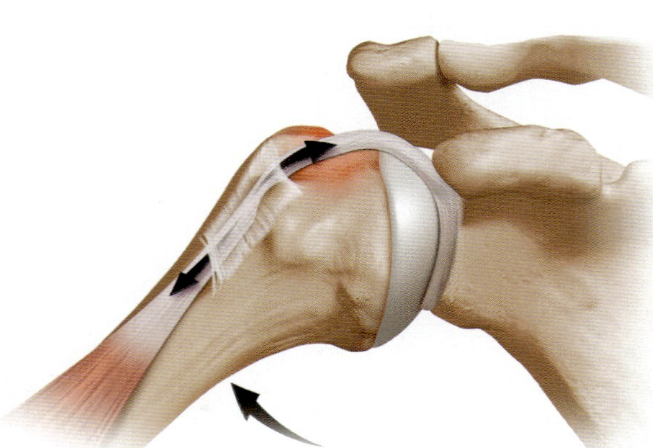

Figure 15.3 Schematic of a biceps tenodesis high in the bicipital groove. **A:** Prior to tenodesis, the biceps tendon crosses the glenohumeral joint. **B:** Movement of the glenohumeral joint results in relative motion of the biceps tendon within the bicipital groove.

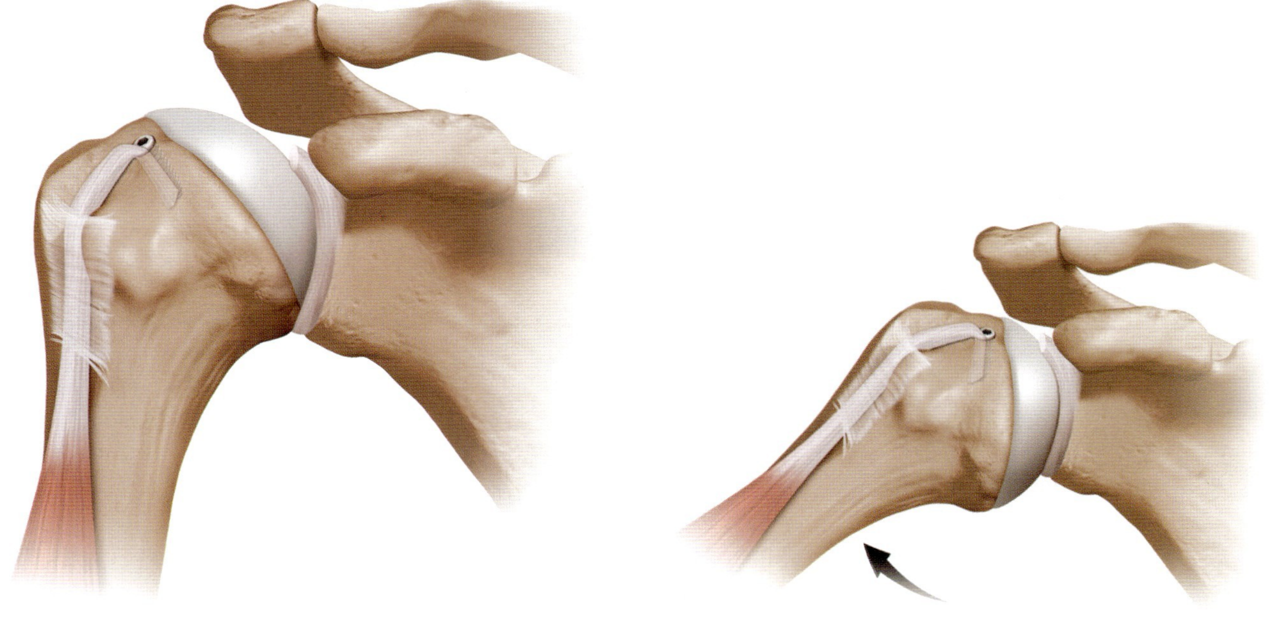

Figure 15.3 *(Continued)* **C:** Following a biceps tenodesis high in the bicipital groove, the tendon no longer crosses the glenohumeral joint. **D:** Because the tendon no longer crosses the glenohumeral joint, movement of the joint does not result in any relative motion within the bicipital groove, so pain generation within the groove from relative motion is eliminated.

of the humerus in the subpectoral area, as we are aware of humeral shaft fractures that have occurred through these holes due to their stress-riser effect.

After biceps tenodesis, we have the patient wear a sling for 6 weeks, but we begin stretching exercises right away (elevation, external rotation, and internal rotation). We delay strengthening until 3 months post-op to allow mature healing at the tendon–bone interface.

We occasionally perform biceps tenotomy instead of tenodesis. We do this in elderly inactive patients, and in low-demand patients with fat arms in whom we feel there will not be any adverse cosmetic consequences to tenotomy. Occasionally we will offer tenotomy to high-demand patients who do not want to comply with 6 weeks of immobilization, but we are careful to counsel these patients on the potential for persistent biceps cramping and deformity after tenotomy.

In summary, we reserve SLAP repair for high-demand overhead athletes, particularly baseball players. Virtually all other symptomatic patients with stable shoulders have their SLAP lesions managed by biceps tenodesis.

REFERENCE

1. Denard PJ, Lädermann A, Burkhart SS. Long-term outcome following arthroscopic repair of type II SLAP lesions: results according to age and worker's compensation status. *Arthroscopy;* In press.

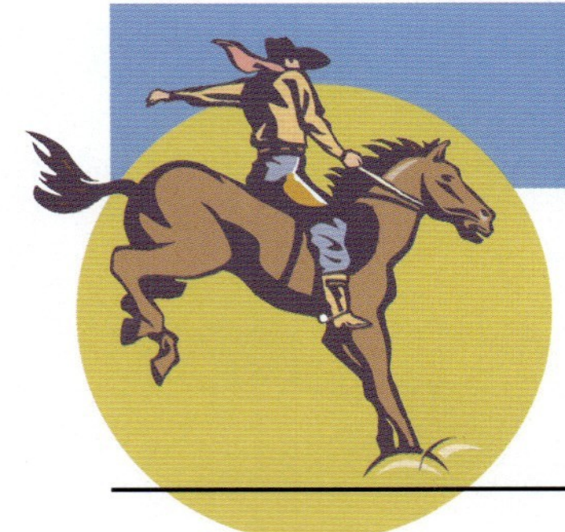

16

SLAP Lesions

WESTERN WISDOM

Don't sit in the saddle if you're afraid of getting throwed.

Since their initial description by Snyder in the late 1980s, the etiology, diagnosis, and treatment of superior labral tears (SLAP lesions) have been controversial. Furthermore, misdiagnosis and overtreatment of SLAP lesions, particularly in older individuals, have led to mixed results in the literature. Care must be taken to ensure that inappropriate surgical intervention is avoided, particularly in cases where a SLAP lesion is identified in passing.

The appropriate diagnosis of a SLAP lesion is based on clinical history, physical exam, and confirmatory arthroscopic findings. The classic patient is a young overhead athlete (age <30), with minimal daily symptoms but with disability while performing overhead athletics. Throwers often report pain when attempting to throw as well as inability to throw hard. This is known as the "dead arm syndrome." Such patients will commonly have confirmatory physical exam findings (O'Driscoll sign, O'Brien sign, and reduction of pain with the Jobe relocation test) and classic arthroscopic findings of a SLAP lesion (see below). In addition, the absence of other pathology (e.g., full-thickness tears of the rotator cuff, chondromalacia, impingement) is further indicative that the SLAP lesion is the cause of the patient's symptoms.

In patients over the age of 35, with an atraumatic onset of symptoms, generalized pain, which is worsened with overhead activities (not necessarily athletics), and other concomitant modifiers (worker's compensation claim, litigation) or associated conditions (e.g., full-thickness tear of the rotator cuff), the diagnosis of a SLAP lesion should be guarded. While an anatomic SLAP lesion may exist on arthroscopic evaluation, many of these patients will have equivocal physical examination findings and the tear of the superior labrum may not be the cause of the symptoms. Other concomitant diagnoses should be considered (e.g., rotator cuff tear). We believe that patients over the age of 35 with an unstable biceps root may have a *degenerative SLAP lesion*. However, in these patients, SLAP repair is usually not indicated and one may choose to perform a biceps tenodesis if biceps tendinopathy is suspected.

ARTHROSCOPIC DIAGNOSIS

When a superior labral tear is suspected preoperatively, the superior labrum is carefully evaluated arthroscopically for injury. We base the *arthroscopic* diagnosis of a SLAP lesion on five specific findings:

1. Drive through sign
2. Superior sublabral sulcus >5 mm
3. Bare sublabral footprint
4. Displaceable biceps root
5. Positive peel-back sign

In general, we require that three of these five characteristics must be present in order to definitively diagnose a SLAP lesion.

A drive-through sign occurs while viewing through a posterior portal when the arthroscope can be easily "driven" from the superior glenohumeral joint to the axillary recess with minimal resistance (Fig. 16.1). This is indicative of the *pseudolaxity* that may occur with SLAP lesions.

The width of the normal sublabral sulcus of the superior labrum ranges from approximately 3 to 5 mm and may increase with age. Therefore, if the width of the sublabral sulcus is increased and is associated with exposed bone (bare sublabral footprint), this is indicative of detachment of the superior labrum from the superior glenoid. Since

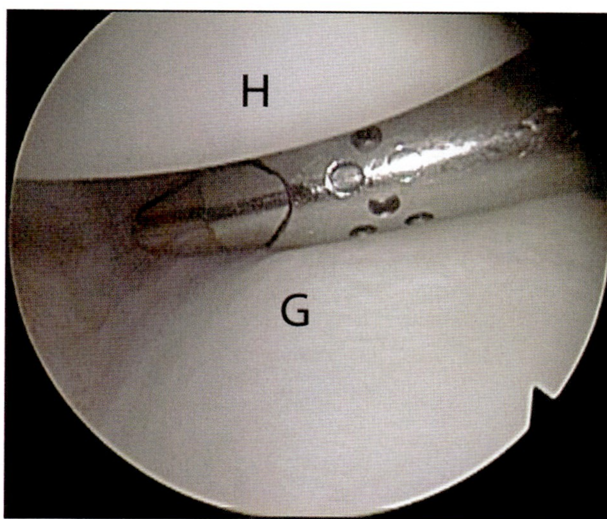

Figure 16.1 Right shoulder, anterosuperolateral viewing portal. The drive-through sign is demonstrated by an instrument that is easily passed from superior to inferior, with minimal resistance from the humeral head, in this patient with a SLAP lesion. G, glenoid; H, humerus.

the superior aspect of the glenoid under the labrum (the normal sublabral sulcus) is normally covered with articular cartilage (Fig. 16.2A), a bare sublabral footprint with exposed bone (further supported by associated undersurface labral fraying) is again indicative of detachment of the superior labrum from the glenoid (Fig. 16.2B). When this detachment is significant, stability of the biceps root may be affected and the root of the biceps may be easily translated medially with a probe (displaceable biceps root) (Fig. 16.3).

Finally, dynamic stability of the superior labrum and biceps root is evaluated by placing the arm in the functional throwing position of 90° of abduction and full external rotation. In patients with an intact superior labrum, the biceps root and superior labrum remain centered on the superior glenoid and the intra-articular portion of the biceps tendon merely changes its angular position relative to the superior labrum (Fig. 16.4). However, in patients with tears of the superior labrum (particularly if involving the posterior superior labrum), as the arm is brought into external rotation, the torsional force from the biceps tendon lifts the superior labrum off the glenoid and the labrum begins to "peel-back" off the glenoid, falling medially off the glenoid rim (Figs. 16.5 and 16.6). This is considered a positive peel-back sign and is indicative of an unstable superior labrum. Typically, a positive peel-back sign occurs in overhead athletes who have posterosuperior labral disruption in addition to disruption of the biceps root attachment into the bone. However, degenerative SLAP lesions usually do not display a positive peel-back sign.

INDICATIONS FOR REPAIR

In patients with an arthroscopic diagnosis of a SLAP lesion (i.e., satisfying three of the five criteria above), the decision to proceed with SLAP repair is largely based on the patient's age, activity, and preoperative symptoms. In patients with the primary complaint of instability and associated Bankart or reverse Bankart lesions, a concomitant SLAP lesion is universally repaired to provide a stable base for labral repair and enhance stability. Furthermore, in young patients with difficulty with overhead sports, particularly in the absence of other major concomitant diagnoses, the SLAP lesion is repaired.

All other patients should be carefully reviewed for the preoperative suspicion of a SLAP lesion. In older patients

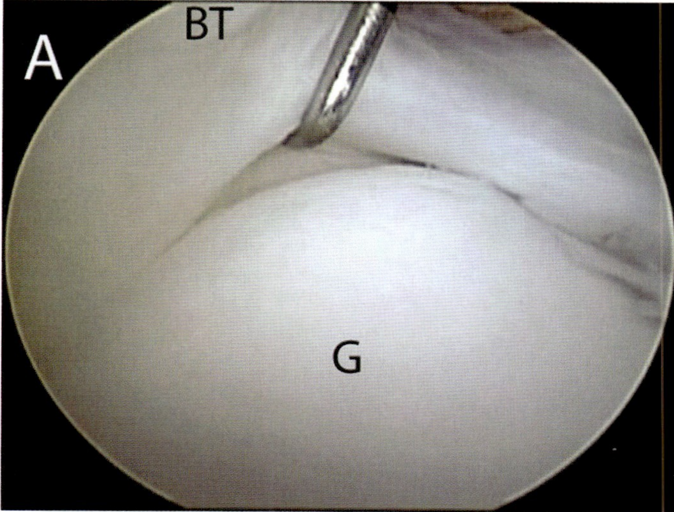

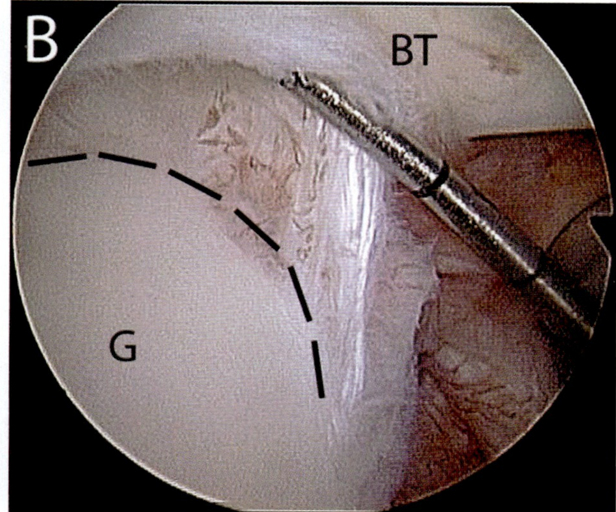

Figure 16.2 Right shoulder, posterior viewing portal demonstrating **(A)** normal superior sublabral sulcus; **(B)** an abnormal sublabral recess >5 mm with exposed bone (glenoid rim outlined by *dashed lines*) BT, biceps tendon; G, glenoid.

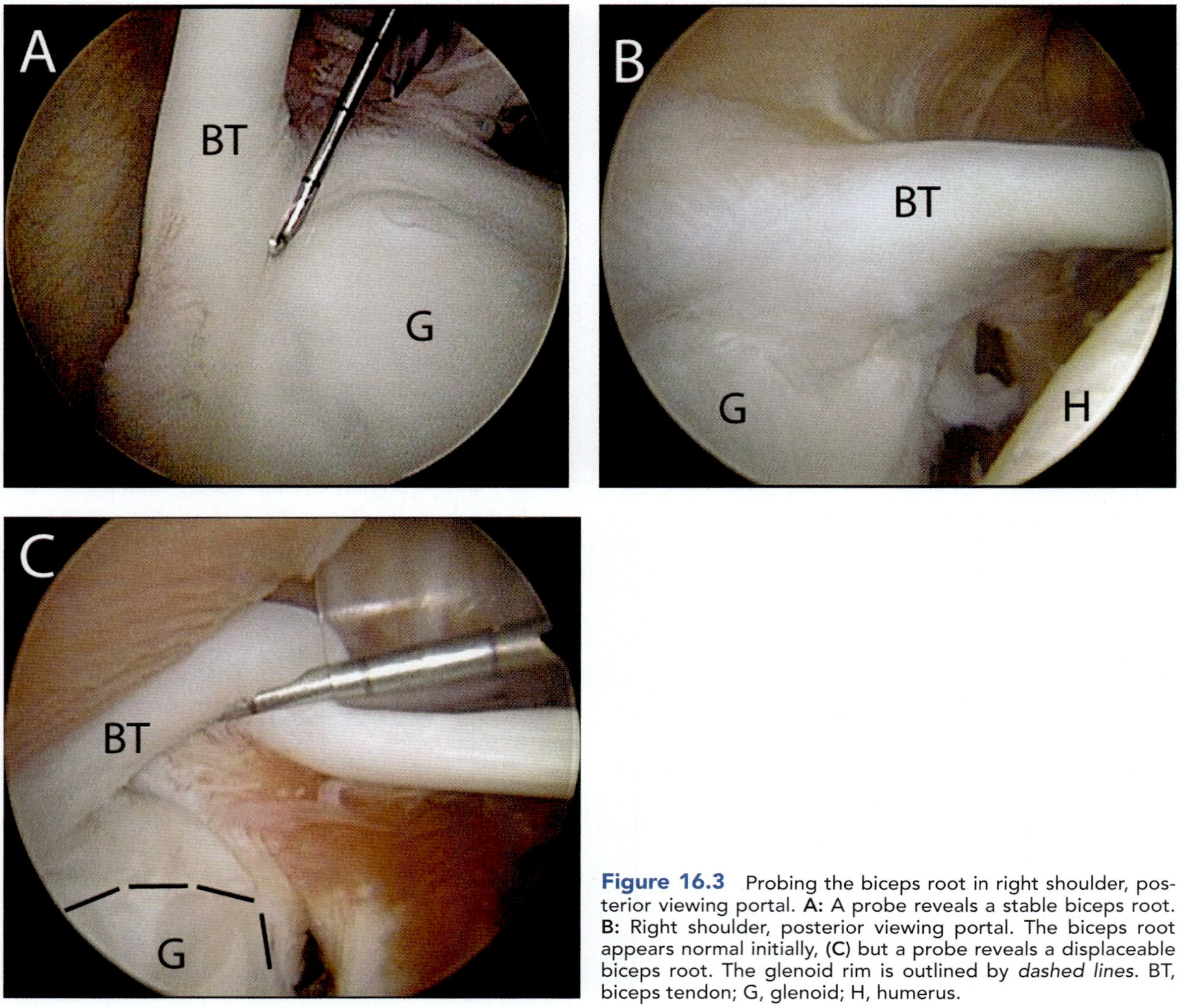

Figure 16.3 Probing the biceps root in right shoulder, posterior viewing portal. **A:** A probe reveals a stable biceps root. **B:** Right shoulder, posterior viewing portal. The biceps root appears normal initially, **(C)** but a probe reveals a displaceable biceps root. The glenoid rim is outlined by *dashed lines*. BT, biceps tendon; G, glenoid; H, humerus.

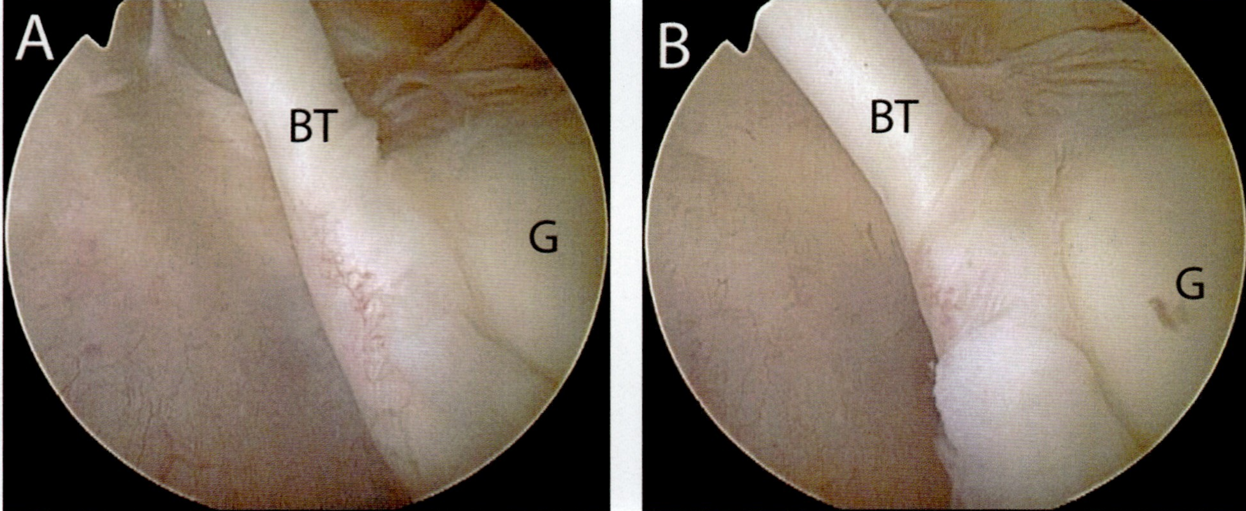

Figure 16.4 Right shoulder, posterior viewing portal demonstrates a negative peel-back **(A)** prior to peel-back maneuver; **B:** peel-back maneuver demonstrates an angle change of the biceps without displacement. BT, biceps tendon; G, glenoid.

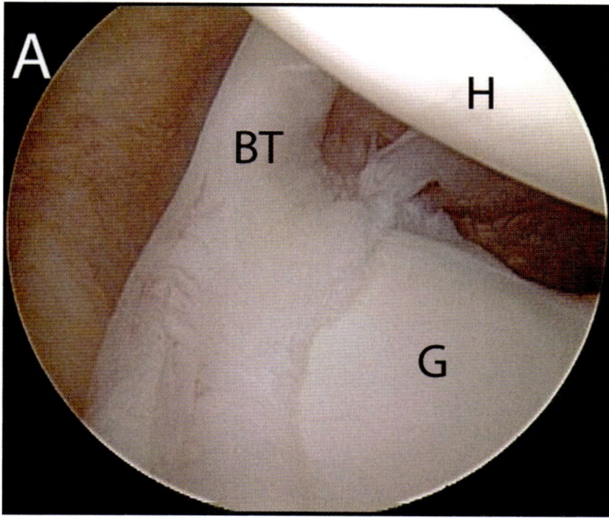

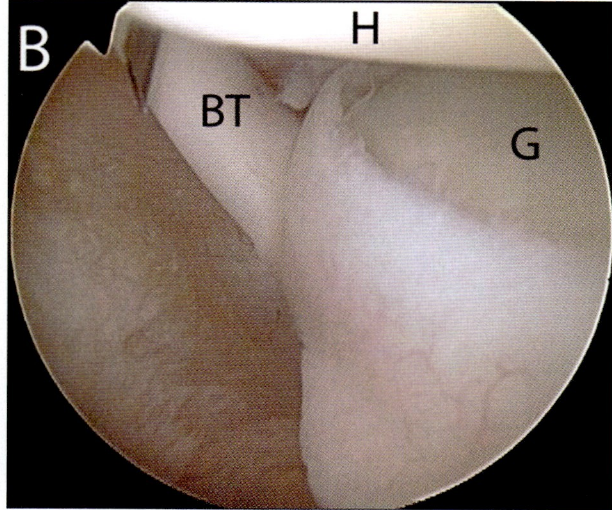

Figure 16.5 Right shoulder, posterior viewing portal demonstrates a positive peel-back sign (**A**) prior to peel-back maneuver; **B:** peel-back maneuver results in medial displacement of the superior labrum and biceps root. BT, biceps tendon; G, glenoid; H, humerus.

where pain is the primary complaint, particularly in the presence of other concomitant diagnoses (e.g., rotator cuff tear), alternative treatment of the SLAP lesion may be indicated (e.g., biceps tenodesis or biceps tenotomy).

TYPE II SLAP REPAIR (KNOTTED ANCHORS)

Standard posterior, anterior, and anterosuperolateral portals are established. However, in preparation for SLAP repair, it is important to create the anterior portal just superior to the lateral half of the subscapularis tendon to ensure a 45° of approach to the glenoid and adequate spacing for a second high anterior (anterosuperolateral) portal. Standard diagnostic arthroscopy is performed, evaluating for commonly associated lesions including partial-thickness rotator cuff tears or associated labral injuries (e.g., Bankart, reverse Bankart lesions). Pathology of the superior labrum is evaluated according to the criteria described above.

Once a SLAP lesion has been diagnosed, a separate anterosuperolateral portal is created just anterior to the supraspinatus tendon and directly above the biceps tendon to provide a 45° angle of approach to the superior glenoid rim (Fig. 16.7). This portal is usually 5 to 10 mm lateral to the anterolateral corner of the acromion. Through an anterior working portal, the superior glenoid neck is debrided with a shaver or ring curettes in order to remove

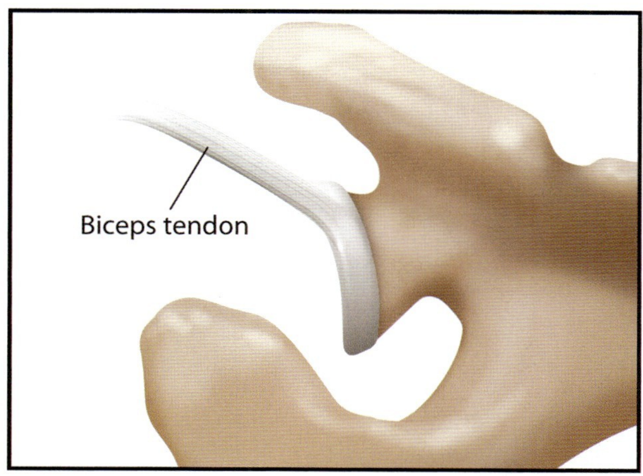

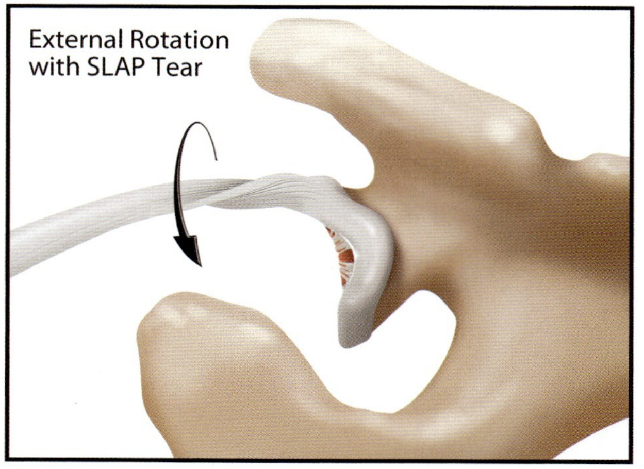

Figure 16.6 Schematic of the peel-back maneuver for demonstration of a superior labrum anterior and posterior (SLAP) tear. **A:** Appearance of the biceps root with the arm at the side. **B:** Placing the arm in 90° of abduction and maximal external rotation creates a torsional force on the biceps root. In the setting of a SLAP tear, the biceps root and the labrum just posterior to the biceps root displace medially during this maneuver.

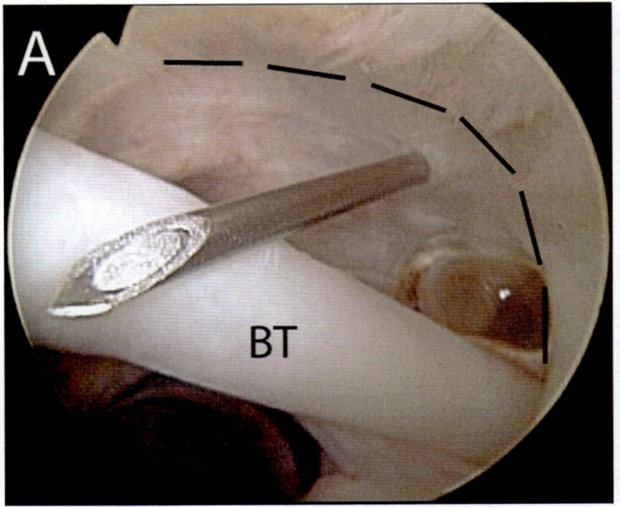

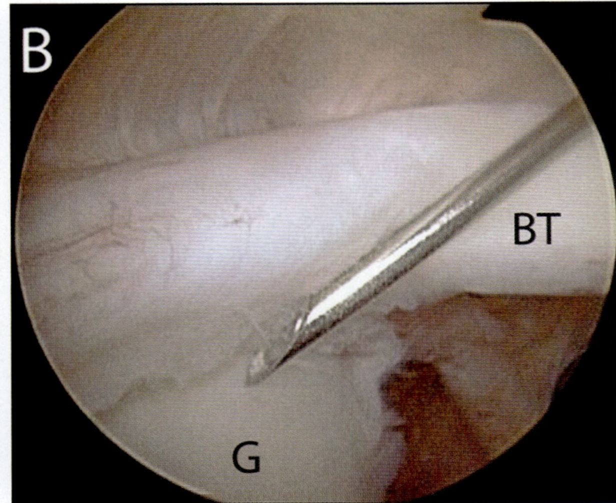

Figure 16.7 Right shoulder, posterior viewing portal. **A:** An anterosuperolateral portal is established anterior to the supraspinatus ridge (outlined by *dashed lines*) with a spinal needle, and **(B)** provides a 45° angle of approach to the superior glenoid rim. BT, biceps tendon; G, glenoid.

any overlying cartilage and to create a bed of bare bone (Fig. 16.8). If the tear extends anteriorly or posteriorly, debridement from an anterosuperolateral portal may be necessary to gain access around the "corner" of the glenoid.

Most SLAP lesions, particularly those with unstable biceps roots that display a positive peel-back sign, will require two anchors, one directly under the biceps root and one more posterior in the posterosuperior glenoid rim. Smaller lesions may require only one anchor, usually under the biceps root. The anterior anchor (3.0 mm Bio-Composite SutureTak, Arthrex, Inc., Naples, FL) is placed first through the anterosuperolateral portal just at the articular bone junction (Fig. 16.9). Unlike Bankart or reverse Bankart lesions, creation of a "bumper" is not required and therefore reduction of the labrum to the articular junction is desirable for a "water tight" anatomic repair.

Although sutures may be passed directly in a retrograde fashion (Fig. 16.10), this technique can make a large hole through the labrum. Our current preference is to use a percutaneous shuttling technique with a small curved needle (Micro SutureLasso; Arthrex, Inc., Naples, FL) through the labrum, passing simple sutures that encircle the labrum. If the superior glenohumeral ligament is avulsed, just anterior to the biceps, a separate anchor is used for its repair.

To pass a suture posterior to the long head of the biceps, a Micro SutureLasso is inserted percutaneously through a modified Neviaser portal piercing the labrum posterior to the biceps tendon (Fig. 16.11). The suture shuttle and the

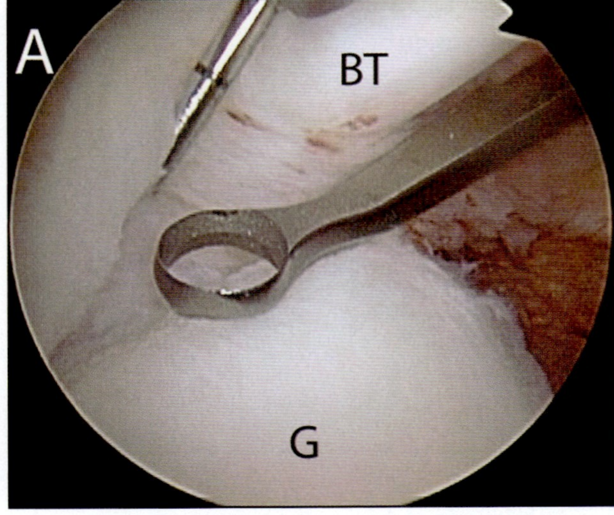

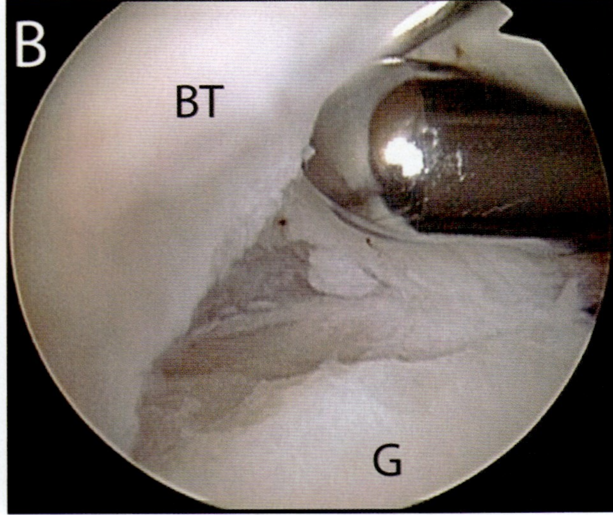

Figure 16.8 Right shoulder, posterior viewing portal. Preparation of bone bed for SLAP repair is accomplished with **(A)** a ring curette and **(B)** a shaver to expose an adequate bone bed for healing. BT, biceps tendon; G, glenoid.

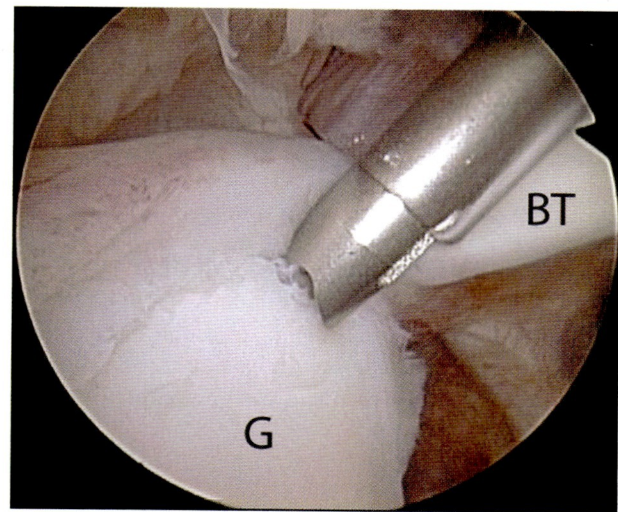

Figure 16.9 Right shoulder, posterior viewing portal. An anterior anchor is placed through an anterosuperolateral portal for SLAP repair. BT, biceps tendon; G, glenoid.

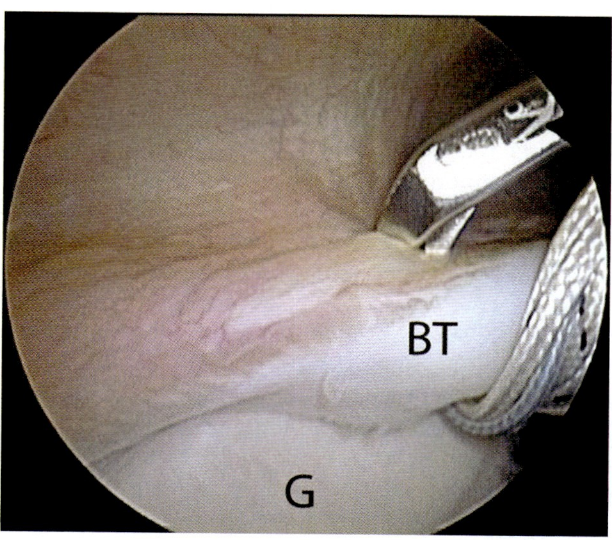

Figure 16.10 Right shoulder, posterior viewing portal demonstrating retrograde pass of sutures for SLAP repair with a 45° BirdBeak instrument (Arthrex, Inc., Naples, FL). BT, biceps tendon; G, glenoid.

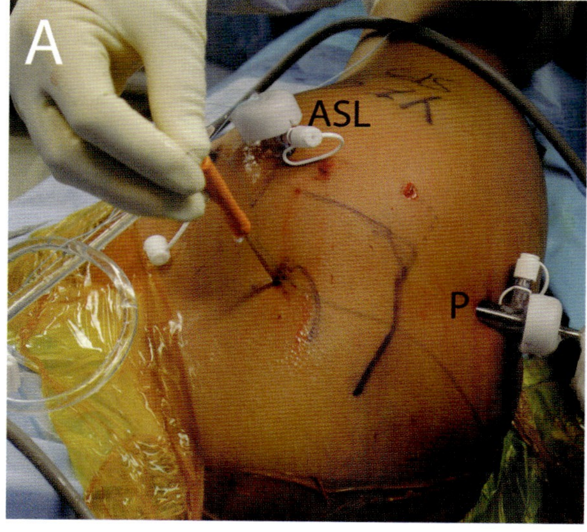

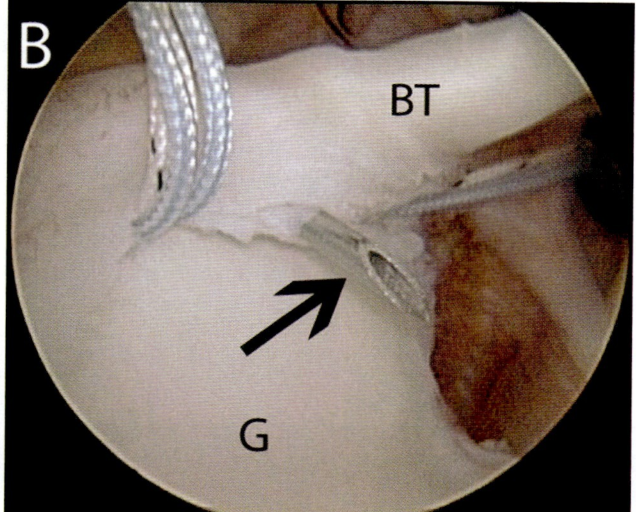

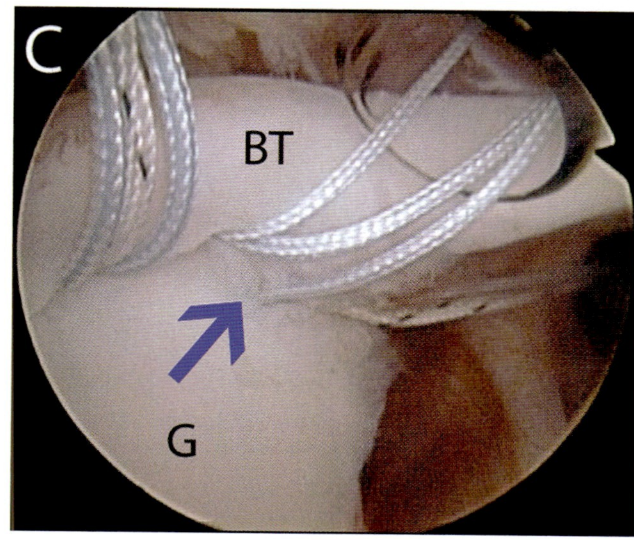

Figure 16.11 Micro SutureLasso (Arthrex, Inc., Naples, FL) shuttling technique for SLAP repair in a right shoulder. **A:** External view shows a Micro SutureLasso percutaneously placed through a modified Neviaser portal. **B:** Arthroscopic view from a posterior portal shows the needle (*black arrow*) piercing the labrum. **C:** After retrieval of the shuttling wire, a suture from the anterior anchor (*blue arrow*) is passed to encircle the labrum. ASL, anterosuperolateral portal; BT, biceps tendon; G, glenoid; P, posterior portal.

suture are then retrieved through the anterior or anterosuperolateral portal. It is important when placing these sutures not to incarcerate the biceps tendon. Sutures should be placed so that they secure the labrum, stabilizing the long head of the biceps tendon, but do not capture the tendon itself. Furthermore, in patients with cord-like middle glenohumeral ligaments or Buford complexes, it is important to avoid closing the anterior sulcus, as this can significantly restrict external rotation. The sutures are not tied until the posterior anchor is placed to avoid early binding of the soft tissue to bone which limits subsequent suture passage.

When the tear extends posteriorly into the posterosuperior quadrant, a second anchor is required. Due to the rounded shape of the superior glenoid, the anterosuperolateral portal often does not provide the correct angle of approach to the posterosuperior glenoid for anchor placement (Fig. 16.12). A separate Port of Wilmington portal may be required. This is created approximately 1 cm lateral and 1 cm anterior to the posterolateral corner of the acromion (Fig. 16.13A). When created, this portal provides a 45° angle of approach to the posterosuperior corner of the glenoid (Fig. 16.13B). The BioComposite SutureTak Spear is then inserted transmuscular through the rotator cuff (Fig. 16.13C). Although only a small 4.5-mm puncture is created through the rotator cuff, it is important to create this portal medial to the rotator cable avoiding the avascular crescent region of the rotator cuff. A cannula is not required since only anchors are inserted through this portal via the Spear guide.

Sutures are then passed for the posterosuperior anchor with a Micro SutureLasso percutaneously inserted through a modified Neviaser portal or a posterosuperior portal. Once all sutures have been passed, the sutures may be tied (Fig. 16.14).

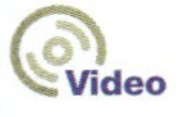

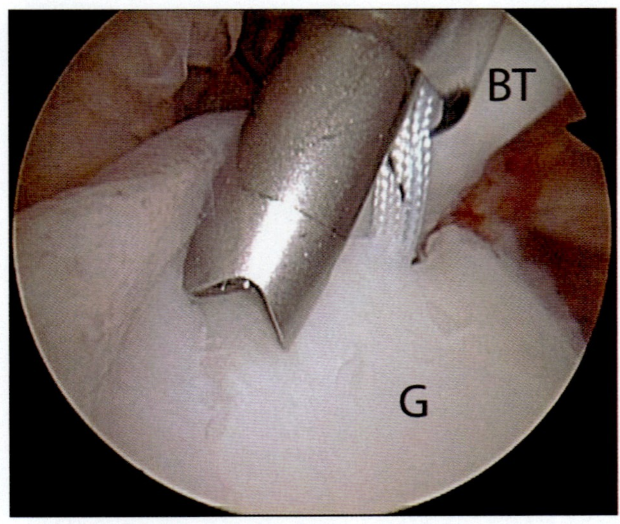

Figure 16.12 Right shoulder, posterior viewing portal. The angle of approach from an anterosuperolateral portal is too oblique for placement of a posterior anchor during SLAP repair. A Port of Wilmington portal is required (Fig. 16.13). BT, biceps tendon; G, glenoid.

TYPE II SLAP REPAIR (KNOTLESS TECHNIQUE)

As an alternative to the technique described above, a knotless type II SLAP repair may be performed based on surgeon preference. Knotless repair has the potential advantages of avoiding sutures knots within the glenohumeral joint. However, since only two suture limbs may be accommodated in a 2.9-mm BioComposite PushLock anchor (Arthrex, Inc., Naples, FL), we sometimes pass the suture limbs as mattress stitches rather than a single simple stitch. This maximizes fixation strength, labrum to bone contact, and may better recreate the meniscoid-like superior labrum attachment.

Standard posterior, anterior, and anterosuperolateral portals are created. In the knotless technique, sutures are passed first through the labrum prior to anchor insertion. It is important to place the anterosuperolateral portal high in the rotator interval to provide a correct angle of approach for anchor insertion.

The sutures posterior to the long head of the biceps tendon are passed first. A Micro SutureLasso is inserted percutaneously through a modified Nevaiser portal and passed through the labrum (Fig. 16.15). A Nitinol loop suture shuttle is retrieved out the anterior portal and used to shuttle a #2 FiberWire through the labrum (Fig 16.16). Alternatively, shuttling at this stage can be avoided by passing a #2 FiberStick (Arthrex, Inc., Naples, FL) directly through the Micro SutureLasso. To complete the mattress stitch, the Micro SutureLasso is used to penetrate the labrum 5 to 8 mm posterior to the first pass. A suture shuttle is passed through the labrum, and the suture limb that exits the from the superior aspect of the labrum is shuttled through the labrum completing the mattress stitch (Fig 16.17)

The sutures are retrieved out the anterosuperolateral portal. The drill guide is inserted through the anterosuperolateral portal and a bone socket is drilled for a PushLock anchor. Extracorporeally, the sutures are then fed through the distal suture eyelet of a PushLock anchor. The sutures are then tensioned and the anchor is inserted into the bone, securing labrum fixation to bone (Fig. 16.18). If a proper angle of approach cannot be achieved from the anterosuperolateral portal, the posterior anchor is placed through a Port of Wilmington portal.

To secure the anterior superior labrum (superior glenohumeral ligament attachment), a mattress stitch is again placed just anterior to the biceps tendon. Using a similar technique, a Micro SutureLasso is percutaneously inserted and the suture shuttle or a #2 FiberStick is advanced through the labrum and retrieved out the anterosuperolateral portal. The SutureLasso is used again to penetrate the labrum approximately 5 to 8 mm inferior to the initial stitch and a suture shuttle is used to complete the mattress stitch. The sutures are retrieved out the anterosuperolateral portal, and the bone socket is drilled through the anterosuperolateral

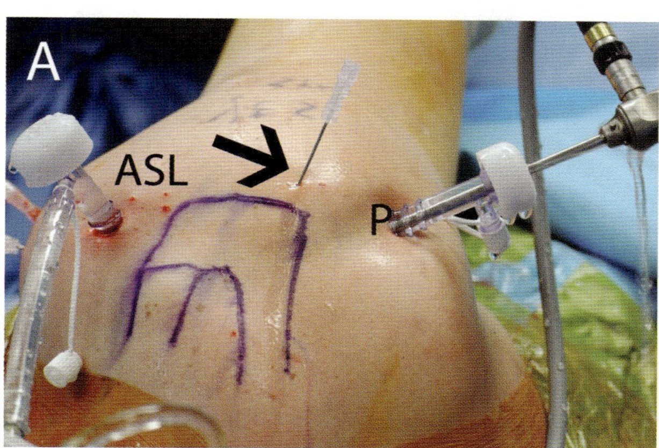

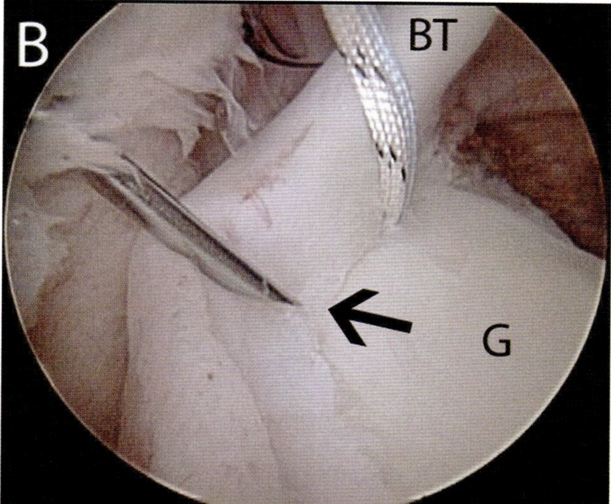

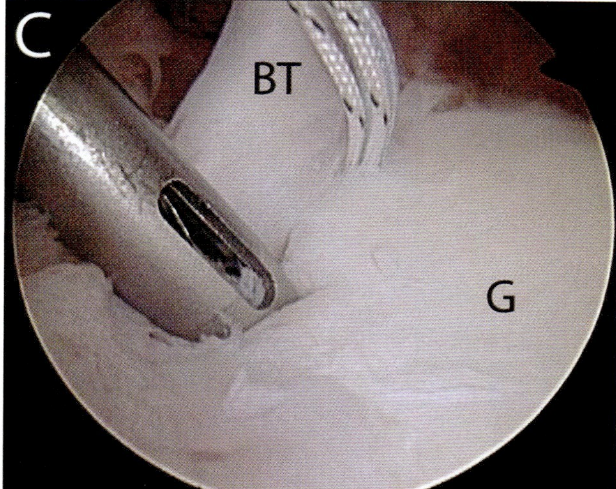

Figure 16.13 Port of Wilmington portal for posterior anchor in SLAP repair. **A:** An external view shows placement of a spinal needle (*black arrow*) 1 cm lateral and 1 cm anterior the posterolateral corner of the acromion in a right shoulder. **B:** Arthroscopic view from a posterior portal demonstrating the spinal needle's (*black arrow*) trajectory. **C:** Placement of a posterior anchor for SLAP repair through the Port of Wilmington portal. ASL, anterosuperolateral portal; BT, biceps tendon; G, glenoid; P, posterior portal.

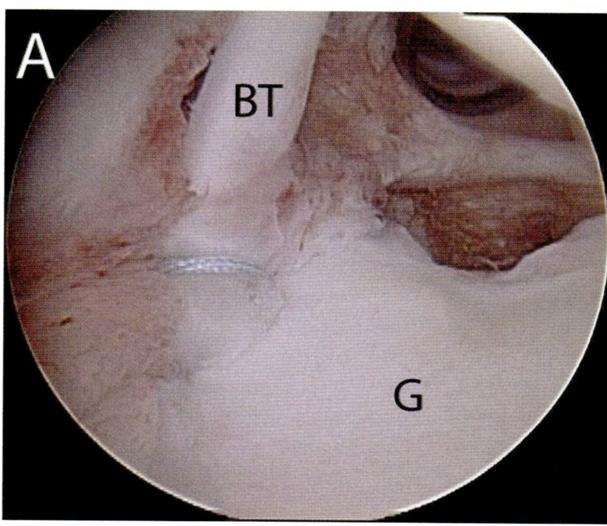

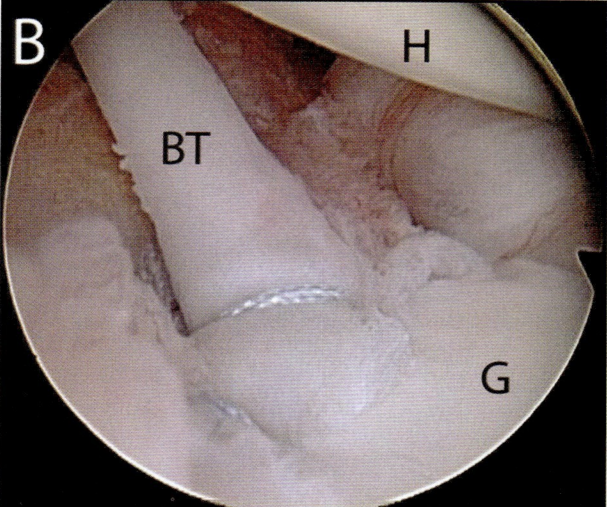

Figure 16.14 Final repair of a SLAP lesion in a right shoulder viewing from posterior. **A:** Sutures encircle the labrum to stabilize the biceps root. **B:** Retesting of the peel-back maneuver demonstrates a stable construct that does not displace medially. BT, biceps tendon; G, glenoid; H, humerus.

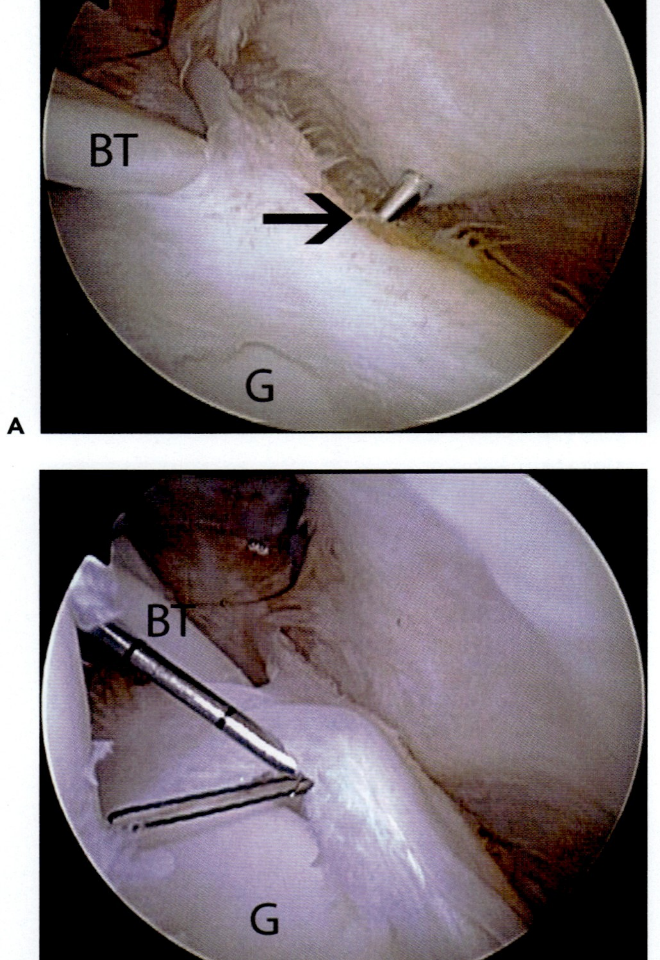

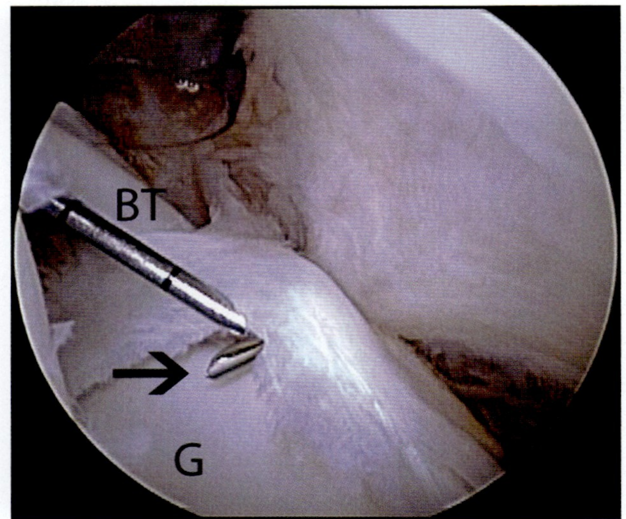

Figure 16.15 Left shoulder, posterior viewing portal, demonstrates use of a Micro SutureLasso (Arthrex, Inc., Naples, FL) to pass a suture shuttle through the superior labrum. **A:** A Micro SutureLasso (*black arrow*) is inserted through a modified Neviaser portal. **B:** The Micro SutureLasso (*black arrow*) penetrates the superior labrum. **C:** A Nitinol loop is advanced through the labrum for subsequent suture shuttling. BT, biceps tendon; G, glenoid.

portal. The sutures are retrieved out the anterosuperolateral portal, and using a similar procedure, the sutures are tensioned and the anchor inserted into the bone hole.

Video The final construct is evaluated for reduction and stability.

SPINOGLENOID CYST DECOMPRESSION WITH TYPE II SLAP REPAIR

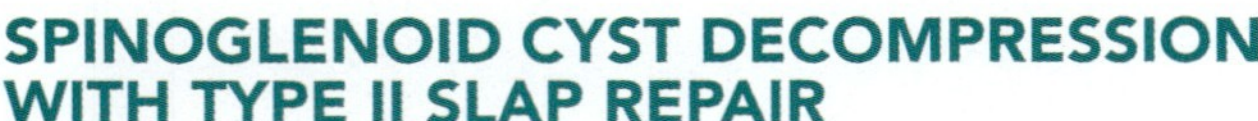

In some cases, type II SLAP lesions may be associated with the formation of a paralabral cyst. Paralabral cysts associated with type II SLAP lesions are usually formed in the posterior superior quadrant of the labrum and are classical spinoglenoid cysts (Fig. 16.19). When large, spinoglenoid cysts may encroach upon the suprascapular nerve and result in suprascapular neuropathy (Fig. 16.20). Unlike suprascapular neuropathy due to compression at the suprascapular notch, suprascapular neuropathy from a spinoglenoid cyst usually results in isolated infraspinatus atrophy and weakness and spares the supraspinatus. Although spontaneous decompression of spinoglenoid cysts may occur, when suprascapular neuropathy is present, decompression of the spinoglenoid cyst is indicated with repair of the superior labral tear. Furthermore, decompression alone has been associated with inferior outcomes compared to decompression combined with repair of the SLAP lesion.

It is important to consider however, that not all paralabral cysts are associated with SLAP lesions. Many paralabral cysts are the result of degenerative tears of the labrum and osteoarthritis and do not cause suprascapular neuropathy. These cysts usually present more inferiorly along the glenoid, are smaller, and are associated with glenohumeral arthritis (Fig. 16.21).

The standard portals for a SLAP repair are established and a diagnostic arthroscopy is performed to confirm a type II SLAP lesion and evaluate for evidence of the spinoglenoid cyst. When large, a spinoglenoid cyst may be

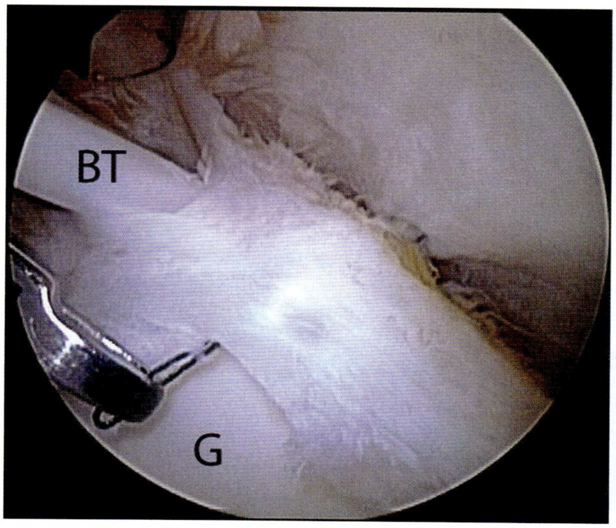

Figure 16.16 Left shoulder, posterior viewing portal, demonstrates shuttling of a suture through the superior labrum. **A:** A Nitinol loop previously passed through the labrum (Fig. 16.15) is retrieved out an anterior working portal. **B:** Appearance of the Nitinol loop prior to suture shuttling. One end has been retrieved out an anterior working portal (**left in image**), while the other end remains in a modified Neviaser portal (**right in image**). **C:** A #2 TigerWire suture (Arthrex, Inc., Naples, FL) has been shuttled through the labrum. BT, biceps tendon; G, glenoid.

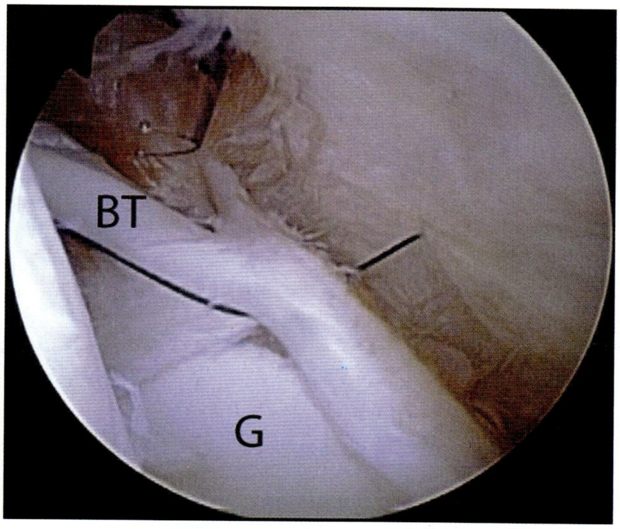

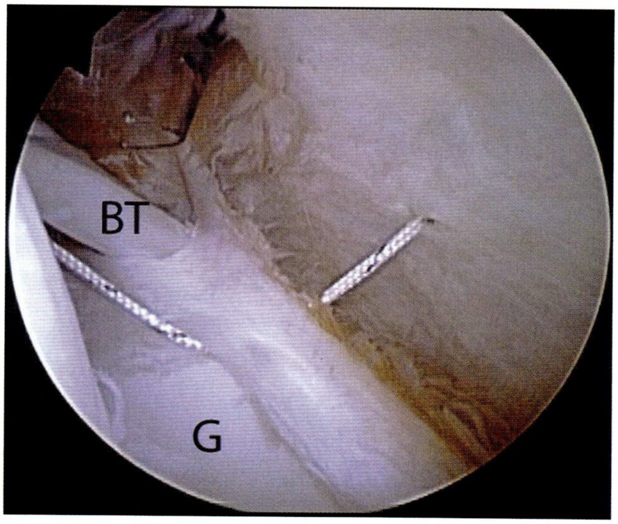

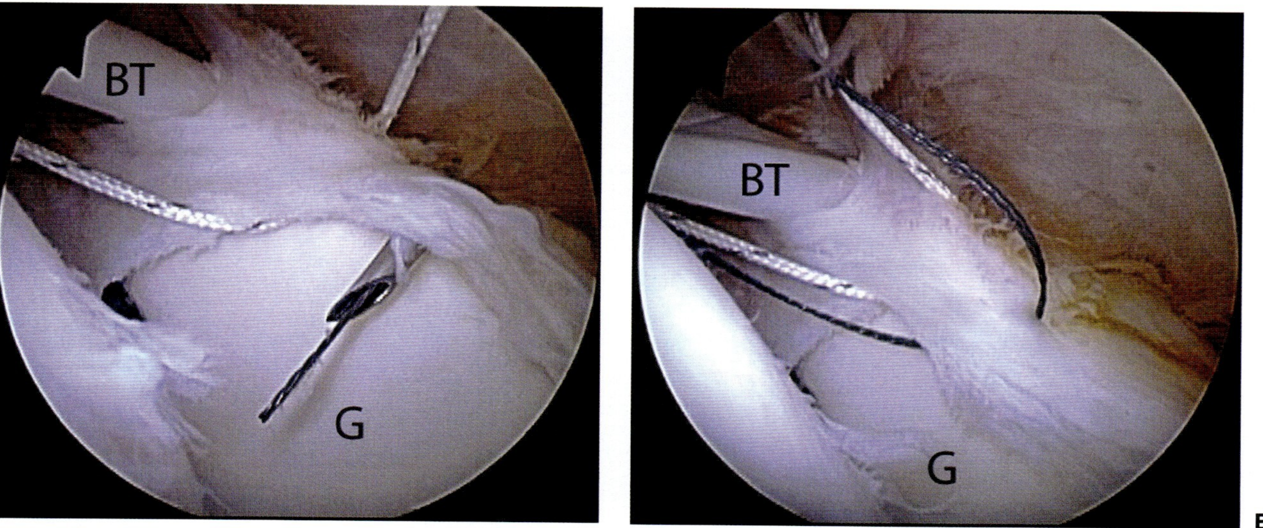

Figure 16.17 Left shoulder, posterior viewing portal, demonstrates completion of a mattress stitch in the superior labrum. **A:** A suture has previously been shuttled through the superior labrum (Fig. 16.16). A Micro SutureLasso (Arthrex, Inc., Naples, FL) penetrates the superior labrum posterior to the first suture and a Nitinol loop is passed through the labrum. **B:** The superior suture limb from the previously placed #2 TigerWire suture (Arthrex, Inc., Naples, FL) and the superior end of the Nitinol loop are retrieved out the same portal. Extracorporeally, the suture limb will be threaded through the Nitinol loop.

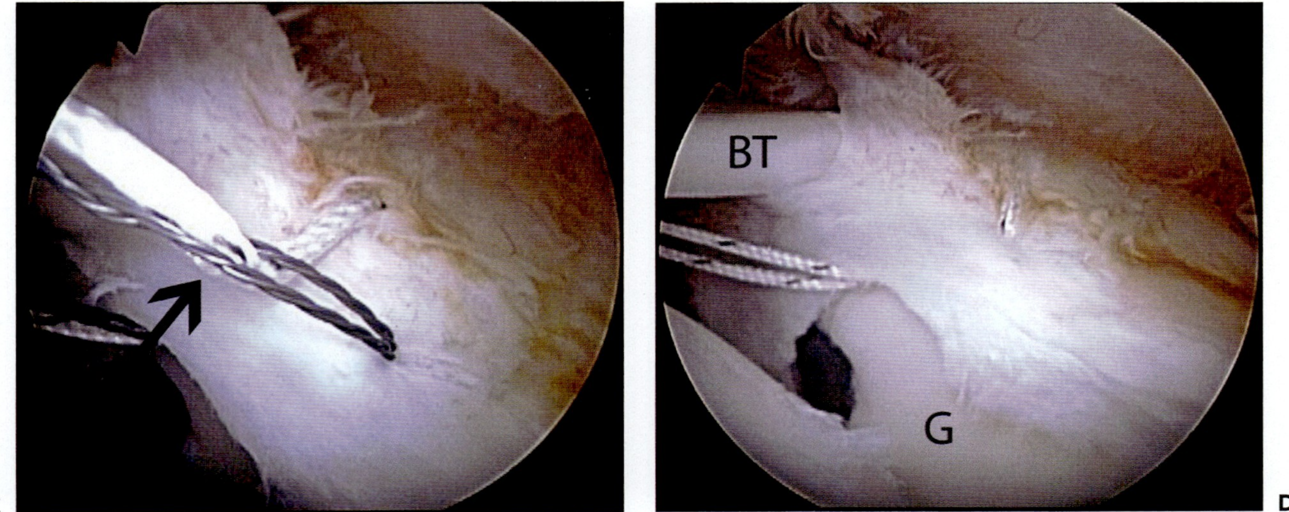

Figure 16.17 *(Continued)* **C:** Pulling the inferior end of the Nitinol loop shuttles the suture (*black arrow*) back through the labrum to create a mattress stitch. **D:** Appearance of the mattress stitch in place. BT, biceps tendon; G, glenoid.

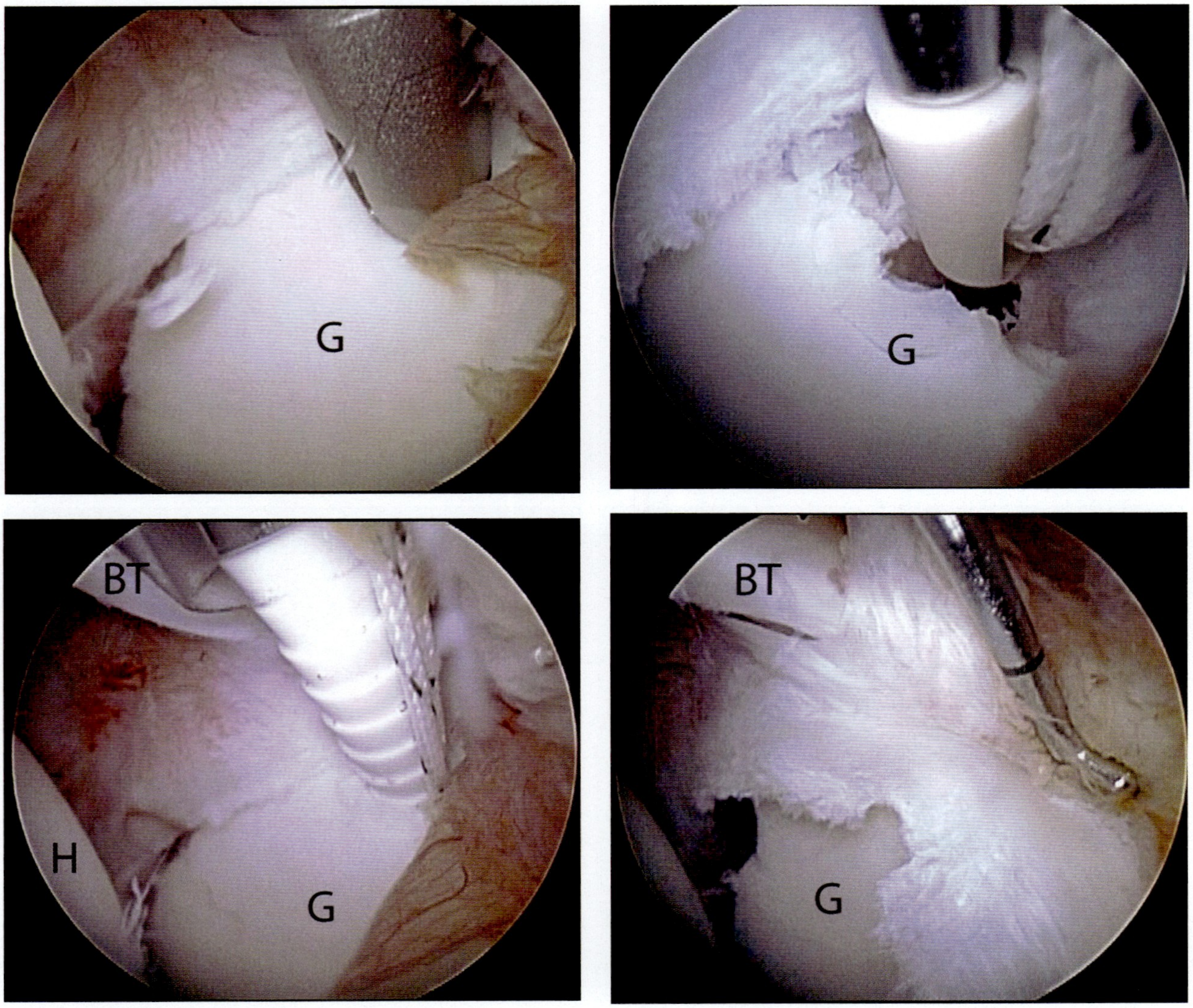

Figure 16.18 Left shoulder, posterior viewing portal, demonstrates placement of a PushLock anchor (Arthrex, Inc., Naples, FL) for a knotless repair of a SLAP lesion. **A:** A Spear guide inserted through an anterosuperolateral portal is placed on the superior glenoid rim so that a bone socket can be created for the PushLock anchor. **B:** Extracorporeally, previously passed suture limbs (Fig. 16.17) are threaded through the eyelet of the PushLock anchor. Then, the eyelet is seated into the bone socket. **C:** The anchor is impacted into the bone socket. **D:** Final appearance of this low-profile knotless mattress stitch technique. BT, biceps tendon; G, glenoid; H, humerus.

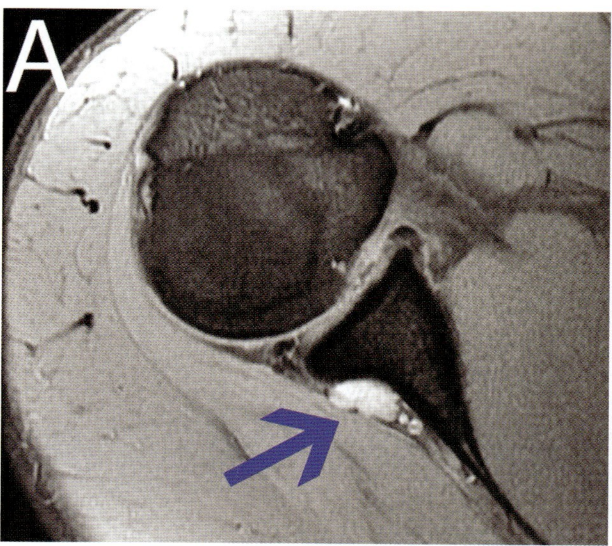

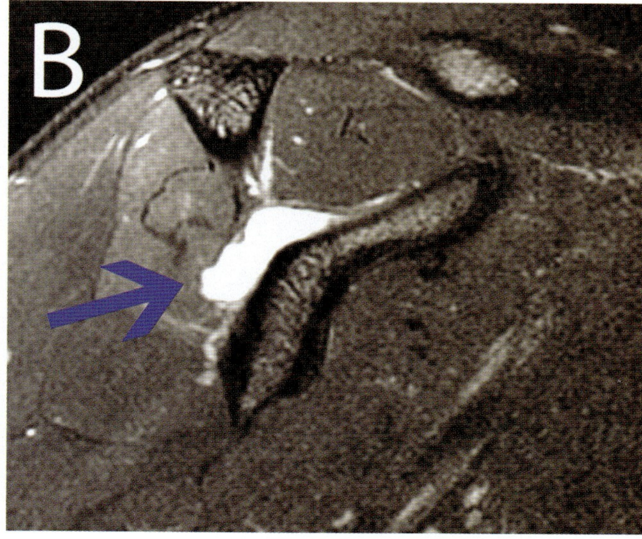

Figure 16.19 MRI of a right shoulder with a spinoglenoid cyst resulting in suprascapular neuropathy. **A:** Axial view shows a cyst posterior (*blue arrow*) to the glenoid. **B:** Sagittal view shows the cyst (*blue arrow*) at the spinoglenoid notch.

detected as a bulge underneath the capsule allowing for an intra-articular transcapsular decompression. However, usually the cyst is easiest to decompress under the labral tear itself.

Prior to SLAP lesion repair, the cyst should be located and decompressed. Careful evaluation of the MRI is necessary to locate the approximate location of the cyst. The SLAP lesion is initially debrided and elevated off the superior and posterosuperior labrum. Using an elevator from the anterior or anterosuperolateral portal, the superior and posterior superior labrum is carefully elevated off the glenoid neck until the cyst is encountered (Fig. 16.22). We commonly view through an anterior portal and insert instruments through the anterosuperolateral portal, providing a superior view and access to the posterior superior labrum. Once the cyst has been located, the cyst is decompressed using a combination of elevator, switching stick, and shaver. Identification of the suprascapular nerve itself is unnecessary and is best avoided to avert iatrogenic injury.

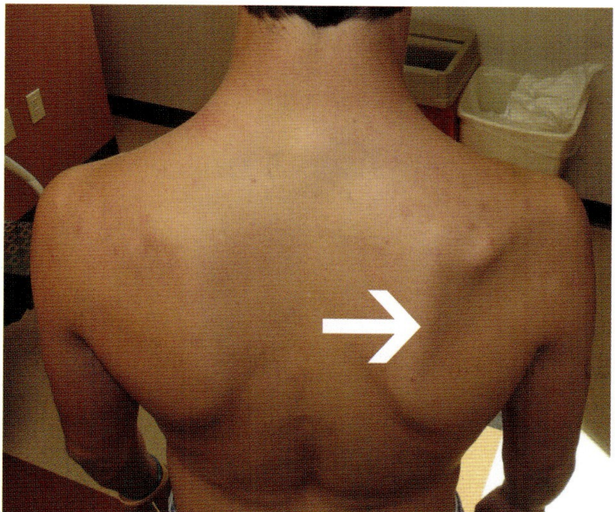

Figure 16.20 Clinical photo demonstrating infraspinatus atrophy (*white arrow*) in the right shoulder that resulted from a spinoglenoid cyst (Fig. 16.19). Note the lack of supraspinatus atrophy on the right. The supraspinatus is preserved because the compression of the suprascapular nerve occurs at the spinoglenoid notch, distal to the supraspinatus innervation.

Using the techniques as described above, the type II SLAP lesion may now be repaired. It is important to obtain a "water-tight" closure to ensure that reaccumulation of fluid within the cyst does not occur.

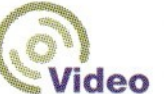

BICEPS TENODESIS FOR THE DEGENERATIVE SLAP LESION

We have observed symptomatic *degenerative SLAP lesions* in patients over the age of 35. These can be painful both with sports and with daily activities, and the pain pattern mimics impingement and rotator cuff symptoms.

On physical exam, patients exhibit biceps tension signs, the most reliable of which is the O'Driscoll sign, or Mayo shear sign. The O'Driscoll test involves placing the shoulder in the provocative position of combined abduction and external rotation, and then applying a downwardly directed lateral shear force (Fig. 16.23). This maneuver is quite painful in the patient with a degenerative SLAP lesion.

Arthroscopically, the peel-back test is usually negative. However, there is a displaceable biceps root on probing, with varying degrees of degeneration and failed footprint

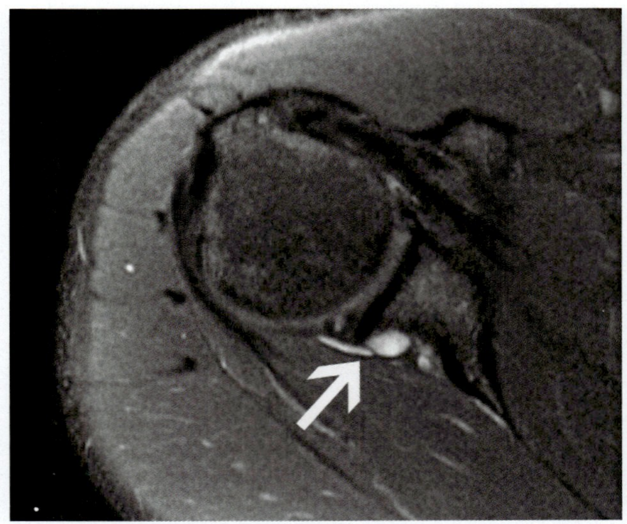

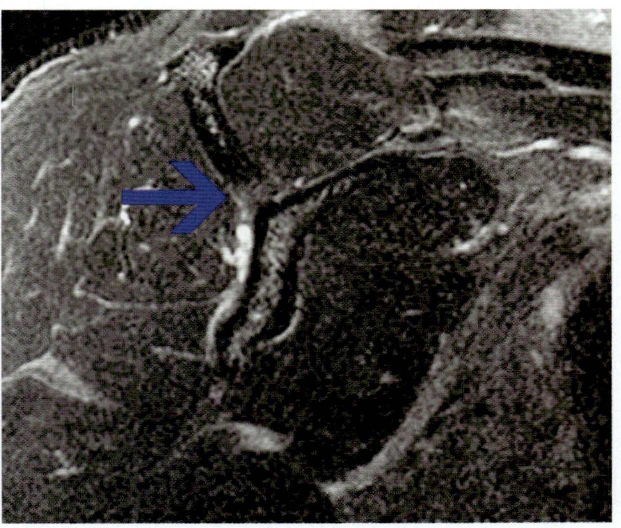

Figure 16.21 Paralabral cyst. **A:** Axial T2 magnetic resonance image demonstrates a paralabral cyst (*white arrow*) associated with glenohumeral arthritis. **B:** Sagittal T2 image of the same shoulder. Note the lack of a cyst at the spinoglenoid notch (*blue arrow*). Unlike a spinoglenoid cyst (Fig. 16.19), this paralabral cyst will not result in compression of the suprascapular nerve.

contact beneath the superior labrum. Probing the root of the biceps with a hooked probe reveals that there is virtually no carry-through of biceps root fibers to the bone of the supraglenoid tubercle (Fig. 16.24).

In patients over the age of 35, we have noted that postoperative stiffness after SLAP repair is more frequent than in younger people and the final outcome is less predictable (Unpublished data). Therefore, in this older category, we prefer to do biceps tenodesis rather than SLAP repair. We do a standard BioComposite Tenodesis screw construct at the top of the bicipital groove. Occasionally, we combine the tenodesis with a repair of the superior labrum (without its biceps root), but we do this only in high-level, high-demand athletes. Lower-demand patients do quite well with biceps tenodesis without concomitant repair of the superior labrum.

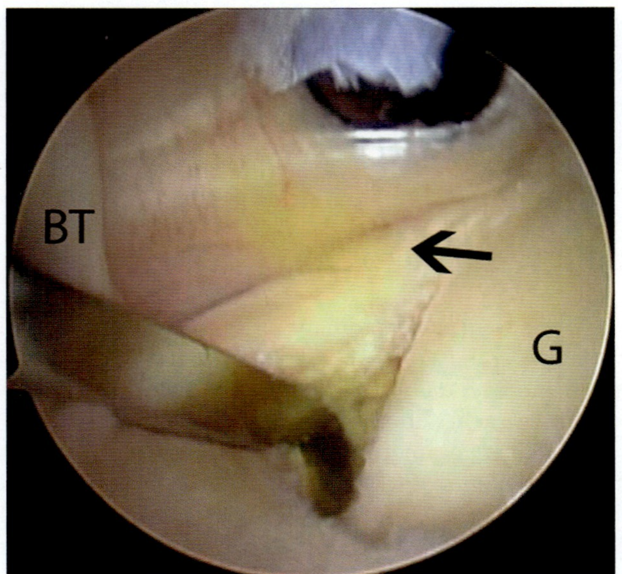

Figure 16.22 Right shoulder, anterior glenohumeral viewing portal demonstrating decompression of a spinoglenoid cyst with an arthroscopic elevator introduced from an anterosuperolateral portal. Decompression of the cyst is confirmed with extravasation of *cystic yellow fluid* (*black arrow*) into the glenohumeral joint. BT, biceps tendon; G, glenoid.

TYPE IV SLAP REPAIR

Type IV SLAP lesions are relatively rare and involve extension of the superior labral tear into the biceps tendon. The decision to repair these lesions or to debride and perform a biceps tenodesis (or tenotomy) is based on a number of factors including the age of the patient, location of the tear (i.e., red on red, red on white, white on white), extent of involvement of the biceps tendon, and concomitant degenerative changes or fraying of the superior labrum and biceps. It is important to recognize what is the primary indication for surgery. In patients with the primary complaint of instability, preservation of the biceps and superior labrum may be indicated to maximize the labral repair and optimize stability, especially if the bucket-handle portion of the tear extends inferiorly. In contrast, if the primary complaint is pain, debridement of the labrum, and release of the biceps tendon (+/– tenodesis) will likely provide a more reproducible result.

When a type IV SLAP lesion is encountered in addition to other labral pathology, and repair is indicated, repair of

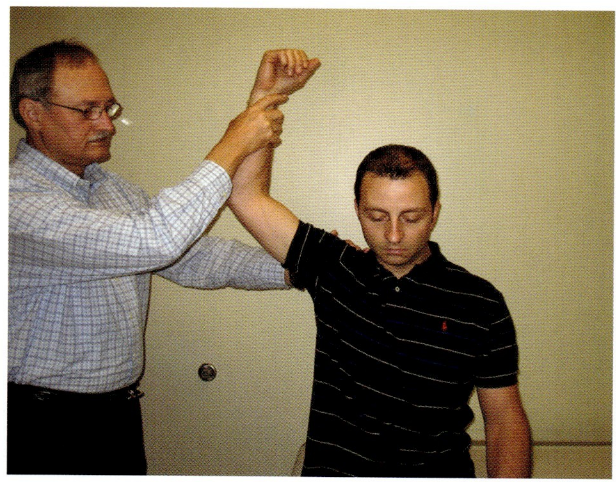

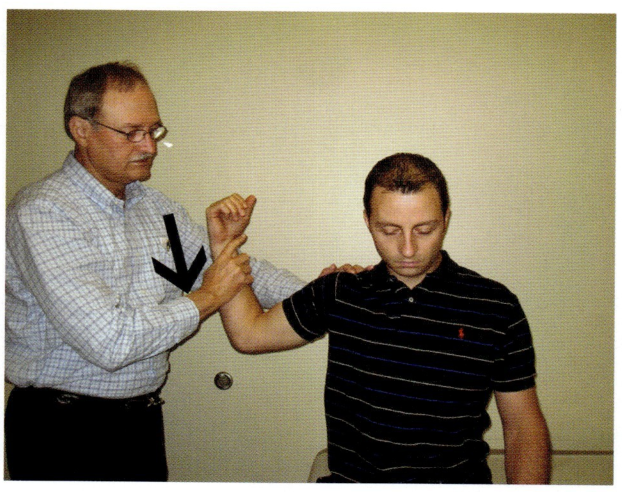

Figure 16.23 O'Driscoll sign (Mayo Shear sign). **A:** Starting position. The arm is placed in 90° of external rotation and approximately 120° of abduction with the elbow positioned slightly behind the plane of the scapula. **B:** Ending position. While stabilizing the shoulder, the arm is adducted (*black arrow*) to approximately 60°. Pain during this maneuver is considered a positive O'Driscoll sign for a proximal biceps lesion.

the SLAP lesion is performed first to help reduce the displaced bucket-handle portion of the labrum out of the joint and to provide a stable superior labral base for subsequent inferior repair. Standard anterior, posterior, and anterosuperolateral portals are established and the extent of labral and biceps tearing is assessed (Fig. 16.25A). The labral edges and biceps tendon are lightly debrided to provide a healing bed.

The superior glenoid neck is debrided to a bleeding bone surface (Fig. 16.25B). Depending on the amount of labral displacement, the bone may be debrided either through the tear or while reducing the labrum to the bone. Care must be taken to ensure that inadvertent injury to the labrum or cartilage does not occur.

To repair the type IV SLAP lesion, the labrum must be reduced back to the residual labrum attachment and also secured to the bone. We sometimes place one anchor just under the biceps root and one anchor more posteriorly (i.e., through a Port of Wilmington portal) (3.0-mm BioComposite SutureTak). Usually the anterior anchor is placed first. Depending on the displacement of the bucket-handle portion of the labrum, the SutureTak Spear may be used to reduce the labrum back to the superior glenoid while drilling, or the anchor may be inserted through the bucket-handle tear.

A Micro SutureLasso is passed through the residual labral tissue and one limb of the suture is shuttled through. The

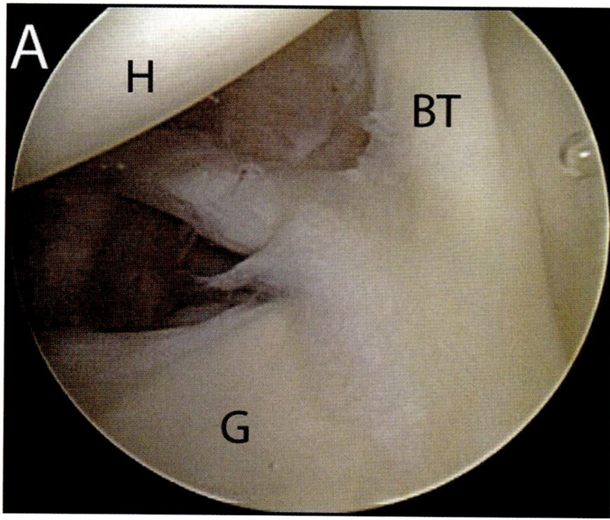

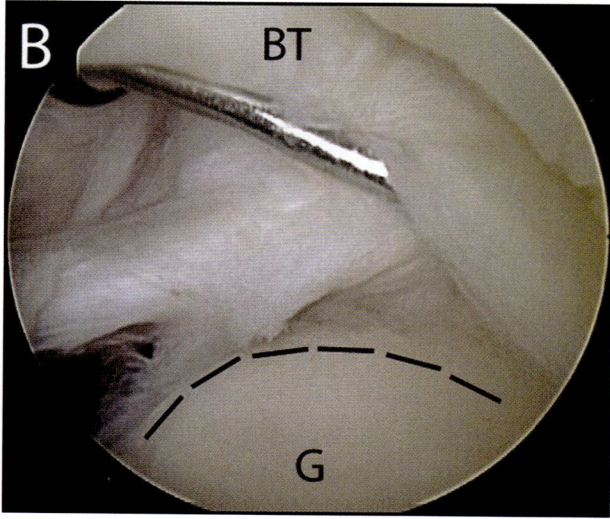

Figure 16.24 Degenerative SLAP lesion in a left shoulder viewed from a posterior portal. **A:** The biceps root shows moderate degenerative changes. **B:** Probing reveals a displaceable biceps root. The glenoid rim is outlined by *dashed lines*. BT, biceps tendon; G, glenoid; H, humerus.

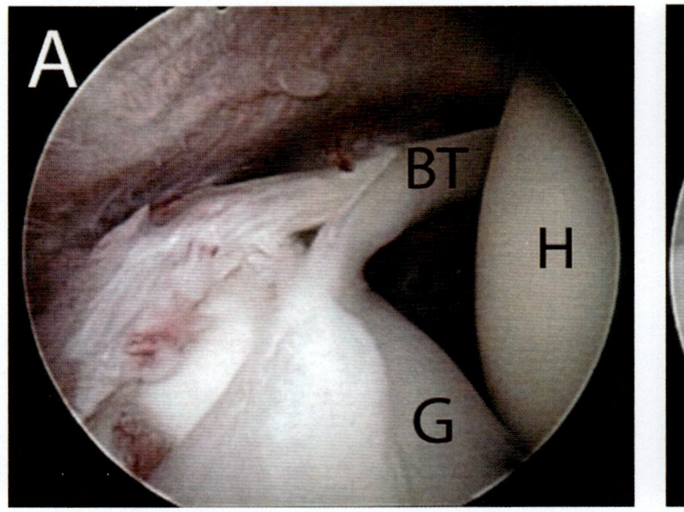

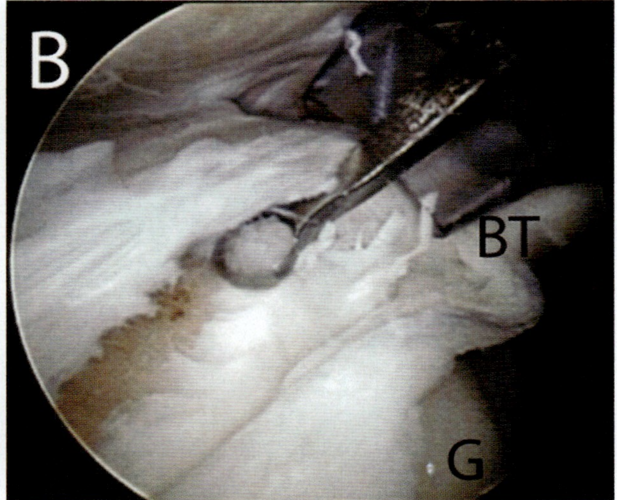

Figure 16.25 Right shoulder, posterior viewing portal demonstrates **(A)** a type IV SLAP lesion. **B:** Repair begins by preparing the bone bed. BT, biceps tendon; G, glenoid; H, humerus.

other limb of the suture is then retrieved so that it captures the bucket-handle portion of the tear. Alternatively, one may choose to pierce this portion of the labrum as well. A similar procedure is repeated for the second suture pair, passing the suture anterior to the biceps tendon.

A posterior anchor is placed through the Port of Wilmington portal (as previously described). Using the SutureLasso, sutures are passed through the residual labral tissue and the suture limbs are retrieved to capture the displaced labrum.

Once all sutures have been passed, the sutures are tied, reducing the labrum to the residual labral rim and securing the labrum to bone. The initial stitch to be tied is the one just posterior to the long head of the biceps tendon. This is the key stitch to tie since it will result in reduction of the labrum and bone. Care is taken during tying to anatomically reduce the labrum and biceps tendon. If necessary, an arthroscopic grasper may be inserted through the anterior portal to ensure anatomic reduction of the labrum. The remaining sutures are then tied.

Even in patients with tears extending deeply into the long head of the biceps tendon, labral reduction usually results in reduction of the long head of the biceps tendon. However, occasionally one or two side-to-side stitches are necessary to secure the biceps tendon. A Scorpion (Arthrex, Inc., Naples FL) suture passer or spinal needle inserted through the anterior or anterosuperolateral portal may be used to pass a #2 FiberWire stitch through the biceps tendon (Fig. 16.26).

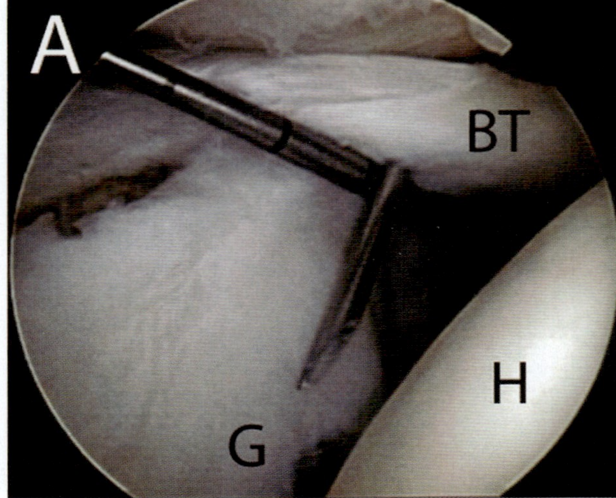

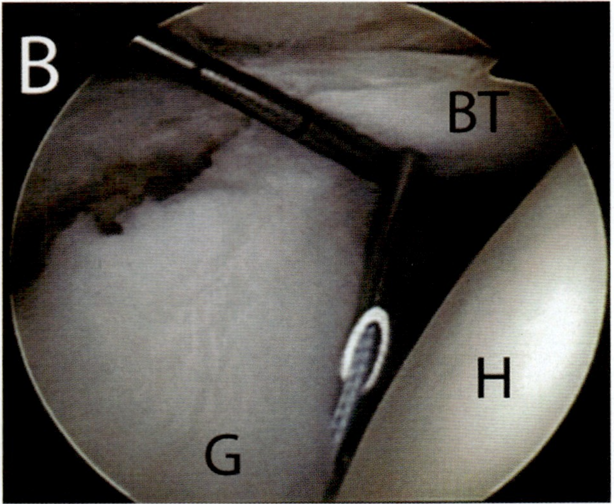

Figure 16.26 Right shoulder, posterior viewing portal. **A:** An instrument is used to reduce the biceps portion of a type IV SLAP lesion. Then, a spinal needle is passed between the two ends of the biceps tendon. **B:** A suture (FiberStick; Arthrex, Inc., Naples, FL) is threaded through the spinal needle. BT, biceps tendon; G, glenoid; H, humerus.

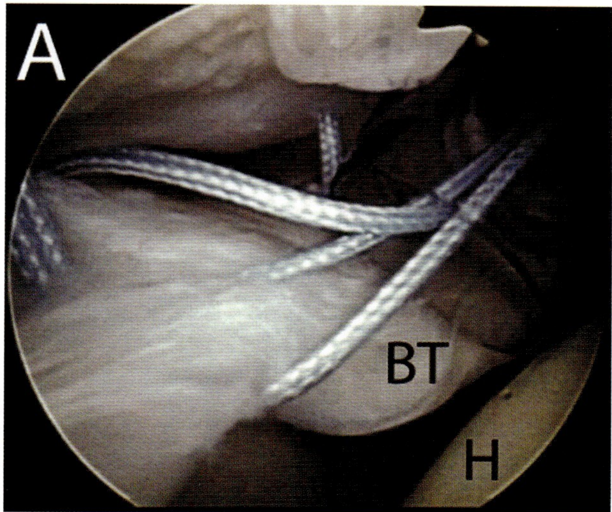

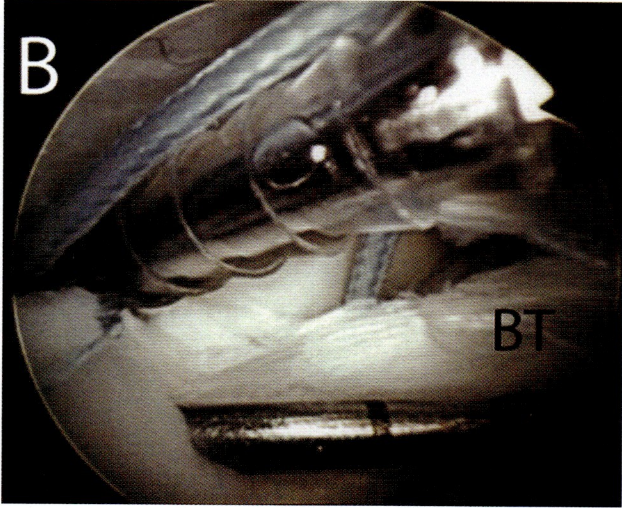

Figure 16.27 Right shoulder, posterior viewing portal. **A:** Sutures have been passed in a simple configuration to capture both limbs of a type IV SLAP lesion such that the free ends exit the defect. **B:** Once passed, the sutures are secured with a PushLock (Arthrex, Inc., Naples, FL) anchor placed in between the defect in the two labral limbs. BT, biceps tendon.

An alternative to the technique described above is to use a knotless anchor technique (PushLock or SwiveLock). In this case, a Micro SutureLasso or spinal needle is used to place #2 FiberWire suture that passes through both the stable medial rim and the bucket-handle segment of labrum. The stitch is placed in a simple configuration such that the sutures tails exit the defect between the labral limbs. The suture limbs are then threaded through the eyelet of the anchor and the anchor is inserted through the defect between the labral limbs (Figs. 16.27 and 16.28).

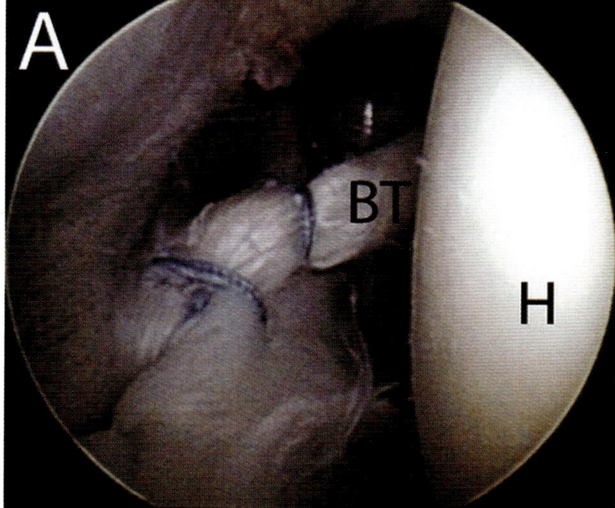

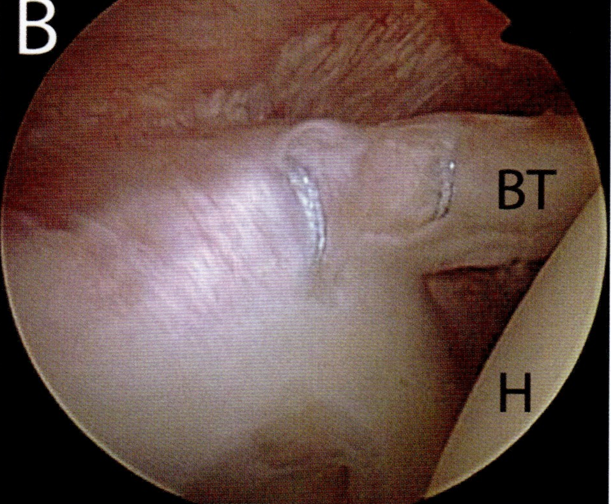

Figure 16.28 Right shoulder, posterior viewing portal demonstrates **(A)** completed repair of a type IV SLAP lesion using a knotless technique (compare to Fig. 16.24). **(B)** Second-look arthroscopy in the same patient demonstrates a healed repair. BT, biceps tendon; G, glenoid; H, humerus.

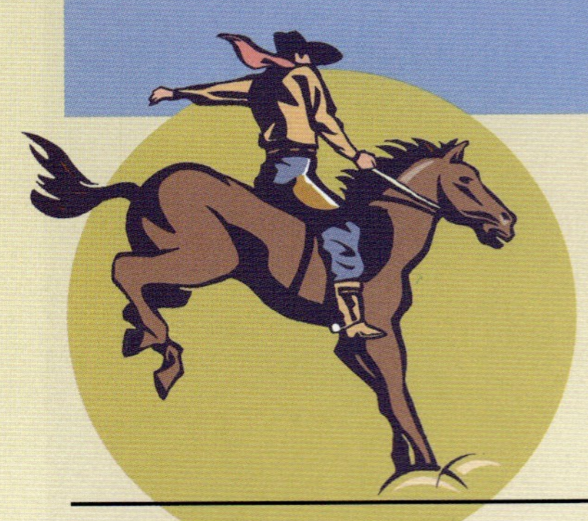

SECTION IV

ASSORTED TOPICS

COWBOY PRINCIPLE 6

If someone would pump water into it, a dry creek would be a river.

Sometimes you've got to accept things you can't change. Sometimes you've got to change things that you can't accept. Enough said.

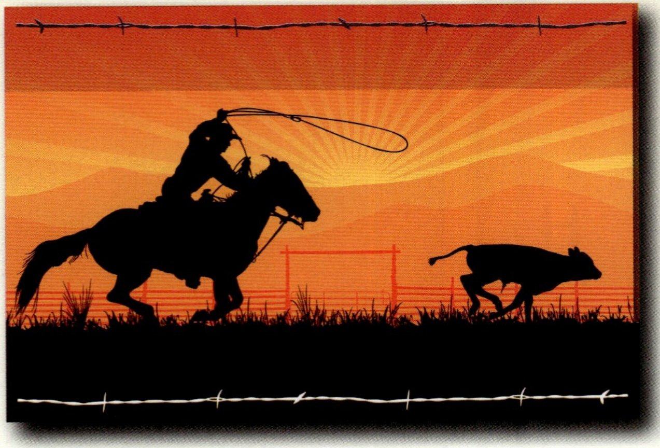

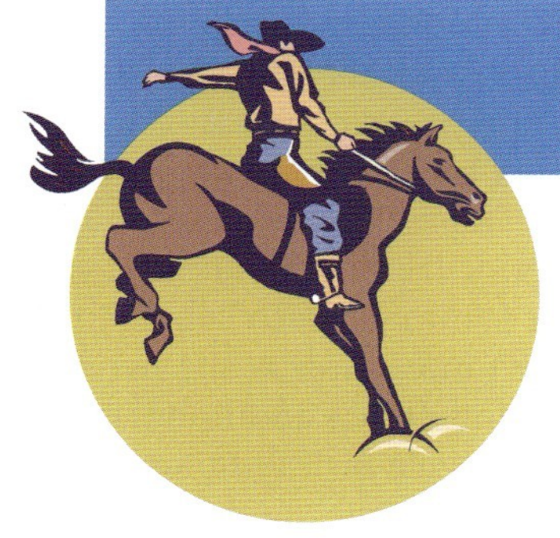

17 Suprascapular Nerve Release

WESTERN WISDOM

A self-centered, self-made man worships his creator.

Recently, there has been increased interest in disorders of the suprascapular nerve. While the suprascapular nerve provides sensory branches to the acromioclavicular (AC) and glenohumeral joints, its primary function is to innervate the supraspinatus and infraspinatus muscles. During its convoluted course from the upper trunk of the brachial plexus to its distal infraspinatus branches, the nerve may be compressed at either the suprascapular notch or the spinoglenoid notch (Fig. 17.1).

As the suprascapular nerve enters the supraspinatus fossa, it passes through the suprascapular notch, medial to the base of the coracoid and under the transverse scapular ligament. Although many anatomic variations have been described, the suprascapular artery (SA) and vein classically pass superficial to the transverse scapular ligament, while the suprascapular nerve travels under the transverse scapular ligament. The course under the ligament limits excursion of the nerve and predisposes to traction injury at the suprascapular notch. As it crosses the floor of the supraspinatus fossa, the nerve provides motor branches to the supraspinatus muscle and progresses toward the spinoglenoid notch.

The spinoglenoid notch is formed by the lateral aspect of the base of the scapular spine and is roofed laterally by the spinoglenoid ligament. Because of its distal attachment to the posterior capsule, tension of the spinoglenoid ligament is a dynamic function. The ligament is most taut with the arm in adduction and internal rotation. After it passes the spinoglenoid ligament, the suprascapular nerve turns sharply medially and innervates the infraspinatus muscle with several terminal motor branches.

During its course, the suprascapular nerve is particularly vulnerable to injury at regions where local anatomy limits its excursion. While various etiologies may exist (e.g., fracture, dislocation, hardware, prominent veins, traction), the most common neuropathies encountered in clinical practice are associated with paralabral cysts and large or massive rotator cuff tears.

Suprascapular neuropathy frequently occurs in association with a superior or posterosuperior labral tear. In this scenario, labral detachment forms a one-way synovial valve creating a paralabral spinoglenoid ganglion cyst. While no critical size limit has been described, presumably the larger the cyst, the greater the mass effect and the more likely suprascapular nerve compression may result. Since the nerve compression is usually distal to supraspinatus innervation, only the infraspinatus muscle is affected. In this situation, arthroscopic treatment of the mass effect along with labral repair is all that is required (i.e., arthroscopic spinoglenoid cyst decompression combined with labral repair), and formal suprascapular nerve decompression is unnecessary (1). Aspiration alone, however, does not reliably prevent cyst recurrence and is associated with inferior outcomes compared to labral repair (2).

While suprascapular neuropathy in association with spinoglenoid cysts has been recognized for several years, recent interest in the presence of suprascapular neuropathy in association with large or massive rotator cuff tears has emerged. In contrast to compression at the spinoglenoid notch, primary suprascapular nerve entrapment at

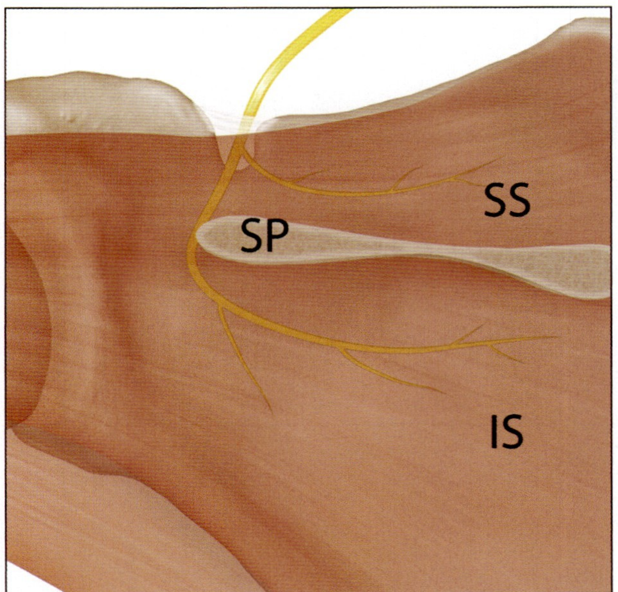

Figure 17.1 Schematic of the path of the suprascapular nerve as viewed from posterior. The nerve passes through the scapular notch beneath the transverse scapular ligament and provides innervation to the supraspinatus muscle. The nerve then courses around the scapular spine to provide innervation to the infraspinatus muscle. IS, infraspinatus; SP, scapular spine; SS, supraspinatus.

the suprascapular notch affects both the supraspinatus and the infraspinatus muscles. In a cadaveric rotator cuff tear model, progressive medial retraction of the rotator cuff led to increased traction and angulation of the suprascapular nerve indicating potential nerve compression (3). Recent clinical studies have suggested that suprascapular neuropathy as documented by electromyography (EMG) and nerve conduction velocity (NCV) studies may be present in nearly 30% of large to massive rotator cuff tears and contribute to both pain and muscular atrophy (4). This has led some authors to perform routine suprascapular nerve decompression at the suprascapular notch in patients with massive rotator cuff tears.

SURGICAL TREATMENT

It is important to remember that not all patients with suprascapular neuropathy require surgical decompression. Most patients with neuropathy secondary to traction or overuse with no focal mass lesion, may respond well to a course of nonoperative treatment. In contrast, patients with mass lesions or massive tears of the rotator cuff may benefit from early surgical intervention to maintain muscular strength and prevent progression of muscle atrophy. Although spontaneous resolution of paralabral ganglions has been reported, only a short course of nonoperative treatment should be considered if significant neurologic deficit is detected.

It is important to remember, however, that in patients with a paralabral cyst or with a rotator cuff tear, the treatment of the primary pathology is usually all that is necessary and formal release of the suprascapular nerve may be unnecessary. For example, in patients with isolated infraspinatus involvement with a paralabral cyst secondary to a posterior or posterosuperior labral tear, arthroscopic glenohumeral decompression of the cyst, with labral repair will usually suffice. Formal decompression of the nerve is only required if EMG/NCV testing detects addition pathology (e.g., supraspinatus involvement) or if symptoms persist despite cyst decompression.

Some authors have recommended routine suprascapular nerve release in conjunction with repair of a massive rotator cuff tear based on the high prevalence of suprascapular neuropathy on EMG/NCVs in these patients. However, the benefit of this remains unproven at the time of this writing. It is our experience that routine suprascapular nerve release is unnecessary (Fig. 17.2). In fact, nerve recovery has been documented following arthroscopic rotator cuff repair without formal nerve release (4,5). Furthermore, routine suprascapular nerve release was rarely performed in conjunction with open or mini-open rotator cuff repair and its popularity has increased only recently with the description of a relatively easy arthroscopic technique. Therefore, due to the potential risk of iatrogenic nerve injury, we perform suprascapular nerve release in association with rotator cuff repair only in cases of persistent postoperative suprascapular neuropathy, or in some cases where only partial repair of the rotator cuff is possible (i.e., infraspinatus and supraspinatus are largely irreparable) and nerve traction may potentially persist. Even so, we hardly ever perform suprascapular nerve release in the case of a partial repair of a massive rotator cuff tear.

SURGICAL TECHNIQUE

Suprascapular Nerve Release at the Transverse Scapular Notch

Although once mastered arthroscopic suprascapular nerve release is a relatively quick and safe procedure, this should not be used as an endorsement for irresponsible indications for arthroscopic release. We have seen cases of severe neuropathic pain after suprascapular release and recommend judicious use of this procedure.

When indicated, we decompress the suprascapular nerve at the suprascapular notch through a subacromial approach. The subacromial space is initially viewed through a posterior subacromial portal and a standard lateral portal is established. All bursal and fibrofatty tissue is cleared off the surface of the supraspinatus and the undersurface of the acromion, and the scapular spine is exposed (Fig. 17.3). The AC joint is identified and confirmed by palpation or by using a spinal needle (Fig. 17.4A). A modified Neviaser portal is then established posterior to the AC joint (Fig. 17.4B).

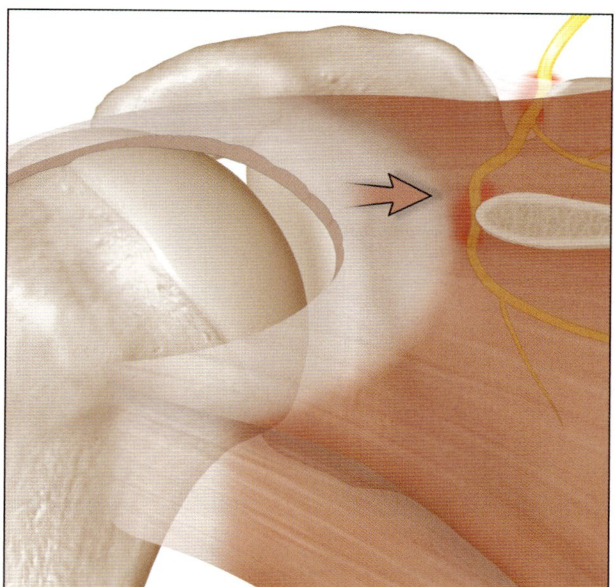

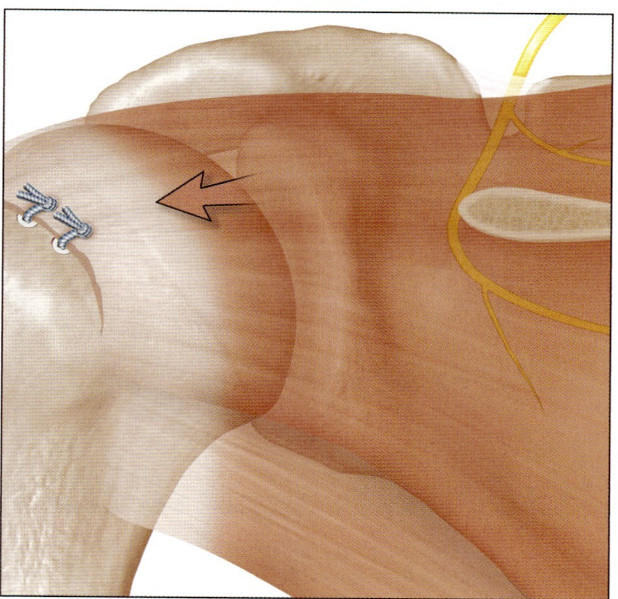

Figure 17.2 **A:** A massive retracted rotator cuff tear can result in compression of the suprascapular nerve at the scapular notch and at the base of the scapular spine. **B:** Repair of the rotator cuff tear relieves the medial compression of the nerve. The arrows denote that the muscular forces resulting in suprascapular nerve compression **(A)** have been reversed by cuff repair **(B)**, thereby relieving the nerve compression.

Once the position of the AC joint has been confirmed, the inferior and posterior aspect of the lateral clavicle is cleared until the lateral edge of the trapezoid portion of the coracoclavicular (CC) ligament is identified. The dissection is continued medially along the posterior aspect of the CC ligaments until the medial border of the CC ligament is identified. This is the medial border of the conoid portion of the CC ligament (Fig. 17.5A).

Through a modified Neviaser portal, a probe or switching stick is used to sweep the anterior edge of the supraspinatus muscle belly in a posterior direction to allow visualization of the conoid ligament as it traverses inferiorly toward the coracoid (Fig. 17.5B). To maximize visualization, a combination of a 70° arthroscope and lateral viewing portal may be utilized. This allows the arthroscopist to look over the supraspinatus muscle belly and down onto the superior transverse ligament and suprascapular nerve.

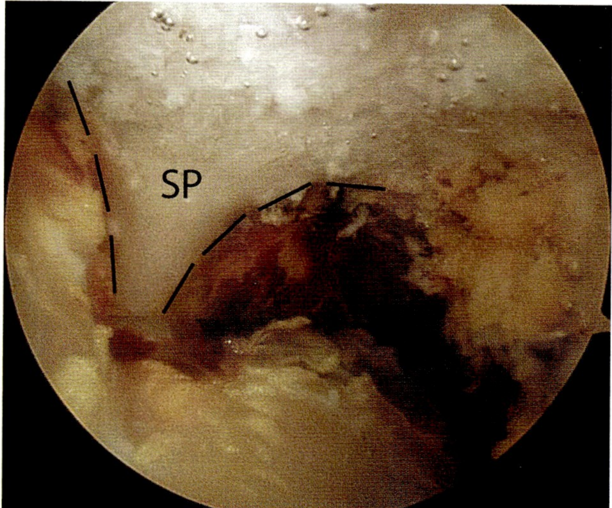

Figure 17.3 Left shoulder, lateral subacromial viewing portal. In the first step of suprascapular nerve release, the scapular spine (outlined by *dashed lines*) is indentified. SP, scapular spine.

As the conoid ligament is followed inferiorly, the confluence of the conoid ligament, trapezoid ligament, and the superior transverse ligament will be identified. The superior transverse scapular ligament can be identified traveling horizontally across the arthroscopic field (Fig. 17.5C). The probe is used to sweep the overlying soft tissues and suprascapular artery (SA) medially away, allowing visualization of the entire length of the superior transverse scapular ligament (Fig. 17.6). During exposure of the superior transverse scapular ligament, we use only blunt dissection with minimal use of the shaver to avoid iatrogenic injury to adjacent neurovascular structures. The probe may be used to palpate the inferior aspect of the ligament as well and therefore the suprascapular notch.

Although the suprascapular nerve can be identified inferior to the ligament surrounded by fibrofatty tissue, routine neurolysis is rarely performed. However, gentle traction on the perineural fat surrounding the nerve may help reveal the suprascapular nerve and its motor branches. Blunt dissection is utilized to clear sufficient tissue from the under surface of the ligament to ensure safe division of the ligament. Using needle localization, a separate portal is then created in the midportion of the supraspinatus fossa and an arthroscopic scissor is used to carefully incise the ligament. It is safest to incise the ligament at its most lateral insertion toward the coracoid, avoiding the more medial

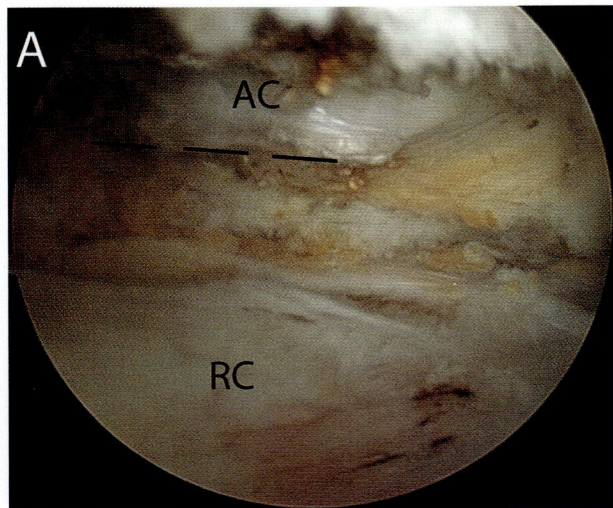

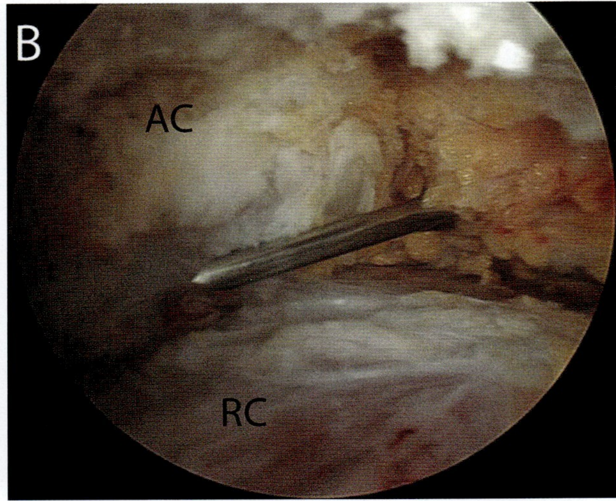

Figure 17.4 Left shoulder, lateral subacromial viewing portal. **A:** Following exposure of the scapular spine, the acromioclavicular joint is identified (*Dashed black lines mark* the inferior border of the distal clavicle.) **B:** A modified Nevaiser portal is established posterior to the acromioclavicular joint to assist in medial dissection. AC, acromioclavicular joint; RC, rotator cuff.

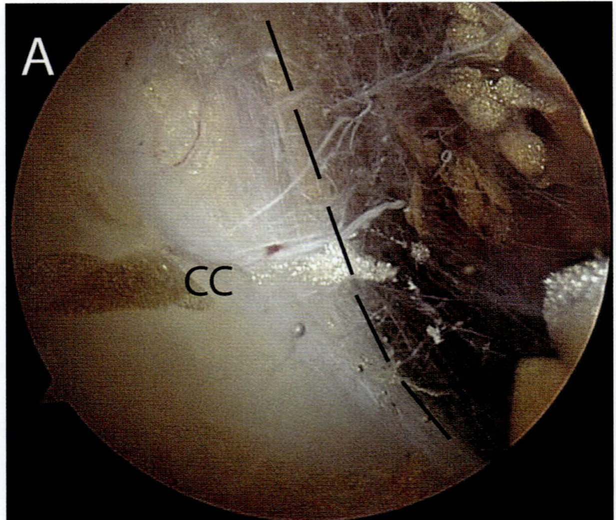

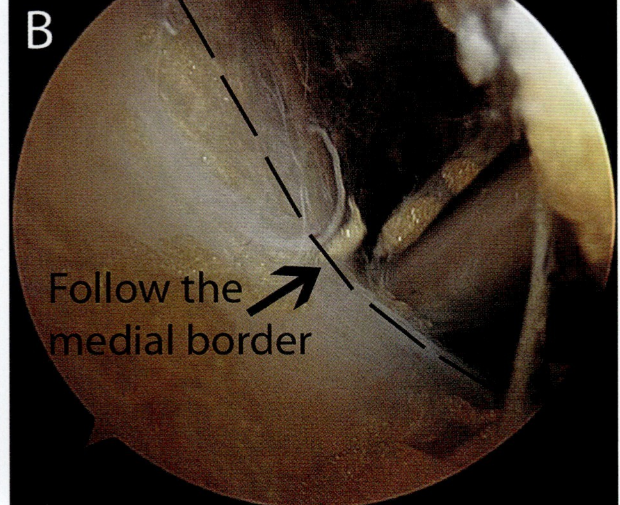

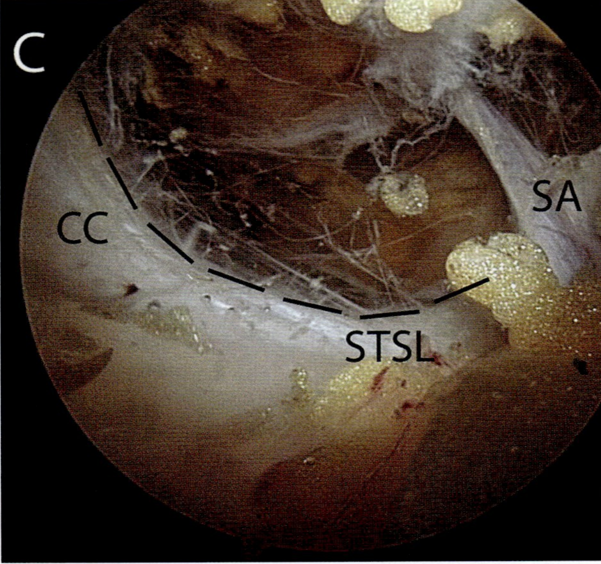

Figure 17.5 Left shoulder, lateral subacromial viewing portal with a 70° arthroscope demonstrating use of the CC ligaments to locate the suprascapular notch. **A:** After locating the acromioclavicular joint, the dissection is continued medially until the conoid ligament (medial border outlined by *dashed lines*) is visualized. **B:** The medial border (*dashed lines*) of the conoid ligament is followed as an instrument sweeps the supraspinatus muscle posteriorly. **C:** Following the medial border of the conoid ligament will lead to the superior transverse scapular ligament (outline by *dashed lines*). CC, conoid ligament; SA, suprascapular artery; STSL, superior transverse scapular ligament.

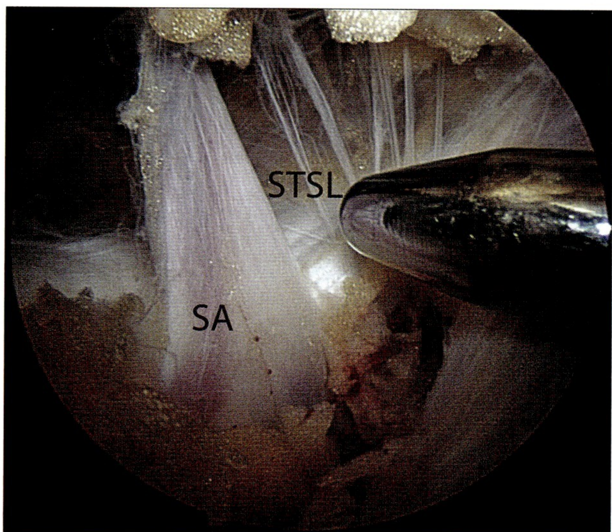

Figure 17.6 Left shoulder, lateral subacromial viewing portal with a 70° arthroscope. The suprascapular artery (SA) is visualized passing above the superior transverse scapular ligament (STSL). The suprascapular nerve lies beneath the STSL.

SA and nerve (Fig. 17.7A). A probe is then used to ensure that no residual fibers remain and that the suprascapular nerve is no longer under tension (Fig. 17.7B).

Video

PARTIAL ROTATOR CUFF REPAIR WITH SUPRASCAPULAR NERVE RELEASE

In patients with massive tears of the rotator cuff that are not repairable by direct tendon repair to bone or by margin convergence, complex releases may be required for rotator cuff repair. These may include a combination of capsular releases, and interval slides. In general, if a rotator cuff tear is significantly immobile, we proceed with capsular release first and then to interval slides. Usually, the vast majority of tears are completely repairable when mobilized using capsular releases and a modified double interval slide.

However, in chronic tears, particularly in older individuals with poor tendon quality, complete repair may not be possible. Almost universally, however, the posterior infraspinatus tendon is repairable following capsular release and a posterior interval slide. This tendon is advanced laterally and anteriorly and repaired to balance the force couples and provide a stable fulcrum of motion. Occasionally in these scenarios, however, the supraspinatus tendon may still have insufficient mobility or its tissue quality is so poor that repair is futile. In this scenario, only a partial repair is performed and the supraspinatus (previously released by a posterior interval slide) is sutured side to side to the infraspinatus in an effort to reestablish the rotator cable.

In this situation, the suprascapular nerve may still be under tension due to the medially retracted supraspinatus tendon. The arthroscopist may therefore elect to also perform a suprascapular nerve release at the suprascapular notch. In this scenario, visualization and suprascapular nerve release is often easier because of atrophy of the supraspinatus muscle. However, we are not united in support of suprascapular nerve release in the face of a massive rotator cuff tear that is only partially repairable. Some of us believe that retraction of the infraspinatus is more important as a culprit of suprascapular neuropathy than

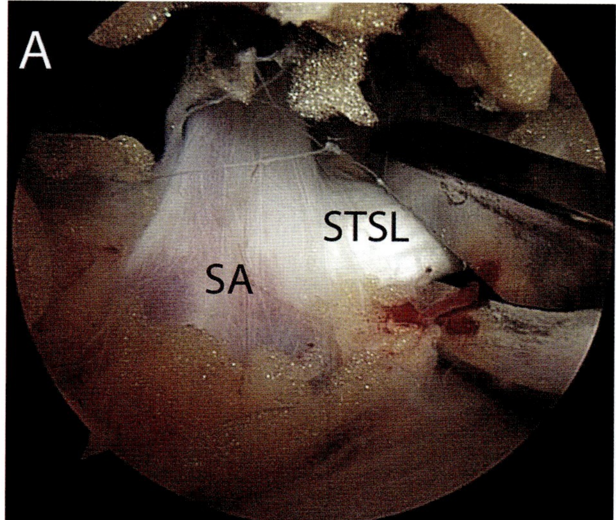

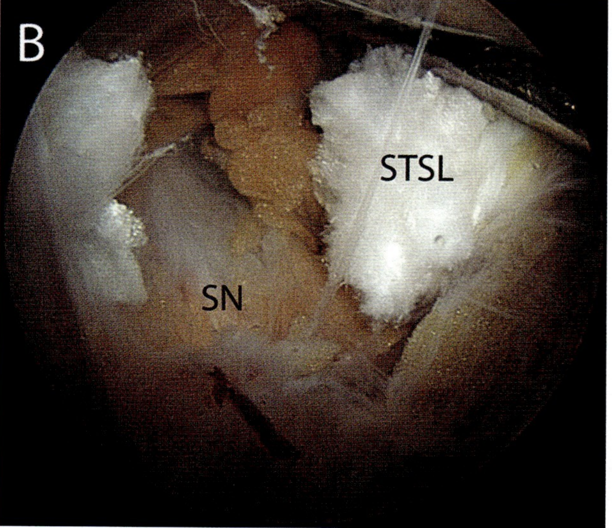

Figure 17.7 Left shoulder, lateral subacromial viewing portal with a 70° arthroscope. **A:** Arthroscopic scissors are used to release the superior transverse scapular ligament. The suprascapular artery is visualized superior to the ligament. Although the ligament is usually cut lateral to the artery, in this case the ligament was cut medial to the artery because there was more space on that side. **B:** The suprascapular nerve has been decompressed and is clearly seen. SA, suprascapular artery; SN, suprascapular nerve; STSL, superior transverse scapular ligament.

retraction of the supraspinatus because medial retraction of the infraspinatus can tension the nerve as it courses around the scapular spine. Under this theory, suprascapular nerve release is only likely to benefit the rare patient with an irreparable infraspinatus tendon tear. Finally, partial cuff repair without suprascapular nerve release has an enviable record of success in improving strength and diminishing pain (4).

If suprascapular nerve release is elected following partial repair, the CC ligaments are identified traversing inferiorly from the clavicle toward the base of the coracoid. The medial aspect of the conoid ligament is followed inferiorly toward its confluence with the superior transverse scapular ligament. Through a modified Neviaser portal, the SA and overlying soft tissues are retracted medially revealing the superior transverse scapular ligament. The superior transverse scapular ligament is then incised using an arthroscopic scissor.

REFERENCES

1. Youm T, Matthews PV, El Attrache NS. Treatment of patients with spinoglenoid cysts associated with superior labral tears without cyst aspiration, debridement, or excision. *Arthroscopy*. 2006;22:548–552.
2. Piatt BE, Hawkins RJ, Fritz RC, et al. Clinical evaluation and treatment of spinoglenoid notch ganglion cysts. *J Shoulder Elbow Surg*. 2002;11:600–604.
3. Albritton MJ, Graham RD, Richards RS II, et al. An anatomic study of the effects on the suprascapular nerve due to retraction of the supraspinatus muscle after a rotator cuff tear. *J Shoulder Elbow Surg*. 2003;12:497–500.
4. Costouros JG, Porramatikul M, Lie DT, Warner JJ. Reversal of suprascapular neuropathy following arthroscopic repair of massive supraspinatus and infraspinatus rotator cuff tears. *Arthroscopy*. 2007;23:1152–1161.
5. Mallon WJ, Wilson RJ, Basamania CJ. The association of suprascapular neuropathy with massive rotator cuff tears: a preliminary report. *J Shoulder Elbow Surg*. 2006;15:395–398.

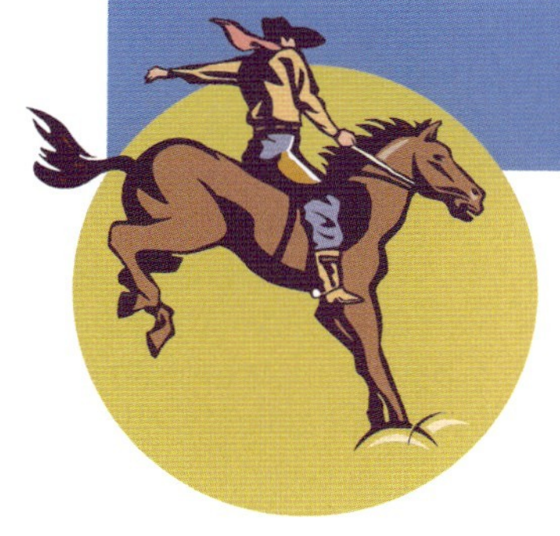

18

The Acromioclavicular Joint

WESTERN WISDOM

The man who knows the least repeats it the most.

The acromioclavicular (AC) joint often gets overshadowed by the more glorious glenohumeral articulation. While its complexity and function are less intricate than those of the glenohumeral joint, pathology of this small joint can be extremely symptomatic. Pathology of the AC joint can be the result of acute trauma or more commonly can be due to overuse or intrinsic degeneration of the joint. Traumatic AC joint problems include AC joint separations (partial or complete), distal clavicle fractures, and rarely acromial fractures. Chronic problems include AC joint arthropathy, distal clavicle osteolysis (DCO), and symptomatic os acromiale. AC joint pathology is often related to activities such as weightlifting, contact sports, repetitive overhead lifting at work, and multiple other causes.

CHRONIC PROBLEMS

AC joint arthropathy can be quite symptomatic. Consistent physical exam findings in these patients include tenderness to palpation of the AC joint and pain with cross body adduction of the arm. In general, we utilize three criteria when deciding to perform a distal clavicle resection. These include a positive finding of pain on cross body adduction exam, tenderness to palpation at the AC joint, and workers' compensation cases. If two out of three of the above criteria are met, we proceed with an arthroscopic distal clavicle resection. The technical pearls of this procedure were thoroughly covered in *A Cowboy's Guide to Advanced Shoulder Arthroscopy*, so they will not be reviewed at length here. However, some of the important considerations include the following:

1. Appropriate placement of an anterior portal over the lateral half of the subscapularis while visualizing intra-articularly will usually set up a perfect trajectory for instruments to perform the distal clavicle excision (Fig. 18.1).
2. Thorough debridement within the subacromial space all the way to the spine of the scapula should be performed. This allows for appropriate positioning of the arthroscope to best visualize the AC joint from a posterior portal (Fig. 18.2).
3. The inferior, anterior, and posterior AC joint capsule should be excised. This will not lead to instability as long as the superior joint capsule and superior AC joint ligaments are preserved during the procedure. Over 50% of anterior–posterior AC joint stability is provided by the superior ligaments and we have not seen any complications as a result of removing the other portions of the capsuloligamentous envelope.
4. Excision proceeds from inferior to superior in an anterior to posterior direction. One centimeter of the distal clavicle is excised, being careful to preserve the superior AC joint capsule (Fig. 18.3).
5. Care is taken to assure that complete resection is performed. The most commonly unresected portions of the distal clavicle include the superior lip and the posterior edge. It is beneficial to use a 70° arthroscope to thoroughly visualize the entire joint during resection (Fig. 18.4).

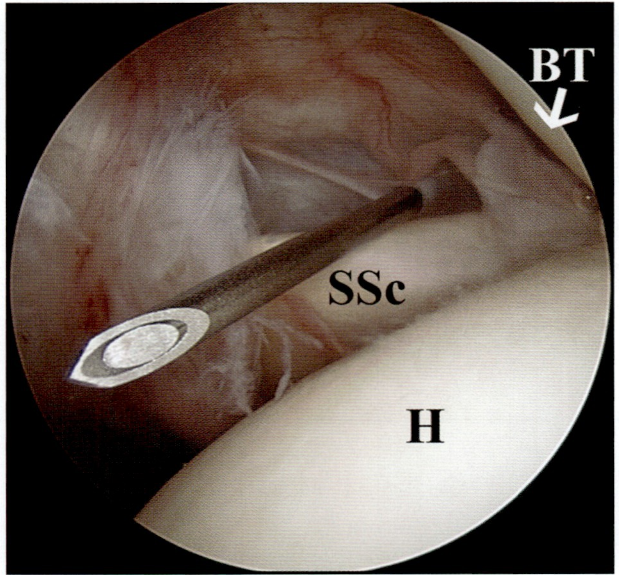

Figure 18.1 Right shoulder, posterior viewing portal, demonstrates spinal needle localization of the anterior portal that enters the glenohumeral joint over the lateral aspect of the subscapularis tendon. In addition to the intra-articular angle of approach, this placement usually provides a good angle of approach for distal clavicle excision. BT, biceps tendon; H, humerus; SSc, subscapularis tendon.

6. It is also important to recognize that the clavicular facet of the acromion can have a moderate amount of inferior–medial to superior–lateral slope, thus enhancing the need for the use of a 70° scope. We have termed this obliquity the "ski-slope" acromion (Figs. 18.5 and 18.6).

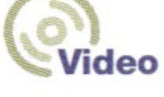

DISTAL CLAVICLE OSTEOLYSIS

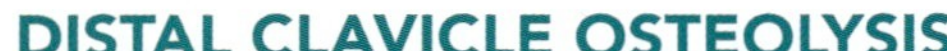

DCO is a condition often found in younger patients who put high stresses on the AC joint, such as weightlifters, wrestlers, and football players. The etiology is not entirely understood but is presumed to involve disruption in the blood supply to the distal clavicle. With conservative treatment, symptoms often resolve with time and activity modifications. However, in cases of persistent symptoms, an arthroscopic distal clavicle excision can reliably alleviate symptoms.

SYMPTOMATIC OS ACROMIALE

An os acromiale can be classified into three types—preacromion, mesoacromion, and metaacromion (Fig. 18.7). The mesoacromion variant is most common. The cleft in a mesoacromion usually lines up with the posterior border of the clavicle as viewed on an axillary radiograph or magnetic resonance image (MRI) (Figs. 18.8 and 18.9). Os acromiale pain can be confused with AC joint symptoms. It is important to recognize the presence or absence of an os acromiale when addressing anterior or superior shoulder pain. Recognition of this pathology will avoid mistakenly diagnosing AC joint pain and inappropriately performing a distal clavicle resection. This is particularly relevant because excision of a mesoacromion after a previous distal clavicle excision can result in a relatively large bone defect in the anterior shoulder and may compromise deltoid function or predispose toward deltoid detachment.

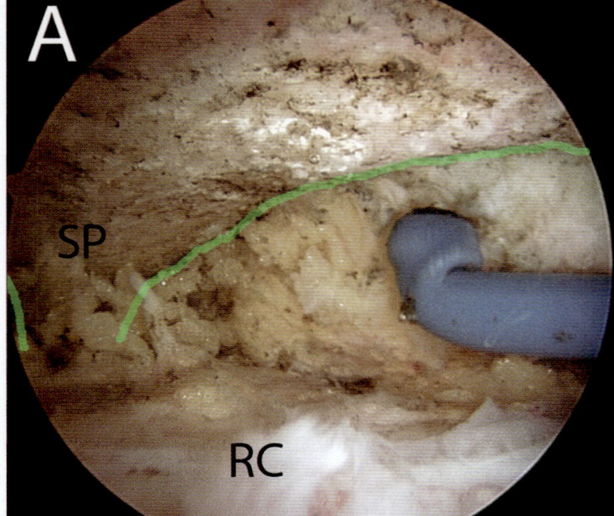

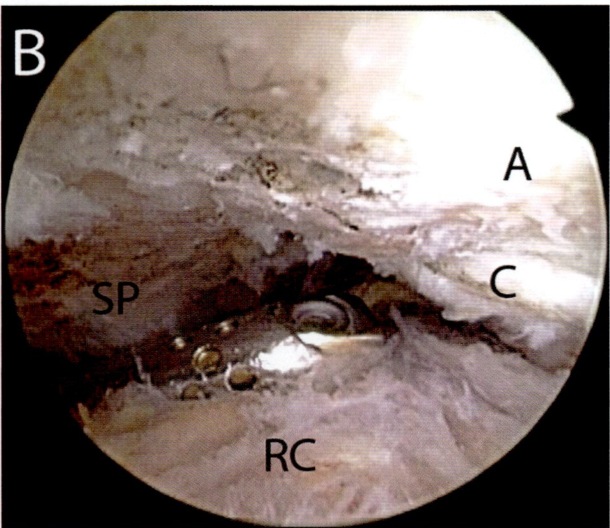

Figure 18.2 **A:** Right shoulder, lateral subacromial viewing portal, demonstrates skeletonization of the scapular spine (outlined by *green line*) in preparation for a distal clavicle resection. **B:** Clearing the soft tissue between the scapular spine and the AC joint provides a space for the arthroscope to view the AC joint from a posterior subacromial portal. A, acromion; C, distal clavicle; RC, rotator cuff; SP, scapular spine.

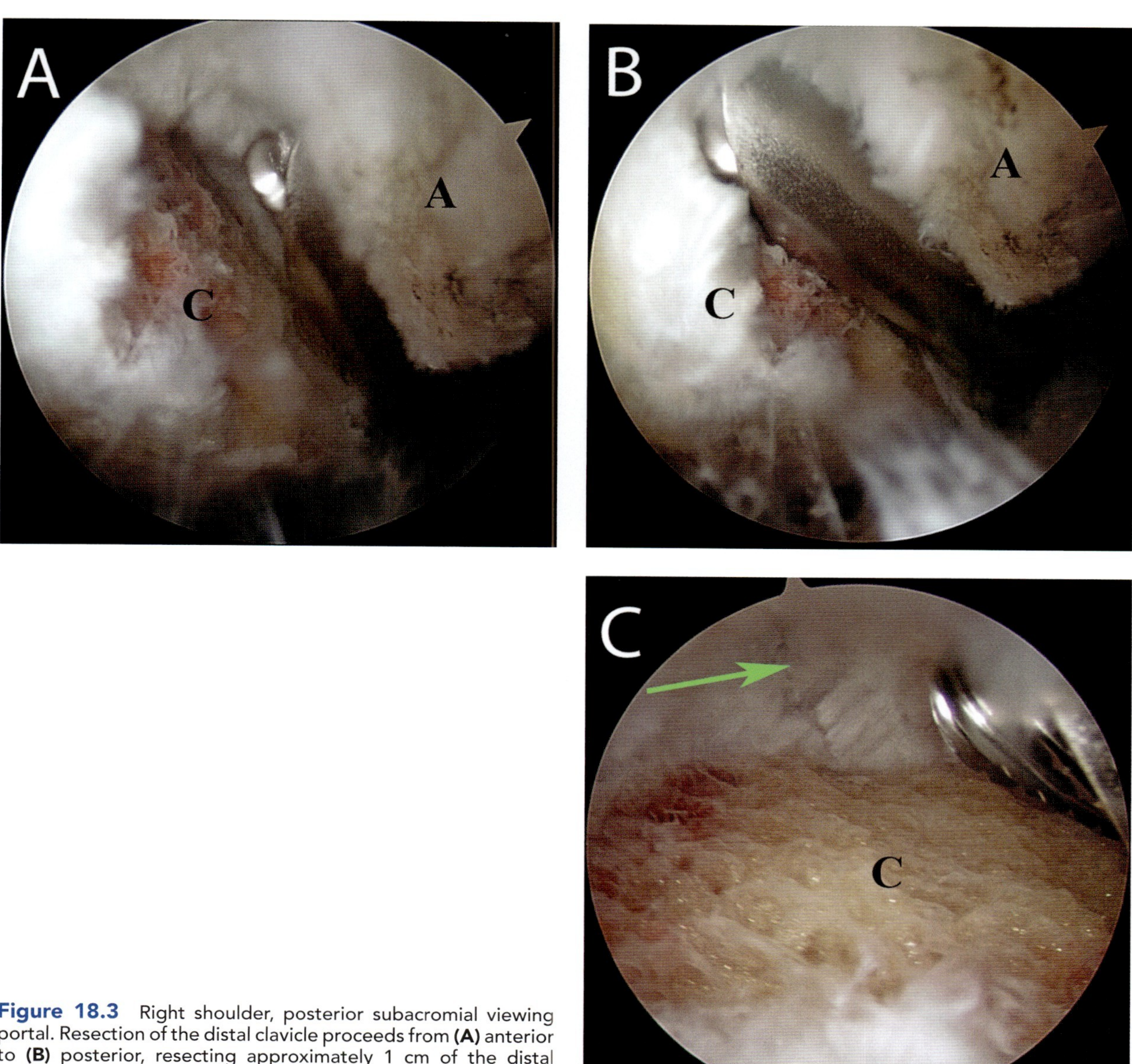

Figure 18.3 Right shoulder, posterior subacromial viewing portal. Resection of the distal clavicle proceeds from **(A)** anterior to **(B)** posterior, resecting approximately 1 cm of the distal clavicle. **C:** Care is taken to preserve the superior AC ligaments (*green arrow*). A, acromion; C, distal clavicle.

Typically, when we treat a patient with both a symptomatic mesoacromion and AC joint arthritis, we excise only the os acromiale segment. In fact, excision of the os acromiale fragment also addresses the AC joint arthropathy since the distal clavicle will no longer have any bone to articulate against. When an os acromiale occurs in association with a rotator cuff tear, we perform an acromioplasty, just as if there were not an os acromiale, so as not to compromise the coracoacromial arch. The complication rate from attempted fusion of an os acromiale is so high that we never attempt to fuse an os acromiale.

Os Acromiale Excision

The subacromial space is cleared through a lateral portal while viewing with a 30° arthroscope from a posterior portal. Electrocautery is used to skeletonize the undersurface of the acromion and expose the synchrondosis of the os acromiale segment (Fig. 18.10). The mesoacromion is then excised with a burr beginning laterally and working medially (Fig. 18.11). Care is taken to preserve the periosteal layer between the superior acromion and the deltoid muscle (Fig. 18.12). The excision is continued until all

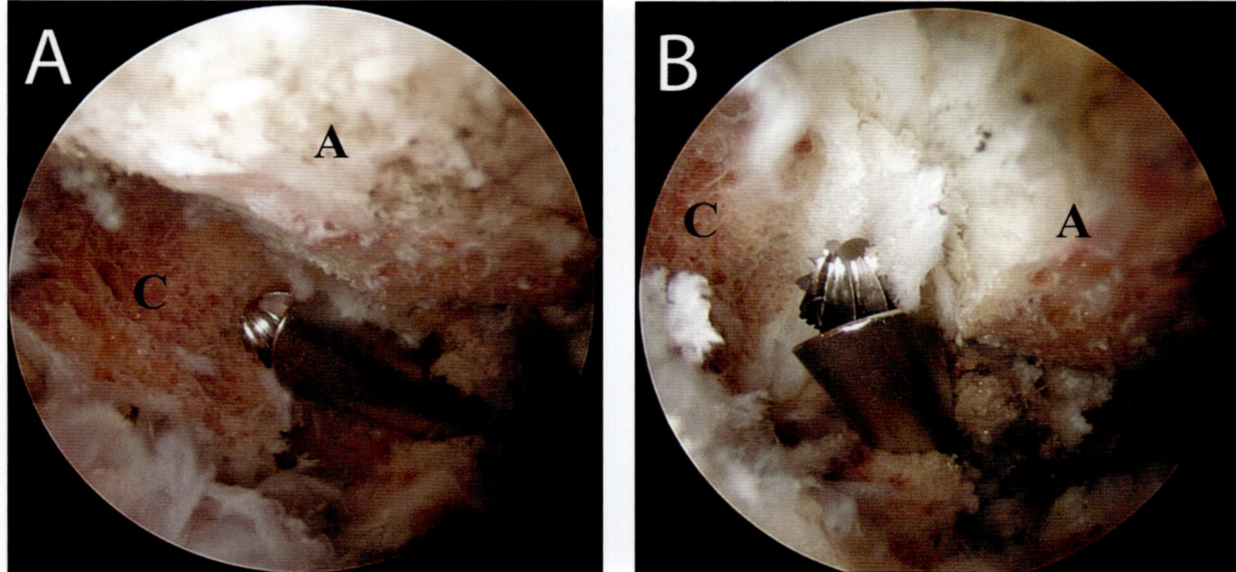

Figure 18.4 Right shoulder, posterior subacromial viewing portal, demonstrates comparative field of view of the AC joint obtained with **(A)** a 30° arthroscope and **(B)** a 70° arthroscope. A, acromion; C, distal clavicle.

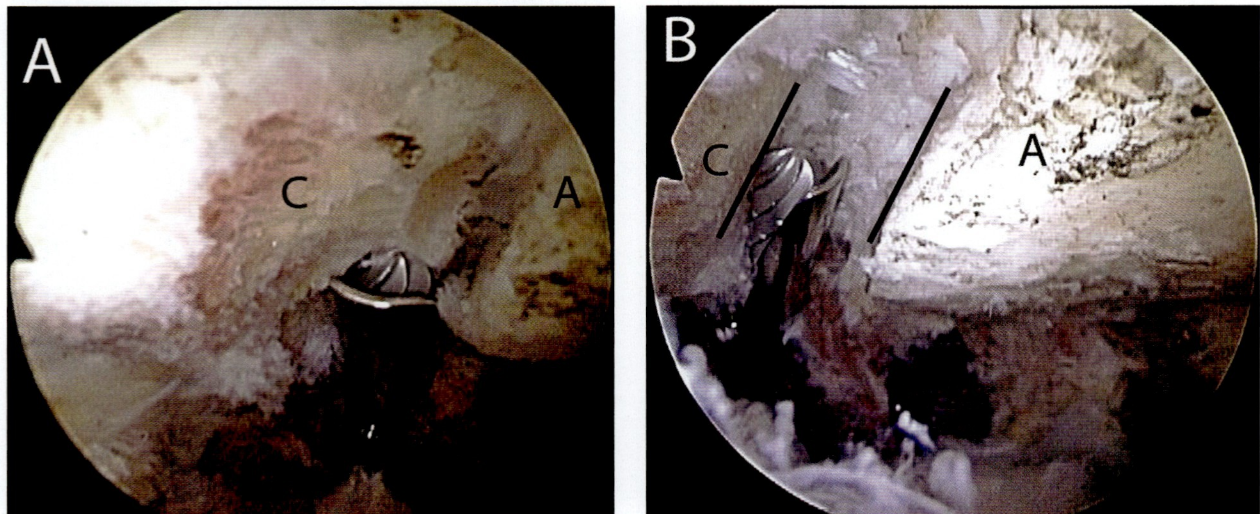

Figure 18.5 **A:** Right shoulder, posterior subacromial viewing portal with a 30° arthroscope. In this case, there is a reverse obliquity to the AC joint that prevents visualization of the superior aspect of the joint with a 30° arthroscope from a posterior subacromial portal. A 70° arthroscope is required to perform the resection from this portal. **B:** View with a 70° arthroscope postresection of the distal clavicle. Note: The obliquity of the AC joint (*black lines*) and that the superior aspect of the joint is clearly visualized. A, acromion; C, distal clavicle.

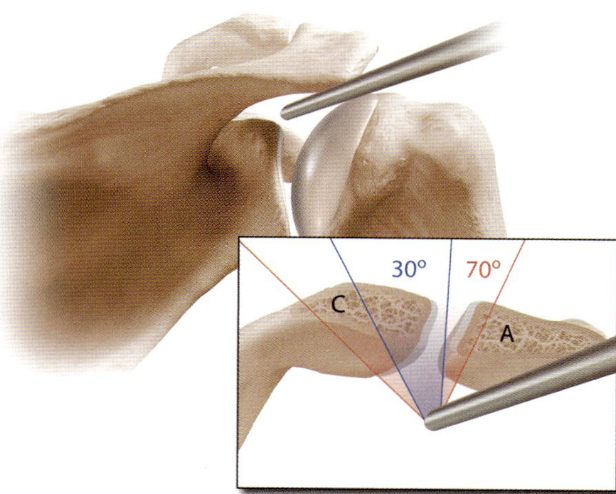

Figure 18.6 Schematic illustration of the view of the AC joint from a posterior portal. A 30° arthroscope provides a limited field of view (*shaded in blue*). The field of view with this arthroscope may not be sufficient to visualize the superior aspect of the joint, particularly when there is an oblique orientation of the joint. The 70° arthroscope provides a larger field of view (*shaded in red*) and with this arthroscope the superior aspect of the joint can always be visualized. A, acromion; C, distal clavicle.

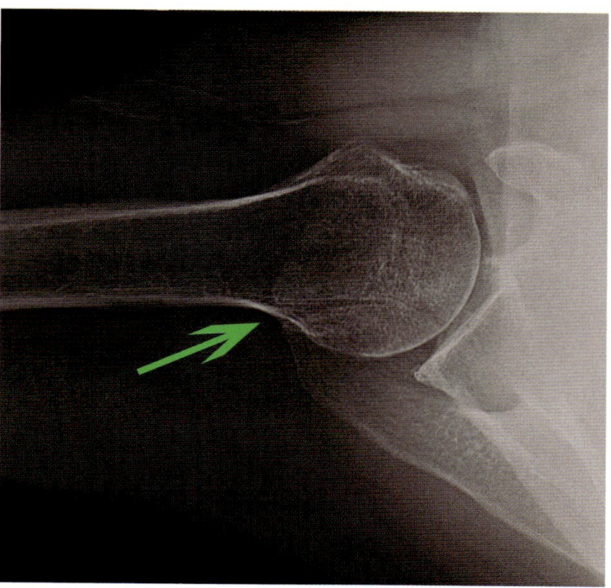

Figure 18.8 Axillary radiograph of a right shoulder demonstrates a mesoacromion (*green arrow*).

visible os acromiale bone is removed. The arthroscope is moved to the lateral portal to confirm a complete excision (Fig. 18.13). Any residual os acromiale can be excised using a burr introduced from an anterior portal (Fig. 18.14). Video

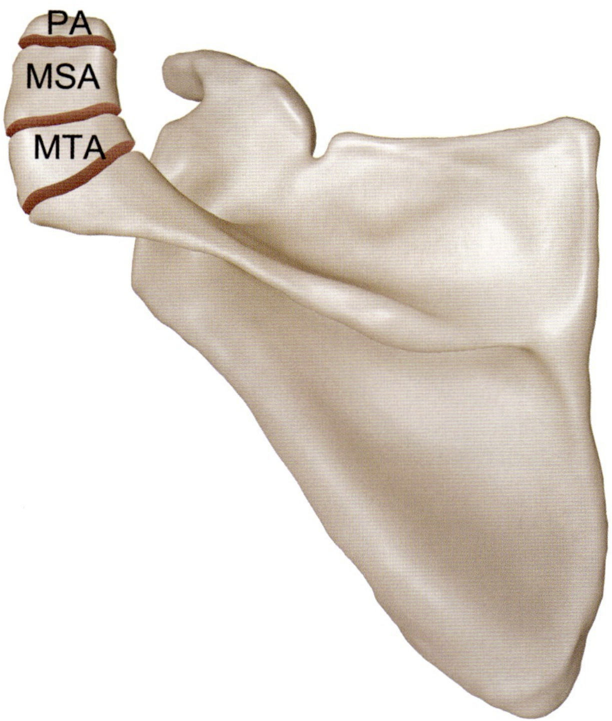

Figure 18.7 Schematic of the different types of os acromiale. MSA, mesoacromion; MTA, metaacromion; PA, preacromion.

ACUTE AC JOINT INJURIES

AC joint separations are common injuries and have been divided into six subtypes (Fig. 18.15). Conservative treatment is appropriate for grade I and II separations as these injuries typically improve with time and modification of activities. Conversely, grade IV through VI separations respond poorly to conservative care and are thus usually managed operatively. The major area of controversy surrounding AC separations is the management of grade III injuries. Historically, several studies suggested that nonoperative management of grade III injuries is equivalent or

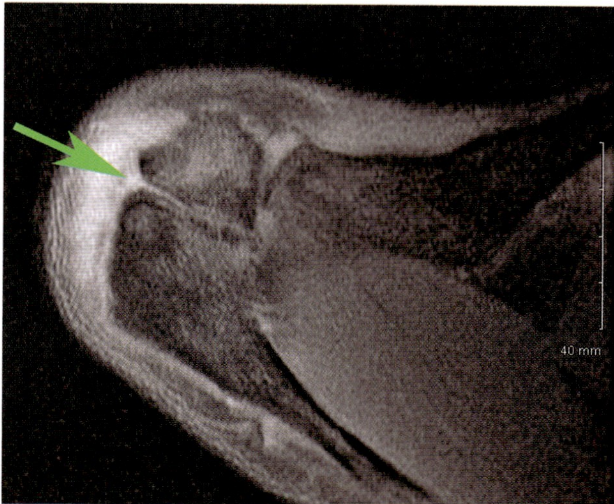

Figure 18.9 Axial MRI of a right shoulder demonstrates a mesoacromion (*green arrow*).

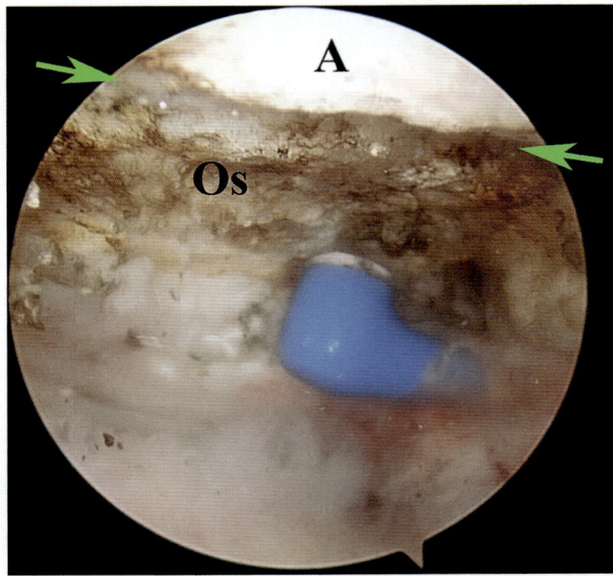

Figure 18.10 Right shoulder, posterior subacromial viewing portal demonstrates use of an electrocautery to skeletonize an os acromiale (borders marked by *green arrows*). A, acromion; Os, os acromiale.

superior to operative management (1,2). However, there are several limitations to these studies. In these older studies, the patient population was likely less active with lower athletic demands compared to current patients. Additionally, several of these studies were published prior to the creation or routine use of validated patient-directed outcome measures. Third, the fixation methods employed during these older operative repairs have been shown to be woefully inadequate from a biomechanical standpoint. Finally, the technique for repair of an AC joint separation has evolved from historical open methods to the current age where a less invasive arthroscopic technique is reproducible.

Due to the above factors, we now commonly offer operative management to many active patients with grade III AC separations. While operative management is not indicated for every patient, we believe that a significant proportion of patients will benefit from reconstruction. Specifically, patients with physically demanding occupation or athletes who participate in overhead sports, or patients with hobbies that require significant use of the shoulder, may benefit appreciably from AC joint reconstruction after a grade III separation.

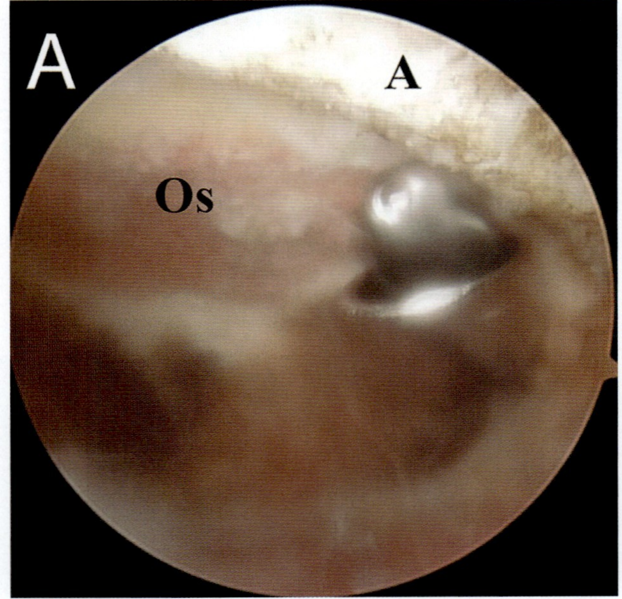

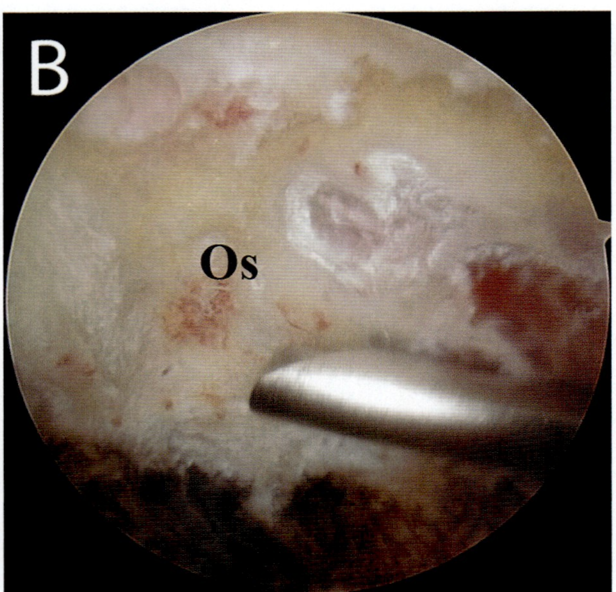

Figure 18.11 **A,B:** Right shoulder, posterior subacromial viewing portal, demonstrates resection of an os acromiale with a burr working from lateral to medial and posterior to anterior. A, acromion; Os, os acromiale.

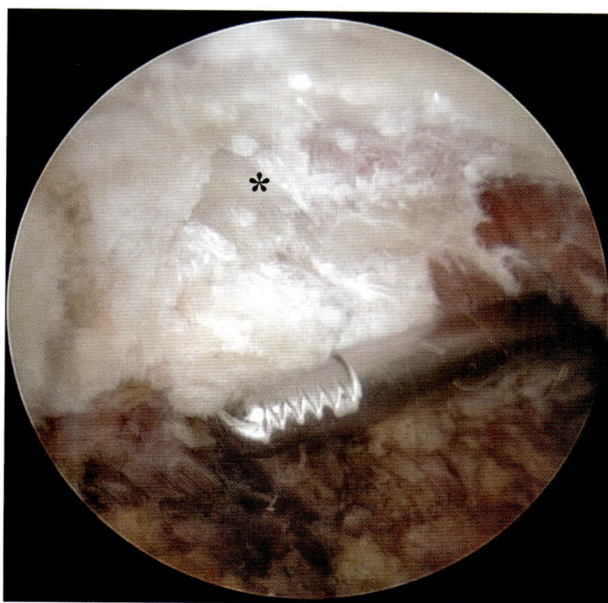

Figure 18.12 Right shoulder, posterior subacromial viewing portal. During resection of an os acromiale, care is taken to preserve the origin of the deltoid on the acromion (*asterisk*).

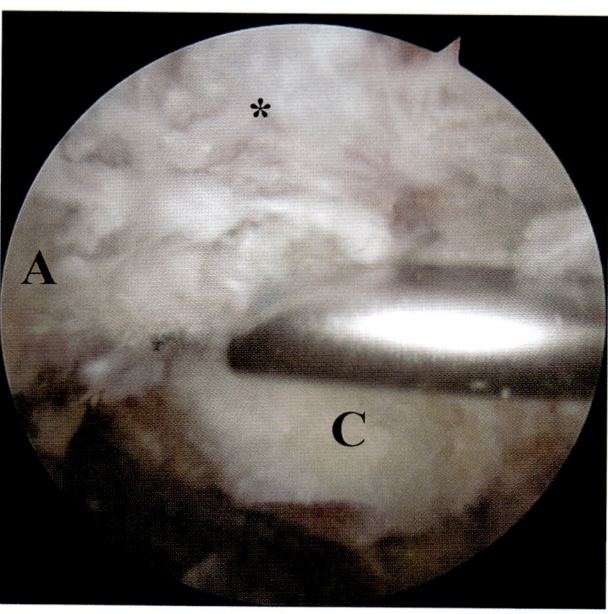

Figure 18.14 Right shoulder, lateral subacromial viewing portal, demonstrates fine-tuning of an os acromiale excision with a burr introduced from an anterior portal. A, acromion; C, distal clavicle; *asterisk*, deltoid origin.

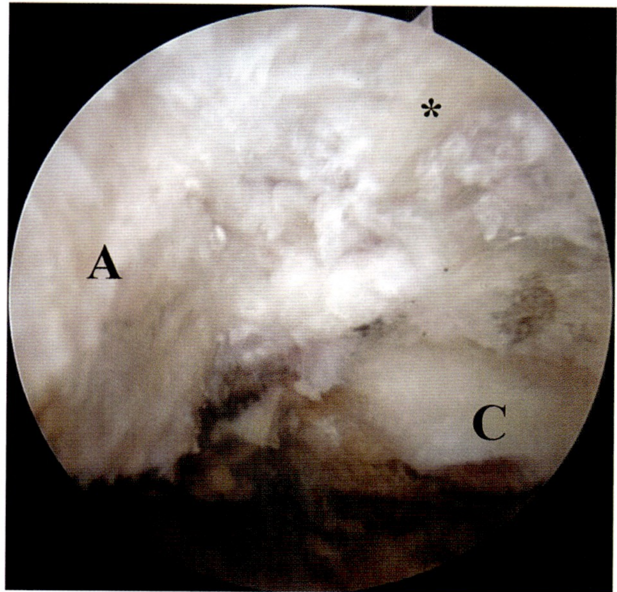

Figure 18.13 Right shoulder, lateral subacromial viewing portal. After preliminary resection of an os acromiale from a posterior portal, the arthroscope is moved to a lateral portal to confirm of a complete os acromiale excision. Note: The deltoid origin on the acromion (*asterisk*) has been preserved. A, acromion; C, distal clavicle.

There are several consequences to a misaligned AC joint. Cosmesis is often a concern to patients but should not be a strong indication for surgical intervention except in the most unusual of circumstances. We remind each patient that surgery for cosmesis alone just trades a lump for a scar. More important to consider is the potential functional compromise. Overhead athletes may have chronic issues of pain to varying degrees. Similar to a shortened midshaft clavicle fracture, an AC joint separation can lead to scapular protraction that has biomechanical ramifications on the shoulder. Commonly, this will manifest as posterior trapezial and scapular pain as a result of this muscle being under constant tension in an abnormal anatomical position. High-demand patients also often report fatigue with repeated activities as well as shoulder impingement. Common physical examination findings include impingement signs, coracoid tenderness, and scapular dyskinesis as a result of scapular protraction (Fig. 18.16).

Another consideration in patients with acute AC joint separations is the degree of associated pathology in the shoulder. In two recent studies of patients with grade III separation and an average patient age of 38 and 35 years, the incidence of additional associated shoulder pathology was 14% to 18% (3,4). Also for patients in an older age group, the actual incidence may be even greater. In a review of pooled data from the BRASS group (Burkhart's Research Association of Shoulder Specialists), over 100 patients undergoing AC joint reconstructions were reviewed and we noted approximately a 35% risk of associated pathology. In light of this information, patients with a grade III AC joint separation should receive a thorough exam and MRI should be considered early in their workup to rule out any associated pathology, particularly if a nonoperative treatment course is not proceeding as expected.

While multiple techniques for AC joint reconstruction have been described in the literature, the most widely utilized historically has been the Weaver-Dunn reconstruction. This procedure, however, is a nonanatomic reconstruction

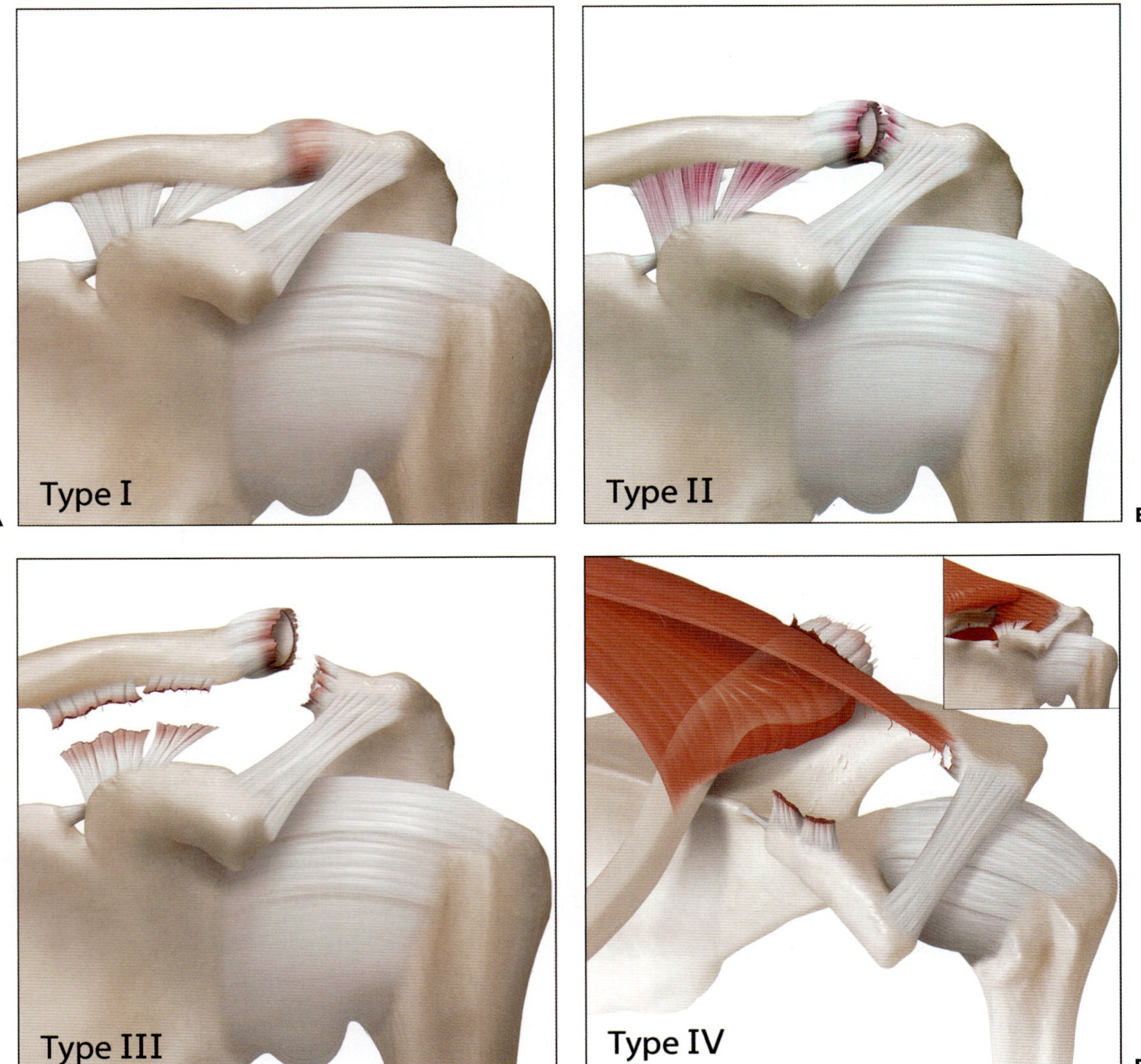

Figure 18.15 Schematic of the six types of AC joint separations. **A:** A grade I injury involves a strain of the AC ligaments only. **B:** A grade II injury includes disruption of the AC ligaments, but the CC ligaments are intact. **C:** In a grade III injury, the AC and CC ligaments are disrupted, but the deltoid fascia remains intact and displacement of the coracoid relative to the clavicle is <100%. **D:** In a grade IV injury, the AC and CC ligaments are disrupted and the clavicle is displaced posteriorly into or through (**inset**) the trapezius muscle.

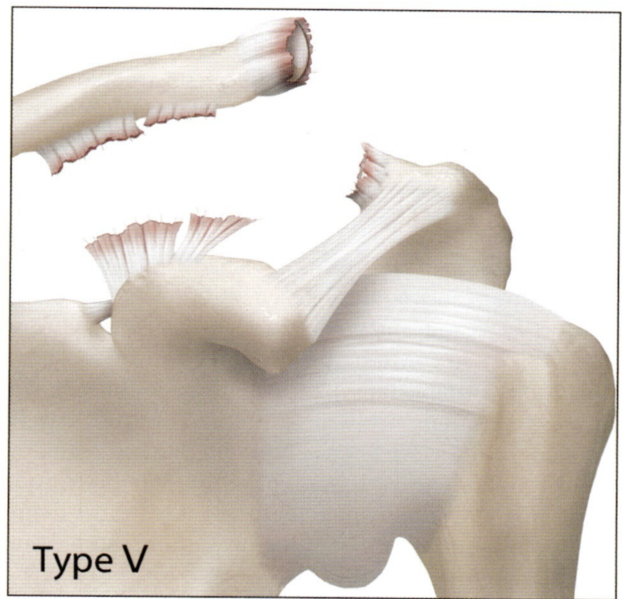

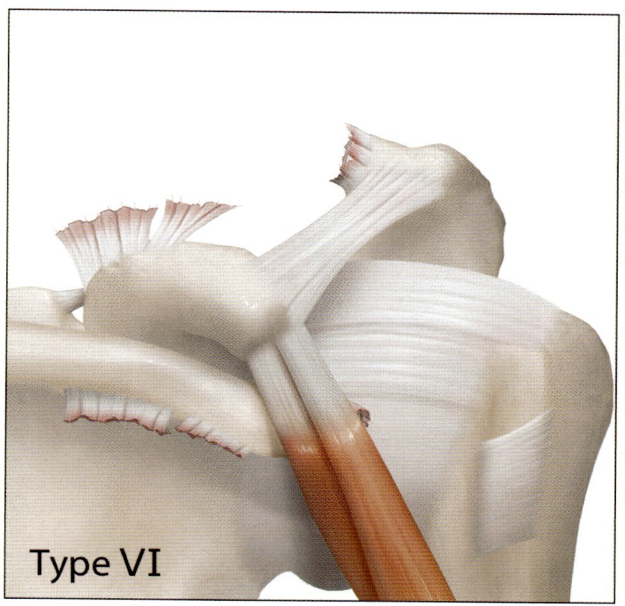

Figure 18.15 (*Continued*) **E:** In a grade V injury, the AC and CC ligaments are disrupted and the CC displacement is >100% relative to the contralateral distance. **F:** In a grade VI injury, the clavicle is displaced inferior to the coracoid.

and also has significant biomechanical limitations. Cadaveric studies have shown that while intact coracoclavicular (CC) ligaments fail at 725 N of load, the transferred CA ligament (i.e., the Weaver-Dunn procedure) offers only 145 N until failure (5). Having performed many Weaver-Dunn procedures in the past, we can also clinically attest that there is a high variability in the quality of the coracoacromial ligament. Sometimes, it is stout and offers excellent tissue to repair, while at other times it is thin and inadequate for AC joint reconstruction. This inconsistency likely contributes to the poor outcomes with the Weaver-Dunn reconstruction (6).

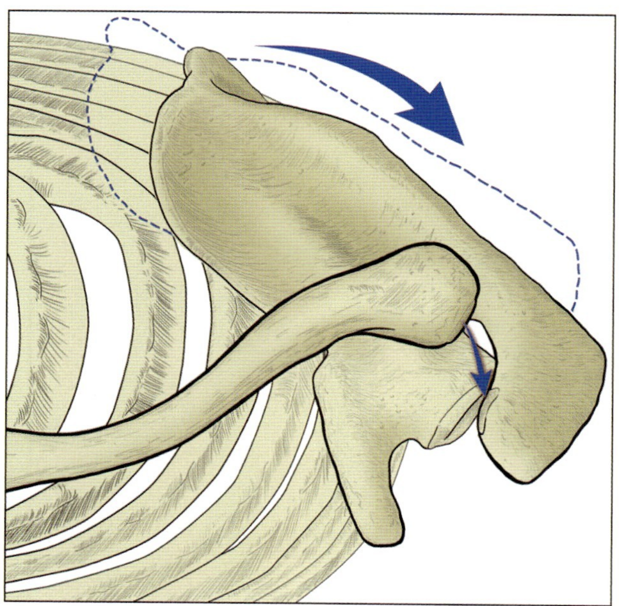

Figure 18.16 Following disruption of the Acromioclavicular joint, the scapula protracts (*blue arrows*). This can result in impingement and scapular dyskinesis, as well as coracoid tenderness as a result of pectoralis minor contracture.

Recently, reconstructive procedures have been described that not only are biomechanically superior to the Weaver-Dunn procedure but also more closely restore the normal anatomy and biomechanics of the AC joint. Most of these procedures however still require an open incision and a complex open dissection. As the entirety of this book will attest—this is just not the cowboy way!

With recent instrumentation and implant advancements, an all-arthroscopic AC joint reconstruction method for both acute and chronic AC joint separations is now possible. There are several advantages to an arthroscopic approach. As noted above, when an AC joint separation occurs, there is a substantial risk of associated intra-articular pathology that cannot be evaluated or easily addressed with an open approach to the AC joint separation. Though unproven at this point in time, we believe that performance of a shoulder arthroscopy to identify associated pathology prior to AC joint reconstruction may prove to be an essential component for obtaining satisfactory outcomes. Furthermore, while a preoperative MRI can identify intra-articular pathology, the gold standard for diagnosis remains the arthroscope. With an arthroscopic approach, soft tissue damage is decreased compared to an open approach, and

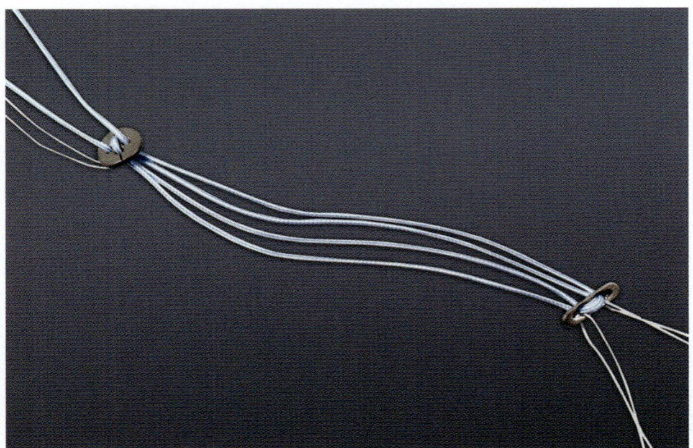

Figure 18.17 The TightRope (Arthrex, Inc., Naples, FL) is indicated for reconstruction of an acute acromioclavicular separation. The oblong button (**right**) is seated beneath the coracoid and the round button (**left**) is placed on the clavicle. The buttons are connected by a #5 FiberWire suture.

this may decrease postoperative stiffness. And, of course, the incidence of wound infection is dramatically decreased with an arthroscopic approach.

Selection of Procedure

In those patients in which an AC joint reconstruction is chosen, we utilize a TightRope (Arthrex, Inc., Naples, FL) or GraftRope device (Arthrex, Inc., Naples, FL). The newest advance is a device called the "Dog Bone" (Arthrex, Inc., Naples, FL). This device allows for reconstruction of acute AC joint injuries utilizing much smaller bone tunnels, thus decreasing the risk of clavicle or coracoid fractures.

The Dog Bone and the TightRope are indicated in acute injuries (<6 weeks), in which the CC ligaments have the potential to heal. The TightRope includes a continuous loop of #5 FiberWire suture attached to an oblong coracoid button and a round clavicle button. The coracoid button is passed antegrade through 4-mm bone tunnels (Fig. 18.17). In contrast, the Dog Bone construct comprises two loops of FiberTape passed retrograde through 3-mm tunnels and then attached to both a coracoid Dog Bone implant and a clavicle Dog Bone implant. Thus, the Dog Bone implant never has to pass through bone tunnels (Fig. 18.18). We anticipate that the bone tunnel diameter will decrease even further in the near future as smaller cannulated drills are developed.

For chronic injuries that are older than 6 weeks, we prefer the GraftRope. This device is similar to the TightRope but is larger and allows a tissue graft (allograft or autograft) to be secured in the center of the implant. This is necessary in chronic cases when healing of the native CC ligaments cannot be relied upon (Fig. 18.19). Because placement of the graft requires a larger hole, the clavicle and coracoid tunnels must be drilled to 6 mm rather than the 4-mm

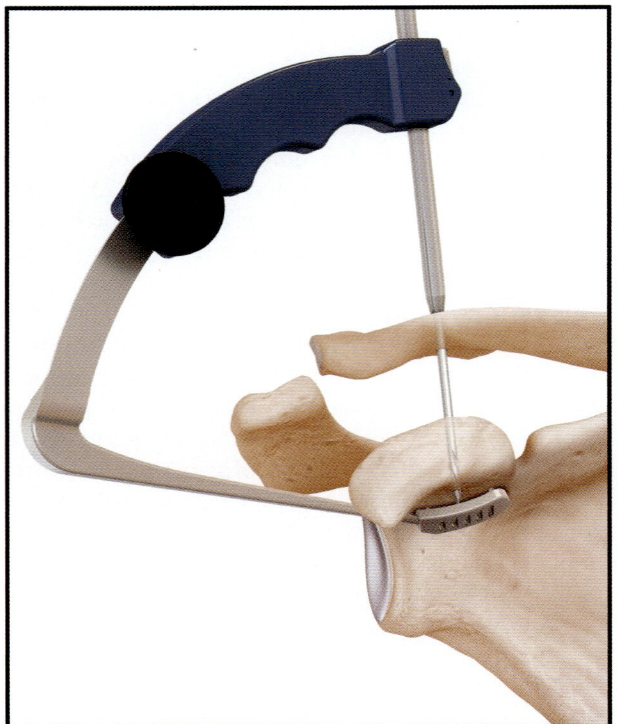

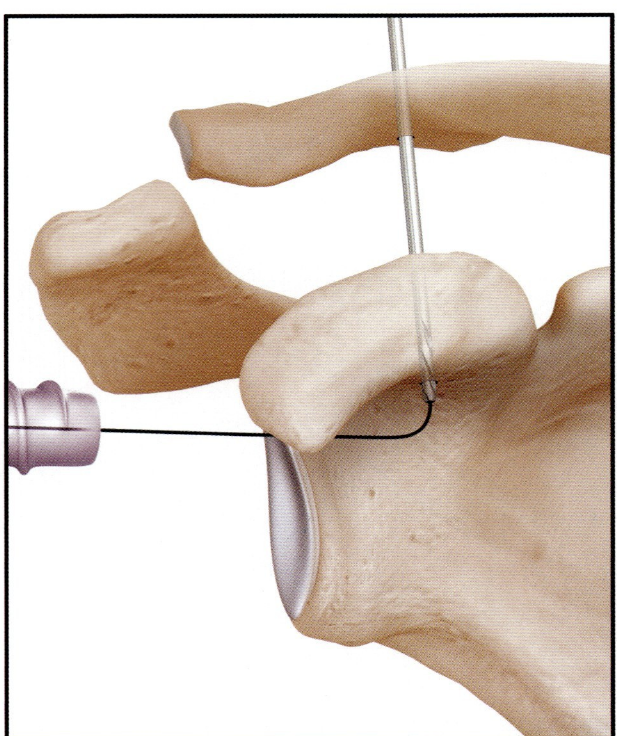

Figure 18.18 Schematic of Dog Bone (Arthrex, Inc., Naples, FL) CC reconstruction. **A:** A Constant Guide is used for placement of a cannulated drill through the clavicle and coracoid. **B:** A Nitinol shuttling wire is passed from superior to inferior through the cannulated guide drill and retrieved out an anterior working portal.

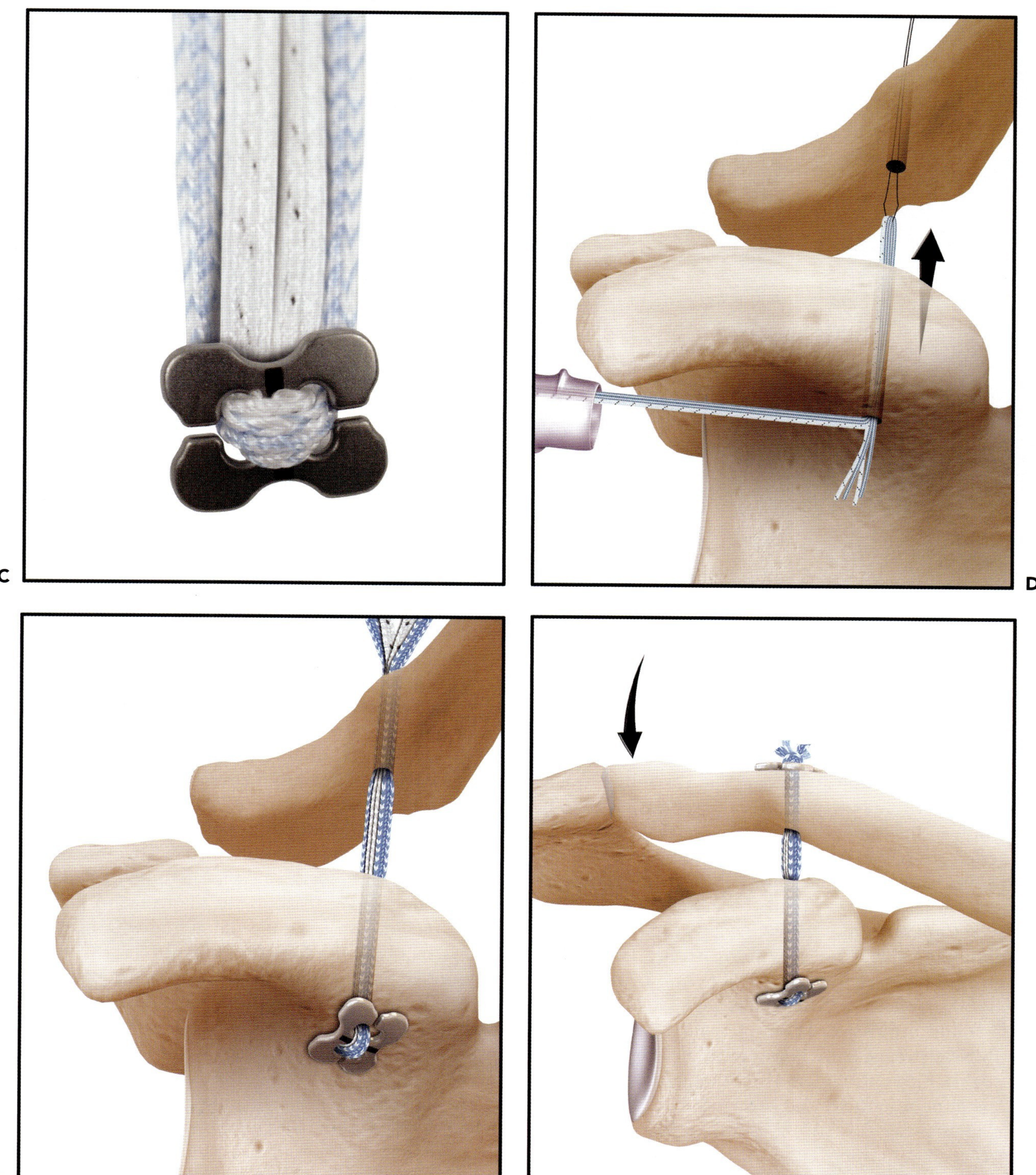

Figure 18.18 (*Continued*) **C:** Two FiberTape sutures are loaded on the Dog Bone device. **D:** The suture limbs are threaded through the Nitinol shuttling wire and the wire is pulled superiorly (*arrow*) to shuttle the sutures through the bone tunnels. **E:** The Dog Bone is positioned under the base of the coracoid with the *black line* aligned perpendicular to the base. **F:** A second Dog Bone is loaded onto the FiberTape sutures that exit the clavicle bone tunnel. The acromioclavicular joint is then reduced (*arrow*) and the sutures are tied to complete the reconstruction.

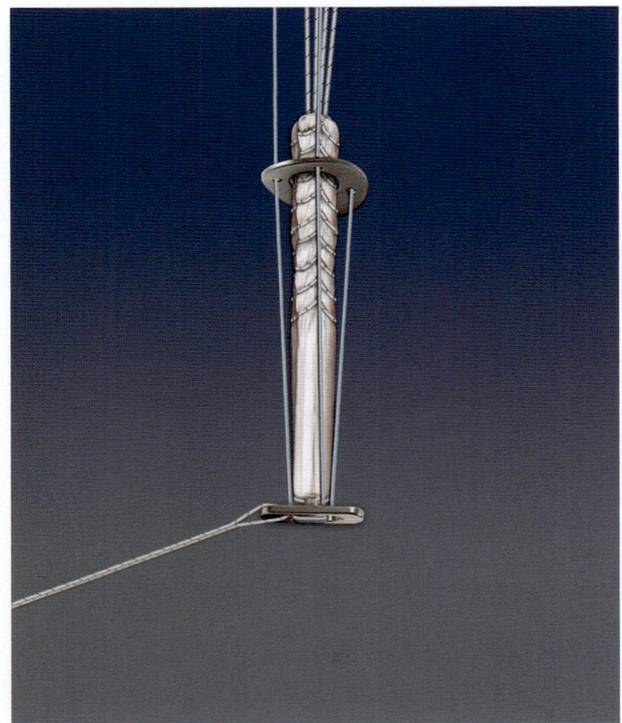

Figure 18.19 The GraftRope (Arthrex, Inc., Naples, FL) is conceptually similar to the TightRope (Arthrex, Inc., Naples, FL) but accommodates a graft and is indicated for reconstruction of a chronic acromioclavicular separation. An allograft or autograft is doubled over and secured to a coracoid button. The round clavicle button (**top**) has a hole in the middle to accommodate the tails of the graft.

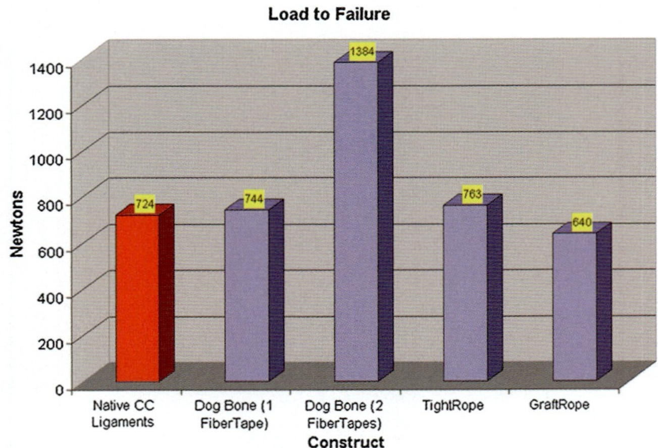

Figure 18.20 Graphical representation of the load to failure of CC reconstruction with various constructs.

tunnels required for the TightRope. The remaining modification of the GraftRope systems is a larger clavicle button with a hole in the center that accommodates the graft and an interference screw. To minimize the morbidity of graft harvest, we typically use an allograft for reconstruction. However, for patients who prefer an autograft, an ipsilateral flexor carpi radialis or hamstring graft can be used.

Biomechanically, these new arthroscopic techniques have greatly enhanced the strength of AC joint reconstructions. While the native CC ligaments have a load to failure of 725 N and the Weaver-Dunn procedure offers a meager 145 N of strength, the newer constructs are dramatically superior. Specifically, the TightRope fails at 763 N, the GraftRope at 640 N, and the Dog Bone reconstruction is almost twice as strong as any other construct at 1,384 N load to failure (Fig. 18.20). Also of interest in this testing is that while the failure mechanism for the TightRope and GraftRope procedures was bone fracture (coracoid), the failure mechanism for the Dog Bone construct was suture breakage. This is a result of the much smaller bone tunnels that are created during the Dog Bone reconstruction procedure. Because of these compelling strength data and the minimal invasiveness of these procedures, we now perform AC joint reconstructions with these devices.

Arthroscopic Acute AC Joint Reconstruction Technique: Dog Bone Construct

We perform the entire procedure in the lateral decubitus position and have not found the beach chair position necessary. The limb is prepped and draped in the standard fashion with care to be sure that the majority of the clavicle is accessible. A standard diagnostic arthroscopy is performed and any associated labral or rotator cuff pathology is identified and addressed, paying special attention to keeping the soft tissue swelling to a minimum. This requires both speed and a reasonably low pump pressure. If associated pathology cannot be addressed quickly, we suggest performing the AC joint reconstruction first and fixing the associated problem(s) afterward. Correct portal placement is critical to the procedure. Specifically, anterosuperolateral (ASL) and anterior portals are utilized and should be far enough apart to allow for triangulation during the reconstruction. We place the ASL portal with an angle of approach in line with the subscapularis (Fig. 18.21). Working through the ASL portal while viewing through the posterior portal, the superior border of the subscapularis is identified and a generous window is created in the rotator interval with electrocautery. Usually, the tip of the coracoid can be easily palpated in this area (Figs. 18.22 and 18.23).

The dissection begins while using a 30° arthroscope to maintain orientation. Once the coracoid is identified, a 70° arthroscope is used for enhanced medial visualization. The coracoid is skeletonized along its entire posterolateral surface, from coracoid tip to coracoid base (Fig. 18.24). Sometimes, the base of the coracoid can be well visualized with a 70° arthroscope from the posterior portal. However, it is critical to have a panoramic view of the coracoid arch and base, and a 30° arthroscope from the ASL portal may provide better visualization (Fig. 18.25). The best viewing portal may vary from case to case or from step to step and the surgeon should not hesitate to switch portals if visualization is inadequate.

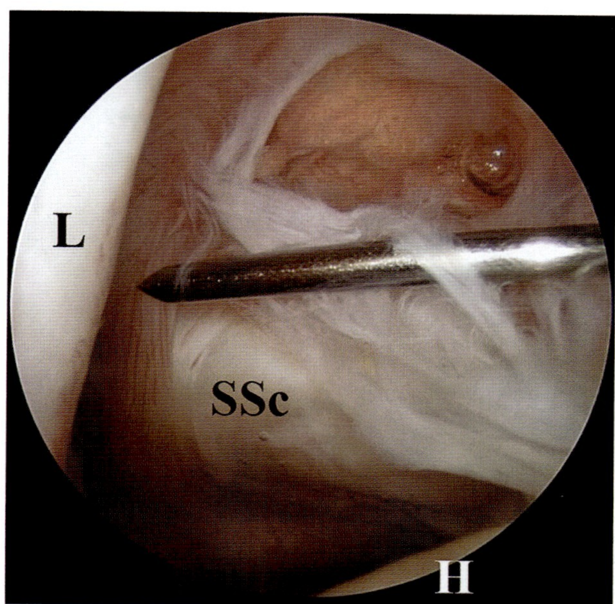

Figure 18.21 Right shoulder, posterior viewing portal, demonstrates use of a spinal needle to determine an adequate angle of approach for an ASL portal that is in line with the trajectory of the subscapularis tendon. H, humerus; L, labrum; SSc, subscapularis tendon.

The coracoid anatomy can be separated into three regions—the base, the neck, and the tip (Figs. 18.26 and 18.27). Once excellent visualization is achieved, a probe is used to palpate the medial, lateral, anterior, and posterior coracoid margins. This step provides a good sense of the undersurface dimensions of the coracoid (notice how much larger the base dimensions are compared to the neck) and will facilitate placement of the implant (Fig. 18.28). Optimal placement of the coracoid tunnel is in the middle of the base of the coracoid, and this spot is marked with electrocautery. Appropriate tunnel placement is the most critical step in the case and cannot be overemphasized. A helpful tip is to view the undersurface of the coracoid from the ASL portal and follow the plane of the subscapularis straight to the coracoid. Tunnel placement in the coracoid base should be posterior to the midsubscapularis plane. Avoiding a coracoid fracture is critical with this procedure and making the tunnel at the base will diminish the risk of fracture as there is much more bone in this area and thus the margin for error is greater. Also, if the tunnel is placed more anteriorly, not only is the bone more narrow, but the force per unit area on the coracoid also becomes greater, thus increasing fracture risk. Since the Dog Bone construct utilizes small 3-mm bone holes, the risk of fracture is significantly decreased but nonetheless, optimal tunnel placement is still a critical step.

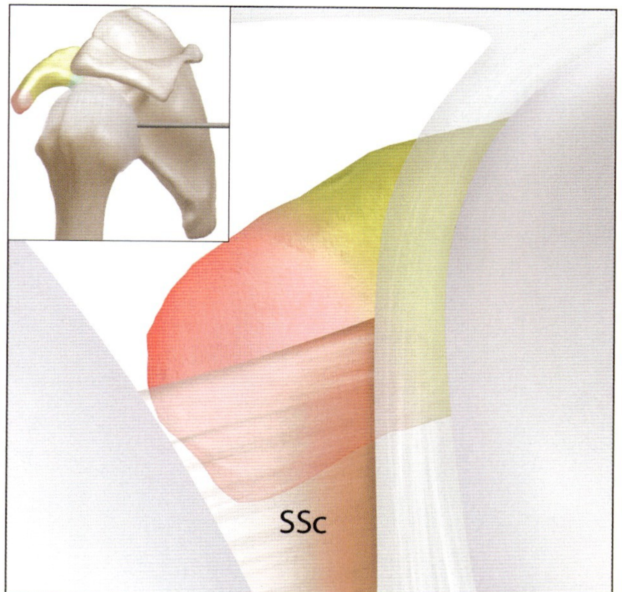

Figure 18.22 When viewing from a posterior glenohumeral portal, the coracoid tip (colored in *red*) can be identified anterior to the upper subscapularis tendon. A 30° arthroscope allows visualization of the coracoid tip primarily. A 70° arthroscope is required to visualize the coracoid base. The **inset** demonstrates the posterior glenohumeral viewing portal. SSc, subscapularis tendon.

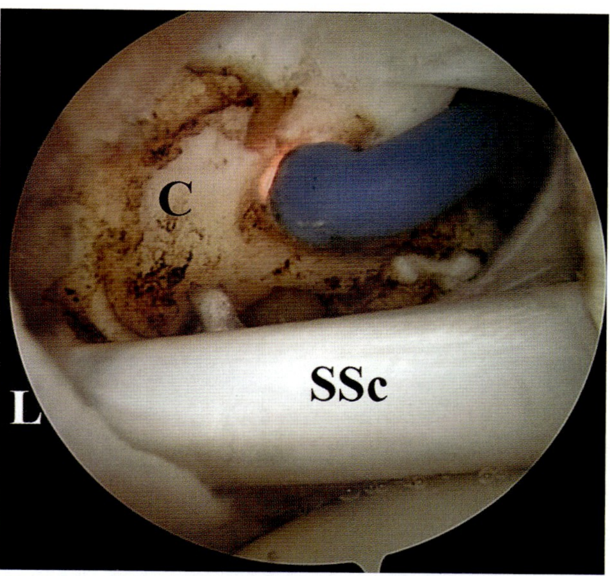

Figure 18.23 Right shoulder, posterior viewing portal, demonstrates use of an electrocautery to skeletonize the tip of the coracoid after a window has been created in the rotator interval. C, coracoid; L, labrum; SSc, subscapularis tendon.

Once adequate coracoid exposure is attained, the coracoid aiming guide is inserted through the anterior portal and placed underneath the base of the coracoid. The left or right (as appropriate) coracoid aiming guide (Constant Guide) is inserted through the anterior portal. Usually, the anterior portal offers a good angle of approach. However, if the tip of the coracoid inhibits proper placement, then the ASL portal may be better for guide insertion. The downside of placement of the guide through the ASL portal is that it limits viewing to the posterior portal only. The center of the aiming guide is positioned underneath the base of the

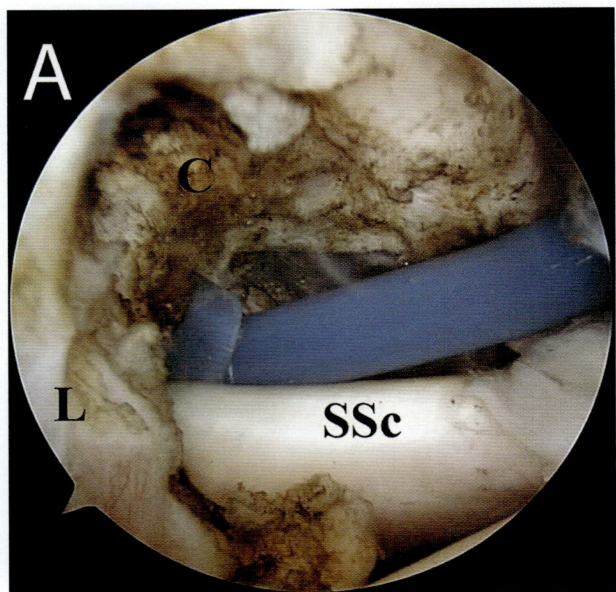

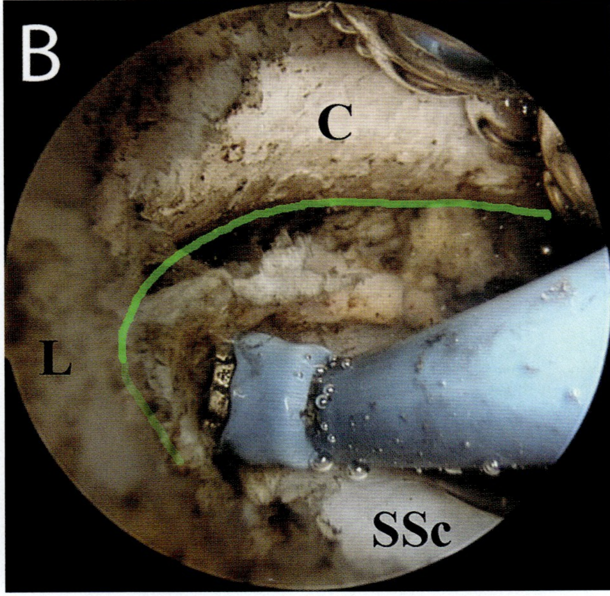

Figure 18.24 **A:** Right shoulder, posterior viewing portal with a 70° arthroscope. After identifying the coracoid tip, dissection is carried medially, staying on bone, until **(B)** the base of the coracoid is identified. The *green line* outlines the inferolateral undersurface arc of the coracoid, with the subscapularis passing underneath this arc. C, coracoid; L, labrum; SSc, subscapularis tendon.

coracoid at the predetermined location (Fig. 18.29). Use the post on the tip of the aiming guide to get a feel for the coracoid anatomy and place the guide under the center of the coracoid base.

A small incision is then made over the clavicle, centered approximately 3.5 cm lateral to the AC joint. We usually make a horizontal incision, but a vertical incision can be made toward the coracoid if one suspects a possible need for conversion to an open procedure. Sharp dissection is carried down to the clavicle, the periosteum is elevated, and small Hohmann retractors are placed on the anterior and posterior borders of the clavicle. The Guide Pin Sleeve of the aiming guide is placed on the surface of the middle of the clavicle between these retractors (Fig. 18.30). An assistant holds this position while the position of the aiming guide under the coracoid is rechecked and

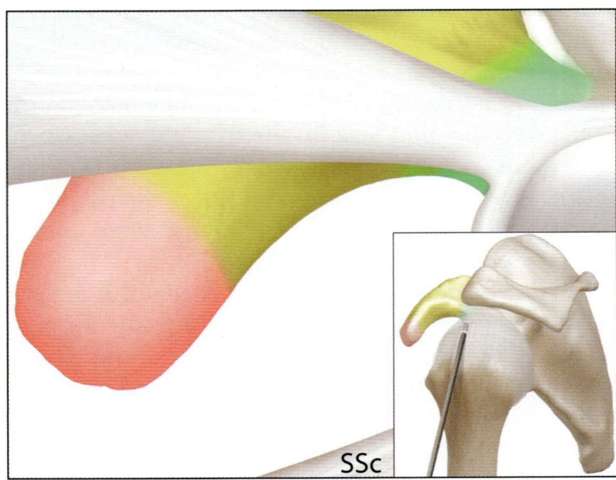

Figure 18.25 Schematic of the view of the coracoid from an ASL portal with a 30° arthroscope. With a 30° arthroscope in this portal, the base of the coracoid (*shaded in green*) can be visualized. The inset demonstrates the position of the arthroscope. SSc, subscapularis tendon.

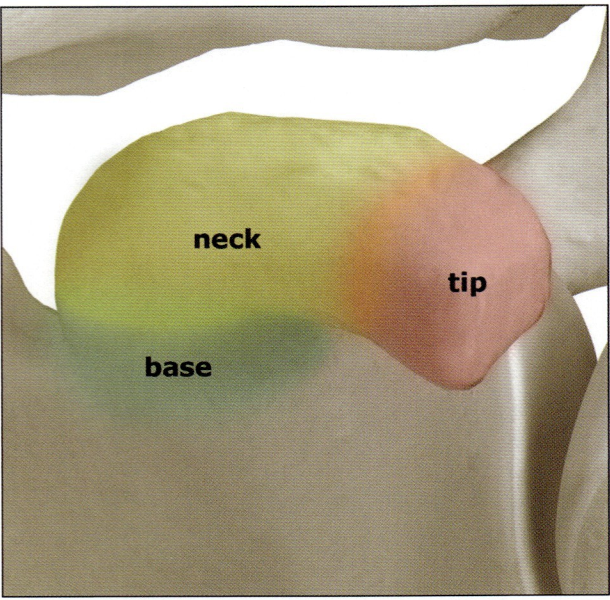

Figure 18.26 The coracoid can be divided into tip, neck, and base segments.

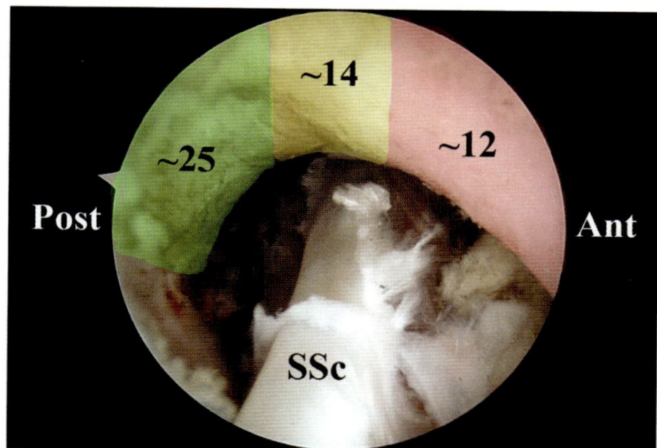

Figure 18.27 Right shoulder, ASL viewing portal, demonstrates the regions of the coracoid, which can be separated into the base (*green*), neck (*yellow*), and tip (*pink*). The coracoid is thickest at the base (~25 mm wide) and narrows anteriorly to a width of 12 mm. Thus, the most robust fixation will be achieved in the coracoid base. SSc, subscapularis tendon; Post, posterior; Ant, anterior.

adjustments are made if needed. The assistant then holds the arthroscope, while the surgeon holds the aiming guide and drills a 3-mm cannulated drill to penetrate through four cortices (two for the clavicle and two for the coracoid) (Fig. 18.31). If four distinct cortices are not felt, the position of the guide should be checked for malposition. At times, poor bone quality makes it difficult to feel four distinct cortices, but it is important to confirm the position before proceeding. Proper drill position is confirmed from multiple portal positions. Viewing the undersurface of the coracoid from the anterior portal helps confirm that the drill has been centered in the medial-to-lateral dimension so as to avoid fracturing the coracoid. Another useful technique to assure adequate bone on both sides of the drill is to place a calibrated probe through the ASL portal and palpate the distance between the drill and the medial coracoid cortex as well as the lateral coracoid cortex (Fig. 18.32).

Next, the looped end of a Nitinol suture passing wire is advanced through the cannulation of the drill (Fig. 18.33). A toothed grasper is introduced through the anterior portal to retrieve the Nitinol wire so that the looped end exits the anterior portal and the crimped end exits the clavicle through the cannulated drill. The drill and aiming sleeve are then removed by hand. It is important to do this step by hand as use of the driver may cut the Nitinol wire. This is an excellent opportunity to visualize the entire coracoid tunnel to make sure that the medial or the lateral cortices have not been violated, and that the tunnel is entirely within the bone (Fig. 18.34).

Next, the two strands of FiberTape are passed through the bone tunnels from inferior to superior. These FiberTape

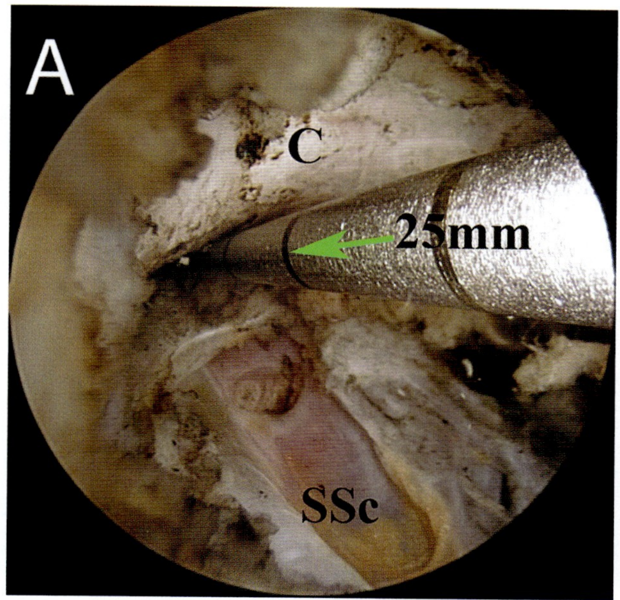

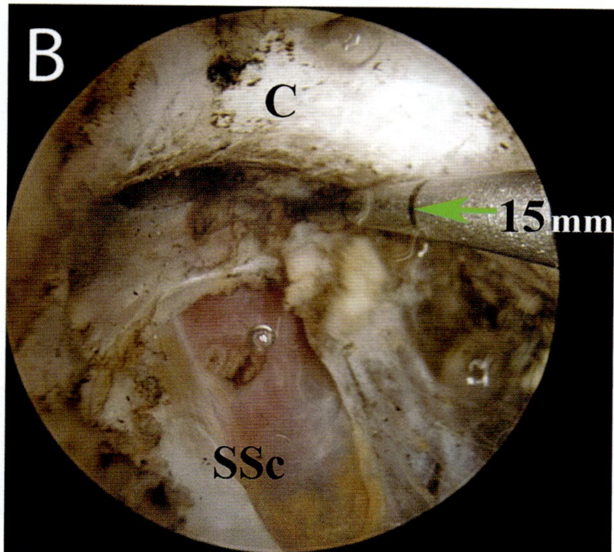

Figure 18.28 **A:** Right shoulder, posterior viewing portal with a 70° arthroscope, demonstrates use of a probe to measure the medial to lateral width of the coracoid. In this case, the base of the coracoid width is approximately 25 mm (*green arrow*). **B:** At the neck of the coracoid, the width is 15 mm. C, coracoid; SSc, subscapularis tendon.

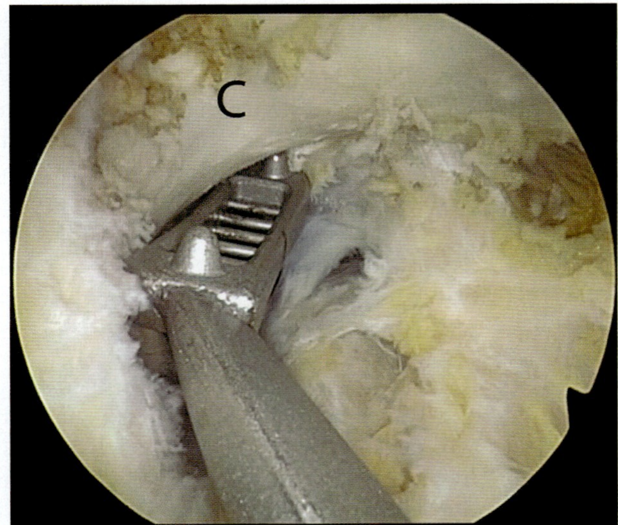

Figure 18.29 Right shoulder, posterior viewing portal with a 70° arthroscope, demonstrates placement of a Constant Guide (Arthrex, Inc., Naples, FL) at the base of the coracoid. C, coracoid.

loops are merged into two FiberWire strands to allow for easier passage into the coracoid and clavicle tunnels. The FiberWire portion of the implant is loaded into the loop of the Nitinol wire (Fig. 18.35) and end of the Nitinol wire

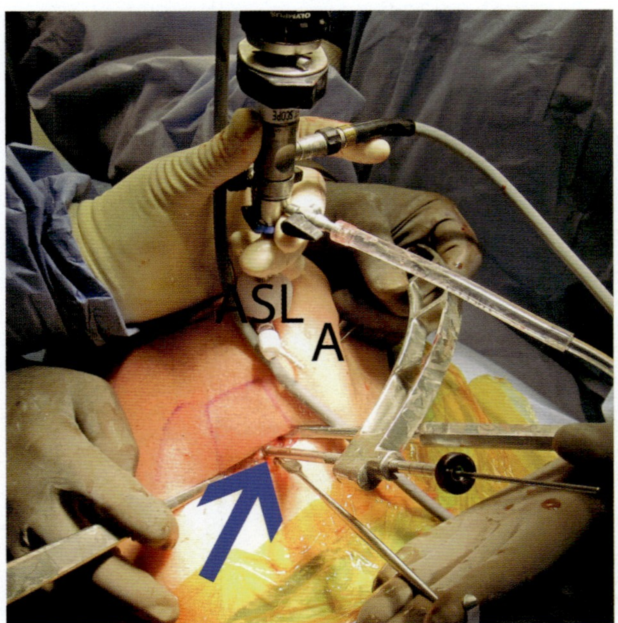

Figure 18.30 Left shoulder, lateral decubitus position, demonstrates placement of a Constant Guide (Arthrex, Inc., Naples, FL) for arthroscopic acromioclavicular joint reconstruction. The drill stop tip of the aiming guide has been inserted through an anterior portal and positioned at the base of the coracoid. The Guide Pin Sleeve (*blue arrow*) is centered on the distal clavicle. Then, a guide pin is advanced through the clavicle and coracoid while viewing from an ASL portal with a 30° arthroscope (as in this case), or from a posterior portal with a 70° arthroscope. A, anterior portal; ASL, anterosuperolateral portal.

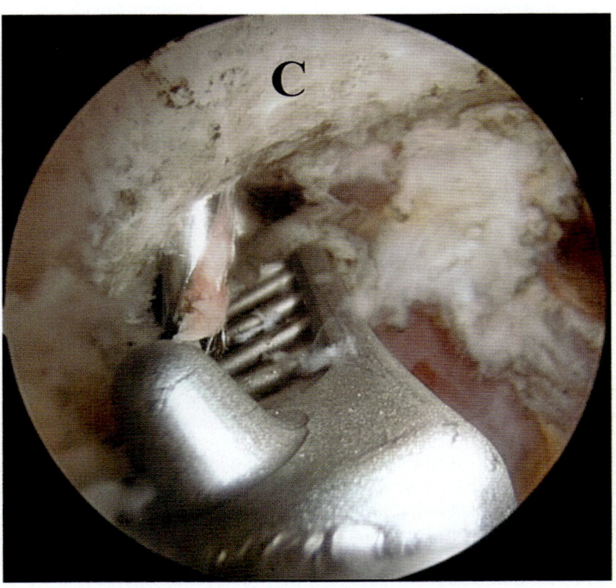

Figure 18.31 Arthroscopic view of drill placement for acromioclavicular joint reconstruction in a right shoulder viewed from a posterior portal with a 70° arthroscope. C, coracoid.

that exits the clavicle can be pulled to shuttle the FiberTape into the bone tunnels (Fig 18.36). However, before the FiberTape is pulled all the way into the anterior portal, the Dog Bone implant must be attached to the FiberTape (Fig. 18.37). The slots in the implant allow the FiberTape to be loaded onto the Dog Bone. The concave side of the Dog Bone will sit against the undersurface of the coracoid.

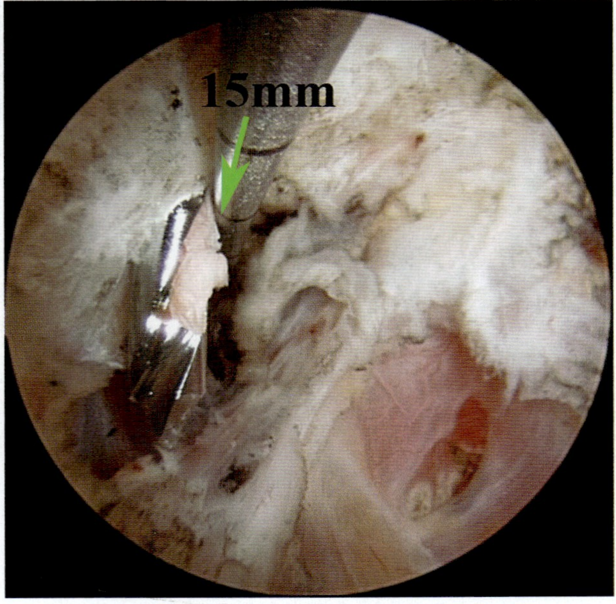

Figure 18.32 Right shoulder, posterior viewing portal with a 70° arthroscope, demonstrates use of a probe to confirm that a drill is centered on the coracoid base. In this case, the drill is 15 mm (*green arrow*) from the medial border that is approximately centered on the coracoid base.

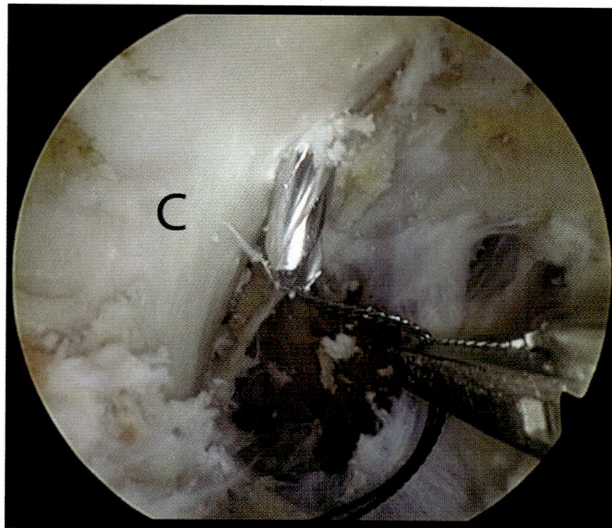

Figure 18.33 Right shoulder, posterior viewing portal with a 70° arthroscope. A Nitinol wire has been threaded through a cannulated drill that was drilled to create bone tunnels in the clavicle and coracoid. C, coracoid.

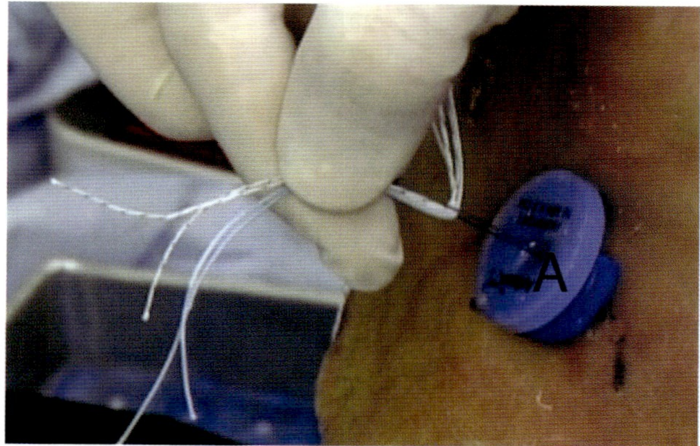

Figure 18.35 External view of a right shoulder. A Nitinol loop has been retrieved out an anterior portal. Sutures are threaded through the loop for shuttling through coracoid and clavicle bone tunnels. A, anterior portal.

Therefore, it should be loaded on the FiberTape such that the concave side faces inward and the convex side (which is marked with an etched black line) faces outward. Once the Dog Bone is loaded, the FiberTape loops are pulled the rest of the way into the shoulder to engage the Dog Bone implant underneath the base of the coracoid (Figs. 18.38 and 18.39).

A second Dog Bone is then loaded onto the FiberTape strands that exit the superior aspect of the clavicle tunnel. The clavicle is compressed distally to reduce the AC joint and the FiberTape sutures are tied over the clavicle Dog Bone. The etched black line on the implant should be aligned with the axis of the clavicle (Fig. 18.40).

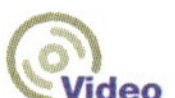

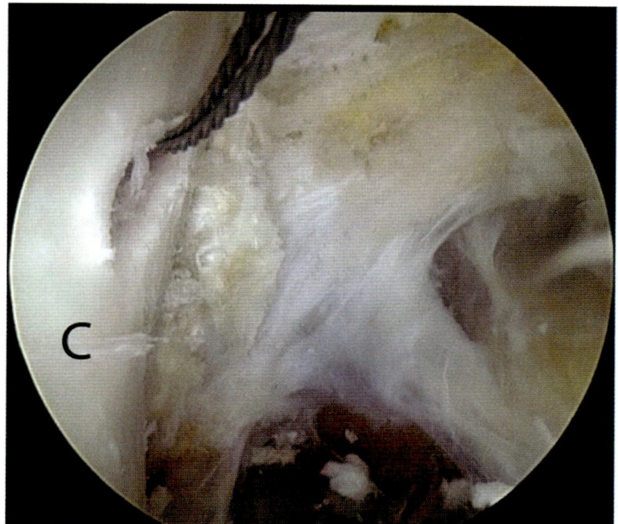

Figure 18.34 Right shoulder, posterior viewing portal with a 70° arthroscope. A Nitinol wire has been threaded through a cannulated drill and then retrieved out an anterior working portal. The drill has also been removed. C, coracoid.

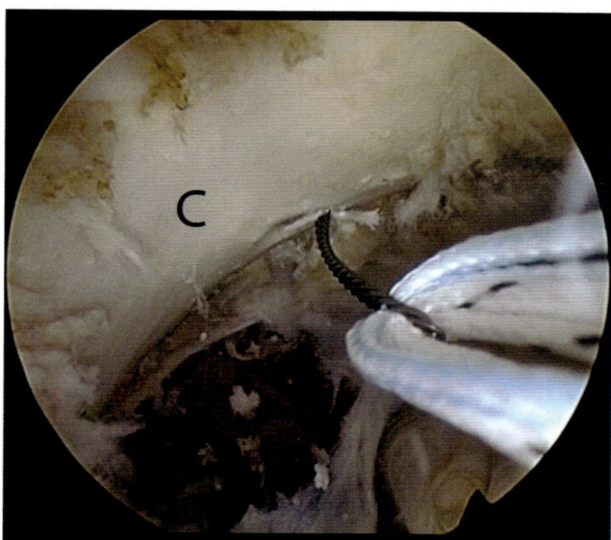

Figure 18.36 Right shoulder, posterior viewing portal with a 70° arthroscope. FiberTape sutures (Arthrex, Inc., Naples, FL) looped through a Nitinol wire are shuttled from inferior to superior through coracoid and clavicle bone tunnels. C, coracoid.

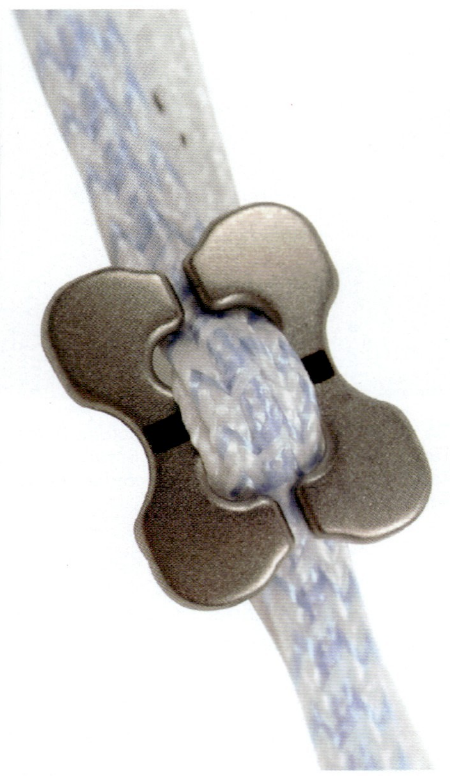

Figure 18.37 Photo of the Dog Bone (Arthrex, Inc., Naples, FL) loaded with FiberTape (Arthrex, Inc., Naples, FL) sutures.

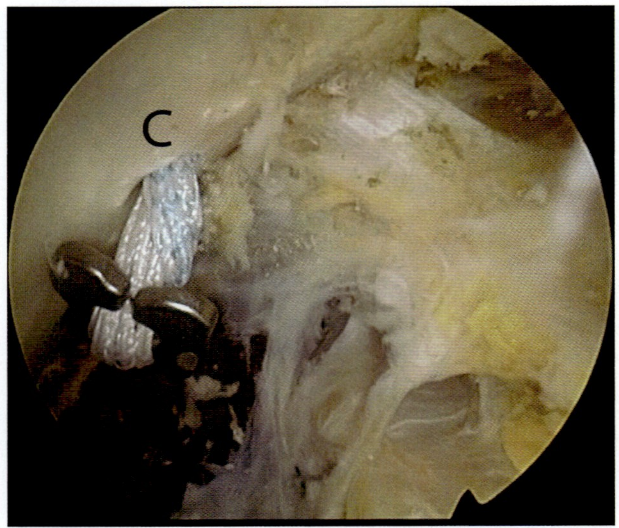

Figure 18.38 Right shoulder, posterior viewing portal with a 70° arthroscope. The Dog Bone (Arthrex, Inc., Naples, FL) has been shuttled into the shoulder, adjacent to the base of the coracoid. C, coracoid.

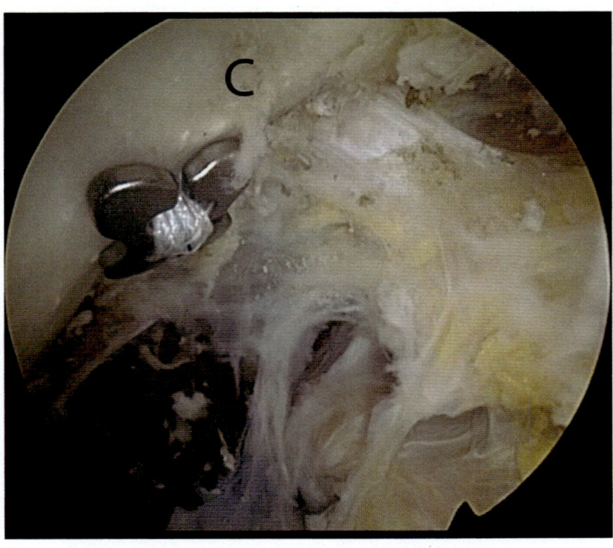

Figure 18.39 Right shoulder, posterior viewing portal with a 70° arthroscope, demonstrates the final position of the Dog Bone (Arthrex, Inc., Naples, FL) at the base of the coracoid. C, coracoid.

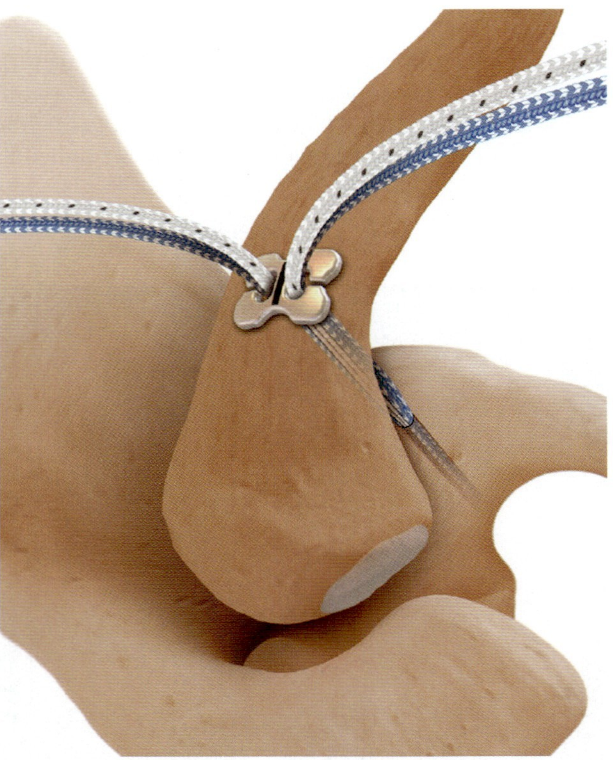

Figure 18.40 Illustration of the Dog Bone (Arthrex, Inc., Naples, FL) positioned on the superior clavicle. Note that device is positioned so that the etched *black line* is parallel with the clavicle.

Arthroscopic AC Joint Reconstruction Techniques: TightRope and GraftRope

The TightRope and GraftRope procedures are very similar to the Dog Bone reconstruction with some notable exceptions. Patient positioning, portal placement, visualization, coracoid preparation, and clavicle incisions are identical to the Dog Bone procedure.

Instead of drilling the tunnels with a single pass of a 3-mm cannulated guide pin, however, the TightRope and GraftRope procedures require that a 2.4-mm guide pin is inserted and then overreamed with either a 4-mm (TightRope) or a 6-mm (GraftRope) reamer (Fig. 18.41). With the GraftRope procedure, the middle of the graft should be tied to the coracoid button and the ends of the graft are prepared with a whipstitch (Fig. 18.42). Instead of passing the looped end of the Nitinol through the cannulation, the crimped end should be passed through the cannulation and then grasped with a suture grasper and pulled out the anterior portal. The pull suture of the coracoid button (oblong button) is passed through the Nitinol loop and pulled through the tunnels in an antegrade direction and out the anterior portal (Fig. 18.43). It is important to avoid breaking the leading sutures. If resistance is encountered, a grasper from the anterior portal can help pull the coracoid button down through the coracoid. It is often necessary to change the trajectory of the pull on the sutures from a lateral trajectory to more of a downward trajectory by using a forked probe or grasper to create a pulley effect (Fig. 18.44). Fraying of the leading sutures is another indicator that the trajectory should be manipulated with a grasper. Once the coracoid button has been positioned under the coracoid, a Kingfisher grasper (Arthrex, Inc., Naples, FL) introduced through the anterior portal can align the button in the sagittal plane (Fig. 18.45).

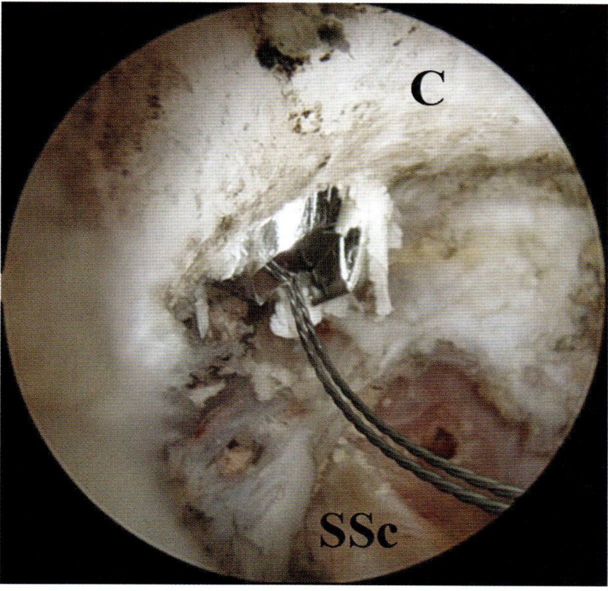

Figure 18.41 Right shoulder, posterior viewing portal with a 70° arthroscope. A guide pin has been overreamed with a cannulated reamer, and a Nitinol wire has been threaded through the cannulated reamer and retrieved out an anterior portal. C, coracoid; SSc, subscapularis tendon.

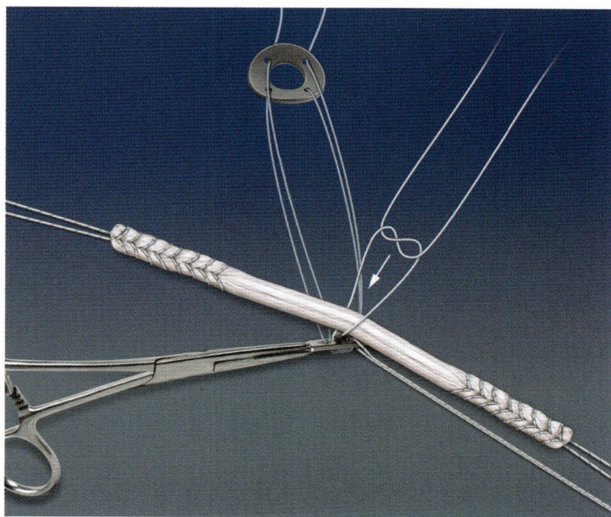
Figure 18.42 Illustration of GraftRope (Arthrex, Inc., Naples, FL) preparation. The ends of an allograft or autograft are prepared with a whipstitch. Then, the center of the graft is tied to the coracoid button. This will double-over the graft and the limbs will exit through the round coracoid button (**top of image**).

The next step is to reduce the AC joint. The arm is removed from traction and an assistant pushes down on the clavicle and up on the arm while the surgeon pulls on the two limbs of the #5 FiberWire to pull the clavicle button down to the dorsal cortex of the clavicle. It is helpful to pull each suture individually in an alternating manner and even to use the index finger to help the clavicle button sit flush on the dorsal cortex of the clavicle (Fig. 18.46). The reduction of the AC joint can be confirmed with fluoroscopy (Fig. 18.47). Alternatively, the reduction of the AC joint can be viewed arthroscopically within the subacromial space. With an anatomic reduction, the undersurface of the distal clavicle should align well with the undersurface of the acromion just as is encountered in normal subacromial visualization (Fig. 18.48). Once an adequate AC joint reduction is confirmed, the #5 FiberWire sutures are tied to finalize the security of the implant.

With the GraftRope procedure, an autograft or allograft is prepared with the implant so that the graft is doubled over at the coracoid end and the tails of the graft will exit the clavicle. The free limbs of the graft are tensioned and a 1.1-mm flexible Nitinol wire is passed in between the limbs of the graft. A 5.5 mm × 12 mm PEEK interference screw is then passed over this Nitinol wire and secured in the clavicle (Fig. 18.49). The free limbs of the graft are then cut flush with the clavicle button, being careful not to cut the FiberWire sutures holding the button down. Next, the surgeon can proceed with traditional arthroscopic distal clavicle excision if appropriate. However, we usually do not excise the distal clavicle.

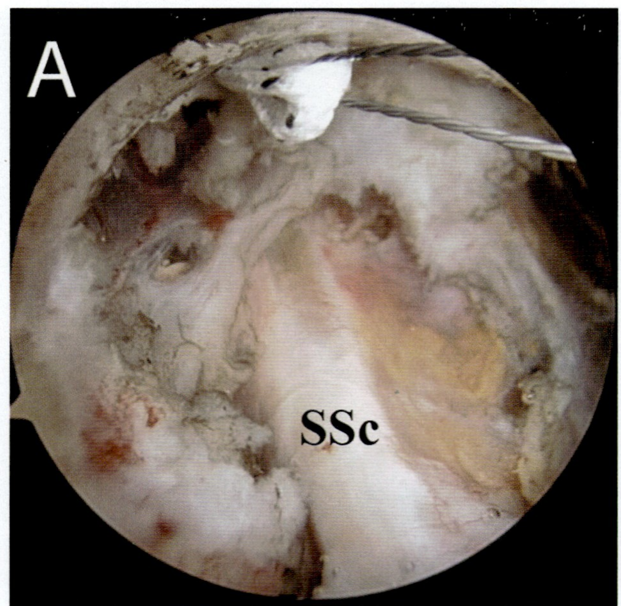

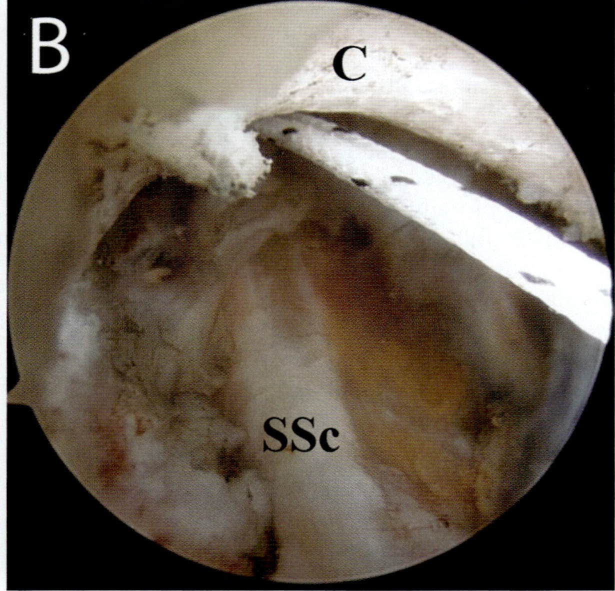

Figure 18.43 **A,B:** Right shoulder, posterior viewing portal with a 70° arthroscope, demonstrates use of a Nitinol wire to shuttle sutures through the clavicle and out the base of the coracoid. C, coracoid; SSc, subscapularis tendon.

Avoiding Pitfalls

There is currently no information that we are aware of regarding the rate of complications after arthroscopic AC joint reconstruction. We have found that it is a very safe procedure if performed meticulously with particular attention to exposure of the coracoid and proper tunnel placement.

For some surgeons, operating arthroscopically near the coracoid is intimidating. A thorough understanding of the anatomy around the coracoid is important for any arthroscopic shoulder surgeon but even more so where AC joint reconstruction is considered. Improper tunnel placement can occur for a multitude of reasons. Pitfalls and keys for avoiding improper tunnel placement are:

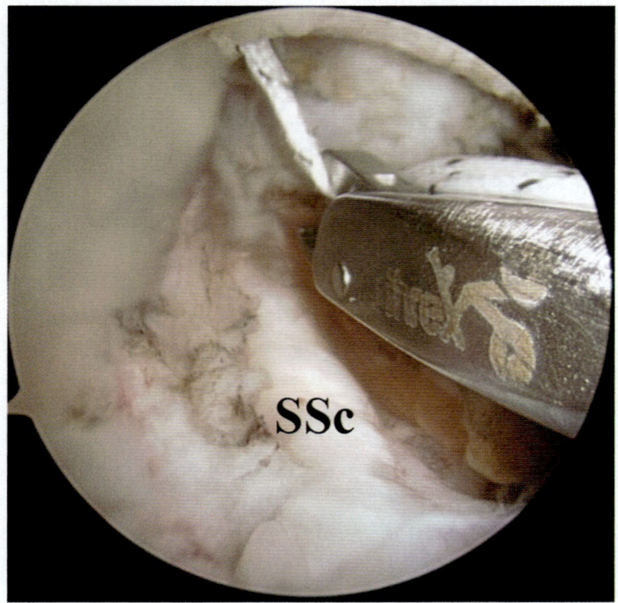

Figure 18.44 Right shoulder, posterior viewing portal with a 70° arthroscope, demonstrates use of a grasper to medialize the shuttling sutures so that the trajectory of pull is in line with the bone tunnels. SSc, subscapularis tendon.

1. Inadequate visualization. If you can't see underneath the coracoid, the implant should not be passed blindly. As noted previously, a thorough exposure of the base of the coracoid is most important. The importance of finding the best portal for visualization, the best angle scope (30° vs. 70°), and the proper placement of the working portal cannot be overemphasized.
2. Improper understanding of the anatomy. Initially, the tendency for surgeons is to place the coracoid tunnel at the arch (or neck) of the coracoid. Since the coracoid thins out quickly from proximal to distal, the base is the safest portion of the anatomy for placing bone tunnels. As noted, the medial to lateral width in the distal region is significantly thinner than the width at the base. Thus, while the 2.4-mm guide pin may be bicortical, when overreaming with a 4.0-mm or 6.0-mm reamer, one may violate the medial or lateral cortex if the guide pin has been placed eccentrically in the coracoid base. Violation of the cortex will result in lack of fixation of the coracoid button, and thus failure of the construct.

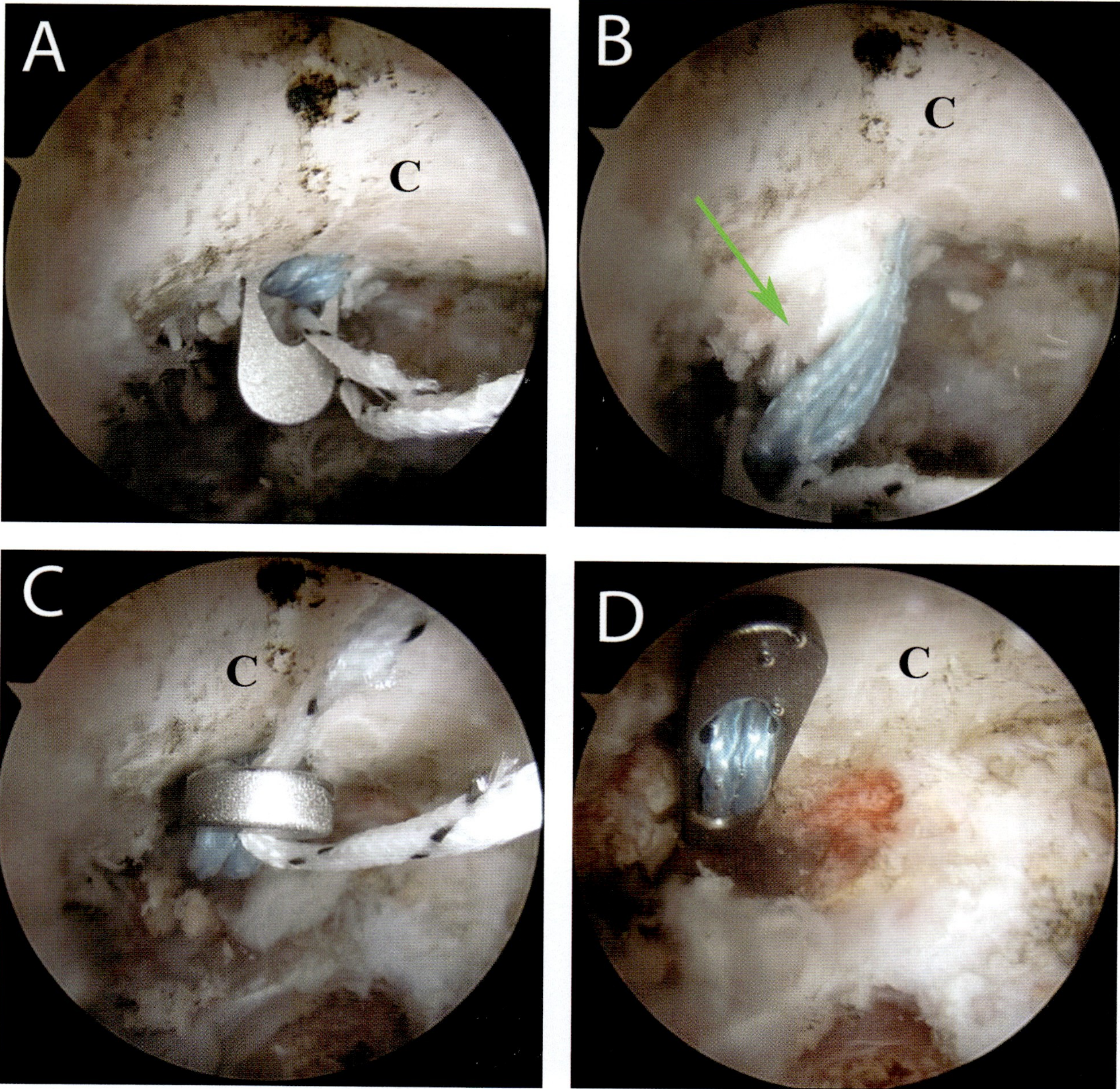

Figure 18.45 Right shoulder, posterior viewing portal with a 70° arthroscope, demonstrates positioning of a coracoid button for TightRope (Arthrex, Inc., Naples, FL) fixation of an acromioclavicular joint separation. **A:** White pull sutures are used to shuttle a coracoid button through bone tunnels in the clavicle and coracoid. **B:** The coracoid button is advanced until the trailing end (*green arrow*) is visible. **C:** Relaxing the pull on the white suture and pulling on the coracoid button sutures (*blue*) flips the coracoid button so that it is perpendicular to the bone tunnel. **D:** Final view of a well-positioned coracoid button. C, coracoid.

3. Improper placement of the clavicular tunnel. The tunnel should be placed approximately 3 cm medial to the AC joint and centered on the clavicle from an anterior to posterior perspective. Inadequate exposure of the anterior and posterior borders of the clavicle can result in the tunnel being placed too anterior or too posterior. If the reamer violates the anterior or posterior borders of the clavicle, fixation may not be achieved or will be at risk for failure.
4. Difficulty passing the graft. It is imperative that the surgeon test the graft size and make sure that it slides easily through a 6-mm tunnel. In fact, the isolated graft should probably fit through a 5- or 5.5-mm tunnel since the final construct will be larger with the incorporation of the #5 FiberWire suture. Once the graft is attached to the implant, be sure the entire construct will fit through a 6-mm tunnel relatively easily. If not, trim the graft to make it thinner.

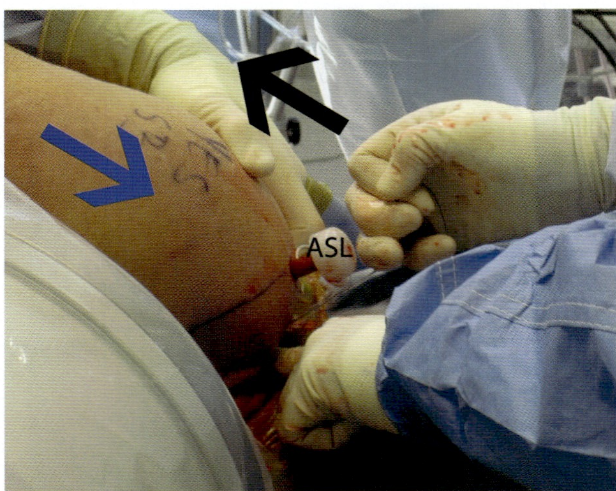

Figure 18.46 Left shoulder, lateral decubitus position, demonstrates reduction of an acromioclavicular joint separation using a TightRope device (Arthrex, Inc., Naples, FL). An assistant provides superior force to the arm (*blue arrow*) and an inferior force to the distal clavicle (*black arrow*), while the surgeon (**right**) seats the clavicle button on the distal clavicle cortex. ASL, anterosuperolateral portal.

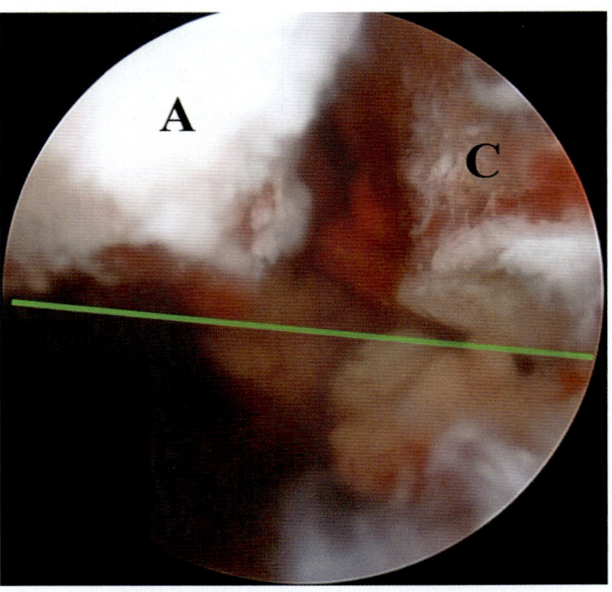

Figure 18.48 Left shoulder, posterior subacromial viewing portal, provides arthroscopic confirmation of a reduced (*green line*) acromioclavicular joint separation. A, acromion; C, distal clavicle.

5. Graft and implant get stuck in the tunnels before passage is complete. First of all, if the surgeon sizes the graft correctly, this is unlikely to occur. Secondly, it is critical to change the vector of pull on the FiberWire coracoid button pull suture. Use an instrument with smooth edges to change this vector. The suture grasper works well for this.
6. Do NOT break the pull suture. If you break the pull suture during implant passage, then the coracoid button will become wedged underneath the clavicle. This makes for a lousy CC ligament reconstruction since there is no coracoid fixation! If you notice that the pull sutures are becoming frayed, then pull on one side of the pull suture to get the frayed part OUT of the pull zone. If the sutures are extremely frayed, they can be replaced with a *suture through a suture* technique.

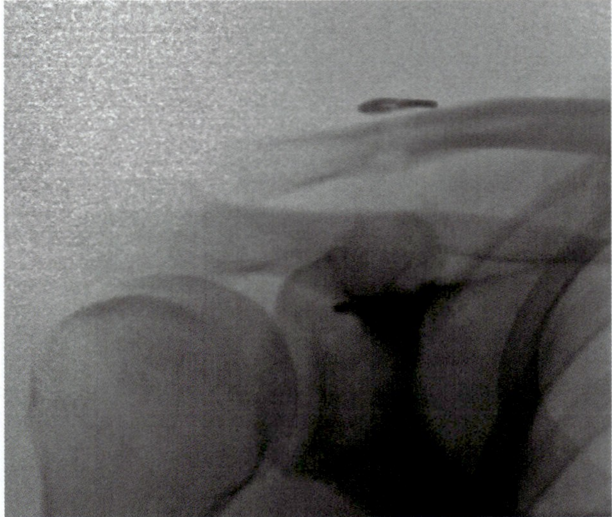

Figure 18.47 Intraoperative fluoroscopic view of TightRope (Arthrex, Inc., Naples, FL) fixation of an acromioclavicular joint separation confirms reduction and implant position.

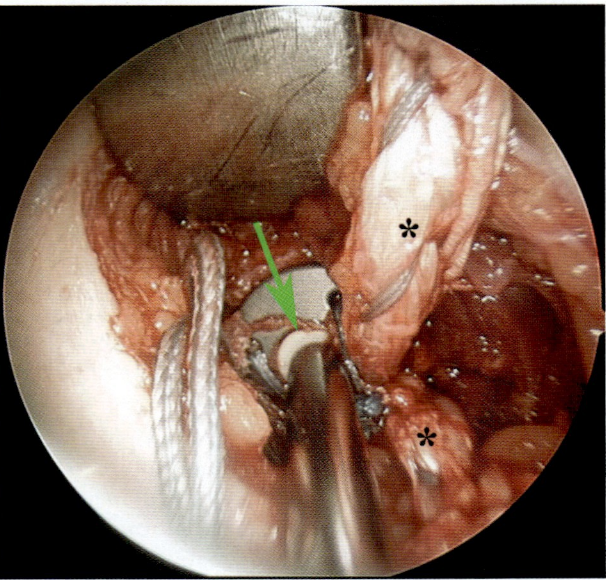

Figure 18.49 Intraoperative photo of GraftRope (Arthrex, Inc., Naples, FL) fixation for a chronic acromioclavicular joint separation. After arthroscopic graft placement, an interference screw (*green arrow*) is placed in the distal clavicle to compress the graft limbs (*asterisk*) to bone.

REFERENCES

1. Bjerneld H, Hovelius L, Thorling J. Acromio-clavicular separations treated conservatively. A 5-year follow-up study. Acta Orthop Scand. 1983;54: 743–745.
2. Glick JM, Milburn LJ, Haggerty JF, et al. Dislocated acromioclavicular joint: follow-up study of 35 unreduced acromioclavicular dislocations. *Am J Sports Med.* 1977;5:264–270.
3. Pauly S, Gerhardt C, Haas NP, et al. Prevalence of concomitant intraarticular lesions in patients treated operatively for high-grade acromioclavicular joint separations. *Knee Surg Sports Traumatol Arthrosc.* 2009;17:513–517.
4. Tischer T, Salzmann GM, El-Azab H, et al. Incidence of associated injuries with acute acromioclavicular joint dislocations types III through V. *Am J Sports Med.* 2009;37:136–139.
5. Motamedi AR, Blevins FT, Willis MC, et al. Biomechanics of the coracoclavicular ligament complex and augmentations used in its repair and reconstruction. *Am J Sports Med.* 2000;28:380–384.
6. Tienen TG, Oyen JF, Eggen PJ. A modified technique of reconstruction for complete acromioclavicular dislocation: a prospective study. *Am J Sports Med.* 2003;31:655–659.

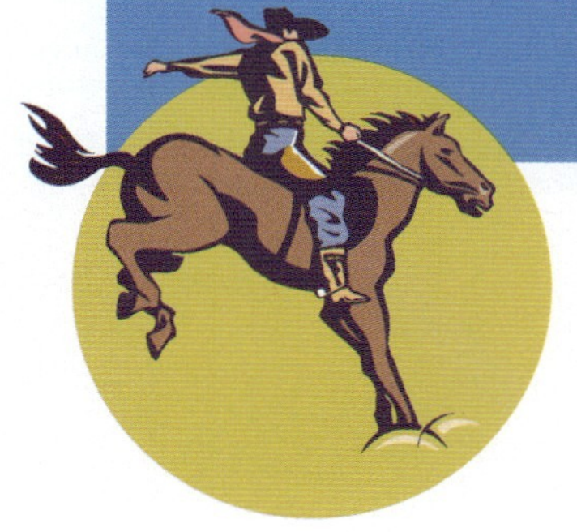

19

Arthroscopic Treatment of Fractures about the Shoulder

WESTERN WISDOM

A loud mouth and a quiet brain can always be found under the same hat.

Historically fractures about the shoulder have been managed in an open manner. However, with the advent of advancing technology and evolving techniques, many injuries can now be managed with arthroscopic reduction and internal fixation (ARIF).

Priority number one is (and will always remain) to accomplish the most optimal result for every patient we encounter. A well-performed open fracture fixation is preferable to a mediocre arthroscopic procedure. However, if the arthroscopic technique can be done well and reliably, it offers significant advantages. First and foremost is the advantage of minimally invasive techniques. Similar to the philosophy of percutaneous fixation of periarticular fractures of the lower extremity, minimizing soft tissue dissection with an arthroscopic technique may preserve greater blood supply and thus lead to improved healing with a lower risk of infection. With glenoid osteosynthesis, the greatest benefit of an arthroscopic approach is the ability to obtain and maintain a reduction without the subscapularis tenotomy that is required to obtain access to the joint during an open approach. Paralleling the advantages of arthroscopic rotator cuff repair over open rotator cuff repair, arthroscopic fixation of tuberosity fractures may lead to decreased postoperative stiffness and lower incidence of infection. Based on these advantages, we have gradually increased the number and types of fractures we manage arthroscopically. As one's skills improve, increasingly complex fractures may be managed arthroscopically.

GLENOID FRACTURES

Glenoid fractures may result from high-energy axial or off-axis load injuries, or they may occur in association with traumatic anterior shoulder dislocations. Acute lesions, particularly those that are large, often benefit from operative management. The size and quality of the bone fragment is usually the determining factor in the decision of whether to use screw fixation or to incorporate the fragment in a Bankart repair with suture anchors (see Chapter 12 "Repair of Anterior Instability without Bone Loss" for full discussion). After initial closed reduction of an anterior dislocation (which is typically rather easy because of the glenoid fracture), postreduction radiographs should be obtained to determine the status of the glenoid and humeral head after the reduction (Fig. 19.1). We also obtain a computed tomography (CT) scan, preferably with three-dimensional (3D) reconstructions, on these traumatic injuries (Fig. 19.2).

For younger active patients (<30 years old), we fix almost all glenoid fractures, either with suture anchors or with screws. In older patients, we consider acute screw fixation of glenoid fractures that are >20% of the glenoid width. Thankfully new techniques and technology have made glenoid fractures more amenable to arthroscopic repair. Our surgical planning for these fractures takes several factors into consideration:

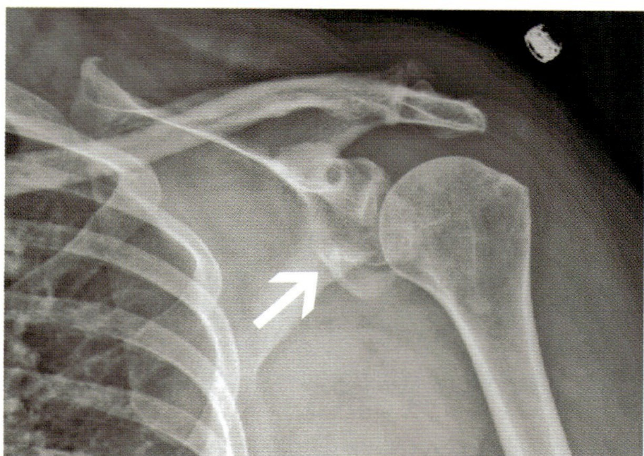

Figure 19.1 Anteroposterior (AP) radiograph of a left shoulder demonstrates a large displaced anteroinferior glenoid fracture (*white arrow*).

1. Size of the fracture fragment. For screw fixation to be a feasible option, the fragment typically must measure at least 1.5 cm in length from superior to inferior. Fractures amenable to screw fixation often include approximately the anterior one-third of the glenoid (Fig. 19.3). While screw fixation with only one centrally positioned screw is a potential option, it is desirable to obtain a second point of fixation to eliminate the potential for rotational instability. If placement of a second screw is not possible, additional fixation can be accomplished with a suture anchor and a cerclage suture around the fragment.
2. Comminution of the fracture. Simple fracture fragments with minimal comminution are obviously the most amenable to screw fixation.
3. Patient age and gender. In younger patients, higher bone quality typically results in fractures that are more amenable to screw fixation (and are often less comminuted as a result of bone quality). Likewise, men tend to have better bone quality than women, with fractures more amenable to screw fixation.
4. Fracture age. Acute fractures (<6 weeks) have not had time to remodel and are thus more likely to be reducible in an anatomic position. A chronic fracture is likely to have begun to heal in a malunited position and during the process of fracture mobilization, the fragment may be damaged, thus making anatomic screw fixation much more difficult.

Bony Bankart Fracture Repair

Diagnostic arthroscopy is performed via the standard posterior portal. Typically, joint visualization is initially obscured by fracture hematoma. An arthroscopic shaver is used to evacuate the fracture hematoma and fully visualize the fracture fragment. The anterior portal is placed as low as possible to maximize the potential to reach the inferior glenoid through this portal (Fig. 19.4). Next the anterosuperolateral (ASL) portal is established. This will be an important viewing portal as well as a working portal (Fig. 19.5). It is important to utilize arthroscopic cannulas in all three intra-articular portals. This will allow for easy exchange of the arthroscope and instruments into whichever portal offers optimal visualization/instrumentation. Any associated pathology is then identified. However, since it is important to address the fracture prior to excessive swelling and fluid extravasation, one should delay any additional procedures until after the bony Bankart lesion is addressed.

Once the bony Bankart is identified, it must be mobilized. Use a 15° arthroscopic elevator (Arthrex, Inc., Naples, FL) from the anterior portal or the ASL portal to fully elevate and mobilize the fracture fragment. Unless the fracture

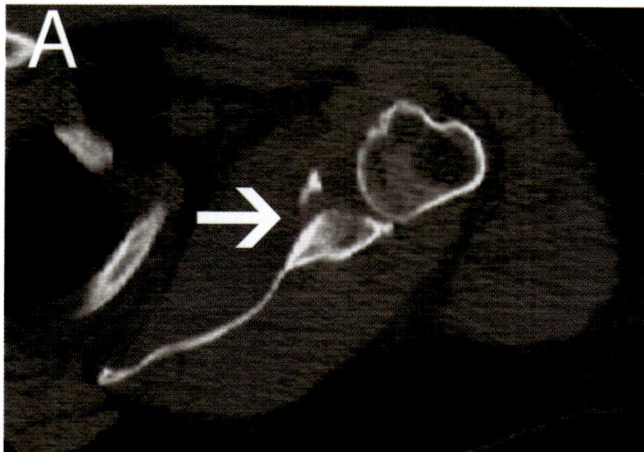

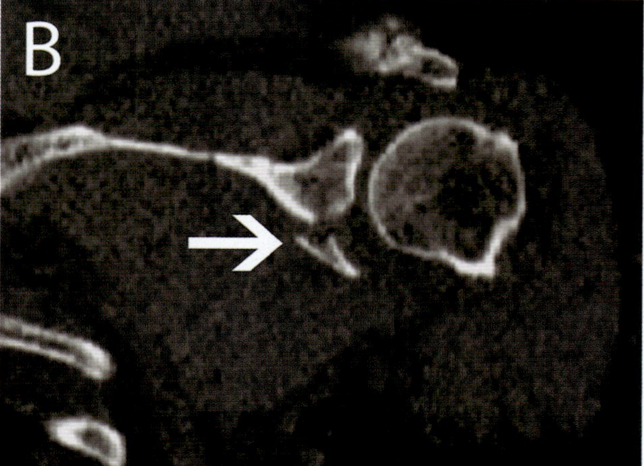

Figure 19.2 **(A)** Axial and **(B)** coronal reconstruction CT views of the same left shoulder as in the previous figure demonstrate a relatively large and displaced anteroinferior glenoid fracture (*white arrow*).

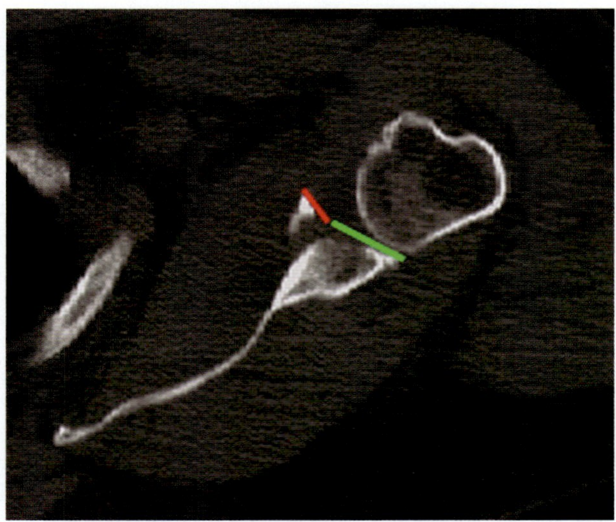

Figure 19.3 The axial view of the CT scan demonstrates that the displaced fracture fragment (*red line*) measures approximately one-third of the anterior to posterior diameter of the glenoid (*red line plus green line*).

is extremely fresh (a week or less), some fibrous and perhaps even bony healing may have already occurred. Just as with a typical Bankart lesion, complete mobilization of the tissue is essential in order to reestablish the normal tension of the anterior band of the inferior glenohumeral ligament (Fig. 19.6). If the fracture is more than a few weeks old, significant bony union may have already occurred in a malunited position. If this is the case, the arthroscopic elevator may be used to perform an osteotomy through the fracture callus. Care should be taken to maximize the size of the fracture fragment and minimize any additional comminution during the osteotomy (Fig. 19.7A). After the fracture fragment has been thoroughly freed, the bone should be freshened to remove any soft tissue to maximize the amount of bone healing that will occur (Fig. 19.7B). A helpful trick with these injuries, as well as with regular Bankart lesions, is to place one traction suture at the superior edge of the displaced labrum. This traction suture can be delivered out the ASL portal and will help in determining when adequate mobilization of the lesion has been achieved (Fig. 19.8).

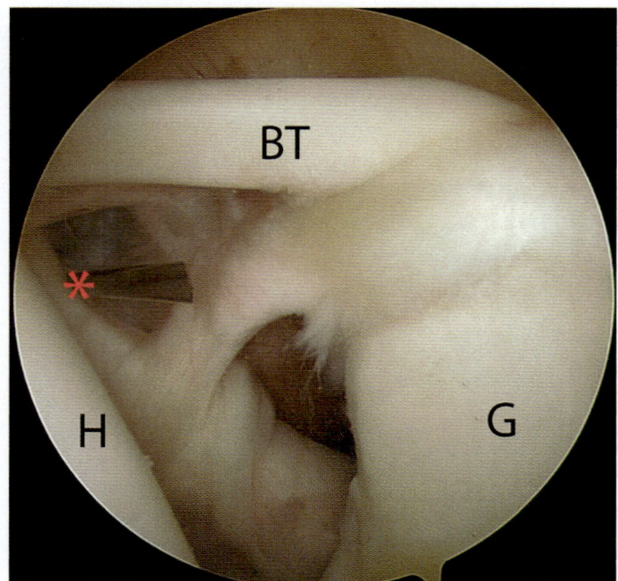

Figure 19.4 Posterior view of a left shoulder demonstrates a spinal localization needle entering (*asterisk*) the glenohumeral joint over the lateral half of the subscapularis. Notice that the spinal needle is aimed upward toward the superior glenoid and thus starts on the skin relatively low. BT, biceps tendon; G, glenoid; H, humerus.

Once sufficient mobilization has been achieved, a provisional reduction is performed with a grasper. The reduction and fragment are evaluated for proposed fixation sites. The fracture fragment may not fit perfectly into the glenoid defect like a puzzle piece, as some mild comminution or cartilage damage occurs in almost every case and will obscure the fracture margins. With a little fragment manipulation, one should be able to confidently determine the correct position for the fragment even if it does not key in perfectly.

Next is perhaps the most critical portion of the procedure. For optimal screw fixation of a fracture fragment, success is largely dependent on obtaining the proper angle of approach. Specifically, the screws should intersect the fracture line at as close to a right angle as possible. This cannot be achieved through a standard anterior portal. Therefore, we find it critical to create a 5 o'clock portal for this procedure (see Chapter 1 "Advanced Shoulder Arthroscopy Essentials" for portal descriptions). An optimal angle should be confirmed with a spinal needle before proceeding (Fig. 19.9). Because the goal is screw fixation perpendicular to the fracture rather than anchor placement, the guide wire will usually enter the skin more medial than the anterior portal.

A 1.6-mm guidewire for the Nesting Guide Sleeve System (Bone Loss Set; Arthrex, Inc., Naples, FL) (Fig. 19.10) is inserted adjacent to the localization spinal needle. Once the guidewire is appropriately positioned, the spinal needle is removed. A small incision is made and the Nesting Guide Sleeve is then inserted over the guidewire, passing bluntly through the subscapularis, and then into the intra-articular space. This device is sufficiently rigid to assist in fracture reduction as well (Fig. 19.11).

In order to allow the screw head to sit directly on bone, electrocautery is used to create a small window along the anterior edge of the fracture fragment. If anterior labrum is still attached to the glenoid fragment (which is typically the case with bony Bankart fractures), it is left in place, and this window is created anterior to the labrum (Fig. 19.12). The screw should be positioned over the anterior edge of the glenoid (medially) beneath the labrum so that the screw head will not make any contact with the humeral

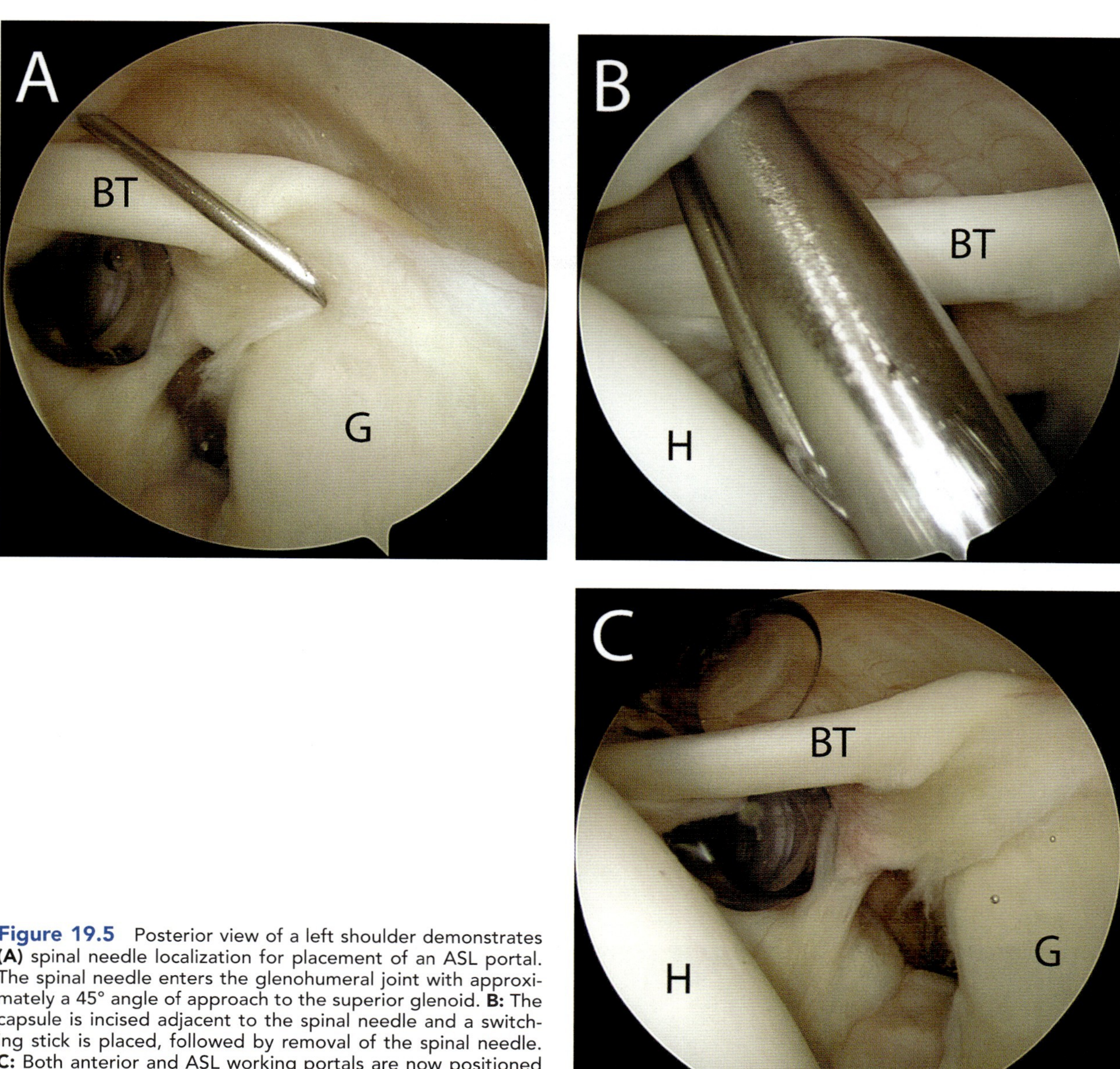

Figure 19.5 Posterior view of a left shoulder demonstrates **(A)** spinal needle localization for placement of an ASL portal. The spinal needle enters the glenohumeral joint with approximately a 45° angle of approach to the superior glenoid. **B:** The capsule is incised adjacent to the spinal needle and a switching stick is placed, followed by removal of the spinal needle. **C:** Both anterior and ASL working portals are now positioned appropriately within the glenohumeral space. BT, biceps tendon; G, glenoid; H, humerus.

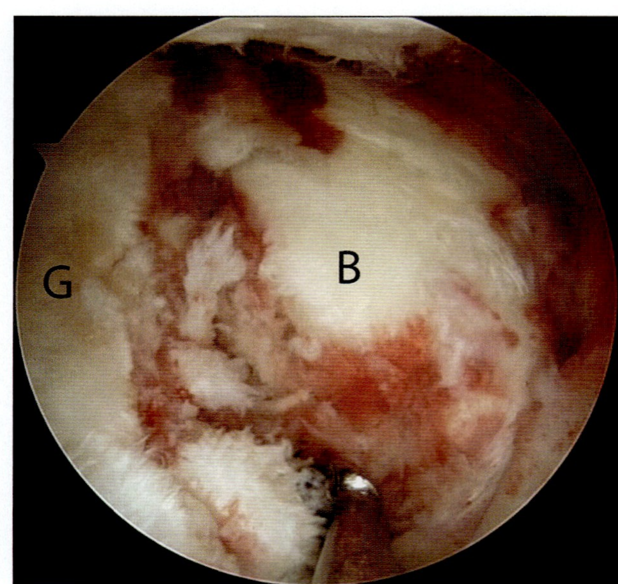

Figure 19.6 Left shoulder viewed from the ASL portal shows an anterior glenoid fracture (**right**). B, bony Bankart lesion; G, glenoid.

head. If the screw must be positioned more laterally, then the labrum should be elevated, the screw placed, and then the labrum positioned over the top of the screw head.

Utilizing the previously placed traction suture and the Nesting Guide, the fracture is reduced. Inferior screw fixation is performed first. While visualizing from the ASL portal, the guidewire is advanced, oriented perpendicular to the fracture plane. The screw length is measured with the screw sizer. Although the screws are self-drilling and self-tapping, we generally predrill the near cortex of the fracture fragment to avoid torque and fracture displacement with screw insertion. A 2.75-mm drill is used to predrill the near cortex, and a 3.75-mm titanium screw of appropriate length is then screwed into place. When the screw head nears the fracture cortex, one should advance the screw slowly and secure the screw "two fingers tight." It is critical not to split the fracture fragment at this point (Fig. 19.13).

Once the inferior screw has been placed, a second point of fixation must be achieved. If the fragment is of sufficient size to allow for a second screw, then this is placed approximately 1 cm superior to the first screw. As an alternative, if there is fear of fracturing the fragment, a PushLock anchor (Arthrex, Inc., Naples, FL) may be used superiorly as a second point of fixation. A bone socket is created for the PushLock anchor superior to the bony fragment, thus averting the risk of damaging the fragment. Often, the traction suture previously placed in the superior corner of the labrum is ideal for fixation at the PushLock anchor site (Fig. 19.14). The fixation is then assessed for stability and reduction. For rehabilitation after ARIF of glenoid fractures, we have patients follow the same protocol as that of a standard Bankart repair, with the exception that we delay strengthening until 3 months postoperatively (see Chapter 20, "Postoperative Rehabilitation").

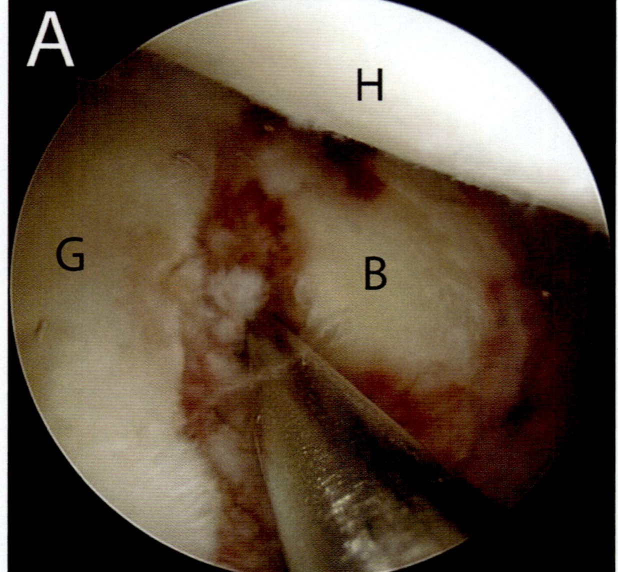

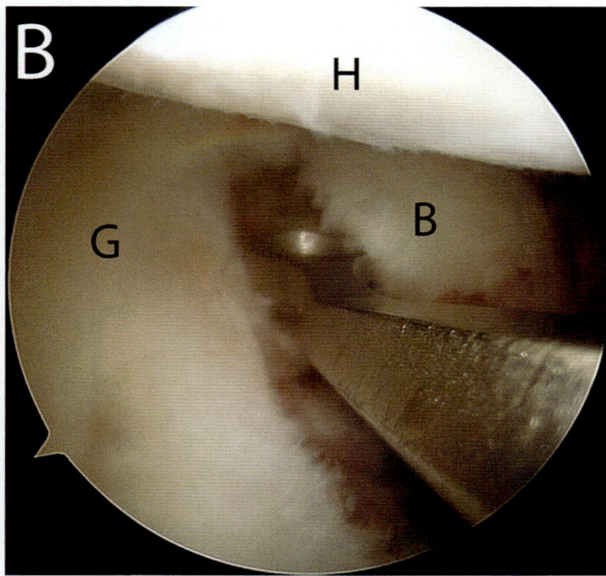

Figure 19.7 Left shoulder, ASL viewing portal. **A:** Using a 15° arthroscopic elevator (Arthrex, Inc., Naples, FL), the bony Bankart lesion is mobilized being careful to avoid obscuring the fracture margins. **B:** A ring curette is used to remove fibrous tissue and expose bone. B, bony Bankart lesion; G, glenoid; H, humerus.

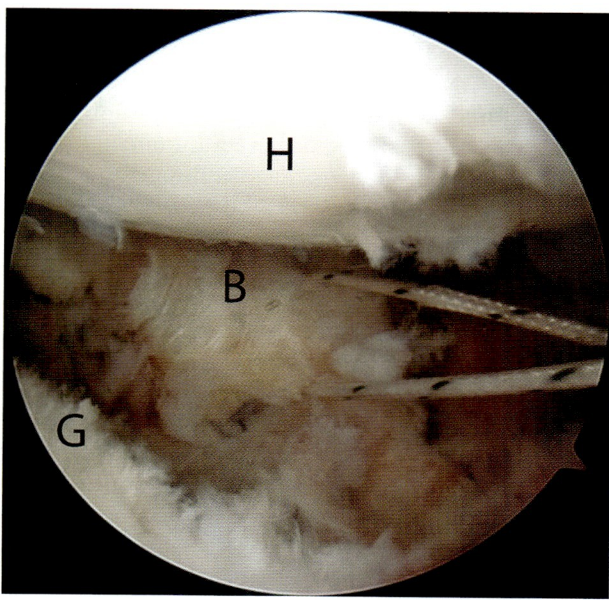

Figure 19.8 Left shoulder, ASL viewing portal. A traction suture is placed at the superior margin of the bony Bankart fragment. This is pulled out the anterior (in this case) or the ASL portal to assist with fracture reduction during the repair. B, bony Bankart lesion; G, glenoid; H, humerus.

Other Glenoid Fractures

Although the bony Bankart fracture is clearly the most common glenoid fracture encountered, other patterns can be seen as well (Fig. 19.15). The general principles of fixation

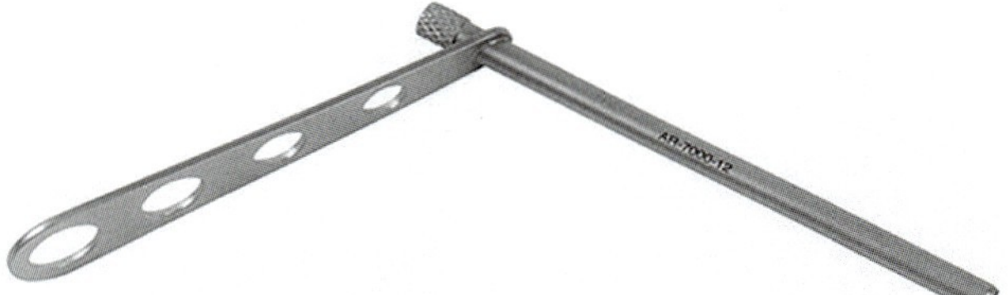

Figure 19.10 Nesting Guide Sleeve (Bone Loss Set; Arthrex, Inc., Naples, FL).

as outlined above should be followed no matter where the fracture occurs:

1. Secure fixation in two locations to avoid rotational instability.
2. Hardware (and thus arthroscopy portals) should be placed as perpendicular to the fracture plane as possible.
3. Respect the quality and size of the fracture fragment and plan fixation accordingly.
4. If the screw head impinges lateral to the glenoid rim, cover the exposed metal with capsular advancement to suture anchors, and then remove the screws at 6 to 9 months postoperatively.

With appropriate attention to these principles, almost any glenoid fracture can be addressed arthroscopically (Fig. 19.16). ARIF of glenoid fractures is a technique that is here to stay and clearly has tremendous benefits in comparison to open reduction and internal fixation.

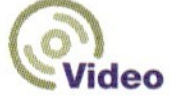

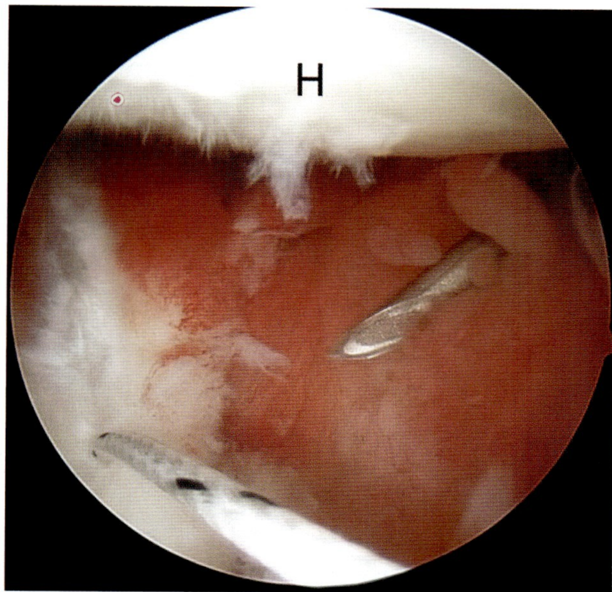

Figure 19.9 Left shoulder, view from the ASL portal demonstrating spinal needle localization of a 5 o'clock portal that enters the joint through the subscapularis. This 5 o'clock portal is necessary to achieve an angle of approach perpendicular to the fracture line. H, humerus.

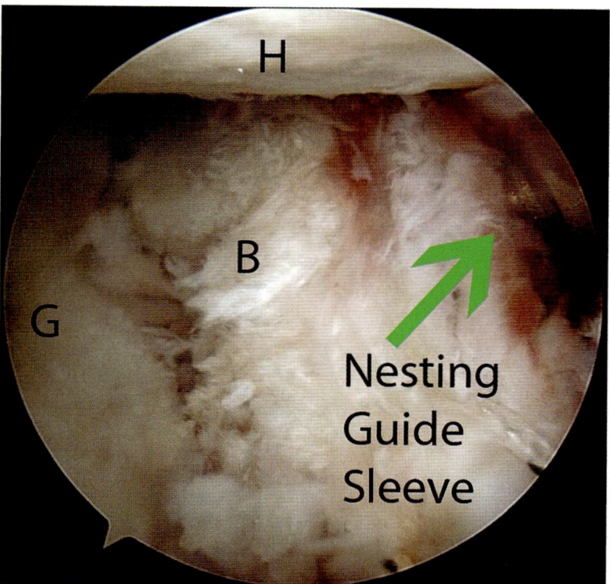

Figure 19.11 Left shoulder, ASL viewing portal. The glenoid fracture is reduced with the assistance of the superior traction suture (lower right corner). A Nesting Guide Sleeve (*green arrow*) (Arthrex, Inc., Naples, FL) is positioned and also helps reduce the fracture. Then a guidewire can be inserted to secure the reduction. B, bony Bankart lesion; G, glenoid; H, humerus.

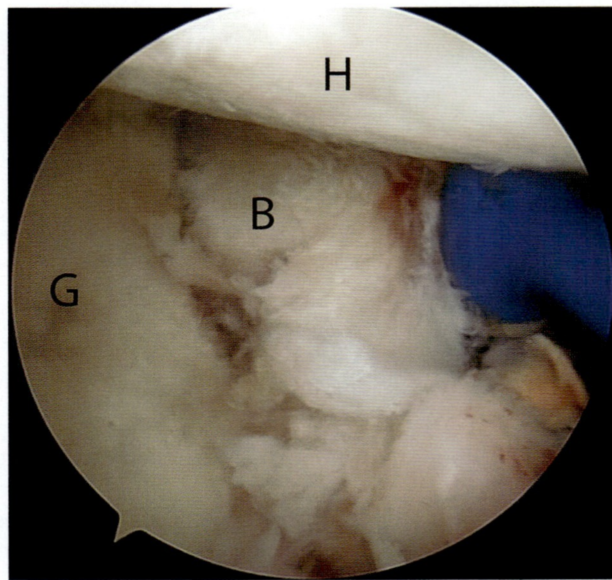

Figure 19.12 Left shoulder, ASL viewing portal. An electrocautery device is utilized through an anterior portal to clear the soft tissues around the guidewire. B, bony Bankart lesion; G, glenoid; H, humerus.

PROXIMAL HUMERUS FRACTURES

Successful management of proximal humerus fractures relies upon maintaining rotator cuff function. It is therefore no surprise that arthroscopy has a definite role in proximal humerus fractures. We have found that arthroscopy is useful in two settings. The first is an acute isolated fracture of the greater or lesser tuberosity (Fig. 19.17). Displacement of these fractures (>5 mm) leads to dysfunction of the rotator cuff and may result in mechanical impingement. Arthroscopy can be used to achieve a minimally invasive, anatomic reduction of tuberosity fractures.

Greater Tuberosity ARIF

The patient is placed in the lateral decubitus position and a standard diagnostic arthroscopy is performed via the posterior portal. In the acute setting, visualization often requires significant time to evacuate hematoma. Furthermore, since the anatomy is disrupted, it is important to take a few moments to achieve orientation and fully assess the injury. The key is to locate a known landmark or structure, such as the biceps root, and then reference the dissection from there. Once adequate visualization is obtained, the fracture fragment and fracture pattern are identified (Fig. 19.18). A complete bursectomy is performed subacromially, including the anterior, lateral, and posterior gutters. Visualization will likely be limited subacromially because the tuberosity and cuff are displaced superiorly and encroach upon the undersurface of the acromion. To manage this, a traction suture is helpful. Since the bone can be hard to penetrate, the traction suture is placed medially at the cuff–bone interface (Fig. 19.19) with a penetrator (Arthrex, Inc., Naples, FL) introduced from the posterior portal. Alternatively, sometimes a shuttle technique through the Neviaser portal is required. Pulling laterally on the traction suture increases the working space.

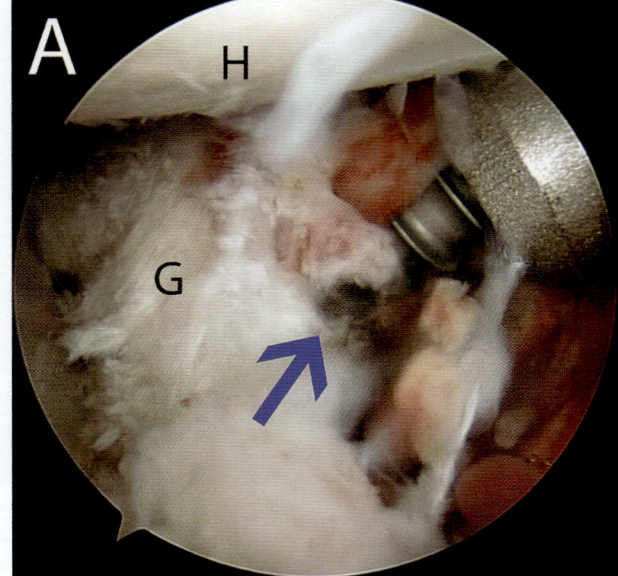

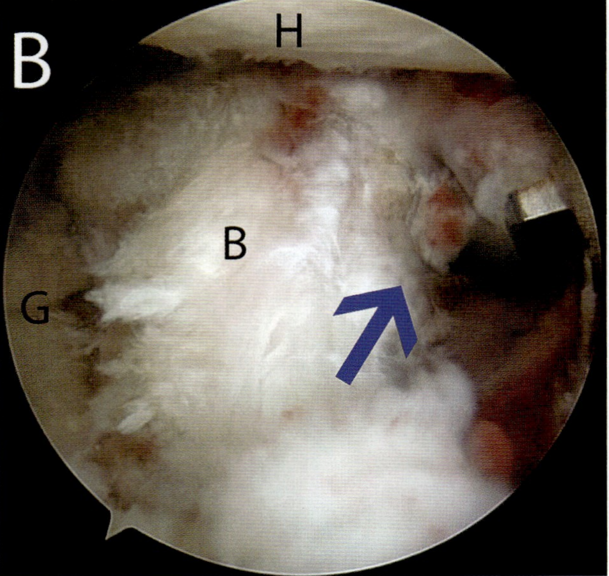

Figure 19.13 Left shoulder, ASL viewing portal. **A:** A 3.7-mm cannulated screw (*blue arrow*) is advanced over a guidewire to secure the glenoid fracture and **(B)** is tightened "two fingers tight."

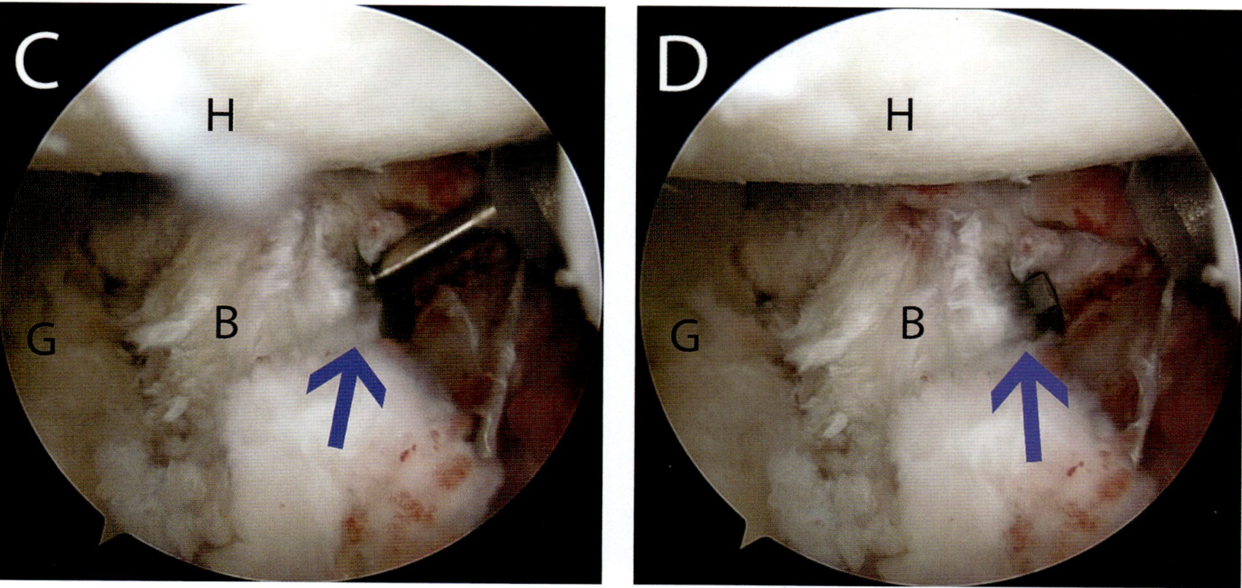

Figure 19.13 *(Continued)* **C:** Once the screw head is fully seated, the guide pin is removed, and the screw head (*blue arrow*) is examined to ensure that it is not prominent **(D).** B, bony Bankart lesion; G, glenoid; H, humerus.

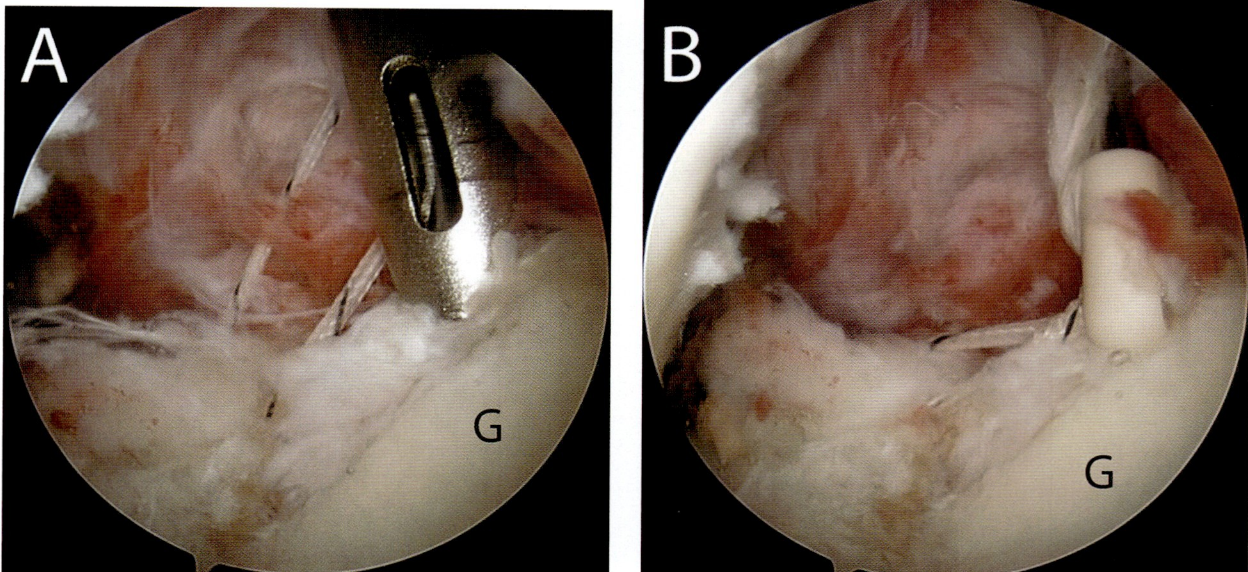

Figure 19.14 Left shoulder, posterior viewing portal. In addition to screw fixation of the glenoid fracture previously (Fig. 19.13), a second point of fixation can be achieved with a PushLock anchor (Arthrex, Inc., Naples, FL). **A:** A bone socket is created superior to the fracture and **(B)** a previously placed traction stitch is threaded through the anchor eyelet for knotless fixation. G, glenoid.

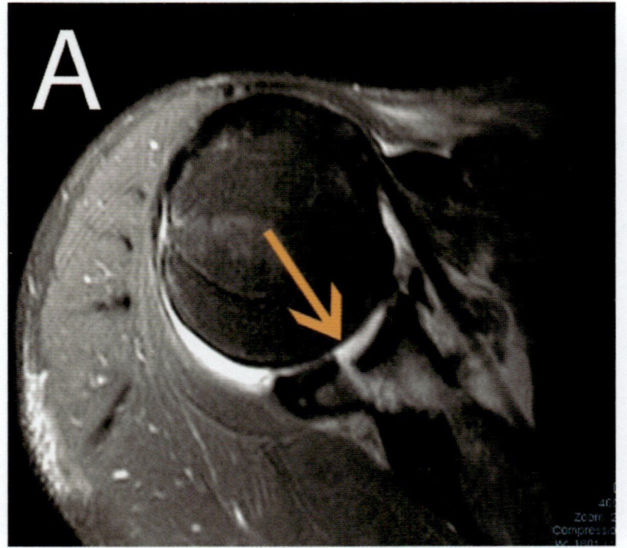

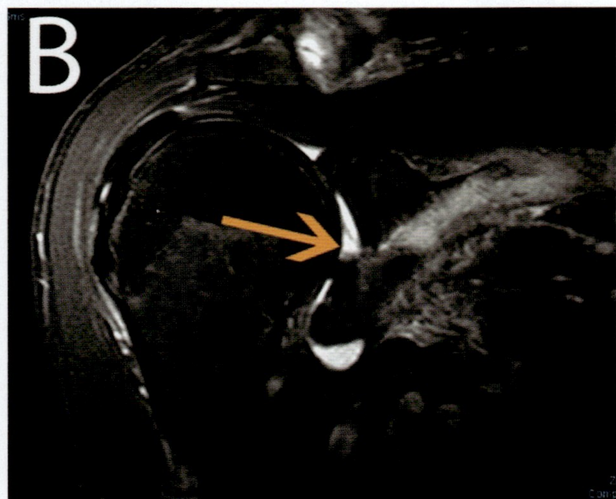

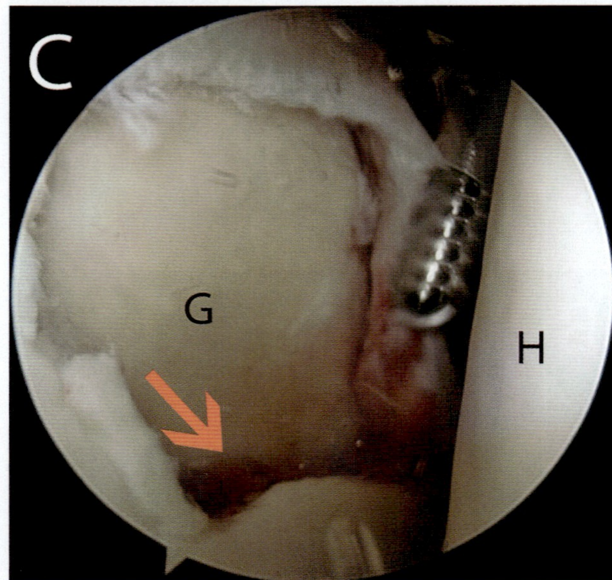

Figure 19.15 **A:** Preoperative axial and **(B)** coronal magnetic resonance imaging views of a right shoulder demonstrate a large glenoid fracture (*orange arrow*) with medial displacement of the superior fragment. **C:** Arthroscopic view from the posterior portal of the same shoulder demonstrates a large fracture (*orange arrow*) in the superior glenoid with medially displacement. G, glenoid; H, humerus.

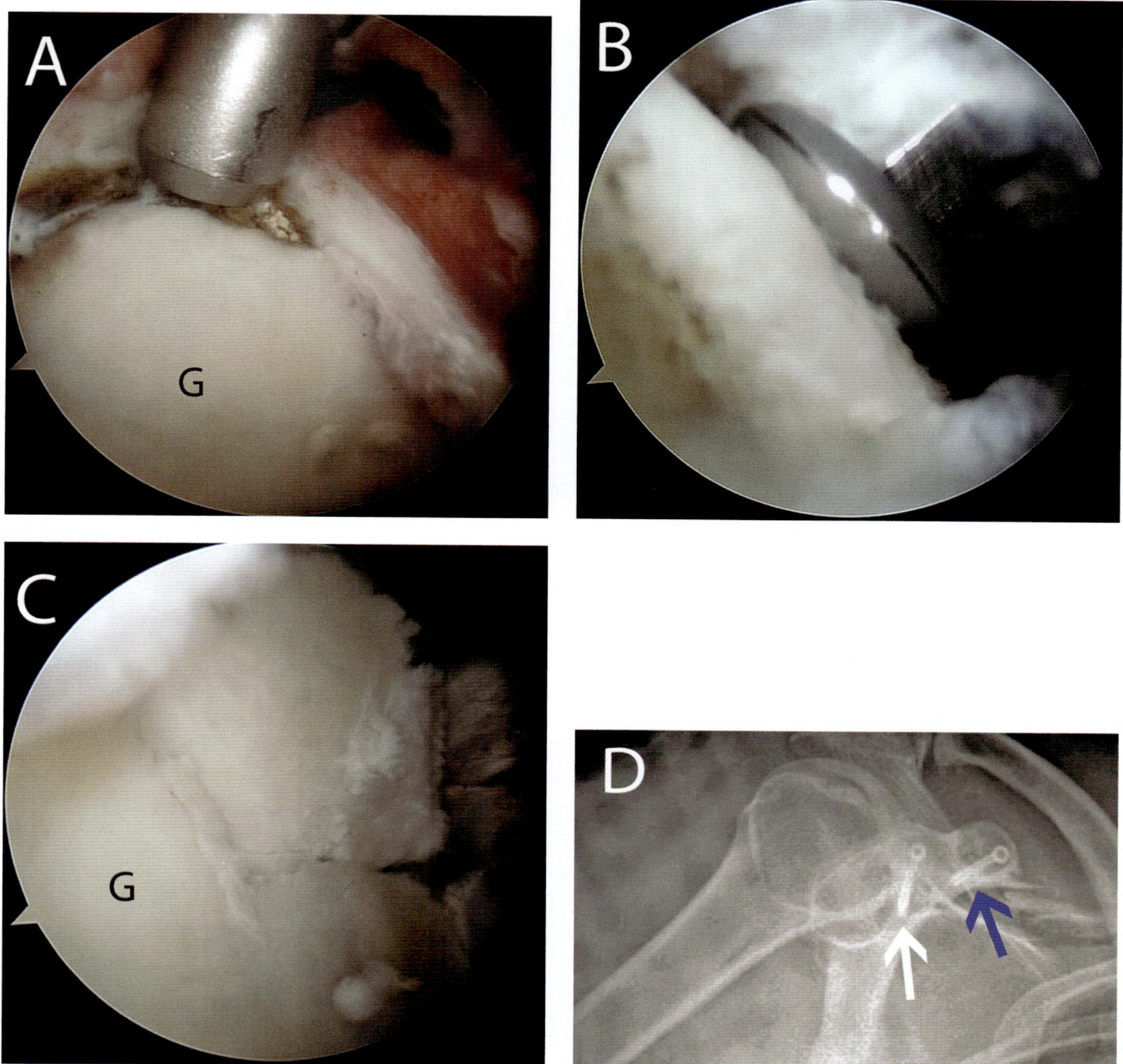

Figure 19.16 Left shoulder, posterior viewing portal demonstrating **(A)** placement of a Nesting Guide Sleeve through a modified anterior/superior portal, **(B)** followed by screw fixation of the glenoid fracture. **C:** After the screw is secured, excellent compression of the fracture is achieved and anatomical alignment of the fracture is restored. **D:** Postoperative radiographs demonstrate good fracture reduction. A *white arrow* demonstrates the first screw placed. A second screw was also placed more medially at the base of the coracoid (*blue arrow*). G, glenoid.

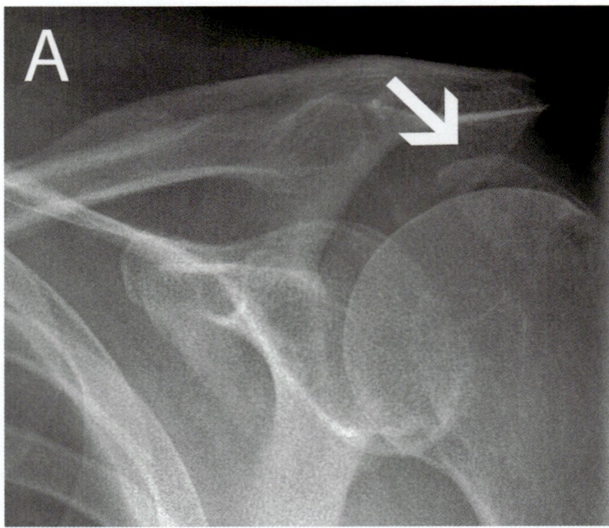

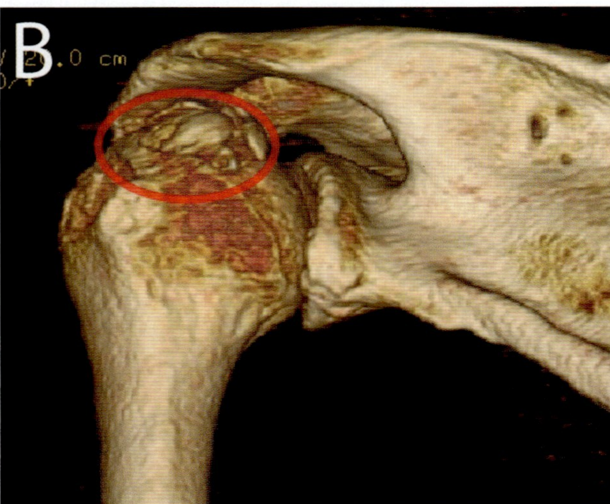

Figure 19.17 **A:** AP shoulder radiograph of a left shoulder demonstrates a fracture of the greater tuberosity (*white arrow*) that is displaced medially. **B:** 3D reconstruction CT image demonstrates the displaced fracture and the amount of fracture comminution (*circled in red*).

A provisional reduction is obtained by securing the inverted mattress traction suture laterally with a SwiveLock C anchor (Arthrex, Inc., Naples, FL) (Fig. 19.20). Alternatively, a 1.6-mm guidewire can be inserted percutaneously to secure the tuberosity. In either case, placement of the anchor or wire should take into consideration the final construct. Even if the reduction is not perfect, getting it secured will free up the surgeon's hands, increase the subacromial space, and make the remaining procedure much more simple. The reduction can be fine-tuned later. Now that the fragment is at least in a near anatomical position, we typically proceed with a transtendon SpeedBridge technique (see Chapter 4, "Complete Rotator Cuff Tears") (Fig. 19.21). Two 4.75-mm BioComposite SwiveLock C anchors (Arthrex, Inc., Naples, FL) are placed medially at the articular margin of the humeral head. These are placed in a transtendon manner

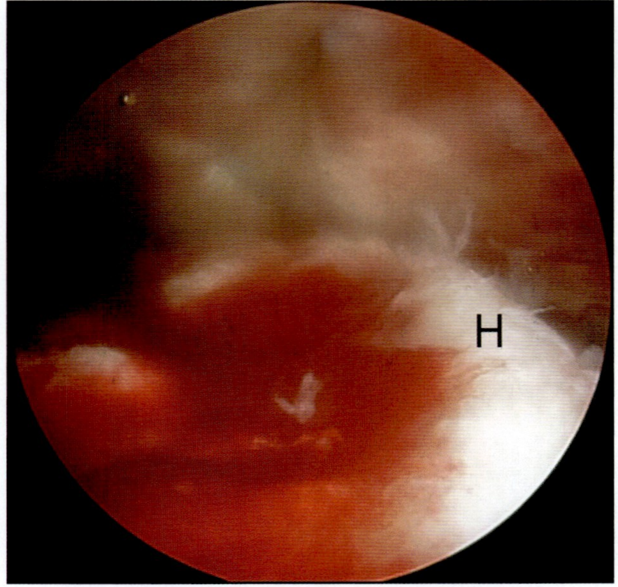

Figure 19.18 Left shoulder, subacromial view from a posterior portal demonstrates the fracture bone bed on the greater tuberosity of the humerus. Fracture hematoma lies on the bone bed. H, humerus.

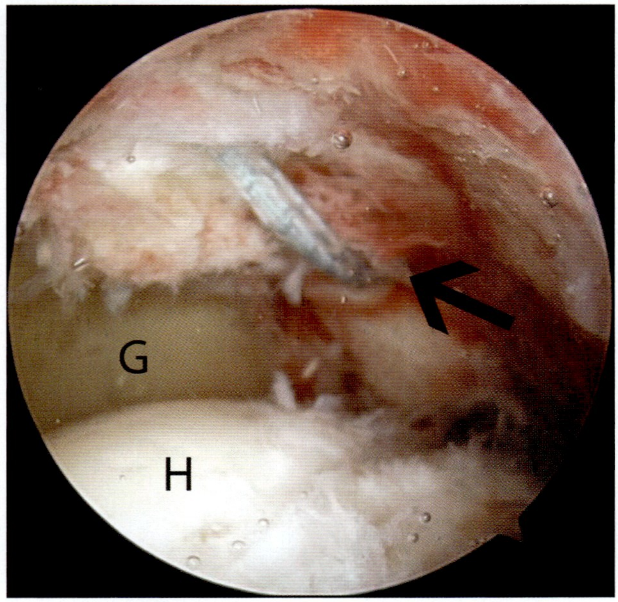

Figure 19.19 Left shoulder, view from the lateral portal demonstrates a traction stitch (*black arrow*) passed through the fragment at the rotator cuff–fracture junction. G, glenoid; H, humerus.

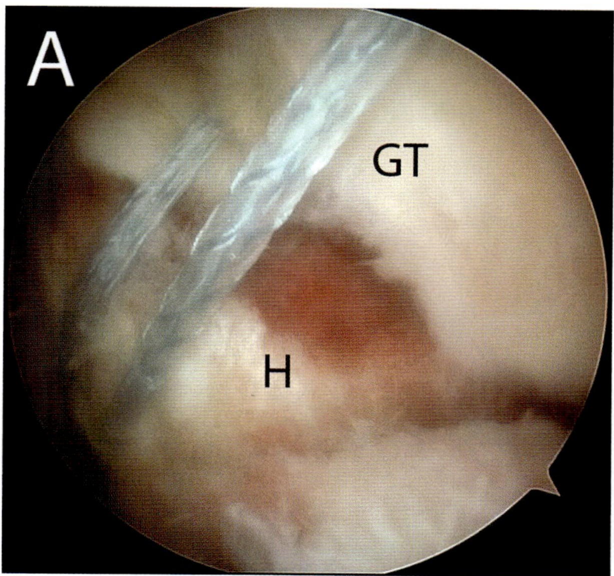

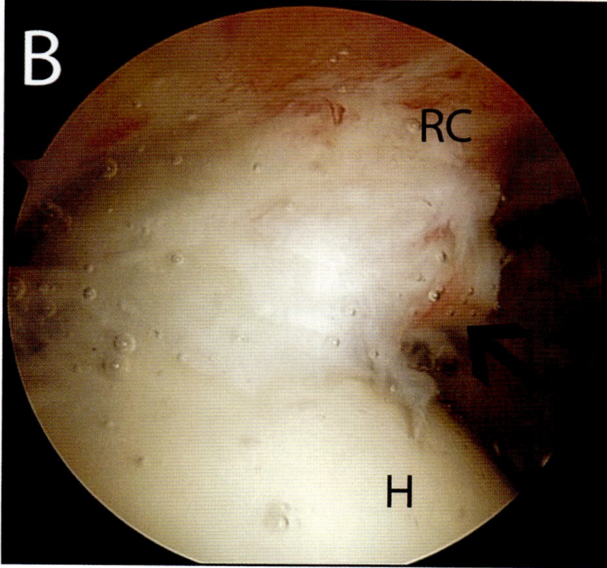

Figure 19.20 Provisional reduction of greater tuberosity fracture. **A:** Left shoulder, lateral subacromial viewing portal. Initial fixation is achieved by pulling the traction suture limbs laterally and securing them with a SwiveLock anchor (Arthrex, Inc., Naples, FL) laterally in the metaphyseal bone of the proximal humerus. **B:** After this initial reduction, the intra-articular view demonstrates improvement; however, a large bony fragment (*black arrow*) is sitting too proud. GT, greater tuberosity; H, humerus; RC, rotator cuff.

while visualizing intra-articularly (Fig. 19.22). The arthroscope is reinserted in the subacromial space, and the medial FiberTape limbs are secured laterally with two additional lateral SwiveLock C anchors. Compression of the fracture is achieved by tensioning the FiberTape suture prior to seating the eyelet for the SwiveLock anchor. Usually, simply removing the slack in the suture adequately reduces the fracture fragment. A switching stick or other blunt instrument can be utilized to assist with the fracture reduction. Abduction of the arm is also helpful to decrease tension on the reduction. Once both anchors are secured laterally, the reduction is evaluated subacromially and intra-articularly. The eyelet sutures from the SwiveLock C anchors are not removed until reduction is felt to be satisfactory since these can be used for additional sites of fixation if necessary (Fig. 19.23). The final reduction can also be confirmed with intraoperative fluoroscopy (Fig. 19.24).

Video

Rehabilitation after such a repair is identical to rotator cuff repair rehabilitation with the exception that radiographs are obtained at frequent intervals postoperatively until healing is observed. Passive motion is delayed until 6 weeks postoperatively and strengthening is delayed until 4 months postoperatively to minimize the chance of redisplacement of the fracture.

Tuberoplasty and Rotator Cuff Retensioning for Greater Tuberosity Malunion

The second role for arthroscopy in proximal humerus fractures is managing sequelae including posttraumatic or postsurgical stiffness (see Chapter 21, "Shoulder Stiffness") and malunion. The most common malunion deformities following proximal humerus fractures are varus of the humeral head in relation to the shaft and posterosuperior displacement of the greater tuberosity. Both deformities lead to dysfunction of the rotator cuff by altering the normal length–tension relationships of the muscle-tendon units. As the Blix curve describes, maintenance of length is required for a muscle to generate adequate tension. Rotator cuff tear models have shown that muscle retraction leads to loss of force generation. Similarly, an alteration of the function of the rotator cuff in relation to malunion of the proximal humerus has been attributed to shortening of the muscle tendon unit and to changes in muscle force vectors. Reestablishment of this biomechanical relationship is required to restore rotator cuff function. It is with this philosophy that we have performed tuberoplasty and rotator cuff advancement in the setting of a head-shaft varus malunion or a malunion of the greater tuberosity (Figs. 19.25 to 19.27). We have observed a substantial amount of improvement in range of motion and a high degree of patient satisfaction and return to activity with this approach (1). We have this technique particularly rewarding in younger adults without glenohumeral arthritis. In this setting the advanced shoulder arthroscopist may avoid procedures such as osteotomy or hemiarthroplasty, which have both been associated with unpredictable outcomes.

A diagnostic arthroscopy is performed and associated pathology is identified and addressed if necessary. Preoperative passive range-of-motion loss is addressed

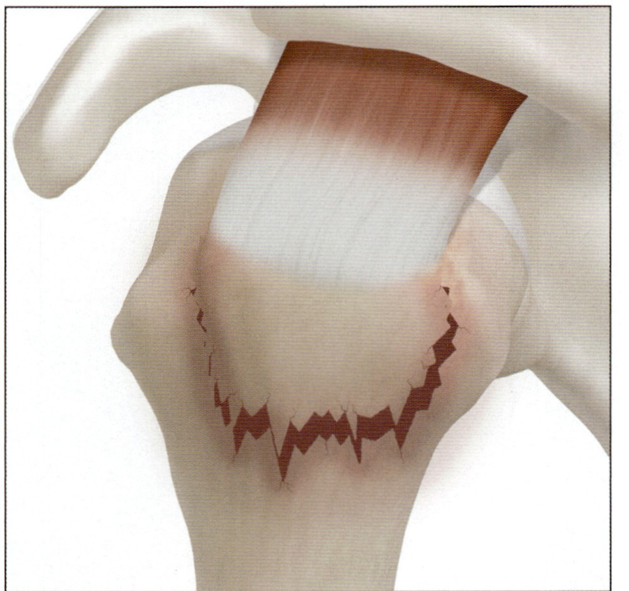

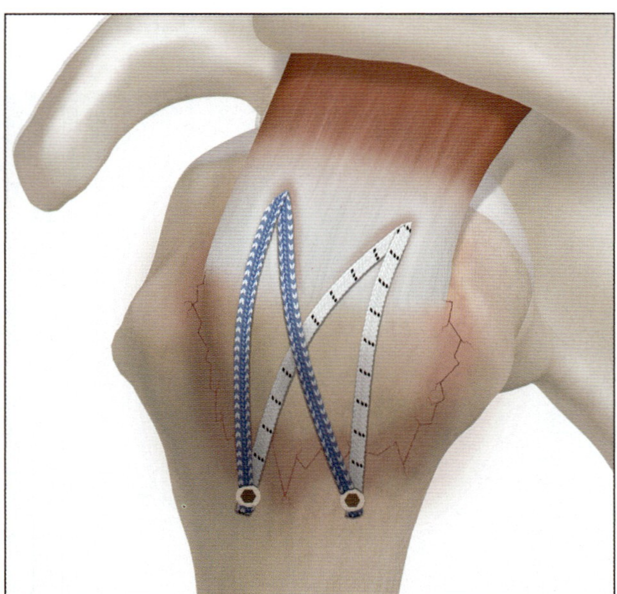

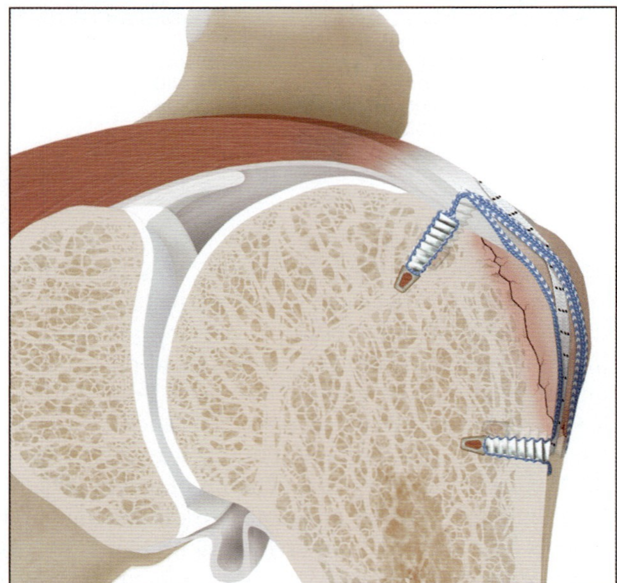

Figure 19.21 Schematic of a SpeedBridge (Arthrex, Inc., Naples, FL) repair of a greater tuberosity fracture. **A:** A displaced greater tuberosity fracture can result in dysfunction of the rotator cuff due to loss of the normal length–tension relationship, as well as impingement due to superior migration of the fracture fragment. **B:** Arthroscopic reduction can be performed with a SpeedBridge technique. Two medial BioComposite SwiveLock C anchors preloaded with FiberTape are linked to two lateral BioComposite SwiveLock C anchors to anatomically reduce the fracture fragment. **C:** Coronal view of the repair construct.

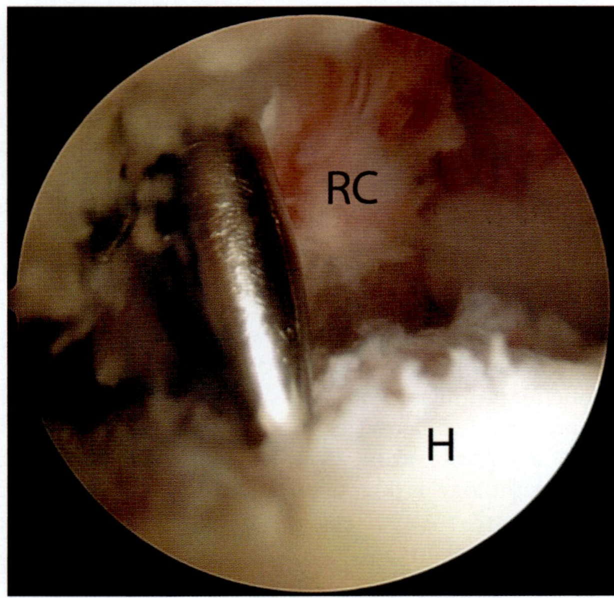

Figure 19.22 While visualizing intra-articularly from a posterior glenohumeral portal in a left shoulder, a SwiveLock C anchor preloaded with FiberTape (Arthrex, Inc., Naples, FL) is passed transtendon into the intact greater tuberosity bone. This photo demonstrates the placement of the punch for the posteromedial anchor. A second anchor will be placed anterior to this one. H, humeral head; RC, rotator cuff.

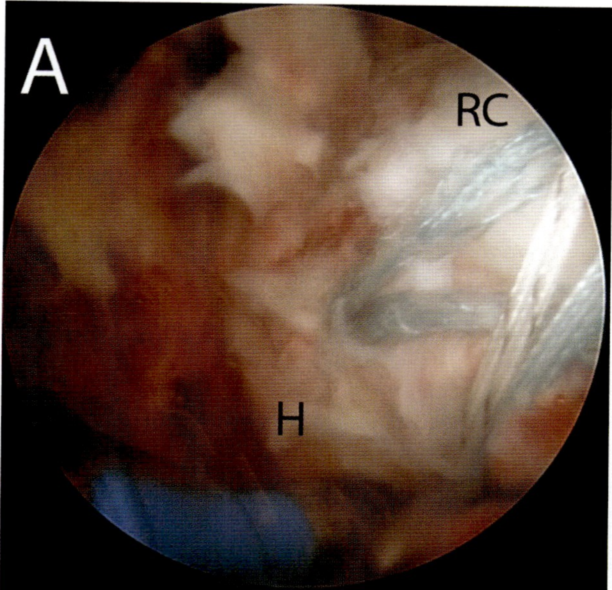

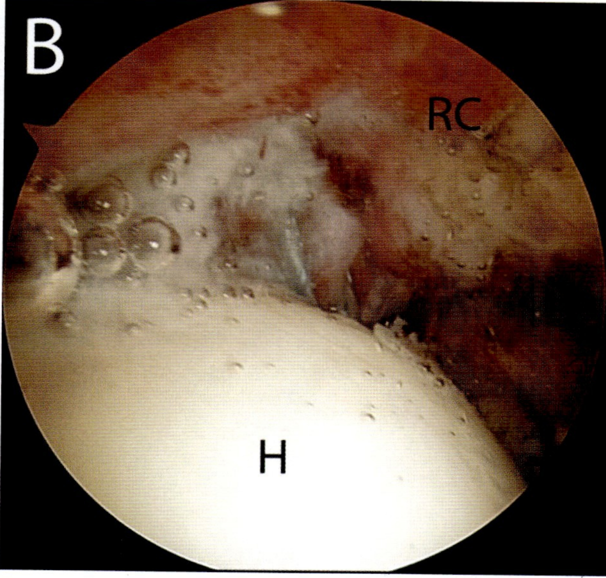

Figure 19.23 Final SpeedBridge repair of greater tuberosity fracture in a left shoulder viewed from **(A)** a posterior subacromial portal with a 70° arthroscope, and **(B)** a posterior glenohumeral portal. H, humerus; RC, rotator cuff.

with a complete capsular release (see Chapter 21, "Shoulder Stiffness"). Removal of any hardware is delayed until after the capsular release and manipulation under anesthesia are performed. Biceps pathology is common in this setting and may require tenodesis.

Viewing intra-articularly, the tuberoplasty begins by delineating the anterior and posterior borders of the superior facet of the greater tuberosity with two spinal needles. The needles are placed parallel to the tuberosity as much as possible. Because of the pull of the rotator cuff, the tuberosity is usually malunited posterior and superior to its normal location. The arthroscope is moved to the subacromial space and a bursectomy is performed via a lateral portal. The lateral extent of the rotator cuff insertion is identified with a spinal needle.

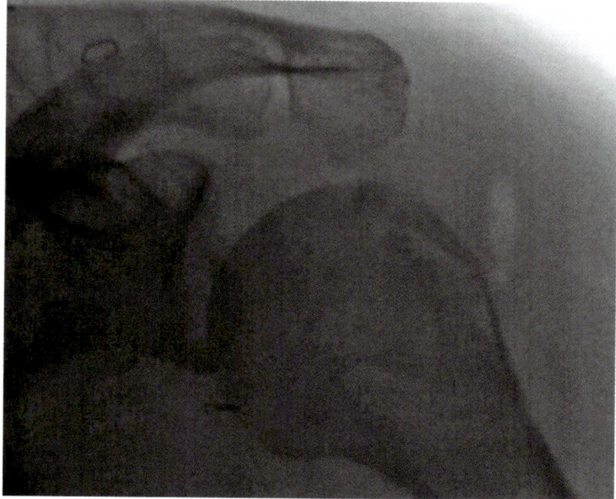

Figure 19.24 Intraoperative fluoroscopic imaging can be used to confirm anatomical restoration of a greater tuberosity fracture repaired with a SpeedBridge technique (Arthrex, Inc., Naples, FL).

The supraspinatus and anterior half of the infraspinatus insertions are elevated from the greater tuberosity with a sharp knife or a pencil tip electrocautery (Fig. 19.28). It is important to stay directly on bone to maximize the amount of tendinous rotator cuff for later repair. Elevation of the rotator cuff consists of the supraspinatus and anterior half of the infraspinatus, which is the part that overlies the proximally migrated tuberosity (Fig. 19.29). Once the rotator cuff is elevated, an electrocautery is used to fully identify the malunited tuberosity fragment. A burr is then used to perform a tuberoplasty (Fig. 19.30). The goal of the tuberoplasty is to remove any areas of potential impingement and restore biomechanical function of the rotator cuff.

Once an adequate tuberoplasty is performed, the procedure proceeds as a rotator cuff repair via a SpeedBridge or SutureBridge technique (Figs. 19.31 and 19.32) (see Chapter 4, "Complete Rotator Cuff Tears"). A standard acromioplasty is then performed. Rehabilitation is also identical to our rotator cuff protocol.

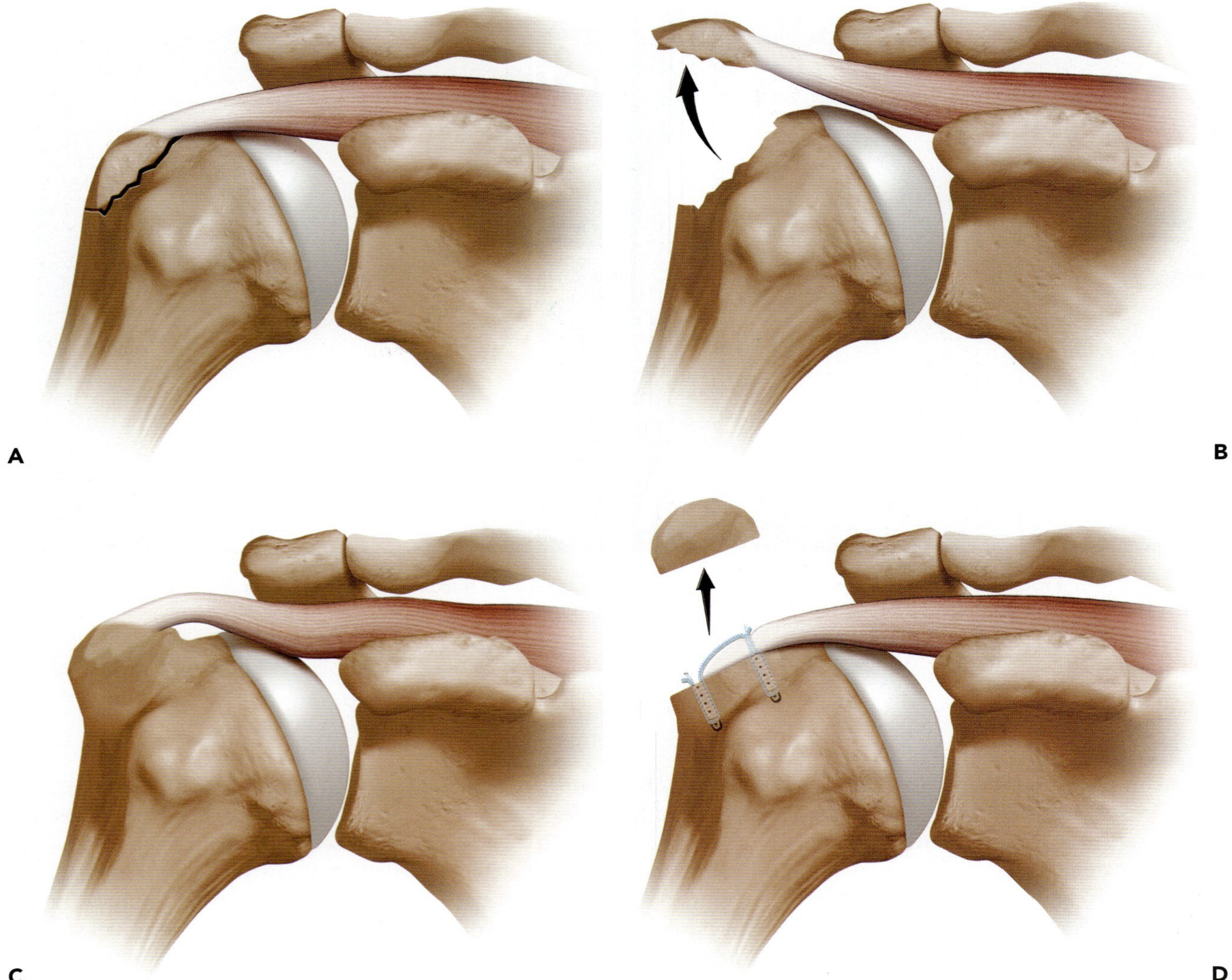

Figure 19.25 Schematic of a tuberoplasty for a greater tuberosity malunion. **A:** Intact greater tuberosity. **B:** Fracture of the greater tuberosity results in superior displacement (*curved black arrow*). **C:** Greater tuberosity malunited superiorly results in dysfunction of the rotator cuff because the length–tension relationship is altered. **D:** The rotator cuff is detached, a tuberoplasty (*straight black arrow*) is performed with a burr, and the rotator cuff is repaired. The repair results in restoration of the normal length–tension relationship of the rotator cuff.

DISTAL CLAVICLE FRACTURES

The vast majority of clavicle fractures occur in the midshaft. Approximately 25% of clavicle fractures occur in the lateral third of the clavicle and are categorized as distal clavicle fractures. These fractures have a relatively high incidence of persistent clinical symptoms and also a substantial risk of fracture nonunion or malunion. These sequelae are related to multiple deforming forces and ligamentous restraints in the distal end of the clavicle. The clavicle is a strut that connects the arm to the trunk through its relationship with the scapula. The coracoclavicular (CC) ligaments, which provide ligamentous connection between the clavicle and coracoid process of the scapular, resist superior translation of the clavicle. The acromioclavicular (AC) joint ligaments link the acromion and clavicle at the AC joint and provide the primary stabilization against anterior and posterior forces. Deforming forces exerted upon the distal clavicle include the weight of the arm that provides an inferior force; the trapezius that exerts superior, medial, and posterior forces; and the sternocleidomastoid that inserts on the proximal clavicle and exerts a superior force.

Distal clavicle fractures can occur in various locations and have been classified into types I through III (Table 19.1; Fig. 19.33). Depending on the location of the fracture, significant bone displacement occurs in up to

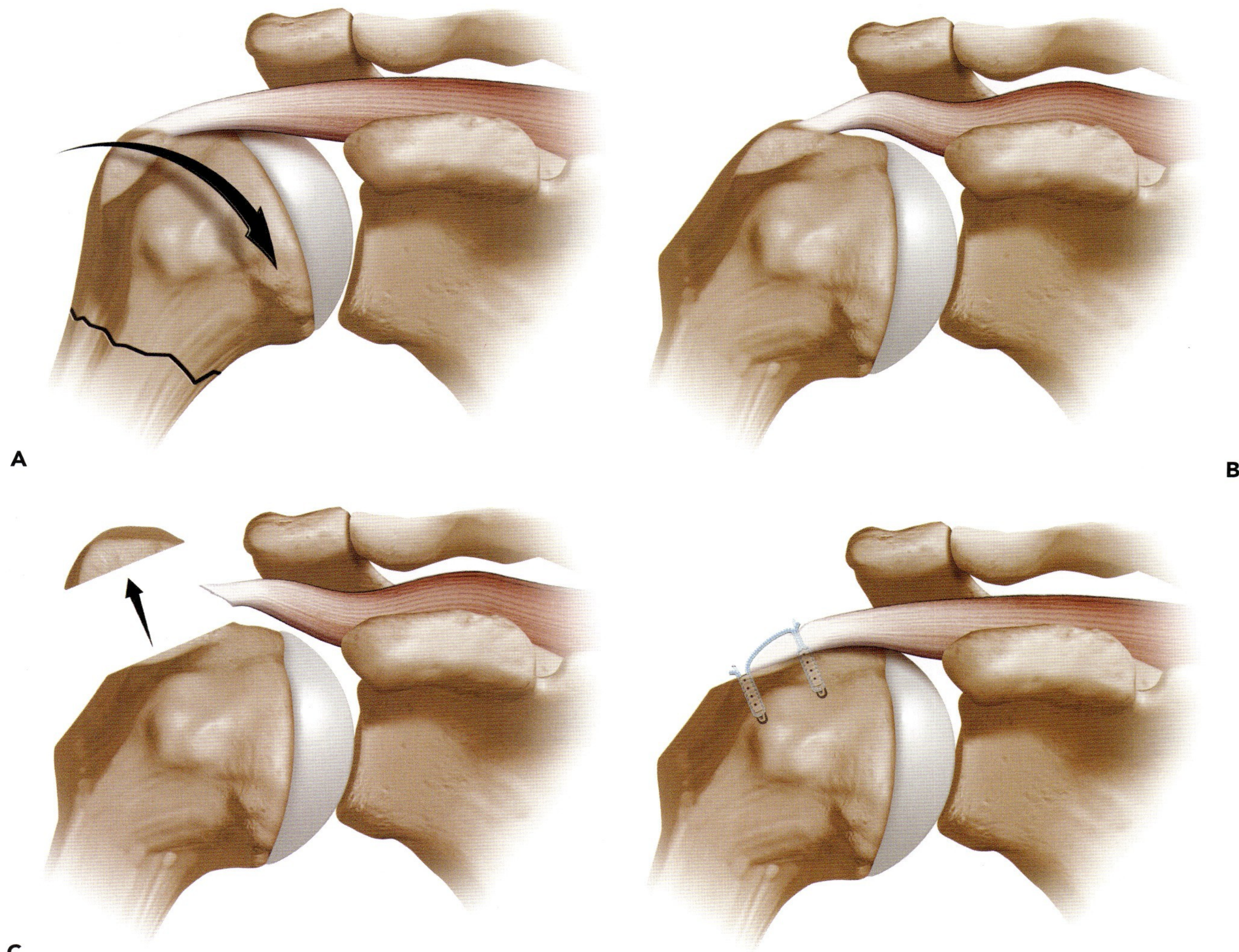

Figure 19.26 Schematic of a tuberoplasty for a varus malunion of a surgical neck fracture. **A:** Intact proximal humerus. **B:** Varus malunion (*curved black arrow*) results in a medialized greater tuberosity and effectively decreases the resting tension in the rotator cuff. As a result, force generation is compromised. **C:** The rotator cuff is detached, and a tuberoplasty (*straight black arrow*) is performed with a burr. **D:** Reattachment of the rotator cuff laterally results in restoration of the rotator cuff length–tension relationship.

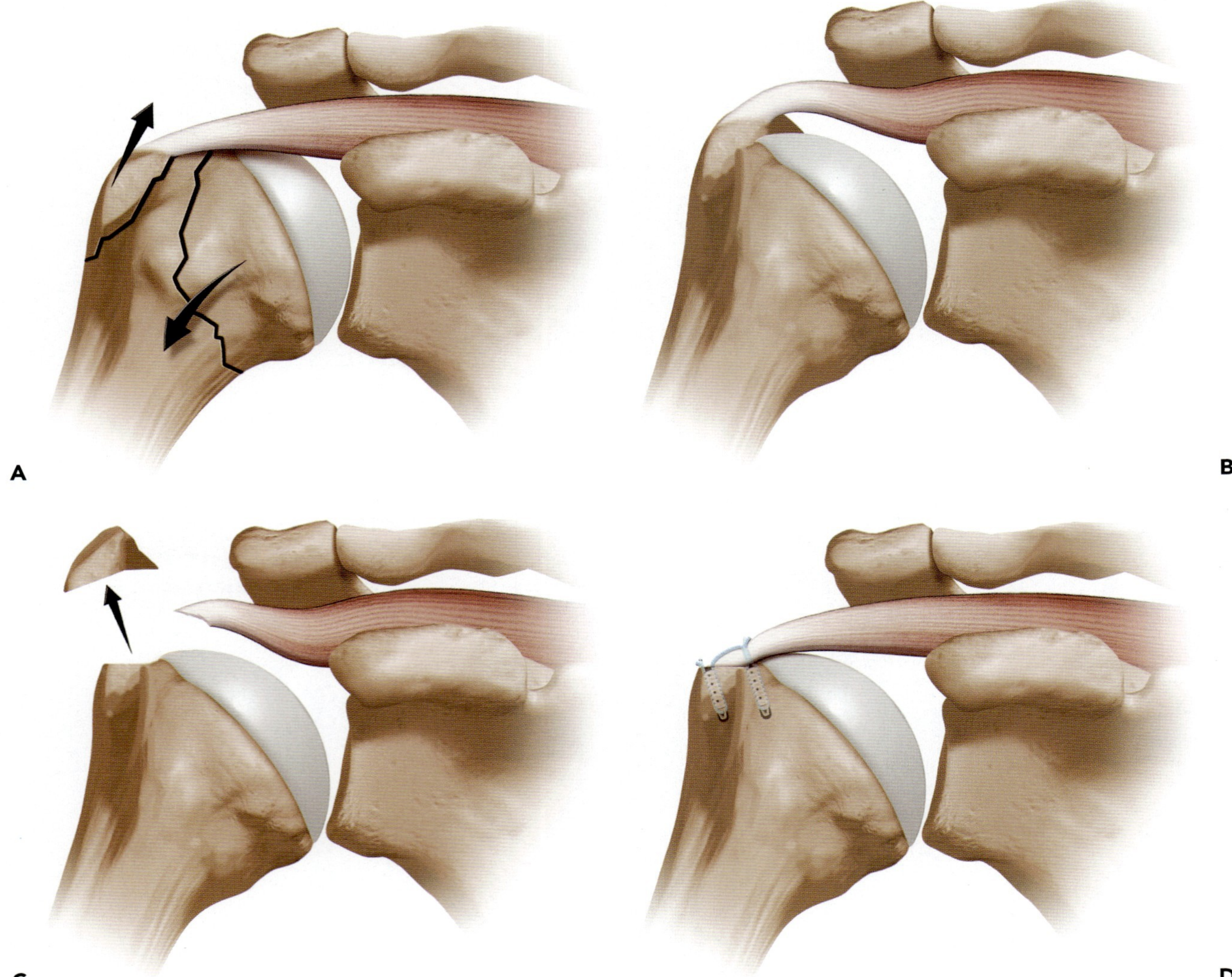

Figure 19.27 Schematic of a tuberoplasty for a valgus malunion of a three-part proximal humerus fracture. **A:** Intact proximal humerus. **B:** Valgus impaction (*curved black arrows*) results in superior displacement of the greater tuberosity and effectively decreases the resting tension in the rotator cuff. As a result, force generation is compromised. **C:** The rotator cuff is detached and a tuberoplasty (*straight black arrow*) is performed with a burr **D:** Reattachment of the rotator cuff laterally results in restoration of the rotator cuff length–tension relationship.

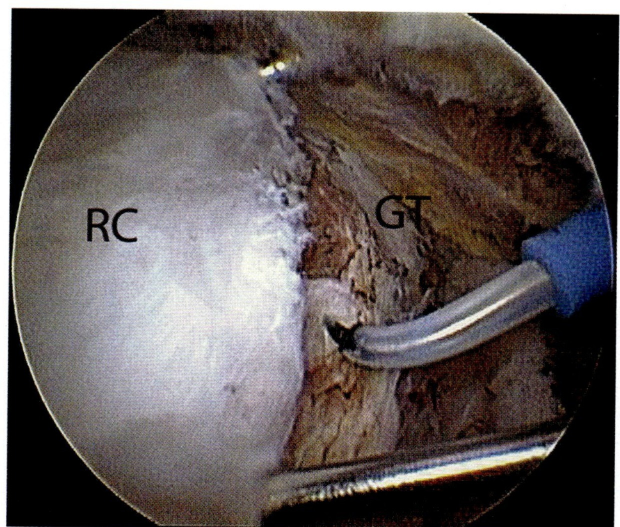

Figure 19.28 Right shoulder, posterior subacromial viewing portal. The anterior and posterior borders of the malunited greater tuberosity are marked with two spinal needles A pencil-tip electrocautery is used to sharply elevate the rotator cuff insertion from the malunited footprint. GT, greater tuberosity; RC, rotator cuff.

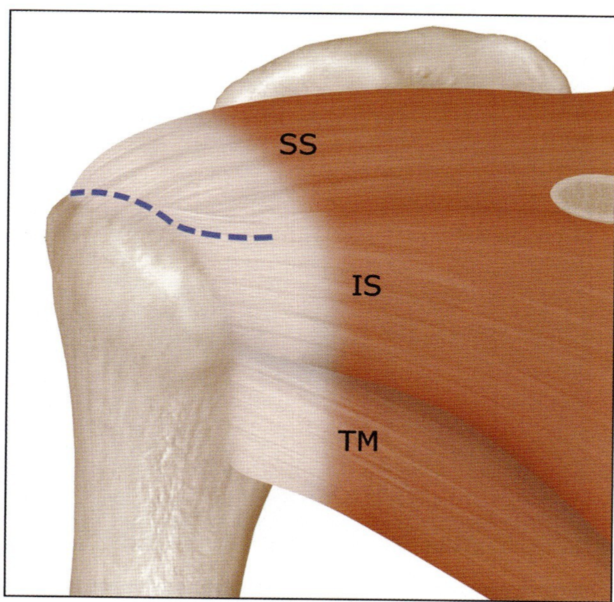

Figure 19.29 Schematic demonstrating the rotator cuff elevation (*dashed blue line*) that is performed to access the greater tuberosity for a tuberoplasty. The entire supraspinatus (SS) is elevated. Additionally, because the anterior half of the infraspinatus (IS) curves anterior to insert on the greater tuberosity, it must also be elevated to expose the greater tuberosity. TM, teres minor.

35% of all distal clavicle fractures. In particular, the location of the fracture will have a tremendous effect on what occurs with the proximal shaft fragment and thus will have a significant effect on the alignment and the outcome of the fracture.

The most common displaced distal clavicle fracture subtype is the type II fracture pattern. With this pattern, the fracture line is medial to (type IIa) or within (type IIb) the CC ligaments, and the proximal clavicle has no ligamentous restraint against inferior displacement of the lateral bone due to the weight of the arm. In addition, muscle attachments exert a superior force on the proximal fragment. This creates substantial fracture displacement and thus makes these fractures much more prone to symptomatic nonunion. While conservative treatment can be attempted, we typically counsel most patients with this fracture pattern that operative fixation is preferable. Fortunately, there now exist minimally invasive options for potential treatment of such fractures.

Type III fractures are not very common but nonetheless can be problematic. The fracture line extends intra-articularly into the AC joint. The fracture fragment itself is often quite small and can be comminuted, thus making osteosynthesis difficult as adequate distal bony fixation can be impossible. Since the CC ligaments are not disrupted, overall the fracture usually maintains a fairly good alignment, and nonoperative treatment may fare acceptably. However, sometimes these fractures remain chronically symptomatic, and an effective option can be simply an arthroscopic excision of the distal clavicle fracture fragment.

Type II Fracture Stabilization

As mentioned, we typically counsel patients toward operative treatment of type II distal clavicle fractures. However, determining the appropriate treatment can be challenging. In our practice, the most important factor with these fractures is the size and quality of the distal clavicle fragment. If the distal fragment is large and the patient is healthy (with good bone quality), then we typically utilize a locking plate (Arthrex, Inc., Naples, FL).

When dealing with a type II fracture where the distal fragment is either highly comminuted or of poor quality, we will elect to perform an arthroscopic-assisted AC joint stabilization procedure and in some cases we will excise the distal clavicle fragments. In the acute setting we will utilize the Dog Bone (Arthrex, Inc., Naples, FL) construct, and in the chronic setting we will utilize the GraftRope device (Fig 19.34). The arthroscopic assistance is also important because a substantial percentage of these injuries also have concomitant intra-articular or subacromial pathology that can be addressed arthroscopically during the same surgery.

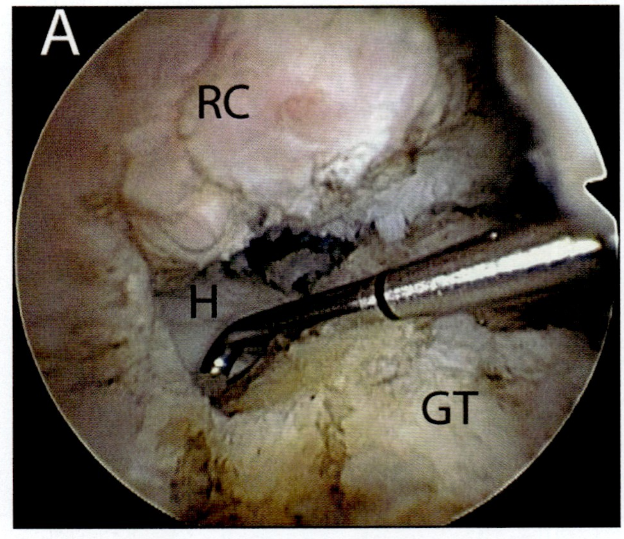

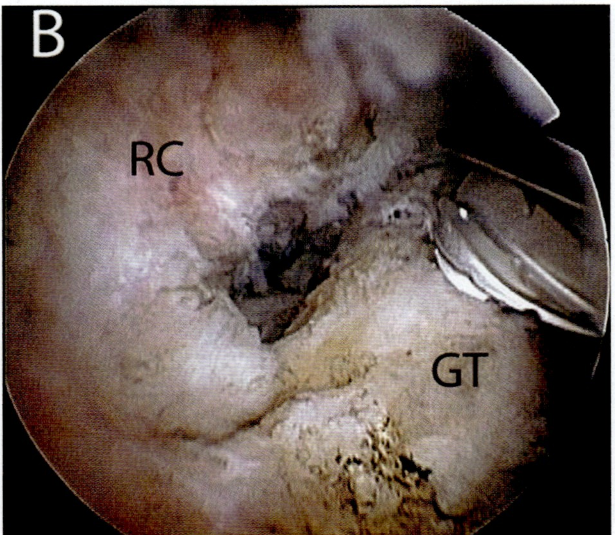

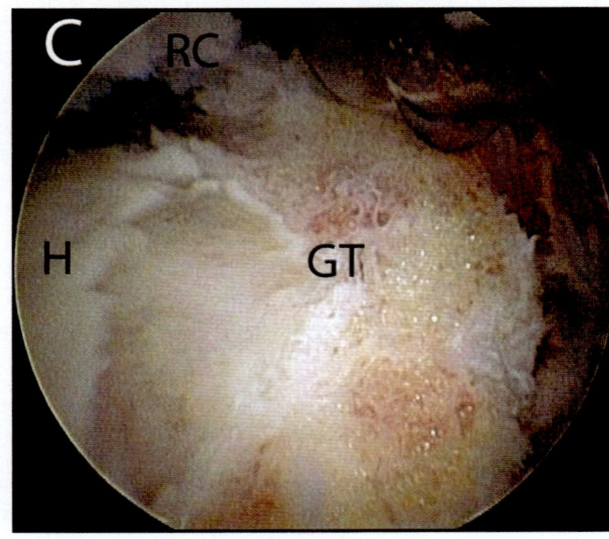

Figure 19.30 Right shoulder, posterior subacromial viewing portal demonstrating arthroscopic tuberoplasty in preparation for retensioning of the rotator cuff. **A:** The greater tuberosity has malunited in a superior position. As shown with the calibrated probe, the top of the greater tuberosity is now nearly 1 cm above the top of the humeral head. **B:** A tuberoplasty of the greater tuberosity is performed with a burr. **C:** The tuberoplasty is complete when the greater tuberosity bone bed is approximately level with the height of the humeral head. H, humerus; GT, greater tuberosity; RC, rotator cuff.

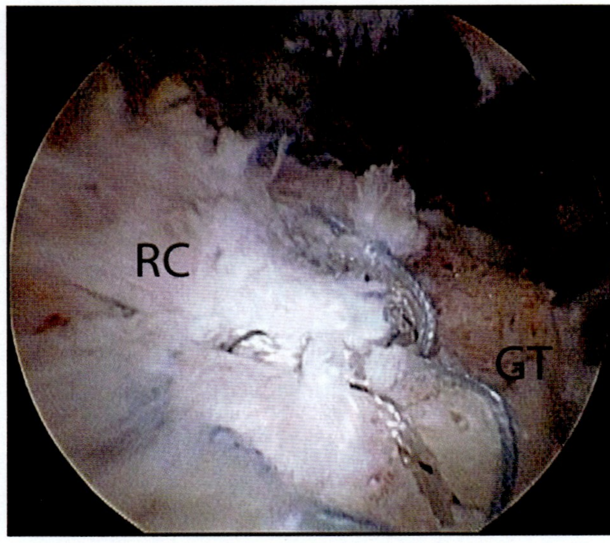

Figure 19.31 Right shoulder, lateral subacromial viewing portal demonstrating rotator cuff retensioned and repaired with a SutureBridge (Arthrex, Inc., Naples, FL) linked double-row footprint restoration technique. GT, greater tuberosity; RC, rotator cuff.

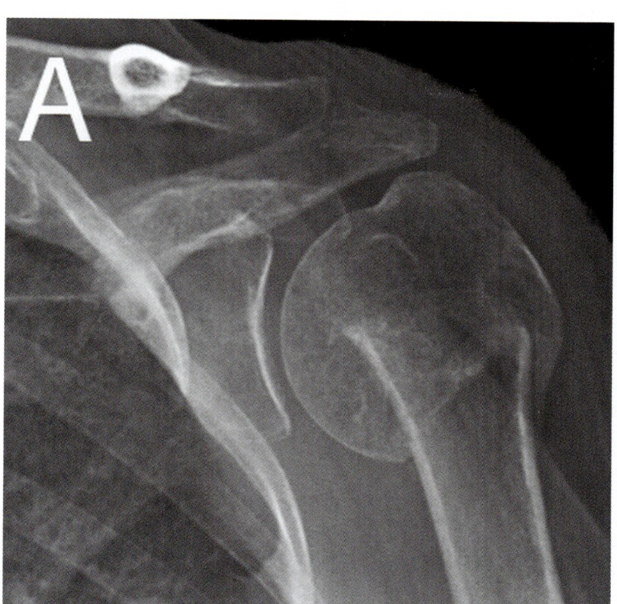

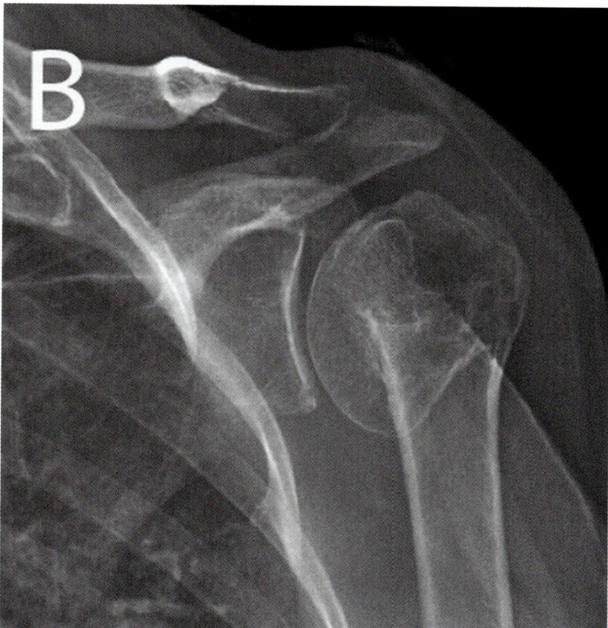

Figure 19.32 **A:** Preoperative AP radiograph of a left shoulder showing a varus malunion. The greater tuberosity is medialized relative to normal anatomy, and the acromiohumeral distance is decreased to 4.6 mm. **B:** Following arthroscopic tuberoplasty and retensioning of the rotator cuff, the acromiohumeral distance is restored (9.5 mm) to normal values.

TABLE 19.1
CLASSIFICATION OF DISTAL CLAVICLE FRACTURES

Type	Description
I	Fracture lateral to CC ligaments; results in little displacement
II	Fracture medial to or between the CC ligaments; affects vertical stability and results in displacement
IIa	Both the conoid and trapezoid attached to the distal fragment
IIb	Fracture line extends through the conoid ligament, and trapezoid ligament still intact and attached to the distal fragment
III	Fracture extends into the articular surface

Percutaneous Fracture Approximation without Osteosynthesis

Another potential technique in the treatment of type II distal clavicle fractures is to simply reduce the clavicle shaft back down into an appropriate position via an arthroscopic Dog Bone or TightRope CC fixation technique as described for AC joint separations (see Chapter 18, "The Acromioclavicular Joint"). With either a type IIa or IIb fracture pattern in a healthy individual, plate osteosynthesis may be unnecessary. A less invasive option is to simply eliminate the fracture gap created with these fracture patterns via a CC fixation technique (Fig. 19.35). In the acute setting, reapproximation of the fracture ends without the soft tissue disruption of an open incision will provide a high likelihood of bony union. Thus the implant only needs to hold the fracture in a reduced position for approximately 12 weeks for union to

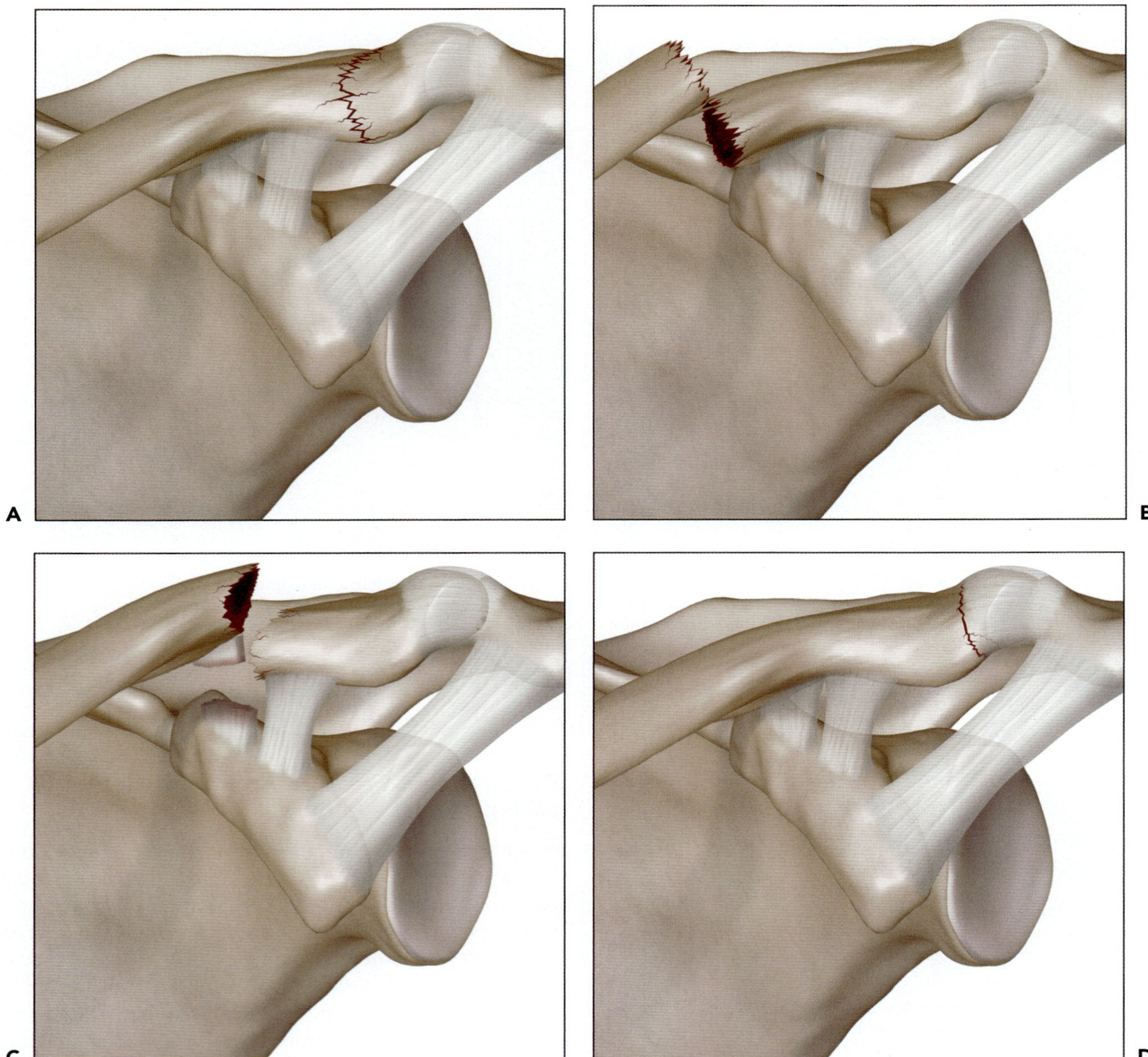

Figure 19.33 Schematic of the different types of distal clavicle fractures. **A:** A type I fracture occurs lateral to the CC ligaments. **B:** A type IIa fracture occurs medial to the CC ligaments. **C:** A type IIb fracture occurs between the CC ligaments. **D:** A type III fracture is intra-articular.

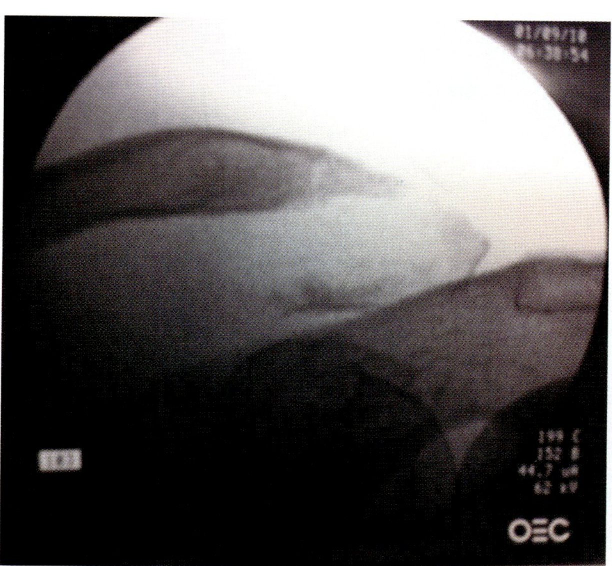

A

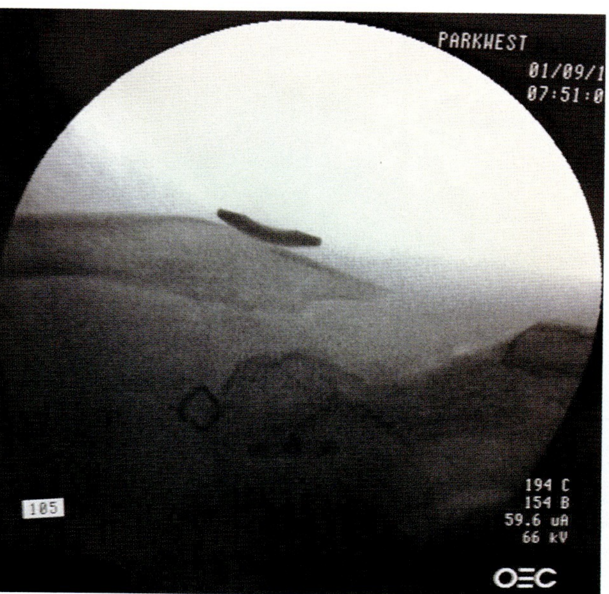

B

Figure 19.34 **A:** Preoperative fluoroscopic image of a left shoulder demonstrates a chronic nonunion of a type II distal clavicle fracture. **B:** Postoperative fluoroscopic image of the same shoulder following excision of the fracture fragments (excised due to the chronicity of the fracture) and stabilization of the distal clavicle with a GraftRope device (Arthrex, Inc., Naples, FL).

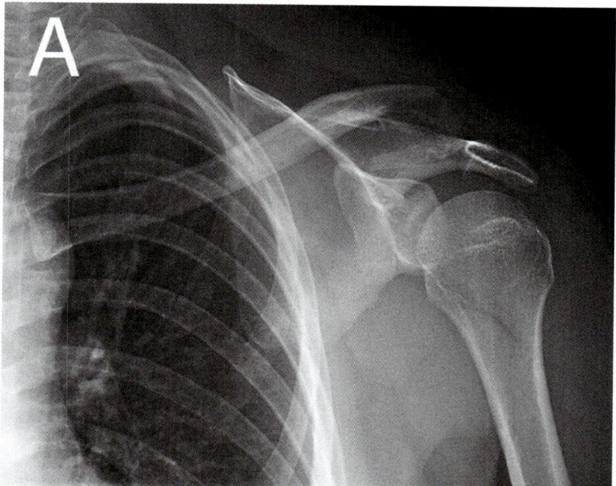

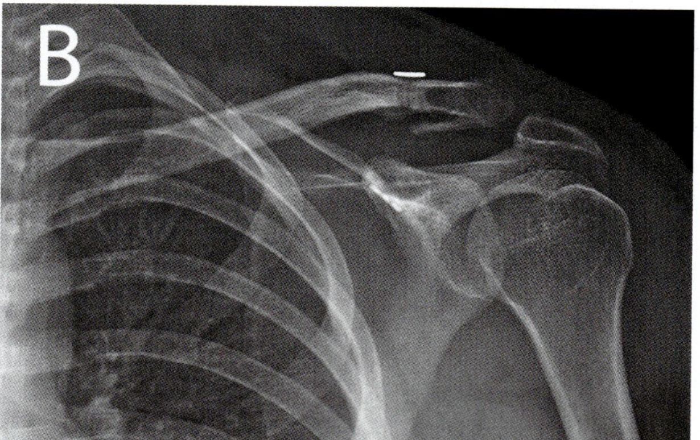

Figure 19.35 **A:** Preoperative radiograph of a left shoulder demonstrating a displaced distal clavicle fracture. **B:** Postoperative radiograph demonstrates reduction of the fracture and fixation with a TightRope device (Arthrex, Inc., Naples, FL).

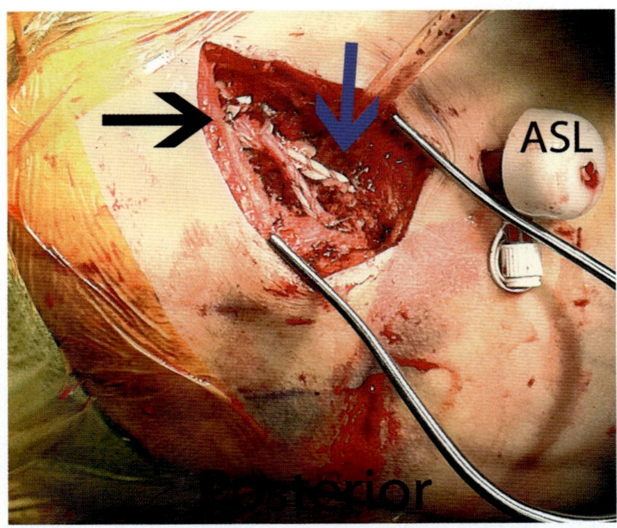

Figure 19.36 External image of a right shoulder demonstrates allograft reconstruction of the AC ligaments following excision of a chronic distal clavicle fracture. A CC reconstruction has been performed with a GraftRope device (*black arrow*). The allograft tendon limbs have been preserved and used laterally (*blue arrow*) to reconstruct the AC joint. ASL, anterosuperolateral portal.

occur. The arthroscopic assistance is also important because a substantial percentage of these injuries also have concomitant intra-articular or subacromial pathology that can be addressed arthroscopically during the same surgery.

Distal Clavicle Fracture Fragment Excision with AC Joint Reconstruction

Distal clavicle fracture fragment excision with AC joint reconstruction is used for chronic fractures (>6 weeks old), malunions, and nonunions. A diagnostic arthroscopy is performed. The distal clavicle fragment is excised via a small open incision. An arthroscopic CC reconstruction is then performed using a GraftRope (Arthrex, Inc., Naples, FL) as described for chronic AC joint separations (see Chapter 18, "The Acromioclavicular Joint"). In addition, however, after the GraftRope and allograft or autograft are secured, a reconstruction of the AC joint ligaments is also performed.

In contrast to the procedure for chronic AC joint separations, the tails of the graft are preserved rather than cut flush with the clavicle. The acromion surface is then roughened with a rongeur to facilitate healing of the graft. Two #2 FiberWire (Arthrex, Inc., Naples, FL) sutures are passed through the clavicular facet of the acromion. The graft tails from the CC reconstruction are then pulled laterally and tied to the #2 FiberWire passing through the acromion. Excess graft tissue is cut. The graft is secured to the acromion in order to reconstruct the superior AC restraint and thus potentially improve anterior–posterior stability of the clavicle in relation to the acromion (Fig. 19.36).

SUMMARY

As arthroscopic techniques have advanced, there are more and more fractures that we are able to effectively manage arthroscopically. The development of the arthroscopic percutaneous fixation techniques has made ARIF even more feasible. Although these procedures are technically demanding, with careful and meticulous attention to detail the surgeon can achieve excellent outcomes.

REFERENCE

1. Lädermann A, Denard PJ, Burkhart SS. Arthroscopic management of proximal humerus malunion with tuberoplasty and rotator cuff re-tensioning. *Arthroscopy* 2012; In press.

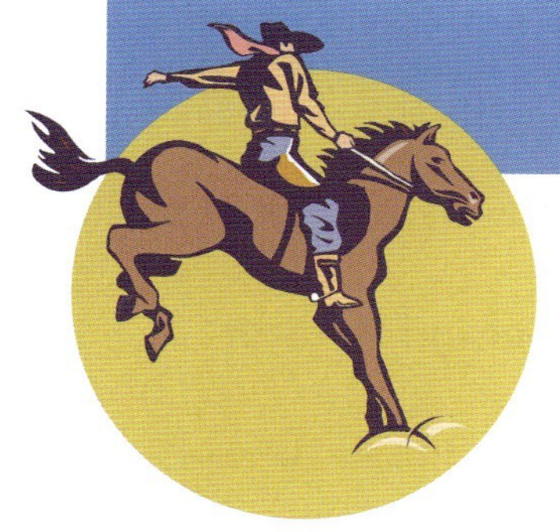

20

Postoperative Rehabilitation

WESTERN WISDOM

A cow outfit is no better than its horses.

Rehabilitation following arthroscopic shoulder surgery is as important as performing a technically sound procedure. Our general philosophy is that stiffness is a complication, but a retear of the rotator cuff or recurrence of instability is a failure. In most cases, stiffness in the postoperative period is transient and resolves with a stretching program (1). The incidence of resistant stiffness (stiffness resistant to stretching) with our rehabilitation protocols is extremely low (2). Moreover, as fully discussed in the next chapter (Chapter 21, "Shoulder Stiffness"), resistant stiffness can reliably be overcome with an arthroscopic capsular release. For these reasons, our protocols are conservative compared to some authors. Our evidence-based rehabilitation protocols emphasize healing first, followed by restoration of range of motion, and then strengthening. All our programs are surgeon directed with the initial exercises performed by the patient. Formal physical therapy is considered when strengthening begins or occasionally earlier if the patient needs additional assistance.

ARTHROSCOPIC ROTATOR CUFF REPAIR REHABILITATION PROTOCOLS

Historically, postoperative stiffness was one of the most devastating complications for open shoulder surgeons since there was no effective open surgical treatment for stiffness. Efforts to avoid stiffness led to the popularization of early passive range of motion following rotator cuff repair (3,4). Recent basic science investigations, however, have shown that early passive mobilization may actually encourage stiffness. Furthermore, early passive motion produces strains on the rotator cuff that can compromise healing. In a rat model of rotator cuff repair, Peltz el al. (5) demonstrated that immediate passive range of motion actually led to increased stiffness compared to a continued immobilization protocol. Sarver et al. (6) reported that immobilization following rotator cuff repair led to stiffness that was transient only. In addition to its role in the development of stiffness, immobilization following rotator cuff repair may lead to increased healing potential. Gimbel and colleagues found that immobilization led to enhanced mechanical properties of repaired rat supraspinatus tendons (7). In a histological evaluation of rotator cuff healing in a primate model, Sonnabend et al. (8) reported that maturation of the repaired rotator cuff requires 12 to 15 weeks. In summary, the above basic science investigations demonstrate that the ideal rehabilitation protocol to prevent stiffness and encourage healing following rotator cuff repair includes an initial period of immobilization.

In addition to the above information, our considerations in the rehabilitation protocol following arthroscopic rotator cuff repair include tear size, subscapularis involvement, concomitant labral repair, and propensity for postoperative stiffness (e.g., adhesive capsulitis and calcific tendonitis). Tear size, concomitant labral repair, and concomitant diagnoses affect the addition of early closed-chain passive forward flexion. Subscapularis tears affect the amount of immediate external rotation. Tear size and revision repairs affect the time to initiation of strengthening.

Partial-thickness Tears and Single-tendon Full-thickness Tears (≤3 cm)

Patients with partial-thickness tears and single-tendon tears are more prone to postoperative stiffness. These patients are placed in a sling for 6 weeks, which they may remove for showering and meals. Elbow flexion and extension and hand and wrist exercises begin immediate post-op. We begin passive external rotation with a stick immediately post-op (Fig. 20.1). If there is an associated full-thickness subscapularis repair of more than 30% of the tendon, we restrict external rotation to 0°. With subscapularis tears of ≤30% of the tendon, we allow 30° of passive external rotation. Closed-chain passive forward flexion stretches via table slides begin immediately post-op (Fig. 20.2). The addition of this exercise alone decreased postoperative stiffness from 13.5% for partial-thickness tears and 7.3% for single-tendon tears in the report by Huberty et al. (9), to 0% in the report by Koo et al. (2) Patients are instructed to perform passive external rotation and table slide exercises twice daily; each stretch is held for 10 seconds, with 10 repetitions per set, for 2 sets.

At 6 weeks post-op, the sling is discontinued. Patients begin passive overhead forward elevation with a rope and pulley (Fig. 20.3) and supine overhead stretches using the opposite arm (Fig. 20.4). Passive external rotation with a stick is continued. Passive internal rotation is delayed until 12 weeks post-op as this places significant strains on the anterior supraspinatus and upper subscapularis.

Strengthening with elastic bands begins at 12 weeks post-op. This is our "4-pack," which includes resisted internal and external rotation with the arm at the side, low row, and biceps curl (Fig. 20.5). The patient starts with the smallest diameter (yellow) elastic band and is encouraged to perform four sets of ten repetitions, twice a day. The patient progresses in band diameter as tolerated (red, then blue). The stretching program is continued during the strengthening phase.

Return to full activity is permitted at 6 months (Table 20.1).

Large, Massive, and Revision Rotator Cuff Repairs

The incidence of postoperative stiffness decreases as tear size increases and also decreases in revision cases. Consequently, for the first 12 weeks post-op, these patients follow the protocol outlined above with the exception that table slides are not performed immediately post-op. Strengthening is initiated at 12 weeks for large tears (3 to 5 cm). Strengthening is delayed until 16 weeks post-op for massive tears (>5 cm), tear involving an interval slide, or for revision repairs. Return to full activity is not allowed until 1 year post-op (Table 20.1).

Subscapularis Tendon Repair

In general, for most subscapularis tears, we delay external rotation beyond neutral until 6 weeks post-op. Other than that, the protocol is for the size of the major tear excluding the subscapularis. If the tear involves only a small portion of the upper subscapularis (≤30%), external rotation is allowed to 20° or 30° in the immediate postoperative period.

Biceps Tenodesis

A biceps tenodesis may be performed in conjunction with a rotator cuff repair. The rehabilitation protocol therefore is usually dictated by the standard protocol for the type of rotator cuff tear that was repaired. In either case,

A
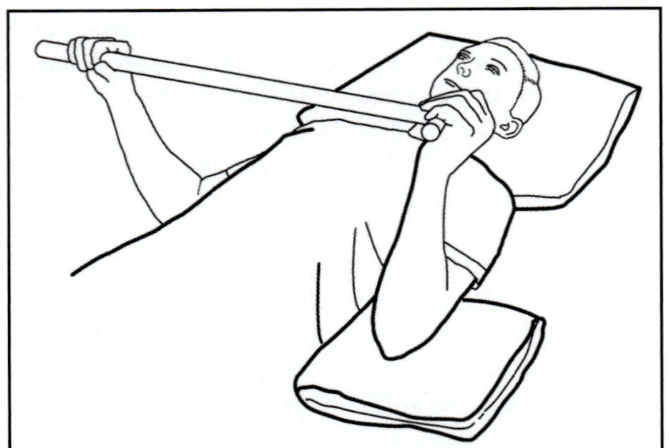
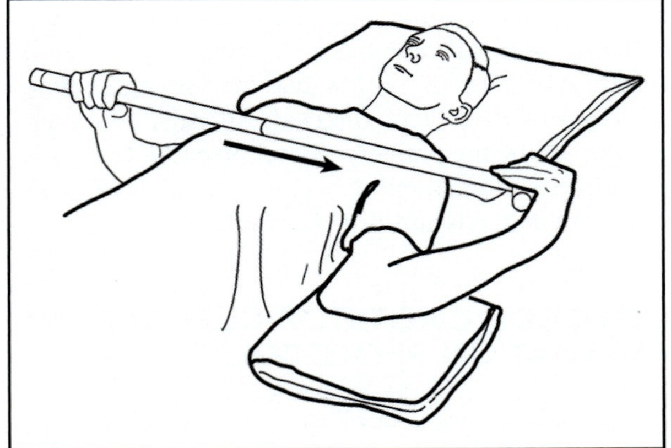
B

Figure 20.1 Passive external rotation is performed with the patient lying supine and the normal arm using a stick to passively externally rotate the operative arm. Note that a towel is placed under the elbow of the operative arm to facilitate the exercise. **A:** Starting position. **B:** Ending position.

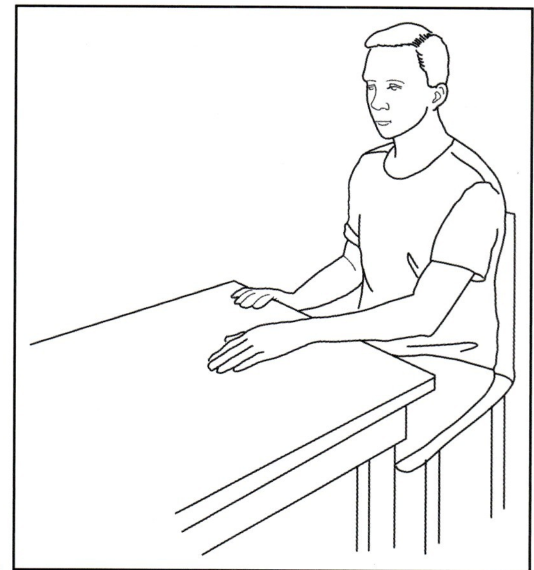

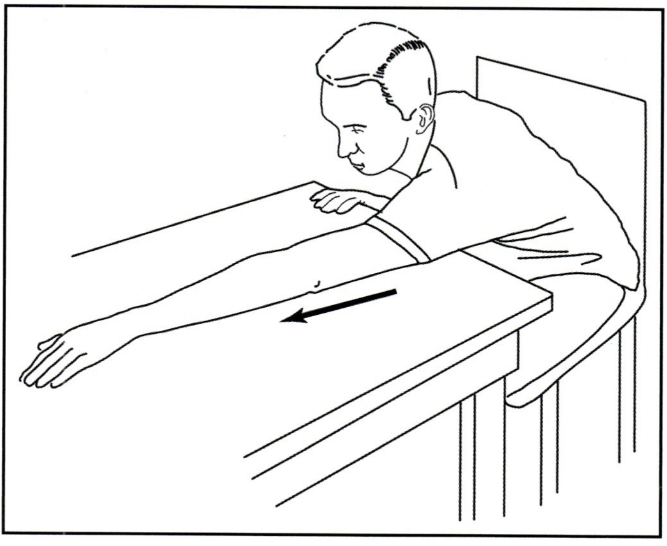

Figure 20.2 Table slide. **A:** Starting position. While seated at a table, the patient places the hand of the affected shoulder on a sliding surface (e.g., a magazine that slides over a smooth table surface). **B:** Ending position. The patient slides the hand forward, maintaining contact with the table, while the head and chest advance toward the table.

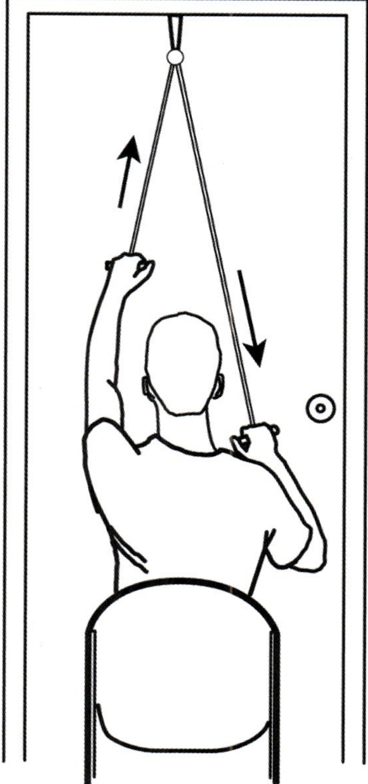

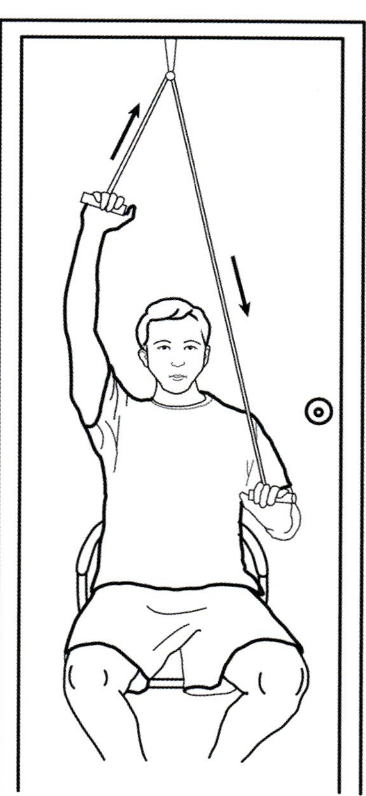

Figure 20.3 Overhead passive forward elevation is performed with a rope and pulley. With the patient seated, the normal arm passively elevates the operative arm via a pulley attached to the top of a door. **A:** The exercise begins with the patient facing the door and can be advanced to **(B)** the patient facing away from the door as rehabilitation progresses.

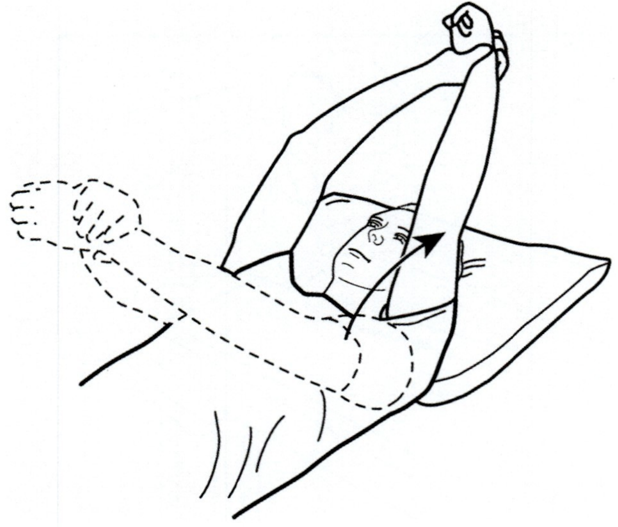

Figure 20.4 Supine passive forward flexion is accomplished by using the opposite arm to stretch the involved shoulder.

active flexion and extension of the elbow without resistance are allowed immediately post-op. In the absence of a rotator cuff repair, immediate closed-chain overhead motion is also encouraged (table slides). Strengthening is delayed until 12 weeks post-op since the patient will involuntarily contract the biceps when he or she is doing resisted internal and external rotation exercises.

Preoperative Adhesive Capsulitis or Calcific Tendinitis

In our initial study, we reported that patients with adhesive capsulitis (16%) or calcific tendinitis (17%) had an increased risk of stiffness following rotator cuff repair (9). Because of this, our rehabilitation protocol for these two categories of patients was modified to include the addition of early table slides. The protocol is therefore the same that is currently used following repair of a partial-thickness tear or single-tendon tear (see previous discussion).

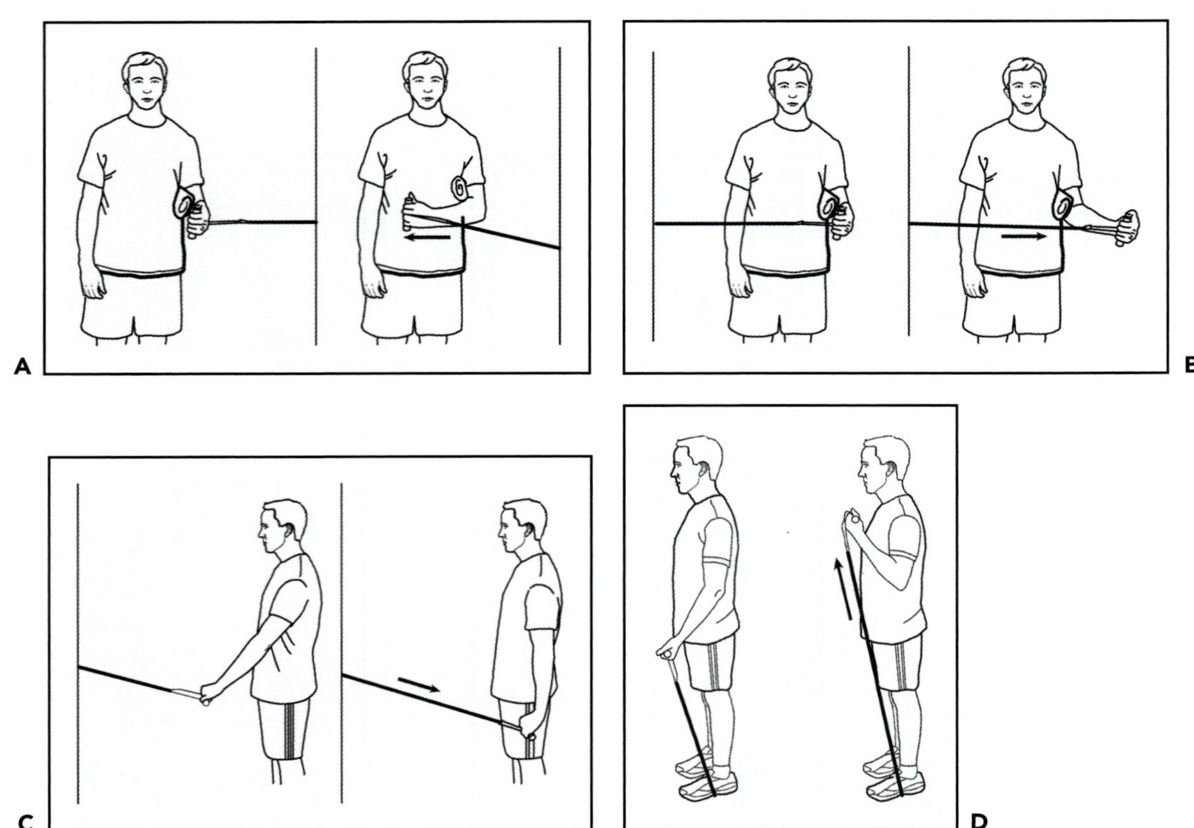

Figure 20.5 Four-pack strengthening exercises. **A:** Resisted internal rotation and **(B)** resisted external rotation are performed with the arm at the side and a towel in the axilla. **C:** One-armed low row. **D:** Biceps curl.

TABLE 20.1
REHABILITATION PROTOCOL FOLLOWING ARTHROSCOPIC ROTATOR CUFF REPAIR

Preoperative:
Surgeon-directed counseling on rehab plan
Give patient therapy kit and instruct on initial use
Therapy kit: Polyvinyl chloride (PVC) cane, rope and pulley, graduated elastic strengthening bands

Immediate postoperative period:
Patient placed in sling with small pillow
Surgeon gives patient and family specifics of rehab plan

Postoperative weeks 0–6:
At initial follow-up, the surgeon directs reinforcement of home rehabilitation plan
Remove sling three times per day for
- Active motion of hand, wrist, and elbow
- Passive external rotation of shoulder with arm at side (using PVC cane)
  - Limited to 45° for small to large posterior-superior cuff tears
  - Limited to 0° (straight ahead) for massive tears and subscapularis tears
- Table slides for partial-thickness and single-tendon tears

Postoperative weeks 7–12:
Discontinue sling and continue previous exercises:
- Advance passive external rotation with cane (limit to that of opposite shoulder)
- Continue with table slides and add rope and pulley overhead stretch
- No strengthening

Postoperative months 3–6:
Continue previous stretching exercises
- Add internal rotation stretches

Begin strengthening program with graduated elastic bands:
- Resisted internal and external rotation with arm at side (deltoid and rotator cuff)
- Curl and low row exercise (biceps and periscapular muscles)
- No heavy overhead lifting and no acceleration of arm in sport

For massive tears and revision repairs, delay strengthening until 4 mo post-op
Patient is given option of using therapist to assist in implementation of strengthening phase of protocol

Postoperative months 6–12:
May progress to light weights in gym
Clearance to full activity given based on exam, usually 6 mo for small tears
Massive cuff tear patients continue overhead lifting restriction and sport restriction until 1 y

Rotator Cuff Repair and Concomitant SLAP Repair

In the case of a combined rotator cuff repair and superior labrum anterior and posterior (SLAP) repair, the protocol generally follows that for small rotator cuff tears. A sling is worn for a 6 weeks post-op. If there is a small rotator cuff tear, table slides and external rotation are begun immediately. In most cases, a SLAP lesion in a patient with a large rotator cuff tear is degenerative and occurs in older patients. For this reason, a biceps tenodesis is usually performed. In the rare situation of a young patient with a large rotator cuff tear and a SLAP repair, passive external rotation stretches are begun immediately, but table slides are delayed until 6 weeks post-op. The sling is discontinued at 6 weeks post-op, overhead stretches are initiated, and strengthening is delayed until 12 weeks post-op. Full return to activity is at 6 months post-op.

Rotator Cuff Repair and Concomitant Bankart Repair

For Bankart repairs, table slides are not started early in order to avoid stress on the inferior capsule. External rotation is also restricted to 0° until 6 weeks post-op. At 6 weeks post-op, the sling is discontinued and passive external rotation begins with a goal of getting half of the external rotation of the normal side by the end of 12 weeks. Strengthening begins at 12 weeks for small rotator cuff tears and at 16 weeks for large rotator cuff tears.

LABRAL REPAIR REHABILITATION PROTOCOLS

SLAP Repair

Patients with an isolated SLAP repair wear a sling for 4 weeks, which is removed for shower and meals. They begin both passive external rotation with a stick and table slides immediately post-op. In addition, if a posterior release is performed, sleeper stretches are started immediately post-op (Fig. 20.6).

The sling is discontinued at 4 weeks and passive forward elevation with a rope and pulley is started. Passive internal rotation sleeper stretches are also initiated at this time if not already started due to a posterior capsular release.

At 6 weeks, doorframe stretches (Fig. 20.7) and strengthening with elastic bands begin. However, biceps strengthening is delayed until 8 weeks post-op. At 8 weeks, closed-chain scapular control exercises and open-chain

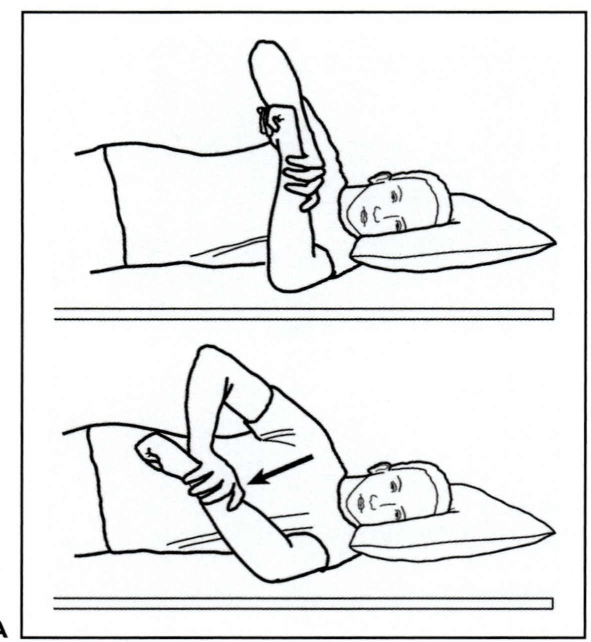

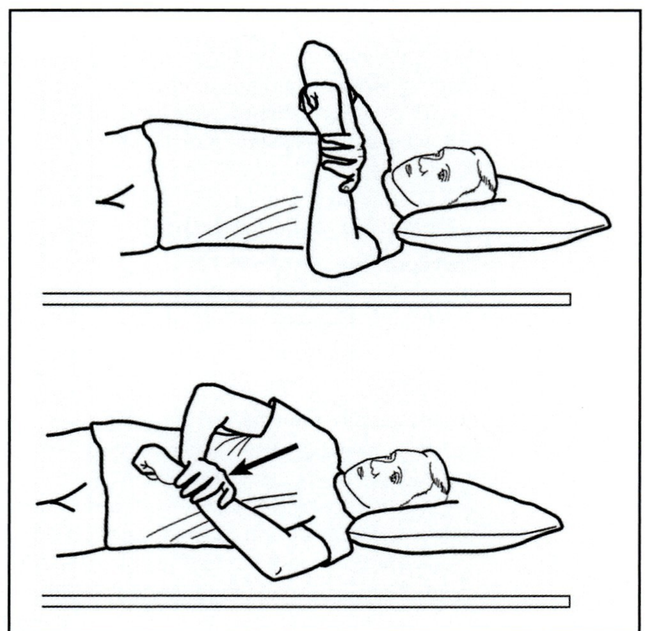

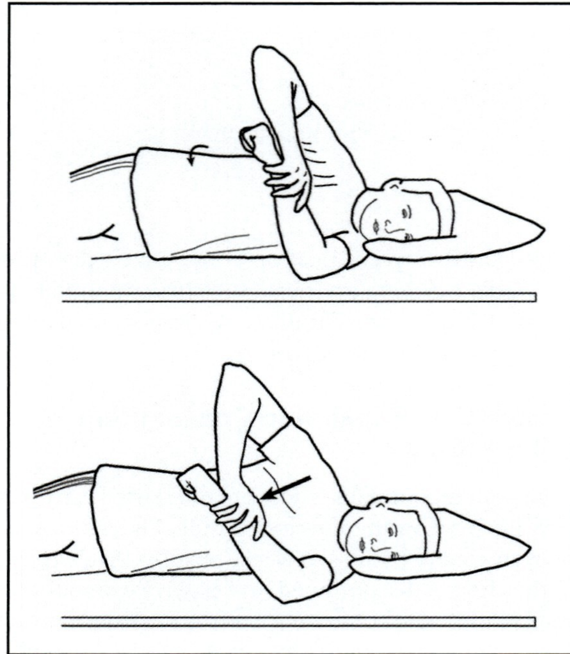

Figure 20.6 Sleeper stretches. These exercises stretch the posterior capsule and are performed with patient lying on the side and using the opposite arm to passive internally rotate the arm. The exercises are performed with the patient **(A)** lying directly on the side, **(B)** leaning back 30°, and **(C)** leaning forward 30°. The different orientations encourage stretching of different portions of the posterior capsule.

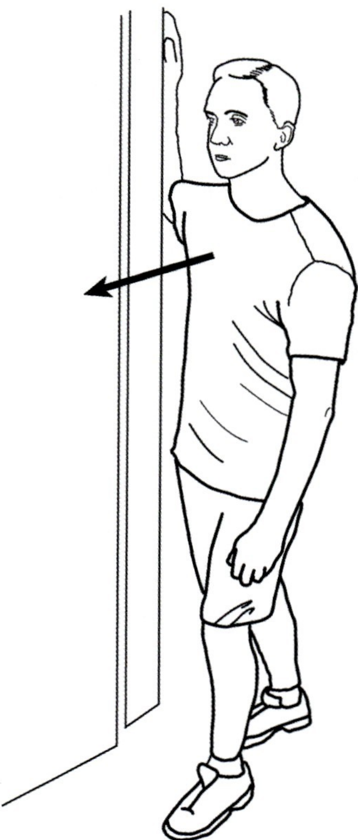

Figure 20.7 The doorframe stretch is performed by placing an abducted arm against a doorframe and leaning the body forward to passive externally rotate and horizontally abduct the arm, so that the elbow passes posterior to the plane of the scapula. The stretch can be performed with the arm at varying degrees of abduction to stretch different portions of the anterior shoulder.

scapular strengthening are also begun. Stretching continues until full motion is recovered.

At 12 weeks post-op, the patient can begin working out in the gym. For baseball players, an interval throwing program begins at 4 months post-op and progresses as previously outlined in *A Cowboy's Guide to Advanced Shoulder Arthroscopy*. Overhead activities that accelerate the arm are not allowed until seven or 8 months post-op (golf, tennis, baseball, etc.).

Bankart Repair

These patients generally wear a sling for 6 weeks unless they are overhead athletes who have undergone surgery on the dominant arm, in which case they use a sling for only 4 weeks. When the sling is discontinued, stretching exercises begin. Full forward flexion is allowed at this point. External rotation is restricted to half that of the normal side. The goal is to have half the external rotation of the normal side at 12 weeks post-op, unless this is a dominant arm in an overhead athlete, in which case more external rotation is allowed. Strengthening begins at 6 weeks post-op unless a remplissage was also performed. If a remplissage was performed, then strengthening must be delayed until 12 weeks post-op since this is essentially a rotator cuff repair. At 4 months post-op, the patient can begin working out in a gym, and full unrestricted activities are allowed at 6 months post-op.

Posterior Instability Repair

The rehabilitation protocol following posterior instability repair is essentially analogous to that for anterior instability. However, passive external rotation is allowed as tolerated. Additionally, passive internal rotation is avoided and the pillow bolster of the sling is reversed to face anteriorly and thus keep the arm at approximately 10° of internal rotation. When the sling is discontinued, internal rotation is not specifically done. The patient is simply allowed to regain internal rotation as the rehabilitation protocol progresses. At 3 months post-op, working out in a gym is allowed with care to avoid "hands-together" bench presses that result in substantial posterior forces. Unrestricted activity is allowed at 6 months post-op.

Combined SLAP Repair and Bankart Repair

In this case, the rehabilitation protocol follows that outlined above for a Bankart repair. Again, strengthening is delayed until 12 weeks post-op if a remplissage was also performed.

OPEN LATARJET RECONSTRUCTION REHABILITATION PROTOCOL

Following open Latarjet reconstruction, the patient is kept in a sling for 6 weeks. At the end of 6 weeks, the sling is discontinued. The patient begins passive overhead forward flexion with a rope and pulley. Passive external rotation with a stick also begins with a goal of getting half the external rotation of the normal side by 12 weeks post-op. At 12 weeks post-op, if the radiographs show the coracoid graft to be in good position, elastic band strengthening exercises are started. At 6 months post-op, if the graft appears to be consolidating, the patient may start weightlifting in a gym. In general, return to full contact activities is delayed until 1 year post-op.

ACKNOWLEDGMENT

We would like to thank John Staley, PT, CSCS, for his contribution to this chapter.

REFERENCES

1. Denard PJ, Lädermann A, Burkhart SS. Prevention and management of stiffness following arthroscopic rotator cuff repair: systematic review and implications for rotator cuff healing. *Arthroscopy.* 2011;27:842–848.
2. Koo SS, Parsley BK, Burkhart SS, et al. Reduction of postoperative stiffness after arthroscopic rotator cuff repair: results of a customized physical therapy regimen based on risk factors for stiffness. *Arthroscopy.* 2011;27:155–160.

3. Cofield RH. Rotator cuff disease of the shoulder. *J Bone Joint Surg Am.* 1985;67:974–979.
4. Harryman DT II, Mack LA, Wang KY, et al. Repairs of the rotator cuff. Correlation of functional results with integrity of the cuff. *J Bone Joint Surg Am.* 1991;73:982–989.
5. Peltz CD, Dourte LM, Kuntz AF, et al. The effect of postoperative passive motion on rotator cuff healing in a rat model. *J Bone Joint Surg Am.* 2009;91:2421–2429.
6. Sarver JJ, Peltz CD, Dourte L, et al. After rotator cuff repair, stiffness—but not the loss in range of motion—increased transiently for immobilized shoulders in a rat model. *J Shoulder Elbow Surg.* 2008;17:108S–113S.
7. Gimbel JA, Van Kleunen JP, Williams GR, et al. Long durations of immobilization in the rat result in enhanced mechanical properties of the healing supraspinatus tendon insertion site. *J Biomech Eng.* 2007;129:400–404.
8. Sonnabend DH, Howlett CR, Young AA. Histological evaluation of repair of the rotator cuff in a primate model. *J Bone Joint Surg Br.* 2010;92:586–594.
9. Huberty DP, Schoolfield JD, Brady PC, et al. Incidence and treatment of postoperative stiffness following arthroscopic rotator cuff repair. *Arthroscopy.* 2009;25:880–890.

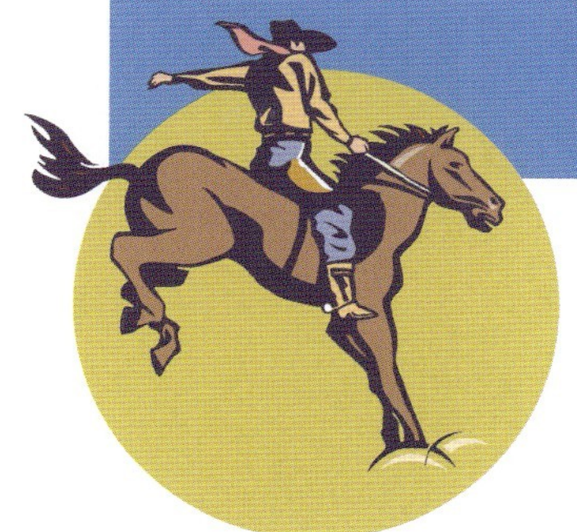

21

Shoulder Stiffness

WESTERN WISDOM

Don't repent. Stop sinning.

A major function of the shoulder is to position the hand in space. When the shoulder is stiff, the hand becomes less functional because its access to the space around it is restricted. That is why stiffness of the shoulder is so disabling: it affects not only the shoulder but also the hand.

Prior to the advent of shoulder arthroscopy, surgical treatment of the stiff shoulder was seldom attempted. Open releases were so painful for patients that vigorous stretching after release was out of the question, and the shoulder would usually stiffen again after open release. Manipulation under anesthesia was the mainstay of treatment, but some shoulders had such thick capsules and dense adhesions that they could not be manipulated, and fracture of the humerus remained a very real possibility during manipulation. The ability to arthroscopically treat stiffness has greatly enhanced our ability to surgically improve shoulder dysfunction.

Stiffness in the nonarthritic shoulder can have two components:

1. Intra-articular restriction due to capsular thickening and shortening
2. Extra-articular restriction due to subacromial and subdeltoid adhesions

TYPES OF STIFFNESS (NONARTHRITIC)

Most nonarthritic stiff shoulders fall into one of three categories:

1. Adhesive capsulitis
2. Postoperative stiffness
3. Posttraumatic stiffness

Adhesive capsulitis usually has only intra-articular restriction due to an inflammatory process affecting the joint capsule, without any subacromial or subdeltoid adhesions.

Postoperative stiffness after rotator cuff repair typically has both intra-articular restriction due to capsular thickening and shortening, as well as subacromial/subdeltoid adhesions. However, postoperative stiffness after labral repair (intra-articular arthroscopic surgery) demonstrates capsular thickening causing intra-articular restriction, but no subacromial adhesions.

Posttraumatic stiffness after fracture of the proximal humerus is most common after surgical treatment of three-part and four-part fractures. In such cases, the source of the stiffness is both intra- and extra-articular, as in other types of postoperative stiffness. Malunion of proximal humerus fractures can cause loss of motion that is not true stiffness. For example, displaced greater tuberosity fractures can cause bony subacromial impingement that blocks overhead motion to varying degrees. Furthermore, varus malunion of humeral neck fractures causes rotational medialization of the greater tuberosity, resulting in shortening of the supraspinatus and infraspinatus muscle-tendon unit in addition to shortening of its moment arm. These biomechanical derangements contribute to loss of motion. Posttraumatic stiffness after glenoid fracture is usually due either to intra-articular adhesions or to posttraumatic arthritis.

ADHESIVE CAPSULITIS

The natural history of untreated adhesive capsulitis passes through freezing, frozen, and thawing stages. Some authors treat adhesive capsulitis differently at different stages.

In contradistinction to stage-specific treatment, we have a standard treatment protocol regardless of the stage of adhesive capsulitis. Our mainstay of treatment is to inject the stiff shoulder three consecutive times at monthly intervals. The injections consist of a mixture of Xylocaine and DepoMedrol and are given into both the intra-articular space and the subacromial space. The patient is placed on a self-administered stretching program that emphasizes restoration of elevation, external rotation, and internal rotation.

If, after 3 months of the above regimen, patients still have significant stiffness, we offer them the choice of continued stretching (but without any further injections), or arthroscopic capsular release and lysis of adhesions.

For patients that choose stretching alone, the duration of the stiffness is usually quite prolonged, often in excess of a year, and it may never fully resolve.

Patients that elect to have arthroscopic capsular release and lysis of adhesions have rapid and dramatic improvements in pain relief as well as range of motion.

In performing the surgery, we first release the rotator interval (including the superior glenohumeral ligament) with a 3-mm electrocautery probe (OPES System; Arthrex, Inc., Naples, FL), while viewing from a posterior portal (Fig. 21.1). Then, we switch the scope to the anterior portal and release the posterior capsule with a pencil-tip cautery (from 11 o'clock down to 7 o'clock in a right shoulder) (Fig. 21.2). Then, we release the axillary pouch, staying at least 5 mm away from the labrum in order to protect the axillary nerve (Fig. 21.3). Next, with the pencil-tip cautery still in the posterior portal, we release the anterior capsule all the way up to the midglenoid notch (Fig. 21.4). Since our posterior working portal has an angle of approach parallel to the glenoid face, it is much easier to release the anterior capsule through this portal than through an anterior portal. The superior capsule is not released, as it

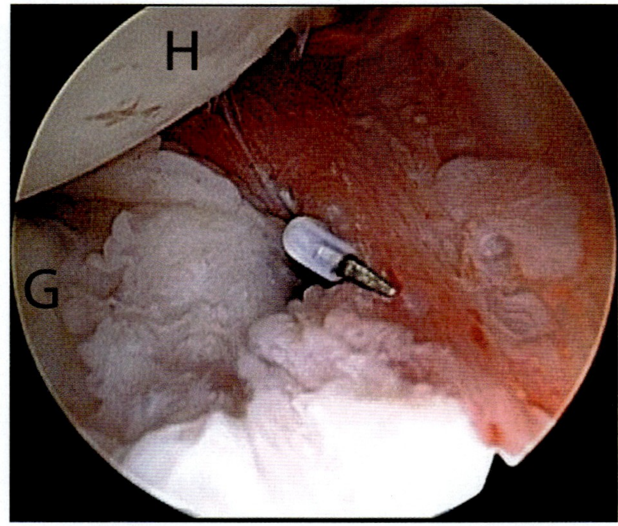

Figure 21.2 Right shoulder, anterosuperolateral viewing portal, demonstrating release of the posterior capsule with a pencil-tip electrocautery. Performing the posterior release prior to the inferior and anterior capsular release provides freedom of movement for the electrocautery device. G, glenoid; H, humerus.

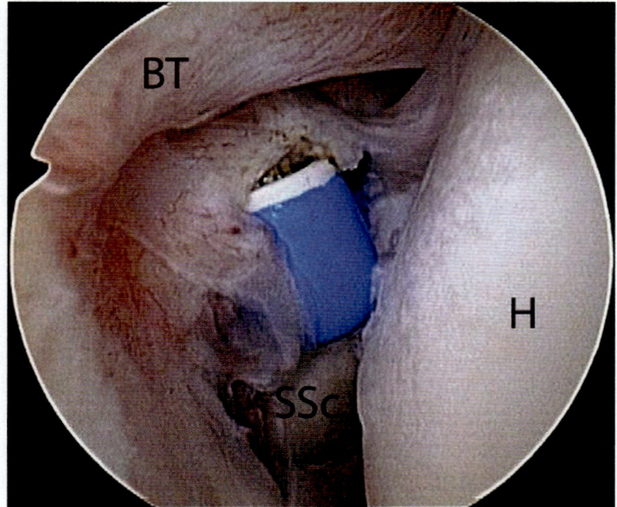

Figure 21.1 Right shoulder, posterior viewing portal demonstrating release of the rotator interval with an electrocautery. This is the first step of a glenohumeral release for stiffness and is performed from the superior border of the subscapularis tendon (SSc) to and including the superior glenohumeral ligament. BT, biceps tendon; H, humerus.

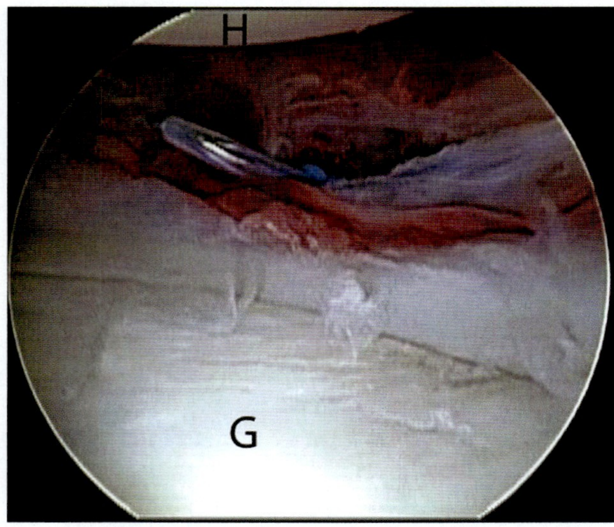

Figure 21.3 Right shoulder, anterosuperolateral viewing portal, demonstrates inferior capsular release with a pencil-tip electrocautery. Note that the electrocautery is at least 5 mm lateral to the labrum in order to avoid iatrogenic injury of the axillary nerve. G, glenoid; H, humerus.

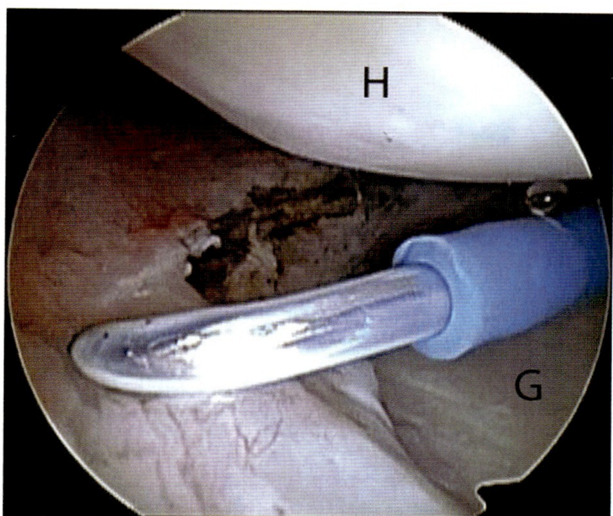

Figure 21.4 Right shoulder, anterosuperolateral viewing portal, demonstrates anterior capsular release performed with a pencil-tip electrocautery introduced through the posterior portal. The posterior portal provides an angle of approach parallel to the glenoid, making it an ideal working portal for the anterior capsular release. G, glenoid; H, humerus.

does not restrict the primary motions of elevation, external rotation, and internal rotation.

After capsular release, we take the arm out of traction and manipulate it through a full range of motion while manually stabilizing the scapula. Even with complete capsular release, manipulation is necessary to stretch the muscles which have become shortened and stiff (*thixotrophy*) because the adhesive capsulitis has restricted their excursion over a prolonged period. Then, the arm is put back into traction and we look into the glenohumeral joint to confirm the adequacy of the capsular release (Fig. 21.5).

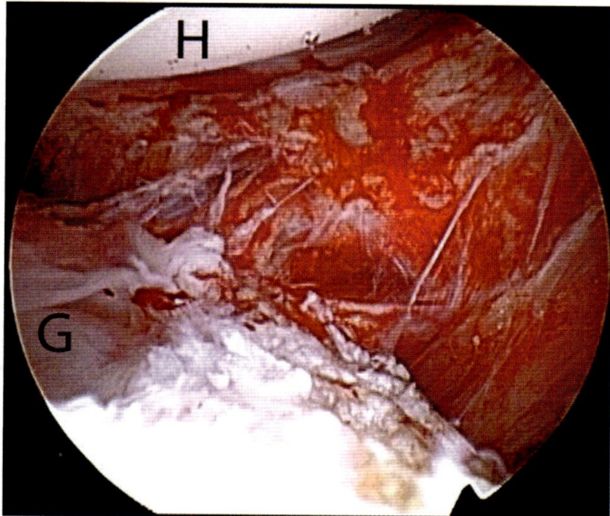

Figure 21.5 Right shoulder, posterior viewing portal. Following capsular release and manipulation under anesthesia, inspection of the axillary recess demonstrates a complete release with visualization of muscle fibers.

Once that is done, we place our arthroscope in the subacromial space. In adhesive capsulitis, the subacromial space is usually normal, in which case we either do nothing or we do an arthroscopic subacromial decompression (if the patient has a type 2 or 3 acromion).

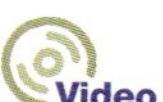

We inject the joint space and the subacromial space with DepoMedrol and Xylocaine. We send the patients to physical therapy 5 days a week for 3 weeks to be sure they maintain their range of motion.

POSTOPERATIVE STIFFNESS

We previously reported on our experience with postoperative stiffness after arthroscopic rotator cuff repair. We employed a conservative program of 6 weeks of postoperative immobilization in a sling for 489 consecutive patients who underwent arthroscopic rotator cuff repair (1). We observed a 4.9% incidence of post-op stiffness that was significant enough to warrant arthroscopic capsular release and lysis of adhesions. In this study, we identified certain categories of patients with rotator cuff tears that were at high risk to develop post-op stiffness. These high-risk categories were cuff-tear patients who also had one of the following pre-op diagnoses:

1. Adhesive capsulitis
2. Concomitant labral repair
3. Calcific tendinitis
4. Single-tendon tear (including single-tendon PASTA lesions)

Based on that study, we instituted a modification to our conservative post-op protocol. In this modified protocol, patients in the high-risk categories for stiffness would do table slides (closed-chain overhead stretches) twice daily (see Chapter 20, "Postoperative Rehabilitation"). Then, we did a second study in which we reviewed a group of 152 patients with this modified protocol and identified 79 patients that were in high-risk categories for developing stiffness (2). All 152 patients were kept in a sling for 6 weeks post-op, and those 79 patients in the high-risk groups did 10 table slides daily. Only one of these patients developed post-op stiffness, confirming the validity and success of this minor modification to our postoperative protocol.

Cause of the Stiffness

In general, patients who develop stiffness after rotator cuff repair have two causes for stiffness: (a) capsular contractures, and (b) subacromial adhesions. If surgery is undertaken, then one must do both an intra-articular capsular release and a subacromial lysis of adhesions.

Interestingly, patients with repair of large and massive cuff tears virtually never get stiff. Furthermore, when patients do develop post-op stiffness after repair of rotator cuff tears of any size, they have almost always completely healed their cuff tears (96% healing in our study). We have found that it useful to explain to patients with post-op stiffness that they have "overhealed" their rotator cuffs and that if post-op releases are done, we can begin early vigorous rehabilitation after release because the cuff will be healed.

In contradistinction to cuff repair patients, those who develop stiffness after labral repair (SLAP or Bankart repair) will have capsular contractures that may require release but will not have subacromial adhesions.

Timing of the Release

In general, we prefer to wait until at least 6 months post-op before performing arthroscopic releases for post-op stiffness.

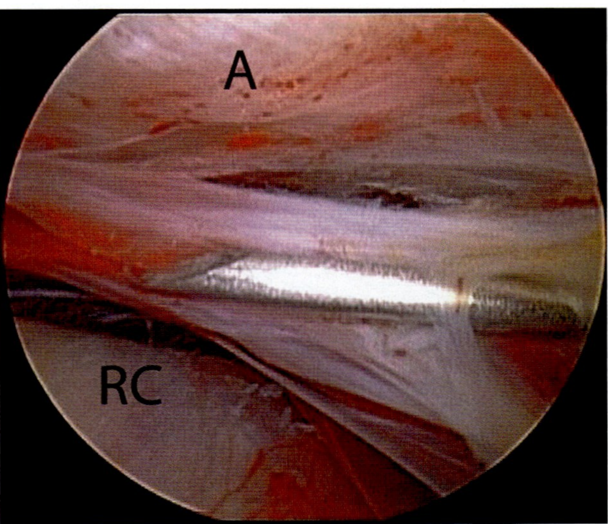

Figure 21.6 Right shoulder, posterior subacromial viewing portal demonstrating dense subacromial adhesions in an individual with postoperative stiffness. A, acromion; RC, rotator cuff.

Technique of Release for Postoperative Stiffness after Rotator Cuff Repair

In general, the sequence of intra-articular capsular release for post-op stiffness following cuff repair is the same as for adhesive capsulitis. We release the rotator interval, but we are careful to preserve the medial sling of the biceps. Then, we switch to an anterior or anterosuperolateral viewing portal and release the posterior, inferior, and anterior capsules with a pencil-tip cautery through a posterior viewing portal.

If the subscapularis had been previously repaired, there may be a component of *subscapularis capture* due to subcoracoid adhesions. This usually necessitates a three-sided release of the subscapularis in order to reestablish lateral excursion of the tendon (see Chapter 6, "Subscapularis Tendon Tears"). This is done prior to releasing the posterior, inferior, and anterior capsules in order to minimize extra-articular fluid extravasation prior to manipulating the shoulder.

Once the capsular and subcoracoid releases have been done, we take the arm out of traction and do a manipulation of the shoulder while stabilizing the scapula. It is important to do the intra-articular releases rather quickly because extra-articular fluid extravasation will greatly reduce the ability to manipulate the shoulder through a full range of motion.

We believe that manipulation after capsular release of a stiff shoulder is very important because these shoulders have an element of muscle stiffness (thixotrophy) due to the fact that the muscle-tendon units have not been fully stretched for a number of weeks or months.

After capsular release and manipulation of the shoulder, we do a subacromial lysis of adhesions. The subacromial adhesions can be quite dense (Fig. 21.6). We begin by exposing the bony landmarks: scapular spine, undersurface of acromion, and AC joint (Fig. 21.7). Then, we use a combination of arthroscopic shaver, electrocautery, and scissors to reestablish the posterior, lateral, and anterior gutters of the subacromial space. The posterolateral gutter, which is the tightest part of the subacromial space, is most effectively visualized with the use of a 70° arthroscope (Figs. 21.8 and 21.9).

Technique of Release for Postoperative Stiffness after Labral Repair

Shoulders with post-op stiffness after labral repair (SLAP or Bankart or posterior Bankart repair) have capsular thickening with intra-articular restriction, but they do not have subacromial adhesions.

Most shoulders with stiffness after labral repair will gradually regain satisfactory motion. However, for those that do not, we do a limited capsular release that is targeted at the specific capsular segments that are tight, using a pencil-tip electrocautery probe. We first release the rotator interval, making a window in the interval that allows visualization of the coracoid tip. Occasionally, there will be adhesions between the coracoid and the subscapularis tendon that cause *subscapularis capture*, limiting the excursion of the subscapularis with external and internal rotation. If subcoracoid adhesions are present between the coracoid and subscapularis tendon, they must be released by using a combination of motorized shaver, electrocautery, arthroscopic scissors, and an elevator.

Next, a capsular release is performed, targeted at the areas that are restricting motion. For example, if external rotation is significantly restricted but internal rotation is normal, then we will release the anterior capsule but not the posterior capsule.

Just as with adhesive capsulitis, we release the capsule while viewing through an anterior or anterosuperolateral

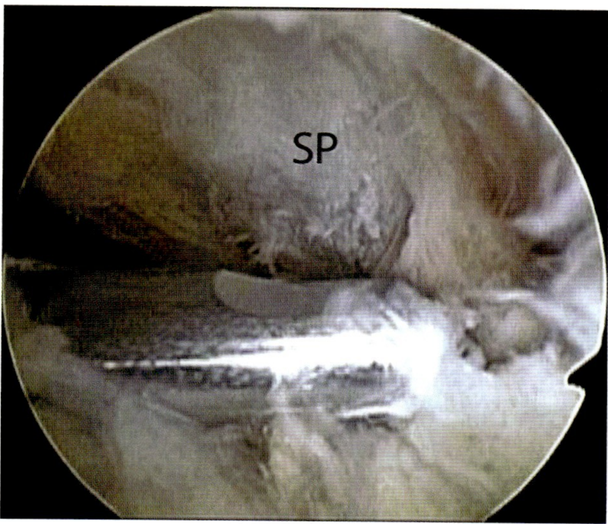

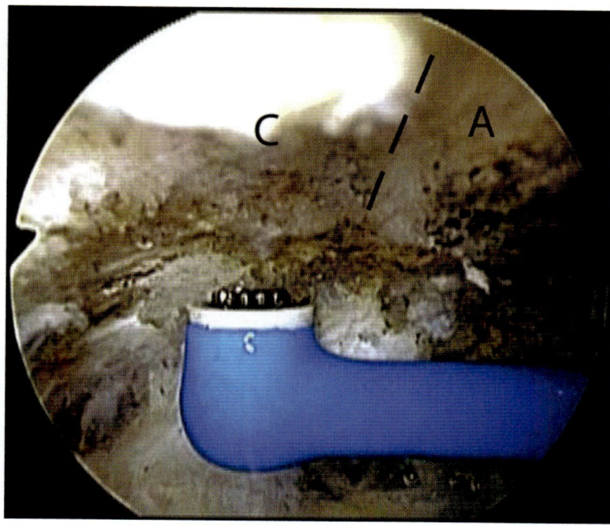

Figure 21.7 Subacromial debridement and lysis of adhesions requires identification of the acromion, scapular spine, and acromioclavicular joint. **A:** Right shoulder, lateral viewing portal demonstrates initial identification of the scapular spine that is surrounded by dense subacromial adhesions. **B:** After a space is cleared anterior, posterior, and lateral to the scapular spine, the arthroscope is placed in the posterior portal and an electrocautery introduced from a lateral portal is used to identify the undersurface of the acromioclavicular joint (*dashed lines*). A, acromion; C, distal clavicle. SP, scapular spine.

portal, with the cautery probe entering through a posterior portal.

The most critical technical point in doing a capsular release for postcapsulorrhaphy stiffness is to preserve the labral bumper. The labral bumper is necessary to provide the concavity necessary to preserve the "suction-cup effect" that helps to provide stability. Therefore, we release the capsule approximately 5 mm lateral to the labrum.

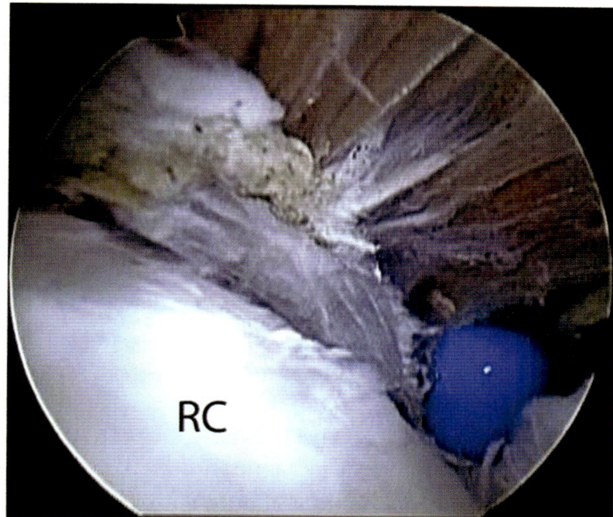

Figure 21.8 Right shoulder, posterior viewing portal with a 70° arthroscope demonstrates reestablishment of the lateral gutter by splitting the internal deltoid fascia with an electrocautery in a patient with postoperative stiffness. RC, rotator cuff.

SPECIAL SITUATIONS

Preoperative Stiffness

Some patients with full-thickness rotator cuff tears will have preoperative stiffness. In such cases, we try to regain passive motion prior to surgery by means of stretching exercises and one or two corticosteroid injections if necessary. If full motion is not regained preoperatively, then we do an anterior, posterior, and inferior capsular release at the time of arthroscopic cuff repair, without any modification of our standard postoperative protocol (i.e., for repair of two- or three-tendon tears, we do not do early range of motion). Most of these shoulders will regain full motion in the postoperative period. For those that are still quite stiff at 6 months post-op, we perform an arthroscopic release.

Stiffness after Hemiarthroplasty or after ORIF for Fracture

Stiffness can be a problem after hemiarthroplasty for three-part and four-part fractures of the proximal humerus. However, an even greater problem is loss of fixation of the tuberosities, leading to tuberosity resorption. Some authors have recommended early passive motion to prevent the stiffness, but we believe the risk of disrupting the tuberosities is too great to justify this approach (3). Therefore, we immobilize the patient for 6 weeks after open reduction and internal fixation or hemiarthroplasty for fracture, before beginning stretches. This helps to ensure healing of the tuberosities. If the shoulder remains stiff by 6 months

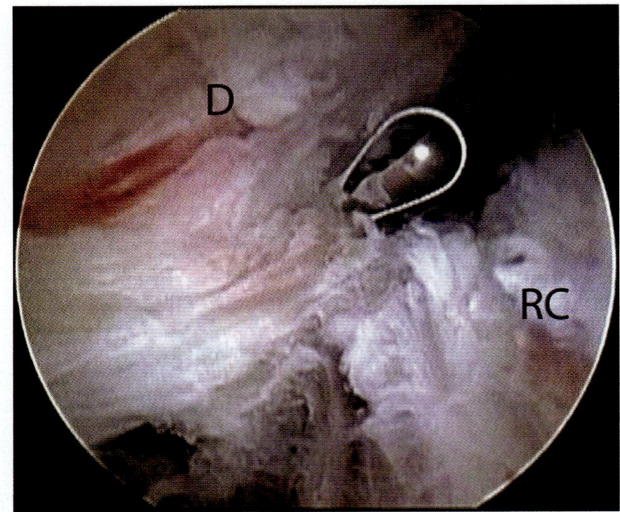

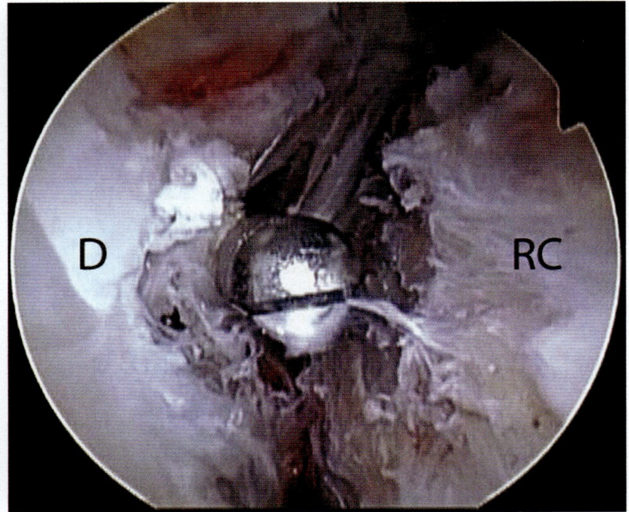

Figure 21.9 Right shoulder, lateral viewing portal demonstrates reestablishment of the posterolateral gutter. **A:** Dense adhesions are seen between the rotator cuff and internal deltoid fascia. **B:** A shaver has been used to debride the adhesions and reestablish the posterolateral space between the rotator cuff and internal deltoid fascia. D, internal deltoid fascia; RC, rotator cuff.

post-op, we do an arthroscopic release followed by immediate range-of-motion exercises. In the case of internal fixation, hardware removal is only considered after the capsular release and manipulation have been performed so as to avoid any stress riser during gentle manipulation.

Malunion of Proximal Humerus Fractures

In cases of humeral neck fracture with varus malunion, loss of motion usually occurs as a result of the rotational medialization of the greater tuberosity. In this position, the tuberosity tends to undergo early painful impingement with attempted elevation of the arm, limiting motion due to pain. Furthermore, elevation is limited on a biomechanical basis because the medial rotation of the insertional footprints of the supraspinatus and infraspinatus causes loss of the optimal length–tension relationships of the muscle-tendon units. In such cases, we have had success at improving function by taking down the insertions of the supraspinatus and infraspinatus tendons with a pencil-tip cautery, followed by tuberoplasty to reduce the impingement profile of the greater tuberosity, and then a lateralized footprint repair of the tendons on the reconfigured greater tuberosity (see Chapter 19, "Arthroscopic Treatment of Fractures about the Shoulder").

In cases of isolated greater tuberosity fracture malunion, in which the tuberosity heals in a "proud" position, we do a similar procedure: take-down of supraspinatus and the anterior half of the infraspinatus, then tuberoplasty, then footprint repair.

Freedom Through Release

Video

With arthroscopic releases, we are able to regain full range of motion in virtually all stiff shoulders. This has created a paradigm shift in postoperative rehabilitation. Before the advent of arthroscopy, most postoperative patients (including rotator cuff repairs and fracture repairs) underwent early stretching and range-of-motion exercises in order to avoid stiffness. This early motion would frequently cause loss of fixation of the rotator cuff or of fracture fragments, resulting in poor outcomes or the need for revision surgery.

Now, with the ability to do arthroscopic releases, the surgeon enjoys the freedom to immobilize the patient as long as necessary to achieve healing. If postoperative stiffness ensues, then an arthroscopic release can be done to restore motion.

Emotional and Psychological Considerations

In considering whether to immobilize patients or to begin early motion postoperatively, it is instructive to take the patient's perspective and consider the emotional and psychological aspects of doing two sequential surgeries for a single pathology (e.g., a rotator cuff tear).

Let's assume that a patient undergoes a rotator cuff repair followed by early range of motion in order to reduce the chance of post-op stiffness. Let's further assume that the early motion overloads the repair construct, resulting in disruption of the repair. When the surgeon tells the patient that he must undergo a second repair for the same tear, the patient is usually devastated because he has to start over at the very beginning. The patient feels that all of the original treatment was wasted, because he has to repeat all of the earliest steps of surgery and rehabilitation.

On the other hand, if the patient has 6 weeks of postoperative immobilization to ensure healing, but then develops postoperative stiffness, the scenario is entirely different. Since most rotator cuff repairs that develop post-op stiffness are completely healed, the surgeon has a very different type of conversation with this patient. Now he can tell the patient that the cuff is healed, that motion can be restored with a simple arthroscopic release, and that the rehabilitation can be expedited immediately post-op because the cuff is solidly healed. In this case, the patient is relieved because he is not starting over (as with a failed cuff repair) and he can rapidly progress with his rehabilitation.

A NEW VIEW OF STIFFNESS

Armed with the ability to restore motion with arthroscopic releases, today's arthroscopic shoulder surgeons view stiffness in an entirely different way from their predecessors, the open shoulder surgeons. The "new view" afforded by arthroscopy is that stiffness of the shoulder is always a temporary condition. Motion can always be restored. The ability to consistently restore motion is a very powerful tool.

REFERENCES

1. Huberty DP, Schoolfield JD, Brady PC, et al. Incidence and treatment of postoperative stiffness following arthroscopic rotator cuff repair. *Arthroscopy*. 2009;25:880–890.
2. Koo SS, Parsley BK, Burkhart SS, et al. Reduction of postoperative stiffness after arthroscopic rotator cuff repair: results of a customized physical therapy regimen based on risk factors for stiffness. *Arthroscopy*. 2011;27:155–160.
3. Barth JR, Burkhart SS. Arthroscopic capsular release after hemiarthroplasty of the shoulder for fracture: a new treatment paradigm. *Arthroscopy*. 2005;21:1150.

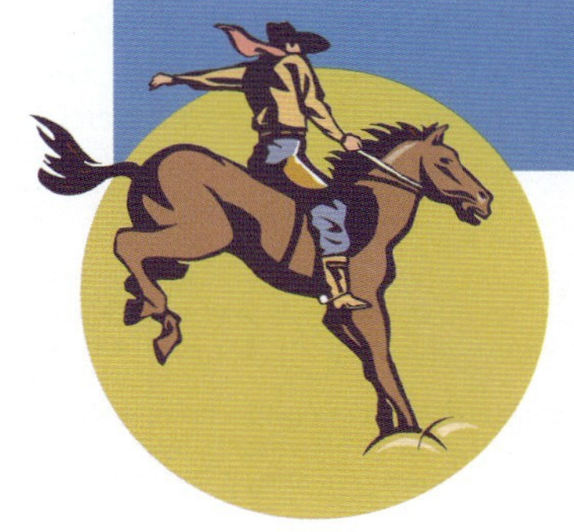

22

Glenohumeral Arthritis

WESTERN WISDOM

Weigh words. Don't count them.

Glenohumeral arthritis may result in considerable disability. The impact of glenohumeral arthritis is comparable to chronic medical conditions such as congestive heart failure, diabetes, and acute myocardial infarction (1). In adults over the age of 60, the majority of glenohumeral arthritis is primary osteoarthritis and treatment algorithms are well defined with shoulder arthroplasty providing the mainstay of operative treatment. In this population, total shoulder arthroplasty (TSA) provides reliable pain relief and functional improvement with satisfactory implant longevity. However, for adults under the age of 60, and particularly for those under 50, diagnoses usually involve more complex pathology and arthroplasty outcomes are less predictable. Treatment decision-making factors that become more important in this young adult population include higher activity levels, greater functional expectations, and implant longevity. In addition, a subset of elderly patients may prefer a minimally invasive procedure that avoids the risks associated with TSA.

For these populations, a wide spectrum of glenohumeral arthritis pathology can successfully be managed arthroscopically. Current arthroscopic management techniques for glenohumeral arthritis include debridement and capsular release with biceps tenotomy or tenodesis, labral advancement, microfracture, and glenoid resurfacing. Additionally, an arthroscopic total shoulder replacement is on the horizon (see Chapter 25, "Future Developments").

PREOPERATIVE EVALUATION AND INDICATIONS

While treatment decision making always requires detailed evaluation of the patient, there are several factors that are more commonly encountered in the younger patient with glenohumeral arthritis that take on increased importance. The etiology of glenohumeral arthritis differs in the young adult compared to the older adult, with younger patients often having diagnoses that are more complex and may result in poorer outcomes. In a study of 1,030 patients, Saltzman et al. (2) reported that primary osteoarthritis was present in 66% of patients over the age of 50 undergoing shoulder arthroplasty compared to only 21% in patients under the age of 50. Young patients were much more likely to carry diagnoses of capsulorrhapy arthropathy, post-traumatic arthritis, avascular necrosis, and rheumatoid arthritis. These diagnoses have been associated with worse functional results compared to arthroplasty for primary osteoarthritis (3).

In elucidating the history, particular attention is paid to social factors. While young patients often have few comorbidities, occupation and hobbies are important to consider. The manual laborer will place more stress on his or her shoulder and is more likely to loosen a polyethylene implant than a sedentary patient of the same age. Similarly, young athletic individuals may participate in sports that place greater demands on their upper extremities than the typical elderly patient.

Glenoid morphology and bone quantity affect outcome and are important to assess on an axillary radiograph. The primary osteoarthritis typical of the older patient

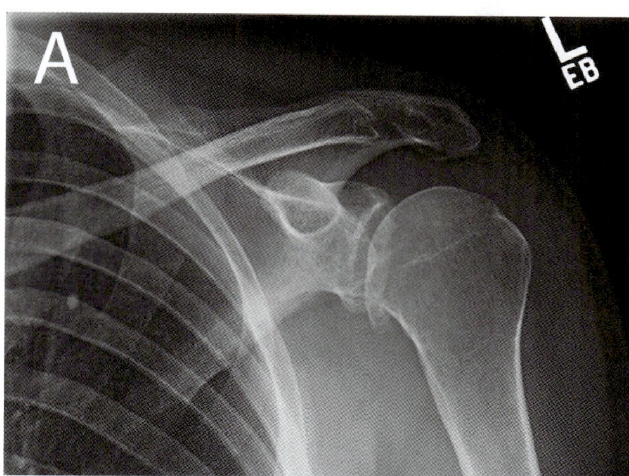

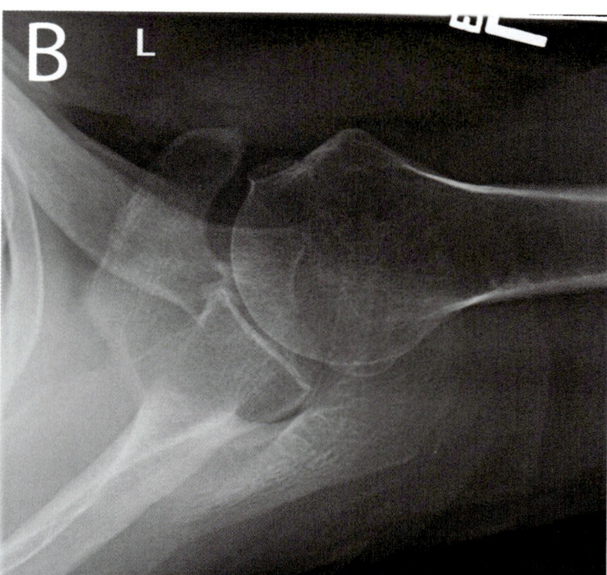

Figure 22.1 Left shoulder plain **(A)** anterior–posterior and **(B)** axillary radiographs in a 40-year-old man with primary glenohumeral arthritis. In this individual with stiffness and relative preservation of the joint space, an arthroscopic capsular release, osteophyte debridement, and biceps tenodesis are likely to provide substantial pain relief and delay the need for total shoulder replacement.

population is characterized by cartilage loss and deformity involving both the humeral head and the glenoid. Younger patients are more likely to have traumatic arthritis and may exhibit asymmetric changes that involve only one side of the glenohumeral joint. Focal cartilage damage affecting a portion of an articular surface can also be seen. Thorough evaluation to determine the location and extent of arthritic change is therefore required in order to provide treatment that has a high likelihood of symptomatic improvement.

For elderly patients desiring a minimally invasive procedure, a capsular release, debridement, and biceps tenotomy or tenodesis can provide substantial pain relief in some cases. For young patients, treatment is based on the location of arthritis and the quality of the joint space. In patients with a relatively preserved joint space and stiffness, an arthroscopic capsular release and debridement alone often provides pain relief (Fig. 22.1). For isolated cartilage lesions, we perform microfracture or labral advancement based on the location of the lesion. For patients with a substantial loss of joint space, however, a biologic glenoid resurfacing procedure is indicated (Fig. 22.2).

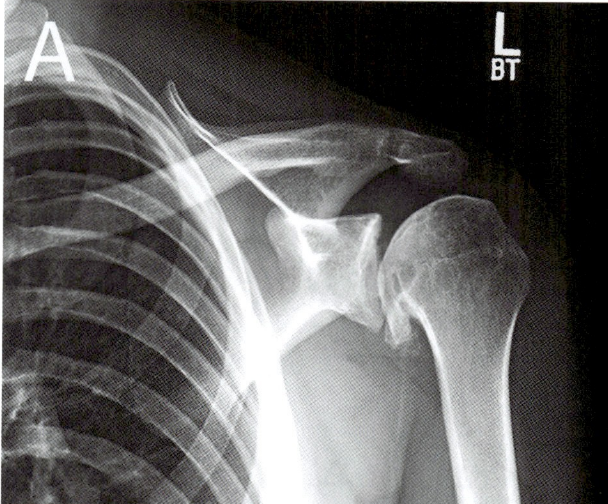

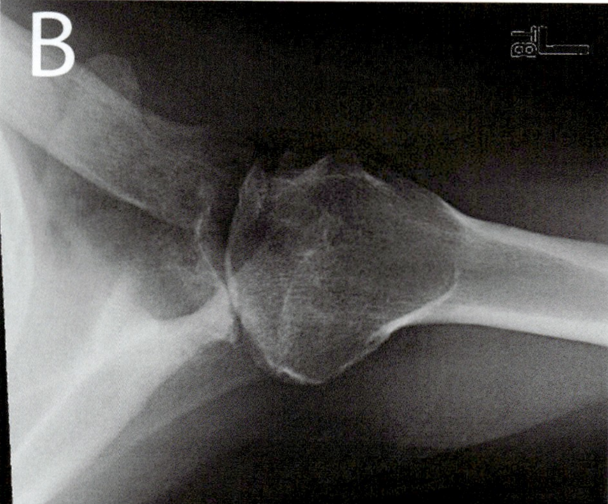

Figure 22.2 Left shoulder plain **(A)** anterior–posterior and **(B)** axillary radiographs in a 22-year-old man with posttraumatic arthritis. Based on the extent of arthritis and decreased joint space, a capsular release alone is unlikely to provide substantial pain relief and a biologic glenoid resurfacing procedure is indicated.

CAPSULAR RELEASE AND GLENOHUMERAL DEBRIDEMENT

The expression "a stiff shoulder is a painful shoulder" is just as true in glenohumeral arthritis as it is in adhesive capsulitis. In the case of glenohumeral arthritis, patients present with capsular stiffness as well as impinging osteophytes that produce a painful mechanical block to motion. We have found that capsular release and osteophyte debridement can restore motion and reduce pain (4). It is our belief that a capsular release results in symptomatic relief by reducing joint contact pressures, particularly near the extremes of motion.

Technique for Capsular Release and Joint Debridement

The patient is placed in the lateral decubitus position and a diagnostic arthroscopy is performed through a posterior viewing portal. Anterior and anterosuperolateral portals are established. The stability of the biceps root is assessed with a probe introduced from an anterior portal. In most cases of glenohumeral arthritis, pathology of the biceps will be present in the form of degenerative tearing or disruption of portions of the biceps root. In elderly patients where cosmesis is not a concern, a biceps tenotomy can be performed at this time. However, in most cases, we prefer a tenodesis high in the groove. If a tenodesis is to be performed, we do this after the capsular release and debridement are completed.

The arthroscope is moved to an anterosuperolateral viewing portal and the extent of any humeral osteophytes is assessed. A 70° arthroscope is often necessary for visualization as the typical location for humeral osteophytes is anteroinferior. A shaver is introduced through an anterior portal or a low anterior (5 o'clock) portal and is used to debride the anteroinferior humeral osteophytes (Fig. 22.3A). Care is taken during the debridement to preserve the humeral capsular attachments and avoid overaggressive resection, which could compromise stability. Any cartilage defects on the humerus and glenoid are debrided to a stable rim (Fig. 22.3B).

After the debridement is completed, a capsular release is performed as previously described (see Chapter 21, "Shoulder Stiffness"). Briefly, the arthroscope is returned to the posterior viewing portal and the rotator interval is released with an electrocautery introduced from the anterior portal (Fig. 22.4A). Then, the arthroscope is placed in the anterosuperolateral portal and the posterior, inferior, and anterior capsules are released 5 mm lateral to the labrum with a pencil-tip electrocautery (Fig. 22.4B). When the release is completed, the arm is removed from traction and a gentle manipulation under anesthesia is performed. The extent of the release is then confirmed arthroscopically.

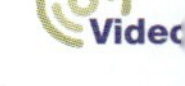

Attention is then turned to the biceps, and a tenodesis is performed high in the groove as previously described (see Chapter 10, "The Biceps Tendon") (Fig. 22.5).

ISOLATED CARTILAGE LESIONS

In addition to stiffness, young patients with a preserved joint space may demonstrate isolated cartilage lesions that can be treated with labral advancement or microfracture.

Labral Advancement

Small (<1 cm) glenoid cartilage lesions near the peripheral margin are amenable to labral advancement. The concept

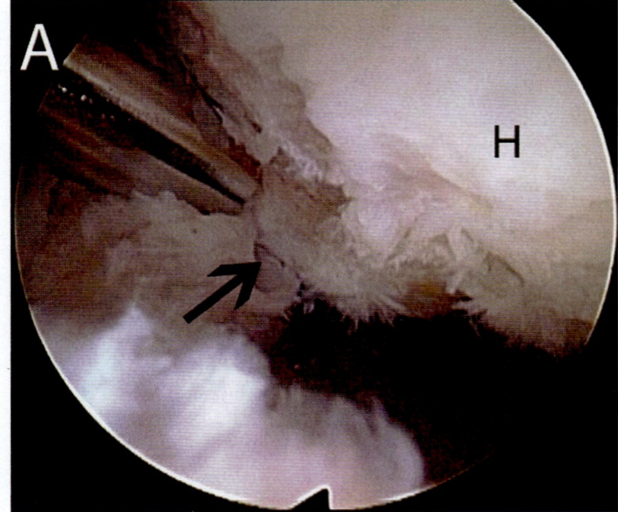

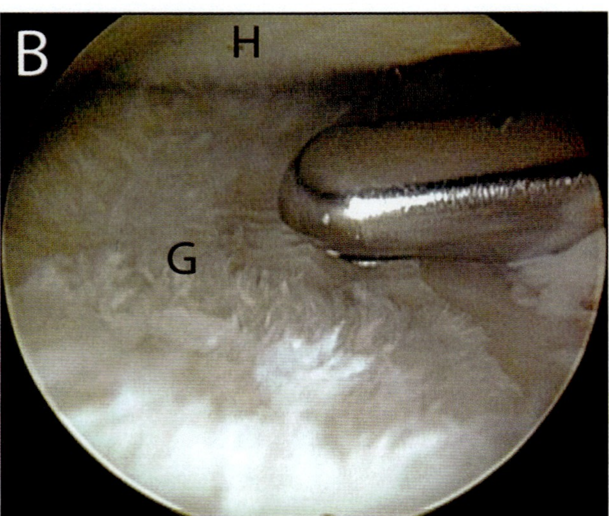

Figure 22.3 Right shoulder, anterosuperolateral viewing portal demonstrates debridement for glenohumeral arthritis. **A:** An anteroinferior humeral head osteophyte (*black arrow*) is debrided with the use of a shaver. Because osteophytes are typically soft, a burr is not usually required for debridement. **B:** A shaver introduced through a posterior portal is used to debride glenoid chondromalacia. G, glenoid; H, humerus

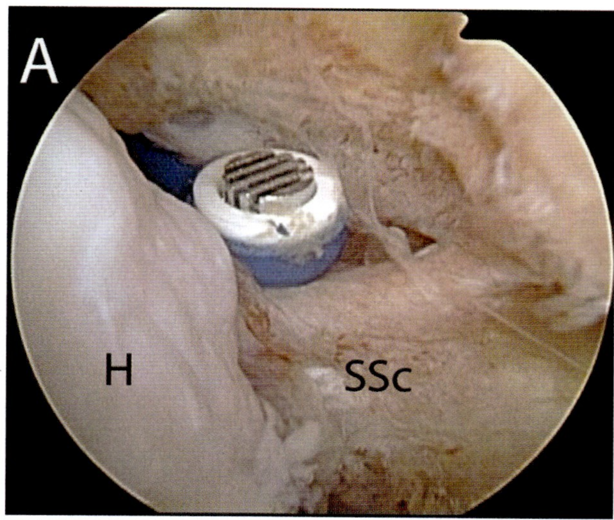

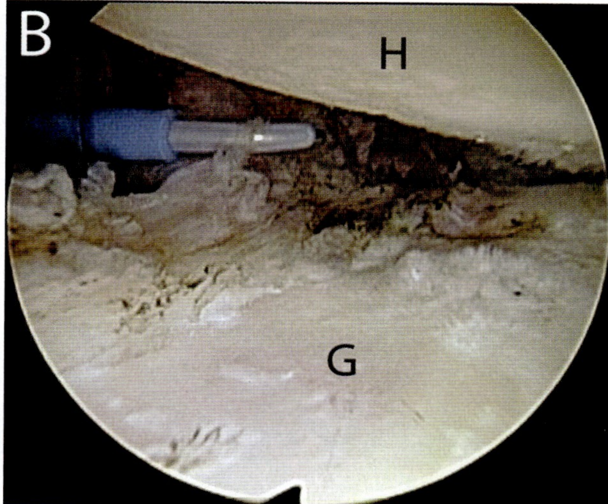

Figure 22.4 Left shoulder demonstrating capsular release in a patient with glenohumeral arthritis. **A:** Posterior viewing portal. The rotator interval is released with an electrocautery. **B:** Anterosuperolateral viewing portal. A pencil-tip electrocautery introduced through the posterior portal is used to release the posterior, inferior (as seen in this figure), and anterior capsules. G, glenoid; H, humerus; SSc, subscapularis tendon.

of labral advancement is to use the labrum to cover a symptomatic cartilage lesion to provide pain relief. We have used this technique with good to excellent outcomes at short-term follow-up in 90% of cases (5).

Peripheral cartilage lesions most typically occur in the setting of a traumatic dislocation and are thus most often performed in conjunction with an anterior or posterior Bankart repair. The technique for labral advancement is very similar to a standard labral repair. The difference is that a greater amount of mobilization is required and anchors are placed slightly further onto the face of the glenoid than usual. After identification of a cartilage defect near the glenoid rim, the adjacent labrum is mobilized with an arthroscopic elevator. Mobilization is completed when the labrum can be adequately advanced onto the glenoid surface to cover the defect. The cartilage is debrided to a stable rim with a shaver and curette. BioComposite Suture-Tak anchors (Arthrex, Inc., Naples, FL) are then placed into the defect and standard suture passing techniques (Suture-Lasso; Arthrex, Inc., Naples, FL) are used to advance the labrum and cover the defect (Fig. 22.6).

Microfracture

Microfracture may have a role in the treatment of symptomatic isolated small- to moderate-sized (<2 cm) articular

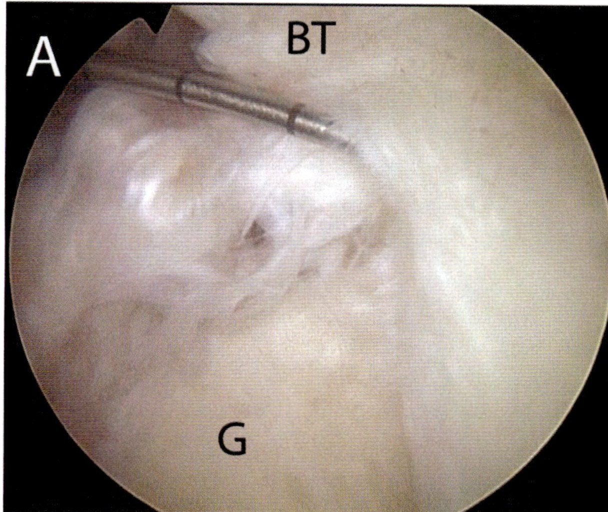

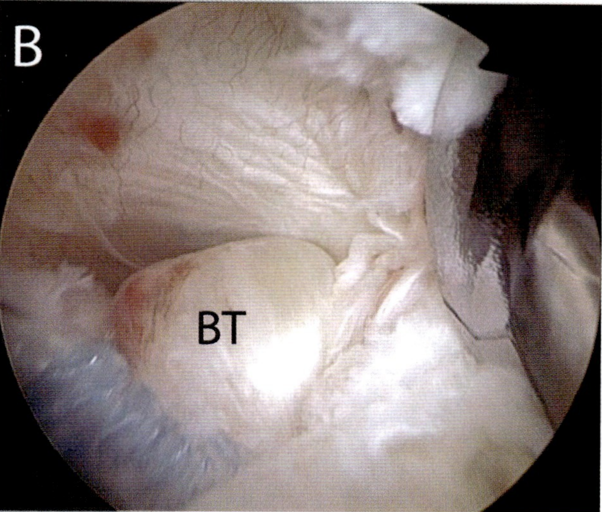

Figure 22.5 Left shoulder, posterior viewing portal demonstrates **(A)** a degenerative biceps root in a patient with glenohumeral arthritis that was **(B)** tenodesed high in the bicipital groove with a BioComposite Tenodesis Screw (Arthrex, Inc., Naples, FL). BT, biceps tendon; G, glenoid.

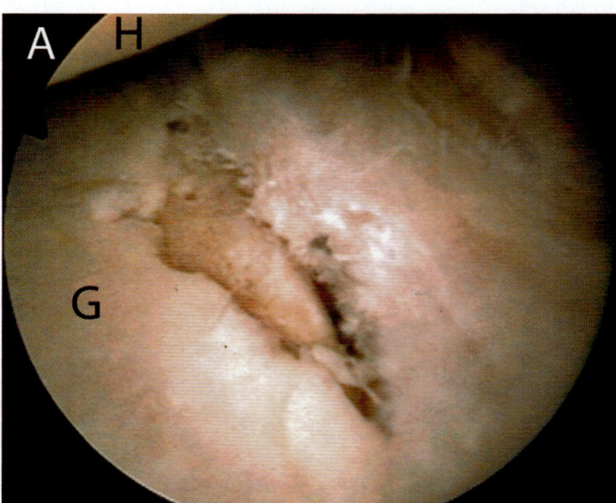

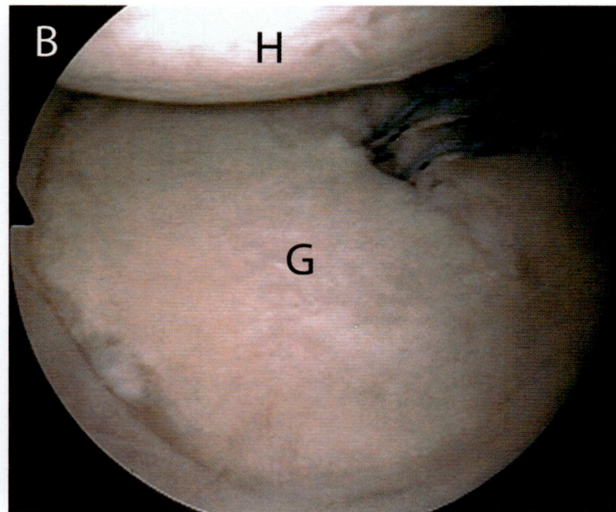

Figure 22.6 Left shoulder, anterosuperolateral viewing portal demonstrates labral advancement for an isolated peripheral glenoid cartilage lesion. **A:** A full-thickness cartilage lesion of the anterior glenoid rim has been debrided to a stable rim. **B:** After mobilizing the labrum, anchors are inserted into the defect and standard suture passing techniques are used to advance the labrum over the cartilage defect. G, glenoid; H, humeral head.

cartilage lesions that occur in the central glenoid or on the humeral side of the joint. There is a lack of high-quality evidence describing outcomes for microfracture in the glenohumeral joint, but we typically reserve the technique for patients <50 years of age given the lower healing potential in older patients.

After identification of the lesion, a stable cartilage rim is created with a shaver and curette. Then, a PowerPick (Arthrex, Inc., Naples, FL) or standard chondral pick is used to create multiple perforations in the bone to allow marrow elements to extrude and encourage fibrocartilage formation. Fluid inflow can be stopped and extrusion of blood from the bone perforations can be used to confirm adequate depth of the microfractures.

GLENOID RESURFACING

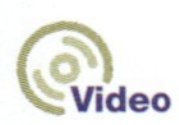

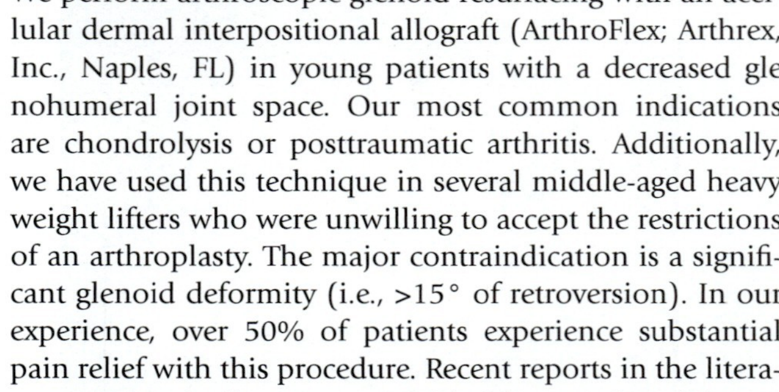

We perform arthroscopic glenoid resurfacing with an acellular dermal interpositional allograft (ArthroFlex; Arthrex, Inc., Naples, FL) in young patients with a decreased gle nohumeral joint space. Our most common indications are chondrolysis or posttraumatic arthritis. Additionally, we have used this technique in several middle-aged heavy weight lifters who were unwilling to accept the restrictions of an arthroplasty. The major contraindication is a significant glenoid deformity (i.e., >15° of retroversion). In our experience, over 50% of patients experience substantial pain relief with this procedure. Recent reports in the literature suggest similar outcomes with this procedure (6).

After a diagnostic arthroscopy through a posterior portal, anterior and anterosuperolateral portals are established. Debridement of impinging osteophytes is performed first as described above since swelling will limit anteroinferior visualization. If visualization is very limited due to capsular stiffness, it may be necessary to perform a capsular release at this point, although this will increase swelling.

Glenoid Preparation

Viewing from an anterosuperolateral portal, the glenoid is prepared with a shaver and curette to remove any remaining cartilage (Fig. 22.7A). If a biconcave glenoid deformity is present, a burr is used to resect the ridge between the two concavities (Fig. 22.7B). Multiple perforations are created with a chondral pick or PowerPick device to create a bone bed suitable for graft healing (Fig. 22.7C). The dimensions of the glenoid are then estimated. A calibrated probe introduced from the posterior portal is used to measure the anterior–posterior width. Measuring the superior–inferior length is more difficult, but an estimate can be made based on a typical superior–inferior length to anterior–posterior width ratio of 3:2.

Graft Preparation

The glenoid graft is then prepared on the back instrument table. The dimensions are outlined and the graft is cut appropriately so that the graft's shiny side will be in contact with the prepared bone bed (Fig. 22.8A). Multiple free #2 FiberWire (Arthrex, Inc., Naples, FL) sutures are then placed circumferentially in the graft, spaced approximately 1 cm apart; a total of three to four are placed both anteriorly and posteriorly depending on the size of the graft. The sutures are placed as simple stitches, with the exception of two most superior stitches at the 10 o'clock and 12 o'clock position that are placed as inverted mattress stitches with

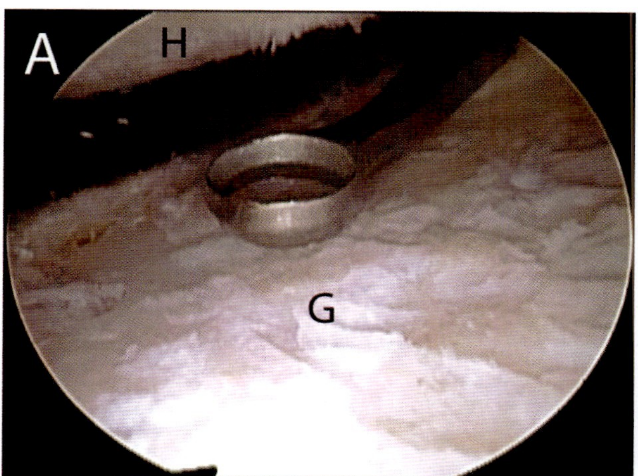

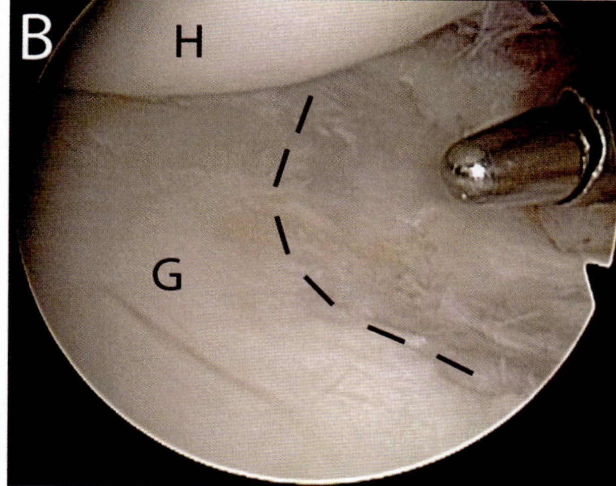

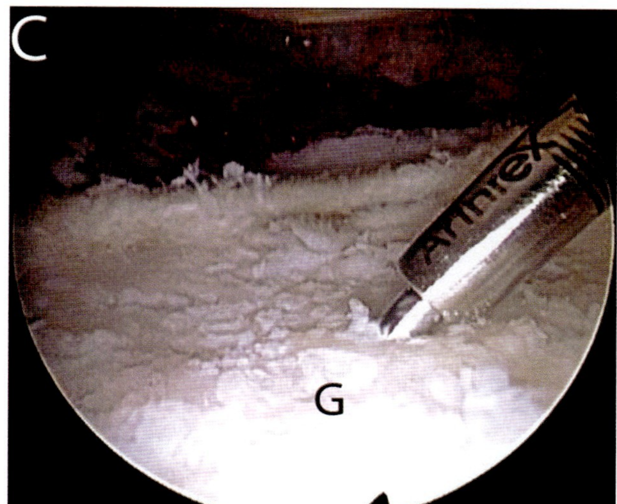

Figure 22.7 Right shoulder, anterosuperolateral portal demonstrating typical steps in glenoid preparation for biological resurfacing. **A:** A curette is used to remove remaining cartilage. **B:** If a biconcave glenoid (biconcavity ridge outlined by *dashed lines*) is present, it may be necessary to burr down the ridge between the two concavities to restore a more normal concavity to the glenoid. **C:** A PowerPick (Arthrex, Inc., Naples, FL) is used to create multiple microfractures in the glenoid to facilitate healing of the dermal allograft to bone. G, glenoid; H, humerus.

the suture limbs exiting the superficial side (i.e., humeral side); as discussed below, this will facilitate suture retrieval as the graft is secured. Due to the elasticity of the graft, suture passage is difficult with a regular needle (and retrograde arthroscopic suture passage with a SutureLasso is difficult for the same reason). We have found that suture passage through the graft is most easily accomplished with a Scorpion suture passer (Fig. 22.8B). Mulberry knots are tied on the end of the simple stitch suture limbs that exit the superficial side of the graft (Fig. 22.8C). These knots are created so that the graft can be shuttled into the glenohumeral joint and will also aid visualization by decreasing the number of long suture limbs in the joint.

Shuttling the graft into the glenohumeral joint and achieving initial graft security is the most difficult portion of the procedure. The diaphragm of an 8.25-mm threaded clear cannula is removed so that the graft can be passed into the glenohumeral joint without obstruction (Fig. 22.9). This cannula is placed in the anterosuperolateral portal. One of two techniques for fixation can then be used depending on whether fixation is labral based or anchor based.

Labral-based Graft Fixation

If there is sufficient labrum for fixation of the graft, our preference is to shuttle and secure the graft via sutures passed through the labrum. Viewing from an anterior portal, a SutureLasso (left curved for a right shoulder) is introduced in the posterior portal and used to pass a Nitinol loop through the labrum at the 7 o'clock position (Fig. 22.10). The loop is retrieved from an anterosuperolateral portal and the most posteroinferior suture limb from the graft is shuttled through the labrum. The suture limb is retrieved just far enough so that it exits the posterior cannula, but is not used to pull the graft in at this time. In order to maintain graft orientation, it is also important that the bottom suture limb (glenoid side) is the one that is shuttled.

The arthroscope is moved to the posterior portal. A SutureLasso (right curved for a right shoulder) is introduced through the anterior portal and used to pass a Nitinol loop through the labrum at the 5 o'clock position. The loop is retrieved from an anterosuperolateral portal and the most anteroinferior suture limb from the graft is shuttled through the labrum. Again, the suture limb is retrieved just

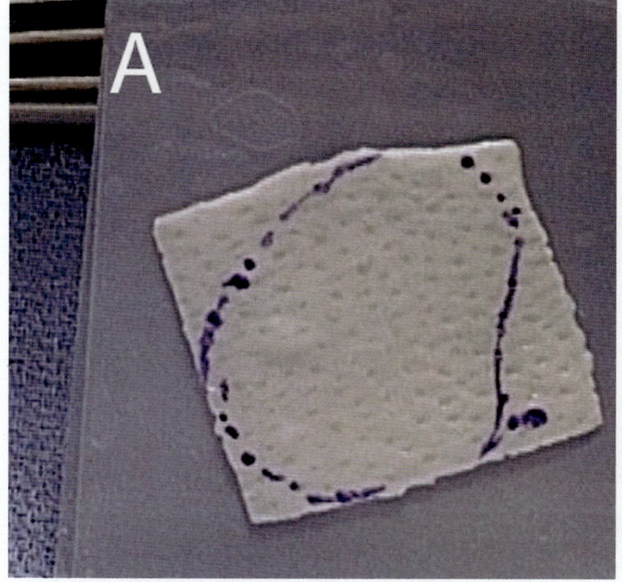

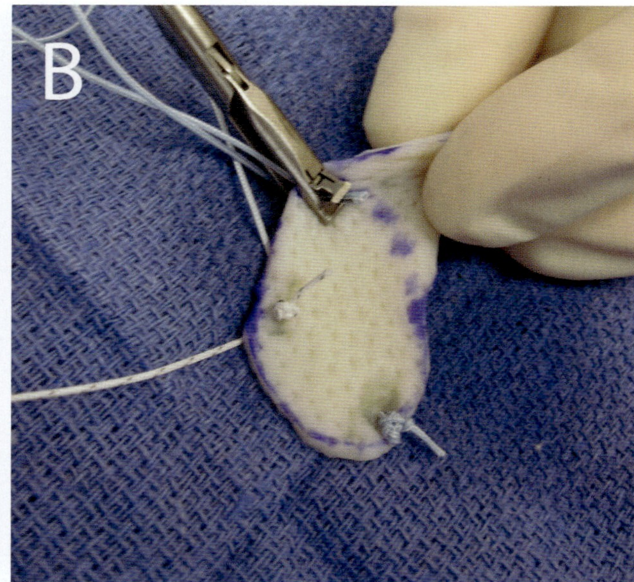

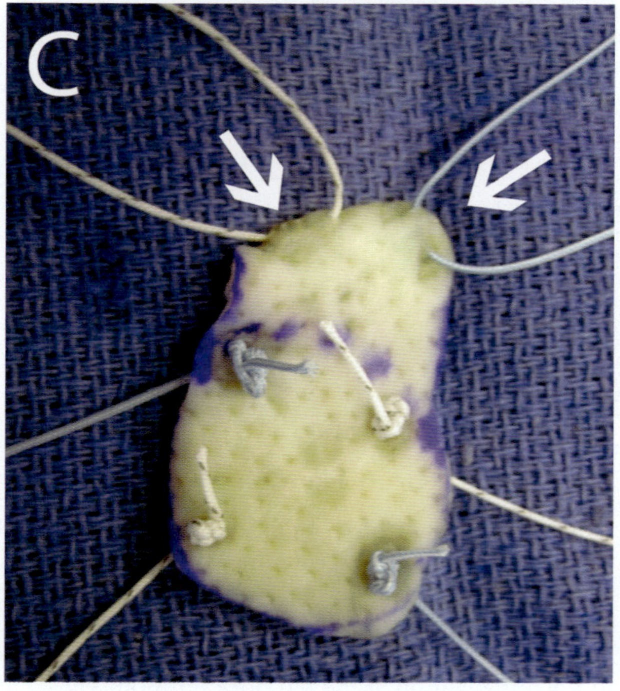

Figure 22.8 Graft preparation. **A:** After the glenoid is sized, an ArthroFlex (Arthrex, Inc., Naples, FL) graft is drawn out to match the size and shape of the native glenoid. **B:** Sutures are easiest to preplace in the graft with a Scorpion (Arthrex, Inc., Naples, FL) suture passer. **C:** Final prepared graft. Mulberry knots are tied in the inferior and middle sutures to assist in graft shuttling. The superior sutures at 10 o'clock and 2 o'clock are placed as inverted mattress stitches (*white arrows*) to facilitate suture retrieval during graft fixation.

enough so that it exits the anterior cannula, but is not used to pull the graft in at this time.

Once the posteroinferior and anteroinferior sutures have been placed, the graft is ready to be shuttled into the joint. The arthroscope is removed from the shoulder. The graft is rolled up on itself to facilitate shuttling into the joint. Then, the suture limbs exiting the anterior and posterior cannulas are simultaneously tensioned to deliver the graft into the joint through the anterosuperolateral portal (Fig. 22.11). Once the graft is delivered into the glenohumeral joint, the anterosuperolateral cannula is replaced with a different cannula that has an intact diaphragm and the arthroscope is reinserted through this portal. The graft is inspected to confirm proper orientation.

To obtain initial security of the graft, the anteroinferior and posteroinferior sutures are tied. The posteroinferior mulberry knot is retrieved out the posterior portal and cut (Fig. 22.12). The posterior sutures are then tied with a Surgeon's Sixth Finger Knot Pusher (Arthrex, Inc., Naples, FL). This step is repeated with the anteroinferior suture. Once these points are secured, the graft will have a reasonable amount of stability and will maintain its orientation within the joint.

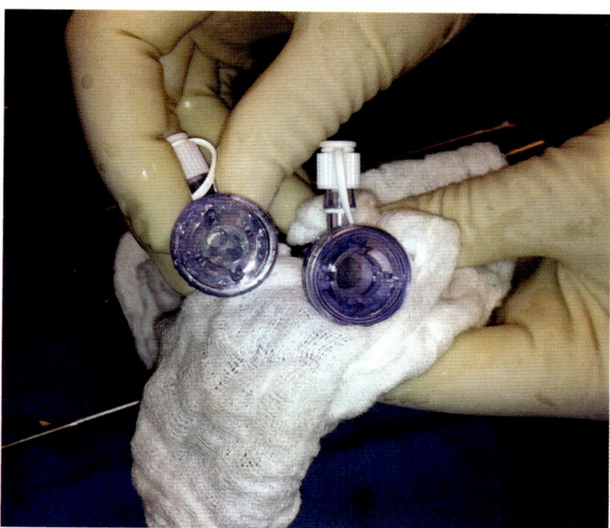

Figure 22.9 External view demonstrating an 8.25-mm cannula in which the diaphragm has been removed (**right**) to facilitate shuttling a glenoid graft into the joint.

The remainder of the graft is then secured with preplaced graft sutures beginning anteriorly and progressing from inferior to superior. A deep-sided anterior suture limb (glenoid side) is retrieved out the posterior portal. A SutureLasso is introduced through the anterior portal and passed through the labrum. A Nitinol loop is retrieved out the posterior portal and used to shuttle the suture through the anterior labrum. Then, the mulberry knot from the suture is retrieved and cut, and static knots are tied. The process continues superiorly until all simple stitches have been passed. Then, the posterior sutures are

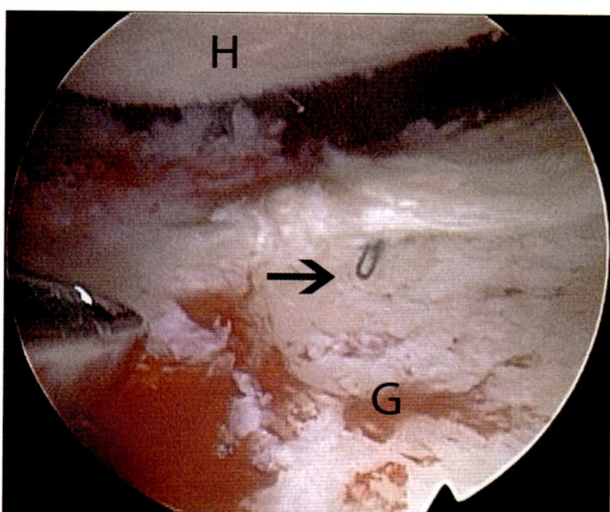

Figure 22.10 Right shoulder, anterosuperolateral portal. A SutureLasso (Arthrex, Inc., Naples, FL) is used to pass a Nitinol loop (*black arrow*) through the posterior labrum in order to shuttle a suture for labral-based fixation of a glenoid resurfacing graft. G, glenoid; H, humerus.

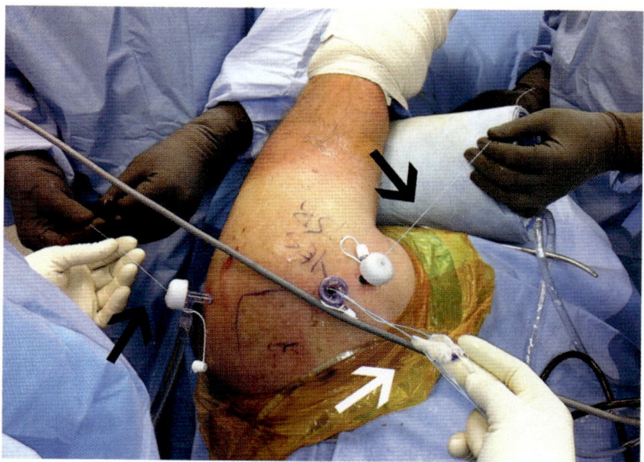

Figure 22.11 External view of a left shoulder demonstrates a glenoid resurfacing graft that is ready to be shuttled into the glenohumeral joint. Note: The graft (*white arrow*) has been rolled on itself to fit through an 8.25-mm cannula. An anteroinferior suture limb placed through the graft was previously passed through the anteroinferior labrum and exits the anterior portal. Similarly, a posteroinferior suture limb placed through the graft was passed through the posteroinferior labrum and exits the posterior portal. Assistants apply traction simultaneously to the suture limbs exiting the anterior and posterior portals (*black arrows*) in order to deliver the graft into the glenohumeral joint.

similarly passed and tied. If the angle of approach allows, suture passage through the labrum can be accomplished in one step by using a Penetrator or BirdBeak (Arthrex, Inc., Naples, FL) to pass underneath the labrum and retrieve a deep-sided suture (Fig. 22.13). As fixation progresses from inferior to superior, it becomes more difficult to retrieve the deep-sided suture limb to shuttle through the labrum. This is why the two most superior sutures were placed as mattress stitches during graft preparation. With this stitch configuration, the sutures are visible on the humeral side

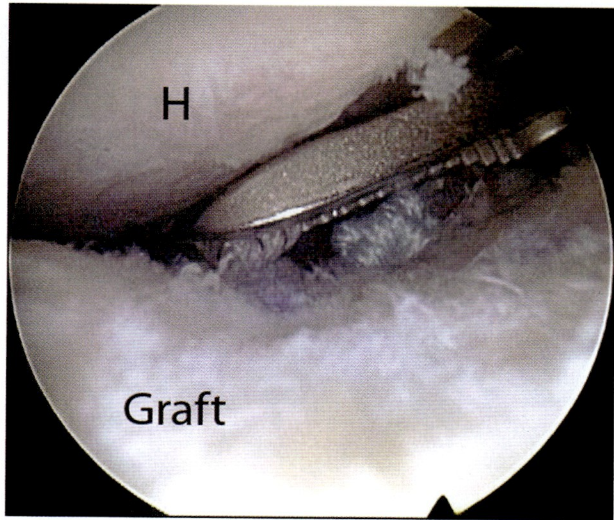

Figure 22.12 Right shoulder, anterosuperolateral viewing portal demonstrates retrieval of a posterior mulberry knot used to shuttle a glenoid resurfacing graft. H, humerus.

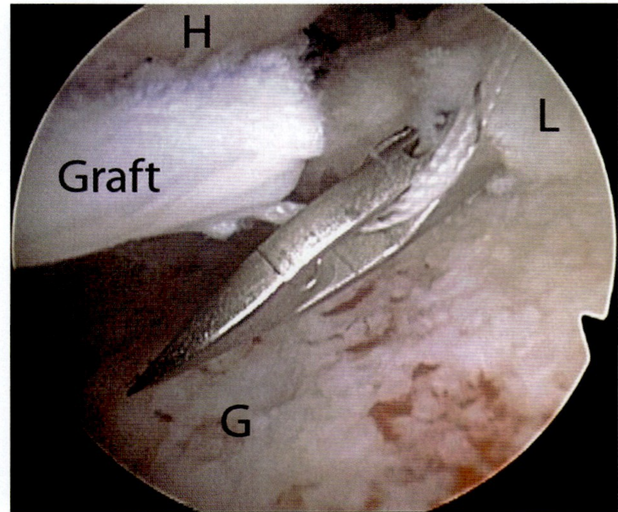

Figure 22.13 Right shoulder, anterosuperolateral viewing portal demonstrates use of a Penetrator (Arthrex, Inc., Naples, FL) to pass a deep-sided resurfacing graft suture underneath the labrum. G, glenoid; H, humerus; L, labrum.

of the graft and retrieval is therefore easier. To secure these stitches superiorly, either PushLock anchors can be used, or both suture limbs are shuttled through the labrum to create a horizontal mattress stitch. The final graft is inspected for stability, contour, and glenoid coverage (Fig. 22.14).

Anchor-based Graft Fixation

If there is insufficient labrum for graft fixation, anchors must be used to shuttle and secure the graft. The graft is prepared in the same manner as previously described with the exception that sutures are not preplaced at the 5 o'clock and 7 o'clock positions. Viewing from an anterior portal, a BioComposite SutureTak anchor is placed posteriorly at the 7 o'clock position and a suture limb is retrieved out the anterosuperolateral portal (with the diaphragm removed). The arthroscope is moved to the posterior portal. A SutureTak anchor is placed anteriorly at the 5 o'clock position and a suture limb is retrieved out the anterosuperolateral portal (Fig. 22.15).

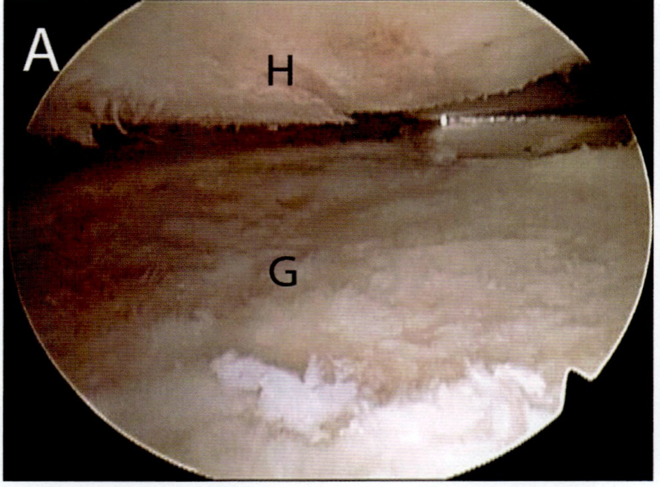

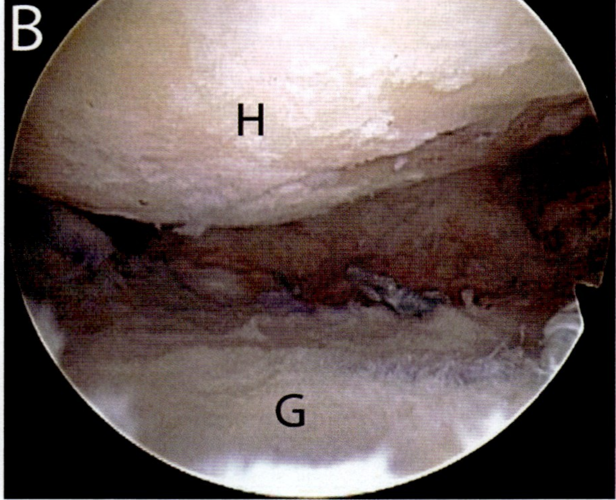

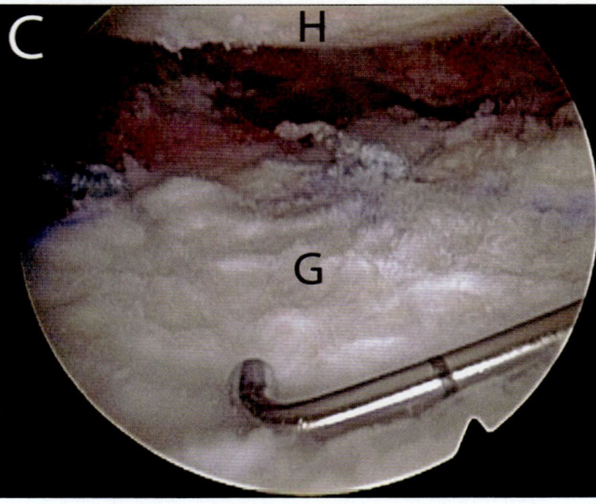

Figure 22.14 Right shoulder, anterosuperolateral viewing portal. **A:** View prior to resurfacing. There are degenerative changes of the glenohumeral joint and decreased glenohumeral joint space. **B:** Same shoulder after capsular release, osteophyte debridement, and biologic glenoid resurfacing with labral-based fixation. Note: The glenohumeral joint space has been increased through capsular release. **C:** Up-close view of the glenoid resurfacing graft. G, glenoid; H, humerus.

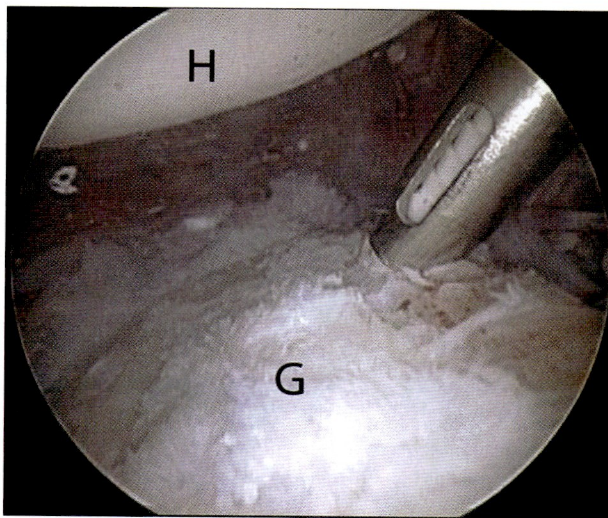

Figure 22.15 Left shoulder, anterosuperolateral viewing portal. In this young patient with multiple prior dislocations and glenohumeral arthritis, there is insufficient labrum for fixation of a resurfacing graft. An anteroinferior anchor is placed in preparation for a glenoid resurfacing graft.

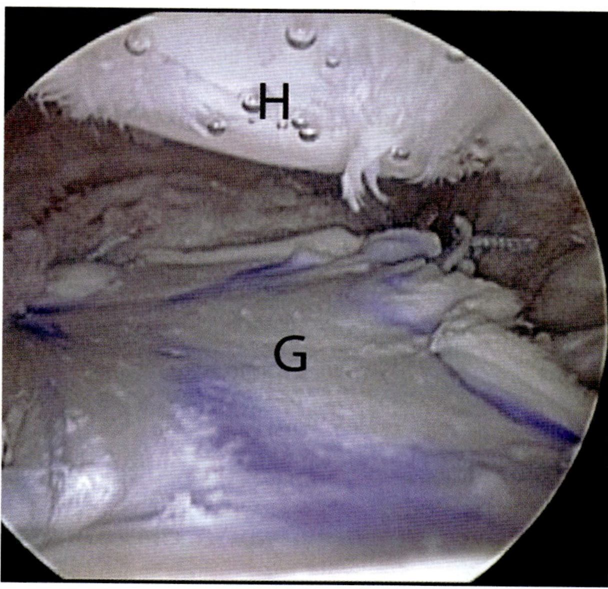

Figure 22.16 Left shoulder, anterosuperolateral viewing portal demonstrates final appearance of a glenoid resurfacing graft secured with anchor-based fixation. Knots are seen inferiorly. The remainder of the graft has been secured with knotless anchors (PushLock; Arthrex, Inc., Naples, FL).

A standard knot pusher or suture retriever is passed down the two sutures that exit the anterosuperolateral portal to ensure that there are not any twists between the anterior and the posterior limbs. The arthroscope is removed from the shoulder. Extracorporeally, a Scorpion is used to pass these anterior and posterior suture limbs from deep (glenoid side) to superficial (humeral side) through the glenoid graft at the 5 o'clock and 7 o'clock positions, respectively. Mulberry knots are tied on the humeral side of the suture limbs.

The graft is rolled on itself and opposite ends of the anterior and posterior suture limbs are simultaneously tensioned to pull the glenoid graft into the joint. The anterosuperolateral cannula is replaced with one with an intact diaphragm, the arthroscope is reinserted through this portal, and the orientation of the graft is confirmed. The posteroinferior mulberry knot is retrieved out the posterior portal and cut. The posterior sutures are then tied with a Surgeon's Sixth Finger Knot Pusher (Arthrex, Inc., Naples, FL). The suture limb the from the double-loaded posterior anchor that was not used for shuttling is then retrieved, passed through the graft with a Scorpion FastPass (Arthrex, Inc., Naples, FL), and a static knot is tied. The step is repeated with the anteroinferior suture.

The remainder of graft fixation is accomplished with a knotless technique. Beginning anteriorly and progressing from inferior to superior, the sutures preplaced in the glenoid graft are retrieved and secured to the glenoid with PushLock anchors (Arthrex, Inc., Naples, FL). Posterior fixation is likewise performed. To achieve fixation superiorly, it is necessary to move the arthroscope to a posterior viewing portal and use techniques similar to those for superior labrum anterior to posterior repair. A Port of Wilmington portal is sometimes required for a proper angle of approach to the posterosuperior anchor. Since this portal may be transtendon, we typically use it for percutaneous anchor placement only without placing a cannula. In the case of knotless fixation, however, it is necessary to retrieve the sutures through the same portal used for anchor placement and anchor insertion is more difficult when passing through soft tissues. To minimize soft tissue damage, a 2.9-mm metal cannula (Arthrex, Inc., Naples, FL) is therefore placed in the Port of Wilmington portal. This small cannula allows unobstructed suture removal and anchor insertion, without creating a large defect in the rotator cuff as would be the case with a 7- or 8.25-mm cannula. After placement of the superior anchors, the graft is circumferentially secured and the final appearance is inspected (Fig. 22.16).

REFERENCES

1. Gartsman GM, Brinker MR, Khan M, et al. Self-assessment of general health status in patients with five common shoulder conditions. *J Shoulder Elbow Surg*. 1998;7:228–237.
2. Saltzman MD, Mercer DM, Warme WJ, et al. Comparison of patients undergoing primary shoulder arthroplasty before and after the age of fifty. *J Bone Joint Surg Am*. 2010;92:42–47.
3. Parsons IM IV, Campbell B, Titelman RM, et al. Characterizing the effect of diagnosis on presenting deficits and outcomes after total shoulder arthroplasty. *J Shoulder Elbow Surg*. 2005;14:575–584.
4. Richards DP, Burkhart SS. Arthroscopic debridement and capsular release for glenohumeral osteoarthritis. *Arthroscopy*. 2007;23:1019–1022.
5. Arrigoni P, Brady PC, Huberty D, et al. Capsulolabral advancement for the treatment of glenoid chondromalacia. *Orthopedics*. 2010;33:480–485.
6. De Beer JF, Bhatia DN, van Rooyen KS, et al. Arthroscopic debridement and biological resurfacing of the glenoid in glenohumeral arthritis. *Knee Surg Sports Traumatol Arthrosc*. 2010;18:1767–1773.

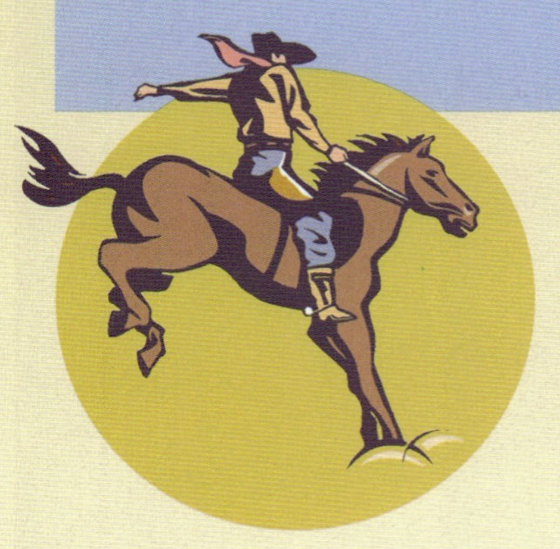

SECTION V

ROUNDTABLE DISCUSSIONS

COWBOY PRINCIPLE 7

The bigger the mouth, the better it looks shut.

Some men talk 'cause they've got somethin' to say. Others talk 'cause they've got to say somethin'.

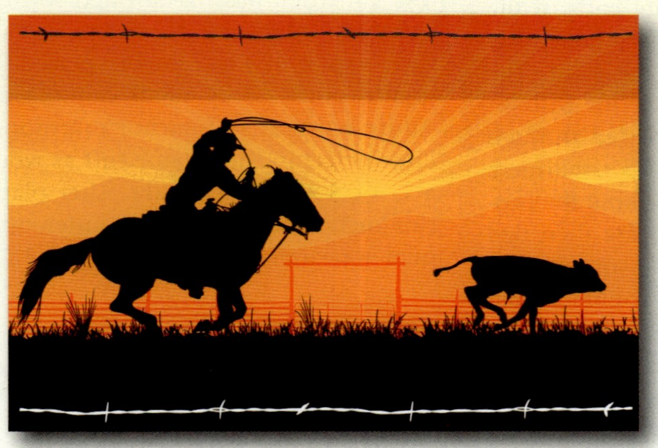

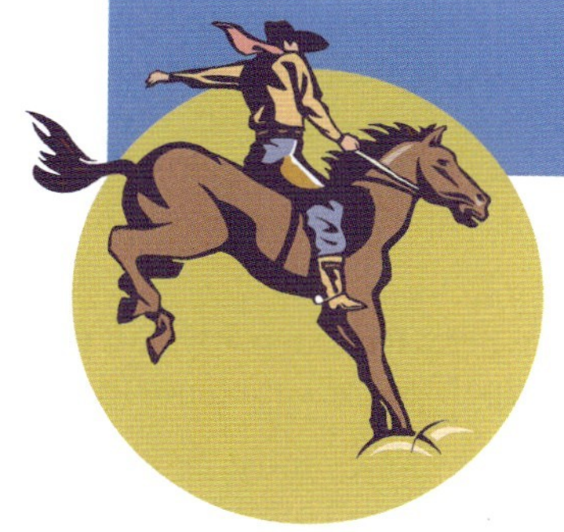

23

Around the Campfire

WESTERN WISDOM

The hottest fire is made by the wood you chop yourself.

As we all know, shoulder arthroscopy has changed the way we treat shoulder disorders and has continued to advance at a rapid pace. Since the first Cowboy's Guide was released in 2006, a number of new techniques have gained increasing popularity necessitating this current companion guide. Furthermore, new scientific evidence has emerged addressing various controversies in shoulder arthroscopy, and this same evidence has created new fields and new questions. In this "campfire chat," we discuss various topics related to arthroscopic shoulder surgery.

SINGLE-ROW VERSUS DOUBLE-ROW REPAIR FOR ROTATOR CUFF TEARS

Ian Lo, MD: Dr Burkhart, when I was a fellow with you in 2001, you showed me a case with 10-year follow-up of a double-row rotator cuff repair. You've obviously been performing double-row rotator cuff repairs for years. What is your current preferred technique for repair of a routine nonretracted tear of the supraspinatus tendon?

Stephen Burkhart, MD: Over many years, my technique of arthroscopic rotator cuff repair has evolved due to both changes in technology and research studies. Although I originally performed classical double-row techniques with medial mattress stitches and lateral simple stitches, my current technique incorporates linkage of the medial and lateral rows. I usually use two SwiveLock suture anchors medially and two SwiveLock suture anchors laterally with FiberTape passed in a SpeedBridge (Arthrex, Inc., Naples, FL) crisscrossing fashion between the two rows of anchors. I also tie the medial safety sutures together in a double-pulley fashion to maximize medial footprint coverage and seal the repair site from joint fluid.

I.L.: You obviously prefer double-row repairs whenever possible. How important is it to link the two rows of suture anchors together?

S.B.: Linking the two rows of suture anchors has multiple advantages. By crisscrossing the sutures and having them span over the rotator cuff surface, this evenly distributes force across each of the suture anchors, maximizes footprint contact area and pressure, and creates a self-reinforcing system. Similar to a Chinese finger trap, a self-reinforcing system tightens as load is applied. In the case of a rotator cuff tear that is repaired using this technique, as tension is applied to the rotator cuff tendon the footprint contact pressures actually increase, further stabilizing the construct and minimizing gap formation.

I.L.: That seems like a very strong construct in theory. However, how do we put that into practice? There seems to be recently a lot of concern about overtensioning the spanning sutures and devascularizing the tendon. Paul, what practical tips are there to maximize fixation and contact pressure while respecting the biology of the tissue?

Paul Brady, MD.: Whenever I'm repairing a rotator cuff I like to think of two things, achieving a stable rotator cuff repair construct and enhancing the biology of the repair as well. It's important to remember that both are critically important in obtaining a healed, functional rotator cuff. In regard to tension, there is medial to lateral tensioning of the torn cuff and there are compressive stabilization forces of the tendon against the bone. While it is critically important to not overtension the repaired tendon from a medial to lateral standpoint, applying compressive force of the repaired tendon against the bone is a good thing. Currently, when I apply compressive forces to the rotator cuff tendon against the bone, I compress until there is tissue indentation, indicating adequate contact pressure against the footprint. Although there is no doubt that overcompressing the sutures is possible, in practice I think that's pretty difficult. Recent studies have shown that even though the transosseous-equivalent technique has the highest contact pressures when compared to other double-row designs, the contact pressures decrease over time as the tendon–bone interface reaches a new steady state level. So that in vivo, I don't think that there is a significant problem with devascularizing the tendon.

It should also be remembered that the tendon itself is a relatively avascular tissue and the majority of the vascular supply, blood vessel ingrowth, and cell migration occurs from the adjacent bone. In fact, blood flow studies have demonstrated that the majority of blood flow comes from the anchors sites. That's why I spend time preparing the bone bed and I like to use cannulated, vented anchors whenever possible (BioComposite SwiveLock C and BioComposite Corkscrew FT; Arthrex, Inc., Naples, FL). These anchors are composed of tricalcium phosphate. I believe that the vents in these anchors allow access channels from the deeper marrow elements to the repair site, enhancing the biological milieu at the repair site while still providing stable fixation.

I.L.: Those are some good tips, Paul. If you usually do double-row repairs, then when do you perform a single-row repair? Is it ever indicated?

P.B.: My major indication for a single-row repair is when the mobility of the tendon is insufficient to perform a double-row repair. I would never advocate overtensioning a repair just to obtain a double-row construct. We already know that tension overload is a major cause of repair failure. If I'm faced with a situation where there is minimal mobility of the tendon despite mobilization techniques, like a double interval slide case, I will perform a single-row rotator cuff repair. The second situation in which I will only utilize a single-row repair is if I have an isolated small bursal-sided partial-thickness tear or an upper subscapularis tear. Sometimes I will only utilize one anchor for such a repair. Also, if there is tendon loss, as when there is a significant tendon stump on the tuberosity, I will do a single-row repair. The key is to place the medial fixation point 2 or 3 mm lateral to the musculotendinous junction. You should never medialize your sutures beyond that point. If the tissue quality is poor, I'll also augment the fixation utilizing a tissue-grasping suturing technique like a modified Mason Allen stitch or MAC stitch.

I.L.: I agree. The other place I will perform a single-row repair is with chronic subscapularis tendon tears. Many times even with a three-sided release, excursion is sufficient for only a single-row repair, which still provides a very secure repair. However, if there is enough excursion, I will still perform a double-row subscapularis repair to maximize the repair construct.

P.B.: That can be a pretty tight space anteriorly. Do you have any tips for double-row repair of the subscapularis?

I.L.: Well, all the standard techniques must be used to maximize the anterior working space. This includes the posterior lever push, internal rotation, and addressing the subscapularis tendon early in the procedure. Then, we perform a transosseous-equivalent technique usually using BioComposite Corkscrew FT anchors medially and BioComposite PushLock or BioComposite SwiveLock C anchors (Arthrex, Inc., Naples, FL) laterally. We pass the medial sutures individually as mattress sutures and tie the sutures. However, when you tie the sutures medially, this usually reduces the tendon to the bone bed and obstructs visualization from a posterior glenohumeral portal. Therefore, to visualize the repair site, I'll use the anterosuperolateral portal as the viewing portal and create accessory anterolateral portals for insertion of the BioComposite PushLock or SwiveLock anchors laterally. The other tip is that if you're running out of lesser tuberosity for anchor insertion, you can cheat slightly into the bicipital groove, which has good bone quality. You just have to be cognizant about the biceps tendon and any previously performed or planned biceps tenodesis.

P.B.: Those are fantastic tips, Ian. I also frequently perform a coracoplasty very early during my subscapularis work. Clearing this space anteriorly can increase visualization significantly as well.

SUBSCAPULARIS REPAIRS

I.L: Speaking of subscapularis tendon tears, Dr Burkhart, you've pretty much developed and championed the field of arthroscopic repair of the subscapularis tendon. Do you always repair a torn subscapularis? Have you ever just debrided a tear of the upper subscapularis?

S.B.: In my mind, the subscapularis tendon is the most important rotator cuff tendon and any pathology should be addressed. It's anatomically a large tendon, it's important in anterior instability, and it forms the anterior moment of the transverse plane force couple. Unrecognized subscapularis tendon pathology that goes unrepaired is a significant cause of poor outcome following rotator cuff repair. With that in mind, I treat the subscapularis tendon similar to the way that you would treat a supraspinatus tendon tear. If a patient had a full-thickness 1-cm tear of the supraspinatus tendon, wouldn't you repair it? Of course, you would.

And you should do the same for the subscapularis. If a patient has a full-thickness tear of the upper 1 cm of the subscapularis tendon, I would repair it. I treat partial tears in a similar fashion. If the partial tear appears to involve greater than one-third of the tendon thickness, especially if I'm worried about incompetence of the medial sling with biceps subluxation, I will repair the partial-thickness subscapularis tendon as well as address the biceps tendon. In active patients, I prefer biceps tenodesis over tenotomy.

I believe that over the long term, debridement of a full-thickness upper subscapularis tendon tear will likely fare similarly to debridement of full-thickness supraspinatus tendon tears. The results will likely deteriorate over time. I would only consider debridement of a subscapularis tendon tear in an elderly patient with limited goals who might not want to have a prolonged rehabilitation period. In this scenario of an elderly low-demand patient, I would probably address the biceps tendon with a biceps tenotomy as well.

I.L.: How about the coracoid, Paul? Do you always perform a coracoplasty when you repair a subscapularis? What are your indications for a coracoplasty?

P.B.: Performing a coracoplasty in conjunction with a subscapularis tendon repair is a common procedure. But it is not performed all the time. First, we should differentiate clearing of the soft tissues off the undersurface of the coracoid and subcoracoid space from actual bony resection of the coracoid tip or coracoplasty. Performing the soft tissue subcoracoid bursectomy is important and I perform this on almost all cases of full-thickness tears of the subscapularis. I perform this routinely since clearing of the soft tissues improves visualization and mobility, and allows for a tension-free repair.

My trigger for a coracoplasty is light. I think the morbidity of a coracoplasty is minimal (much like an acromioplasty) and the potential benefit is great. When clearing the rotator interval tissue, I always expose the coracoid tip in a patient with any subscapularis pathology. If the tip of a shaver, which has a width of 5 mm, fits easily between the coracoid tip and the subscapularis, I do not perform a coracoplasty. If it is tight whatsoever—off with the coracoid tip!

When performing the coracoplasty, I'm careful to both keep the plane of resection parallel to the plane of the subscapularis and maintain the integrity of the coracoacromial arch and the conjoint tendon.

I.L.: Dr Burkhart, let's talk about extremely retracted subscapularis tendon tears. How far medial do you dissect the subscapularis tendon?

S.B.: My routine is to perform a three-sided release of the subscapularis tendon by resecting the rotator interval, skeletonizing the posterolateral coracoid, decompressing the subcoracoid space, releasing the middle glenohumeral ligament, releasing the adhesions between the inferolateral border of the coracoid neck and the superior border of the subscapularis with an arthroscopic elevator, and releasing the adhesions between the anterior glenoid neck and the posterior subscapularis with an arthroscopic elevator. In the vast majority of cases, a three-sided release will provide sufficient mobility for tendon reduction to the anatomic bone bed. I don't believe that more aggressive mobilization is required in routine cases, and medial dissection is potentially dangerous. When I'm performing dissection around the coracoid, I stay on the posterolateral aspect of the coracoid and do not dissect medial to the coracoid or the conjoint tendon. Such medial dissection is unnecessary for subscapularis tendon mobilization and risks injury to the brachial plexus and other important neurovascular structures. Dissection of the axillary or subscapular nerves is unnecessary and does not improve mobility of the subscapularis.

I.L.: Well, that makes sense. What do you do in cases where you have improved mobility but not anatomically to the bone bed?

S.B.: In this scenario, I'll medialize the bone bed by up to 7 mm. I'll do this not only to allow reduction to the bone but also to improve tendon-to-bone contact when there is sufficient mobility. We have shown that we can safely medialize the bone bed by 7 mm to maximize tendon contact without a loss of internal rotation range of motion. In these cases, which are almost always salvage subscapularis tendon cases, I believe it's important to restore the anterior moment and balance the force couples about the shoulder. Furthermore, the only other reasonable alternative is to perform a subcoracoid pectoralis major transfer, which is a major reconstructive procedure and is seldom necessary.

I.L.: Let's just move back to the biceps tendon. How do you decide when to perform a biceps tenodesis and with what technique?

S.B.: In the vast majority of cases of subscapularis tears, even upper subscapularis tears, there is disruption of the medial sling resulting in biceps instability. Therefore, the biceps tendon must be addressed. Failure to address the biceps may result in ongoing biceps instability, and this can disrupt the subscapularis repair. Furthermore, by addressing the biceps tendon early in the procedure, visualization of the subscapularis tear is improved. It's my routine to perform a biceps tenodesis, except in elderly low-demand patients where a biceps tenotomy will suffice. I prefer using a 7- or 8-mm BioComposite Tenodesis screw, performing the tenodesis in the upper portion of the bicipital groove.

PASTA LESIONS

I.L.: Okay, let's move on to another controversial topic, partial-thickness tears of the articular surface of the rotator cuff or the so-called partial articular surface tendon avulsion (PASTA) lesion. Let's suppose you have a tear involving 50% of the tendon thickness. Paul, what's your preferred repair technique?

P.B.: In this type of patient, I prefer to do a transtendon repair. We know from various biomechanical studies that a transtendon repair, which preserves the residual attachment, is stronger under load than a rotator cuff repair following completion of the tear. Also, it may theoretically act as a source of cells for healing and share the load during the early rehabilitation phase. For these reasons, if after debridement of the tendon, there is significant robust tendon remaining that is 25% or more, I prefer to perform a transtendon repair.

I.L.: What's your preferred transtendon technique?

P.B.: If I have a fairly large PASTA lesion, after thorough bone preparation I'll use two suture anchors medially. The anteromedial anchor can usually be placed through the anterosuperolateral portal (thus not violating the cuff during insertion). The posteromedial anchor is passed in a transtendon fashion. I utilize a spinal needle and a shuttle technique (as outlined in the accompanying DVD) to pass two sutures each through four cuff sites. I then tie one color suture from each anchor in a horizontal mattress fashion and the other color sutures are tied in a double-pulley technique. After tying the medial sutures instead of cutting the limbs, I'll pass them laterally and compress them into one or two lateral SwiveLock sites.

I.L.: So you're combining the double-pulley and suture-bridge techniques to repair a PASTA lesion—a so-called PASTA-Bridge technique.

P.B.: Yes, by combining both techniques, you seal the joint off and provide medial footprint compression with the double-pulley technique, and then provide footprint compression for the rest of the lateral rotator cuff using the suture-bridge technique. Although the cuff tear is not full thickness, it is not unreasonable to think that the remaining intact lateral cuff is not healthy and thus applying a transosseous-equivalent type repair could be beneficial.

I.L.: Nice technique. Okay, I always have trouble placing anchors transtendon, since you're essentially passing these anchors blindly through the subacromial space and into the glenohumeral joint and greater tuberosity. Dr Burkhart, do you have any tricks when placing an anchor transtendon?

S.B.: There are a couple of little tricks you can use. First, prior to placing anchors, you should perform a subacromial decompression and clear the subacromial space of bursa. This is performed so that when you do need to retrieve the sutures to tie them they won't be caught up in any bursa and you won't have to unnecessarily shave the subacromial space and risk damaging your sutures. Second, I always use a spinal needle to determine my correct angle of approach and leave this in place to act as a guide. Finally, to ensure that I recreate the same angle of approach with the punch and anchor, I will commonly use a small cannula and place it transtendon through the rotator cuff. This way I can be guaranteed accurate and efficient anchor placement. The small 5-mm hole that is bluntly created by the cannula by spreading of adjacent tendon fibers is really of no clinical significance, especially when the tendon is repaired using the double-pulley suture-bridge technique, or PASTA-Bridge.

I.L.: Those are some great tips. One last question regarding subacromial decompression for a PASTA lesion. Do you perform this in every case with bony resection of the acromion or how do you judge when and how much of a decompression to perform?

S.B.: When I'm addressing the subacromial space with a concomitant PASTA lesion, it's important to evaluate the radiographs preoperatively and to evaluate for evidence of impingement on arthroscopic evaluation. I always perform a bursectomy to assist in identification of the transtendon sutures. Even though we commonly think of PASTA lesions as degenerative lesions, external impingement can contribute to the pathogenesis of a PASTA lesions since indentation of the bursal surface can create high tensile stresses on the undersurface of the cuff and therefore contribute to fiber failure. For this reason, if there is evidence of impingement on arthroscopic evaluation in the subacromial space in addition to a type II or III acromion, I will perform an acromioplasty as part of the treatment of a PASTA lesion.

ROTATOR CUFF GRAFTS

I.L.: Let's move on now, to the other extreme. Let's suppose you have a massive tear of the rotator cuff that is not repairable using standard techniques. What are your options and when would you consider a patch?

S.B.: I believe that rotator cuff patches are a new and expanding field of shoulder surgery and the indications are continuing to evolve. Furthermore, as the technology for graft sterilization and preparation advances, the indications and results will also continue to evolve. Currently, I believe that rotator cuff patches are still somewhat experimental and if a rotator cuff repair is possible using standard or advanced techniques this should be performed first. Many times, a partial repair with restoration of the force couples about the shoulder will result in significantly improved outcomes making a cuff patch unnecessary. Furthermore, in older patients who may not tolerate a prolonged rehabilitation program, a limited goals debridement may provide sufficient pain relief.

So, generally speaking, in my opinion a rotator cuff patch might be a consideration only in the case of a revision procedure in a young, nonsmoking, nonworkers' compensation, motivated patient with an irreparable rotator cuff tear.

I.L.: I agree that rotator cuff patches have a limited place in arthroscopic shoulder surgery. I also believe that repair using native tissues is better than a graft. I use grafts almost exclusively for revision cases and use them for augmentation of large or massive revision cases and for tendon replacement or to bridge a gap in an irreparable rotator cuff tear. However, I caution my patients that the main indication for the use of a graft, especially when used as a tendon replacement or tendon extension, is for relief of pain. Since the length–tendon relationship of the rotator cuff is not restored when the defect is bridged, I do not believe that any significant strength gains will be achieved over and above pain relief alone. This is why I believe it is important to repair as much of the rotator cuff as possible and achieve at least a balanced partial repair to provide a stable fulcrum of motion.

The other important aspect with these grafts is to be slow with their rehabilitation. I'll place these patients in a sling for a minimum of 6 to 8 weeks with only gentle passive range-of-motion exercises. I'll start forward elevation at about 6 to 8 weeks and delay rotator cuff strengthening for 4 months. It takes time for these grafts to heal and remodel and I believe that aggressive rehabilitation risks early graft failure.

BIOLOGICAL ENHANCEMENT OF ROTATOR CUFF HEALING

I.L.: We've talked about the use of grafts for the augmentation of rotator cuff repair. Are there any other techniques you use for the enhancement of rotator cuff healing?

P.B.: I don't use anything routinely in a standard rotator cuff repair. I believe if you have a biomechanically sound repair, which respects the tissue, biological healing will follow. It is important to incorporate the principles of a biomechanically sound repair, which reconstructs the footprint and provides compression. However, we know that the vast majority of healing cells originate from the bone with a lesser contribution from the bursa. For this reason, I prefer to create access channels from the marrow elements to the healing interface. This can be done with chondral picks and a microfracture technique, but the easiest way to do this is by using cannulated vented anchors, which will naturally deliver marrow elements to the bone–tendon interface during the healing process. These anchors also provide excellent tendon fixation to bone at time zero and with healing, as the bone actually grows through the cannulation and vents.

I.L.: Do you do anything special to the bone bed to enhance healing?

P.B.: Thankfully, with the advancement of fully threaded suture anchors, I don't think it's quite so essential that we not decorticate the bone bed. In fact, I prepare the bone bed until two essential goals are achieved. First, I want NO soft tissue present. Secondly, I want to see good bleeding bone. I even turn the pump off occasionally in order to visualize this. Sometimes, this does require an element of decortication of the bone bed and with the enhanced pullout strengths of modern suture anchors, I am not all that concerned about this. Vented anchors are an excellent concept as they will allow for the patient's own marrow contents to extravasate into the repair site. This will allow for natural growth factors and stem cells to enhance the healing process.

I.L.: Those are some great technical pearls, Paul. How about the current enthusiasm about platelet-rich plasma (PRP)? Dr Burkhart, what's the current thinking about PRP?

S.B.: PRP is an exciting new adjunct, which can improve healing in many different situations. However, its use for rotator cuff repair is still in its infancy and there are controversies related to preparation, delivery, amount, and timing to maximize its effect. I currently use PRP in cases where I am worried about the natural healing potential of the patient or to maximize healing in patients where a failure would be catastrophic. For example, in patients over the age of 70, or who are smokers where the inherent tissue quality may be poor and where the healing potential of the patient may be compromised, PRP is a reasonable adjunct for augmenting the healing potential of the patient. The other patient I will use PRP in is a patient with a large or massive tear, especially two- or three-tendon tear where there is significant rotator cuff weakness. In these patients, a retear of the repair would be catastrophic and therefore enhancing the healing environment to maximize the healing rate is essential. Finally, I use PRP in all revision cuff repairs.

I.L.: There are so many different methods of preparation available to the surgeon. What's your preference and why?

S.B.: For me, I need a system that's quick, easy to use, and provides the proper concentration of growth factors to stimulate healing. The Arthrex, double-syringe ACP system (autologous conditioned plasma) is simple, easy to use, requires only 10 ml of blood, and concentrates growth factors from 5 to 25 times. Furthermore, this single-spin technique results in fewer white blood cells than the double-spin techniques, and high white blood cell counts create inflammation that can inhibit healing. When I use the ACP arthroscopically, I will inject the plasma at the bone–tendon interface after the rotator cuff has been repaired, turning off the pump prior to injecting. Usually, 2 to 4 ml of ACP is injected. Obviously, the results are early but in my experience they appear to be promising in these patients.

TENDON FIXATION FOR ROTATOR CUFF TEARS

I.L.: Dr Burkhart, you've been doing arthroscopic rotator cuff repairs for decades now, and in almost all your techniques to repair a rotator cuff, you've used a suture anchor–based technique. There's a resurgence of interest in rotator cuff repair using traditional bone tunnels but performing this arthroscopically. What are your thoughts on this?

S.B.: To me this appears to be a step backward. Although rotator cuff repair using bone tunnels has been used historically, we know that following a rotator cuff tear, the bone is no longer under load and can become osteopenic. This can make secure tendon fixation to bone difficult.

I.L.: What's your preference then in providing secure tendon fixation to bone?

S.B.: I prefer the use of suture anchors, since this provides the most secure fixation under cyclic load, even in osteopenic bone. The problem with bone tunnels is that under cyclic load, the sutures will actually cut through the thin lateral bone of the greater tuberosity like a cheese cutter. When this occurs the suture loop is loosened, there is loss of loop security, and there is loss of tendon to bone contact leading to gap formation. This can occur even at relatively low cycle numbers suggesting that this may occur clinically in the early rehabilitation phase prior to biological healing.

I.L.: What about its use arthroscopically? Are there any specific advantages or disadvantages?

S.B.: Although the use of bone tunnels arthroscopically is advantageous from a cost perspective, I believe the inherent weaknesses of bone tunnels are even more magnified when bone tunnels are placed arthroscopically.

I.L.: What do you mean?

S.B.: Well, we already know that the lateral cortex is the weak link when using bone tunnels. That's why when we placed bone tunnels using an open or mini-open approach, it was important to have the bone tunnels exit laterally in robust bone. However, multiple biomechanical studies have shown that to do this you have to exit in the distal cortical bone. In addition, some surgeons used to support this lateral bone using mini-plates and other augmentation devices. The problem when doing this arthroscopically, is that the majority of devices drill the bone tunnels in the weak metaphyseal bone and drilling the tunnel arthroscopically distally risks injury to the axillary nerve. In fact, I designed and used a jig system for arthroscopic transosseous bone tunnel repair in the early 1990s in which we drilled distally into cortical bone, below the axillary nerve. I did 12 cases with reasonable results, but the system was never released because I thought that drilling below the axillary nerve was too dangerous to recommend as a technique to other surgeons. However, when the lateral bone tunnel exits in the more proximal weak metaphyseal bone, early suture cut-out is almost guaranteed. That's why I've been using suture anchors for about 20 years.

I.L.: What about the suprascapular nerve, Paul? Do you believe that release of the suprascapular nerve is necessary? If so, when?

P.B.: In my opinion, there is only one true indication for a suprascapular nerve release at the transverse scapular notch. That is a patient with pain and weakness with no MRI evidence of rotator cuff tear as well as EMG evidence of abnormality of BOTH the supraspinatus and the infraspinatus. In such a patient, transection of the transverse scapular ligament can be quite successful.

Some have proposed suprascapular nerve release in the setting of rotator cuff tears, particularly massive rotator cuff tears. While indeed it is clear these patients have evidence of suprascapular neuropathy, the cause of this abnormality is the tear and the retraction of the rotator cuff tendons. If the supraspinatus and/or the infraspinatus significantly retract medially, they pull the suprascapular nerve medially with them. However, since the spine of the scapula is immobile, any medial retraction will cause the nerve to become "kinked" around the spine of the scapula. Obviously, this kinking can cause significant symptoms as well as nerve dysfunction.

Releasing the suprascapular nerve at the transverse scapular notch in this setting—in my opinion—is useless. It will not resolve the kinking of the nerve whatsoever. However, if the surgeon is able to reestablish the rotator cuff insertion to the humerus then, in the process of pulling the cuff laterally, the tension and kinking of the suprascapular nerve around the scapular spine is relieved. Over time this will allow for improvement in nerve function as well as decrease in pain.

BICEPS PATHOLOGY

I.L.: Let's move onto another controversial topic, the biceps tendon. I have always had trouble determining when to address the biceps, particularly when associated with other pathology such as rotator cuff tears. Paul, when do you address the biceps tendon?

P.B.: Well, the first requirement is that you must have a high clinical index of suspicion. When I'm presented with a patient where the predominant complaint is pain, and I'm suspicious of rotator cuff pathology, or subscapularis pathology, I will preoperatively discuss with the patient the possibility of concomitant biceps disease and its possible treatment. Arthroscopically, if there are degenerative changes in the biceps tendon, or partial tearing involving more than 30% to 40% of the tendon thickness, or if there is evidence of biceps instability, either subluxation or dislocation, then I believe treatment of the biceps tendon is indicated. The other scenario of course is when there is concomitant subscapularis pathology. In these patients, biceps instability is usually present and failure to address the biceps can lead to persistent instability and failure of your subscapularis repair.

I.L.: What are your indications for a tenotomy versus tenodesis?

P.B.: I prefer a biceps tenodesis for the majority of patients with biceps pathology using a BioComposite

Tenodesis screw. I believe it provides better overall function and better cosmesis. However, in an elderly patient with a large arm, especially in isolated biceps pathology where a tenodesis would significantly alter their rehabilitation program, a biceps tenotomy is a reasonable option. I prefer BioComposite Tenodesis screw fixation since it is the strongest fixation available and has the ability to maintain the tension on the tendon as the fixation is applied.

I.L.: How about the level of the tenodesis? Do you prefer your tenodesis high in the groove, at the midportion, or do you prefer to perform a mini-open subpectoral tenodesis? What factors influence your decision in performing each technique?

P.B.: The level of my tenodesis depends on two factors, the condition of the biceps tendon along its entire length and any associated pathology. If the biceps pathology extends into the groove and is severe, I believe that a biceps tenodesis very low in the groove or a mini-open subpectoral tenodesis is indicated to remove the diseased tissue. However, if the tendon quality is preserved in the bicipital groove, I believe that this allows more choice in regards to the location of the tenodesis. If a supraspinatus tear is present, I position the tenodesis on the anterolateral aspect of the greater tuberosity and use it as a lateral anchor for simple sutures. If an upper subscapularis tear is present without a supraspinatus tear, I perform the tenodesis high in the bicipital groove at the top of the lesser tuberosity bone bed and utilize the sutures in the subscapularis repair.

I.L.: I like your algorithm, Paul. That simplifies it for me. How about in a long head of the biceps rupture? Dr Burkhart, do you ever attempt to repair or tenodesis a biceps rupture?

S.B.: Well, we know that the majority of patients with long head of the biceps ruptures do well with conservative treatment. However, in patients with symptoms of pain, cramping discomfort, perceived weakness, or an unacceptable cosmetic deformity, a biceps tenodesis to restore the tension on the long head of the biceps and minimize the deformity is indicated. In these patients, if the tendon length and quality are sufficient, I prefer repassing the tendon back to a more proximal location rather than a subpectoral tenodesis. This replaces the tendon back into the bicipital groove, restores the tension in the long head of the biceps, reduces the cosmetic deformity, and can improve function. However, in chronically retracted cases, there will not be enough tendon length to allow repassing the tendon for proximal fixation. In such cases, I will do a subpectoral biceps tenodesis.

SLAP LESIONS

I.L.: Let's move on to superior labrum anterior and posterior (SLAP) lesions. Recently, there have been a number of studies on the poor outcomes of arthroscopic SLAP repair, tempering the initial enthusiasm for the treatment of this lesion. Dr Burkhart, what are your indications for SLAP repair versus a biceps tenodesis?

S.B.: The problem with a lot of these studies and a lot of these patients was that there were a number of SLAP lesions that were repaired where the clinical diagnosis was not a SLAP lesion. Many of these lesions were likely asymptomatic and did not require repair. If you have a patient over the age of 35, who is not an overhead athlete, has another primary diagnosis (e.g., rotator cuff tear), or is involved in a workers' compensation or litigation claim, you should rethink the case prior to performing a SLAP repair.

I.L.: Why not just repair the SLAP lesion?

S.B.: The difficulty when repairing SLAP lesions in these patients is that many develop pain and stiffness postoperatively. In these patients, if I feel as though the SLAP lesion may be symptomatic, I will perform a biceps tenodesis as opposed to a primary SLAP repair, which will eliminate pain due to an unstable biceps root but should not overconstrain the joint. Stiffness after biceps tenodesis is exceptionally rare.

I.L.: Those are some good guidelines. What do you do with the superior labrum in the case where you have performed a biceps tenodesis? Do you debride the residual labrum, or repair the labrum?

S.B.: If I have performed a biceps tenodesis in a patient with a SLAP lesion, the superior labrum usually does not need to be formally repaired. This is particularly relevant in cases where there is significant concomitant disease (e.g., full-thickness rotator cuff tear) and a SLAP repair may overconstrain the joint and create stiffness. However, in athletes, especially when the primary diagnosis is instability, repair of the superior labrum in addition to biceps tenodesis is indicated to improve glenohumeral stability. These are unusual cases, but they commonly occur when a tenodesis is performed for the treatment of a type IV SLAP lesion.

I.L.: How about in revision cases? How do you treat the failed SLAP repair?

S.B.: In patients with a failed or recurrent SLAP repair, one of the primary principles is to ensure that there is no other significant concomitant disease that is contributing to the patient's symptomatology, such as stiffness. If the diagnosis, however, is a failed SLAP repair, then a biceps tenodesis is usually indicated. I believe that revision repair of the SLAP lesion is unlikely to be successful. Usually, a biceps tenodesis will improve the patient's symptoms.

The other patients who may present with failed SLAP repairs are overhead athletes. In a handful of baseball players, I have had successful revision repair of failed SLAP repairs. One thing is certain: high-level baseball players will not do as well with biceps tenodesis as with a successful

SLAP repair. In those athletes, the biceps root seems to be essential to stabilize the humerus as it undergoes angular velocities of up to 7,000 degrees per second. On the other hand, overhead athletes whose sport requires lower angular velocities do well with biceps tenodesis. This includes tennis players, football quarterbacks, and recreational baseball players.

THE FIRST-TIME DISLOCATOR

I.L.: Let's move on to classic anterior instability. Paul, what are your indications for arthroscopic stabilization of the first-time dislocator? Do you have any age limits?

P.B.: Well, to me there are a number of factors to consider. The age of the patients is of primary importance. To me a patient under the age of 20 to 22 is a high-risk patient and early stabilization should be considered. We know from prospective randomized studies that the quality of life outcome in this high-risk age group is better with early stabilization.

I.L.: Do sports or activity level affect your decision as well?

P.B.: Absolutely, I do a Bankart repair after a first-time dislocation in patients who are involved in contact sports, combative sports, or activities in which a second dislocation may be catastrophic. For example, in active military recruits or climbers, early stabilization should also be considered. These are softer indications, however, and the patient as a whole should be evaluated.

I.L.: How about radiographic or MRI findings like bony Bankart lesions or Hill-Sachs lesions?

P.B.: These to me are even softer indications. However, if you have a large bony Bankart lesion that is acute, this essentially represents a glenoid fracture and should be treated as such. Fortunately, most bony Bankart lesions and Hill-Sachs lesions in first-time dislocators are not large, and they may be largely ignored. Either way, if you have a patient who has chosen to be treated conservatively, it is important to counsel the patient on returning for follow-up immediately if a second dislocation occurs so that an arthroscopic stabilization can be performed. This will minimize further pathology, either soft tissue or bony, from multiple recurrent instability episodes.

I.L.: How about a first-time dislocation in an overhead athlete's dominant arm? Dr Burkhart, do you believe these should be treated with early stabilization?

S.B.: Yes, I think it is important in such a patient to do an arthroscopic Bankart repair after the first dislocation, before chronic bony lesions can develop.

I.L.: Bone loss with instability has come to the forefront over that last 7 or 8 years. When do you think bone loss is significant enough to require a bone grafting procedure, especially with the newer arthroscopic options such as the remplissage procedure?

S.B.: The first thing we should understand is that bone loss is very common. In fact, if carefully evaluated, probably 80% to 90% of all unstable shoulders have some degree of bone loss, particularly on the glenoid side. However, not all bone loss is significant enough to require a bone grafting procedure. In a patient with glenoid bone loss of >20% to 25%, an arthroscopic Bankart repair will likely fail and a bone grafting procedure is indicated. In this scenario, a Latarjet reconstruction in my hands provides the most reproducible outcome. I prefer this to other options such as an iliac crest bone graft because the coracoid graft is vascular and has the triple blocking effect of the capsular repair, the extension of the articular arc, and the dynamic stability provided by the conjoint tendon. In addition, by rotating the coracoid graft 90° along its long axis, the undersurface of the graft creates an articular arc that is congruent with the natural curvature of the humeral head, and it lengthens the glenoid articular arc.

I.L.: What about large Hill-Sachs lesions? What are your options?

S.B.: In these patients, it's again important to understand that the majority of large Hill-Sachs lesions are associated with major glenoid bone loss. So that in fact, the treatment of the glenoid bone loss takes precedence over the treatment of the Hill-Sachs lesion. In most cases, large Hill-Sachs lesions are associated with glenoid bone loss >20% so that a Latarjet procedure is indicated. When the Latarjet reconstruction is performed, it extends the articular arc of the glenoid so much that the Hill-Sachs lesion no longer can engage the anterior glenoid and the Hill-Sachs lesion essentially becomes irrelevant. It would be exceptionally unusual to have persistent instability despite a Latarjet reconstruction. But if this happened, a humeral head allograft may be necessary.

P.B.: I agree. In rare cases, where there is massive humeral head bone loss without a glenoid defect, humeral head allografting is indicated. I prefer fresh size-matched osteochondral allografts that preserve the viability of the articular cartilage.

I.L.: What about the remplissage procedure? Where does this arthroscopic procedure fit it?

P.B.: The remplissage procedure has been a very useful adjunct to an arthroscopic Bankart repair in cases where the glenoid bone loss is borderline: about 15% to 20% glenoid bone loss. I use the remplissage procedure in a "belt-and-suspenders-type" approach in cases where I have performed a Bankart repair but am still worried about the bone loss; for example in a case with 15% bone loss on the glenoid side and a defect on the humerus that is >4 mm deep. In this scenario, by filling the defect with the infraspinatus to make the Hill-Sachs lesion extra-articular, in addition to providing a capsulodesis effect from the remplissage, I believe that the repair will be more stable with a lower recurrence rate.

I perform this procedure essentially using a transtendon double-pulley technique, placing anchors superiorly and inferiorly along the edge of the Hill-Sachs lesion and then tying sutures anchor to anchor. This provides contact of the capsule and tendon all along the rim of the Hill-Sachs lesion.

The other scenario in which I will perform the remplissage procedure is when there is a bony Bankart lesion. Even in cases with significant bone loss, we know that by reconstruction of the glenoid by preserving and repairing the bony Bankart lesion we can arthroscopically restore stability. In these cases, I will commonly augment the bony Bankart repair with a remplissage procedure.

I.L.: Thanks, Paul. Dr Burkhart, any tips for bony Bankart repair? How do you routinely perform an arthroscopic bony Bankart repair?

S.B.: A couple of things are important to preoperatively assess prior to arthroscopic bony Bankart repair. First of all in many cases, unless the bony Bankart lesion is acute, the size of the bony fragment is usually smaller than the actual amount of bone loss. That's why in many cases, a suture anchor–based technique utilizing sutures that encircle and capture the fragment will successfully repair the bony Bankart lesion. However, if the fragment is >15% to 20% of the articular surface or particularly wide from a medial to lateral standpoint, it is very difficult to capture the fragment with sutures, so screw fixation is indicated in this type of case. I perform this arthroscopically, using a percutaneous, nested guide system (Glenoid Bone Loss Set; Arthrex, Inc., Naples, FL).

I.L.: Dr Burkhart, any final thoughts on the Latarjet procedure?

S.B.: The Latarjet procedure to me has become a very versatile procedure for difficult cases of instability. I have extended its indications over and above bone loss alone. It's a very good alternative in cases of multiple failed instability surgeries or in cases of failed thermal capsulorrhaphy where there is capsular deficiency. In these difficult cases, the Latarjet reconstruction provides excellent stability and the conjoint tendon can provide soft tissue stability substituting for the deficient capsule. Furthermore, the coracoid graft lengthens the articular arc of the glenoid so much that it becomes impossible to translate the humeral head beyond the expanded glenoid, even though the capsule is deficient or absent.

I.L.: Thanks, guys.

SECTION VI

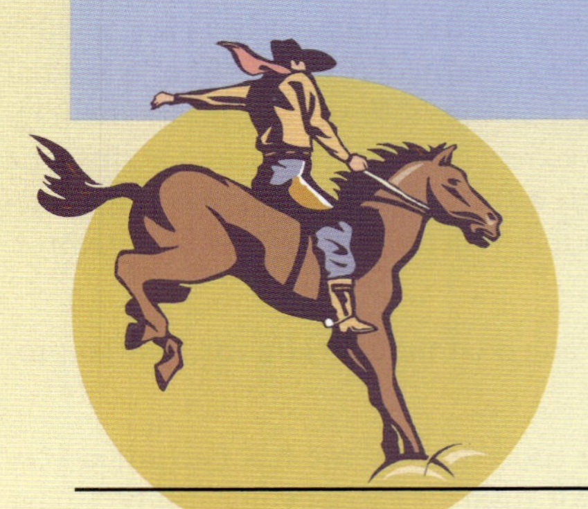

WHAT'S NEW?

COWBOY PRINCIPLE 8

Eagles don't hunt for flies.

We only make progress by discoverin' new tricks or blazin' new trails. All men are created equal, but equal don't mean "the same".

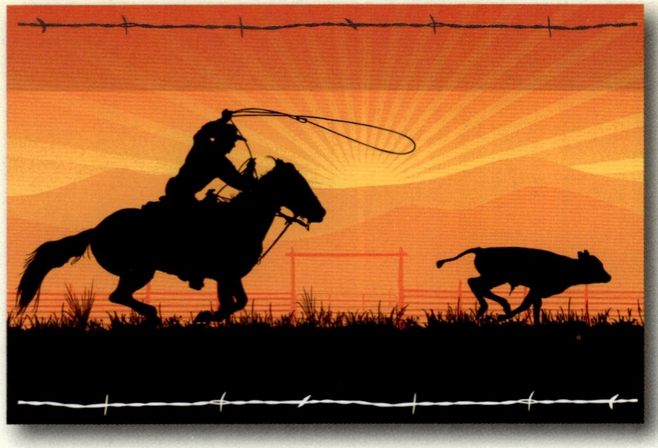

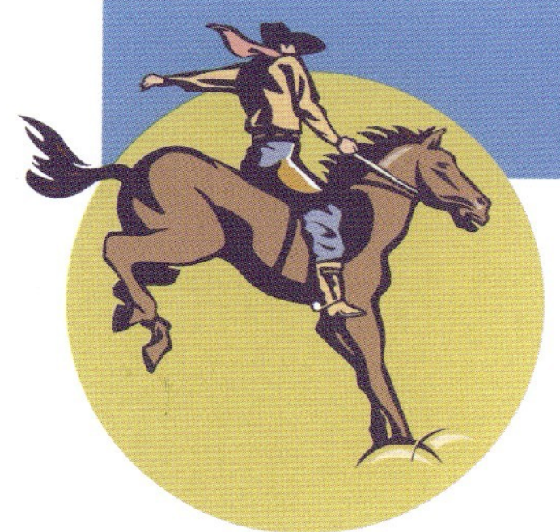

24 Tricks and Tips

WESTERN WISDOM

The wildest broncos are those you rode somewhere else.

This chapter will concentrate on nuggets of useful information that fall into one of three categories of fascinating factoids:

1. Normal arthroscopic anatomy
2. Pathologic arthroscopic anatomy
3. Simple technical tricks for optimized visualization and optimized understanding of what is being visualized

ANATOMIC FACTOIDS

Recognizing Normal Anatomy

Subacromial Anatomy

- The medial border of the subacromial bursa is located at the musculotendinous junction of the supraspinatus. Debriding the medial "curtain" of the subacromial bursa will reveal the supraspinatus muscle belly (Fig. 24.1). Video
- The subacromial "space," in which visualization is easily accomplished, underlies the anterior half of the acromion. The posterior half of the subacromial space is filled with dense fibrofatty tissue that must be debrided in order to visualize the structures in that area.
- The lateral gutter has a "blind pouch" at its lower extent, which is the lower limit of the subacromial bursa. All of the axillary nerve branches lie below that "blind pouch," which represents a good anatomical landmark for the limits of safe dissection in the lateral gutter (Fig. 24.2).

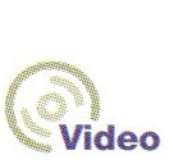

- The scapular spine defines the border between the supraspinatus and infraspinatus muscle bellies. Just lateral to the scapular spine, there is a raphé that continues to define that border (Fig. 24.3).

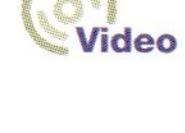

- At the posterior aspect of the greater tuberosity, the tendon of the infraspinatus curls anterolaterally over the top of the supraspinatus tendon and is usually distinctly visible (Fig. 24.4).

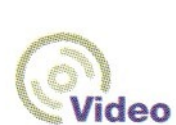

- The anterior border of the supraspinatus is visible as a thickened tendon that borders the thinner rotator interval tissue (Fig. 24.5).

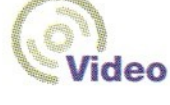

- The teres minor muscle belly extends much further laterally than the infraspinatus muscle belly and can be distinguished as a separate distinct muscle on that basis (Fig. 24.6).

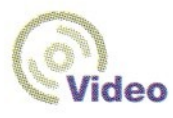

- There is a fat pad overlying the supraspinatus muscle belly, just posterior to the acromioclavicular (AC) joint. This fat pad must be debrided in order to optimally visualize the AC joint (Fig. 24.7).

- When viewed from a posterior viewing portal, the anterior acromion typically has a medial "notch" that lies at the same level as the undersurface of the distal clavicle. This notch is an excellent "target" to aim for when doing an arthroscopic acromioplasty (Fig. 24.8).

Intra-articular Anatomy

- Beneath the superior labrum, the articular cartilage normally extends 2 to 3 mm medial to the corner of the superior glenoid (Fig. 24.9).

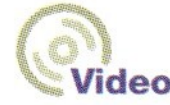

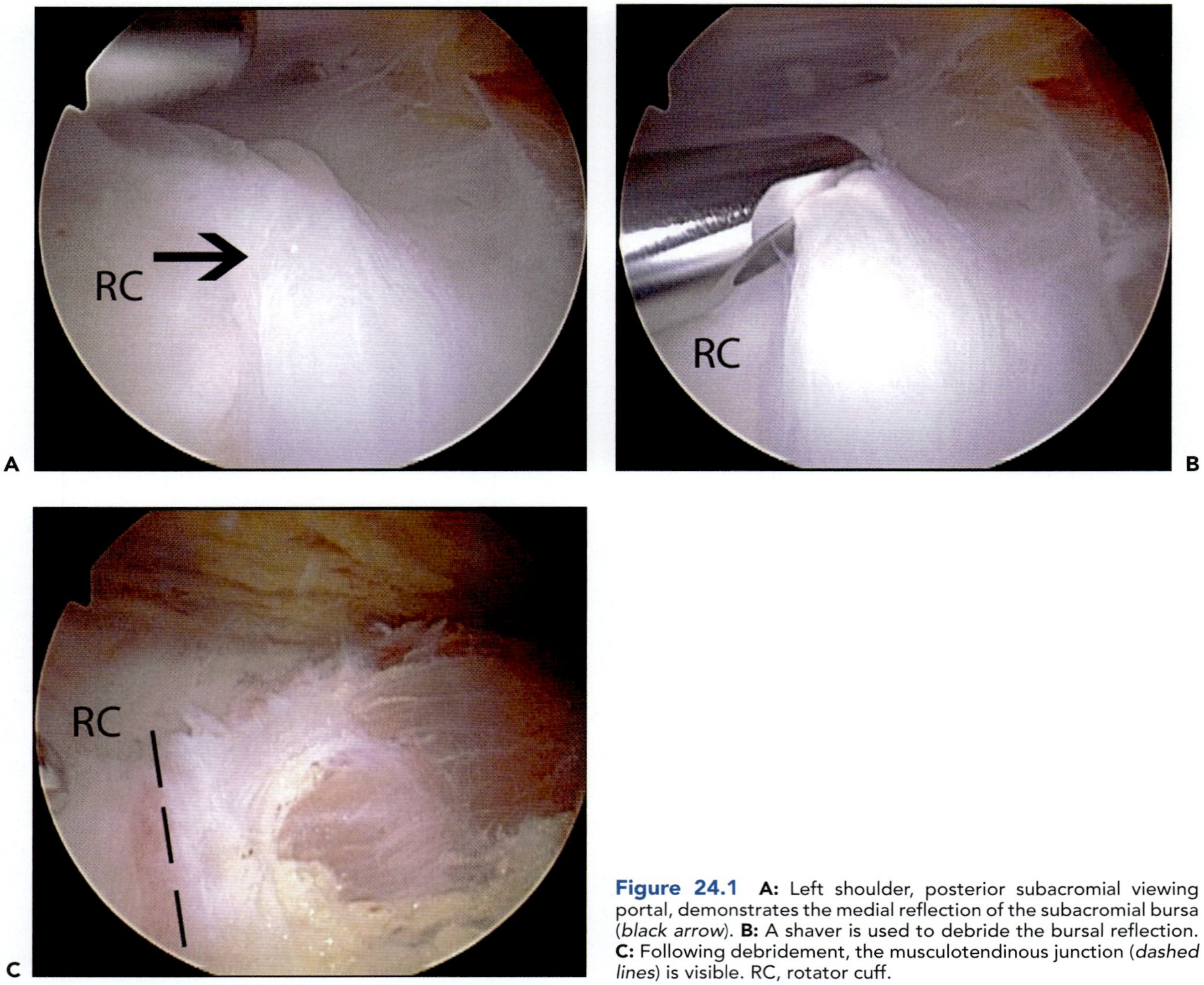

Figure 24.1 **A:** Left shoulder, posterior subacromial viewing portal, demonstrates the medial reflection of the subacromial bursa (*black arrow*). **B:** A shaver is used to debride the bursal reflection. **C:** Following debridement, the musculotendinous junction (*dashed lines*) is visible. RC, rotator cuff.

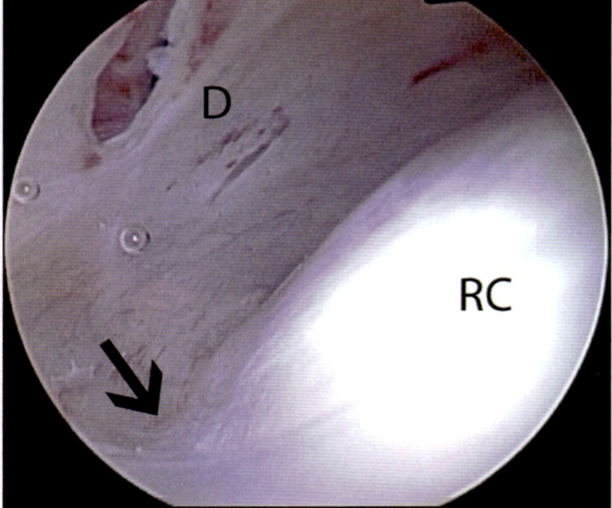

Figure 24.2 Left shoulder, posterior subacromial viewing portal, demonstrates the normal lateral gutter of the subacromial space. The axillary nerve always lies below the lateral bursal reflection (*arrow*). Consequently, lateral dissection should be limited to the level of the lateral bursal reflection. D, internal deltoid fascia; RC, rotator cuff.

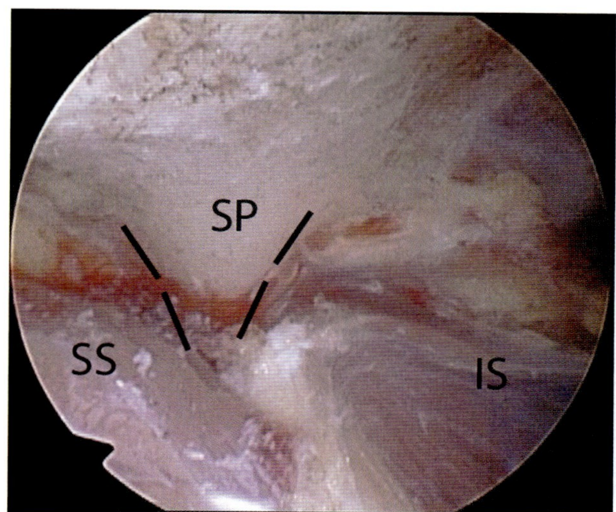

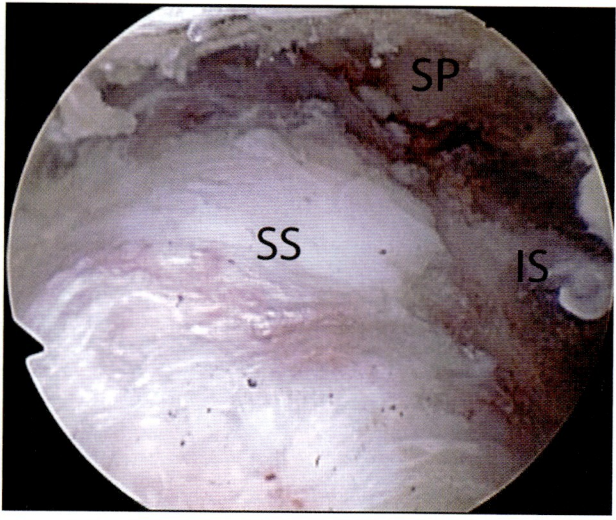

Figure 24.3 **A:** Left shoulder, lateral subacromial viewing portal, demonstrates the scapular spine (outlined by *dashed lines*). The scapular spine defines the interval between the supraspinatus tendon and the infraspinatus tendon. **B:** Profile view in the same shoulder. IS, infraspinatus tendon; SP, scapular spine; SS, supraspinatus tendon.

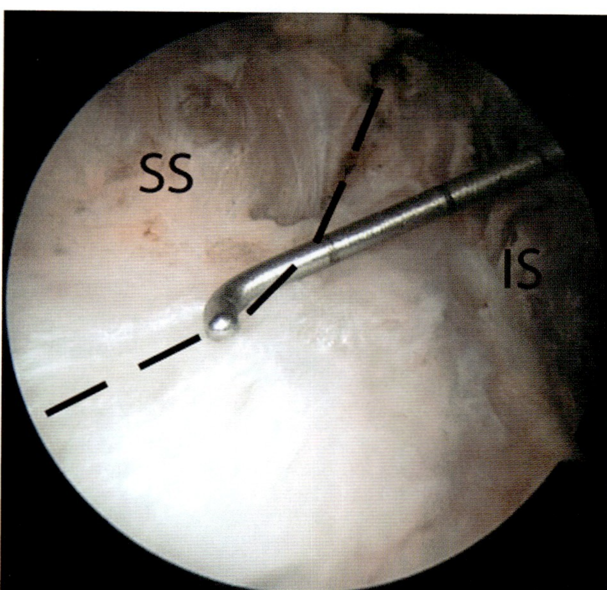

Figure 24.4 Left shoulder, lateral subacromial viewing portal, demonstrates the normal infraspinatus tendon insertion. Note that the anterior insertion of the infraspinatus is not directly lateral to the line of its fibers, but rather curves anterolaterally to its insertion onto the greater tuberosity (*dashed line* indicates anterior margin of infraspinatus). IS, infraspinatus; SS, supraspinatus.

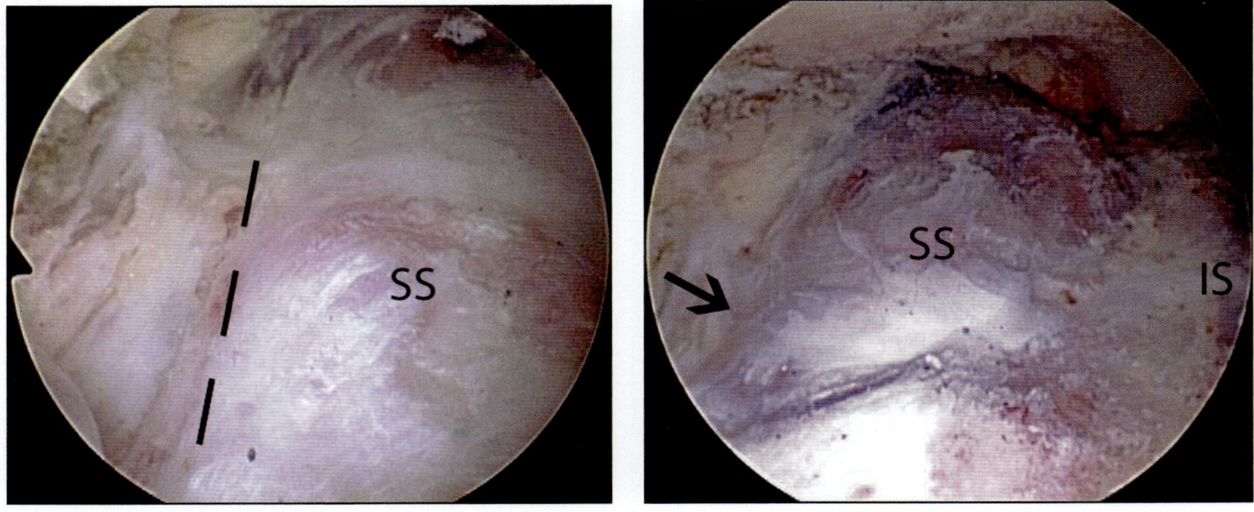

Figure 24.5 **A:** Left shoulder, lateral subacromial viewing portal. The anterior margin of the supraspinatus tendon (*dashed black lines*) has a thickened edge that can be used to define it from the rotator interval. **B:** Same shoulder again demonstrates the thickened anterior border (*black arrow*). IS, infraspinatus tendon; SS, supraspinatus tendon.

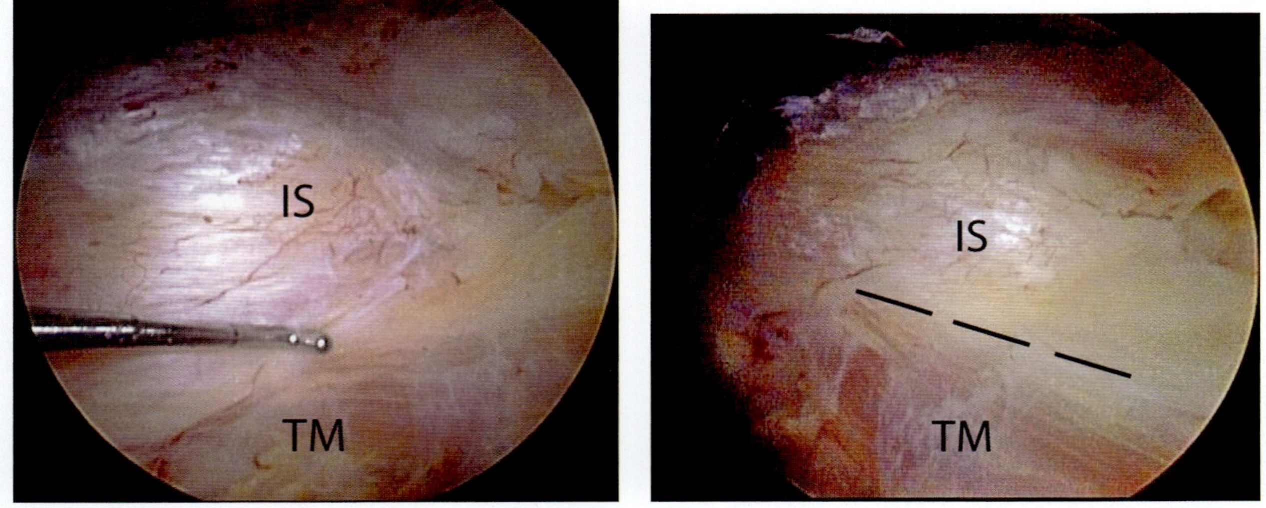

Figure 24.6 **A:** Left shoulder, posterior viewing portal. A probe marks the border between the infraspinatus and teres minor. **B:** Same shoulder, demonstrates how the muscle belly of the teres minor extends further lateral than that of the infraspinatus. The *dashed lines* outline the interval between the infraspinatus and teres minor. IS, infraspinatus tendon; TM, teres minor tendon.

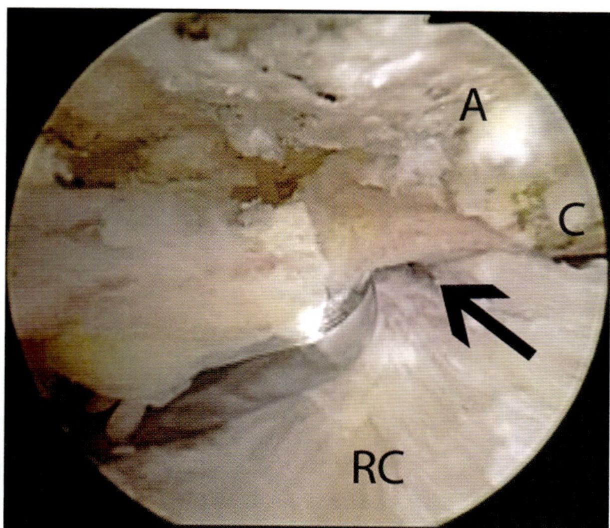

A

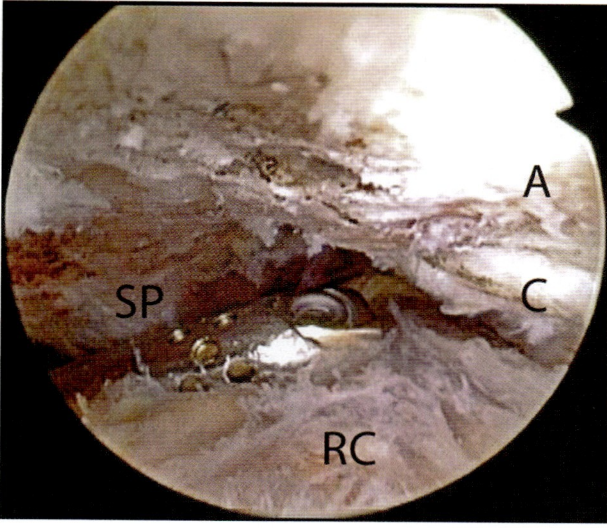

B

Figure 24.7 **A:** Right shoulder, lateral subacromial viewing portal, demonstrates use of a shaver to clear the fibrofatty tissue that lies posterior the AC joint and also covers the scapular spine. This tissue must be removed in order for the AC joint to be viewed from a posterior portal. **B:** Same shoulder following removal of the fibrofatty tissue. An arthroscope introduced from a posterior portal now has an unobstructed view of the AC joint. A, acromion; C, clavicle; RC, rotator cuff; SP, scapular spine.

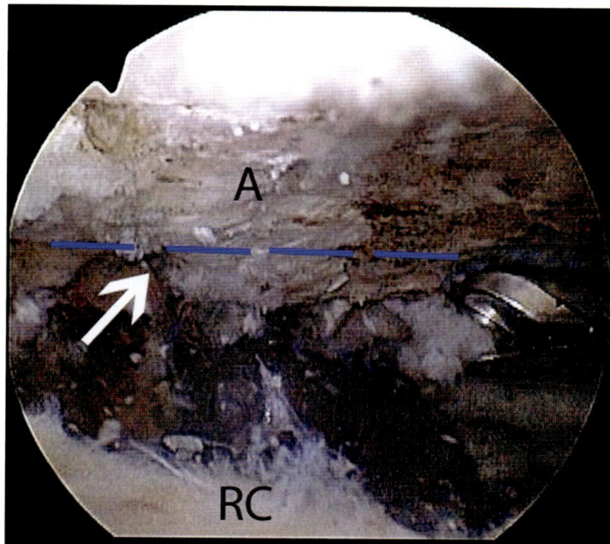

A

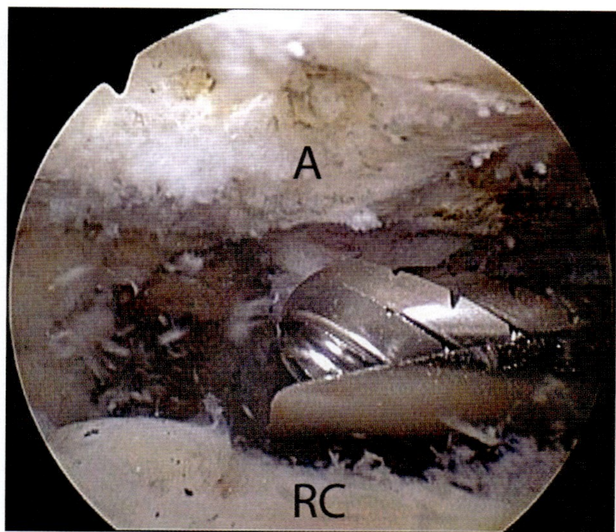

B

Figure 24.8 **A:** Right shoulder, posterior subacromial viewing portal, demonstrates use of a burr to perform an acromioplasty. The medial acromion typically has a notch (*white arrow*) that is level with the distal clavicle. The apex of this notch is often a good landmark for the plane of resection (*dashed blue line*) during an acromioplasty. **B:** Same shoulder demonstrates a flat acromion following the resection to the apex of the notch. A, acromion; RC, rotator cuff.

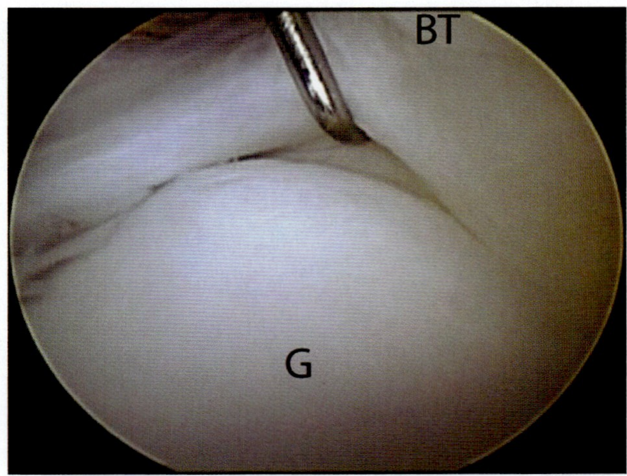

Figure 24.9 Left shoulder, posterior viewing portal, demonstrates a normal superior labral recess. The articular cartilage normally extends 2 to 3 mm medial to the superior glenoid. BT, biceps tendon; G, glenoid.

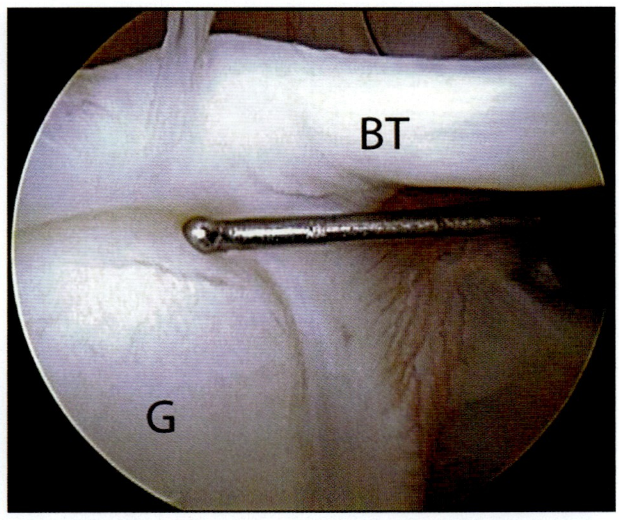

Figure 24.10 Left shoulder, posterior viewing portal. A probe introduced from an anterior working portal demonstrates a stable biceps root. BT, biceps tendon; G, glenoid.

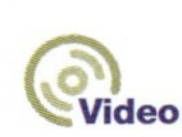

- The root of the biceps should feel stable to palpation with a hook probe, with the tactile feedback that the biceps fibers are well anchored to the bone beneath the biceps (Fig. 24.10).

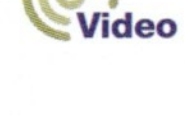

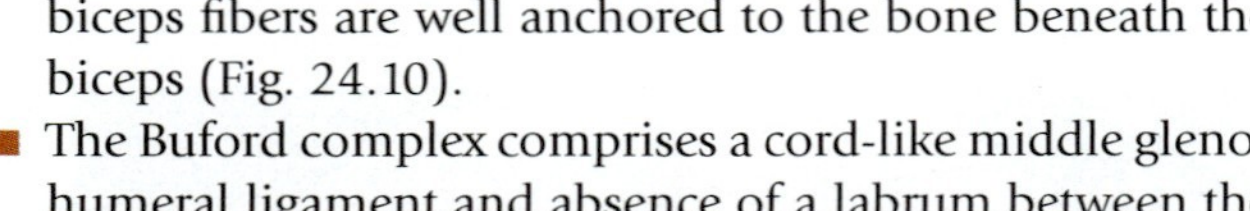

- The Buford complex comprises a cord-like middle glenohumeral ligament and absence of a labrum between the midglenoid notch and the biceps root (Fig. 24.11).
- A sublabral foramen is a normally occurring hole beneath the portion of the labrum that lies between the midglenoid notch and the biceps root. This is distinguishable from the Buford complex because the labrum is present and the middle glenohumeral ligament is a normal band rather than appearing cord-like (Fig. 24.12).

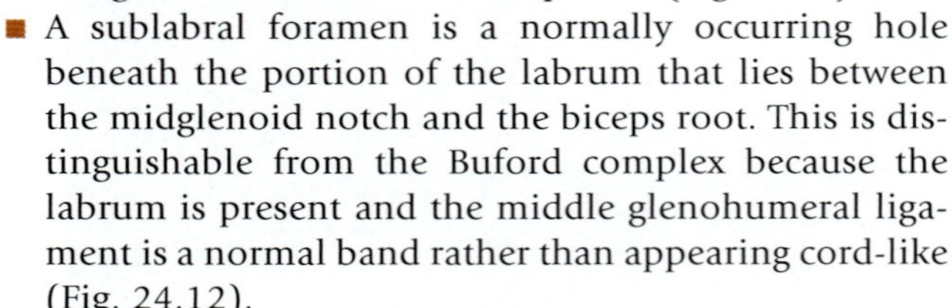

- From an anterosuperolateral viewing portal, the arc of the humeral head should be centered on the bare spot of the glenoid (Fig. 24.13).
- Biceps anomalies do not require treatment. Examples of biceps anomalies are:
  - Bifid long head of the biceps, where one head inserts into the superior labrum and the other head inserts into the rotator cuff (Fig. 24.14).
  - Hypoplastic biceps (Fig. 24.15).
- The axillary nerve lies closest to the glenoid at 5 o'clock and 7 o'clock. It can often be seen in those locations after arthroscopic capsular release (e.g., for adhesive capsulitis) (Fig. 24.16).

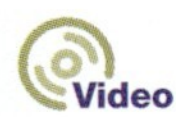

Subscapularis–Biceps–Subcoracoid Space

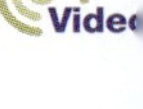

- The normal subscapularis tendon does not have any linear longitudinal splits (Fig. 24.17).
- The coracoid tip generally lies just anterior to the upper border of the subscapularis. A "rolling wave" of indentation of the subscapularis/rotator interval junction can often be seen with internal and external rotation of the humerus. This indentation is caused by the coracoid tip (Fig. 24.18).

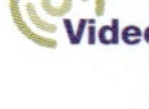

- There is normally a 2 to 3 mm bare strip (i.e., devoid of articular cartilage) just medial to the footprint of the subscapularis (Fig. 24.19).

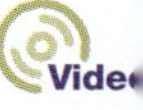

- The subscapularis and proximal bicipital groove are best visualized with a 70° arthroscope. The upper 2.5 cm of the bicipital groove can be visualized in this way (Fig. 24.20).

- When viewed with a 70° scope, the biceps tendon should lie anterior to the plane of the subscapularis tendon (Fig. 24.21).

- To locate and visualize the coracoid, make a window in the rotator interval just above the upper border of subscapularis, palpate the coracoid, then clear the soft tissues from the bone (Fig. 24.22).
- Viewing with a 70° scope through the window in the rotator interval, the entire coracoid can be seen in a panoramic way by rotating the light cable. The normal coracoid tip should not have an osteophyte

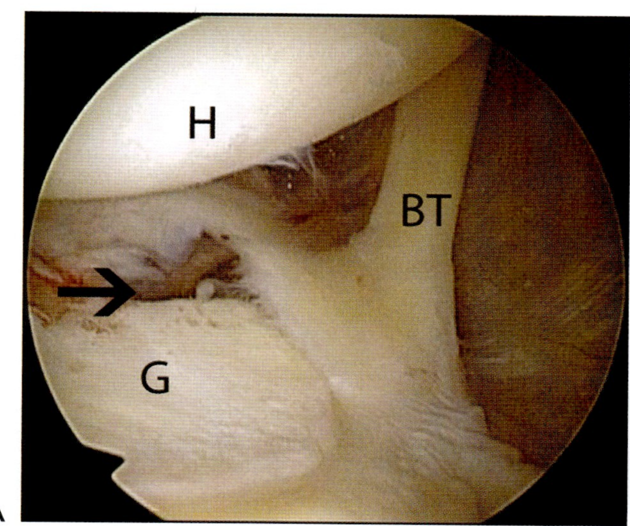

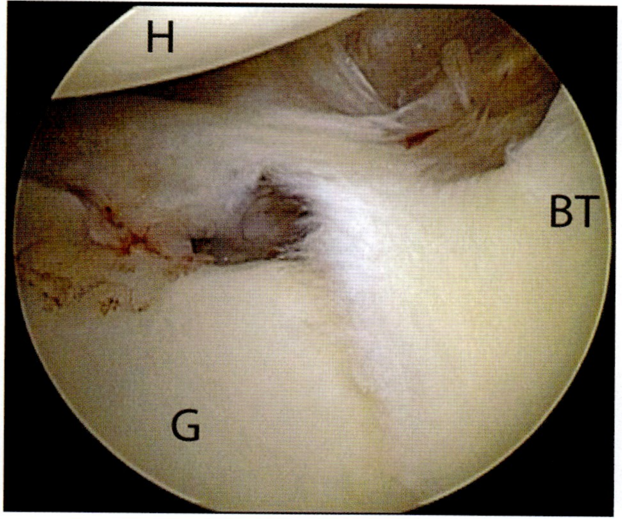

Figure 24.11 Left shoulder, posterior glenohumeral viewing portal, demonstrates **(A)** panoramic and **(B)** up-close views of a Buford complex that is characterized by a cordlike middle glenohumeral ligament with absence of the labrum between the biceps root and the midglenoid notch (*black arrow*). BT, biceps tendon; G, glenoid; H, humerus.

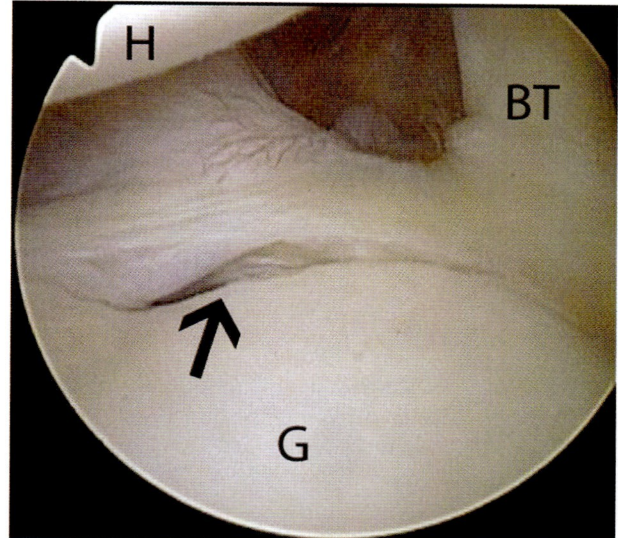

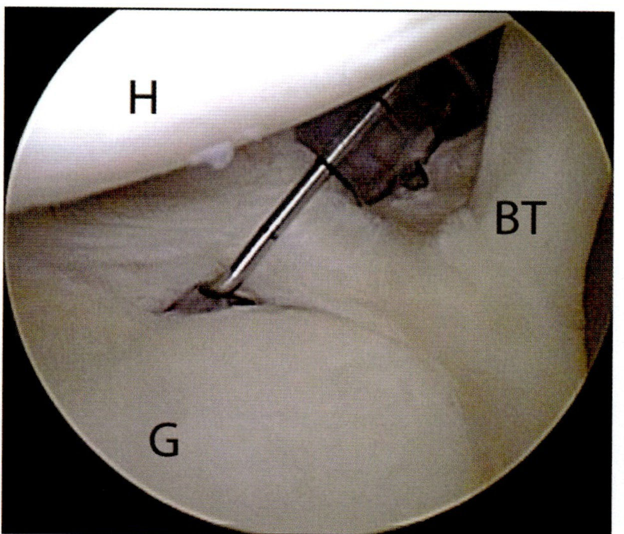

Figure 24.12 **A:** Left shoulder, posterior glenohumeral viewing portal, demonstrates a sublabral foramen (*black arrow*). **B:** Same shoulder. A probe is used to further show this normal anatomic variant. BT, biceps tendon; G, glenoid; H, humerus.

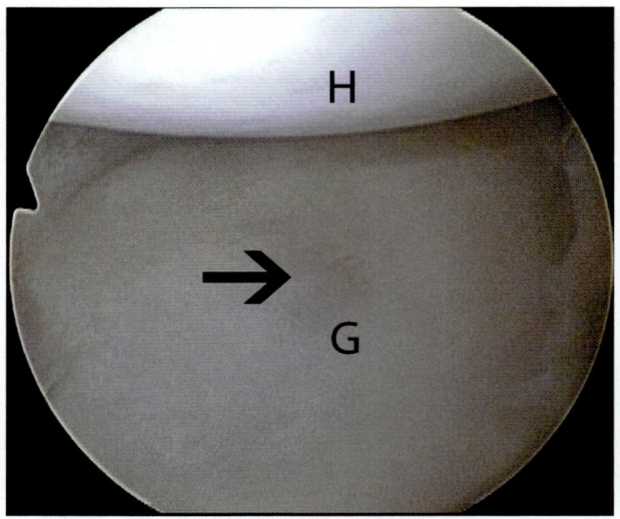

Figure 24.13 Left shoulder, anterosuperolateral viewing portal, demonstrates the normal relationship between the humeral head and the glenoid. The humeral head is centered over the bare spot (*black arrow*) of the glenoid in this individual without a labral tear. G, glenoid; H, humerus.

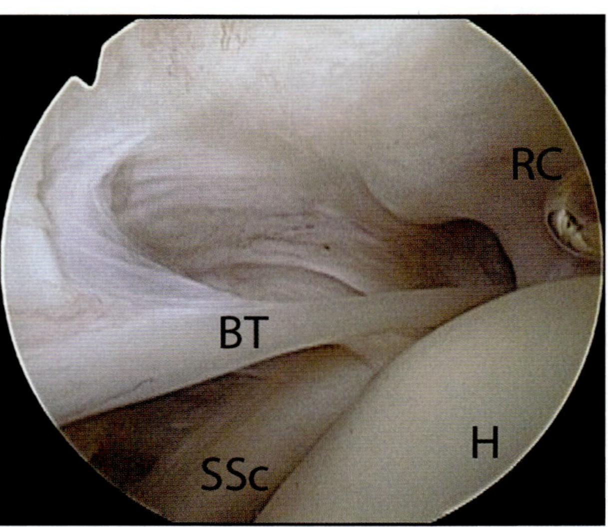

Figure 24.15 Right shoulder, posterior glenohumeral viewing portal, demonstrates a hypoplastic biceps tendon. BT, biceps tendon; H, humerus; RC, rotator cuff; SSc, subscapularis tendon.

projecting posterior to the plane of the conjoined tendon, and the space between the coracoid tip and the subscapularis tendon should be at least 7 mm. This space can be measured by comparison with a shaver or burr of a known diameter (Fig. 24.23).

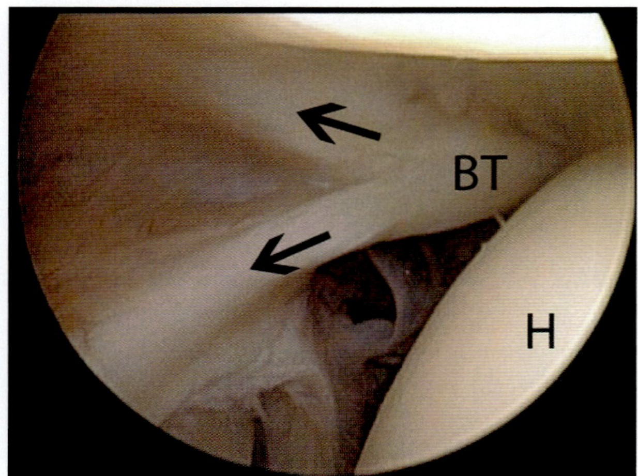

Figure 24.14 Right shoulder, posterior glenohumeral viewing portal, demonstrates a bifid long head of the biceps (*black arrows*), where one head inserts into the rotator cuff, and the other head inserts into the superior labrum. BT, biceps tendon; H, humerus.

Recognizing Pathoanatomy

Subacromial Pathoanatomy

- Extrinsic impingement can occur not only between the acromion and the rotator cuff but also
  - Between the AC joint and the rotator cuff (Fig. 24.24)
  - Between the anterior acromion and the biceps tendon (Fig. 24.25)

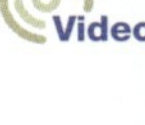

Intra-articular Anatomy

- SLAP lesions in throwers typically demonstrate a positive peel-back sign, in which the biceps root shifts medially during combined abduction and external rotation (Fig. 24.26).
- SLAP lesions in nonthrowers usually do not demonstrate a positive peel-back sign, but have a *displaceable biceps root.* In such cases, a hook probe easily displaces the superior labrum where the biceps inserts, and it feels to the examiner as if there is no carry-through and attachment of the fibers to the biceps root into the bone of the superior glenoid neck (Fig. 24.27).
- PASTA (partial articular surface tendon avulsion) lesions may occur at the infraspinatus attachment, adjacent to the Hill-Sachs lesion, after an anterior dislocation. If

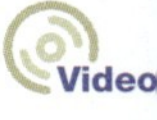

(Text continued on page 443)

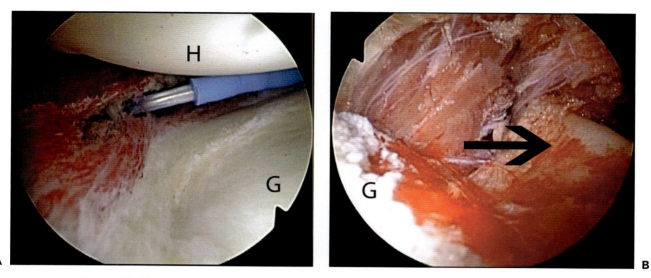

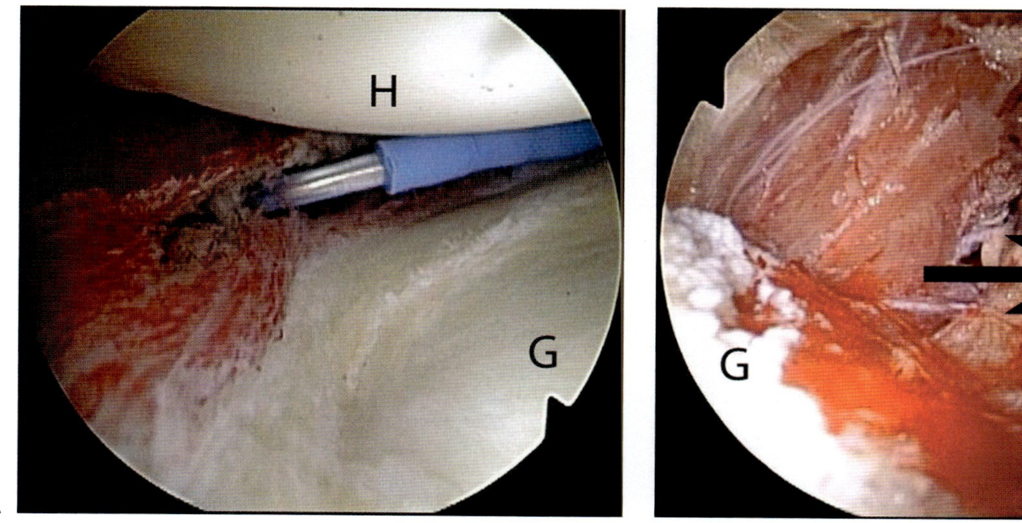

Figure 24.16 **A:** Right shoulder, anterosuperolateral viewing portal, demonstrates use of a pencil-tip electrocautery to perform a capsular release. **B:** Same shoulder, posterior viewing portal. Intra-articular viewing after capsular release and manipulation reveals muscle in the axillary recess and the axillary nerve is also visible at 5 o'clock (*black arrow*). G, glenoid; H, humerus.

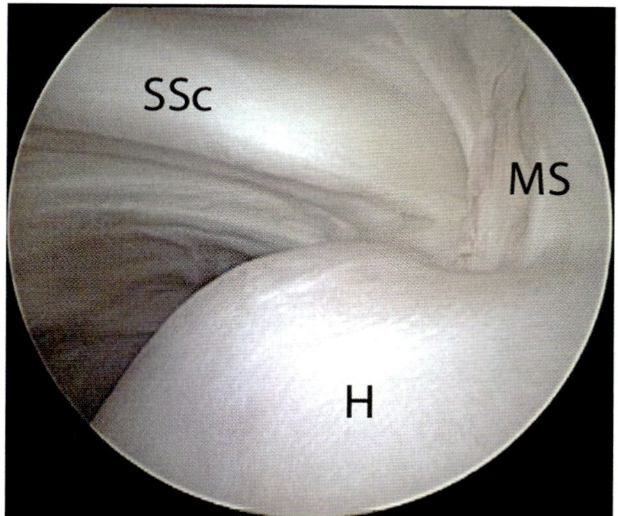

Figure 24.17 Right shoulder, posterior viewing portal with a 70° arthroscope, demonstrates a normal subscapularis tendon. Note: A normal subscapularis tendon does not display any linear longitudinal splits. H, humerus; MS, medial sling of the bicep tendon; SSc, subscapularis tendon.

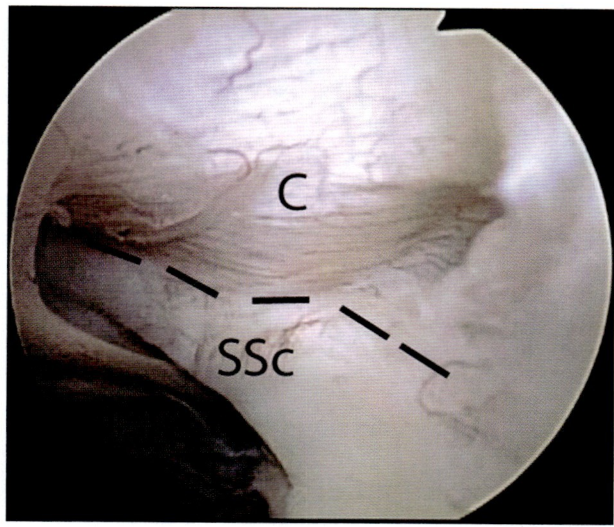

Figure 24.18 Right shoulder, posterior glenohumeral viewing portal with a 70° arthroscope demonstrates subcoracoid impingement. With internal and external rotation, the tip of the coracoid creates an indentation (*dashed black lines*) in the subscapularis tendon. C, coracoid; SSc, subscapularis tendon.

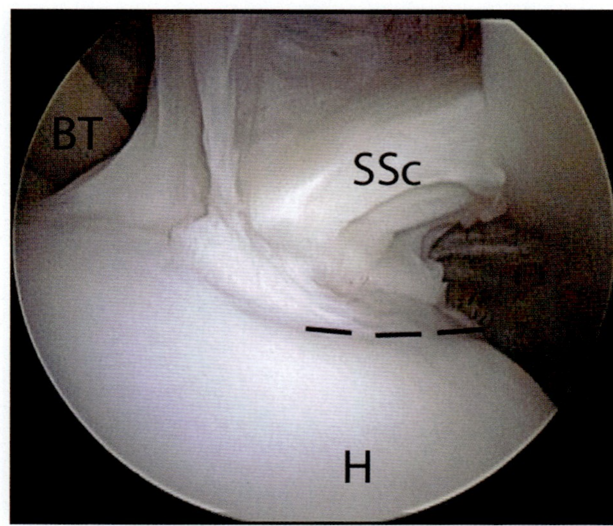

Figure 24.19 Left shoulder, posterior glenohumeral viewing portal with a 70° arthroscope, demonstrates the normal medial footprint of the subscapularis tendon. As shown in this image, there is normally a 2- to 3-mm bare strip just medial to the subscapularis tendon. The *dashed lines* outline the anterior articular margin of the humeral head. BT, biceps tendon; H, humerus; SSc, subscapularis tendon.

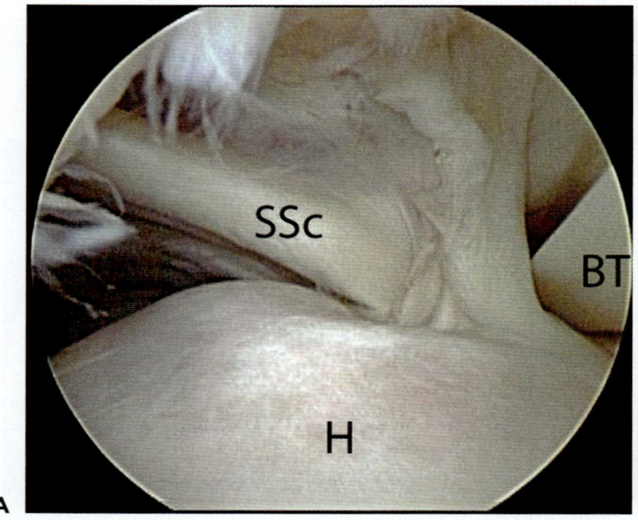

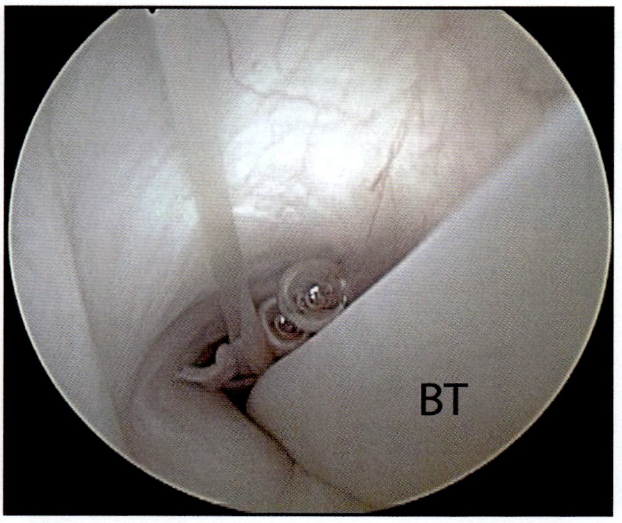

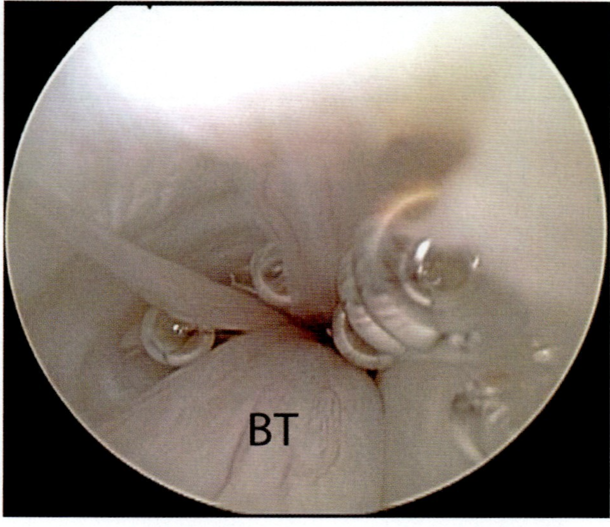

Figure 24.20 **A:** Right shoulder, posterior viewing portal with a 70° arthroscope. The subscapularis tendon and bicipital groove are best visualized with a 70° arthroscope. **B:** By placing a 70° arthroscope adjacent to the biceps tendon, approximately 2.5 cm of the lateral sidewall of the subscapularis (medial bicipital groove) can be seen. **C:** The arthroscope can also be directed over the top of the biceps tendon to provide an aerial view of the bicipital groove. BT, biceps tendon; H, humerus; SSc, subscapularis tendon.

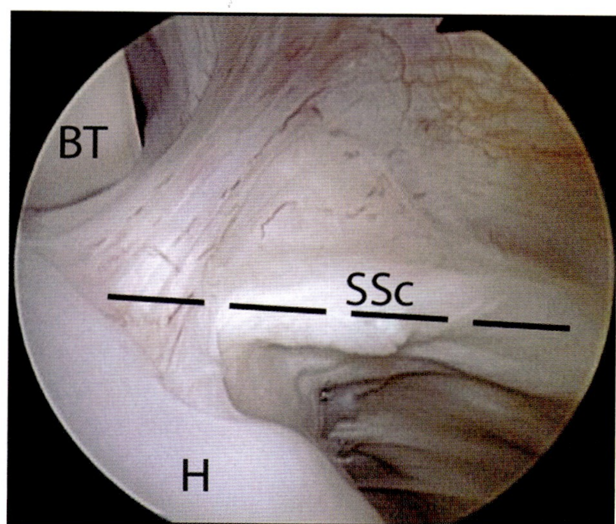

Figure 24.21 Left shoulder, posterior viewing portal. When viewed with a 70° arthroscope, the biceps tendon should lie anterior to the plane of the subscapularis tendon (*dashed black lines*). BT, biceps tendon; H, humerus; SSc, subscapularis tendon.

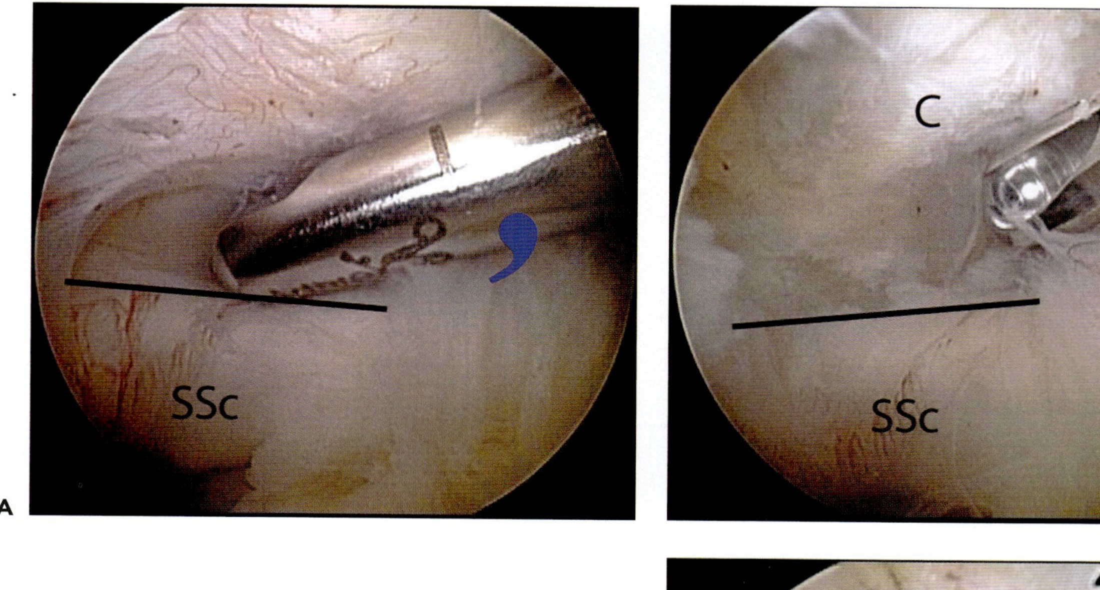

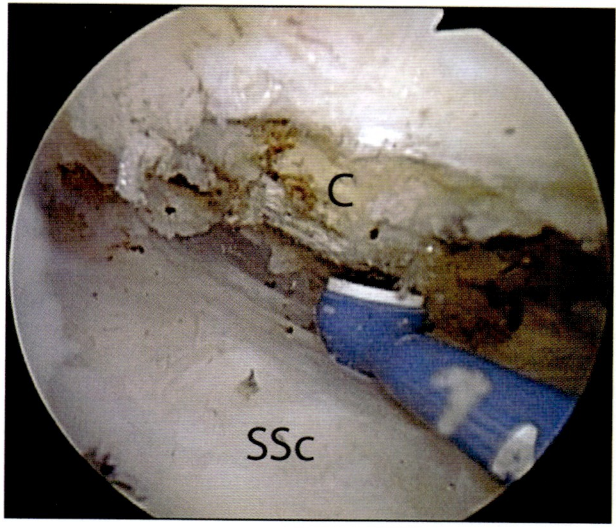

Figure 24.22 Creating a window in the rotator interval. **A:** Right shoulder, posterior viewing portal with a 30° arthroscope, demonstrates use of a shaver to create a window in the rotator interval medial to the comma tissue (*blue comma symbol*) and above the superior border of the subscapularis tendon (*black line*). **B:** The tip of the coracoid is identified. **C:** After the tip of the coracoid is identified, a 70° arthroscope is inserted, and the coracoid tip is skeletonized with an electrocautery. C, coracoid; SSc, subscapularis tendon.

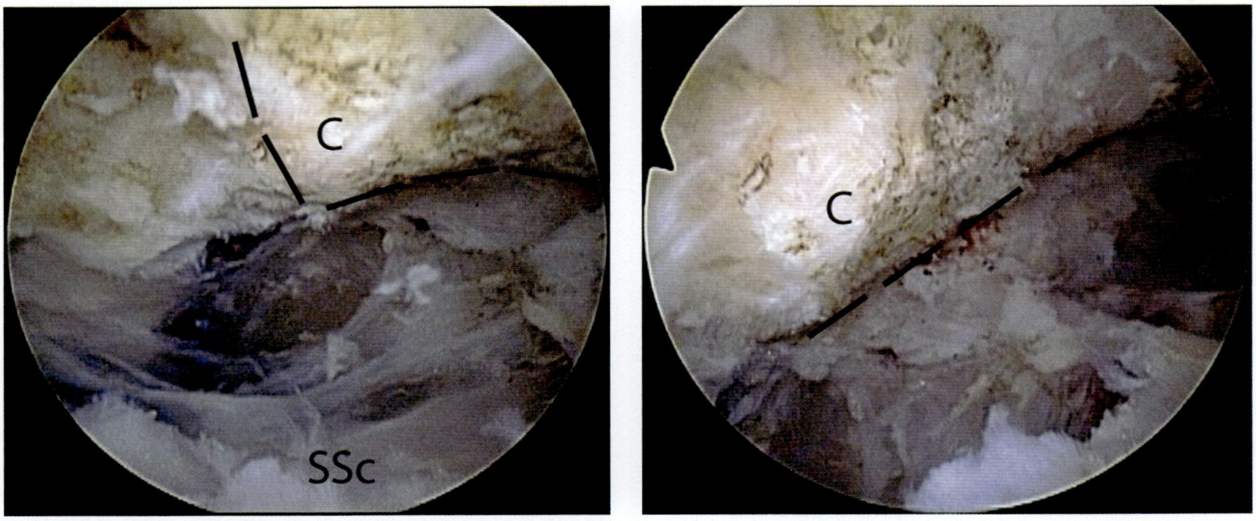

A B C

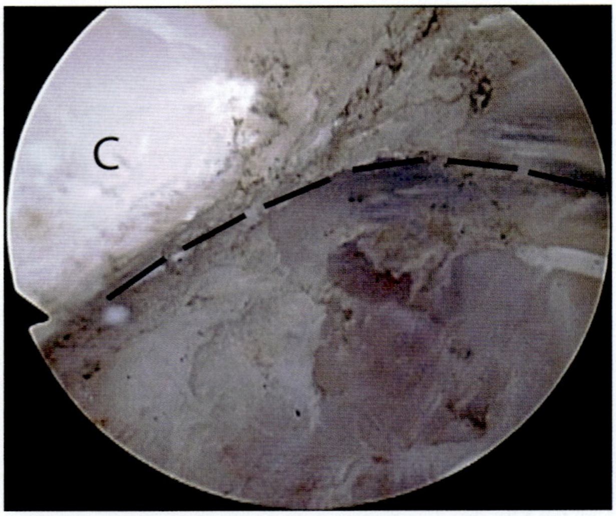

Figure 24.23 **A:** Left shoulder, posterior viewing portal with a 70° arthroscope. The arthroscope has been placed through a window in the rotator interval and the coracoid tip (outlined by *dashed black lines*) is clearly seen. **B:** Rotating the light cable allows one to view follow the view medially all the way to **(C)** the base of the coracoid. The inferior border of the coracoid is outlined by *dashed black lines*. C, coracoid; SSc, subscapularis tendon.

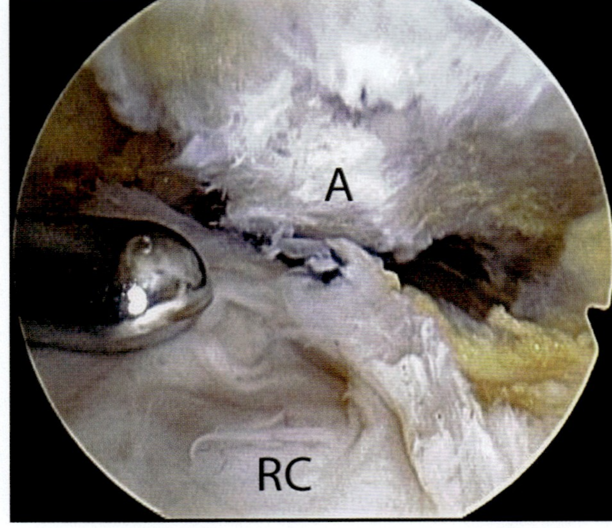

Figure 24.24 Right shoulder, lateral subacromial viewing portal, demonstrates extrinsic impingement upon the rotator cuff by the AC joint. Note the osteophyte on the undersurface of the medial acromion and reciprocal abrasive changes in the medial rotator cuff. A, acromion; RC, rotator cuff.

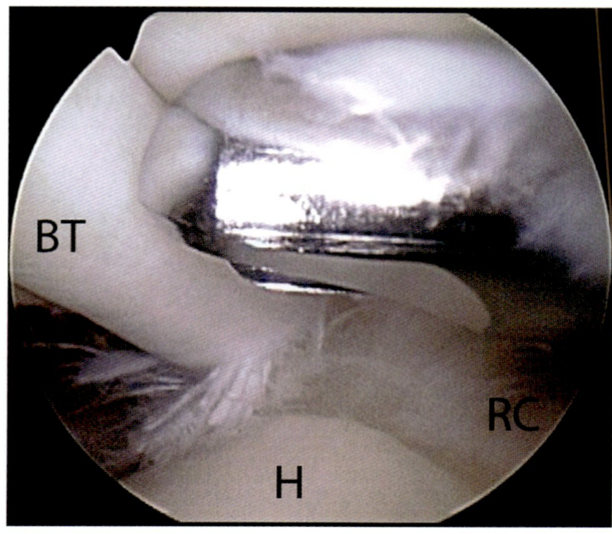

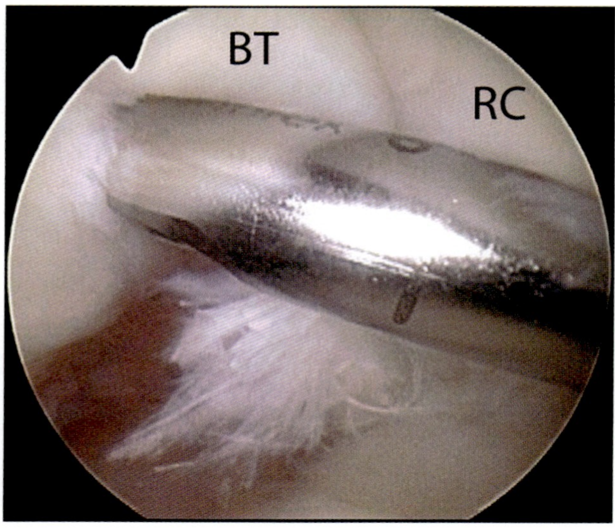

Figure 24.25 **A:** Right shoulder, posterior glenohumeral viewing portal, demonstrates a partial biceps tendon tear. In this case, the partial tear was due to extrinsic impingement from the acromion. **B:** A shaver introduced through the defect in a rotator cuff tear is used to lift the biceps and demonstrate impingement between the biceps tendon and the undersurface of the acromion. BT, biceps tendon; H, humerus; RC, rotator cuff.

the accompanying Bankart lesion satisfies the criteria for arthroscopic repair, the surgeon should consider also doing an arthroscopic remplissage (insetting the infraspinatus into the Hill-Sachs lesion) for deep Hill-Sachs lesions (i.e., ≥4 mm deep) in order to address the infraspinatus tear in addition to augmenting the instability repair (Fig. 24.28).

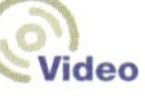

- A Hill-Sachs lesion that engages with the shoulder in a position of <45° of abduction suggests that there has been disruption of the superior glenohumeral ligament (SGHL). The surgeon must specifically look for SGHL tearing in such a case, and then repair it in addition to addressing the Bankart lesion and the bone lesions (Fig. 24.29).

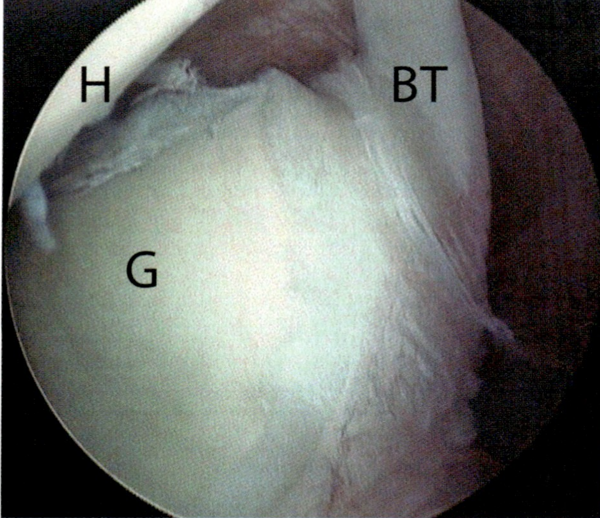

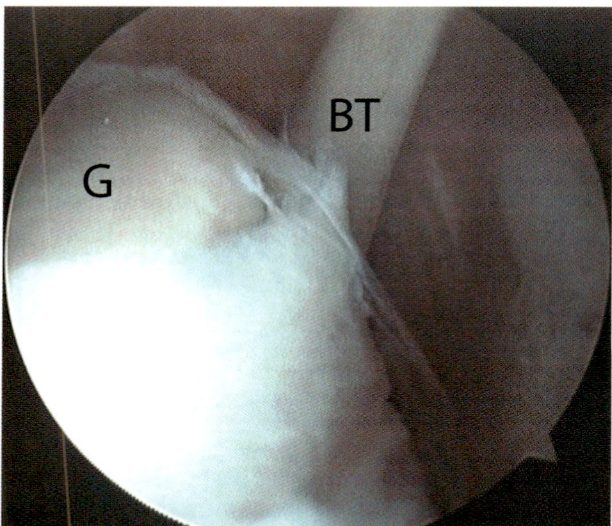

Figure 24.26 Peel-back maneuver **A:** Left shoulder, posterior viewing portal, demonstrates appearance of the biceps root with the arm at the side. **B:** Same shoulder demonstrates a positive peel-back whereby the biceps root displaces medial to the glenoid rim when the arm is placed in 90° of abduction and maximal external rotation. BT, biceps tendon; G, glenoid; H, humerus.

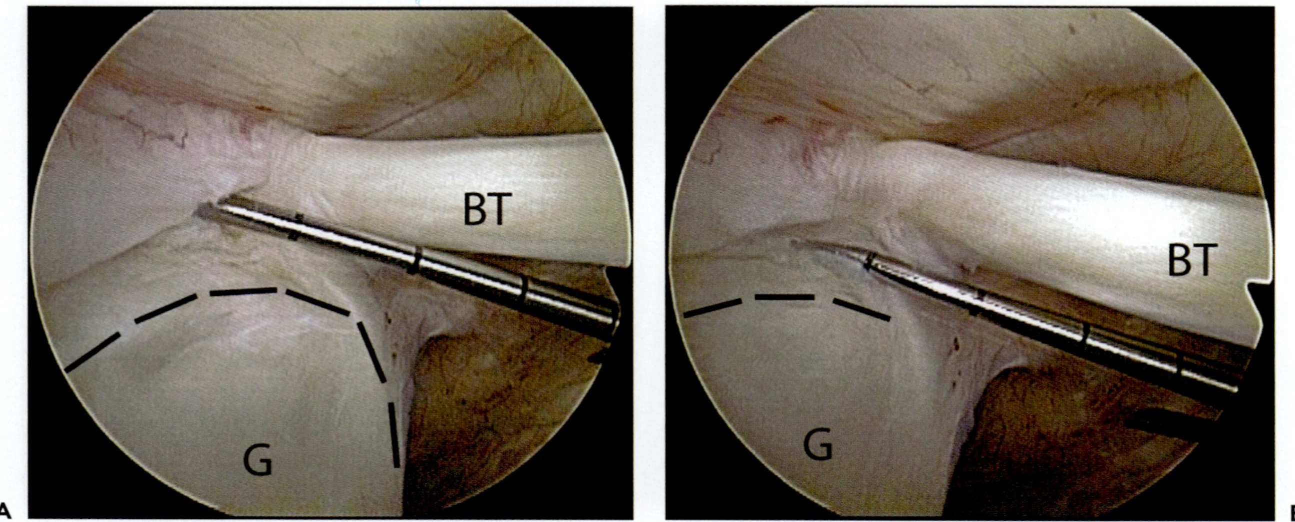

Figure 24.27 **A,B:** Right shoulder, posterior glenohumeral viewing portal, demonstrates a displaceable biceps root. The *dashed black lines* outline the glenoid rim. BT, biceps tendon; G, glenoid.

Subscapularis–Biceps–Subcoracoid Pathoanatomy

- Linear longitudinal splits near the insertion of the subscapularis indicate subcoracoid impingement, with spreading of the fiber bundles due to compression from the coracoid tip. This "battering-ram" effect combines with the roller-wringer effect to cause these tendon splits. Such a finding suggests subcoracoid impingement and the need for a coracoplasty (Fig. 24.30) (Video 24.29).

- Abrasion of the biceps tendon adjacent to the medial sling of the biceps indicates an incompetent sling and, most often, disruption of the upper subscapularis. This finding is best observed with a 70° arthroscope. When present, it demands arthroscopic biceps tenodesis (or tenotomy in low-demand individuals) plus arthroscopic repair of the subscapularis (Fig. 24.31).
- An osteophyte of the coracoid tip that extends posterior to the plane of the conjoined tendon will typically cause subcoracoid impingement. In such a case, the osteophyte should be planed down (coracoplasty) to the plane of the conjoined tendon (Fig. 24.32).

Simple Tricks

- Turbulence control is not a new trick, but it is mentioned again here because of its importance. One should not use an outflow cannula, as this increases turbulence and

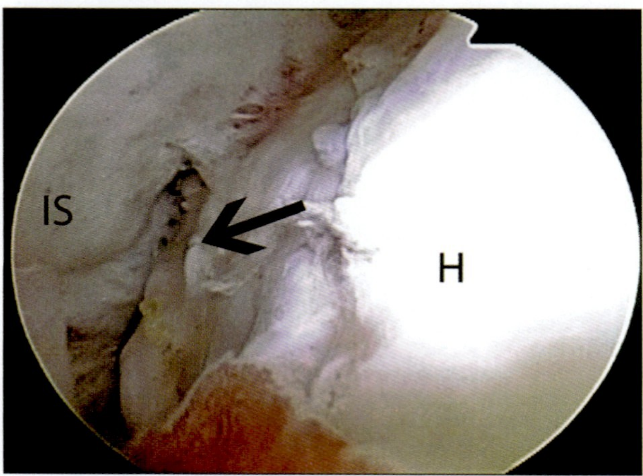

Figure 24.28 Left shoulder, posterior viewing portal with a 70° arthroscope demonstrates a partial articular surface rotator cuff tear (*black arrow*) of the infraspinatus tendon in an individual with a previous anterior dislocation. H, humerus; IS, infraspinatus tendon.

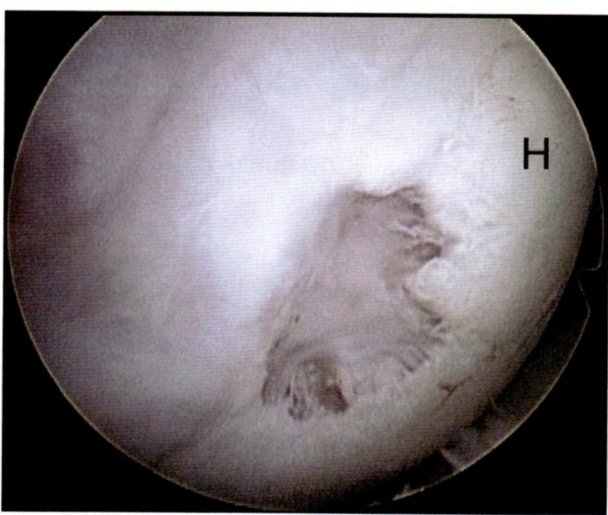

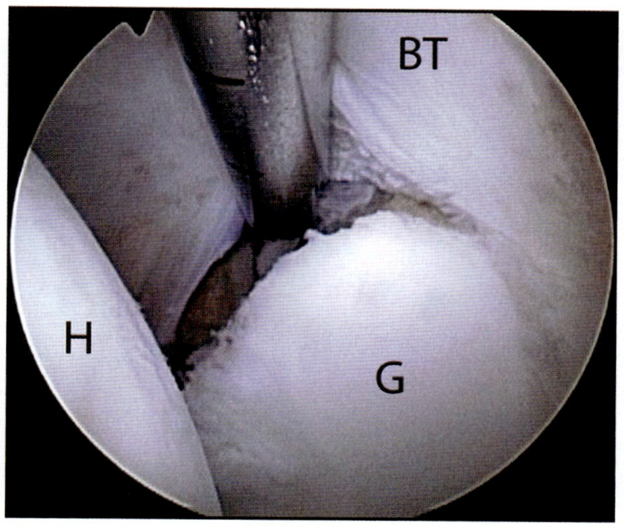

Figure 24.29 **A:** Right shoulder, posterior glenohumeral viewing portal, demonstrates a shallow Hill-Sachs lesion that engages the anterior glenoid rim with 30° abduction plus 70° of external rotation. **B:** Same shoulder, demonstrates disruption of the SGHL just anterior to the biceps tendon insertion. BT, biceps tendon; G, glenoid; H, humerus.

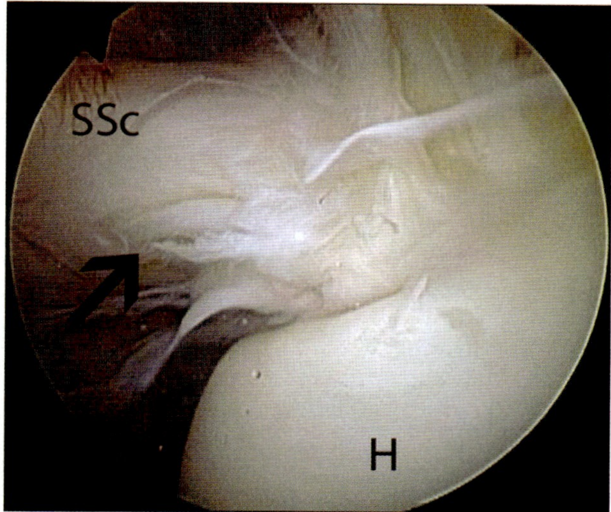

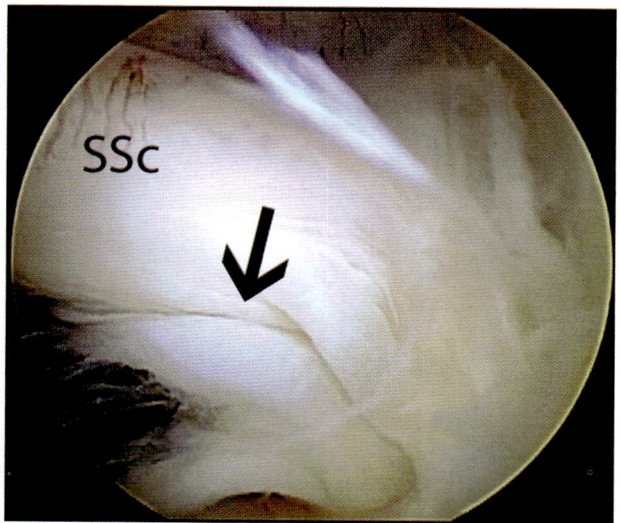

Figure 24.30 **A:** Right shoulder, posterior viewing portal with a 70° arthroscope, demonstrates linear longitudinal splits (*black arrow*) in the subscapularis tendon near its insertion. **B:** Up-close view of the same shoulder. Linear longitudinal splits in the subscapularis tendon are suggestive of subcoracoid impingement. H, humerus; SSc, subscapularis tendon.

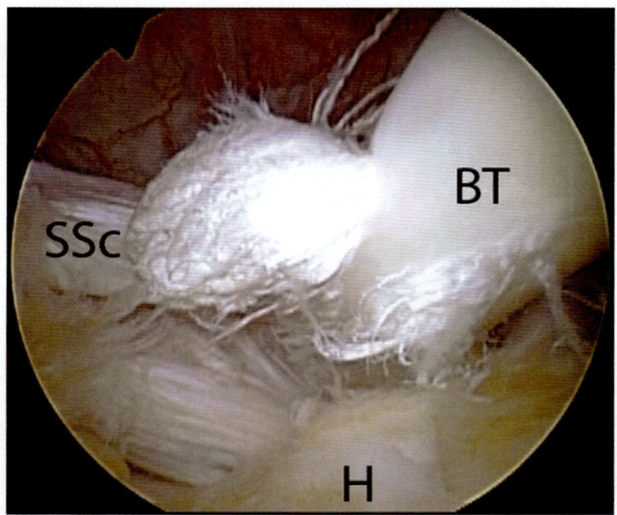

Figure 24.31 Right shoulder, posterior glenohumeral viewing portal with a 70° arthroscope, demonstrates abrasion of the medial biceps tendon. Abrasive changes of the medial biceps tendon are indicative of a subscapularis tendon tear in association with medial subluxation of the biceps. BT, biceps tendon; H, humerus; SSc, subscapularis tendon.

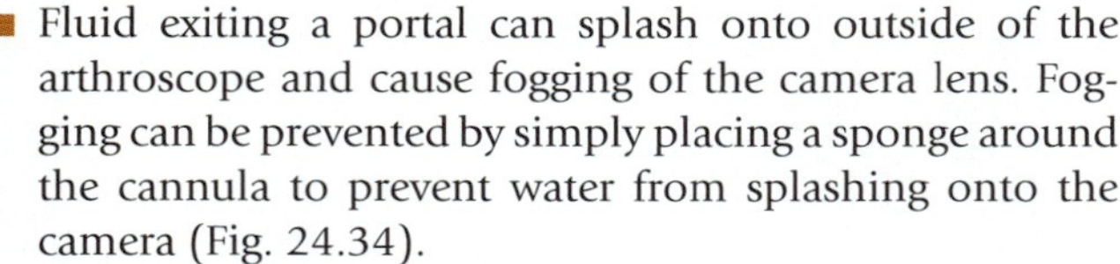

increases bleeding. The first assistant should digitally plug any leaking portals that might be causing turbulence (Fig. 24.33).

- Fluid exiting a portal can splash onto outside of the arthroscope and cause fogging of the camera lens. Fogging can be prevented by simply placing a sponge around the cannula to prevent water from splashing onto the camera (Fig. 24.34).
- In many cases of subacromial impingement and rotator cuff pathology, most of the subacromial space will be filled with fibrofatty tissue and hypertrophic bursa. Even though most of the subacromial space may be filled with soft tissue, there is always a small open space at the anterolateral corner of the subacromial space. If the tip of the arthroscope is inserted into that small open space, clearing the rest of the subacromial space will be much easier. We have found that the most reliable way to get into that small open space is to aim the scope sheath toward the anterolateral corner of the acromion, and then intentionally push the sheath into the anterolateral deltoid muscle. The scope is then

A

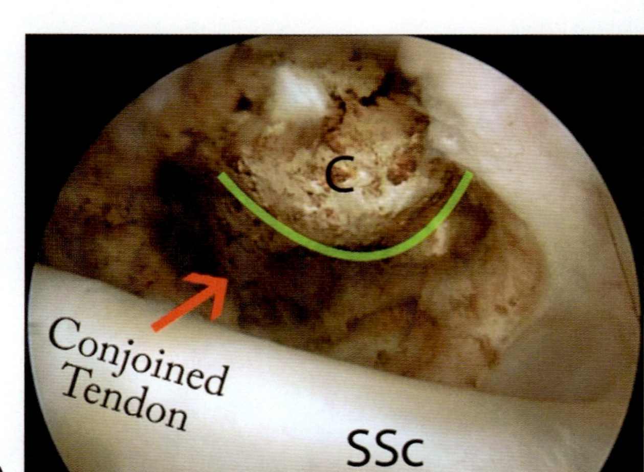

B

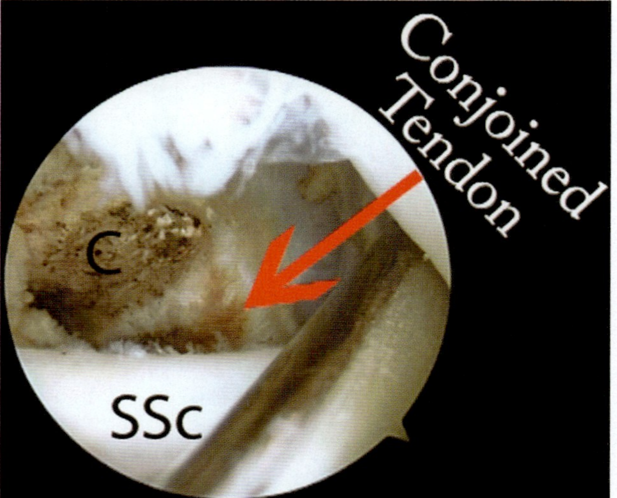

Figure 24.32 **A:** Right shoulder, posterior glenohumeral viewing portal. A window has been created in the rotator interval to expose the coracoid tip. The tip of the coracoid is posterior to the plane of the conjoined tendon, indicating subcoracoid stenosis. **B:** Same shoulder demonstrates appearance postcoracoplasty. The tip of the coracoid no longer projects posterior to the conjoined tendon. C, coracoid; SSc, subscapularis tendon; *red arrow* denotes conjoined tendon; *green line* shows the posterior border of the osteophyte at the coracoid tip.

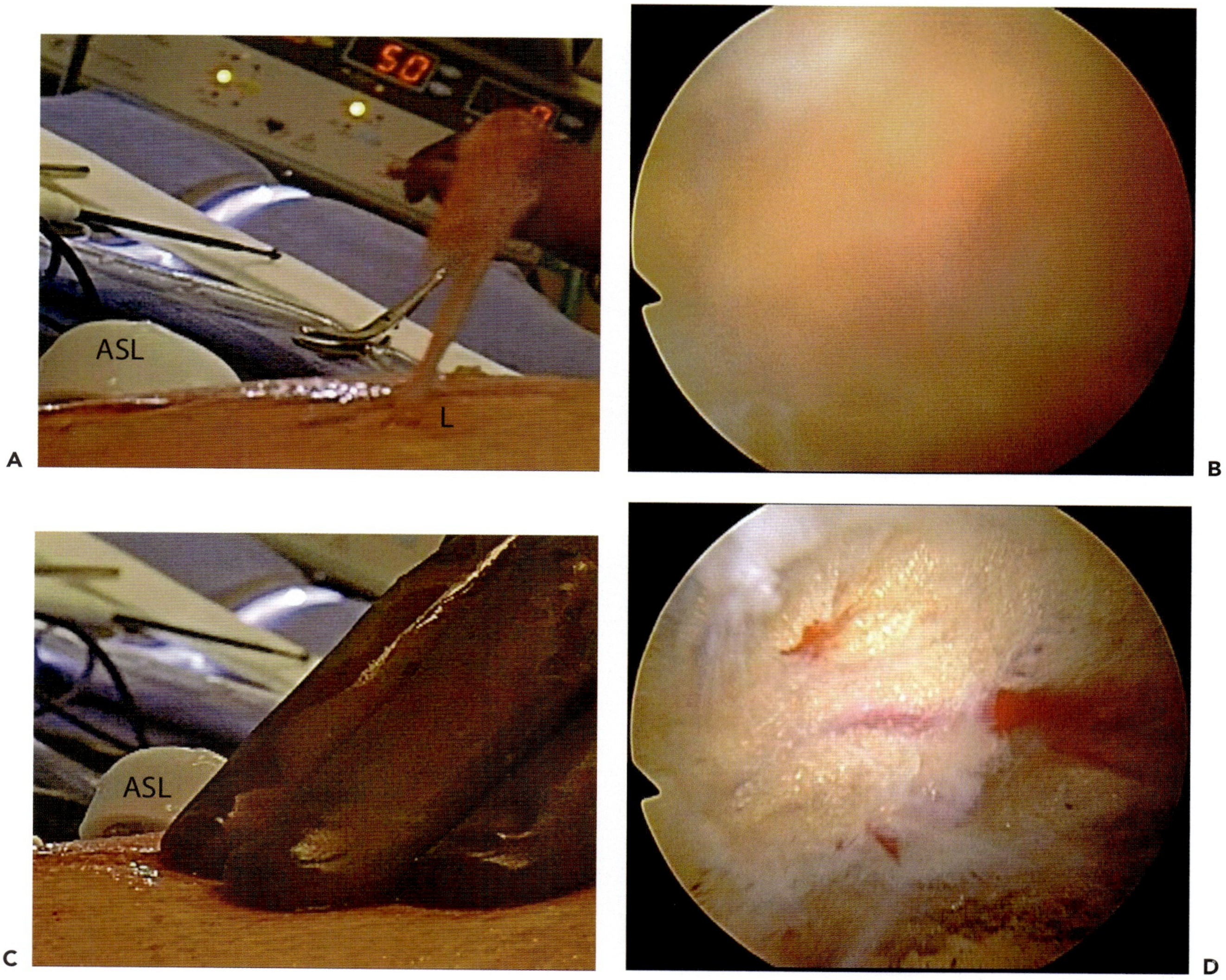

Figure 24.33 **A:** External view of a right shoulder demonstrates fluid escaping from a lateral portal. **B:** Arthroscopic view from a posterior subacromial viewing portal. The turbulent outflow results in bleeding, which limits visualization. **C:** Turbulence is easily controlled by "plugging the hole" with digital pressure. **D:** Turbulence control has halted bleeding from a vessel and the visualization is dramatically improved. ASL, anterosuperolateral portal; L, lateral subacromial portal.

inserted into the sheath while it is still in the muscle. The surgeon views the muscle (musculoscopy) as the scope is slowly pulled back through the muscle until it pops past the internal deltoid fascia. The surgeon will feel and see the difference as soon as the scope pops past the fascia. At that instant, the scope is in the largest available space, so the surgeon must then triangulate to bring a shaver in through a lateral working portal and enlarge the space by debriding the thickened bursa. We have found that this is the most predictable way to get into whatever subacromial space there is, no matter how small (Fig. 24.35).

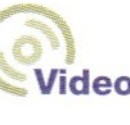

- We recommend dividing the internal deltoid fascia through the lateral portal for three reasons:
  - It allows greater freedom of motion for the working instruments, so that they are not "bound down" and restricted by the internal deltoid fascia.
  - It allows direct identification of the lateral edge of the acromion, which aids in acromioplasty.
  - It creates more space in the lateral gutter, so that placement of lateral-row suture anchors is easier and more precise (Fig. 24.36).
- Tear pattern recognition is greatly enhanced and simplified by clearing the fibrofatty tissue from the scapular spine, then using the scapular spine and its

(Text continued on page 451)

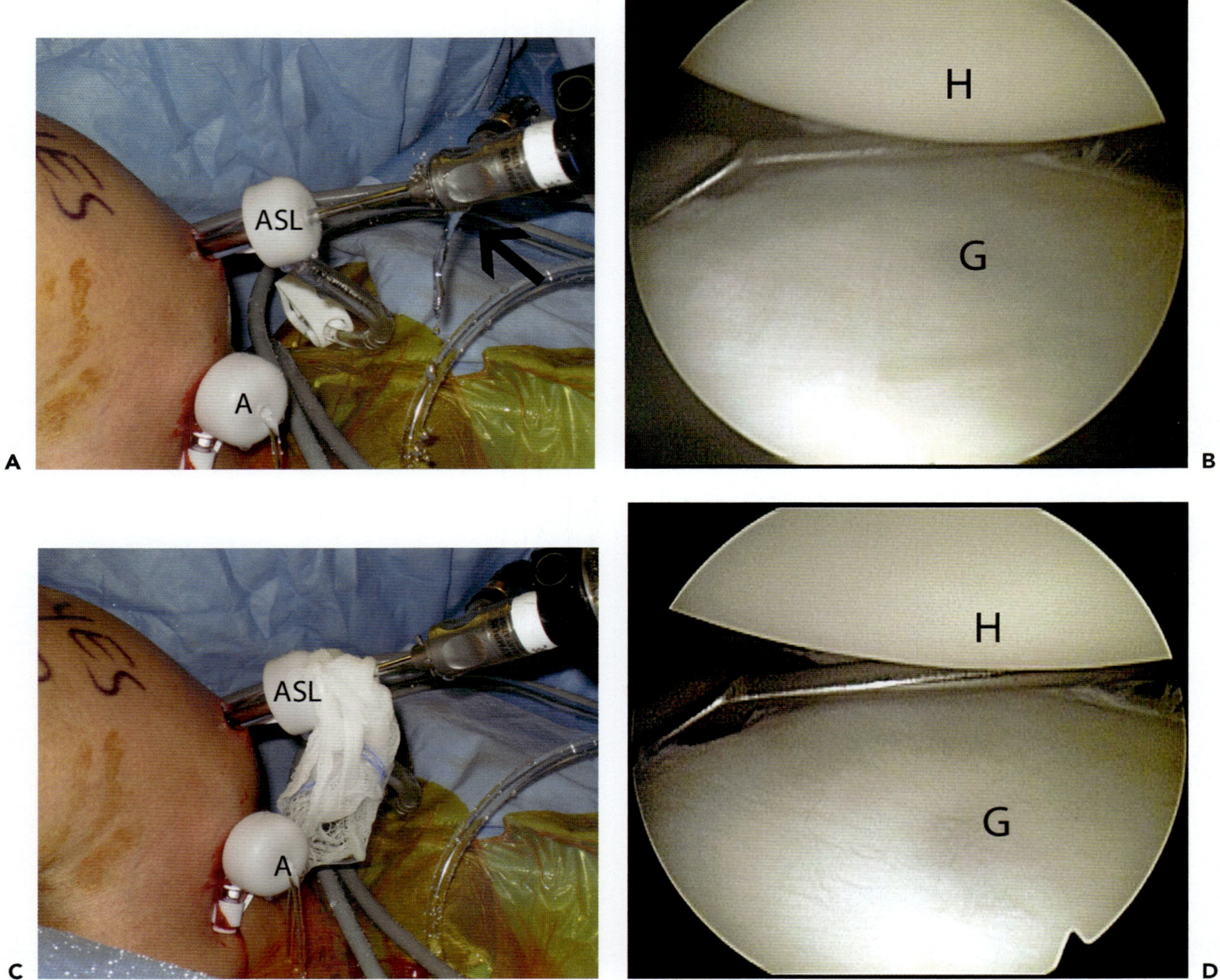

Figure 24.34 **A:** External view of a right shoulder. Water exiting a portal can splash onto the arthroscope (*black arrow*) and cause the camera to fog and limit visualization. **B:** Arthroscopic view from an anterosuperolateral portal demonstrates a "foggy" view. **C:** Placing a sponge around a portal site will prevent water from splashing onto the camera. **D:** Same shoulder with the sponge in place demonstrates a clear view of the glenohumeral joint. A, anterior portal; ASL, anterosuperolateral portal; G, glenoid; H, humerus.

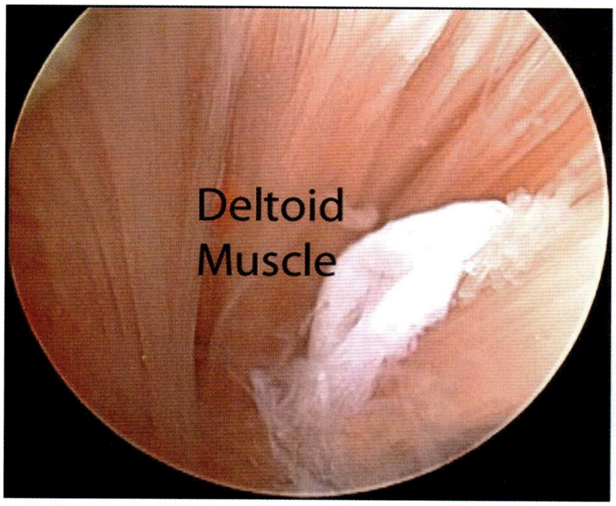

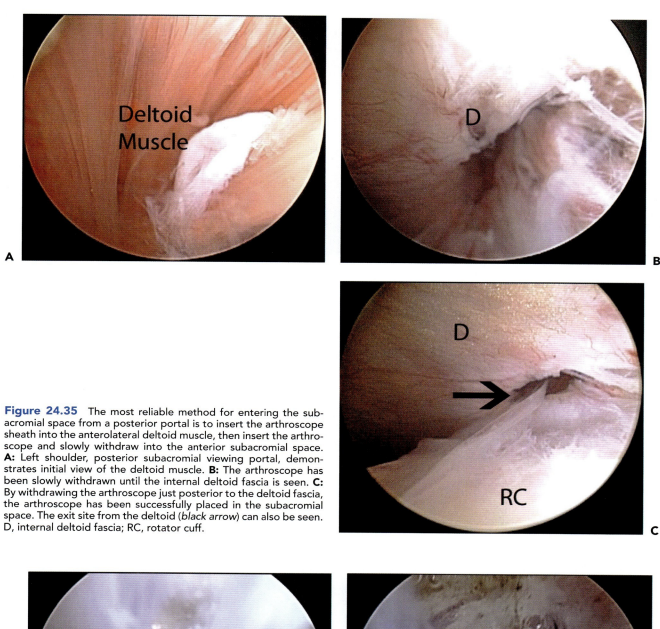

Figure 24.35 The most reliable method for entering the subacromial space from a posterior portal is to insert the arthroscope sheath into the anterolateral deltoid muscle, then insert the arthroscope and slowly withdraw into the anterior subacromial space. **A:** Left shoulder, posterior subacromial viewing portal, demonstrates initial view of the deltoid muscle. **B:** The arthroscope has been slowly withdrawn until the internal deltoid fascia is seen. **C:** By withdrawing the arthroscope just posterior to the deltoid fascia, the arthroscope has been successfully placed in the subacromial space. The exit site from the deltoid (*black arrow*) can also be seen. D, internal deltoid fascia; RC, rotator cuff.

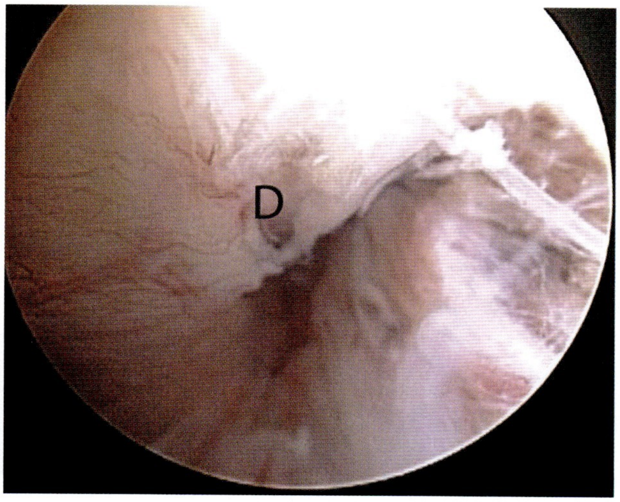

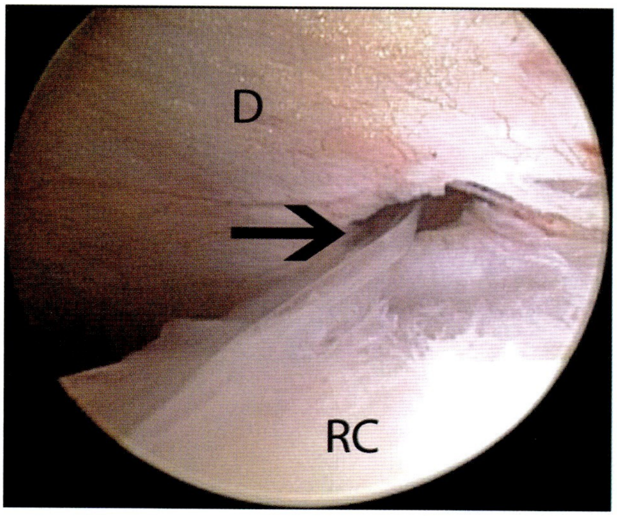

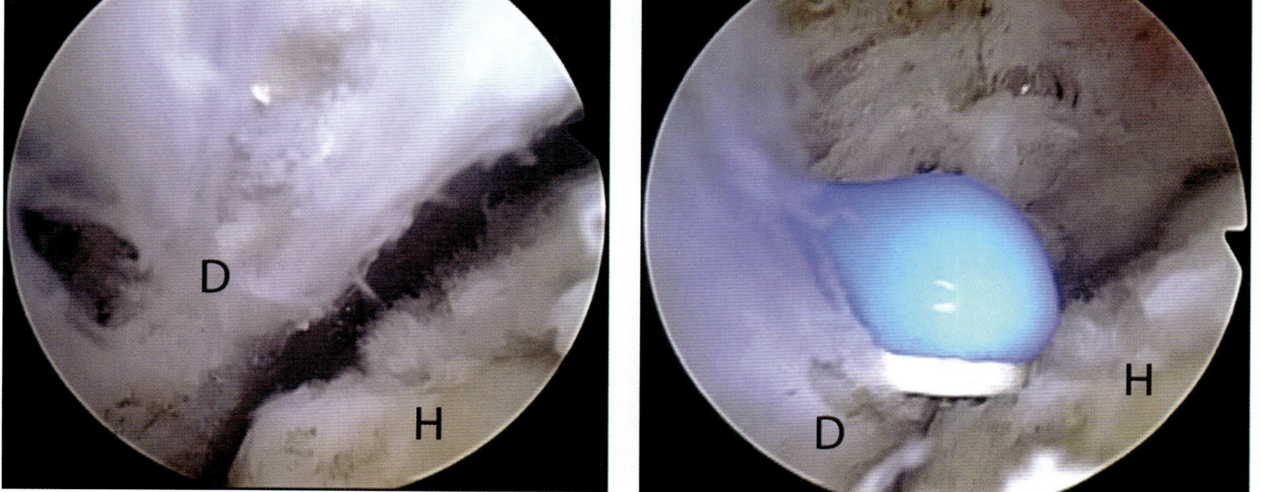

Figure 24.36 **A:** Left shoulder, posterior subacromial viewing portal, demonstrates the view of the lateral subacromial gutter prior to dividing the internal deltoid fascia. The fascia restricts movement of instruments as well as visualization for placement of lateral anchors during rotator cuff repair. **B:** Same shoulder demonstrates division of the internal deltoid fascia with an electrocautery.

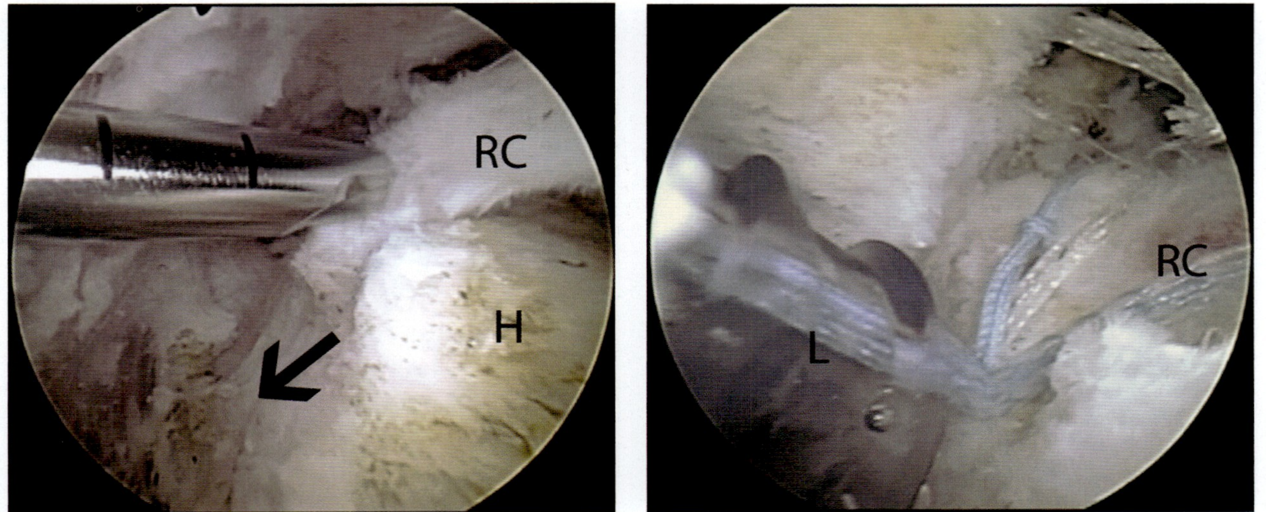

Figure 24.36 *(Continued)* **C:** After dividing the internal deltoid fascia, an instrument has freedom of movement and the lateral gutter (*black arrow*) is well visualized. **D:** Dividing the internal also facilitates placement of lateral anchors during double-row rotator cuff repair. D, internal deltoid fascia; H, humerus; L, lateral subacromial portal; RC, rotator cuff.

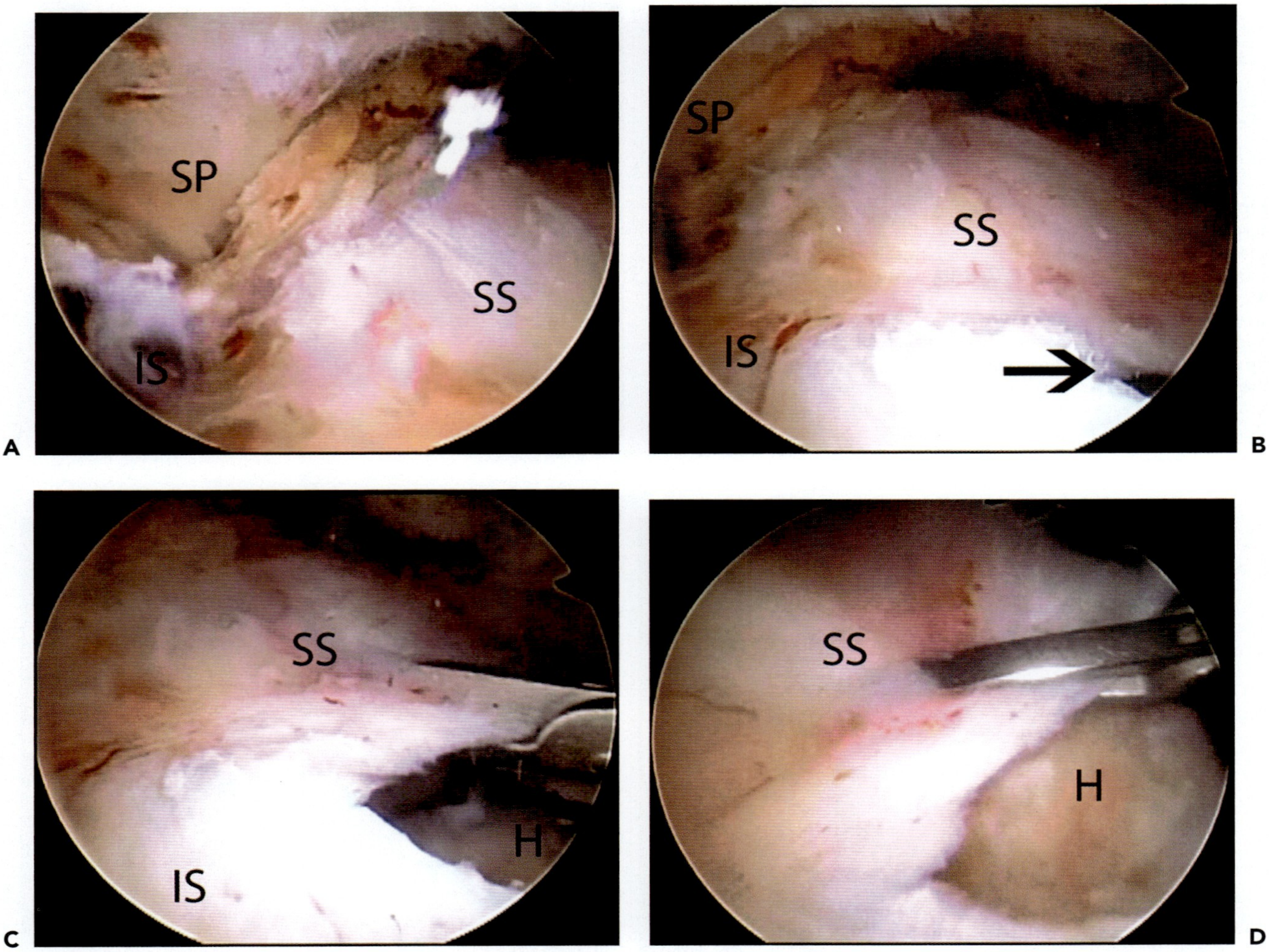

Figure 24.37 Tear-pattern recognition in a right shoulder viewed with a 70° arthroscope from a posterior subacromial portal **A:** The scapular spine has been identified. This landmark is used to define the supraspinatus and the infraspinatus tendons. **B:** Profile view demonstrates the relationship between the two tendons and a rotator cuff tear (*black arrow*). **C:** A grasper is introduced from a lateral portal to assess the tear pattern. **D:** The supraspinatus tendon demonstrates good medial to lateral tendon mobility. H, humerus; IS, infraspinatus tendon; SP, scapular spine; SS, supraspinatus tendon.

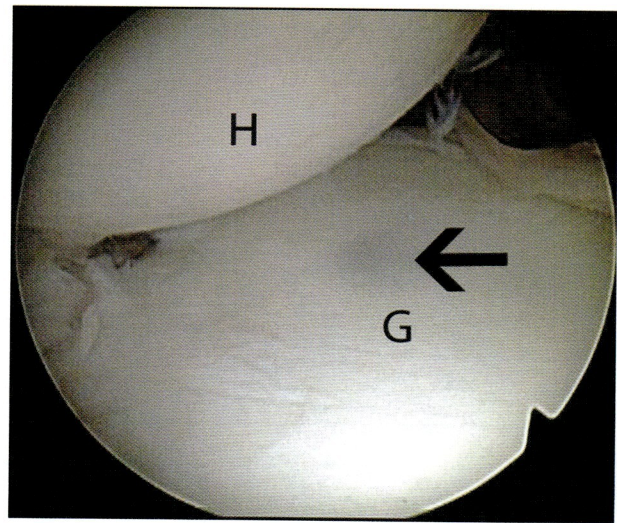

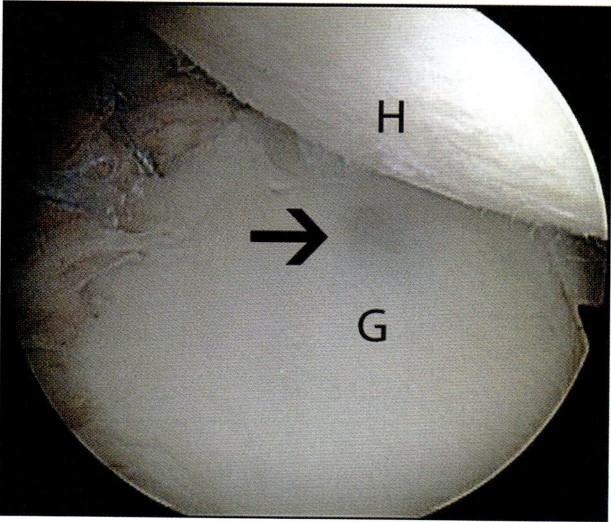

Figure 24.38 **A:** Right shoulder, anterosuperolateral viewing portal, demonstrates anterior subluxation of the humeral head relative to the bare spot (*black arrow*) in an individual with a Bankart lesion. **B:** Same shoulder postarthroscopic Bankart repair shows the humeral head well centered on the glenoid bare spot (*black arrow*), confirming adequate soft tissue tensioning. G, glenoid; H, humerus.

relationship to the muscle-tendon units to determine the tear pattern, which of course is the repair pattern (Fig. 24.37).

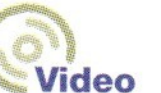

- After performing an arthroscopic Bankart repair, view the shoulder from an anterosuperolateral viewing portal. This gives a panoramic view of the shoulder along the long axis of the glenoid. After a satisfactory Bankart repair, this viewing portal will show the arc of the humeral head to be centered on the bare spot of the glenoid. If the humerus remains anteriorly subluxed, then the anterior capsulolabral sleeve has not been adequately tensioned (Fig. 24.38).

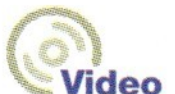

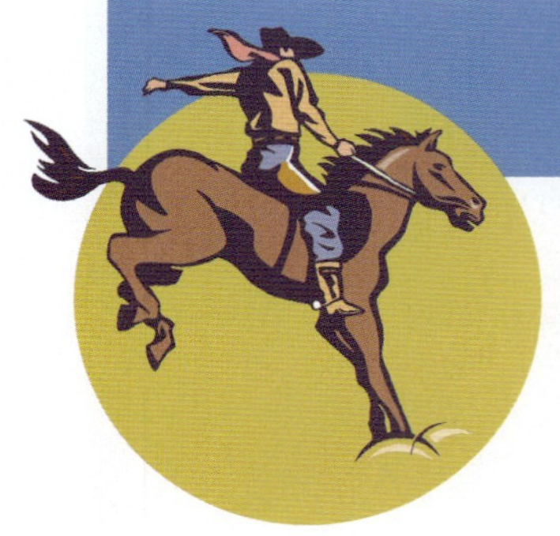

25

Future Developments

WESTERN WISDOM

When the boss wants a long talk, you're in for a long listen.

The senior author (SSB) has been fortunate to participate in the development of shoulder arthroscopy from the very beginning. This experience has produced a unique perspective on where we have been and where we might be going. Naturally, we never really know where the future will take us until we get there, but certain clues can lead us into close proximity.

WHERE WE'VE BEEN

We believe that the development of arthroscopic shoulder surgery was rapidly accelerated when we began to think of the shoulder in mechanical terms. From the standpoint of the rotator cuff, the ability to model the shoulder in terms of balanced force couples and transmission of a distributed load across a cable-like band (suspension bridge analogy) helped us to understand how to repair the mechanical derangements that were brought about by disruption of the rotator cuff insertions. Basic biomechanical research and bench testing allowed us to develop implants and instruments to arthroscopically create mechanical constructs that were significantly stronger than the disruptive forces to which these constructs were subjected.

In the realm of instability, we recognized the critical importance of glenoid and humeral bone deficiency. Significant bone deficiencies have biomechanical consequences, and the adverse consequences of bone loss can be so severe that they cannot be overcome by simple repair. Such biomechanical deficiencies often demand a bone graft to provide a large enough articular arc to restore stability. The development of criteria to recognize and appropriately address bone deficiency in instability has allowed for a biomechanically based algorithm that covers the spectrum from arthroscopic capsulolabral repair to open Latarjet reconstruction with coracoid bone graft (Table 25.1).

WHAT WORKS AND WHAT DOESN'T

Suture anchors were introduced to the orthopaedic market in 1991. The senior author (SSB) was initially skeptical of suture anchor fixation but became convinced of its superiority over transosseous cuff repair after conducting biomechanical studies of these two types of fixation (1,2). These studies demonstrated that suture anchors provided superior fixation in metaphyseal bone, whereas transosseous sutures would routinely cut through that bone in laboratory testing. In fact, it was shown that transosseous bone tunnels needed to be placed in the cortical bone, distal to the metaphyseal bone, to have sufficient strength to avoid bone cut-through of the sutures with cyclic loading.

In the early 1990s, the senior author (SSB) developed a guide system for performing arthroscopic transosseous rotator cuff repair (Fig. 25.1) and actually performed approximately a dozen of these procedures. In order to get good fixation in cortical bone, a new portal was developed that approached the humerus distal to the axillary nerve (3). Although fixation was good at that level and the patients who underwent this procedure generally did well, we abandoned

Happy Trails

TABLE 25.1
ALGORITHM FOR MANAGING ANTERIOR INSTABILITY

1. **Intraoperative arthroscopic assessment**
   Determine glenoid bone loss and Hill-Sachs depth with a calibrated probe
   Assess for an engaging Hill-Sachs lesion
   Evaluate for a SLAP lesion and repair if present
2. **Definitive surgery**
   Glenoid bone loss <25%
      Arthroscopic repair:
         Bankart repair, and
         Remplissage for Hill-Sachs ≥4 mm in depth
   Glenoid bone loss ≥25%
      Open Latarjet after arthroscopic SLAP repair if present
   Deep (>4 mm) Engaging Hill-Sachs without substantial glenoid bone loss
      Open Latarjet for patients with high physical demands vs.
      Arthroscopic Bankart and remplissage for patients with low physical demands
   Engaging Hill-Sachs with glenoid bone loss ≥25%
      Open Latarjet

it in favor of suture anchors because the approach below the axillary nerve seemed potentially too dangerous and the fixation was no better than with suture anchors.

We never even considered changing the transosseous tunnel's exit point to a more proximal and accessible location in metaphyseal bone, above the level of the axillary nerve, because the suture anchor's fixation strength was far superior to transosseous fixation in metaphyseal bone. Once we had identified the strongest fixation construct (suture anchor fixation), there was no logical reason to use the weaker construct (metaphyseal transosseous fixation). We simply switched over to the stronger suture anchor techniques.

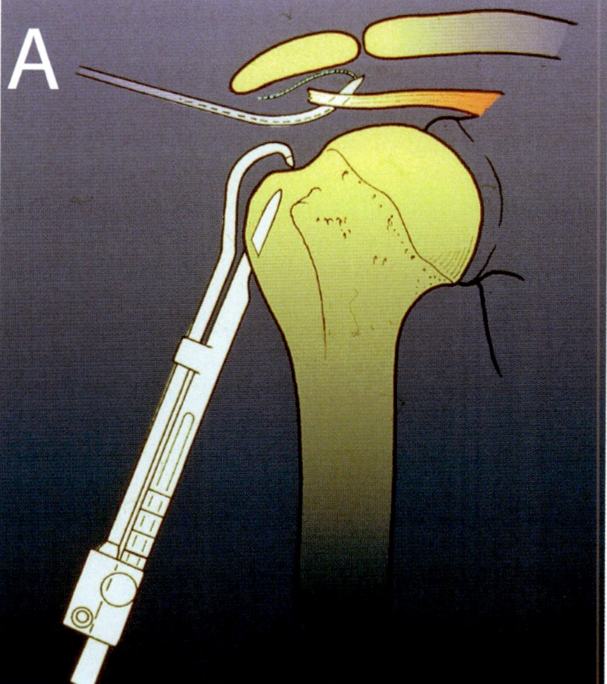

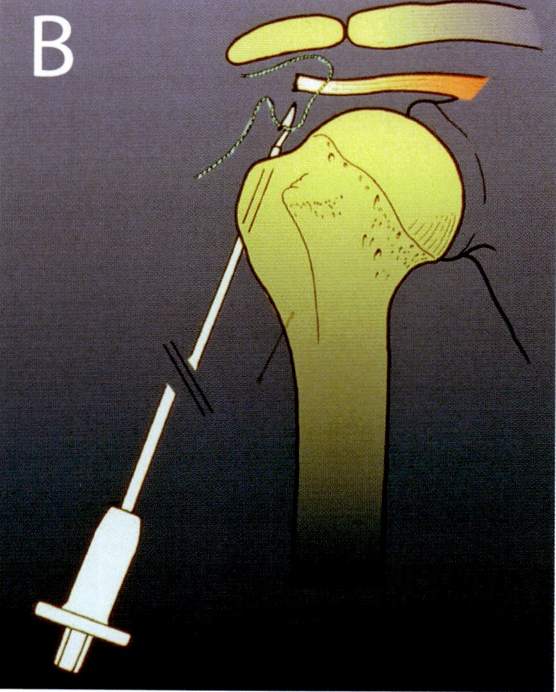

Figure 25.1 Schematic of a transosseous guide system for rotator cuff tear developed by one of the authors (SSB) in the early 1990s. **A:** A suture is passed through the rotator cuff and a bone tunnel is created using a subaxillary nerve lateral portal. **B:** The previously placed rotator cuff suture is retrieved through the bone tunnel with a snare device.

Today, some surgeons are advocating a return to "the gold standard" of metaphyseal transosseous bone tunnel fixation. There are a couple of things wrong with the logic of that position. First of all, it would be a giant step backward, reverting to a procedure that was the "gold standard" of Dr. Charles Neer more than 50 years ago. Secondly, it ignores the biomechanical research that has shown the inferiority of that technique. Finally, from a personal perspective, we've "been there and done that," and we abandoned that technique for a stronger and more reliable suture anchor technique.

BIOMECHANICAL WORKS IN PROGRESS

There is an intriguing biomechanical enhancement technology that has begun in arthroscopic shoulder surgery, and that involves the augmentation of current fixation techniques with self-reinforcing systems.

Self-regulating systems have been around for a long time in the automotive industry, where there are self-balancing engine components and self-centering mechanical systems. However, *biomechanical* self-regulating mechanisms have only recently been identified and utilized. Specifically, the suture-bridge technique of rotator cuff fixation by means of linked bridging sutures between two rows of suture anchors exhibits self-reinforcement characteristics (4).

The term *self-reinforcing* refers to the fact that, the harder one tries to make the system fail, the stronger it becomes. One example of a self-reinforcing system that most surgeons are familiar with is the Chinese finger trap (Fig. 25.2). In the case of the Chinese finger trap, the harder one pulls in an attempt to disengage it from the finger, the tighter it grips the finger. In effect, it harnesses a potentially destructive force to make itself stronger. This is a very useful characteristic, particularly for a biologic repair construct such as a rotator cuff repair.

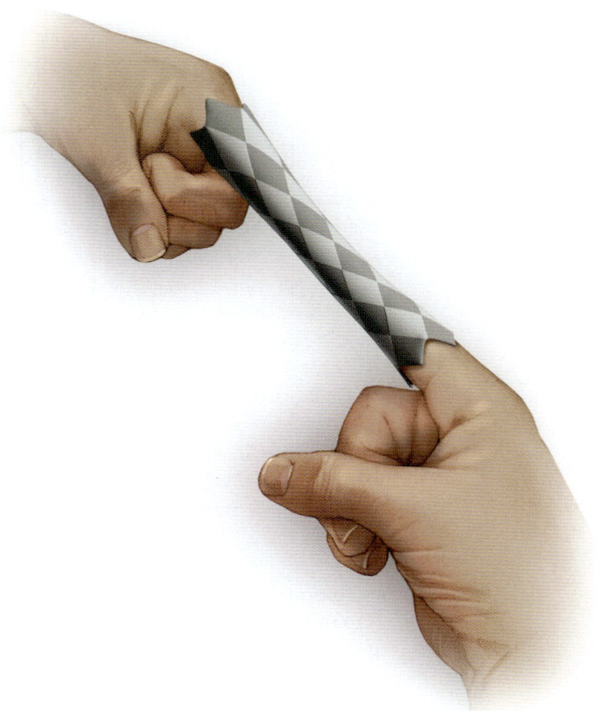

Figure 25.2 A linked double-row rotator cuff repair can be likened to a Chinese figure trap in which a distractive force (tensile load to the rotator cuff) results in further compression of the fingers (rotator cuff footprint).

We first noted the self-reinforcing attributes of bridging double-row rotator cuff repair about 4 years ago while testing this fixation technique on cadavers in the biomechanics lab (5). We noted that the yield load approached the ultimate load, in contradistinction to nonlinked double-row repairs. The reason this happens is that the suture-bridge fixation functions much like a Chinese finger trap.

In the unloaded situation, the suture bridge forms a rectangle of fixation around a segment of rotator cuff tendon (Fig. 25.3A). Under load, this rectangle changes shape into a parallelogram with a decreased height of the construct and an increased normal force perpendicular to the tendon. The increased normal force translates into increased friction at the tendon–bone interface because of the relationship $f = \mu N$. As the normal force increases, the frictional force increases. Also, because the height of the parallelogram continues to decrease under load, the tendon becomes wedged progressively more tightly under the sutures (Fig. 25.3B). We think that the improved clinical results that are being reported with suture-bridge techniques are at least partly due to the enhanced fixation afforded by this self-reinforcing mechanism.

Self-reinforcement and biologic enhancement are incremental enhancing technologies that are layered onto the base technology of strong mechanical fixation. We feel certain that there are other self-reinforcing and self-regulating techniques that will be discovered to enhance fixation and thereby improve healing.

Another area that is rapidly developing in the realm of enhanced arthroscopic technology is that of arthroscopic shoulder arthroplasty. Dr. Werner Anderl in Vienna, Austria, has been performing arthroscopic resurfacing of the humerus (Partial Eclipse; Arthrex, Inc., Naples, FL). In addition, he is developing techniques for arthroscopic transhumeral glenoid preparation (Fig. 25.4). Components are introduced through the rotator interval and secured by screws using a transhumeral retrograde screwdriver. This revolutionary arthroscopic technology should soon lead to a new era in shoulder arthroplasty.

Equally exciting is a new technique of arthroscopic biologic resurfacing of the glenoid and humeral head with large osteochondral allografts. This technique, which is being pioneered by Dr. Reuben Gobezie, is essentially a biologic arthroscopic total shoulder arthroplasty. This technique, if successful, has the potential to cure an arthritic shoulder, which would be truly revolutionary.

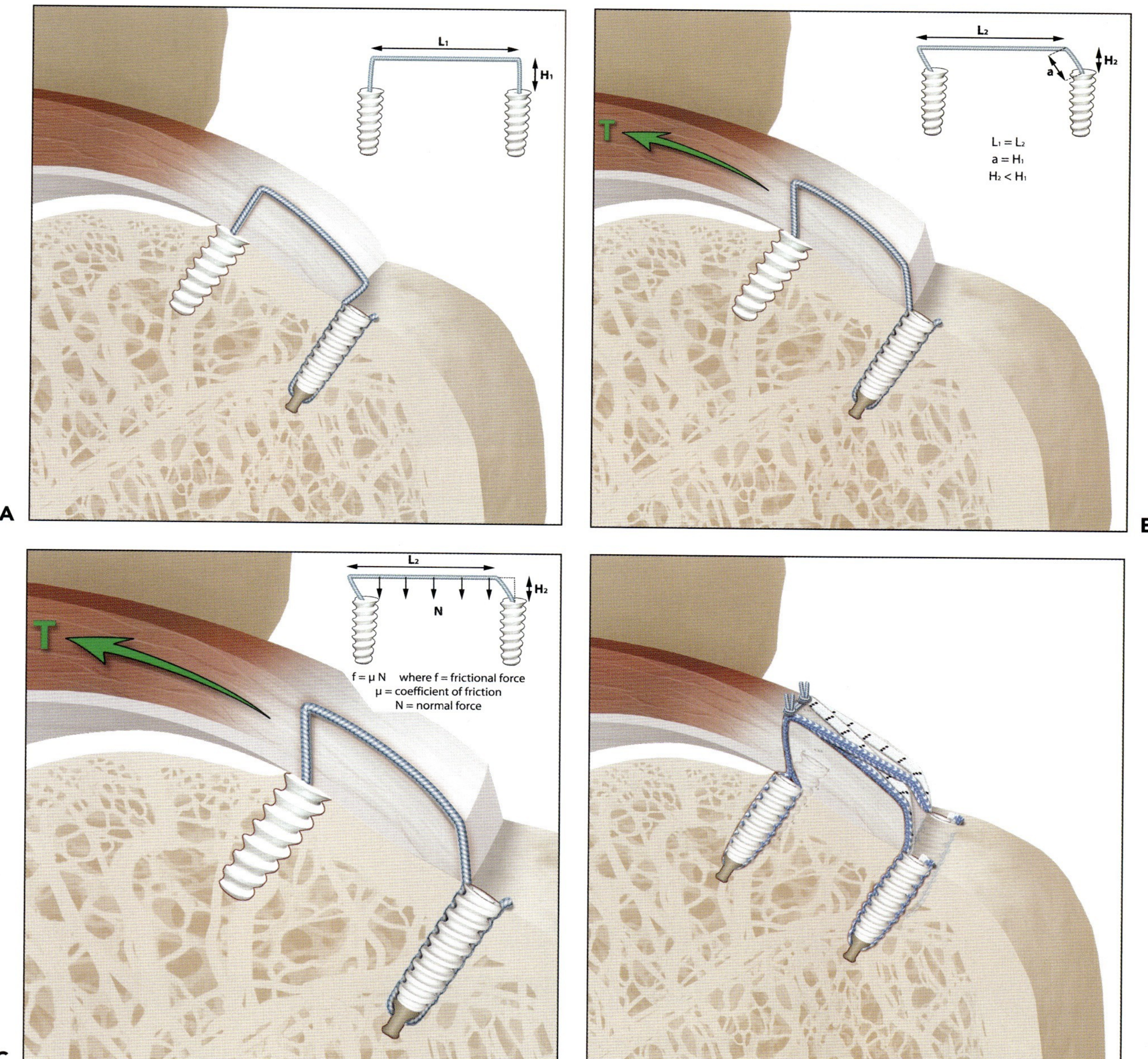

Figure 25.3 Schematic of self-reinforcing suture-bridge technique. **A:** Linked double-row construct before loading. Inset: Free-body diagram of the construct. H1, thickness of rotator cuff before loading; L1, length of tendon beneath suture. **B:** Loading of the linked double-row construct results in compression of the rotator cuff footprint. Inset: Free-body diagram of the construct. T, tensile loading force; L2, length of tendon beneath suture; a, length of suture between tendon edge and lateral anchor; H2, thickness of compressed rotator cuff under tensile load. **C:** Up-close view of the linked double-row construct after loading. Inset: Free-body diagram showing distributed normal force (N) resulting from elastic deformation of tendon beneath the suture. The frictional force (f) increases as the normal force (N) increases under load. **D:** Linked double-row construct with two medial anchors linked to two lateral anchors provides maximal footprint compression under loading. Additionally, a medial double-mattress stitch in this case provides a seal to joint fluid.

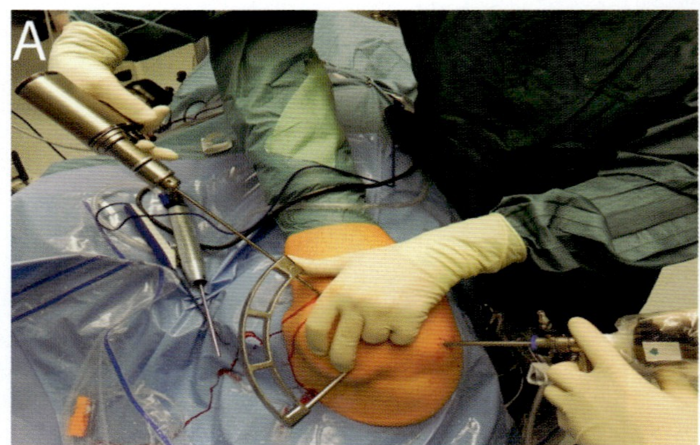

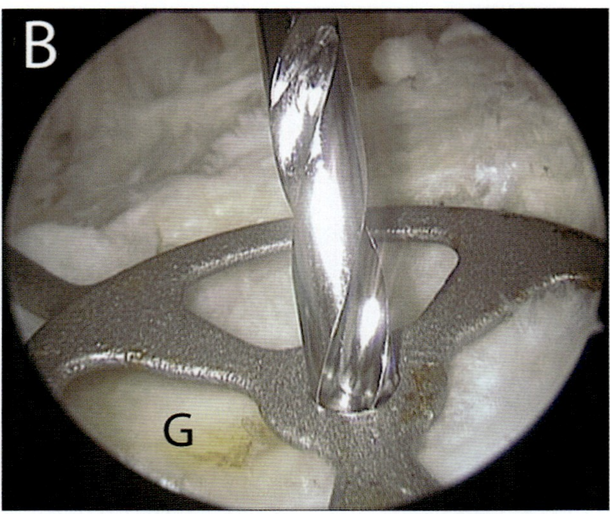

Figure 25.4 Arthroscopic-assisted shoulder arthroplasty. **A:** Transhumeral drilling performed under arthroscopic visualization can be used to prepare the proximal humerus or glenoid for prosthetic implantation. **B:** Arthroscopic photo from a posterior portal demonstrates the use of transhumeral drilling for glenoid (G) preparation. (Photos courtesy of Werner Anderl, MD)

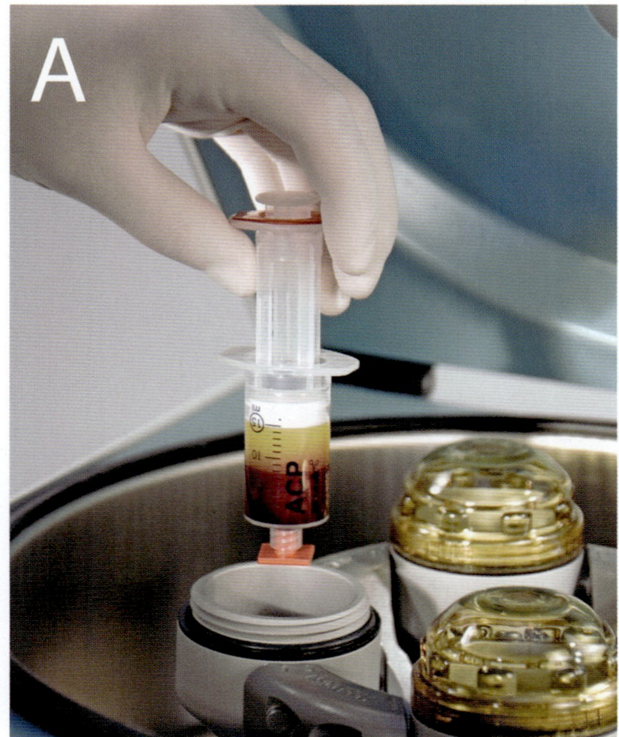

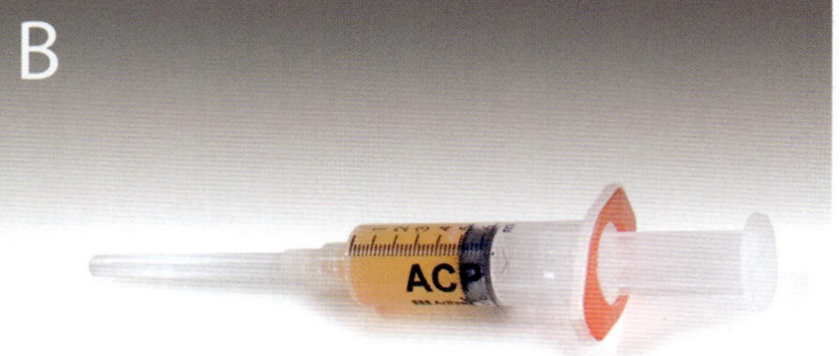

Figure 25.5 Platelet-rich plasma (ACP; Arthrex, Inc., Naples, FL) is one current adjunct used for biological enhancement in shoulder arthroscopy. **A:** Blood obtained from the patient is placed in a centrifuge to separate the plasma rich in growth factors from the red blood cells. **B:** After isolating it from the red blood cells, the platelet-rich plasma can be injected as a biological enhancement during shoulder arthroscopy (e.g., rotator cuff repair.).

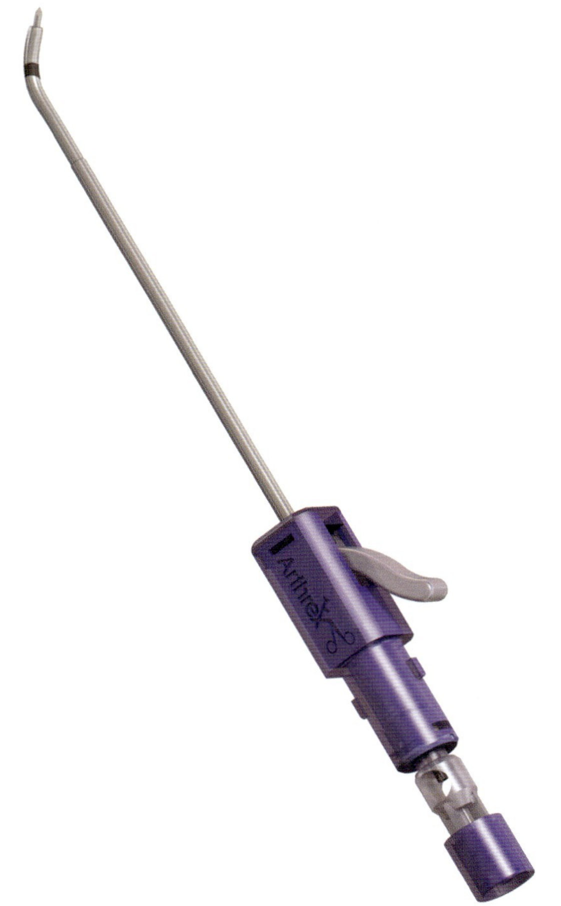

Figure 25.6 The PowerPick device (Arthrex, Inc., Naples, FL) can be used during rotator cuff repair for biologic enhancement by creating vents in the greater tuberosity that allow access of the marrow elements to the surface to encourage tendon to bone healing.

BIOLOGIC ENHANCEMENT

Biologic enhancement technology has already begun, in the form of platelet-rich plasma preparations (Fig. 25.5) and techniques of bone bed preparation (microfracture variants) (Fig. 25.6) and implant design (vented and cannulated suture anchors) (Fig. 25.7) to encourage open access of blood and bone marrow elements to the tendon–bone interface, as well as ingrowth of bone into the vents in the anchors.

Biologic enhancement is in its infancy. Even though a variety of platelet-rich plasma preparations are available, much needs to be learned about how to optimally apply this technology. A great deal of work is currently being done to secure growth factors at the repair site. Perhaps a time-release preparation will ensure that the proper cascade of factors will occur at the proper time to enhance healing. Further research should clarify whether patients need repeated postoperative injections to introduce specific growth factors at the correct time to optimize healing.

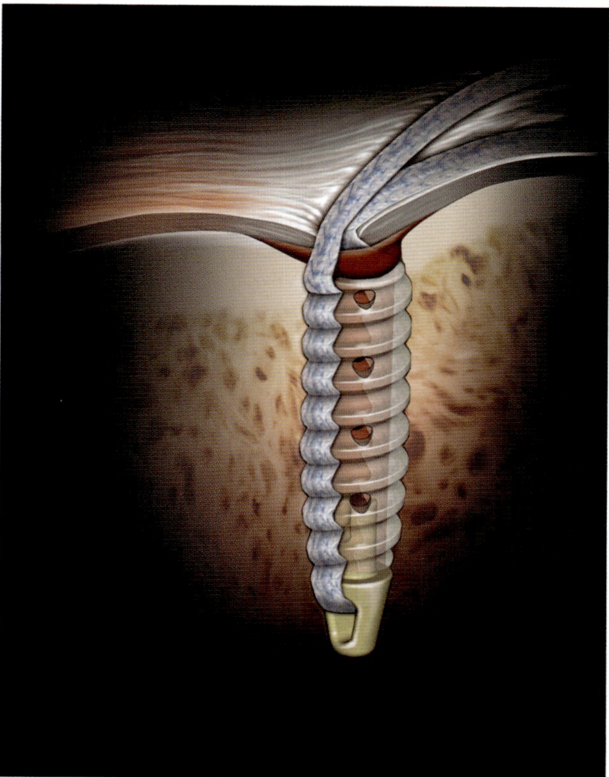

Figure 25.7 Illustration of biologic enhancement of rotator cuff repair with a vented BioComposite SwiveLock C anchor (Arthrex, Inc., Naples, FL). Vents in this anchor allow bone ingrowth within the vent channels.

In addition to the biologic enhancement technologies that you have probably heard of, there are various disparate technologies that you have probably not heard of that may have a profound effect on the future of shoulder surgery (6).

Stem Cell Technologies

Despite the political rhetoric, stem cell research has moved far beyond embryonic stem cells to a process called transdifferentiation. In this process, adult cells, usually from human skin, are transformed into a new kind of stem cell called induced pluripotent stem (iPS) cells. These iPS cells are fundamentally identical to embryonic stem cells, and can be programmed to grow into other cell types such as heart cells or pancreatic islet cells or articular cartilage cells. Scientists at Rice University and at the University of California at Davis have used iPS cells from a mouse to grow its entire distal femur in the lab. Imagine doing this in humans, so that the patient's own skin cells are used to grow a younger version of his own shoulder in the lab, which can then be surgically implanted as a biologic autologous joint replacement. In similar fashion, focal chondral defects could be treated arthroscopically by implanting laboratory-grown autografts.

Synthetic Biology

Manipulating genomes has become so commonplace today that even high schoolers do it. Craig Venter, who decoded the human genome for a fraction of the cost and in a fraction of the time that the US government had allotted, is pushing the boundaries of synthetic biology. Venter and his associates at the J. Craig Venter Institute in California have made a bacterial genome from scratch and have even turned one type of microbe into another. Venter expects to create the first artificial life form within the next year, which will essentially be a "designer bacteria." His next step is to engineer a "designer algae" that will secrete high-grade hydrocarbons that can easily be refined into transportation fuels. ExxonMobil has so much faith in this concept that they have funded Venter's project with $300 million.

Other researchers have created synthetic organelles, and even an entirely new organelle known as the synthosome, to make enzymes for synthetic biology. One can envision the day when synthosomes that produce enzymes and proteins that are useful in the repair process of tendons could be used to enhance rotator cuff healing or to reverse the changes of tendon degeneration.

RNA Interference (RNAi)

Synthetic biology and stem cell strategies can be categorized under the umbrella of regenerative medicine, which has the power to restore damaged or senescent tissues, but does not attack the cause of disease. This is where RNA interference (RNAi) fits in.

RNAi is able to turn off specific genes by blocking their messenger RNA, thus preventing them from creating proteins. RNAi provides the ability to control any of the genes in our bodies as well as the proteins they produce. This is a very powerful function. With its ability to create proteins blocked, the gene is effectively silenced. RNAi could be used to turn off the gene that allows cancers to develop capillary networks. It could turn off the protein production responsible for Alzheimer's disease. In the shoulder, RNAi could be used to turn off the genes responsible for articular cartilage degeneration or rotator cuff degeneration. This strategy could be augmented by cell therapies in which iPS cells are introduced into the damaged tissue to initiate healing with young healthy cells generated by the patient's own DNA.

For the first time, science is looking not just to treat symptoms, but to actually stop the gene functions that cause disease. This is truly revolutionary. The challenge right now is in the delivery of RNAi preparations to cells. These molecules are large and fragile, so they do not penetrate cell membranes easily. Right now, a number of delivery mechanisms are under investigation, and their successful development will assure the future of RNA interference.

Nanotechnology/Biotechnology Convergence

"The role of the infinitely small is infinitely large."

—Louis Pasteur

One nanometer is one one-billionth of a meter. The nanotechnology range is generally considered to be under 100 nm, which gets down to molecular and atomic levels.

Until recently, a large part of nanotechnology's resources were directed toward the creation of molecular machines. Boston College chemistry professor T. Ross Kelly reported that he had constructed a chemically powered nanomotor out of 78 atoms. Another molecular-sized motor fueled by solar energy was built out of 58 atoms by Ben Feringa at the University of Groningen in The Netherlands. Carbon nanotubes have been used to construct nanoscale conveyor belts.

DNA is also proving to be very versatile for building molecular structures. A tiny biped robot constructed from DNA was developed at New York University. It has legs that are only 10 nm long. The robot can walk down a DNA walking track. DNA was chosen as the construction material because of its ability to attach and detach itself in a controlled manner.

Nanoscale scaffolds have been used to grow biological tissues such as skin. Future therapies could use these tiny scaffolds to grow any type of tissue needed for repairs inside the body.

One fascinating application of nanotechnology is to harness nanoparticles to deliver treatments to specific sites in the body. Nanoparticles can guide drugs into cell walls and through the blood–brain barrier. Scientists at McGill University in Montreal demonstrated a "nanopill" with structures in the 25 to 45 nm range. The nanopill is small enough to pass through the cell wall and deliver medication directly to targeted structures inside the cell.

Ray Kurzweil, in his book *The Singularity is Near,* envisions nanoscale robots, or nanobots, that will be able to travel through the bloodstream, going in and around our cells and performing various services, such as removing toxins, correcting DNA errors, repairing and restoring cell membranes, modifying the levels of hormones and neurotransmitters, and a myriad of other tasks.

THE BOTTOM LINE

Shoulder surgery is changing, and it is changing at a faster rate than ever before. The convergence of biomechanical and biologic enhancement with nanotechnology and biotechnology will produce breathtaking advancements that, only a few years ago, would have seemed to fit more properly in the realm of science fiction than of science.

But this is not science fiction. We are living and practicing during the most dynamic, most fluid, and most exciting time in the history of shoulder surgery. So let's make the most of it.

REFERENCES

1. Burkhart SS, Johnson TC, Wirth MA, et al. Cyclic loading of transosseous rotator cuff repairs: tension overload as a possible cause of failure. *Arthroscopy*. 1997;13(2):172–176.
2. Burkhart SS, Diaz Pagan JL, Wirth MA, et al. Cyclic loading of anchor-based rotator cuff repairs: confirmation of the tension overload phenomenon and comparison of suture anchor fixation with transosseous fixation. Arthro*scopy*. 1997;13(6):720–724.
3. Burkhart SS, Nassar J, Schenck RC, Jr, et al. Clinical and anatomic considerations in the use of a new anterior inferior subaxillary nerve arthroscopy portal. *Arthroscopy*. 1996;12(5):634–637.
4. Park MC, Tibone JE, ElAttrache NS, et al. Part II: biomechanical assessment for a footprint-restoring transosseous-equivalent rotator cuff repair technique compared with a double-row repair technique. *J Shoulder Elbow Surg*. 2007;16(4):469–476.
5. Burkhart SS, Adams CR, Burkhart SS, et al.A biomechanical comparison of 2 techniques of footprint reconstruction for rotator cuff repair: the SwiveLock-FiberChain construct versus standard double-row repair. *Arthroscopy*. 2009;25(3):274–281.
6. Burkhart SS. Expanding the frontiers of shoulder arthroscopy. *J Shoulder Elbow Surg*. 2011;20(2):183–191.

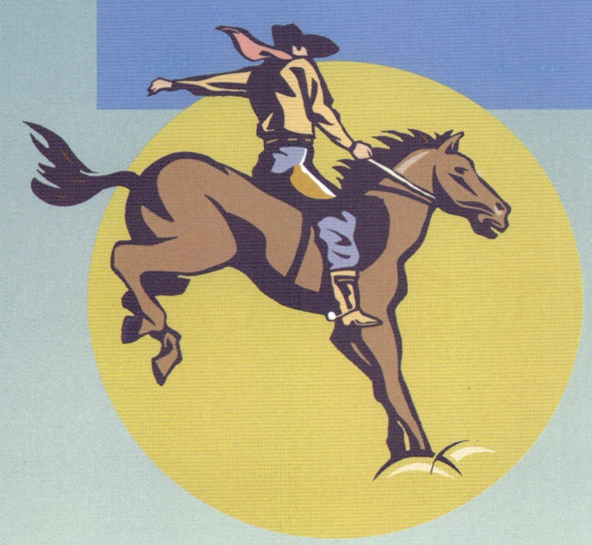

PART II

THE SHOULDER RODEO

COWBOY PRINCIPLE 9

A good bronc rider is light in the head and heavy in the seat.

After the gate opens and it's just you and the bronc, instinct and ingenuity pave the only road to survival. So cinch up your riggin's and hang on.

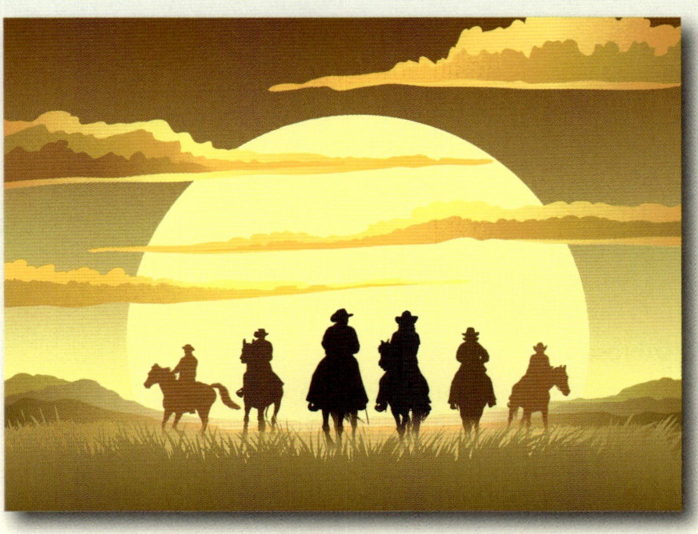

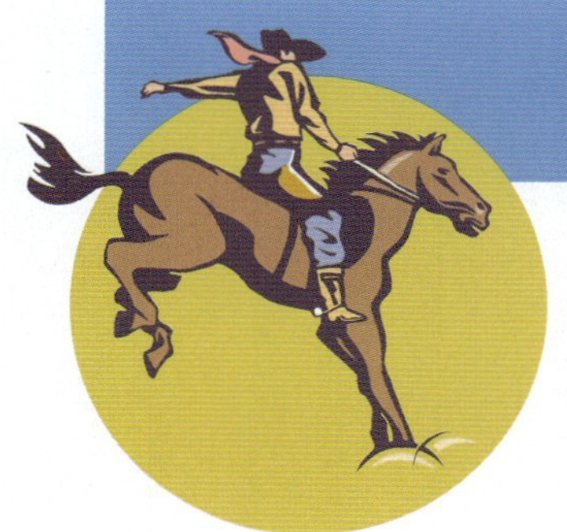

26 Rotator Cuff Cases

WESTERN WISDOM

Followin' the crowd is the quickest way to get nowhere.

CASE 1: MASSIVE TRAUMATIC ROTATOR CUFF TEAR WITH INTRATENDINOUS DISRUPTION NEAR THE MUSCULOTENDINOUS JUNCTION

History:

- 43-year-old contractor who fell through a hole in the attic of a home he was building
- Tried to break his fall by grabbing a support beam
- Hyperabduction injury to left shoulder

Exam:

- Pain with elevation above 90°
- Very weak resisted external rotation

Imaging:

- X-rays are normal.
- MRI shows complete retracted tears of supraspinatus and infraspinatus, with tendon disruption near the musculotendinous junction, and a large tendon stump attached to the greater tuberosity.

Arthroscopic Findings:

- Large retracted traumatic disruption of supraspinatus (SS) and infraspinatus (IS) tendons
- Short tendon leader still attached to SS and IS muscles
- Large viable tendon stump still attached to greater tuberosity (Fig. 26.1A)

Procedures Performed:

- Arthroscopic repair with suture anchors reinforced by a FiberTape rip-stop load-sharing tendon-to-bone construct (Fig. 26.1B)

Key Points:

- With a large distal tendon stump, simple sutures between tendon ends will not provide good fixation and will not hold.
- If the distal stump were removed and the proximal musculotendinous segment were advanced to the bone bed, the muscle-tendon unit would likely be overtensioned.
- In order to accomplish the two goals of strong fixation and normal length–tension relationship of the muscle-tendon unit, we perform an augmented suture anchor repair using a FiberTape rip-stop load-sharing tendon-to-bone construct. Multiple knotted sutures around the FiberTape rip-stop enhance the tendon fixation.

CASE 2: "RESCUE ANCHOR" TECHNIQUE FOR AUGMENTING SUTURE ANCHOR REPAIR IN SOFT BONE

History:

- 67-year-old female
- Chronic pain and weakness in dominant shoulder for 4 years
- Temporary relief from injections

Exam:

- Very weak resisted external rotation

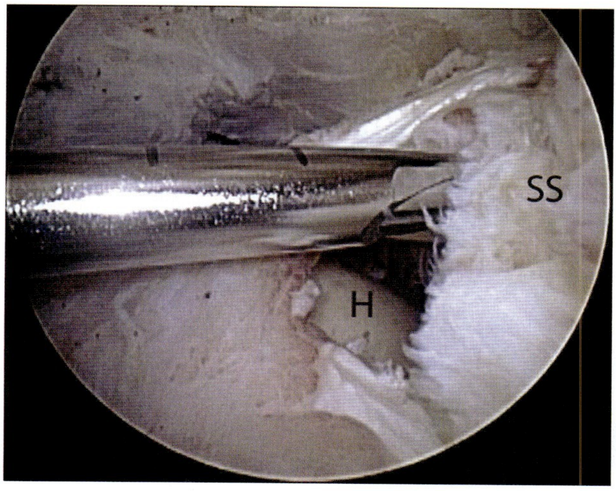

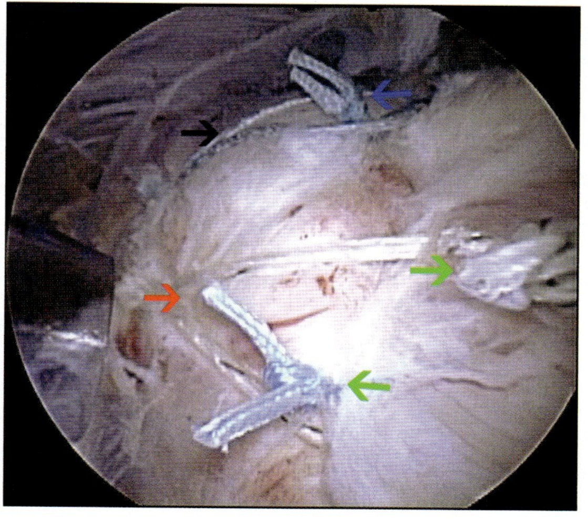

Figure 26.1 **A:** Left shoulder, posterior subacromial viewing portal, demonstrates a medial rotator cuff tear with a lateral tendon stump. **B:** Same shoulder. Two rip-stop sutures have been placed; the anterior FiberTape (Arthrex, Inc., Naples, FL) rip-stop (*black arrows*) encircles simple stitches (*blue arrows*) based from the anteromedial anchor, and the posterior rip-stop (*red arrows*) encircles simples stitches (*green arrows*) based from the posteromedial anchor. H, humeral head; SS, supraspinatus tendon.

- Normal bear-hug and belly-press tests
- Active elevation 30° and passive elevation 180° (pseudoparalysis)

Imaging:

- X-rays show marked osteopenia of proximal humerus.
- MRI shows retracted tear of supraspinatus and infraspinatus, with good quality muscle on T-1 parasagittal sections.

Arthroscopic Findings:

- Large crescent-shaped tear of SS and IS, easily reducible to bone bed with relatively small amount of tension (Fig. 26.2A)

Procedures Performed:

- Arthroscopic suture anchor repair of the rotator cuff, augmented by "rescue anchor" technique (Figs. 26.2B and 26.3)

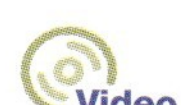

Key Points:

- In osteopenic bone, a suture anchor may begin to tip medially, even under low loads, resulting in a loose anchor with a "reverse deadman angle."
- A laterally placed "rescue anchor" (SwiveLock) can restore an anatomic footprint reduction by anchoring FiberWire suture into the relatively stronger metaphyseal cortex (lateral to the corner of the greater tuberosity).

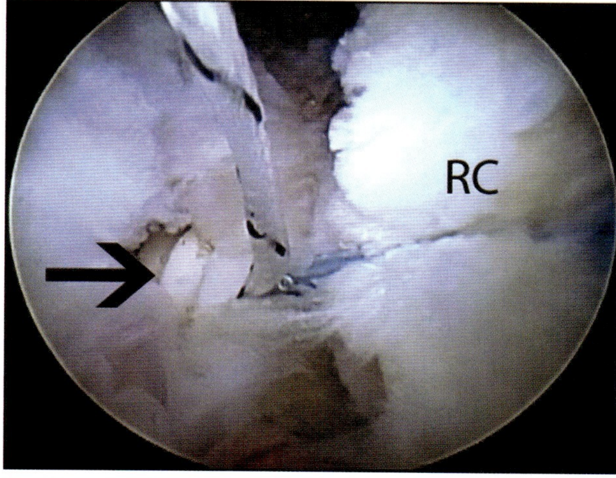

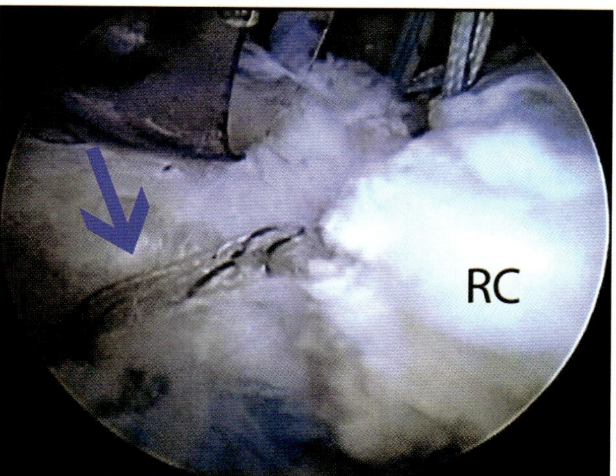

Figure 26.2 **A:** Left shoulder, posterior subacromial viewing portal. After knot tying, an anchor placed for a rotator cuff repair has tilted medially (*black arrow*). **B:** Same shoulder demonstrates a rescue anchor (*blue arrow*) that has been used to reinforce the medial anchor. RC, rotator cuff.

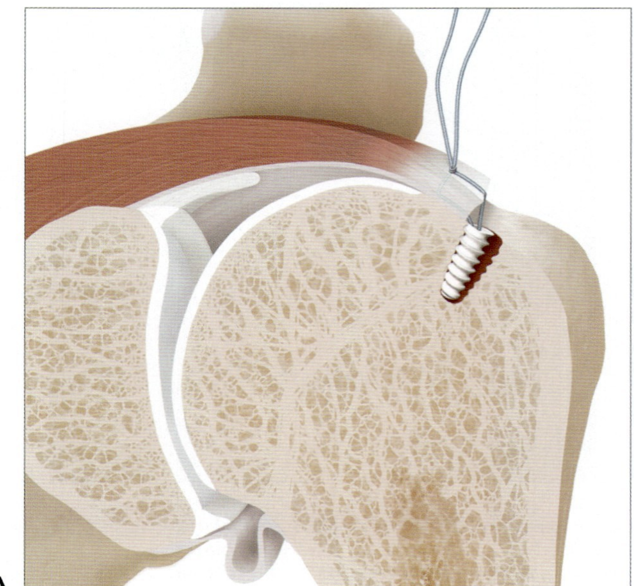

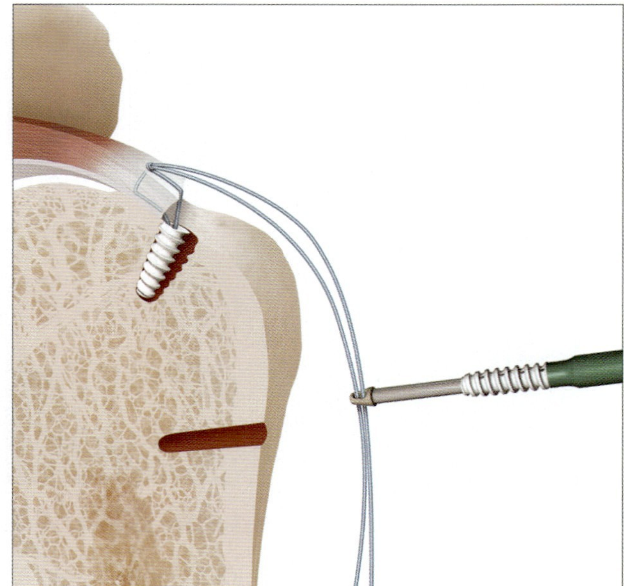

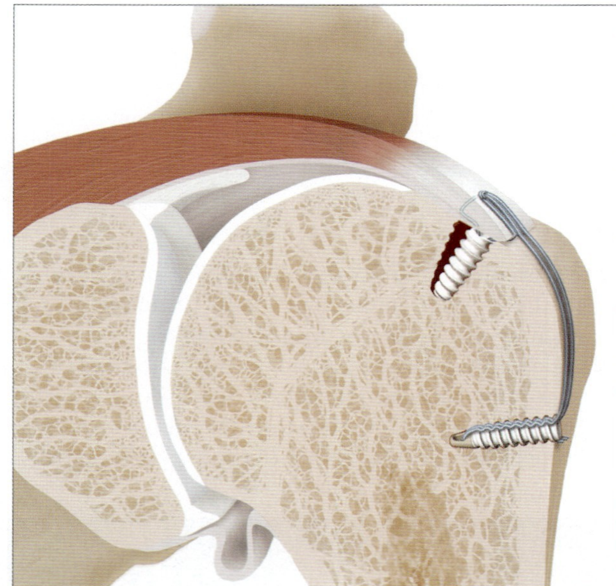

Figure 26.3 Schematic of the "rescue anchor" technique for a loose anchor. **A:** An anchor has been placed in the greater tuberosity for rotator cuff repair. However, while securing the rotator cuff the anchor has tilted medially under tension in poor quality bone. **B:** Although the tear is not amenable to double-row fixation because of limited mobility, a lateral anchor can be used to salvage the construct. The suture tails passed through the rotator cuff are left long and secured in the lateral greater tuberosity with a knotless SwiveLock anchor (Arthrex, Inc., Naples, FL). **C:** The lateral anchor effectively shares the load of the medial anchor.

CASE 3: MASSIVE RETRACTED ROTATOR CUFF TEAR WITH HETEROTOPIC OSSIFICATION OF THE TORN TENDON

History:

- 59-year-old physician
- Head-on motor vehicle accident; struck by drunk driver
- Closed head injury, unconscious for 10 days
- Multiple fractures
- After he regained consciousness, his physician noted that the patient had pain and weakness in his right shoulder

Exam:

- Very weak external rotation
- Active elevation 30°; passive elevation 135° (pseudoparalysis).

Imaging:

- X-rays and computed tomography (CT) showed multiple areas of heterotopic bone, including massive calcification of the tendons of the torn supraspinatus and infraspinatus (Fig. 26.4A).

Arthroscopic Findings:

- Massive retracted tear of SS and IS with ossification of virtually the entire length and breadth of the tendons

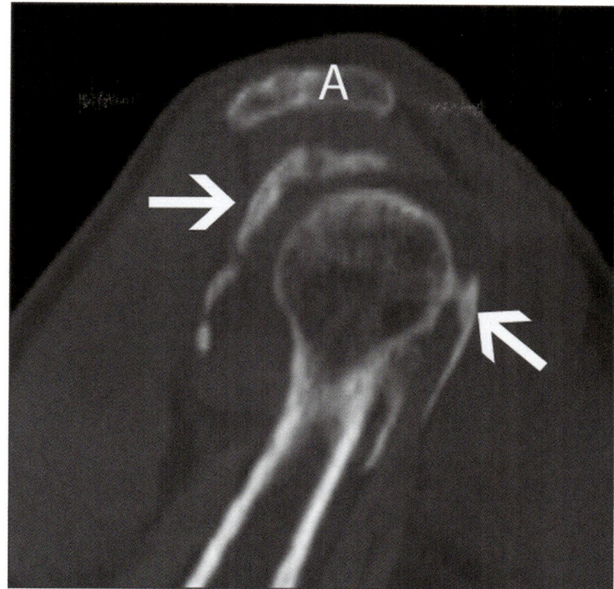

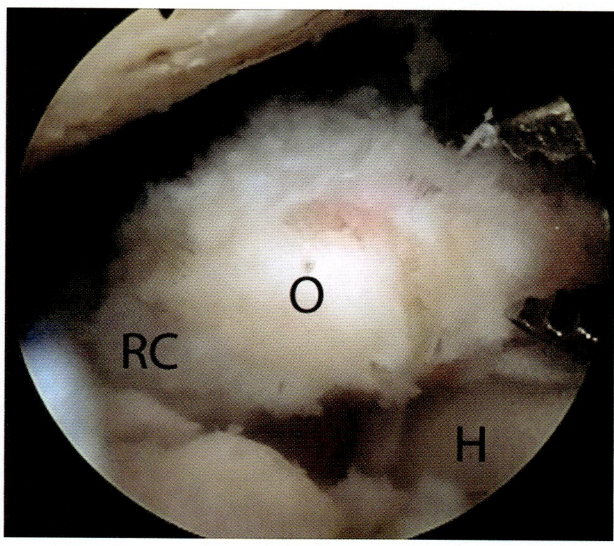

Figure 26.4 **A:** Right shoulder. Sagittal reconstruction of a CT scan, demonstrates ossification within the rotator cuff (*white arrows*). **B:** Arthroscopic photo of the same shoulder from a posterior viewing portal. An osteotomy through the ossification and a posterior interval slide has been performed in preparation for a rotator cuff repair. A, acromion; H, humerus; O, ossification; RC, rotator cuff.

- Tear was very immobile at the posterior interval and appeared to require a posterior interval slide to allow enough excursion for repair to the greater tuberosity (Fig. 26.4B)

Procedures Performed:

- Posterior interval slide performed through ossified tendon by using a 3/8″ osteotome to osteotomize the tendon in the interval between SS and IS, while traction was being applied to the SS and IS
- Bone-to-bone (ossified tendon) fixation obtained by means of suture anchors, with sutures passed through holes bored in the ossified tendons.

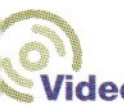

Key Points:

- If the heterotopic bone had been excised, there would have been no remaining tendon for the repair.
- The posterior interval slide was performed using all the usual principles, except that the actual release between the two tendons was done with an osteotome rather than a scissor (osteotomy of the rotator cuff!).
- Since fixation is bone to bone, one can anticipate good healing if fixation is good. The patient's function dramatically improved by 4 years post-op, with active elevation of 135° and strong overhead function.

CASE 4: REVISION REPAIR OF RETRACTED ADHESED SUBSCAPULARIS TENDON

History:

- 55-year-old man
- Failed previous arthroscopic subscapularis tendon repair by another surgeon
- Open biceps tenodesis performed at the time of primary surgery
- Persistent pain and difficulty with activities of daily living

Exam:

- Positive bear-hug and belly-press tests
- Limited active and passive range of motion in all planes

Imaging:

- MRI shows a recurrent retracted subscapularis tendon tear.

Arthroscopic Findings:

- Retracted adhesed tear of the subscapularis tendon
- Unable to identify comma sign on initial assessment due to adhesions and retraction (Figs. 26.5A, B)

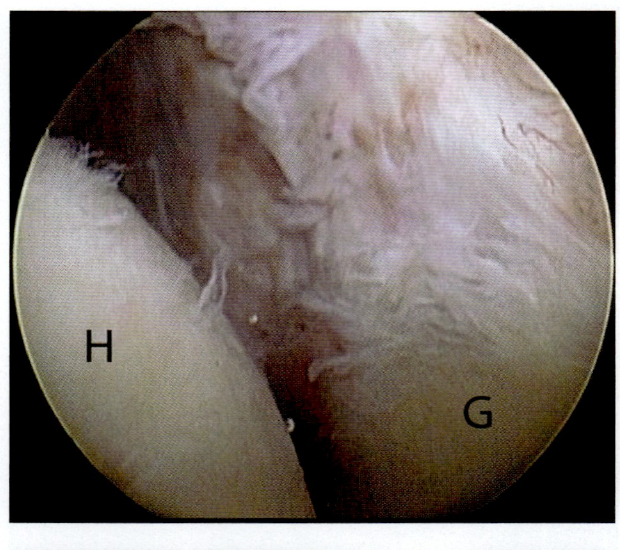

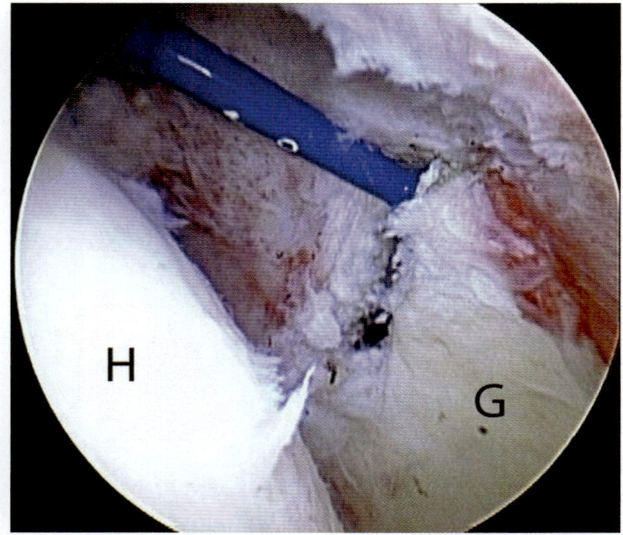

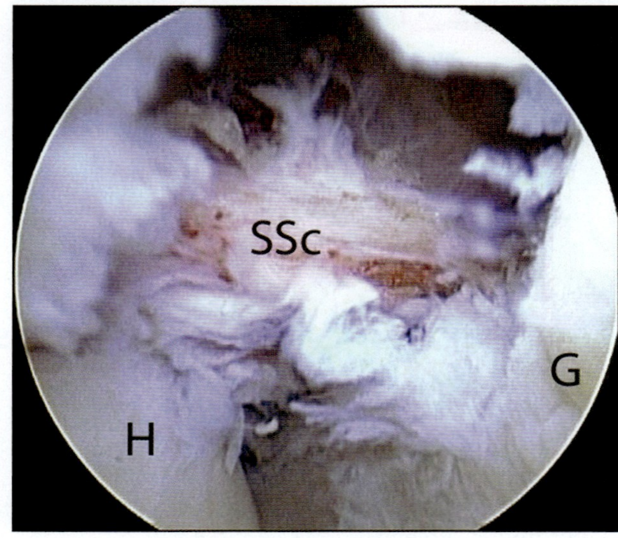

Figure 26.5 **A:** Left shoulder, posterior viewing portal, demonstrates a retracted adhesed subscapualris tendon tear. Note the absence of an identifiable comma sign due to the adhesions. **B:** A plane is developed above the midglenoid notch so that dissection can proceed toward the base of the coracoid for identification of the subscapularis tendon. **C:** Appearance postsubscapularis tendon repair. G, glenoid; H, humerus; SSc, subscapularis tendon.

Procedures Performed:

Video
- Revision subscapularis tendon repair (Fig. 26.5C)
- Capsular release

Key Points:

- If the comma sign is not visible, the normal anatomic landmarks must be used to identify a retracted subscapularis tendon.
  - Normally, the top of the subscapularis tendon crosses the glenoid at the midglenoid notch.
  - The subscapularis can always be located beneath the base of the coracoid.
- A plane must be developed between the subscapularis tendon and the glenoid at the midglenoid notch.
- Dissection then proceeds medially toward the base of the coracoid.
- A three-sided release of the subscapularis should be performed.
- It is acceptable to medialize the lesser tuberosity footprint by 5 to 7 mm to obtain a tendon to bone repair.

CASE 5: ARTHROSCOPIC SUTUREBRIDGE ROTATOR CUFF REPAIR WITH BONE GRAFTING OF GREATER TUBEROSITY CYST

History:

- 47-year-old RHD female, operating room nurse
- Retracting during general surgery case and developed shoulder pain
- Second injury 6 weeks later tripping at work, injuring shoulder

- Minimal improvement with physical therapy

Exam:

- Full range of motion (145/40/T12)
- Positive impingement signs
- Pain with resisted forward elevation and external rotation

Imaging:

- Full-thickness supraspinatus tear
- Greater tuberosity cyst 1.3 × 1.3 × 1.1 cm

Arthroscopic Findings:

- Full-thickness tear supraspinatus tendon
- Greater tuberosity cyst at desired location of posteromedial anchor (Fig. 26.6A)

Procedures Performed:

Video
- Arthroscopic identification and bone grafting of cyst
- Arthroscopic double-row rotator cuff repair (Fig. 26.6B)

Key Points:

- While most cysts can largely be ignored, large or massive cysts may compromise anchor fixation.
- Large cyst requires bone grafting to restore bone stock.
- Cyst is identified and approached through the exposed footprint of the rotator cuff insertion.
- Arthroscopic bone grafting using morcelized allograft is used to sequentially fill and compress the bone graft following cyst preparation.
- Double-row rotator cuff repair is performed avoiding the cyst if possible and sealing the bone graft from the glenohumeral and subacromial spaces.

CASE 6: ARTHROSCOPIC REVISION SUBSCAPULARIS REPAIR WITH DERMAL ALLOGRAFT REPLACEMENT OF THE POSTERIOR SUPERIOR ROTATOR CUFF

History:

- 38-year-old male, LHD, truck driver
- Original injury: slipped on ice suffering massive rotator cuff tear
- Original surgery elsewhere, arthroscopic rotator cuff repair utilizing suture anchors
- Continued with ongoing pain, loss of motion, decreased strength
- Attempted return to work 1 year postoperatively → unable

Exam:

- Painful range of motion (160/20/T12)
- Strength out of 5 in forward flexion, abduction, external rotation
- Intermediate Napoleon test

Imaging:

- MRI shows a massive recurrent rotator cuff tear involving supraspinatus, infraspinatus, and subscapularis

Arthroscopic Findings:

- Rotator cuff tear involving supraspinatus, infraspinatus, and subscapularis (Figs. 26.7A, B)

Procedures Performed:

- Arthroscopic subscapularis repair

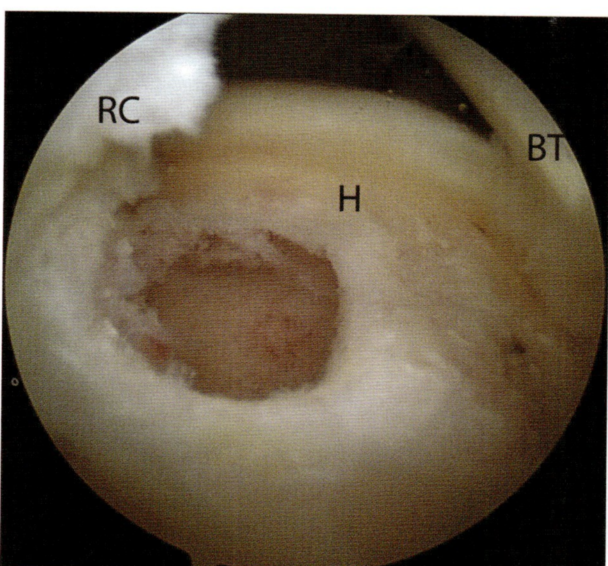

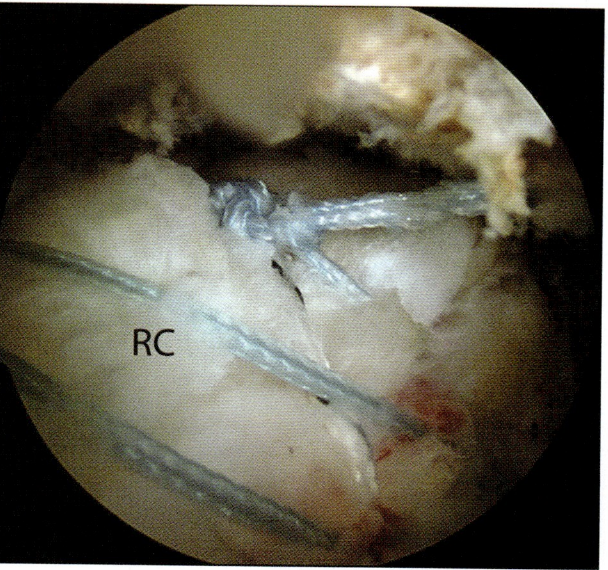

Figure 26.6 **A:** Right shoulder, lateral subacromial viewing portal, demonstrates a full-thickness rotator cuff tear and a large cyst in the greater tuberosity at the desired site of a posteromedial anchor. **B:** Same shoulder. Posterior subacromial viewing portal demonstrates appearance after a double-row rotator cuff repair. BT, biceps tendon; H, humerus; RC, rotator cuff.

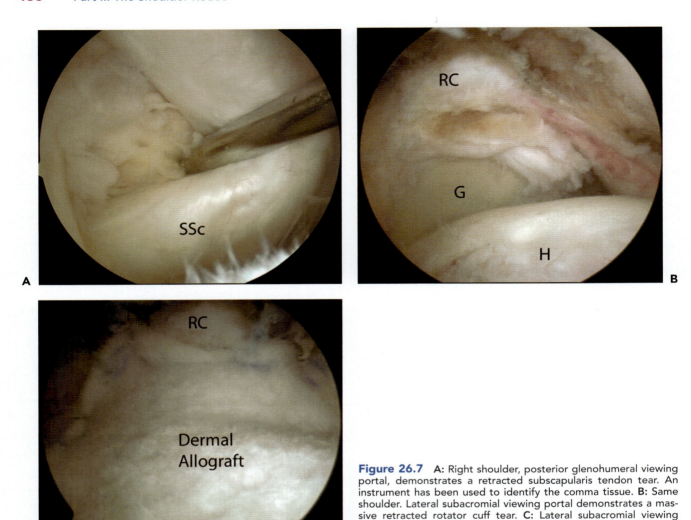

Figure 26.7 **A:** Right shoulder, posterior glenohumeral viewing portal, demonstrates a retracted subscapularis tendon tear. An instrument has been used to identify the comma tissue. **B:** Same shoulder. Lateral subacromial viewing portal demonstrates a massive retracted rotator cuff tear. **C:** Lateral subacromial viewing portal demonstrates posterosuperior rotator cuff dermal allograft replacement. G, glenoid; H, humerus; RC, rotator cuff; SSc, subscapularis tendon.

- Arthroscopic biceps tenodesis

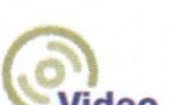

- Arthroscopic dermal allograft rotator cuff replacement (Fig. 26.7C)

Key Points:

- Balance the force couples utilizing partial rotator cuff repair (i.e., subscapularis).
- Biceps tenodesis to protect the subscapularis repair
- Human dermal allograft replacement for the residual rotator cuff defect
- Multisuture fixation for graft fixation to the residual rotator cuff defect and bone
- Careful suture management is critical.

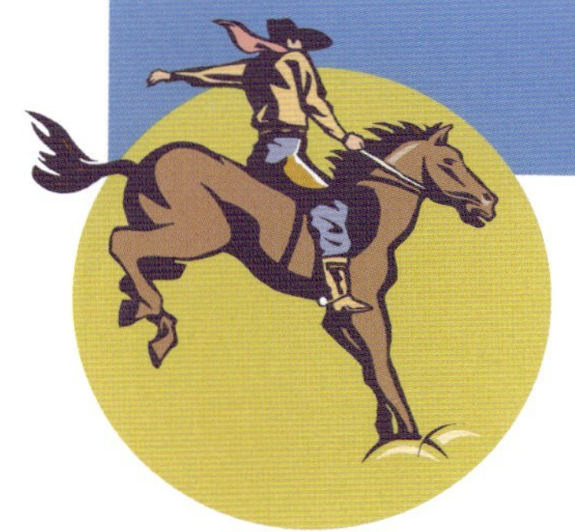

27

Instability Cases

WESTERN WISDOM

On the darkest night, the stars are brightest.

CASE 1: COMBINED REVERSE HAGL (RHAGL) LESION AND POSTERIOR BANKART LESION

History:

- 21-year-old man who fell onto outstretched arm during a soccer game
- Patient had the sensation of the arm momentarily slipping out of joint.

Exam:

- Apprehension in position of combined flexion, adduction, and internal rotation; positive posterior load and shift; 2+ posterior drawer at 45° abduction

Imaging:

- X-rays are normal; MRI shows posteroinferior labral disruption.

Arthroscopic Findings:

- Posterior Bankart lesion; reverse HAGL (RHAGL) lesion (Fig. 27.1A)

Procedures Performed:

- Arthroscopic posterior Bankart repair with suture anchors in glenoid
- Arthroscopic RHAGL repair with suture anchors in humerus (Fig. 27.1B)

Video

Key Points:

- Visualization of muscle deep to posterior capsule is pathognomonic of RHAGL lesion.
- Humeral bone bed for RHAGL repair (posterior) is much more accessible than humeral bone bed for HAGL repair (anterior) due to (a) the retroversion of the proximal humerus (presenting a favorable angle for anchor insertion; and (b) the fact that there is no posterior bone structure equivalent to the coracoid that would block access to the bone bed.
  - Prepare a 2- to 3-mm bare strip of bone at the glenoid margin for insertion of suture anchors.
  - Insert glenoid suture anchors through a posterolateral portal.
  - Insert humeral suture anchors through a posterior portal.

CASE 2: COMBINED HAGL LESION AND BANKART LESION

History:

- 42-year-old man who fell 4 feet from ladder onto outstretched left arm. He felt the shoulder dislocate
- After 5 minutes, a coworker pulled on the arm and reduced it.
- After 4 weeks in a sling followed by 6 weeks of physical therapy, the patient continues to have pain and apprehension with any overhead activities.

Exam:

- Positive apprehension in abduction plus external rotation
- Positive load and shift test
- Normal strength

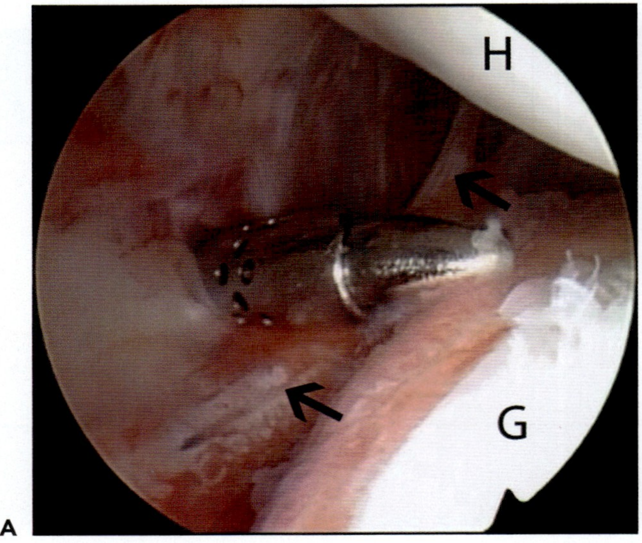

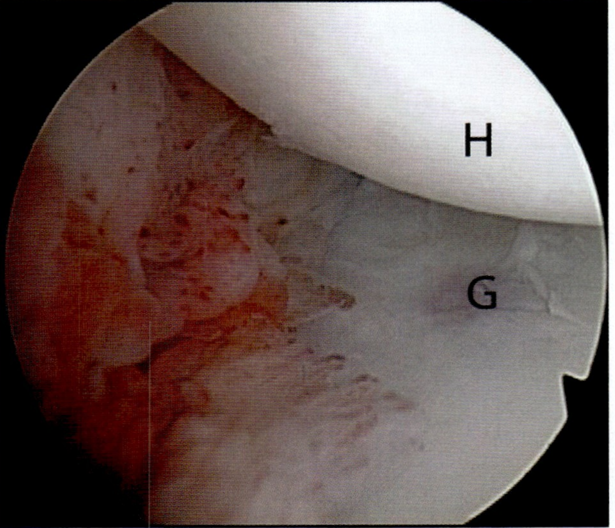

Figure 27.1 **A:** Left shoulder, anterosuperolateral viewing portal, demonstrates a reverse HAGL (RHAGL) (*black arrows*). **B:** Appearance following suture anchor repair. G, glenoid; H, humerus.

Imaging:

- X-rays show small Hill-Sachs lesion.
- MRI shows Bankart lesion (nondisplaced).

Arthroscopic Findings:

- Bankart lesion
- HAGL lesion
- Shallow Hill-Sachs lesion (Fig. 27.2A)

Procedures Performed:

- Arthroscopic Bankart repair
- Arthroscopic HAGL repair (Fig. 27.2B)

Key Points:

- Bankart lesion and HAGL lesion can both occur simultaneously from a single anterior dislocation event, and must both be looked for.
- The key to diagnosing a HAGL lesion is identifying exposed muscle deep to the anterior capsule.
- Fix the Bankart lesion first, then the HAGL lesion.
- Use a spinal needle to identify the proper angle of approach for the humeral suture anchors for HAGL repair. We call this the "killer angle" because of its acute obliquity to the humeral surface that is a result of: (a) the anatomic position of the humeral bone bed, which

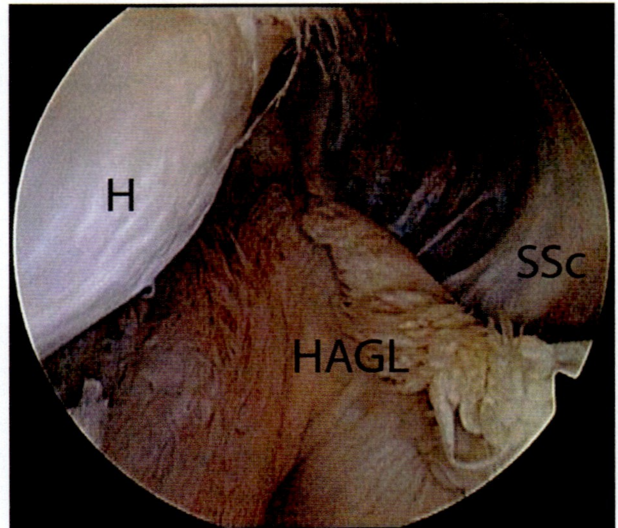

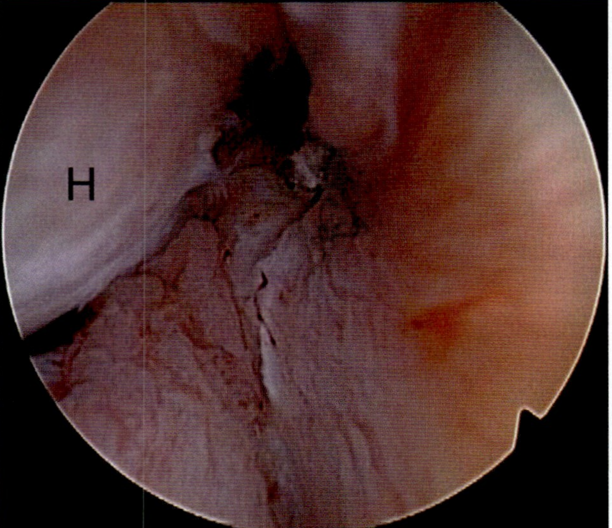

Figure 27.2 **A:** Left shoulder, anterosuperolateral viewing portal, demonstrates a humeral avulsion of the glenohumeral ligaments (HAGL). **B:** Appearance postrepair. H, humerus; SSc, subscapularis tendon.

is rather inferior; and (b) the necessity to pass the instruments and implants inferolateral to the coracoid, which lies directly in the way of a direct pass. This necessitates a transtendon approach through the subscapularis.
- There will be only a 5° to 10° "window" of allowable angle of approach to permit successful insertion of suture anchors into the humerus. We believe that achieving this "killer angle" of approach is one of the most difficult maneuvers in arthroscopic shoulder surgery. If the surgeon is unable to successfully achieve this angle, he must proceed to an open repair of the HAGL lesion.

CASE 3: COMBINED ANTERIOR INSTABILITY (AFTER FAILED BANKART REPAIR) AND TEAR OF UPPER SUBSCAPULARIS TENDON WITH SUBLUXATION OF LONG HEAD OF BICEPS

History:

- 32-year-old man who tripped at work and fell onto outstretching right arm
- He felt the shoulder "slip out"
- History of arthroscopic Bankart repair 1 year earlier

Exam:

- Apprehension and pain with combined abduction and external rotation
- Positive bear-hug test
- Positive belly-press test

Imaging:

- X-rays show Hill-Sachs lesion.
- MRI shows Bankart lesion, torn upper subscapularis tendon, and medial subluxation of biceps.

Arthroscopic Findings:

- Recurrent Bankart lesion (Fig. 27.3A)
- 3 mm × 7 mm area of grade 4 glenoid chondromalacia adjacent to Bankart lesion
- Shallow nonengaging Hill-Sachs lesion (Fig 27.3B)
- Tear of upper 40% of subscapularis (Fig 27.3C)
- Medial subluxation of long head of biceps

Procedures Performed:

- Arthroscopic revision Bankart repair (Fig 27.4A)
- Arthroscopic subscapularis repair (Fig 27.4B)
- Arthroscopic biceps tenodesis

Key Points:

- Order of steps should be
  - Exteriorize the biceps and place whipstitch in preparation for tenodesis. Do this first, before swelling makes it impossible.
  - Repair the Bankart lesion, advancing the capsule over the cartilage defect of the anteroinferior glenoid to achieve a biologic resurfacing.
  - Repair subscapularis with FiberTape-SwiveLock technique.
  - Perform biceps tenodesis with BioComposite Tenodesis screw.
- The Bankart lesion is repaired before the other structures because it represents the tightest working space.
- Knotless repair of tears up to 50% of the superior-to-inferior dimension of the subscapularis with FiberTape-SwiveLock is our preferred technique. For tears of greater than 50% of the inferior-to-superior dimension, we prefer to tie knots with double-loaded BioComposite Corkscrew suture anchors.
- In cases with peripheral glenoid cartilage loss, capsulolabral advancement should be done to provide biologic resurfacing of the damaged glenoid.

CASE 4: TRAUMATIC ANTERIOR AND POSTERIOR BANKART LESIONS SUPERIMPOSED ON PREEXISTING HYPERLAXITY

History:

- 24-year-old female
- Former college swimmer
- Injured shoulder diving for a ball in a softball game

Exam:

- 3+ generalized laxity
- Shoulder is painful with any motion; cannot get a meaningful exam

Imaging:

- X-rays normal
- MRI shows nondisplaced Bankart lesion; no Hill-Sachs lesion.

Arthroscopic Findings:

- Anterior and posterior Bankart lesions (Figs. 27.4A, B)
- Patulous posterior and inferior capsule

Procedures Performed:

- Arthroscopic Bankart repair
- Arthroscopic posterior Bankart repair
- Arthroscopic capsular plication incorporated into capsulolabral repair to suture anchors (Fig. 27.4C)

Key Points:

- Perform anterior Bankart repair before posterior Bankart repair, since working space is more limited anteriorly.

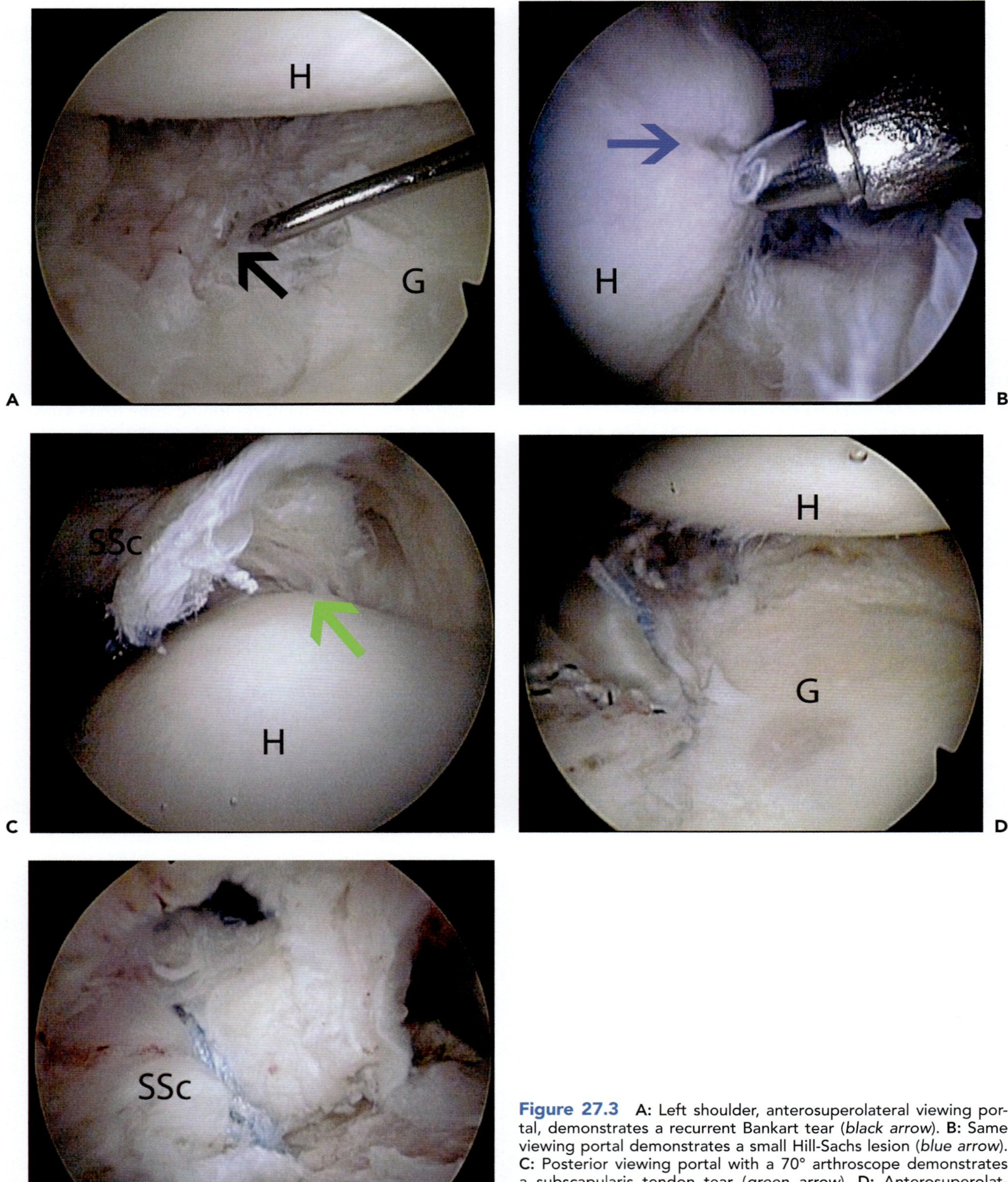

Figure 27.3 **A:** Left shoulder, anterosuperolateral viewing portal, demonstrates a recurrent Bankart tear (*black arrow*). **B:** Same viewing portal demonstrates a small Hill-Sachs lesion (*blue arrow*). **C:** Posterior viewing portal with a 70° arthroscope demonstrates a subscapularis tendon tear (*green arrow*). **D:** Anterosuperolateral viewing portal demonstrates appearance post-Bankart repair. **E:** Posterior viewing portal with a 70° arthroscope demonstrates appearance postsubscapularis tendon repair. G, glenoid; H, humerus; SSc, subscapularis tendon.

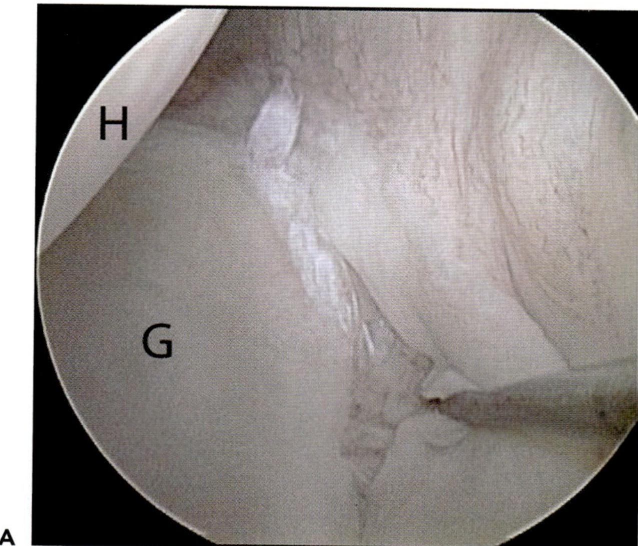

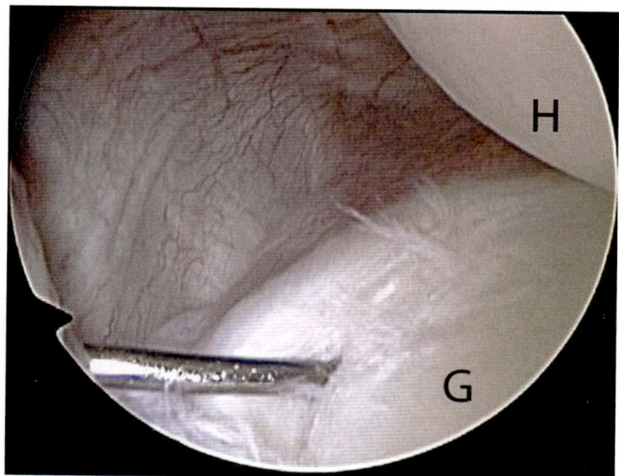

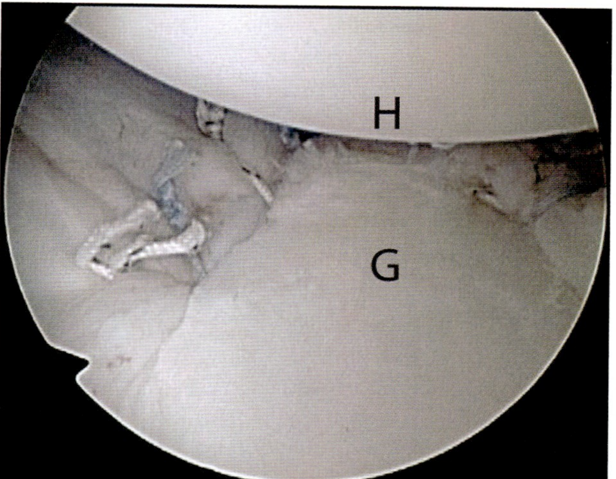

Figure 27.4 **A:** Left shoulder, anterosuperolateral viewing portal, demonstrates a Bankart lesion. **B:** Same shoulder and view demonstrates a posterior Bankart lesion with posterior capsular redundancy. **C:** Appearance post-Bankart repair and posterior Bankart repair with capsular plication. G, glenoid; H, humerus.

- In hyperlax individuals, plicate capsule to suture anchors using a two-pass technique to gather two separate segments of capsule and more precisely reduce the capsular volume.
- Use a posterolateral portal for placing the posterior glenoid anchors.
- Prepare a 2-mm bare strip of glenoid in order to shift the capsule slightly onto the face of the glenoid.
- Close the posterior portal at the conclusion of the case after all cases of posterior instability repair.

CASE 5: COMBINED ANTERIOR AND POSTERIOR BANKART LESIONS WITH LOSS OF PERIPHERAL GLENOID ARTICULAR CARTILAGE

History:

- 42-year-old retired rodeo cowboy
- Shoulder has popped out many times during rodeo events; it was always self-reduced after momentary subluxations
- Cannot do a bench press

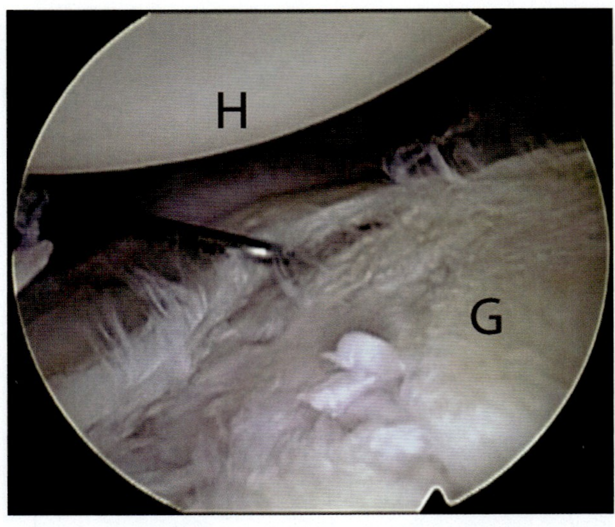

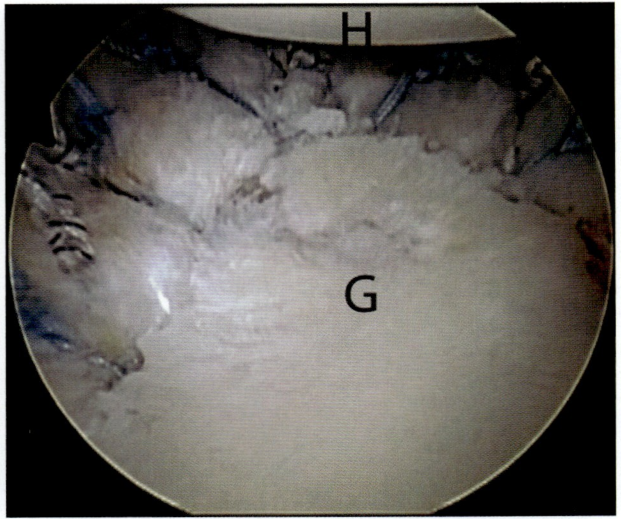

Figure 27.5 **A:** Right shoulder, anterosuperolateral viewing portal, demonstrates a Bankart lesion and articular cartilage damage. **B:** Appearance post-Bankart repair and capsulolabral advancement. G, glenoid; H, humerus.

Exam:

- Equivocal apprehension tests, both in combined abduction-external rotation and in combined adduction-internal rotation.

Imaging:

- X-rays normal
- MRI shows anterior and posterior Bankart lesions.

Arthroscopic Findings:

- Horseshoe-shaped labral disruption anteroinferiorly and posteroinferiorly
- Full-thickness cartilage loss along periphery of lower glenoid (Fig. 27.5A)

Procedures Performed:

- Suture anchor repair of anterior and posterior Bankart lesions, with peripheral glenoid resurfacing by advancement of capsulolabral sleeve over the areas of peripheral cartilage loss (Fig. 27.5B)

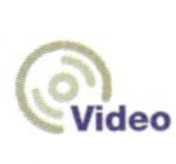

Key Points:

- Although the patient had some early arthritic changes, his primary symptom was a sensation of instability (not pain), so capsulolabral repair was indicated.
- A 6 o'clock anchor can be placed through a posterolateral working portal.
- Pass and tie the inferior and anterior sutures before the posterior ones, as the tightest space is anteroinferior.
- If biologic resurfacing of the peripheral glenoid is to be done by capsulolabral advancement, the capsulolabral sleeve must be mobilized adequately to allow for that degree of advancement.
- At the conclusion of the procedure, the humeral head should be centered over the bare spot of the glenoid (when viewing through an anterosuperolateral viewing portal)

CASE 6: SIGNIFICANT GLENOID AND HUMERAL BONE LOSS AFTER MULTIPLE DISLOCATIONS AND 3 FAILED INSTABILITY SURGERIES

History:

- 33-year-old secretary
- Recurrent anterior instability after three failed Bankart repairs (two arthroscopic, one open)
- Shoulder comes out in her sleep.

Exam:

- Positive apprehension, even in low positions (<45°) of abduction combined with external rotation

Imaging:

- X-rays show large Hill-Sachs.
- MRI and CT confirm large amount of attritional glenoid bone loss (Fig. 27.6A).

Arthroscopic Findings:

- Very narrow glenoid (loss of 50% of width of inferior glenoid), which was underestimated on CT. We call such

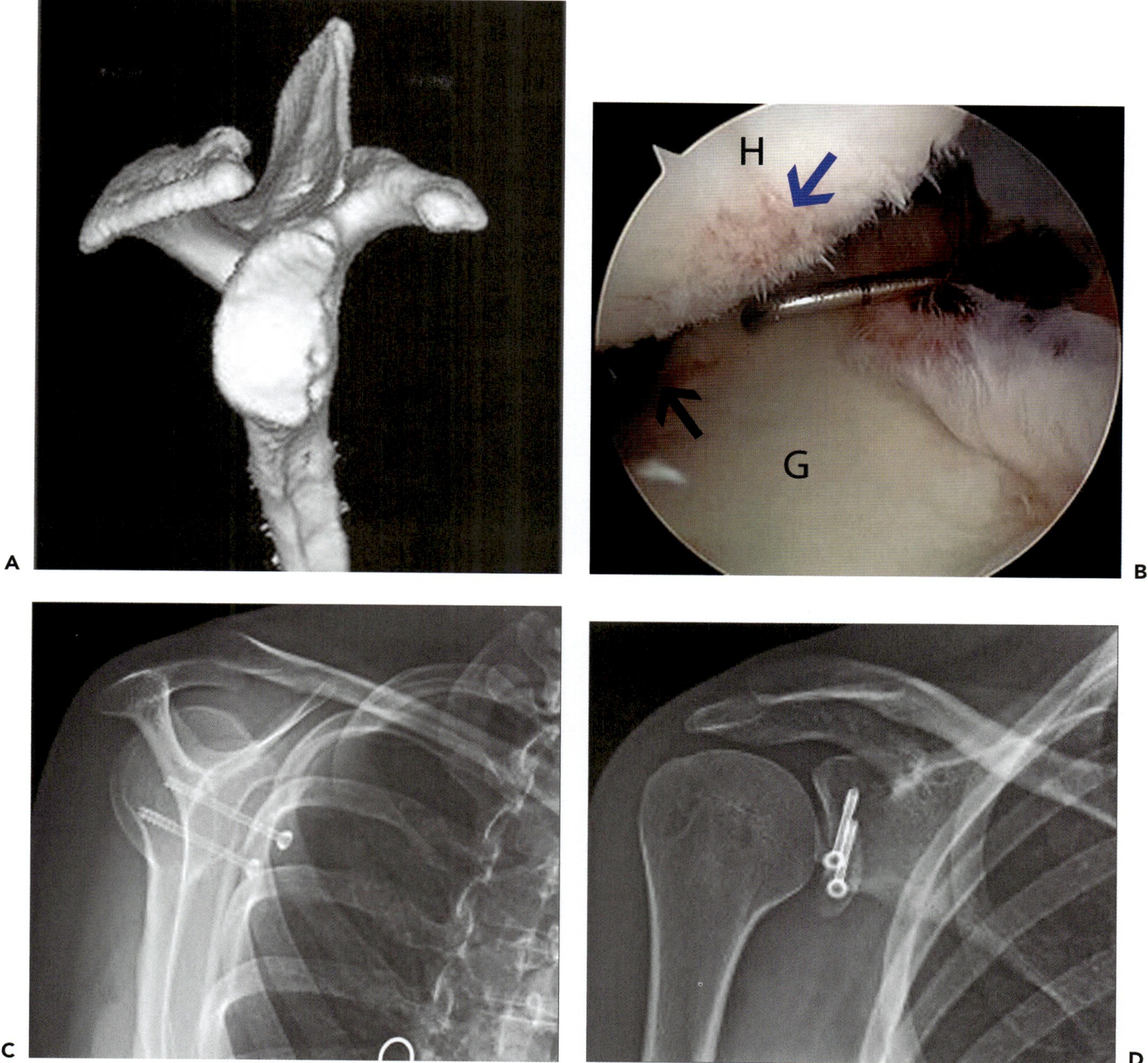

Figure 27.6 **A:** Sagittal 3D reconstruction computed tomography scan of a right shoulder demonstrates substantial glenoid bone loss. **B:** Arthroscopic appearance of the same shoulder viewed from an anterosuperolateral portal demonstrates glenoid bone loss (*black arrow*) and an engaging Hill-Sachs lesion (*blue arrow*). **C:** Scapular-Y and **(D)** postoperative radiograph following Latarjet reconstruction. G, glenoid; H, humerus.

a very narrow glenoid a "banana glenoid" due to its width, which is the same inferiorly and superiorly.

- Deep Hill-Sachs lesion engages at 45° abduction plus external rotation of 45° (Fig. 27.6B).

Video

Procedure Performed:

- Open Latarjet reconstruction with coracoid bone graft (Figs. 27.6C, D)

Key Points:

- "Banana glenoids" always require bone grafting to increase the width of the inferior glenoid.
- A Hill-Sachs lesion that engages easily at low angles of abduction will usually be a large lesion that is associated with a significant glenoid bone deficiency in addition to the Hill-Sachs lesion.

CASE 7: LOCKED POSTERIOR DISLOCATION

History:

- 37-year-old male cabinet maker
- Fell off his son's junior dirt bike 2 months earlier, landed on left arm, and felt something "slip" in shoulder
- Went to ER, had 2 AP x-rays taken, and was told he had sprained his shoulder

Exam:

- Active and passive elevation 60°
- Passive external rotation 0°
- Pain with motion, but he has continued to work at his usual job as a cabinet maker

Imaging:

- Original x-rays (in ER) suggested posterior dislocation, but the diagnosis was missed by the ER physician.
- New x-rays and MRI confirm locked posterior dislocation (Fig. 27.7A).

Arthroscopic Findings:

- Locked posterior dislocation (Fig. 27.7B)
- Humeral avulsion of middle and inferior glenohumeral ligaments (MGHL and IGHL)
- Large reverse Hill-Sachs lesion
- Posterior Bankart lesion

Procedures Performed:

- Arthroscopic reduction of dislocation

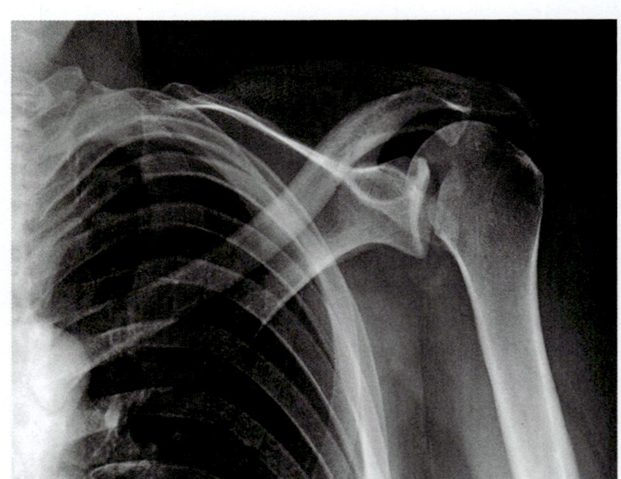

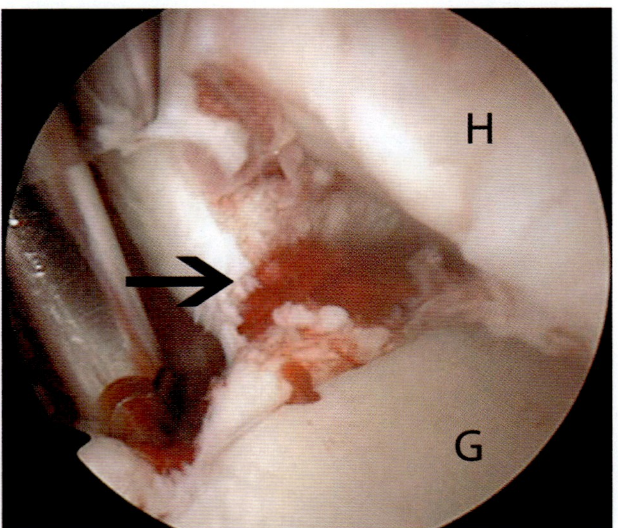

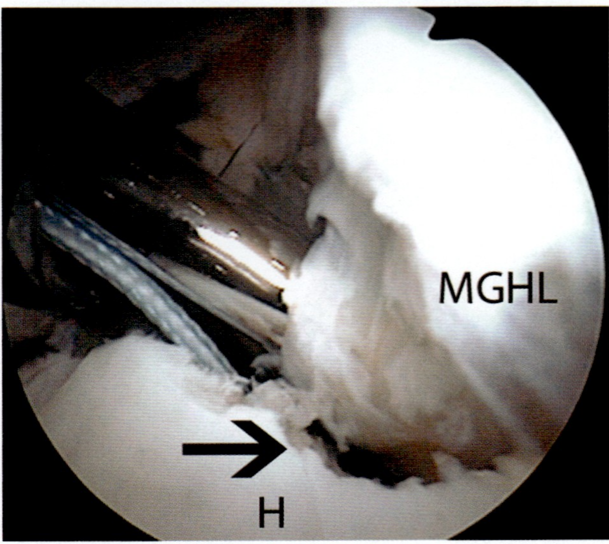

Figure 27.7 **A:** Anterior–posterior plain radiograph of a left shoulder demonstrates a locked posterior glenohumeral dislocation. **B:** Arthroscopic view of the same shoulder from an anterosuperolateral viewing portal demonstrates the locked posterior dislocation and a large reverse Hill-Sachs lesion (*black arrow*). **C:** Posterior viewing portal with a 70° arthroscope demonstrates insetting of the middle glenohumeral ligament into the reverse Hill-Sachs lesion (*black arrow*). G, glenoid; H, humerus; MGHL, middle glenohumeral ligament.

- Arthroscopic posterior Bankart repair
- Inset repair of MGHL and IGHL into reverse Hill-Sachs lesion (Fig. 27.7C)

Key Points:

- In order to put the scope into a shoulder that has a locked posterior dislocation, the best initial portal to place is anterosuperolateral, where the available space is largest; the posteriorly dislocated humeral head blocks the establishment of a posterior portal.
- Once the dislocated humeral head is visualized, an arthroscopic elevator is inserted through a posterosuperior portal to aid in wedging the humeral head laterally enough for reduction. This force is augmented by an assistant pulling the humeral head laterally with a hand in the axilla. Once the humerus is lateralized, external rotation will aid in reduction.
- In this case, the reverse Hill-Sachs lesion was so deep that we did not want to do a reverse remplissage (transfer) of the subscapularis into the reverse Hill-Sachs; this would have dramatically changed the force vector of the subscapularis. Fortunately, his MGHL and IGHL were very robust and could be repaired directly into the humeral bone defect. This accomplished the same goals as remplissage (filling the bone defect and converting it to an extra-articular defect) without changing the force vector of the subscapularis.

CASE 8: RECURRENT ANTERIOR INSTABILITY WITH POOR-QUALITY CAPSULE AFTER TWO FAILED REPAIRS (ONE ARTHROSCOPIC AND ONE OPEN)

History:

- 23-year-old man; active duty military
- Recurrent anterior instability after two failed Bankart repairs
- Multiple subluxations per day

Exam:

- Full range of motion
- Normal strength
- Positive apprehension in 90-90 position

Imaging:

- X-rays normal
- CT shows no significant bone loss.
- MRI suggests deficient anterior capsule.

Arthroscopic Findings:

- Severely deficient and friable anterior capsule; no tissue adequate for anterior repair (essentially absent anterior capsule) (Fig. 27.8A)
- No significant bone loss

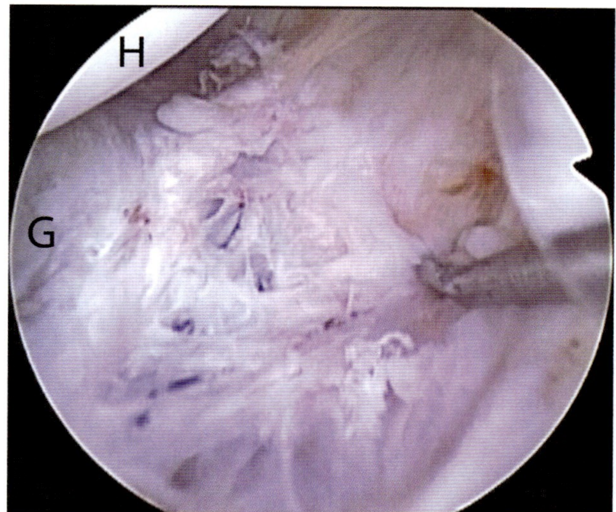

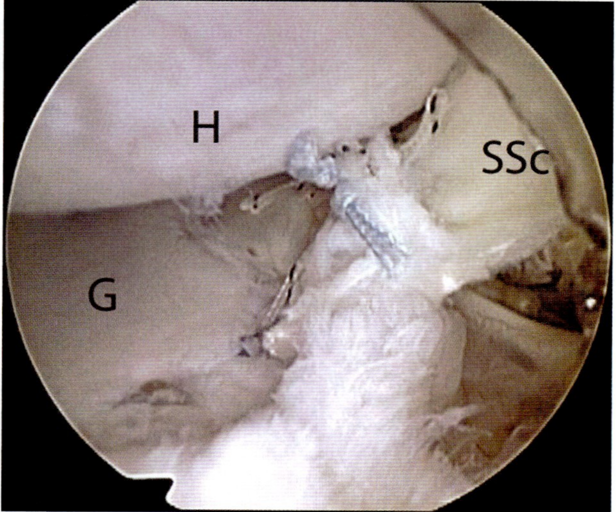

Figure 27.8 **A:** Left shoulder, anterosuperolateral viewing portal, demonstrates severe capsulolabral deficiency. **B:** Same shoulder postsubscapularis split tendon flap augmentation of Bankart repair. G, glenoid; H, humerus; SSc, subscapularis tendon.

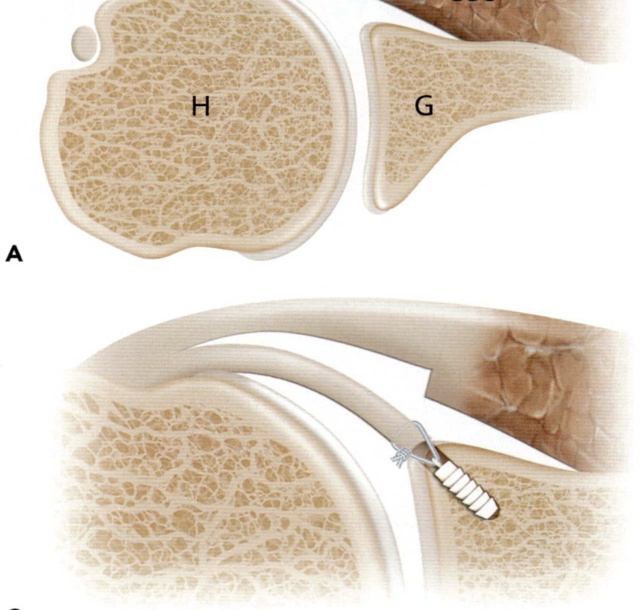

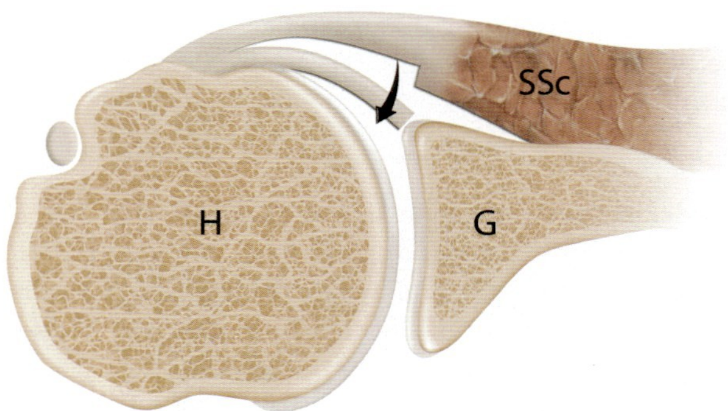

Figure 27.9 Schematic drawing of Bankart augmentation with a split subscapularis tendon transfer. **A:** A flap of the posterior portion (*dashed line*) of the superior half of the subscapularis tendon is created. **B:** The subscapularis flap is mobilized in a "trap-door" fashion such that the capsular surface of the subscapularis tendon is reflected from medial to lateral as a separate lamina (*arrow*) while the outer surface in left unaltered. **C:** The subscapularis flap is tenodesed to the anterior glenoid suture anchors in order to augment capsulolabral deficiency.

Procedures Performed:

- Plication and advancement of inferior capsule
- Split subscapularis tendon flap to replace anterior capsule, fixed to anterior glenoid rim with suture anchors (Fig. 27.8B)

Key Points:

- The split subscapularis tendon flap is a longitudinal flap that is based off the humeral insertion, comprises half the width of the tendon, and is fixed to the glenoid with suture anchors (Fig. 27.9).
- The other half of the subscapularis tendon remains attached to, and dynamized by, the subscapularis muscle, maintaining subscapularis function.
- This procedure is a reasonable option for the shoulder with capsular deficiency that does not have bone deficiency.

CASE 9: BANKART REPAIR WITH A CHONDRAL FLAP

History:

- 17-year-old male football player sustained an anterior dislocation of his dominant arm during a game

Exam:

- Positive apprehension sign and anterior load and shift
- No signs of hyperlaxity or evidence of nerve damage

Imaging:

- Plain radiographs showed no evidence of a bony defect.
- MRI revealed a Bankart tear.

Arthroscopic Findings:

- Bankart tear with a loose chondral flap anteriorly (Fig. 27.10A, B)
- No evidence of glenoid bone loss or a significant Hill-Sachs lesion

Procedures Performed:

- Bankart repair and repair of chondral flap (Fig. 27.10C, D)

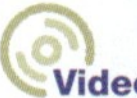

Key Points:

- Chondral flaps are amenable to repair in young individuals.
- The flap is repaired first with an absorbable suture and a knotless anchor (PushLock; Arthrex, Inc., Naples, FL).
- Following stabilization of the chondral flap, the Bankart repair proceeds using standard techniques.

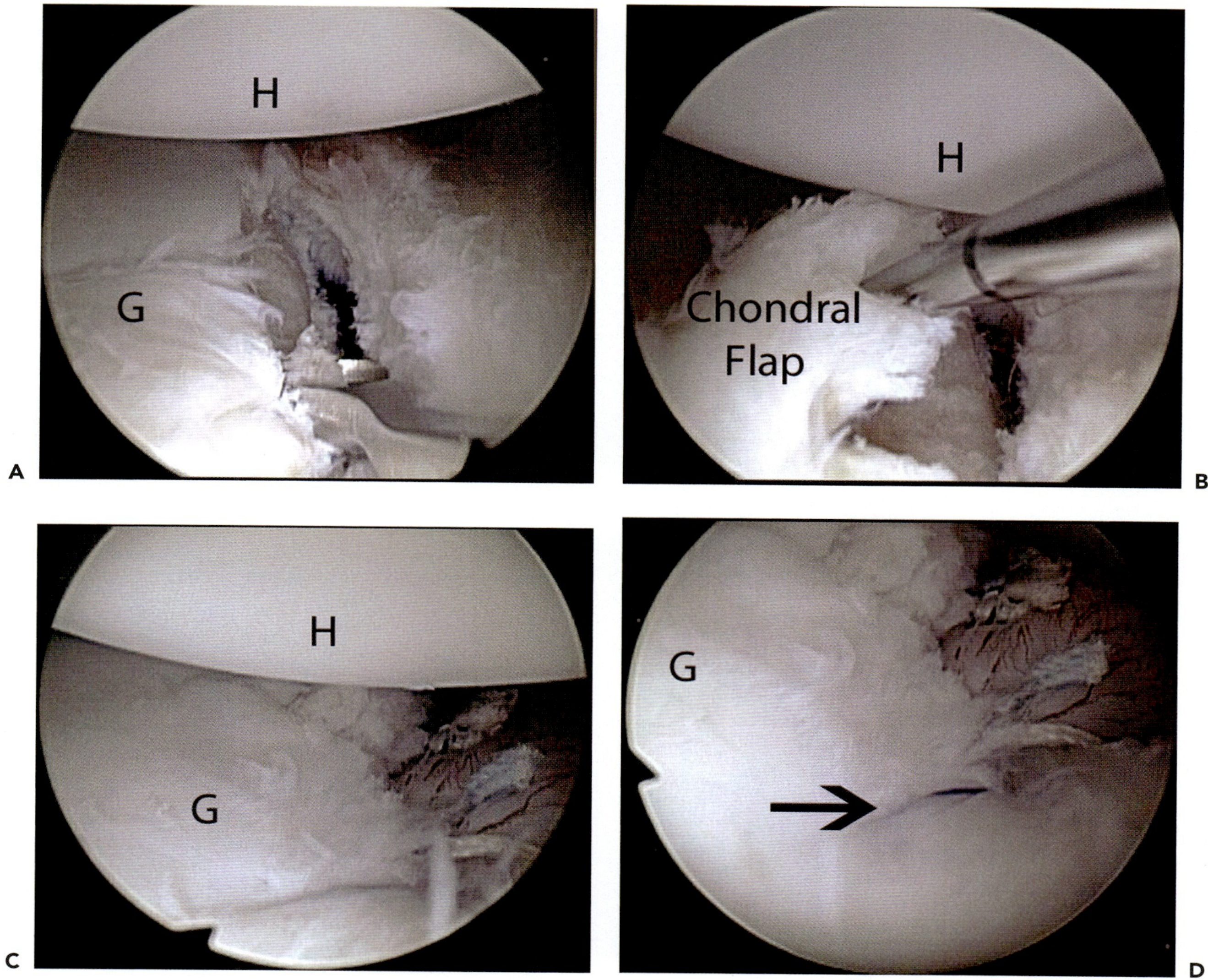

Figure 27.10 **A:** Left shoulder, anterosuperolateral viewing portal, demonstrates a Bankart lesion that has been mobilized for repair. **B:** Same shoulder. A probe is used to demonstrate a loose chondral flap. **C:** Same shoulder demonstrates the final Bankart repair with reduction of the chondral flap. **D:** Up-close view demonstrates the absorbable suture (*black arrow*) used to secure the chondral flap. G, glenoid; H, humerus.

CASE 10: ARTHROSCOPIC HAGL REPAIR USING KNOTLESS FIXATION

History:

- 29-year-old male, RHD, information technologies specialist
- Initial instability episode playing ultimate frisbee, requiring reduction
- One other episode playing ultimate frisbee
- History of epilepsy, well controlled

Exam:

- Full range of motion (165/30/T12)
- Pain with apprehension testing, relieved with relocation maneuver

Imaging:

- No evidence of significant bone loss
- Possible superior labrum anterior and posterior (SLAP) lesion on MRI
- Humeral avulsion of the glenohumeral ligaments (HAGL) on MRI

Arthroscopic Findings:

- SLAP lesion (Fig. 27.11A)
- HAGL lesion (Fig. 27.11B)

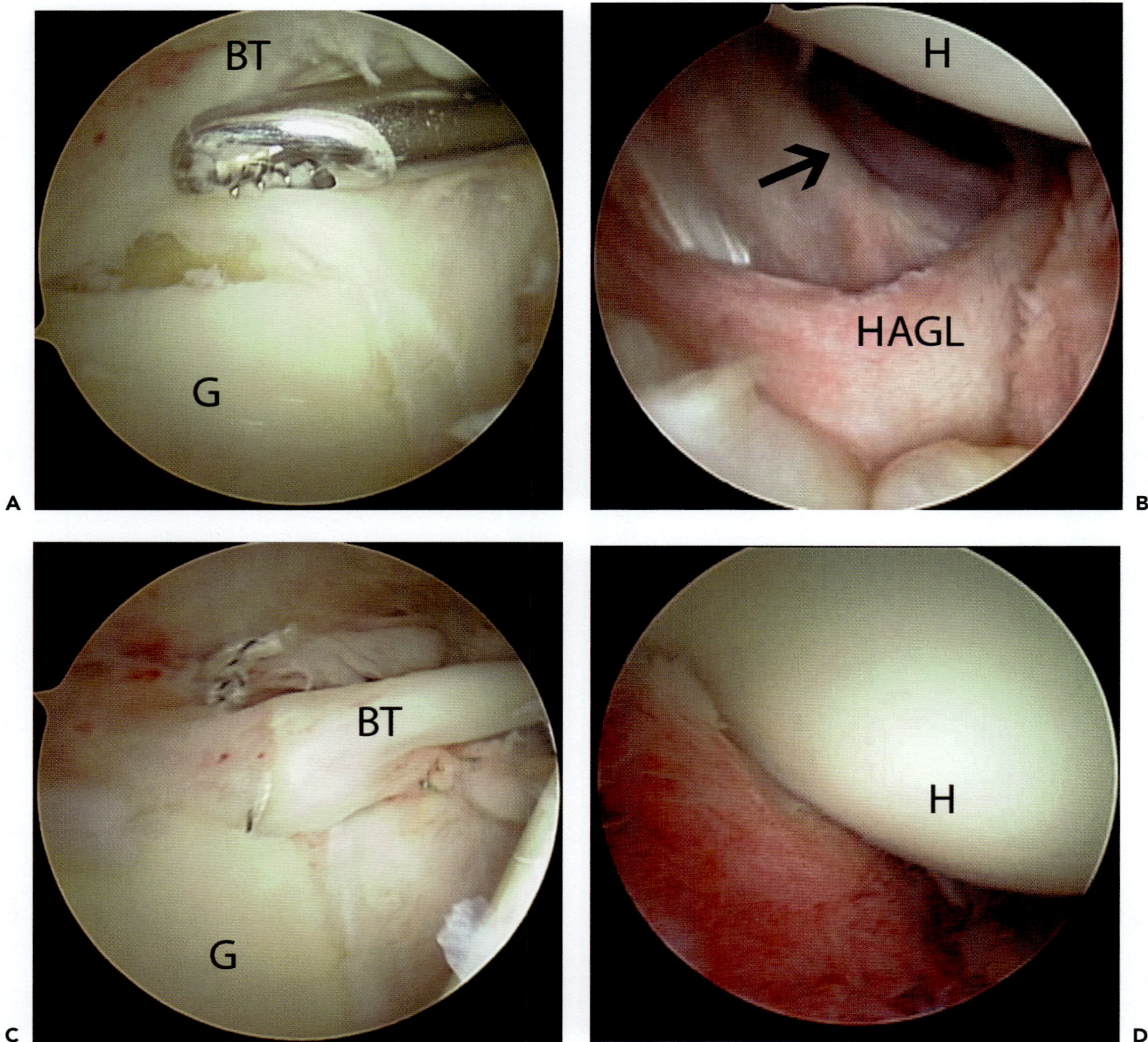

Figure 27.11 **A:** Right shoulder, posterior viewing portal, demonstrates a SLAP lesion for which the bone bed had been prepared for repair. **B:** Same shoulder viewed from an anterosuperolateral portal demonstrates a HAGL. Note the exposed muscle belly (*black arrow*) anterior to the retracted capsule. **C:** Posterior viewing portal demonstrates the repaired SLAP lesion. **D:** Anterosuperolateral viewing portal demonstrates HAGL lesion repair that was performed with knotless anchors. BT, biceps tendon; G, glenoid. H, humerus.

Procedures Performed:

- Arthroscopic SLAP repair (Fig. 27.11C)
- Arthroscopic HAGL repair using knotless technique (Fig. 27.11D)

Video

Key Points

- In non-Bankart instability, careful evaluation of the glenohumeral joint is required to detect capsular avulsion or tearing.
- Repair proceeds while viewing through an anterosuperolateral portal utilizing 30° or 70° arthroscopes.
- Bone preparation and suture passage may be performed using a standard anterior inferior portal.
- Anchor insertion through a medial 5 o'clock (killer angle) portal provides the correct angle of approach for anchor insertion.
- Repair proceeds from inferior to superior.

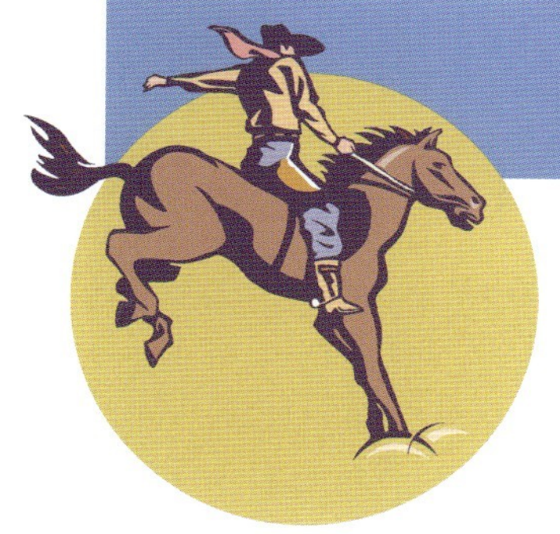

28

Assorted Cases

WESTERN WISDOM

A diamond is a chunk of coal that made good under pressure.

CASE 1: ANTEROINFERIOR GLENOID FRACTURE WITH LARGE BONE FRAGMENT

History:

- 45-year-old man
- Fell 6 feet from ladder
- Taken to local ER
- Anterior dislocation reduced, but shoulder repeatedly redislocates

Exam:

- Neurovascular status intact
- Pain with any range of motion of shoulder

Imaging:

- X-rays show large anteroinferior glenoid fracture.
- 3-D CT images show a large main fracture fragment with some surrounding comminution.

Arthroscopic Findings:

- Depressed fracture fragment that can be elevated to anatomic position (Fig. 28.1A)

Procedures Performed:

Video

- Arthroscopic reduction and internal fixation with two screws
- Arthroscopic labral repair (Fig. 28.1B)

Key Points:

- To elevate the fracture fragment, one must partially detach the labrum from the margins of the fragment. In addition, the labral detachment must be medialized enough to allow for insertion of the screws. However, enough soft tissue attachments should be left intact so that the fragment is not devascularized.
- If the screw heads are "proud," advance the capsulolabral sleeve to the main glenoid to "pad" the screw heads, and schedule arthroscopic removal of the screws at 6 to 9 months post-op (after the fracture has healed).

CASE 2: LOOSE AND FRACTURED GLENOID COMPONENT IN TOTAL SHOULDER REPLACEMENT

History:

- 61-year-old male self-employed machinist and lathe operator
- Had total shoulder replacement 21 years earlier for post-traumatic arthritis following a glenoid fracture (sustained in a motor vehicle accident)
- Had some mild aching pain the past 2 years
- Felt a painful pop in his shoulder 2 days ago while lifting a steel rod
- Owns his own machine-shop business and says he cannot afford to take off work more than 3 days

Exam:

- Pain with any shoulder motion
- Unable to elevate the arm >60° due to pain

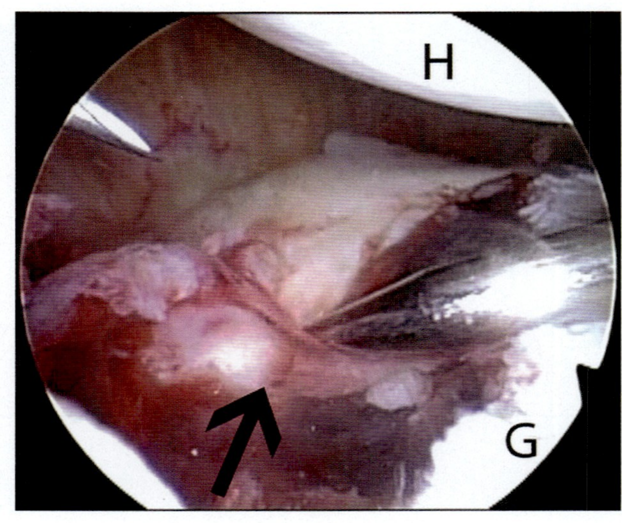

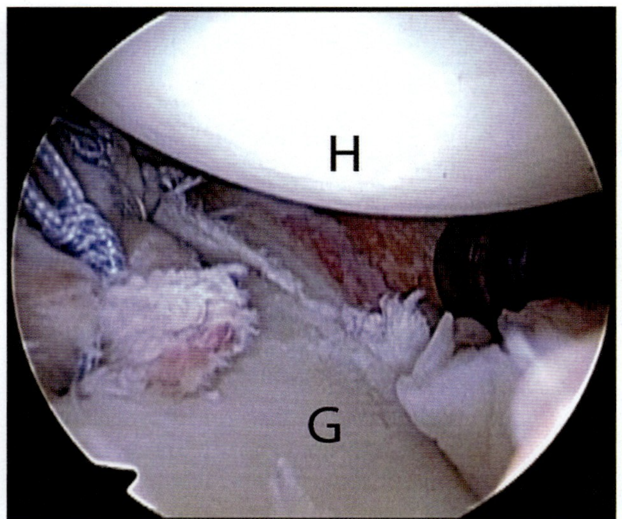

Figure 28.1 **A:** Right shoulder, anterosuperolateral viewing portal, demonstrates a large bony Bankart fracture (*black arrow*). **B:** Appearance postscrew fixation and capsulolabral repair. G, glenoid; H, humerus.

Imaging:

- X-rays show loosening and fragmentation of polyethylene and cement of glenoid component; humeral component is intact.
- CT scan confirms the x-ray impression.

Arthroscopic Findings:

- Multiple loose fragments of polyethylene and methyl methacrylate cement (Fig. 28.2A)

Procedures Performed:

- Arthroscopic excision of loose fragments, debridement of fibrous interface, and contouring of glenoid (Fig. 28.2B)

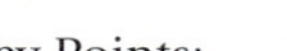

Key Points:

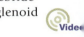

- Large fragments of polyethylene can be reduced in size by using a ¼ or ⅜″ osteotome, thereby facilitating removal through arthroscopic portals.

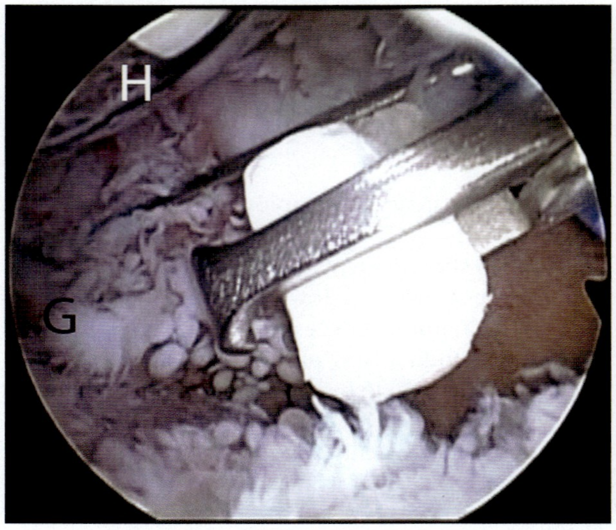

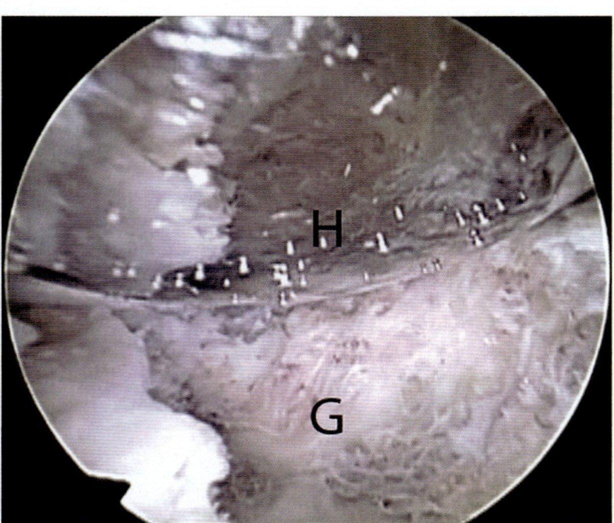

Figure 28.2 **A:** Left shoulder, anterosuperolateral viewing portal, demonstrates removal of a loose polyethylene fragment in an individual with a previous total shoulder replacement. **B:** Appearance postarthroscopic removal of polyethylene component and debris. G, glenoid; H, humerus.

- Glenoid component removal is the ultimate salvage procedure for a failed total shoulder replacement, so it seemed to be the only alternative in this patient whose main goal was to return to his heavy occupation as soon as possible; he returned to regular activity as a machinist 2 days post-op.

CASE 3: PAINFUL SUBCORACOID INTRATENDINOUS OSSICLE

History:

- 17-year-old female Olympic swimmer
- Pain with freestyle stroke and breaststroke for 6 months
- Unable to compete due to pain

Exam:

- Normal strength
- Pain with horizontal adduction (active and passive)
- Pain with forward flexion above 90°
- Palpable ossicle through anterior deltoid

Imaging:

- X-rays (Fig. 28.3A) and MRI confirm intratendinous subcoracoid ossicle at subscapularis insertion.

Arthroscopic Findings:

- Large ossicle located by unroofing bursal surface of subscapularis tendon

Procedures Performed:

- Arthroscopic excision of ossicle, debridement of osteophyte, and repair of subscapularis tendon (Fig. 28.3B)

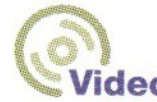

Key Points:

- The palpable ossicle is localized first with a needle and then removed by unroofing the superficial tendon with a pencil-tip electrocautery electrode.
- After ossicle excision, the subscapularis is repaired.
- Patient is asymptomatic and competing at her previous level at 5 years post-op.

CASE 4: CALCIFIC TENDINITIS IN A PATIENT WITH VERY POOR-QUALITY BONE

History:

- 48-year-old female housewife
- 4-month history of severe shoulder pain
- No injury

Exam:

- Pain with any motion of shoulder

Imaging:

- X-rays and MRI show large calcification in supraspinatus tendon (Fig. 28.4A).

A

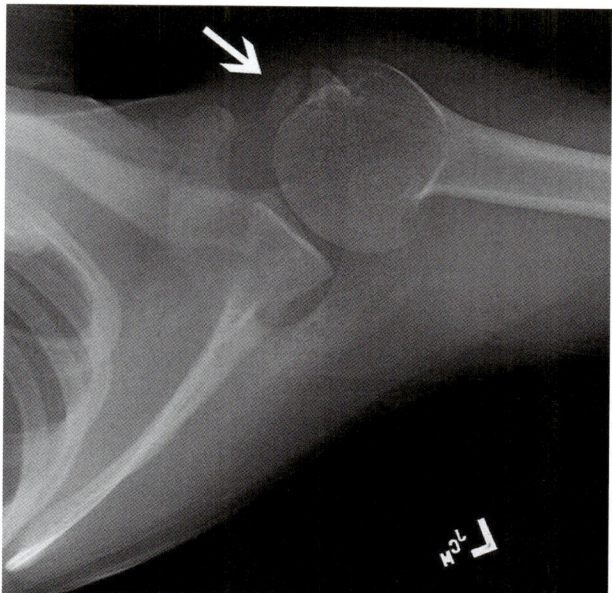

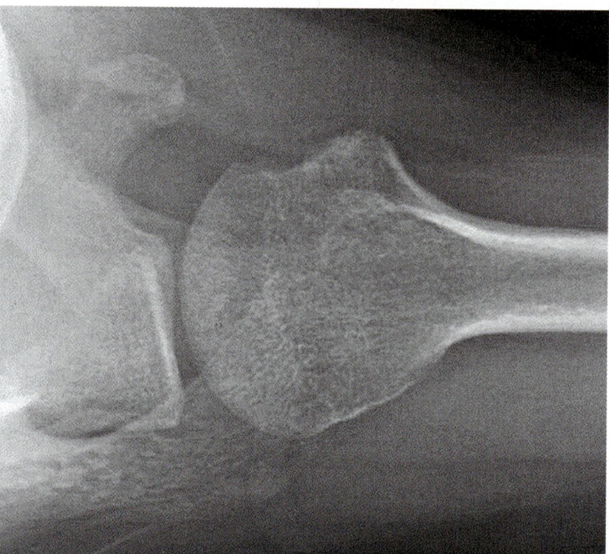

B

Figure 28.3 **A:** Preoperative axillary plain radiograph in a left shoulder demonstrates an ossicle (*white arrow*) within the subscapularis tendon and an adjacent osteophyte on the lesser tuberosity. **B:** Postoperative radiograph following arthroscopic excision of the ossicle and debridement of the osteophyte.

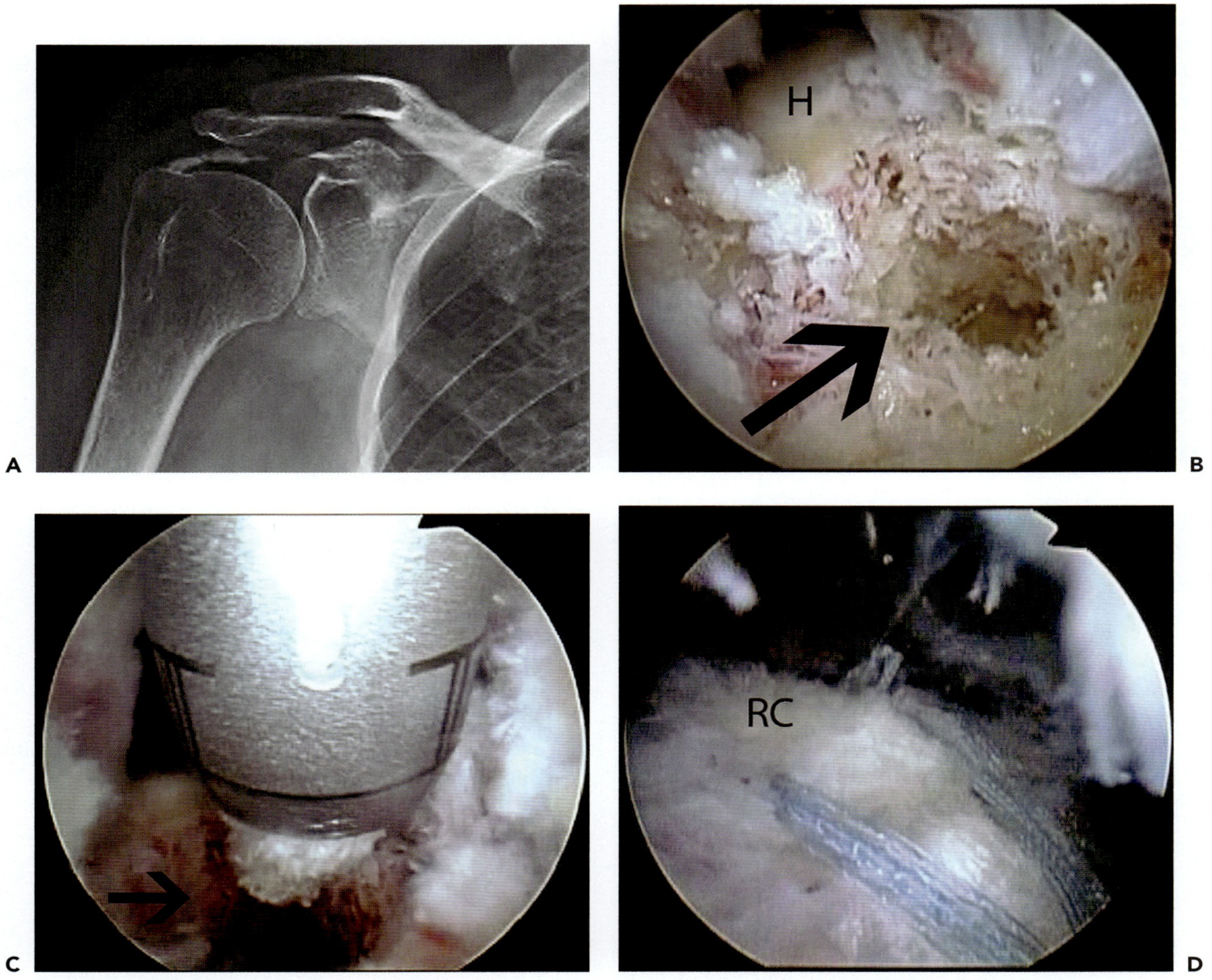

Figure 28.4 **A:** Preoperative radiograph of a right shoulder demonstrates calcific tendinitis. **B:** Arthroscopic appearance of the same shoulder viewed from a lateral subacromial portal demonstrates a bone defect (*black arrow*) in the proximal humerus. **C:** Same shoulder demonstrates allograft cancellous grafting of the bone defect (*black arrow*) with an OATS harvester tube (Arthrex, Inc., Naples, FL). **D:** Appearance from a posterior viewing portal following rotator cuff repair with a SpeedFix technique (Arthrex, Inc., Naples, FL).

Arthroscopic Findings:

- After calcium is removed, there is a 2 cm × 3 cm defect in the supraspinatus tendon.
- The bone in the greater tuberosity is very soft and is even invaded by the calcific deposits (Fig. 28.4B).

Procedures Performed:

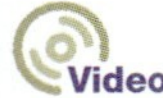

- After multiple anchor configurations pulled out of the soft bone, we did an arthroscopic allograft of the bone socket using OATS harvesters (Arthrex, Inc., Naples, FL) (Fig. 28.4C), then fixed the cuff with a SpeedFix construct (FiberTape plus SwiveLock suture anchors) (Arthrex, Inc., Naples, FL) (Fig. 28.4D).

Key Points:

- Many patients with calcific tendinitis have concomitant osteopenia; in patients who have calcific deposits invading the cancellous bone of the greater tuberosity, the osteopenia is even worse.
- For proper healing, the calcific deposits should be completely excised and the rotator cuff defect must be repaired.
- In cases with very soft bone, a SpeedFix repair that bypasses the weak cancellous bone in favor of the stronger metaphyseal corticocancellous bone can be very strong and is virtually always possible to perform securely, even in very osteoporotic bone where other fixation techniques are impossible.

PART III

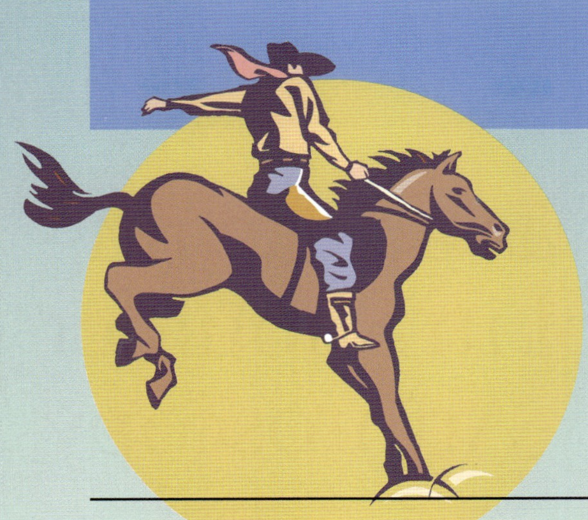

HISTORICAL VIGNETTES

COWBOY PRINCIPLE 10

Every jackass thinks he has horse sense.

If you can laugh at yourself, you will never cease to be amused.

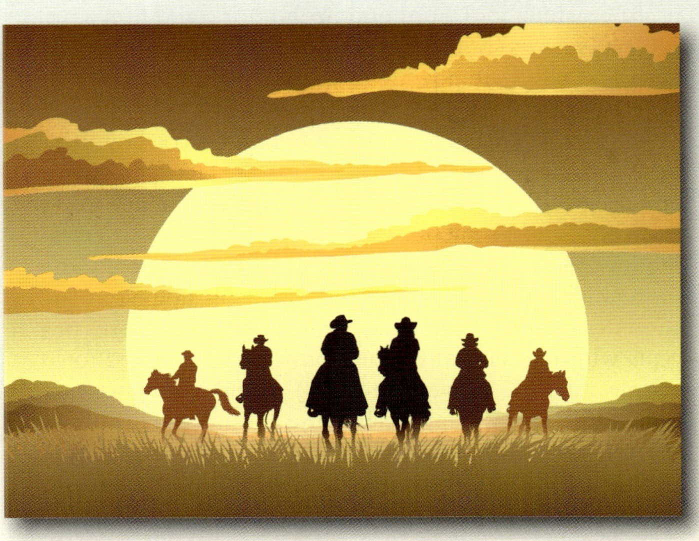

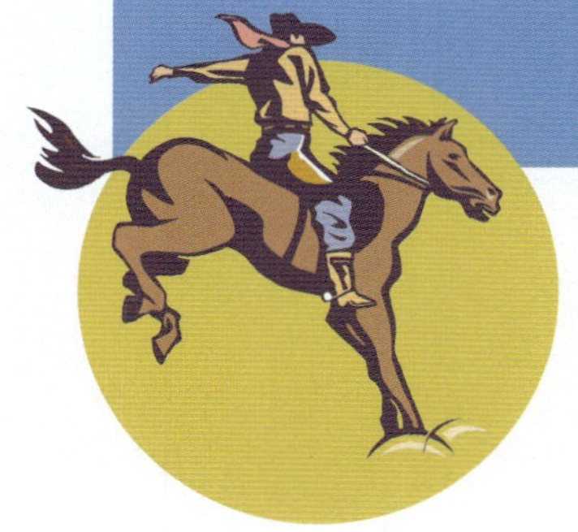

29

Humor as a Teaching Tool in Shoulder Arthroscopy

Stephen S. Burkhart, MD

WESTERN WISDOM

Horse sense is what keeps horses from bettin' on what people will do.

In the early 1990s, the shoulder establishment was laughing at arthroscopic shoulder surgeons, whom they viewed as a pitiful little band of dreamers whose goal of achieving strong arthroscopic repairs for instability and rotator cuff tears would always remain hopelessly out of reach. I recognized that humor, particularly when it was endogenous and self-deprecating, got people's attention and could be a useful teaching tool. Furthermore, humor could turn a dry subject (such as shoulder biomechanics) into a fun experience. So there were now two reasons to employ humor in my teaching efforts.

So, as Will Rogers or some other famous cowboy must have said, "If you can't beat 'em, join 'em." I took his advice and decided to encourage people to laugh at me just to get them to listen to me. As a mechanical engineer by training (prior to medical school), I knew that there were some mechanical concepts that were accepted as dogma in the shoulder that were absolutely wrong. Replacing those concepts with mechanically sound principles (balanced force couples, margin convergence, etc.) would fundamentally change the way we approached the shoulder, particularly the rotator cuff. But getting people to listen and getting people to understand such dry and esoteric topics was not going to be easy.

When I was a kid in the 1950s, there was a black-and-white television show every Saturday morning that was called "Watch Mr. Wizard." Mr. Wizard was an amateur scientist named Don Herbert. In the show, he would teach complex scientific concepts to the kids in his neighborhood by means of simple experiments that could be conducted in his kitchen or his garage, using everyday tools and utensils from his home. To me, the show was fascinating, and it made science understandable and fun. Part of the fun was Mr. Wizard's style; he employed a great deal of good-natured humor and he encouraged the kids to develop their own conclusions based on the experiments he showed them.

In late 1991, I was preparing a talk for the AANA (Arthroscopy Association of North America) Specialty Day Meeting, to be held a few months later at the AAOS (American Academy of Orthopaedic Surgeons) venue in San Francisco. I had been assigned the topic "Biomechanics of the Rotator Cuff." As I tried to develop my ideas, I drew a blank.

Sitting at my desk, frustrated by the impossible task of making a dull subject interesting, I hit upon an idea. I would be the eccentric, good-humored, self-deprecating "Mr. Wizhart" (Wizhart/Burkhart—get it?). My kids (Zack and Sarah) and I filmed a black-and-white "Mr. Wizhart" segment on "Minimal Surface Area" and its effect on the behavior of rotator cuff tears. At the meeting in San Francisco, I didn't tell anyone what I was going to do. When I was introduced, I went to the podium and stated that I would show a self-explanatory video on the biomechanics

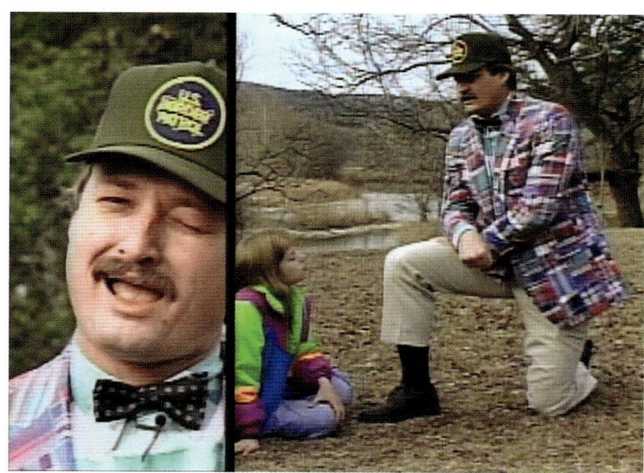

Figure 29.1 Mr. Wizhart.

of the rotator cuff. I turned on the video. Initially there was a stunned silence as the goofy introductory music began to play. Then there was a loud collective roar of laughter from the audience as Mr. Wizhart began to teach them. Orthopaedic surgeons do not usually laugh at lectures, even when the speaker tells a joke. So when I heard wave after wave of belly laughs, I knew I was onto something. The arthroscopic shoulder surgeons had a message, and they had a voice—and now they had an eager audience (Fig 29.1).

My kids and I went on to create a total of four Mr. Wizhart videos. I can't bear to see them simply discarded on the trash heap of time, so I have decided to preserve them here. I take full responsibility for the content and the style. Please don't blame my coauthors for any of this. I hope you enjoy it.

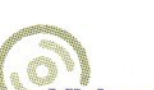

Index

Note: Page numbers followed by t indicate table. Page numbers in *italics* indicate figure.

R